Medicine BMA
& Surgery

an integrated textbook

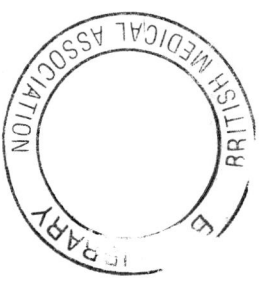

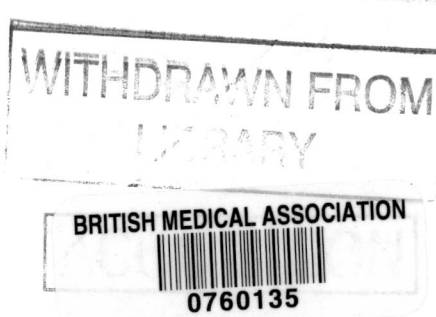

Dedication

To Irene, a loving wife, devoted mother, loyal companion, synergistic partner and a brilliant career strategist.

E.L.

Commissioning Editor: Laurence Hunter
Development Editor: Ailsa Laing / Ruth Swan
Project Manager: Elouise Ball
Designer: Sarah Russell
Illustrations Manager: Gillian Murray
Illustrator: Richard Prime

Medicine &Surgery

an integrated textbook

Edited by

Eric Kian Saik Lim

MB ChB MSc MD FRCS (C-Th)

Consultant Thoracic Surgeon,
Royal Brompton Hospital, London,
Senior Lecturer in Thoracic Surgery,
National Heart and Lung Institute,
Imperial College School of Medicine,
London, UK

Associate Editor for Medicine

Yoon Kong Loke MB BS MRCP MD

Senior Lecturer in Clinical Pharmacology,
School of Medicine, Health Policy and Practice,
University of East Anglia,
Norwich, UK

Associate Editor for Surgery

Alastair Thompson
ALCM BSc(Hons) MBChB MD FRCS(Ed)

Professor of Surgical Oncology,
Department of Surgery and Molecular Oncology,
Ninewells Hospital and Medical School,
Dundee, UK

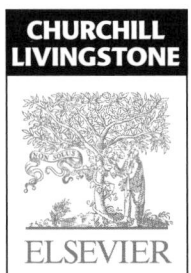

CHURCHILL
LIVINGSTONE

ELSEVIER

EDINBURGH LONDON NEW YORK OXFORD PHILADELPHIA ST LOUIS SYDNEY TORONTO 2007

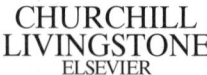

CHURCHILL
LIVINGSTONE
ELSEVIER

An imprint of Elsevier Limited

First published 2007

ISBN-13: 978-0-443-07260-4

British Library Cataloguing in Publication Data
A catalogue record for this book is available from the British Library

Library of Congress Cataloging in Publication Data
A catalog record for this book is available from the Library of Congress

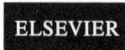

Working together to grow
libraries in developing countries

www.elsevier.com | www.bookaid.org | www.sabre.org

ELSEVIER   BOOK AID International   Sabre Foundation

ELSEVIER your source for books, journals and multimedia in the health sciences
www.elsevierhealth.com

The publisher's policy is to use **paper manufactured from sustainable forests**

Printed in China

Preface

Traditionally, the study of medicine and surgery has been undertaken with two textbooks, one for each discipline. As a student, you are soon aware of the considerable overlap for many topics, and the more perceptive will appreciate that medicine and surgery are simply therapeutic options in the management of disease. As medical education develops, increasing integration of the two disciplines is becoming more apparent in undergraduate teaching, clinical attachments and examinations.

It is a delight to be able to produce a hybrid textbook that has evolved symbiotically with modernising medical curricula. We hope this book will ease the boundaries of tradition that separate medicine and surgery. The many advantages of an integrated approach include reducing the amount of reading by elimination of repetition (and inconsistencies) that may arise from two textbooks, and the ability to provide a unified approach to clinical problems faced by clinicians and students. Perhaps the greatest asset is to illustrate when and which medical or surgical treatment should be used.

Each chapter has been written by a team of surgeons and physicians, in a standard format to allow instant familiarity with the layout of the entire book. We have tried to avoid a dictatorial approach, but rather reveal the decision-making process, a mind set that a student needs to acquire when becoming a doctor. To further bridge the gap between an undergraduate textbook and clinical practice, we ensure that recommendations are concordant with national or international guidelines and utilise where possible a current, evidence-based approach. To help the student adjust to ward and clinical practice, instructions on practical procedures and surgical details have been provided in sufficient detail to facilitate the acquisition of informed consent.

This textbook has been the labour of many young authors; we hope that the end result is a cost-effective solution that reduces studying time and improves on the understanding and approach to the management of disease.

Eric Lim   2007
Yoon Kong Loke
Alastair Thompson

Acknowledgements

Firstly I would like to acknowledge the help and mentoring of Mr Andrew Raftery (Consultant Surgeon, Northern General Hospital, Sheffield), who believed that a medical student would have the ability to co-author a book on differential diagnosis, for cultivating my interests in writing and guiding me from planning through to completion of our first book together. I am indebted to Laurence Hunter (Commissioning Editor, Elsevier) for his help, encouragement, support and belief that a Senior House Officer would have the ability to edit a textbook of Medicine and Surgery.

I am grateful to Mike Rubens (Consultant Radiologist, Royal Brompton Hospital) for permission to use images from the Brompton Hospital diagnostic imaging bank, and the radiographers at the Royal Brompton Hospital for helping me acquire these images at all hours of the day and at weekends (especially Bruce Barton, for sitting with me painfully extracting images from the 'hundreds' machine). I am also indebted to Dr John Pilling (Consultant Radiologist, Norfolk and Norwich University Hospital) for permission to use images from the Norfolk and Norwich University Hospital diagnostic imaging archive.

Many thanks to all the Surgical Care Practitioners at Papworth Hospital (especially Deirdre Evans) for taking the extra effort to acquire operative photos. I would also like to acknowledge Dr Arun Kumar (SpR Anaesthetics, Papworth Hospital, Cambridge) and Dr Andrew Klein (Consultant Anaesthetist, Papworth Hospital, Cambridge) for acquisition of most of the trans-oesophageal images from the TOE machines. Sincere gratitude to Mr Stephen Large (Consultant Cardiothoracic Surgeon, Papworth Hospital, Cambridge) and the operating team – Mr Tom Routledge (SpR Cardiothoracic Surgery, Papworth Hospital, Cambridge) and Dr Yuri Gupta (SHO Cardiothoracic Surgery, Papworth Hospital, Cambridge) – for the images of aortic dissection taken (painstakingly) in the early hours of the morning for the book.

I also acknowledge Dr Amparo Galindo (Imperial College, London, UK) and especially Ni Ni for taking such good care of Ethan and Euan, channelling their energies and keeping them entertained whilst this book was edited.

I would like to thank Mr Derek Cramer (Pulmonary Function Unit, Royal Brompton Hospital) for reviewing the section on the definition of pulmonary function. I also acknowledge the contribution and advice of Mr Ashu Gandhi (Consultant Endocrine Surgeon, Manchester) for the section on hyperparathyroidism.

I am especially touched by the patients who contributed to this textbook, some of whom were in the terminal stages of disease, all of whom generously gave their permission to be photographed in order to contribute to the education of the next generation of doctors and other healthcare professionals.

A big 'thank you' and apologies to the significant contributors whom I have failed to acknowledge personally (send me an email!).

Eric Lim, 2007

How to use this book

Much thought and effort has gone into the structure and layout of this book, to ensure that students are able to easily glean the necessary information. Generally, each chapter is system based and starts with an applied basic science section, symptoms, clinical examination, investigations and manifestations of disease. Then, diseases may be grouped and presented individually.

There are three levels of information presented uniformly for each disease. The first level of presentation for common diseases is the most comprehensive, headed with epidemiology, pathology, scope of disease, clinical features, initial investigations, further investigations, initial management, medical management, surgical management and prognosis. The second level of presentation is for less common diseases and has the headings epidemiology, pathology, clinical features, investigations, management and prognosis. Finally, the third level of information is presented for rare disease and usually consists only of one paragraph.

The layout has been arranged to allow the reader to open any page and instantly recognise the chapter (located at the top banner of the page and associated with a chapter-specific image), the layout of the diseases in the section (top right list) and the disease presented on the page (the bold item on the top right list). In addition, the reader can pick out any line of text and look at the associated icon to determine the context in which the information is provided.

The icons and headings relate to the following:

Epidemiology

The epidemiology section describes the incidence and prevalence of disease, where possible it is presented with 100 000 as the base unit (eg incidence of 3 per 100 000 per year or prevalence of 200 per 100 000). Epidemiological data tends to be best reported for Western countries, which explains the unavoidable bias towards the West. In addition, where pertinent, information is provided on the geography, age and gender distribution of disease.

Pathology

The subsection on pathology mainly relates to the aetiology and pathogenesis of disease.

Scope of disease

A "Scope of disease" section is presented before the clinical features to remind readers that diseases can present as the primary condition (e.g. heartburn with gastro-esophageal reflux) or as a result of a secondary complication (e.g. dysphagia from strictures secondary to gastro-esophageal reflux). With most common cancers, this section is divided into local, metastatic and paraneoplastic manifestations.

Clinical features

The clinical features section relates mainly to the symptoms and examination features of the disease and any associated complications.

Initial investigations

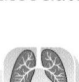

Initial investigations refer to a recommended list for all patients who present with clinical features suggestive of the underlying disease.

Further investigations

Further investigations refer to investigations not usually performed for all patients with clinical features suggestive of the underlying disease, as well as more invasive or specific investigations for patients with specific indications or associated complications.

Initial management

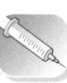

The section on initial management provides information and instruction on simple first-line measures on the management of disease or the important first steps of emergency management.

Medical management

Medical management refers to all non-surgical management and usually describes risk-factor modification and drug treatment, although it may include any other intervention performed by physicians, such as insertion of a Sengstaken tube or percutaneous coronary revascularisation.

Surgical management

Surgical management describes the surgical management, procedure, results and complications, usually in sufficient detail to obtain informed consent.

Prognosis

The prognosis section is used to describe the natural history of untreated disease as well as the results of treatment.

⚡ CLINICAL ALERT

The clinical alert boxes are used to highlight life threatening or emergency procedures.

There are two levels for presentation of images, central and marginal. The central images are larger and illustrate important images, whereas the marginal images usually illustrate interesting but not necessarily critically important images. In addition, the margins are also used to display sequential operative photos.

We hope that you will be able to quickly adapt to and enjoy the layout and structure of this textbook.

Specialist Advisors

General Practice

Jeremy Webb
General Practitioner, Orchard House Surgery, Newmarket;
Deputy Director Cambridge Graduate Course in Medicine,
School of Clinical Medicine, University of Cambridge

Intensive Care Medicine

Mark Griffiths
Consultant Physician, Adult Intensive Care Unit,
Royal Brompton Hospital, London

Pathology

James Lowe
Professor and Hon Consultant in Neuropathology,
University of Nottingham Medical School, Nottingham

Microbiology

Kathleen Bamford
Reader and Consultant Medical Microbiologist,
Hammersmith Hospital, London

Radiology

Simon Padley
Consultant Radiologist, Chelsea and Westminster Hospital,
London

Clinical Pharmacology and Therapeutics

Yoon Kong Loke
Senior Lecturer in Clinical Pharmacology,
School of Medicine, Health Policy and Practice,
University of East Anglia, Norwich

Contributors

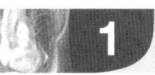 **1** Diseases of the cardiovascular system

Eric Lim Consultant Thoracic Surgeon, Royal Brompton Hospital, London
Senior Lecturer in Thoracic Surgery, National Heart and Lung Institute, Imperial College School of Medicine, London, UK

Ziad Ali Specialist Registrar Surgery, Addenbrooke's Hospital, Cambridge

Kevin Varty Consultant Vascular Surgeon, Addenbrooke's Hospital, Cambridge

John Wallwork Professor of Cardiac Surgery, Papworth Hospital, Cambridge

Philip Poole-Wilson British Heart Foundation Simon Marks Chair of Cardiology, National Heart & Lung Institute, Imperial College School of Medicine, London

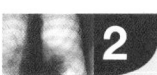 **2** Diseases of the respiratory system

Eric Lim Consultant Thoracic Surgeon, Royal Brompton Hospital, London
Senior Lecturer in Thoracic Surgery, National Heart and Lung Institute, Imperial College School of Medicine, London, UK

Mitra Shahidi Specialist Registrar Respiratory Medicine, Royal Brompton Hospital, London

Michael Polkey Consultant Physician and Reader in Respiratory Medicine, Royal Brompton Hospital, London

Peter Goldstraw Professor of Thoracic Surgery, Royal Brompton Hospital, London

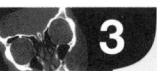 **3** Diseases of the ear nose and throat

Jeevendra Kanagalingam Specialist Registrar ENT, Royal National Throat, Nose and Ear Hospital, London

Azhar Shaida Consultant Otolaryngologist, Royal National Throat, Nose and Ear Hospital, London

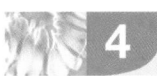 **4** Diseases of the gastrointestinal system

Roger Ackroyd Consultant Surgeon, Royal Hallamshire Hospital, Sheffield

David S Sanders Consultant Gastroenterologist, Royal Hallamshire Hospital, Sheffield

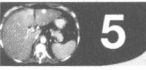 **5** Diseases of the liver, biliary system and pancreas

Christopher Callaghan Specialist Registrar in Surgery, Addenbrooke's Hospital, Cambridge

Wing-Kin Syn Specialist Registrar Gastroenterology and Hepatology, Queen Elizabeth Hospital, Birmingham

Monzur Ahmed Consultant Gastroenterologist, Good Hope Hospital, Birmingham

Paul Gibbs Lecturer and Hon Consultant Hepatobiliary and Transplant Surgeon, Addenbrooke's Hospital, Cambridge

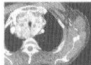 **6 Diseases of the endocrine system**

Marcus Simmgen Consultant Endocrinologist, St George's Hospital NHS Trust, London

Yoon Kong Loke Senior Lecturer in Clinical Pharmacology, School of Medicine, Health Policy and Practice, University of East Anglia, Norwich

Kevin Shotliff Consultant Endocrinologist, Chelsea and Westminster Hospital, London

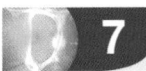 **7 Diabetes and other metabolic diseases**

Kevin Shotliff Consultant Endocrinologist, Chelsea and Westminster Hospital, London

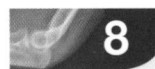 **8 Diseases of the bones and joints**

Andrew Östör Consultant Rheumatologist, Addenbrooke's Hospital, Associate Lecturer, School of Clinical Medicine, University of Cambridge

Nick Carrington Consultant Orthopaedic Surgeon, York Hospitals NHS Trust, York

Brian Hazleman Consultant Rheumatologist, Addenbrooke's Hospital, Cambridge

Nick Harris Consultant Orthopaedic Surgeon, Leeds General Infirmary, Leeds

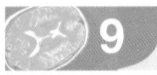 **9 Diseases of the nervous system and voluntary muscle**

Fiona McKevitt Specialist Registrar Neurology, Royal Hallamshire Hospital, Sheffield

Jeremy Rowe Consultant Neurosurgeon, Royal Hallamshire Hospital, Sheffield

Marios Hadjivassiliou Consultant Neurologist, Royal Hallamshire Hospital, Sheffield

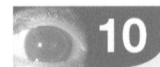 **10 Diseases of the eye**

Jodhbir S Mehta Fellow, Moorfields Eye Hospital NHS Trust, London

Ben Burton Locum Consultant, Moorfields Eye Hospital NHS Trust, London

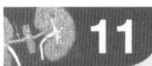 **11 Diseases of the kidney and urinary system**

Sampi Mehta Specialist Registrar Urology, Royal Hallamshire Hospital, Sheffield

Fiona Dallas Consultant Nephrologist, Cumberland Infirmary, Carlisle

Derek Rosario Senior Lecturer and Honorary Consultant Urologist, Royal Hallamshire Hospital, Sheffield

Albert Ong Reader in Nephrology & Hon Consultant Nephrologist, Academic Nephrology Unit, Sheffield Kidney Institute, University of Sheffield

 **12 Diseases of the haematological system**

Mike Greaves Professor of Haematology, Department of Medicine and Therapeutics, Aberdeen Royal Infirmary, Aberdeen

Dominic Culligan Consultant Haematologist, Aberdeen Royal Infirmary, Aberdeen

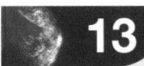 **13 Diseases of the breast**

John A Dewar Consultant Clinical Oncologist, Ninewells Hospital and Medical School, Dundee

Alastair M Thompson Professor of Surgical Oncology, Department of Surgery and Molecular Oncology, Ninewells Hospital and Medical School, Dundee

Colin A Purdie Consultant Histopathologist, Department of Pathology, Ninewells Hospital and Medical School, Dundee

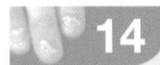 **14 Diseases of the skin**

Hiva Fassihi Specialist Registrar in Dermatology, St John's Institute of Dermatology, Guys and St Thomas' NHS Trust, London

Ian White Consultant Dermatologist, St John's Institute of Dermatology, Guys and St Thomas' NHS Trust, London

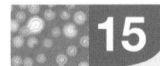 **15 Infectious diseases**

Kathleen Bamford Reader and Consultant Medical Microbiologist, Department of Infectious Diseases and Microbiology, Hammersmith Hospital, London

Contents

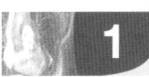

1   Diseases of the cardiovascular system

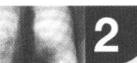

2   Diseases of the respiratory system

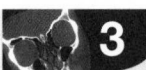

3 Diseases of the ear, nose and throat

4 Diseases of the gastrointestinal system

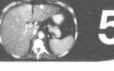

5 Diseases of the liver, biliary system and pancreas

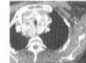

6 Diseases of the endocrine system

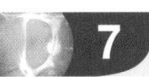

7 Diabetes and other metabolic diseases

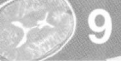

8 Diseases of the bones and joints

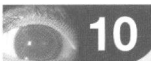

9 Diseases of the nervous system and voluntary muscle

10 Diseases of the eye

11 Diseases of the kidney and urinary system

12 Diseases of the haematological system

13 Diseases of the breast

14 Diseases of the skin

15 Infectious diseases

Diseases of the cardiovascular system

1

Eric Lim, Ziad Ali, Kevin Varty, John Wallwork, Philip Poole-Wilson

PART 1A Diseases of the heart and great vessels

SECTION 1.1 Introduction

Applied basic sciences of the cardiovascular system

Anatomy

The heart

The heart is a four-chambered muscular pump with a valve that guards the outlet of each chamber. The heart is a pyramidal structure situated obliquely in the thorax. The base of the pyramid (which can be considered as lying on its side) that consists of both the atria faces the spine, and the apex points approximately to the 5th intercostal space at the midclavicular line (where the apex beat is situated).

The anterior aspect of the heart is made up of the right atrium and ventricle. Deoxygenated blood travels from the venae cavae into the right atrium, across the tricuspid valve into the right ventricle, across the pulmonary valve and into the pulmonary arteries. Bacteria originating from the venous circulation (e.g. from contaminated syringes in intravenous drug use) predispose to right-sided endo-carditis. Moving backwards, when the right heart pressure

rises (from pulmonary hypertension, right ventricular failure, tricuspid regurgitation) blood pools back into the venae cavae leading to an elevated jugular venous pressure (JVP) and hepatomegaly.

The right atrium and ventricle are supplied by the right coronary artery. In approximately 70%, the right coronary branches into the posterior interventricular artery (posterior descending artery), and this is termed a right dominant coronary system; in the remaining 30%, the coronary system is either left- or co-dominant. Infarction of the right coronary artery can lead to right ventricular failure. Right coronary infarction is usually detected by abnormalities in the inferior leads (II, III and aVF) of the electrocardiogram (ECG).

The left atrium is situated on the most posterior aspect of the (medial facing) base of the heart, and blood in the left atrium travels across the mitral valve into the left ventricle, and then across the aortic valve into the aorta.

The mitral valve has two leaflets, the anterior and posterior. The most common site of valve prolapse is the middle aspect of the posterior leaflet. The mitral valve complex consists of the leaflets, annulus, cordae tendineae, papillary muscles and left ventricle. Failure of any single component can lead to mitral valve dysfunction, and usually mitral regurgitation. A better understanding of mitral valve function has led to the ability to repair the individual components and restore mitral valve competence.

The aortic valve is a semilunar valve with three cusps. The aortic valve complex consists of the valve leaflets, the sinuses of Valsalva (the dilated portion of the aorta that faces the valve leaflets), the annulus, the proximal ascending aorta and the left ventricular outflow tract. Abnormalities of any of the components can similarly lead to aortic valve dysfunction, for example aortic regurgitation can be due to dilatation of the proximal ascending aorta without any aortic valve leaflet abnormality.

The coronary artery supplies most of the blood to the left heart. The left main artery branches into the anterior intraventricular (left anterior descending) and the circumflex artery. The anterior intraventricular artery supplies the septum and the branches (diagonal arteries) supply the left ventricular free wall. Branches of the circumflex artery (obtuse marginals) also supply the left ventricular free wall. Infarction of the anterior intraventricular artery leads to abnormalities in the anterior and septal leads of the ECG, left ventricular dysfunction and cardiogenic shock if sufficiently extensive. Infarction of the circumflex artery leads to abnormalities in the lateral leads of the ECG and left ventricular dysfunction.

The pericardium

The pericardium consists of two layers, a fibrous outer layer and an inner serous layer attached to the surface of the heart forming the epicardium. Normally there is approximately 50 mL of clear straw-coloured pericardial fluid within the pericardium. Normal intrapericardial pressure is either negative or zero. Pericardial constraint facilitates coupling of the ventricles; however, when a pericardial effusion accumulates, the increase in pressure will eventually impair diastolic relaxation of the ventricles and cause cardiac tamponade.

Physiology

Pre-load

At rest, the heart pumps approximately 5 litres of blood per minute. The degree of tension of the heart muscle before it begins to contract is the pre-load. End diastolic pressure is normally considered to be the measure of the pre-load. Within physiological limits, as pre-load increases, cardiac output increases. This is because the digitations of the actin and myosin filaments within the myocyte are optimized by the increase in length. In severe haemorrhage, the pre-load is reduced because of volume losses, cardiac output is suboptimal, and circulatory shock ensues when peripheral vasoconstriction can no longer sustain the blood pressure. Fluid administration will increase the pre-load and restore ventricular performance. In the setting of heart failure, cardiac output is low and once the optimum filling pressure (pre-load) is achieved, further distension results in reduced cardiac output, as the actin and myosin filaments are distended to a point of sub-optimal coaptation. Further

volume replacement lowers the cardiac output and causes back pressure on the left ventricle eventually resulting in pulmonary oedema.

Contractility

Intrinsic contractility of the myocardium is influenced by sympathetic stimulation, and the treatment of circulatory shock (in selected patients) includes the administration of inotropic agents such as adrenaline. Drugs that inhibit the sympathetic system in general also impair contractility, and include beta-blockers (β-blockers). The role of β-blockers in heart failure is complex, as overall survival benefit is thought to be achieved by attenuating the adverse effects of intrinsic sympathetic overstimulation. The contractility of the heart can be assessed visually and is most commonly quantified as the ejection fraction on transthoracic echocardiography (p. 8). The normal ejection fraction is approximately 60%.

Afterload

Afterload is the load against which the heart must exert a contractile force. The systolic pressure is normally considered to be a measure of the afterload, although the systemic vascular resistance is often (loosely) considered. The cardiac output is increased with a lower afterload, and this can be achieved by reducing the systemic vascular resistance and hence systolic pressure. Inodilators are a class of phosphodiesterase inhibitors (milrinone, enoximone) that increase cardiac contractility whilst decreasing systemic vascular resistance (afterload) to improve cardiac output.

Blood pressure

Blood pressure is influenced by the relationship between the pre-load, contractility and afterload. The mean blood pressure is calculated by adding a third of the pulse pressure to the diastolic blood pressure. The relationship between arterial pressure, cardiac output and vascular resistance is:

$$\text{Arterial pressure} = \text{cardiac output} \times \text{total peripheral resistance} \quad [1]$$

$$\text{Cardiac output} = \text{stroke volume} \times \text{heart rate} \quad [2]$$

Since stroke volume is influenced by pre-load and contractility, blood pressure increases if there is an increase in pre-load, contractility, heart rate or total peripheral resistance. Often, manipulations of a combination of these factors are undertaken in the intensive care unit (ICU) when managing a patient with low blood pressure.

With chronic hypertension, the kidney plays a major role in maintaining the blood pressure. This is achieved by changes in the extracellular fluid volume and the renin–angiotensin system. Renin is secreted by the juxtaglomerular cells in response to low blood pressure (secretion is normally reduced in conditions of high blood pressure) and converts angiotensinogen to angiotensin I; angiotensin I is converted to angiotensin II by the angiotensin-converting enzyme (ACE). Angiotensin II is a powerful vasoconstrictor that acts directly on the kidneys, causing salt and water retention, and also stimulates the release of aldosterone that has the same effect on the kidneys.

Antihypertensive medication can lower the blood pressure by a number of mechanisms. With equations [1] and [2] in mind, antihypertensive agents can lower the pre-load (diuretic agents decrease the extracellular volume), reduce contractility (β-blockers, non-dihydropyridine calcium antagonists), reduce heart rate (β-blockers), reduce total peripheral resistance (dihydropyridine calcium antagonists) and inhibit the renin–angiotensin system (ACE inhibitors).

Pressure and volume loading

The physiological response of the left ventricle to pressure overload is concentric hypertrophy. Common conditions that lead to pressure overload include aortic stenosis and chronic hypertension. In mitral stenosis, the chronic pressure overload imposed by the narrowed mitral valve orifice leads to left atrial dilatation, and this predisposes to abnormal electrical pathways and atrial fibrillation. In the right heart, chronic pulmonary hypertension predisposes to dilatation of the thin-walled right ventricle.

With volume overload, the response of the left ventricle is to dilate; therefore, in mitral or aortic regurgitation, the left ventricle dilates to accommodate the regurgitant volume. Initially the dilatation improves the contractility, but later in the disease process gradual dilatation is associated with ventricular impairment as the ventricular function approaches the far right-hand aspect of the Starling curve (Fig. 1.1). Therefore, when deciding the timing of intervention for aortic and mitral regurgitation, measurements of left ventricular end diastolic diameter are important, as increasing dimension is associated with disease progression.

Symptoms of cardiac disease

Chest pain

Chest pain is a common symptom of cardiac disease. Cardiac ischaemia causes angina, a tight and crushing retrosternal pain that may radiate to the jaw and down into the arm. Angina may be precipitated by effort, emotion, food or cold weather. It is usually relieved by rest or glyceryl trinitrate (GTN). If angina occurs at rest for more than 20 minutes, a diagnosis of myocardial infarction should be presumed until proven otherwise. The severity of angina is classified according to the Canadian Cardiovascular Society grade (p. 20).

Other cardiovascular causes of chest pains include pericarditis, often described as a sharp pleuritic chest pain that may radiate to the back (trapezius ridge pain) and is relieved by sitting forwards. The pain of aortic dissection has a tearing quality and is usually described as the most severe pain to be experienced by the patient. It originates in the chest and may radiate to the back or abdomen.

Shortness of breath

Cardiac failure is an important cause of dyspnoea. Its severity is often measured in relation to the New York Heart Association (NYHA) functional class (p. 16). Symptoms of left ventricular failure are dyspnoea, orthopnoea and paroxysmal nocturnal dyspnoea. Orthopnoea refers to shortness of breath when lying flat, and is thought to be due to the redistribution of the interstitial oedema of the lungs. It is relieved by sitting upright, presumably facilitating gravitational redistribution to the lung bases. Paroxysmal nocturnal dyspnoea is sudden onset of dyspnoea whilst sleeping that wakes the patient suddenly and is also relieved by sitting upright. Concomitant symptoms of right ventricular failure are peripheral oedema and abdominal distension (hepatomegaly, ascites).

Palpitations

Palpitation is an awareness of the heartbeat. Arrhythmia is the usual underlying cardiac cause (page 58). A variety of complaints are used to describe palpitations, including 'fluttering', 'pounding' and 'skipping a beat'. Symptoms may also be experienced in the neck. Important aspects are the frequency, regularity of palpitation (e.g. fast and irregular) and precipitating factors.

Knowledge of precipitating factors is important. Palpitations can be a normal manifestation of anxiety or panic reactions. However, it is vitally important that an organic cause is excluded as it is common for anxiety disorders to coexist in a patient with supraventricular tachycardia. Exercise is associated with excess catecholamines and also a precipitator of arrhythmia (supraventricular tachycardia, atrial fibrillation and ventricular tachycardia usually originating from the right ventricle). Excessive caffeine, smoking and alcohol intake are also thought to be precipitators of arrhythmia.

A history of any underlying heart disorder is important, as arrhythmia is associated with ischaemic heart disease (ventricular arrhythmia), hypertensive heart disease (atrial fibrillation), heart failure (ventricular arrhythmia) and heart valve disease.

Early age of onset of arrhythmia (childhood or teenage years) suggests the presence of a congenital abnormality such as a bypass tract that can lead to supraventricular tachycardia.

Syncope

Syncope is often due to vasovagal reaction (simple faint) but can also be a symptom of serious underlying disease. Cardiac outflow obstruction, which occurs with aortic stenosis and hypertrophic obstructive cardiomyopathy, can result in syncope on effort as the cardiac output is not increased on demand. Orthostatic hypotension causes a transient decrease in cerebral perfusion and if sufficiently severe can lead to loss of consciousness. This may result from the use of antihypertensive medications, and especially diuretics, in the elderly. In carotid sinus syndrome, the receptors of the carotid sinus are more sensitive than normal; thus minor stimulation, such as turning the head or pressure from a tight collar, may elicit the carotid sinus reflex and precipitate syncope.

Applied basic sciences of the cardiovascular system

Symptoms of cardiac disease

Examination of the cardiovascular system

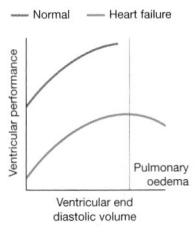

Fig. 1.1 Relationship between ventricular performance and end-diastolic volume.

Examination of the cardiovascular system

Inspection

The first impression can yield a lot of information: by standing at the end of the bed it is easy to appreciate dyspnoea at rest, evidence of cyanosis, the nodding of the head with severe aortic regurgitation (de Musset's sign), and cachexia of severe cardiac failure.

Inspection of the fingers may reveal clubbing (cyanotic heart disease, endocarditis), splinter haemorrhages, Osler's nodes (painful erythematous lesions on the pulps of the fingers) and Janeway lesions (flat erythematous lesions on the palms of the hands). Peripheral infarctions of the digits can be due to emboli from atrial fibrillation or prosthetic heart valves.

Palpation

The peripheral pulse reveals the rate and rhythm (pulse volume should be assessed at the carotids). In addition the character of the pulse may be bounding in aortic regurgitation, giving a water hammer quality. Symmetry of the pulses is important and may be affected by aortic dissection and coarctation (radio-femoral delay). The blood pressure is obtained and a narrow pulse pressure (less than half the diastolic pressure) may be indicative of aortic stenosis.

The JVP is examined: elevation occurs with congestive cardiac failure, tricuspid valve disease and pericardial tamponade.

The precordium is palpated, and the apex beat located. The apex beat is displaced by conditions that lead to cardiomegaly (congestive heart failure, aortic valve disease, mitral regurgitation). A thrill (palpable murmur) will occur with the associated heart valve disease.

Auscultation

The heart is auscultated in the apex with the bell and diaphragm of the stethoscope and then over the second right intercostal space (aortic area), the second left intercostal space (pulmonary area), down the left border of the sternum (for the diastolic murmur of aortic regurgitation) and over the tricuspid area. A summary of the heart valve lesions and corresponding murmurs is provided in Table 1.1.

Peripheral examination

At the end of the examination it is also important to auscultate the lung bases for pulmonary oedema and to examine the liver for hepatomegaly and the legs for peripheral oedema.

Table 1.1	Summary of cardiac murmurs			
Valve disease	**Murmur**	**Location of greatest intensity**	**Other features**	
Systolic murmurs				
Aortic stenosis	Ejection systolic	Right second interspace	Radiates to the carotids	
Mitral regurgitation	Pansystolic	Apex	Radiates to the axilla	
Tricuspid regurgitation[a]	Pansystolic	Left lower sternal edge	Elevated JVP, right ventricular heave, pulsatile hepatomegaly	
Ventricular septal defect[b]	Pansystolic 'tearing'	Left sternal edge		
Coarctation of the aorta[b]	Systolic	Over precordium (collateral flow) and the back	Radio-femoral delay	
Diastolic murmurs				
Aortic regurgitation[a]	Early diastolic	Left sternal edge	Accentuated by expiration	
Mitral stenosis[a]	Mid diastolic rumbling	Apex	Accentuated by expiration with the patient turned to the left	

[a] Uncommon conditions
[b] Rare conditions

Blood tests

Serum cardiac markers

The cardiac enzymes (creatine kinase and lactase dehydrogenase) have largely been superseded by troponin (T or I) as the serum cardiac marker of choice (troponin is a peptide). The almost absolute specificity of troponin to cardiac muscle has led to the recent re-definition of myocardial infarction using elevated serum troponin as the primary diagnostic criterion. Troponin is detected in the serum approximately 4–10 hours after the onset of myocardial infarction, peaks at 12–48 hours and remains elevated for 4–10 days.[1] CK-MB (myocardium-bound fraction of creatine kinase) is a suitable alternative when troponin assay is not available. CK-MB is elevated 4–8 hours after myocardial infarction, peaks at approximately 12 hours and returns to normal after 2–3 days. CK-MB remains elevated for a much shorter time than troponin, is a useful indicator for early re-infarction and provides an estimate of the size of the infarct.

Electrocardiogram

The standard 12 lead ECG is obtained by the analysis of electrical current generated by the heart and analyzed in two planes. The first plane is the coronal plane of the limb leads. There are six different leads (Fig. 1.2a). Lead I is created by making the left arm positive and the right arm negative, giving the angle of orientation of 0°. The angles of orientation of the subsequent leads are created similarly, giving rise to different angles (Table 1.2). By extrapolation, the entire coronal axis can be analyzed in multiples of 30° (Fig. 1.2a). The electrical axis of the heart is analyzed in the coronal plane and the normal axis is defined to lie within −30° to +120°.

The precordial leads look at the heart in a horizontal plane (Fig. 1.2b). Each lead is made positive in turn: V1 is in the 4th intercostal space to the right of the sternum, V4 is in the 5th intercostal space to the left of the sternum, and V6 lies in the midaxillary line.

Grouping of the leads allows the different aspects of the heart to be analyzed. The main regions are the anterior, inferior and left lateral surfaces (Table 1.3). Each small square on the ECG represents 0.04 seconds and each large square (5 small squares) is 0.20 seconds.

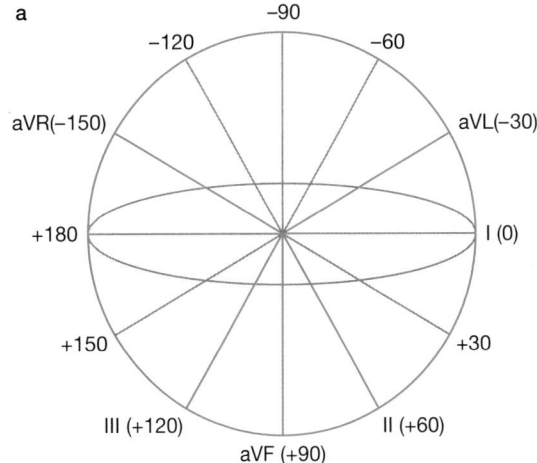

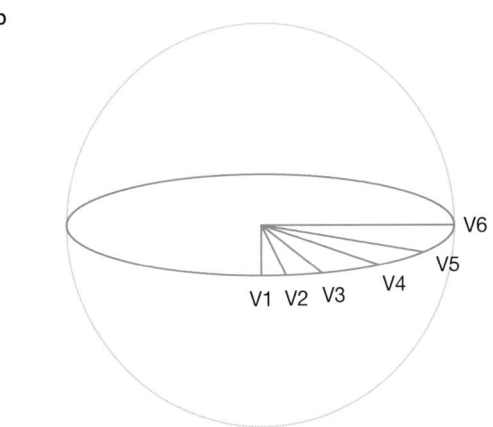

Table 1.2	Electrical axis of the limb leads of the ECG		
Lead	**Positive electrode**	**Negative electrode**	**Angle of orientation**
I	Left arm	Right arm	0°
II	Legs	Right arm	60°
III	Legs	Left arm	120°
aVL*	Left arm	All other leads	−30°
aVR*	Right arm	All other leads	−150°
aVF*	Legs	All other leads	90°

The limb leads are in multiples of 60° from 0°
* The augmented limb leads are in multiples of 30° from 0°
Extrapolating from all the leads, the angle of orientation of the entire coronal axis can be analyzed in multiples of 30°

Fig. 1.2a Orientation of the limb leads. The standard leads are in black, and the extrapolations that can be used are in grey.
Fig. 1.2b Orientation of the precordial leads.

Table 1.3	Grouping of the leads of the ECG	
Group	**Lead combination**	
Anterior	V_1, V_2, V_3, V_4	
Left lateral	I, V_5, V_6	
Inferior	II, III, aVF	

P wave

The P wave (Fig. 1.3) results from atrial depolarization. The current flows from right atrium to left atrium and in a slightly inferior direction; it is therefore positive in the left and inferior leads. The duration of the P wave is 0.12–0.20 seconds (3–5 small squares). A short P wave is usually due to an accessory pathway into the ventricle that bypasses the normal conduction, hence shortening the P wave. Two such common pathways are the bundle of Kent in Wolff–Parkinson–White syndrome and James fibres in Lown–Ganong–Levine syndrome, the pre-excitation syndromes.

QRS complex

The QRS complex (Fig. 1.3) is caused by depolarization of the ventricles. From the atrio-ventricular node, the conducting system (the sites of fastest conduction) comprises the bundle of His, which divides into the right and left bundle branches and finally the terminal Purkinje fibres. The QRS duration is normally less than 0.12 seconds (3 small squares) and the QRS axis normally lies within −30° to +90°. Left axis deviation is associated with left ventricular enlargement (loosely termed hypertrophy, but the ECG cannot distinguish between myocardial hypertrophy and ventricular dilatation). Right axis deviation is much less common and is associated with right ventricular dilatation.

The ST segment

The ST segment (Fig. 1.3) represents the time from ventricular depolarization to repolarization. The height of the ST segment is affected by ischaemia and infarction. It was previously thought that ST segment elevation was associated with infarction whilst ST segment depression was associated with ischaemia. It is now recognized that either configuration can be associated with infarction and troponin release.

T wave and QT interval

The T wave (Fig. 1.3) is due to repolarization of the ventricles. Peaked T waves can result from hyperkalaemia. The QT interval (from the onset of the Q to the end of the T wave) measures the duration from the start of depolarization to the end of repolarization (Fig. 1.3). The normal QT interval varies with the heart rate, therefore the corrected QT interval is normally estimated as QT interval divided by the square root of the R to R interval of a successive beat and is normally less than 0.45 seconds. Drugs (antihistamines, tricyclic antidepressants) and electrolyte abnormalities (hypokalaemia, hypocalcaemia) that prolong the QT interval predispose to a form of ventricular tachycardia (torsade de pointes) with a risk of progression to ventricular fibrillation.

Conduction blocks

First-degree heart block is defined as a prolonged PR interval (more than 0.20s) without any dropped beats (Fig. 1.4a). This is a common finding and may be associated with drugs such as β-blockers. In general, first-degree heart block is a benign rhythm due to delay in conduction at the AV node or bundle of His.

Second-degree heart block occurs when not every atrial impulse passes through the AV node into the ventricles. There are two types of second degree heart block: Mobitz type I (or Wenckebach block) that occurs within the AV node and causes the PR interval to become progressively longer resulting in a dropped beat (Fig. 1.4b), and Mobitz type II conduction block that occurs below the AV node where a dropped beat occurs after 2 to 3 normal beats without a prolonged PR interval (Fig. 1.4c). Mobitz type II second degree heart block is usually associated with more serious underlying disease compared to Mobitz type I block.

Complete heart block occurs when the atria and ventricles are conducting independently of each other (Fig. 1.4d). The ventricle usually generates an escape rhythm at a rate of 40 beats per min. A wide QRS results (Fig. 1.4d) as the 'new' pacemaker originates within the ventricular tissue and not the conducting system.

Partial conduction block can also occur below the bundle of His, resulting in right or left bundle branch block. It is associated with a normal heart rate with a wide QRS complex (more than 0.12 s). A right bundle branch block results in an RSR′ pattern in lead V1 and left bundle branch block is associated with notched R waves in V6; the pattern is not usually as pronounced as in right bundle branch block.

Cardiac enlargement

Left ventricular hypertrophy (more accurately, enlargement) is suggested when the sum of the S wave amplitude

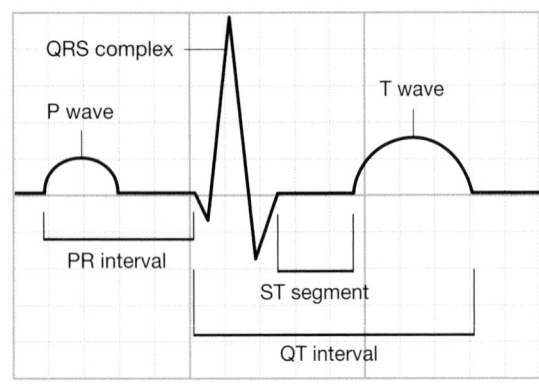

Fig. 1.3 Standard ECG complex.

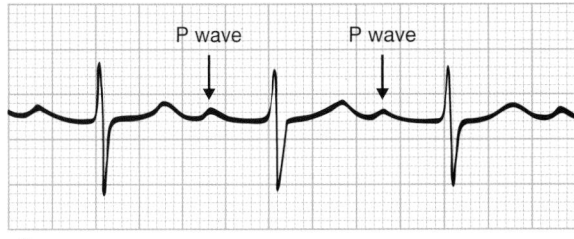

a

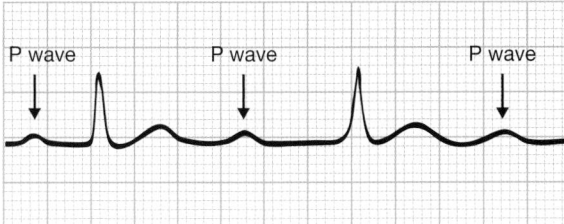

b

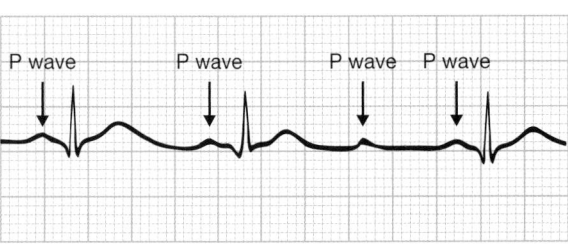

c

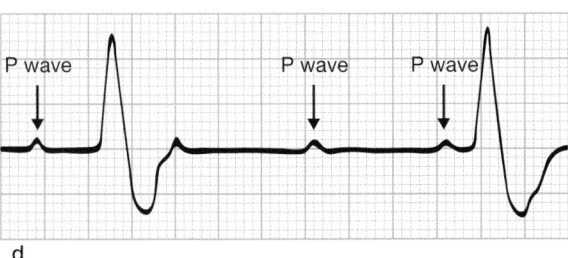

d

Fig. 1.4 Conduction blocks. (a) First-degree heart block. (b) Second-degree heart block (Mobitz type I (Wenckebach) block. (c) Second-degree heart block (Mobitz type II block). (d) Third-degree (complete) heart block.

in V1 (or V2) and the R wave amplitude in V6 (or V5) is more than 35 mm, usually with accompanying left axis deviation. Right ventricular hypertrophy is less common and suggested by an R wave that is taller than the S wave in V1 and right axis deviation.

Exercise electrocardiogram

Exercise ECG is often used to determine the presence of coronary artery disease. The resting ECG is often normal in patients with stenotic coronary disease, therefore myocardial ischaemia is induced by stress (exercise or with pharmacological agents such as dobutamine) and the corresponding ST segment and T wave changes are screened to evaluate the presence of flow-limiting coronary disease. Exercise testing is contraindicated in patients

with uncontrolled angina, heart failure, and symptomatic aortic stenosis.

The most common method of investigation is the Bruce protocol. The patient walks on the treadmill at an initial speed of 1.7 mph and an incline of 10 degrees; every three minutes the speed and incline are increased, for example stage 2 is a speed of 2.5 mph and an incline of 12 degrees. The test continues until the target end point is reached (2 mm ST segment depression), until completion if no demonstrable ECG change suggestive of ischaemia occurs, or if a complication develops (ST segment elevation, hypotension, moderate angina, arrhythmia).

Diagnostic imaging

Chest X-ray (CXR)

The standard films for the evaluation of cardiac disease are the postero-anterior (PA) and the lateral plain chest X-ray (Fig. 1.5). In this section we focus on cardiac abnormalities. The right heart border consists of the superior vena cava and right atrium, whilst the left heart border consists of the aortic arch, pulmonary artery, left atrial appendage and the free wall of the left ventricle.

Cardiomegaly is defined when the transverse diameter of the heart is more than 50% of the transverse diameter of the chest. This is an approximate definition; common causes are congestive cardiac failure, mitral regurgitation, aortic valve disease and pericardial effusion (globular cardiac silhouette).

Other radiological features of congestive cardiac failure are bilateral patchy consolidation (pulmonary oedema), upper lobe venous diversion, Kerley B lines (linear shadows at the peripheral 2 cm of the lung fields) and bilateral pleural effusions (page 164).

Isolated enlargement of the left atrium (mitral stenosis) results in a double right heart shadow (the second shadow

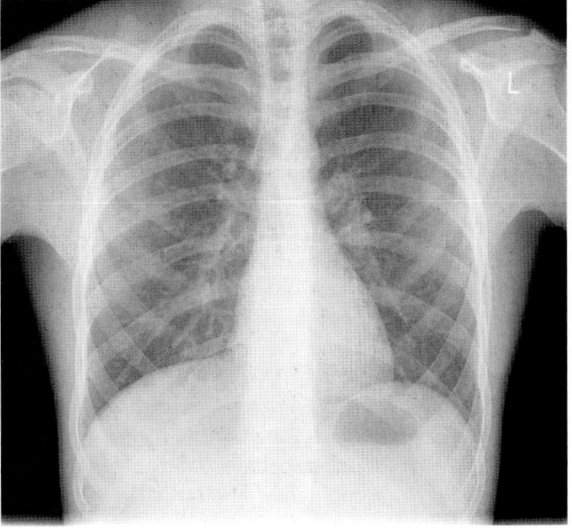

Fig. 1.5 Plain chest film.

RECENT ADVANCES

Cardiac MRI (Fig. 1.6) has moved from research tool to mainstream imaging and is an important technique for three-dimensional assessment of cardiac structure, myocardial function, myocardial perfusion and myocardial viability.[2] Cardiac gated CT is able to detect coronary calcification and is currently being evaluated as a tool for quantification and risk stratification of coronary artery disease.[3]

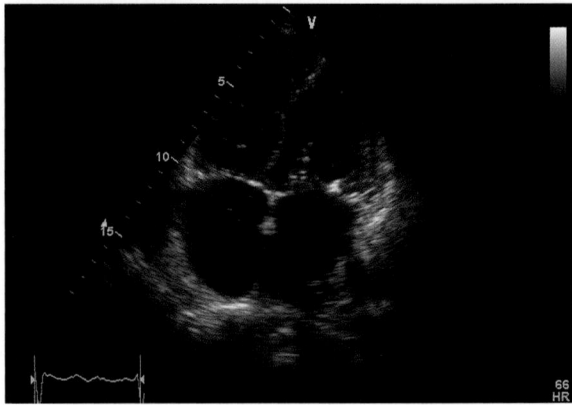

Fig. 1.7 Transthoracic echocardiogram—a four-chamber view.

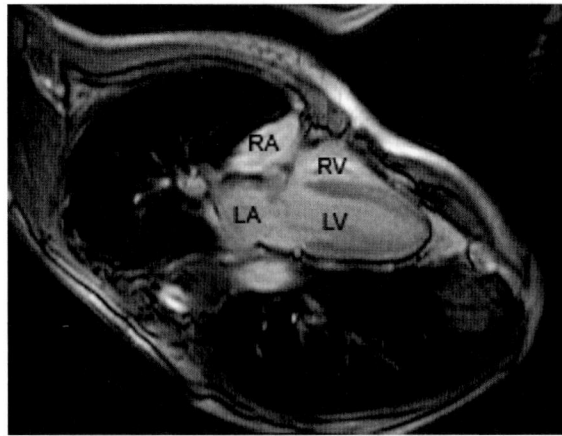

Fig. 1.6 Cardiac MRI. In this scan of all four chambers of the heart, the cross-section is viewed as if looking from the feet up to the head.

is the left atrial border, p. 1), tenting of the left heart border (enlarged atrial appendage) and, in very large atria, splaying of the carina (due to pressure from the left atrium).

Echocardiography

Transthoracic echocardiography is a widely used non-invasive investigation that has the ability to visualize the anatomy and function of the heart valves, myocardium and pericardium. It is the investigation of choice for the evaluation of heart valve disease.

The standard view on transthoracic echocardiography is the apical four-chamber view (Fig. 1.7), where the probe is positioned over the apex and the structure and function of all four cardiac chambers can be visualized. Additional views are the parasternal short and long axis views. In addition, continuous wave and colour flow Doppler modalities can quantitate the presence and severity of valve stenosis and regurgitation.

Transoesophageal echocardiography can be performed as a day case procedure or intraoperatively. The echocardiogram probe is introduced into the oesophagus and visualizes the heart along the length of the oesophagus and from within the stomach. In contrast to transthoracic echocardiography, the probe visualizes cardiac structures from deep to superficial. The standard views are the midoesophageal four-chamber view and the transgastric short axis view. In addition, numerous other views are able to visualize the structures of the heart. The advantage of transoesophageal echocardiography lies in the visual-

ization of the left atrium (situated immediately anterior to the oesophagus) and the mitral valve. The right heart structures, situated furthest away from the probe, are better visualized by transthoracic echocardiography.

Dobutamine stress echocardiogram

Dobutamine stress echocardiography is a useful investigation for detecting inducible myocardial ischaemia. A resting echocardiogram is performed to assess wall motion and is then repeated after exercise or pharmacologically induced stress. New regional wall motion abnormalities correspond to areas of ischaemia. The overall sensitivity is 82% and specificity is 84% for the detection of areas of significant coronary disease.

 INFORMATION ON ECHOCARDIOGRAPHY

Cheitlin MD, Armstrong WF, Aurigemma GP, et al. ACC/AHA/ASE 2003 guideline update for the clinical application of echocardiography: summary article: a report of the American College of Cardiology/American Heart Association Task Force on Practice Guidelines (ACC/AHA/ASE Committee to Update the 1997 Guidelines for the Clinical Application of Echocardiography). Circulation 2003; 108: 1146–1162.

Cardiac radionuclide imaging

A cardiac radionuclide image (cardiac scintigraphy) is obtained by injecting a radionuclide into the peripheral circulation and imaging with a gamma camera. The emitted gamma rays are focused using a collimator, and the anatomical origin and time of isotope decay is transformed into an image.

The radiopharmaceuticals used for single photon myocardial perfusion imaging include thallium-201 (^{201}Tl, a potassium analogue) and technetium-99m (^{99m}Tc). The tracers used for positron emission tomography (PET) include oxygen-15, carbon-11 and fluorine-18, which may be coupled to physiologically active molecules such as fatty acids (^{11}C labelled fatty acids), and deoxyglucose (^{18}F-labelled deoxyglucose).

Myocardial perfusion imaging

Planar and single photon emission computed tomography (SPECT) images are widely acquired for the assessment of the presence and severity of coronary disease, detection of myocardial viability, myocardial wall mass and global ventricular function.

The presence of coronary disease and myocardial viability can be assessed on rest and stress images that are induced by exercise or pharmacological agents such as dobutamine. Typically, ^{99m}Tc is the myocardial perfusion agent of choice. The patient is usually subjected to pharmacological or exercise stress. Just before termination of the protocol, the isotope is injected and its myocardial fixation represents blood flow in the stressed state. The ^{99m}Tc MIBI (2-methoxy isobutyl isonitrile) attaches to the myocardium in proportion to the instantaneous regional perfusion. Approximately 60 minutes later, images are obtained using SPECT and reformatted to represent images perpendicular to the long and short axis of the heart.

In some departments, the ^{99m}Tc MIBI injection is repeated the next day at rest, and rest scans are compared for discordant or concordant areas of activity (Fig. 1.8). A discordant deficit indicates a region of ischaemia, whilst a concordant deficit (no isotope visible on the stress or exercise study) is due to the presence of an infarct or scarred non-viable myocardium. It is possible to use different isotopes and perform the two phases of the same study on the same day.

Analysis of ventricular function

In addition to areas of regional ischaemia or infarction, it is possible to analyze the ventricular function. Gated SPECT myocardial perfusion images that are synchronized with the ECG (to determine the onset of systole and diastole) are used to estimate the area of the ventricle in systole and diastole. The cross-sectional areas are used to calculate the three-dimensional ventricular volume and hence the ejection fraction. An alternative method is to use a first-pass radionuclide angiogram, where the ejection fraction is estimated based on the change in radioactivity over time.

Myocardial infarct avid imaging

Radionuclide imaging can also be used to assess the presence of myocardial necrosis using tracers such as ^{99m}Tc pyrophosphate that localize to infarcted myocardium. The

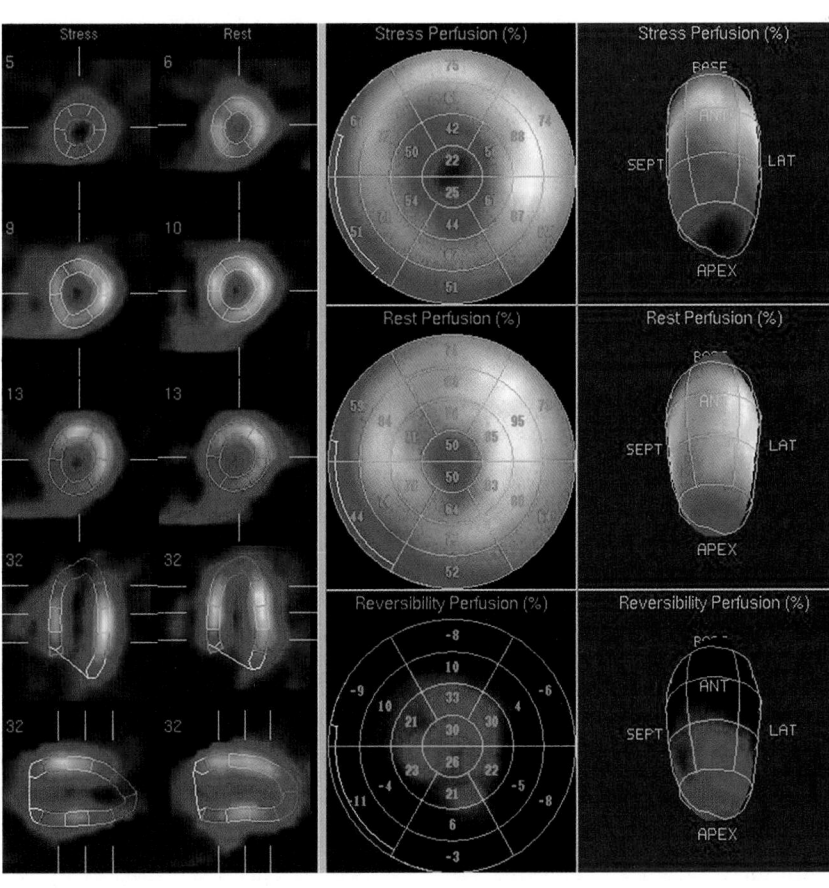

Fig. 1.8 Cardiac SPECT scan. The presence of reversible ischaemia is indicated by the orange-lighted cardiac segments at rest.

most intense localization usually occurs 48–72 hours after infarction. However, serum troponin has largely superseded this radionuclide technique to detect myocardial infarction.

 INFORMATION ON RADIONUCLIDE IMAGING

Klocke FJ, Baird MG, Lorell BH, et al. ACC/AHA/ASNC guidelines for the clinical use of cardiac radionuclide imaging—executive summary: a report of the American College of Cardiology/American Heart Association Task Force on Practice Guidelines (ACC/AHA/ASNC Committee to Revise the 1995 Guidelines for the Clinical Use of Cardiac Radionuclide Imaging). Circulation 2003; 108: 1404–1418.

REFERENCES

(1) *Wu AHB, Apple FS, Gibler WB, Jesse RL, Warshaw MM, Valdes R Jr. National Academy of Clinical Biochemistry Standards of Laboratory Practice: recommendations for the use of cardiac markers in coronary artery diseases. Clinical Chemistry 1999; 45: 1104–1121.*
(2) *Constantine G, Shan K, Flamm SD, Sivananthan MU. Role of MRI in clinical cardiology. Lancet 2004; 363: 2162–2171.*
(3) *Schoepf UJ, Becker CR, Ohnesorge BM, Yucel EK. CT of coronary artery disease. Radiology 2004; 232: 18–37.*

SECTION 1.3   Diagnostic procedures

Diagnostic cardiac catheterization

Cardiac catheterization is a technique that can be used to measure intracardiac pressures and perform coronary or ventricular angiography. Percutaneous coronary intervention and radiofrequency ablation are extensions to this technique in which angioplasty, stenting or the treatment of arrhythmia is performed through the same approach.

Indications

The main indication for diagnostic cardiac catheterization is the identification and assessment of the severity of coronary artery disease. It may also be a complementary investigation to assess cardiac haemodynamic measurements and the severity of heart valve disease.

Patient preparation

Cardiac catheterization is usually performed as a day case. Informed consent is required and patients are admitted preoperatively to screen for relative contraindications such as coagulopathy and extensive femoral arterial disease.

Procedure

The patient is positioned supine in the cardiac catheterization suite, and an X-ray image intensifier is used. Right or left heart catheterization can be performed. The approach to the right heart is via the jugular, subclavian or femoral vein. The left heart is usually approached via the femoral artery. A needle is used to puncture the vessel and a guidewire is introduced. The original needle is removed and a sheath is introduced into the vessel using the guidewire. Once the sheath is securely in the vessel, the guidewire is removed.

For right heart catheterization, the cardiac catheter is introduced into the sheath and advanced to the right atrium, right ventricle and pulmonary artery where haemodynamic measurements or the injection of contrast media can be performed.

For left heart catheterization, the catheter is advanced to the ascending aorta, through the aortic valve and into the left ventricle (Fig. 1.9). Haemodynamic measurements can be performed and contrast media injected into the ventricle to obtain a ventriculogram or into the left main

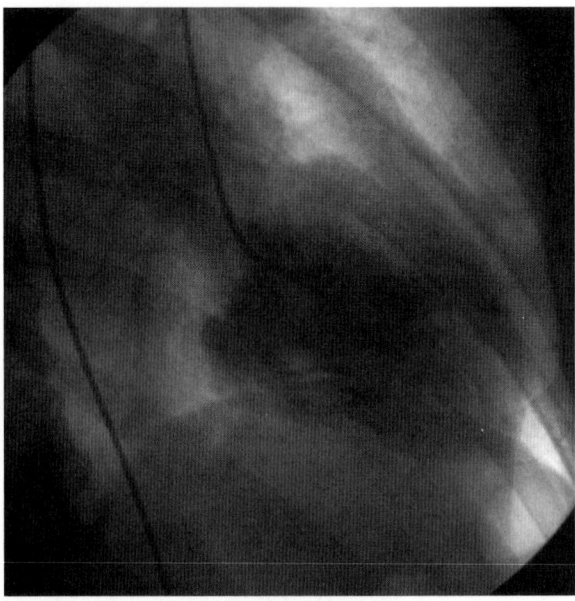

Fig. 1.9 A left ventricular angiogram illustrating reflux of contrast into the left atrium due to mitral regurgitation.

and right coronary arteries for coronary angiography. An arch aortogram can also be performed if necessary to visualize the aortic arch.

Complications

There is a 0.11% risk of mortality, 0.05% risk of myocardial infarction and 0.07% risk of stroke with coronary angiography.[1]

Post procedure care

After the procedure, sustained pressure over the groin is usually required for left heart catheterization where the

femoral artery has been punctured. Patients are monitored for femoral arterial bleeding and complications such as myocardial infarction and stroke.

> **REFERENCE**
>
> **(1)** *Scanlon PJ, Faxon DP, Audet A-M, et al. ACC/AHA guidelines for coronary angiography: executive summary and recommendations: a report of the American College of Cardiology/American Heart Association Task Force on Practice Guidelines (Committee on Coronary Angiography) Developed in collaboration with the Society for Cardiac Angiography and Interventions. Circulation 1999; 99: 2345–2357.*

SECTION 1.4   Therapeutic procedures

Permanent pacing and implantable cardioverter defibrillators

Indications

The main indications for a permanent pacemaker are symptomatic bradycardia associated with (complete and bifascicular) heart block, acute myocardial infarction, sinus node dysfunction or neurocardiogenic syncope. The disease specific indications are listed in Table 1.4.

An implantable cardioverter defibrillator looks like and can function as a pacemaker; however, it can also deliver low-energy synchronized cardioversion and high-energy defibrillation shocks that are successful in terminating 99% of ventricular fibrillation attacks. The implantation proce-

Table 1.4	**Indications for a permanent pacemaker***

Acquired atrioventricular block

Third degree or advanced second-degree heart block with any of the following features:
- Symptomatic bradycardia
- Arrhythmia or other medical condition that requires medications that cause symptomatic bradycardia
- Documented asystole of more than 3 seconds, or any escape beat less than 40 bpm
- After catheter ablation of the atrioventricular junction
- Atrioventricular block after cardiac surgery that is not expected to recover
- Neuromuscular diseases with atrioventricular block

Second-degree heart block with associated symptomatic bradycardia

Chronic bifascicular and trifascicular blocks

Intermittent third-degree atrioventricular block

Type II second-degree atrioventricular block

Alternating bundle branch block

After myocardial infarction

Persistent second-degree atrioventricular block with bilateral bundle branch block or third-degree atrioventricular block below the His–Purkinje system

Transient advanced (second- or third-degree) infranodal atrioventricular block and associated bundle branch block

Persistent and symptomatic second- or third-degree atrioventricular block

Sinus node dysfunction

Sinus node dysfunction with documented symptomatic bradycardia, including frequent sinus pauses that produce symptoms

Symptomatic chronotropic incompetence

Carotid sinus syndrome and neurocardiogenic syncope

Recurrent syncope caused by carotid sinus stimulation

* Selected class I indications from Gregoratos G, Abrams J, Epstein AE, et al. ACC/AHA/NASPE 2002 guideline update for implantation of cardiac pacemakers and antiarrhythmia devices: summary article: a report of the American College of Cardiology/American Heart Association Task Force on Practice Guidelines (ACC/AHA/NASPE Committee to Update the 1998 Pacemaker Guidelines). Circulation 2002; 106: 2145–2161.

dure is similar to that of a pacemaker but the indications differ and are listed in Table 1.5.

Patient preparation

Informed consent is required and patients are required to starve from midnight in case general anaesthesia is required.

Procedure

Under local anaesthesia, a small incision is sited below the clavicle and a subcutaneous pocket is created. Access to the subclavian vein is obtained and the pacemaker leads are advanced under fluoroscopic (X-ray) control from the subclavian vein to the brachiocephalic vein, superior vena cava and into the right atrium and right ventricle. Dual chambered pacemakers require the implantation of a pacemaker lead in the right atrium and right ventricle. The leads are tested to ensure good electrical contact and then connected to the pacemaker, which is then placed into the subcutaneous pocket. The defect is closed in layers.

Complications

Complications that can arise include bleeding and infection. Rarely, perforation of the heart can occur. Pacemaker-related complications include fracture and dislodgement of the pacing leads.

Table 1.5	Indications for an implantable cardioverter defibrillator
Cardiac arrest due to ventricular fibrillation or ventricular tachycardia not due to a transient or reversible cause	
Spontaneous sustained ventricular tachycardia in association with structural heart disease	
Syncope of undetermined origin with clinically relevant, haemodynamically significant sustained ventricular tachycardia or ventricular fibrillation induced at electrophysiological study when drug therapy is ineffective, not tolerated, or not preferred	
Non-sustained ventricular tachycardia in patients with coronary disease, prior myocardial infarction, left ventricular dysfunction, and inducible ventricular fibrillation or sustained ventricular tachycardia at electrophysiological study that is not suppressible by a class I antiarrhythmic drug	
Spontaneous sustained ventricular tachycardia in patients without structural heart disease not amenable to other treatments	

Post procedure care

After the pacemaker has been implanted, a CXR is performed to screen for pneumothorax. Post procedure ECG is required and a pacemaker check is performed prior to discharge.

SECTION 1.5 Manifestations of heart disease

Acute heart failure

Acute heart failure is defined as the rapid onset of symptoms or signs due to abnormal cardiac function.

Epidemiology

The overall incidence is not precisely known, but acute heart failure is associated with 13% of patients admitted to hospital with acute coronary syndrome.[1]

Pathology

The causes of acute heart failure are listed in Table 1.6, the most common being coronary artery disease. The pathophysiological changes associated with acute heart failure are reduced cardiac output with poor tissue perfusion and increased pulmonary capillary wedge pressure (a surrogate marker of increased left atrial pressure from reduced forward blood flow). In patients without pre-existing chronic heart failure, the JVP may not be elevated (acute left ventricular failure), the heart size is normal (cardiomegaly is a chronic process), and the sudden increased back pressure leads to severe pulmonary oedema.

Table 1.6	Causes of acute heart failure
Acute decompensation of existing heart failure	
Acute coronary syndromes	
Acute heart valve disease	
Arrhythmia	
Hypertensive crises	
Myocarditis	
Cardiac tamponade	
High-output cardiac failure	

Scope of disease

Reduced organ perfusion from acute heart failure results in a multisystem disorder as detailed below.

Clinical features

Acute heart failure can result in a number of clinical presentations. Acute decompensated heart failure is associated with mild dyspnoea without evidence of pulmonary oedema or cardiogenic shock.

Patients with pulmonary oedema (as confirmed by chest X-ray) usually present with severe dyspnoea and on examination may be cyanosed with diffuse pulmonary crepitations.

Patients with cardiogenic shock usually have hypotension and a low urine output associated with a pulse rate of more than 60 bpm.

Less common manifestations of acute heart failure include hypertensive acute heart failure (symptoms and signs of heart failure with elevated blood pressure and pulmonary oedema) and high-output heart failure.

Initial investigations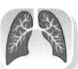

Full blood count
Anaemia is associated with reduced oxygen carriage and may be a precipitating cause.

Urea and electrolytes
Reduced organ perfusion can lead to renal impairment.

Liver profile
Reduced organ perfusion can lead to a deranged liver profile.

Serum cardiac markers
Elevated troponin levels would suggest myocardial infarction (p. 28) as the underlying cause for acute heart failure.

Arterial blood gases
An estimation of Po_2 is useful to guide management. Patients with pulmonary oedema may have type I respiratory failure (low Po_2 and low Pco_2).

Electrocardiogram
An ECG is useful to screen for myocardial ischaemia (p. 8) and arrhythmia.

Chest X-ray
A plain chest film will reveal pulmonary oedema in patients with severe heart failure (Fig. 1.10).

Echocardiogram
A transthoracic echocardiogram is an essential investigation to assess ventricular function, heart valve disease, pericardial disease and mechanical complications of myocardial infarction.

Further investigations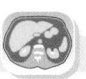

Haemodynamic measurements
Measurements of cardiac output and other haemodynamic indices (pulmonary capillary wedge pressure) can be obtained with a pulmonary artery flotation catheter (Swan–Ganz) and are usually reserved for patients with severe heart failure requiring inotropic support.

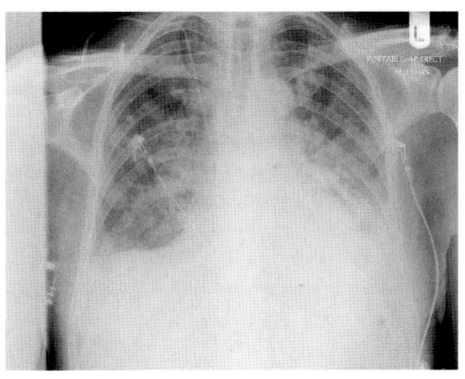

Fig. 1.10 Acute pulmonary oedema. The CXR shows bilateral patchy consolidation, Kerley B lines, and pleural effusions with a relatively normal heart size.

Acute heart failure

Chronic heart failure

Initial management

Oxygen
Maintaining oxygen saturations above 95% is important to improve tissue oxygenation and reduce pulmonary artery pressure (improve right ventricular forward flow). If adequate oxygenation cannot be achieved by supplementary oxygen, continuous positive airway pressure (CPAP) can be employed. With severe heart failure, intubation and ventilation may be required.

Monitoring of oxygen levels can be undertaken by peripheral saturations, or by repeated measurements from an indwelling arterial line.

Morphine
Morphine is indicated in the early stages to induce vasodilatation and alleviate symptoms of dyspnoea.

Nitrates
Intravenous nitrates are administered to relieve pulmonary congestion and improve coronary flow. However, tolerance to treatment usually develops after 24 hours.

Identify and address any precipitating cause
Any precipitating cause such as myocardial infarction, arrhythmia or infection should be addressed. Drugs that are associated with hypotension (ACE inhibitors, β-blockers) should be stopped in the presence of acute heart failure.

Medical management

Diuretics
Loop diuretics are administered to patients with acute heart failure and fluid overload. Volume status is usually assessed using central venous or pulmonary capillary wedge pressure. More rapid removal of fluid can be undertaken using haemofiltration.

Inotropic agents

Inotropic agents may be required to augment cardiac output. Usually pulmonary artery flotation catheter measurements of cardiac output, pulmonary capillary wedge pressure and systemic vascular resistance are performed to guide selection of an appropriate inotropic agent. Adrenaline is a commonly used inotropic agent, and phosphodiesterase inhibitors (enoximone) are also a useful alternative when increased cardiac output is required in addition to lowering of the systemic vascular resistance.

Surgical management

Definitive surgical management is directed to correcting any underlying cause such as acute heart valve regurgitation, correcting any mechanical complication of myocardial infarction, and relief of cardiac tamponade. Mechanical circulatory assistance can be provided whilst the underlying cause is being addressed, or if the underlying cause is reversible, or whilst awaiting definitive treatment (e.g. heart transplantation).

Intra-aortic balloon pump support

The intra-aortic balloon is a 25–50 mL elongated balloon (17–27 cm) that is designed to rest in the aorta, distal to the subclavian artery and proximal to the renal arteries (Fig. 1.11). It is introduced percutaneously (via the femoral artery) and controlled by timed helium inflation during diastole and deflation during systole. The effect of the balloon is to increase aortic pressure during diastole (improving coronary perfusion) and decrease aortic pressure during systole (reducing workload and myocardial oxygen consumption).

The indications of intra-aortic balloon usage are temporary cardiac support during acute ventricular failure/cardiogenic shock or mechanical complications of myocardial infarction (p. 28). In view of the favourable effects on coronary perfusion it is also used in refractory unstable angina (p. 23) and intractable ischaemic ventricular arrhythmia. Contraindications are aortic regurgitation, aortic aneurysm and severe aorto-iliac disease. Complications of usage include lower limb ischaemia, aortic dissection and haemolysis.

Ventricular assist devices

Ventricular assist devices are designed to provide a longer period of cardiac support and require surgical implantation with the use of cardiopulmonary bypass. Ventricular assist devices can augment or take over the role of the heart by diverting the flow of blood from the ventricles into the assist device and back into the aorta (or pulmonary artery for right ventricular assist devices). They can be implanted on the left, right, or both sides of the heart. A multitude of devices are currently employed and differ with respect to construction from pulsatile (pump assisted) to continuous flow (axial and centrifugal flow pumps).

Candidate selection is paramount as this is currently a very expensive treatment option. It is usually used in the setting of temporary assistance for acute cardiac failure in anticipation of full recovery in conditions such as acute myocarditis (bridge to recovery) or as a holding measure prior to heart transplantation (bridge to transplantation). More recently, the scope for ventricular assist devices has been extended to prolong the quality of life in end stage heart failure (destination therapy).

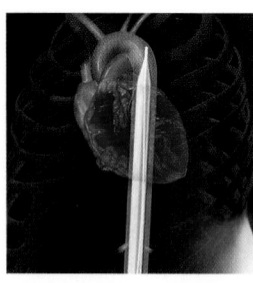

Fig. 1.11 An intra-aortic balloon pump. Image courtesy of Datascope Medical, Huntingdon, United Kingdom.

> **RECENT ADVANCES**
>
> *The first totally implantable artificial heart was implanted at the Jewish Hospital in Kentucky in 2001.[2] The recipient survived 151 days, and at least 4 recipients have now survived past 60 days.*

i **FURTHER INFORMATION**

Nieminen MS, Bohm M, Cowie MR, et al. ESC Committee for Practice Guideline (CPG). Executive summary of the guidelines on the diagnosis and treatment of acute heart failure: The Task Force on Acute Heart Failure of the European Society of Cardiology. European Heart Journal 2005; 26: 384–416.

REFERENCES

(1) *Steg PG, Dabbous OH, Feldman LJ, et al. for the Global Registry of Acute Coronary Events (GRACE) Investigators. Determinants and prognostic impact of heart failure complicating acute coronary syndromes: Observations from the Global Registry of Acute Coronary Events (GRACE). Circulation 2004; 109: 494–499.*
(2) *SoRelle R. Cardiovascular news. Totally contained AbioCor artificial heart implanted July 3, 2001. Circulation 2001; 104: E9005–9006.*

Chronic heart failure

The most encompassing description of heart failure is a state in which the heart fails to maintain an adequate circulation for the needs of the body despite a satisfactory filling pressure. The latter part of the definition excludes all conditions that cause poor venous return such as hypovolaemia. Congestive heart failure refers to concomitant symptoms or signs of fluid overload.

Epidemiology

The epidemiology of heart failure is variable due to the lack of agreement in definition and diagnostic criteria. The overall prevalence is up to 2%, and this increases with age (13% in individuals over 65 years).[1] The overall sex distribution is equal. However, after adjustment for age, heart failure is approximately 1.5 times more common in men (reflecting the epidemiology of myocardial infarction).[2] It is more common in developed countries.

Pathology

Heart failure is not a diagnosis, it is a clinical syndrome produced by a variety of cardiac and some circulatory disorders. Although classified into broad groupings, the pathophysiological effects of each disease often overlap.

Cardiac disorders

Impairment of myocardial function

Diseases of the myocardium (cardiomyopathies) make up the majority of the causes of impairment of myocardial function. Ischaemic cardiomyopathy is the most common cause and accounts for two-thirds of patients with heart failure. The non-ischaemic cardiomyopathies are caused by chronic hypertension, valvular heart disease and myocarditis. In some cases the cause is unknown (idiopathic dilated cardiomyopathy).

Mechanical overload

Acute mechanical overload due to aortic regurgitation (e.g. aortic dissection) or mitral regurgitation (e.g. myocardial infarction) can cause heart failure despite normal heart function. Over a period of time, this usually results in hypertrophy, dilatation and scarring, leading to impaired myocardial function.

Impairment of ventricular filling

Ventricular filling can be impaired by pericardial constriction (pericardial effusion), increased passive stiffness (restrictive cardiomyopathy) and impaired relaxation (consequence of ageing, chronic hypertension). These conditions give rise to diastolic dysfunction and, if sufficiently severe, result in diastolic heart failure (symptoms and signs of heart failure and preserved ejection fraction).

Circulatory disorders

With any degree of impairment, the heart may not be able to maintain adequate circulation for the needs of the body in conditions such as severe anaemia (where oxygen carrying capacity is impaired), large arterio-venous fistulae (due to shunting of blood), thyrotoxicosis and Paget's disease (due to increased metabolic demands of peripheral tissue).

Scope of disease

Whilst heart failure is rarely confined to a single chamber, the pathophysiology, symptoms and signs are usually presented for the left and right sides of the heart to improve understanding.

As the left heart fails, filling pressures rise and the back pressure exerted by the left heart in turn increases pulmonary capillary pressure. The imbalance on Starling forces results in accumulation of fluid in the interstitium of the lung; when the amount is greater than can be ordinarily removed by lymphatic drainage, pulmonary oedema and pleural effusions result.

Increasing back pressure from failure of the right heart results in hepatic congestion, hepatomegaly, ascites and peripheral oedema. A low cardiac output state can result in poor peripheral tissue perfusion, confusion (poor cerebral perfusion) and renal impairment. The combination of mucosal oedema impairing absorption, feeling of fullness from ascites or general anorexia can result in cardiac cachexia.

Clinical features

A spectrum of disease is increasingly recognized, ranging from the risk of heart failure to asymptomatic ventricular dysfunction to clinically apparent congestive heart failure.

The predominant symptoms of left ventricular failure are dyspnoea, orthopnoea and paroxysmal nocturnal dyspnoea. It is important to assess how far patients can walk before breathlessness sets in and how many pillows they require to sleep. Symptoms originating from right heart failure are peripheral oedema, abdominal distension (hepatomegaly, ascites) and anorexia. In addition, patients may have symptoms suggestive of an underlying cause, such as angina (ischaemic heart disease). A positive family history of heart failure at an early age may indicate familial cardiomyopathies, and a history of chronic alcohol abuse is associated with dilated cardiomyopathy.

On inspection, cyanosis, peripheral oedema and ascites may be visible. The JVP is usually raised. A sinus tachycardia may be present from increased sympathetic tone and the blood pressure may be low (severe disease) or elevated (chronic hypertension as an underlying cause). The apex beat may be displaced by cardiomegaly. On auscultation, a third heart sound is characteristic and murmurs can arise from underlying heart valve disease or functional mitral/tricuspid regurgitation (failure of valve coaptation due to ventricular/valve annulus distension). Coarse crepitations can arise from pulmonary oedema. Hepatomegaly and ascites can be confirmed on abdominal examination. Serial body weight estimation is a simple method to monitor fluid status and subsequent response to therapy.

A detailed clinical assessment should identify any precipitating factors (Table 1.7) and underlying causes (Table 1.8) and discriminate between other causes of dyspnoea (p. 112). The severity of dyspnoea is graded according to the NYHA functional class (Table 1.9), and an estimation of volume status (body weight, JVP, pulmonary and peripheral oedema) directs the clinician to the need for subsequent diuretic therapy.

Acute heart failure

Chronic heart failure

Table 1.7	Precipitating factors of heart failure
Non-compliance with existing heart failure therapy	
Inadequate existing heart failure therapy	
Uncontrolled hypertension	
Arrhythmia	
Infection	
Drugs (NSAIDs)	
Myocardial infarction	

Table 1.8	Underlying causes of heart failure

Cardiac disorders

Impairment of myocardial function

Ischaemic heart disease

Ischaemic cardiomyopathy

Myocardial infarction

Ventricular aneurysm

Chronic hypertension

Heart valve disease

Myocarditis

Cardiomyopathies

Mechanical overload

Acute aortic regurgitation

Acute mitral regurgitation

Impairment of ventricular filling

Pericardial effusion

Restrictive pericarditis

Restrictive cardiomyopathy

Infiltrative cardiomyopathy

Circulatory disorders

Anaemia

Large arterio-venous fistulae

Thyrotoxicosis

Paget's disease of the bone

Table 1.9	NYHA functional classification*

Class I

Patients with cardiac disease but without resulting limitations of physical activity. Ordinary physical activity does not cause undue fatigue, palpitations, dyspnoea or angina pain

Class II

Patients with cardiac disease resulting in slight limitation of physical activity. They are comfortable at rest. Less than ordinary physical activity causes fatigue, palpitations, dyspnoea or angina pain

Class III

Patients with cardiac disease resulting in marked limitation of physical activity. They are comfortable at rest. Less than ordinary physical activity causes fatigue, palpitations, dyspnoea or angina pain

Class IV

Patients with cardiac disease resulting in inability to carry on any physical activity without discomfort. Symptoms of cardiac insufficiency or of the anginal syndrome may be present, even at rest. If physical activity is undertaken, discomfort is increased

* Criteria Committee of the New York Heart Association. Diseases of the heart and blood vessels: nomenclature and criteria for diagnosis, 6th edn. Boston: Little, Brown and Company, 1964.

Initial investigations

Full blood count

Haemoglobin estimation can confirm the presence of anaemia.

Urea and electrolytes

As a crude estimation of significant renal impairment, urea and creatinine may be elevated as a result of hypoperfusion. Renal function and serum potassium levels are important measures prior to the initiation of heart failure therapy (diuretics and ACE inhibitors).

Liver profile

Liver enzymes may be raised due to hepatic congestion from right heart failure.

Lipid profile and random plasma glucose

These investigations primarily screen for risk factors of ischaemic heart disease, the most common underlying aetiology for heart failure.

Electrocardiogram

A 12 lead ECG may reveal myocardial ischaemia or a silent infarction (p. 28). Left ventricular hypertrophy may result from chronic hypertension, heart valve disease or cardiomyopathy. Low voltage complexes may be suggestive of

an effusion giving rise to diastolic heart failure. The presence and type of arrhythmia, either precipitating or associated with heart failure, may be revealed. If an arrhythmia is suspected and the ECG is normal, 24 hour monitoring is appropriate.

Chest X-ray

Classical features of congestive heart failure are cardiomegaly, patchy consolidation from pulmonary oedema, pleural effusions, upper lobe venous diversion and Kerley B lines (horizontal lines on the lateral 2 cm of the lung fields thought to be fluid in the septa). However these features are not always present. Absence of these features is not sensitive enough to rule out the diagnosis of heart failure.

Transthoracic echocardiogram

Transthoracic echocardiography is an excellent investigation for the diagnosis and estimation of severity of impaired ventricular function (p. 8). Atrial and ventricular dimensions, wall thickness, contractility and ejection fraction can be quantified. In addition, pericardial effusions and restriction of ventricular motion can be visualized. Increased use of echocardiography has identified patients with ventricular impairment before the syndrome of heart failure develops and improved the identification of diastolic heart failure.

> **RECENT ADVANCES**
>
> *Despite the name, a major source of brain natriuretic peptide (BNP) is the ventricle. Elevated levels of BNP correlate with impairment of left ventricular function, and its use as a marker of heart failure is currently under evaluation.*[1]

Further investigations

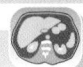

Cardiac enzymes

CK-MB or troponin I should be assessed to diagnose myocardial infarction (p. 28) if there is a history of chest pain or if new ECG abnormalities suggestive of ischaemia are present.

Thyroid stimulating hormone

TSH is a screening investigation for patients with a history or examination findings suggestive of thyroid disease (p. 393).

Cardiac catheterization

Cardiac catheterization (p. 10) is an advanced investigation prior to specific therapy (coronary surgery, heart transplantation). It provides haemodynamic measurements and is able to quantify the exact extent of coronary disease by coronary angiography.

Cardiac biopsy

Myocardial biopsies can be obtained from the right ventricle via access from the internal jugular vein. This procedure is usually reserved for the diagnosis of patients with suspected infiltrative cardiomyopathies (amyloidosis, haemochromatosis).

RECENT ADVANCES

Understanding the progression of heart failure led to the 2001 AHA classification into four stages. Stage A patients are at high risk of developing heart failure but without any structural disorder of the heart. Stage B patients have structural disorders of the heart but without any symptoms of heart failure. Stage C patients have current or past symptoms of heart failure and structural heart disease. Stage D patients have end-stage heart failure requiring specialized treatment.[3]

Initial management

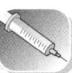

An overview of management is presented in Table 1.10.

Identify and address any precipitating cause

Initial treatment should be directed to any precipitating cause such as myocardial infarction, arrhythmia or infection. Patients should be educated on the importance of compliance with medication. Drugs that may have precipitated heart failure should be stopped.

Identify and address any underlying cause

Blood pressure should be controlled. Specific therapy is required for ischaemic heart disease, heart valve diseases, thyrotoxicosis and rare causes such as haemochromatosis.

Lifestyle modification

Patients should be educated on the importance of regular exercise, dietary salt restriction and control of risk factors

Table 1.10	Management summary

Initial management

1. Treat any precipitating cause

2. Treat any underlying cause

3. Lifestyle modification
   a. Regular exercise
   b. Dietary salt restriction
   c. Stop smoking, blood pressure control as well as lipid and diabetic control
   d. Discourage excessive alcohol intake

Medical therapy

1a. Diuretic

A loop diuretic (furosemide, bumetanide) should be prescribed for patients with evidence of fluid overload

1b. ACE inhibitor

Captopril, enalapril or lisinopril may be used. Patients who develop angio-oedema or severe intractable cough with ACE inhibitors may be placed on an angiotensin receptor blocker (ACE II inhibitor)

1c. β-Blocker

Carvedilol and metoprolol are the two most established β-blockers in this setting

2. Addition of aldosterone antagonist

Spironolactone may be used as a substitute or addition to β-blockade

3. Addition of digoxin

For patients in atrial fibrillation, or as part of quadruple therapy for patients who remain symptomatic despite step 1(a to c)

Surgical therapy

1. High-risk coronary, valve or ventricular restoration surgery to correct underlying cause

2. Cardiac support

For selected patients with acute decompensation

3. Heart transplantation

For patients with end stage irreversible cardiac disease, unacceptable quality of life and high risk of mortality despite optimum medical therapy

for ischaemic heart disease (stop smoking, blood pressure, lipid and diabetic control). Excessive alcohol intake should be discouraged.

Medical management

Currently an ACE inhibitor and β-blocker is the standard therapy for all asymptomatic patients with evidence of left ventricular dysfunction and for patients with symptomatic heart failure.

Diuretic

A loop diuretic is the first agent of choice in treating patients with congestive cardiac failure to rapidly control the pulmonary and systemic symptoms and signs of fluid overload. As a class, this group of drugs inhibits the sodium/potassium/chloride cotransporter in the ascending limb of the loop of Henle, resulting in diuresis and excretion of sodium, potassium and chloride ions. Diuretics should be prescribed in appropriate doses that result in clinical improvement and target weight loss, and continued at a dose for prevention of recurrent fluid retention. The adverse effects include hypokalaemia, hypotension and impairment of renal function.

As a single agent, diuretics are unable to maintain the clinical stability of patients with heart failure and therefore should be prescribed in conjunction with an ACE inhibitor and β-blockers.

ACE inhibitor

Low blood pressure and impaired renal perfusion stimulate renin production as part of a neurohormonal cascade in heart failure. ACE inhibition prevents the conversion of angiotensin I to angiotensin II. This results in reducing the peripheral vascular resistance that the failing heart has to work against and consequently decreasing myocardial oxygen consumption. ACE inhibitors prolong life in patients with heart failure as well as asymptomatic left ventricular dysfunction.[4] The side effects are a dry cough, hypotension, renal impairment and hyperkalaemia.

Angiotensin II receptor blockers (ACE II inhibitors) have recently been discovered. However, the equivalent effects on survival compared with conventional ACE inhibitors cannot be assumed. At present, ACE II inhibitors are used as a substitute in patients who develop angio-oedema or severe intractable cough to conventional ACE inhibitors.

β-Blocker

Activation of the sympathetic nervous system augments the failing heart by increasing contractility and maintains blood pressure by increasing systemic vascular resistance. These effects are deleterious in the long run due to the increasing workload on the heart, causing ventricular hypertrophy and increasing myocardial oxygen consumption. β-Blockers interrupt this process and improve survival in patients with stable heart failure.[5] Carvedilol and metoprolol are the two most established drugs in this class. Initiation of therapy requires careful dose titration due to the possibility of worsening heart failure. Side effects include bradycardia, heart block and hypotension.

Aldosterone receptor blocker

Recent evidence has shown spironolactone to be effective in combination with an ACE inhibitor to reduce morbidity and death in severe heart failure.[6] The precise role of this drug in the management of heart failure is yet to be defined. At present, it is used in conjunction with an ACE inhibitor either as a substitute or addition to β-blockade in selected patients.

Digoxin

The best indication for the addition of digoxin in heart failure is the presence of atrial fibrillation. Digoxin increases the contractility of the heart whilst slowing the ventricular rate. It improves symptoms of heart failure but has little to no effect on survival. It is usually prescribed for patients who remain symptomatic despite diuretic, ACE inhibitor and β-blocker therapy.

> **RECENT ADVANCES**
>
> *New drug classes are currently being developed and tested to interrupt the adverse effects of neurohormonal activation in heart failure. These drugs include vasopeptidase inhibitors, cytokine antagonists and endothelin antagonists. Future therapy may include stem cell transplantation to augment the contractility of the failing ventricle.*

Surgical management

At present, surgical therapy cannot cure heart failure. The aims of surgical therapy are the prevention of heart failure and correction of the underlying cause. In more advanced cases, mechanical circulatory assistance can be provided for the failing heart (p. 14) and ultimately replacement with cardiac transplantation.

High-risk coronary surgery

Surgical revascularization is preferred over percutaneous coronary interventions in the setting of heart failure. Coronary artery bypass surgery improves angina and may prevent progression to worsening heart failure (a concept that is currently being evaluated by ongoing international trials). The risk of surgical mortality in the setting of heart failure is increased; the procedure is detailed on page 22.

Surgical ventricular restoration

As a complication of myocardial infarction, some patients develop ventricular aneurysms due to the thinning and scarring of dead myocardium. Eventually, paradoxical motion occurs in the affected area ballooning outwards with each systolic contraction, forming a ventricular aneurysm and impairing the mechanics of ventricular contraction.

In these patients, resection of the aneurysm and reconstruction of the ventricle can improve overall function. This is usually performed in conjunction with coronary artery surgery. Prior to initiating cardiopulmonary bypass, the ventricle is opened, the margins of the weakly contracting diseased segment are palpated, the diseased area is excised and the defect is geometrically reconstructed, usually with a circular patch. The remainder of the operation is then performed as detailed on page 22.

High-risk valve surgery

Valve disorders can result in heart failure. Conversely, chronic heart failure can result in valve disorder. This usually occurs in the setting of ventricular enlargement causing functional (secondary) mitral regurgitation by annular dilatation or distraction of the papillary muscles.

Valve repair or replacement will reverse or prevent further ventricular impairment if performed sufficiently early. Tertiary referral is usually required for patients with very severe ventricular impairment as they may require postoperative cardiac support or transplantation.

Heart transplantation

Cardiac transplantation is the only established surgical treatment of advanced heart failure, and is reserved for patients with irreversible cardiac disease, unacceptable quality of life and high risk of mortality despite optimum medical therapy.

Prognosis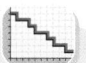

Following the diagnosis of heart failure the 1- and 5-year survival is approximately 74% and 48% respectively.[2]

i FURTHER INFORMATION

Costanzo MR, Augustine S, Bourge R, Bristow M, O'Connell JB, Driscoll D, Rose E. The treatment of heart failure. Task Force of the Working Group on Heart Failure of the European Society of Cardiology. European Heart Journal 1997; 18: 736–753.

REFERENCES

(1) Cowie MR, Mosterd A, Wood DA, Deckers JW, Poole-Wilson PA, Sutton GC, Grobbee DE. The epidemiology of heart failure. European Heart Journal 1997; 18: 208–225.
(2) Levy D, Kenchaiah S, Larson MG, et al. Long-term trends in the incidence of and survival with heart failure. New England Journal of Medicine 2002; 347: 1397–1402.
(3) Hunt SA, Baker DW, Chin MH, et al. ACC/AHA guidelines for the evaluation and management of chronic heart failure in the adult: executive summary. A report of the American College of Cardiology/ American Heart Association Task Force on Practice Guidelines (Committee to revise the 1995 Guidelines for the Evaluation and Management of Heart Failure). Journal of the American College of Cardiology 2001; 38: 2101–2113.
(4) Flather MD, Yusuf S, Kober L, et al. Long-term ACE-inhibitor therapy in patients with heart failure or left-ventricular dysfunction: a systematic overview of data from individual patients. ACE-Inhibitor Myocardial Infarction Collaborative Group. Lancet 2000; 355: 1575–1581.
(5) Lechat P, Packer M, Chalon S, Cucherat M, Arab T, Boissel J-P. Clinical effects of β-adrenergic blockade in chronic heart failure : a meta-analysis of double-blind, placebo-controlled, randomized trials. Circulation 1998; 98: 1184–1191.
(6) Pitt B, Zannad F, Remme WJ, et al. The Randomized Aldactone Evaluation Study Investigators. The effect of spironolactone on morbidity and mortality in patients with severe heart failure. New England Journal of Medicine 1999; 341: 709–717.

SECTION 1.6 Ischaemic heart disease

Chronic stable angina

Angina is the most common manifestation of ischaemic heart disease. It is a syndrome characterized by chest discomfort associated with myocardial ischaemia without necrosis. It is defined as stable if it has not changed in frequency, duration or precipitating cause in the past 60 days.[1]

Epidemiology

The prevalence of angina increases with age and occurs in up to 5% of the 45–54-year age group and up to 20% in the 65–74-year age group.[2] It is twice as common in men as in women, and occurs more commonly in developed countries.

Pathology

Angina results from an imbalance between the oxygen supply and demand of the myocardium, hence the relationship of chest pain with exercise. By far the most common cause is ischaemia resulting from atherosclerotic narrowing of the coronary arteries (p. 1). Haemodynamic compromise usually occurs after a 70% reduction in the luminal diameter of a coronary artery. Reduction of flow may also occur from coronary artery vasospasm.

Angina can also result from reduced oxygen carrying capacity of blood (anaemia) and increased oxygen demand can be due to myocardial hypertrophy (e.g. valvular heart disease).

Scope of disease

The acute complications of angina tend to result from atherosclerotic plaque instability. Ulceration and fissuring of the plaque may lead to acute coronary syndromes presenting as unstable angina (p. 25) or non ST elevation myocardial infarction (NSTEMI, p. 25). Embolus or thrombosis may result in coronary artery occlusion and ST segment elevation myocardial infarction (STEMI). Myocardial ischaemia also predisposes to arrhythmia and sudden death.

Clinical features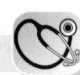

The history is crucial to the diagnosis of angina. It is exemplified by the character, location and duration of chest pain. The most consistent feature in the history is the relationship of chest pain with exercise.

Classic angina is characterized by tight chest discomfort that originates in the precordium and radiates into the jaw, shoulder or left arm. Occasionally it may be described as pressure, an ache, weight or constriction, but rarely as a sharp or stabbing pain. Typically, angina is precipitated by exertion and relieved with rest. Each episode usually lasts from 1 to 3 minutes if the initiating event is discontinued. Other precipitating factors may include emotion, meals, cold weather and lying supine (decubitus angina).

Variants of angina include vasospastic (or Prinzmetal's) angina that occurs without provocation, due to coronary artery vasospasm. It is diagnosed by characteristic ECG changes of ischaemia associated with the attacks of chest pain (p. 3). Classical angina with objective evidence of myocardial ischaemia can manifest with apparently normal coronary arteries on angiography due to micro-vascular disease (syndrome X). Occasionally, the only mani-festation of cardiac ischaemia may be dyspnoea (angina equivalents).

A detailed history should identify risk factors associated with ischaemic heart disease and underlying factors predisposing to angina (anaemia, thyrotoxicosis, infections, drugs) and discriminate between other causes of chest pain. The severity of chronic stable angina is graded according to the Canadian Cardiovascular Society classifi-cation (Table 1.11).

Clinical examination is often normal. However, evidence of risk factors or concomitant manifestations of athero-scleroses may be evident on careful examination. A corneal arcus and xanthelasma is associated with hyperlipi-daemia. The blood pressure may be chronically elevated. Auscultation of the carotid arteries may reveal concomi-tant carotid stenosis. An ejection systolic murmur may suggest aortic stenosis as the underlying cause, while a pansystolic murmur may reflect mitral regurgitation that can result from ischaemia. Peripheral pulses should also be examined for concomitant peripheral vascular disease, known to be strongly associated with coronary artery disease.

Table 1.11	Canadian Cardiovascular Society's classification of angina pectoris

Class I. Ordinary physical activity does not cause angina

For example walking or climbing stairs, angina occurs with strenuous or rapid or prolonged exertion at work or recreation

Class II. Slight limitation of ordinary activity

For example, angina occurs walking or stair climbing after meals, in cold, in wind, under emotional stress or only during the few hours after awakening, walking more than two blocks on the level or climbing more than one flight of ordinary stairs at a normal pace and in normal conditions

Class III. Marked limitation of ordinary activity

For example, angina occurs walking one or two blocks on the level or climbing one flight of stairs in normal conditions and at a normal pace

Class IV. Inability to carry on any physical activity without discomfort

Angina syndrome may be present at rest

From Campeau L. Letter to the editor. Circulation 1976; 54: 522.

Initial investigations

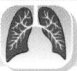

Full blood count
Anaemia can precipitate or exacerbate angina.

Plasma glucose
A random plasma glucose should be obtained to screen for diabetes.

Lipid profile
Serum cholesterol levels have important implications for therapy in primary and secondary prevention of coronary events.

Resting electrocardiogram
The resting ECG in patients with chronic stable angina is normal in more than 50%. This does not exclude the presence of ischaemic heart disease. Evidence of Q waves from previous myocardial infarctions strongly supports the diagnosis of angina. The presence of arrhythmias such as atrial fibrillation may result from myocardial ischaemia.

In the presence of chest pain, however, the ECG is abnormal in more than 50% of patients with angina, with T wave inversion and ST segment depression being the usual findings.

Chest X-ray
The chest film is often normal in patients with chronic stable angina and the clinical utility of this routine inves-tigation is not well established. Characteristic X-ray features of heart failure from myocardial ischaemia may be present (p. 41), and cardiomegaly secondary to valvular heart disease may point to the underlying aetiology.

Echocardiography
Transthoracic echocardiography is not routinely indicated in patients with chronic stable angina. However, it is useful when features of valvular heart disease are present or to assess ventricular function in the presence of symptoms suggestive of congestive cardiac failure.

Further investigations

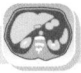

Non-invasive testing
Exercise electrocardiogram
An exercise ECG is useful for the objective documentation of myocardial ischaemia and also to assess the functional capacity and prognosis of patients with established coronary disease. Details of this procedure are given on page 7.

Stress imaging studies
The indications for imaging studies over exercise ECG are usually due to baseline ECG abnormalities such as complete left bundle branch block, pre-excitation (Wolff–Parkinson–White) and patients with pre-existing revascularization where localization of the area of ischaemia is important. Details of pharmacological stress testing with radionuclide

and echocardiographic imaging techniques are given on page 8.

Invasive testing

Coronary angiography

The coronary angiogram is the current gold standard to diagnose coronary artery disease. Currently it is indicated for diagnosis in patients with contraindications to stress testing, risk stratification in patients with angina refractory to medical therapy, diagnosis after successful resuscitation for sudden near cardiac death, patients with symptoms of congestive cardiac failure and high-risk patients identified on non-invasive testing.

RECENT ADVANCES

Imaging modalities that are currently under evaluation are ultra fast CT scanning and magnetic resonance coronary angiography. Intravascular ultrasonography has the ability to measure luminal dimensions and characterize plaque size and distribution.

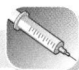

Initial management

There are four main aims in the managements of patients with coronary artery disease: to address underlying conditions that provoke or exacerbate angina; to prevent myocardial infarction and death; to give pharmacological therapy for angina; revascularization.

Identify and address any precipitating factors

Attention should be given to underlying conditions that provoke or exacerbate angina. These include anaemia, hyperthyroidism, tachyarrhythmias and valvular heart disease. Drugs that are known to provoke angina such as vasoconstrictors and vasodilators should be substituted with other similar agents that have a neutral cardiovascular profile.

Lifestyle and risk factor modification[3]

The cessation of smoking should be encouraged as coronary heart disease risk will decline. However, it may be up to 10 years before the baseline risk is achieved compared to non-smokers.

There is a strong relationship between blood pressure and coronary heart disease risk. Hypertension should be controlled, aiming for a systolic pressure of less than 140 mmHg and diastolic pressure of less than 90 mmHg.

A number of primary and secondary prevention trials have shown that cholesterol lowering is associated with a reduced risk of coronary events, and serum levels should be maintained below 5.0 mmol/L.

Although definitive evidence is not yet available on strict glycaemic control and reduction of coronary disease risk, current consensus opinion favours tight blood sugar control in diabetics and patients with impaired glucose tolerance.

Aspirin

The use of aspirin (75–325 mg) is associated with an average 33% reduction in coronary events.[4] It should be prescribed for all patients with angina unless absolutely contraindicated. Under these circumstances, an alternative antiplatelet agent such as clopidogrel should be considered.

Medical management

Sublingual nitrates

Short-acting sublingual glyceryl trinitrate (nitroglycerin) works quickly in treating acute attacks of angina.

β-Blockers

Numerous β-blockers are available and appear equally effective. The mode of action is by decreasing heart rate, contractility and blood pressure, and hence the oxygen demands of the heart. β-Blockers are frequently combined with nitrates to ameliorate reflex tachycardia. Although limited data exist in the setting of chronic stable angina, reduction of mortality after myocardial infarction is established. β-Blockers also improve survival and prevent stroke in patients with hypertension.

Addition of long-acting nitrates

Prophylaxis can be achieved with longer-acting preparations such as isosorbide mononitrate and isosorbide dinitrates. Nitrates improve exercise tolerance and time to onset of angina by reducing pre-load and promoting coronary artery vasodilatation. The main problems with nitrates are headaches (which subside as the patient gets used to the drug), reflex tachycardia and the development of tolerance. There are no long-term studies on the use of nitrates in chronic stable angina.[2]

Addition of calcium antagonists

Calcium antagonists exert a negative inotropic effect by reducing the transmembrane flux of calcium. They can be broadly divided into short-acting dihydropyridine (nifedipine), long-acting dihydropyridine (amlodipine, felodipine) and non-dihydropyridine calcium antagonists (e.g. diltiazem, verapamil). All the calcium antagonists are of similar efficacy in treating chronic stable angina and are excellent first-line agents for vasospastic (Prinzmetal's) angina.

Combination therapy with dihydropyridine calcium channel antagonists and β-blockers has been reported to exert a greater anti-anginal effect and better prevent adverse cardiac events than either agent individually.[5] However, non-dihydropyridine calcium channel antagonists act on the cardiac conduction system to reduce the heart rate, and should not be used together with β-blockers in view of the risk of complete heart block. Controversy currently exists regarding the prescription of short-acting dihydropyridine calcium antagonists (such as nifedipine) as a single agent for the treatment of angina in view of the suggestion of increased adverse events.[6]

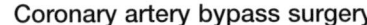

RECENT ADVANCES

A number of agents have been introduced recently for the treatment of angina. Nicorandil (a potassium channel activator) is effective in the treatment of angina, although evidence of comparative efficacy with other anti-anginal agents and reduction of adverse events are awaited.

Revascularization

The indications for revascularization are symptomatic (angina refractory to maximal medical therapy) and prognostic. Prognostic features for revascularization are determined from a coronary artery disease configuration obtained by coronary angiography. The following adverse prognostic features are clearly associated with survival benefit from revascularization:

a. left main stem coronary artery disease
b. triple vessel disease
c. double vessel disease involving the proximal left anterior descending artery.

Percutaneous coronary interventions (PCI)

Catheter-based intervention techniques are employed for patients with suitable anatomy (discrete and short segments of stenosis) without left main involvement, poor ventricular function or diabetes.

Percutaneous transluminal coronary angioplasty (PTCA) is employed by femoral arterial puncture and introduction of a catheter into the aorta and subsequently into the coronary arteries. Balloon dilatation of coronary stenoses is undertaken under radiological guidance (Fig. 1.12a–d). Freedom from angina is achieved in 72% of patients at one year. The mortality rate associated with angioplasty is 1% and the frequency of myocardial infarction is 5%. Other procedural complications are similar to coronary angiography (p. 10). The main disadvantage is the high proportion of restenosis, occurring in 30–40% at 6 months.

The use of coronary stents (Fig. 1.13a–c) has increased due to lower rates of restenosis and re-intervention compared to PTCA. Self-expanding stents are deployed in the coronary arteries using the same approach as PTCA. The in-stent restenosis rate is approximately 22% at 7 months.[7]

RECENT ADVANCES

Other new therapies currently under evaluation are the use of drug eluting stents to minimize restenosis, coronary atherectomy, and laser angioplasty that directly ablates coronary artery plaques.

Surgical management

When revascularization is indicated, coronary artery bypass surgery is preferred for patients with left main stem involvement, diabetes and poor ventricular function as survival advantage has been demonstrated over PCI. Surgery is also advocated for patients with unsuitable anatomy for PCI (long complex stenosis and occluded vessels).

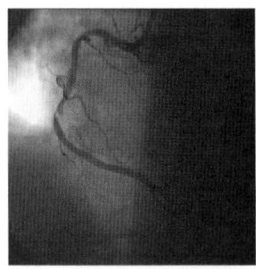

(a)

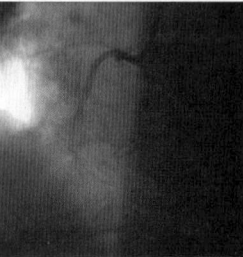

(b)

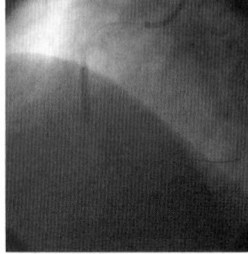

(c)

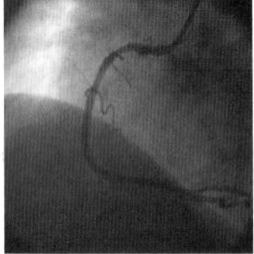

(d)

Fig. 1.12a–d Angiographic views of angioplasty to the right coronary artery.

Coronary artery bypass surgery

The patient is positioned supine and a median sternotomy is performed. The sternum is opened longitudinally with an oscillating saw. The internal mammary artery is harvested (Fig. 1.14a) simultaneously with the long saphenous vein (by a second operator; Fig. 1.14b). The pericardium is opened and cardiopulmonary bypass is instituted. The heart is arrested using cardioplegia solution containing a high concentration of potassium (Fig. 1.14c). The segments of long saphenous veins are reversed and anastomosed to the coronary arteries and aorta (Fig. 1.14d). This will deliver blood directly from the aorta to the coronary arteries, bypassing segmental stenoses. The internal mammary artery is anastomosed directly to the left anterior descending artery as a pedicle graft. Once the cardioplegia solution is washed out of the coronary system, the heart resumes beating. Haemostasis is achieved and the sternum closed with stainless steel wires.

Coronary artery bypass surgery can prolong the quantity and quality of life. The success rate is 95% for complete relief of angina, although this falls to 75% at 5 years. Internal mammary artery patency to the left anterior descending artery is 90% at 10 years, but vein graft occlusion occurs in approximately 15% after the first year and 2–4% per year thereafter. The average mortality rate of this procedure is 3%. Postoperatively, stroke occurs in 3% and transient atrial fibrillation in 30%. Other complications include bleeding and wound infection.

RECENT ADVANCES

Coronary artery surgery can currently be performed without the use of cardiopulmonary bypass (off pump) with the use of specific stabilizers. The advantages and impact on graft patency are currently under evaluation. Coronary revascularization using only arterial grafts (internal mammary and radial arteries) is also under evaluation to determine if graft patency can be improved. Thoracoscopic robotic surgical techniques of coronary surgery without sternotomy or bypass are currently being developed.

Prognosis

The average mortality of patients with chronic stable angina is 2–3% per year with a similar risk of myocardial infarction at 2–3% per year.[8]

ι FURTHER INFORMATION

Management of stable angina pectoris. Recommendations of the task force of the European society of cardiology. European Heart Journal 1997; 18: 394–413

Gibbons RJ, Chatterjee K, Daley J, et al. ACC/AHA/ACP-ASIM guidelines for the management of patients with chronic stable angina. Journal of the American College of Cardiology 1999; 33: 2092–2197.

REFERENCES

(1) *Hurst JW. Cardiovascular diagnosis. The initial examination. Mosby-Year Book, St Louis, 1993, p. 45.*
(2) *Management of stable angina pectoris. Recommendations of the Task Force of the European Society of Cardiology. European Heart Journal 1997; 18: 394–413*
(3) *Wood D, Durrington P, Poulter N, McInnes G, Rees A, Wray R. Joint British recommendations on prevention of coronary heart disease in clinical practice. Heart 1998; 80: Suppl 2.*
(4) *Antiplatelet Trialist Collaboration. A collaborative overview of randomised trials of antiplatelet therapy. BMJ 1995; 308: 81–106.*
(5) *Opie LH. Drugs for the heart, 4th edn. WB Saunders, Philadelphia, 1995.*
(6) *Furberg CD, Psaty BM, Meyer JV. Nifedipine: dose related increase in mortality in patients with coronary heart disease. Circulation 1995; 92: 1326–1331.*
(7) *Serruys PW, de Jaegere P, Kiemeneij F, et al. A comparison of balloon expandable stent implantation with balloon angioplasty in patients with coronary artery disease. Benestent study group. New England Journal of Medicine 1994; 331: 489–495.*
(8) *Brunelli C, Cristofani R, L'Abbate A. Long term survival in medically treated patients with ischaemic heart disease and prognostic importance of clinical and echocardiographic data. European Heart Journal 1989; 10: 292–303.*

RECENT ADVANCES

The previous classification of myocardial infarction into subendocardial/transmural, Q wave/non Q wave infarcts has little clinical significance and is no longer in common use.

The term 'serum/biochemical cardiac markers' has replaced the previous term 'cardiac enzymes' to encompass non-enzyme protein structures (myoglobin) and peptides (troponins).

REFERENCES

(1) *Alpert JS, Thygesen K, Antman E, Bassand JP. Myocardial infarction redefined—a consensus document of the Joint European Society of Cardiology/American College of Cardiology Committee for the redefinition of myocardial infarction. Journal of the American College of Cardiology 2000; 36: 959–969.*

Chronic stable angina

Acute coronary syndrome

Unstable angina/non ST segment elevation myocardial infarction

ST-segment elevation myocardial infarction

Acute coronary syndrome

Acute coronary syndrome is an operational definition that encompasses any clinical symptoms that are compatible with *acute* myocardial ischaemia. It includes unstable angina, non ST elevation myocardial infarction (NSTEMI) and ST elevation myocardial infarction (STEMI), see Figure 1.15.

A spectrum of presentation for acute coronary syndrome is increasingly recognized, starting with unstable angina, a diagnosis that implies ischaemia without infarction. Myocardial infarction refers to myocardial necrosis due to prolonged ischaemia. In view of the sensitivity and specificity of serum cardiac markers, myocardial infarction was redefined in the year 2000 principally on the rise and fall in serum troponin or CK-MB levels.[1] By this definition, elevation of serum cardiac markers differentiates NSTEMI from unstable angina.

Myocardial infarction has been further subdivided based on ST segment morphology on ECG into NSTEMI and STEMI. This clinical classification differentiates between two types of myocardial infarction due to important differences in pathogenesis (unstable angina and NSTEMI are closely related) and differences in clinical management (thrombolysis is beneficial for STEMI, but not for NSTEMI). The development of Q waves corresponds with the progression of myocardial necrosis and is an indicator of an evolving infarct.

Unstable angina/non ST segment elevation myocardial infarction

Unstable angina and NSTEMI are often considered together as the pathogenesis and management approach are similar. The principal differentiating feature is evidence of myocardial necrosis with NSTEMI, a diagnosis established by elevated serum cardiac markers.

Epidemiology

The epidemiology of acute coronary syndromes reflects that of chronic stable angina. The median age for presentation with unstable angina is 66, and it is 1.6 times more common in men. For NSTEMI, the median age of presentation is 68, and it is 2 times more common in men.[1]

Pathology

The most common cause of unstable angina is reduced myocardial perfusion from non-occlusive thrombus or disrupted atherosclerotic plaque in the coronary arteries. Other causes include severe vasospasm (Prinzmetal's angina), severe narrowing without spasm, arterial inflammation and secondary unstable angina (due to diseases or conditions not directly related to the heart such as increased myocardial oxygen requirements from fever, reduced systemic blood flow from hypotension and oxygen delivery from anaemia).

Scope of disease

Patients with unstable angina and NSTEMI are at increased risk of death. Other complications include ventricular failure and cardiogenic shock. Myocardial ischaemia can

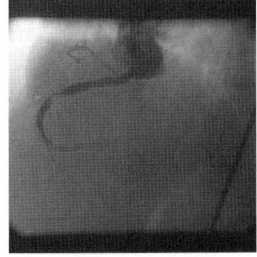
(a)

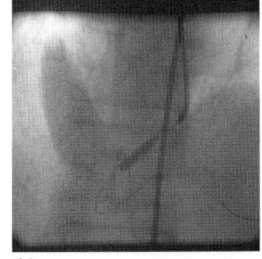
(b)

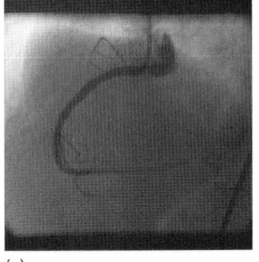
(c)

Fig. 1.13a–c Angiographic views of stenting of the right coronary artery.

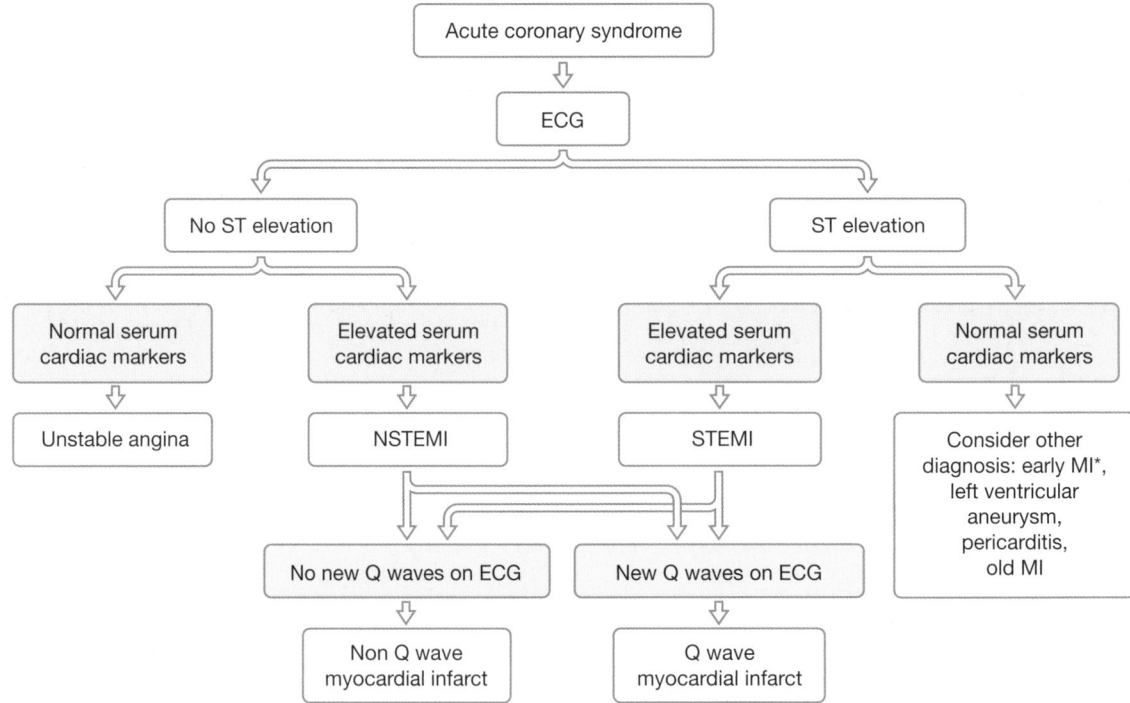

Acute coronary syndrome
↓
ECG
↓
No ST elevation / ST elevation

No ST elevation:
- Normal serum cardiac markers → Unstable angina
- Elevated serum cardiac markers → NSTEMI

ST elevation:
- Elevated serum cardiac markers → STEMI
- Normal serum cardiac markers → Consider other diagnosis: early MI*, left ventricular aneurysm, pericarditis, old MI

NSTEMI / STEMI:
- No new Q waves on ECG → Non Q wave myocardial infarct
- New Q waves on ECG → Q wave myocardial infarct

Fig. 1.15 Diagnosis and progression of acute coronary syndrome. These pathways/diagnoses are not mutually exclusive—one form of acute coronary syndrome can rapidly evolve into another. *Serum cardiac markers may be normal in the first few hours, and require repeat measurements in the 6–8-hour period after the onset of pain.

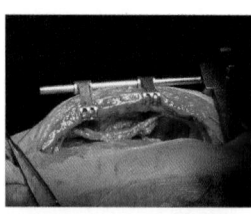

(a)

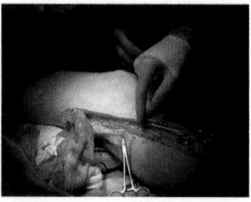

(b)

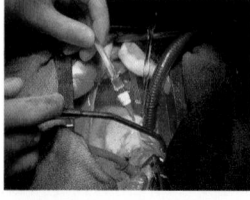

(c)

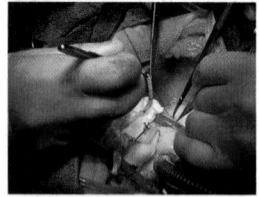

(d)

Fig. 1.14 a–d Coronary artery bypass grafting. Images courtesy of Mr Francis Wells, Consultant Cardiac Surgeon, Papworth Hospital, Cambridge, United Kingdom.

also cause mitral regurgitation and predispose to ventricular arrhythmia.

Clinical features

The characteristic features and assessment of the severity of angina are detailed on page 19–20. Unstable angina is defined as:
1. new onset angina (CCS III or IV in severity), *or*
2. angina that is increasing to CCS III in severity, *or*
3. angina occurring at rest (CCS IV, usually more than 20 min).

On examination, the patient may be sweating with a resting tachycardia (pain, ventricular failure). On auscultation there may be a third heart sound (ventricular failure) and a pansystolic murmur from ischaemic mitral regurgitation.

When assessing a patient with unstable angina it is important to identify any precipitating features of secondary unstable angina and to screen for complications and markers of poor prognosis (third heart sound, left ventricular failure, peripheral vascular disease).

Initial investigations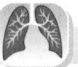

Blood tests

The indications for FBC, U&Es, plasma lipid profile and plasma glucose are similar to those of chronic stable angina (p. 20).

Serum cardiac markers

Serum cardiac markers are useful to determine prognosis and the presence of myocardial necrosis, which differentiates NSTEMI from unstable angina. Previously, CK-MB was the principal marker; currently, increased sensitivity is obtained from cardiac troponin (cTnT and cTnI). If a troponin test is negative within the first 6 hours, it should be repeated between 8 and 12 hours from the onset of chest pain. Elevation of troponin levels persists for 10–14 days.

Electrocardiogram

The ECG is critical to the diagnosis, and also central to the decision making process. Unstable angina is characterized by ST segment depression and T wave inversion that reverts to normal with the resolution of chest pain (Fig. 1.16). The presence of ST elevation and raised cardiac markers indicate STEMI (p. 28), either as the principal diagnosis or progression from unstable angina/NSTEMI.

Chest X-ray

The findings are similar to chronic stable angina (p. 20).

Further investigations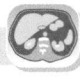

Coronary angiography

Coronary angiography is usually undertaken as an investigation prior to revascularization. It is indicated for high-risk patients in the presence of ongoing ischaemia despite

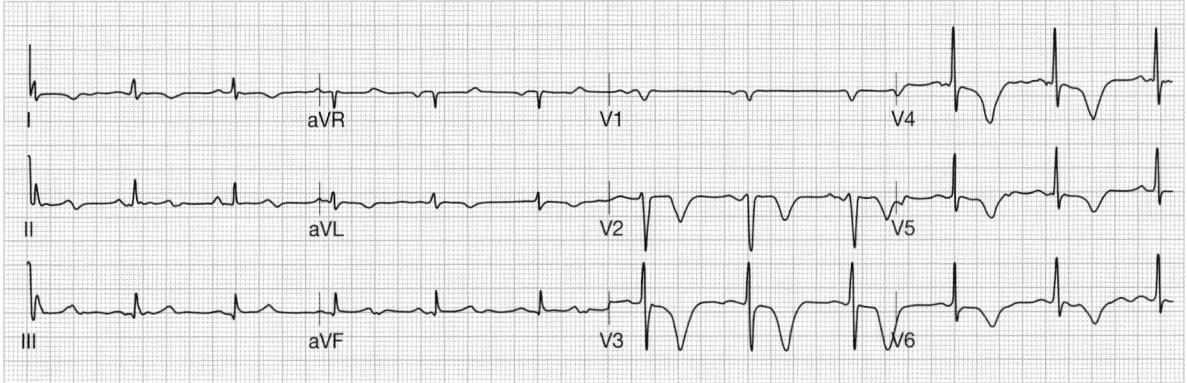

Fig. 1.16 ECG showing anterior ischaemia. The ECG alone does not distinguish between angina, unstable angina and NSTEMI. The differentiation between angina and unstable angina lies in the history, and the differentiation between unstable angina and NSTEMI lies in the serum cardiac markers.

appropriate therapy and for patients with previous percutaneous coronary intervention or coronary surgery.

Initial management

Oxygen
Supplementary oxygen should be provided to all patients to maintain peripheral oxygen saturations of more than 90%.

Nitrates
Immediate sublingual GTN should be administered, followed by intravenous infusion, to alleviate pain and promote coronary vasodilatation. It should not be used if the systolic pressure is below 90 mmHg or the heart rate is less than 50 bpm, and must be used with extreme caution in patients with suspected right ventricular infarction.

Opiate analgesia
If additional analgesia is required, intravenous morphine (or diamorphine) can be administered with an antiemetic (prochlorperazine).

Correct precipitating factors
Attempts should be made to identify and correct any precipitating factor (anaemia, hypoxia).

Admission to coronary care unit
Where available, patients should be admitted to the coronary care unit for continuous monitoring by staff experienced in defibrillation and other aspects of advanced cardiac life support (ACLS).

Medical management

The management aims in unstable angina/NSTEMI are relief of ischaemia and prevention of death and progression to STEMI. There are three groups of drug therapy: antiplatelet, anti-ischaemic and anticoagulation.

Antiplatelet therapy
Aspirin
Aspirin is the first choice therapy and should be administered promptly at a dose of 325 mg. For patients who are intolerant to aspirin, a suitable alternative antiplatelet agent is clopidogrel.

GP IIb/IIIa receptor antagonists
A IIb/IIIa receptor antagonist should be added to aspirin in patients with ongoing ischaemia or patients with high-risk features (Table 1.12).

Anti-ischaemic therapy
Nitrate
A nitrate is usually given to relieve ischaemia and simultaneously to provide pain relief. It is administered as a continuous infusion of GTN.

β-Blocker
In the absence of contraindications (severe asthma, second-degree heart block, severe left ventricular impairment), a β-blocker should be commenced early in the course of disease.

Calcium antagonist
For patients who are intolerant to β-blockers, a calcium antagonist may be used. It is important to avoid a non-dihydropyridine calcium antagonist (nifedipine) as sole therapy due to reflex tachycardia and worsening of symptoms; equally, a dihydropyridine calcium antagonist (verapamil) should not be given to patients with severe left ventricular impairment.

ACE inhibitor
An ACE inhibitor should be prescribed for patients with persisting hypertension despite β-blocker and intravenous nitrate therapy. The rationale for this is based on the favourable effects on survival in extrapolated data from acute myocardial infarction trials.

Table 1.12	Risk of death or non-fatal myocardial infarction in patients with unstable angina		
Feature	High-risk (at least one of the following features must be present)	Intermediate-risk (no high-risk feature but must have one of the following)	Low-risk (no high- or intermediate-risk feature but may have any of the following features)
History	Accelerating tempo of ischaemic symptoms in the preceding 48 h	Prior MI, peripheral or cerebrovascular disease, or CABG, prior aspirin use	
Character of pain	Prolonged ongoing (>20 min) rest pain	Prolonged (>20 min) rest angina, now resolved, with moderate or high likelihood of CAD Rest angina (<20 min) or relieved with rest or sublingual GTN	New-onset or progressive CCS class III or IV angina in the past 2 weeks without prolonged (>20 min) rest pain but with moderate or high likelihood of CAD
Clinical findings	Pulmonary oedema, most likely due to ischaemia New or worsening MR murmur S_3 or new/worsening rales Hypotension, bradycardia, tachycardia Age >75 years	Age >70 years	
ECG	Angina at rest with transient ST segment changes >0.05 mV Bundle branch block, new or presumed new Sustained ventricular tachycardia	T wave inversions >0.2 mV Pathological Q waves	Normal or unchanged ECG during an episode of chest discomfort
Cardiac markers	Elevated (e.g. TnT or TnI >0.1 ng/mL)	Slightly elevated (e.g. TnT >0.01 but <0.1 ng/mL)	Normal

Anticoagulation

Heparin

In unstable angina, intravenous unfractionated heparin reduces the risk of myocardial infarction by 89% and the risk of recurrent angina by 63%.[2] More recently, equivalent efficacy has been proven with low molecular weight heparins that have the additional advantages of subcutaneous administration, lower frequency of heparin-induced thrombocytopenia and no requirement for constant monitoring. However, reversal of a low molecular weight heparin requires fresh frozen plasma, and in the setting of patients who undergo percutaneous coronary intervention or if surgery is contemplated, unfractionated heparin is the preferred agent.

Surgical management

Intra-aortic balloon pump support

The intra-aortic balloon pump (p. 14) is indicated for patients with ongoing ischaemia despite maximal medical therapy and also for patients with haemodynamic instability. This is usually introduced prior to percutaneous coronary intervention or surgery.

Revascularization

An early invasive strategy (coronary angiography and revascularization if required in the acute hospital admission) is recommended for selected patients (Table 1.13). The decision to revascularize and the choice of technique (percutaneous coronary intervention or coronary artery bypass surgery) are the same as for chronic stable angina (p. 22).

Urgent surgery in the setting of unstable angina/NSTEMI carries an increased risk of mortality and bleeding complications in view of the antiplatelet and anticoagulation therapy.

Table 1.13	Indications for early invasive strategy in unstable angina/NSTEMI
Elevation in TnT/TnI (all NSTEMI patients)	
Ongoing angina/ischaemia despite maximum therapy	
New ST segment depression	
Concurrent cardiac failure	
Concurrent ischaemic mitral regurgitation	
Depressed left ventricular function (ejection fraction less than 40%)	
Haemodynamic instability	
Sustained ventricular arrhythmia	
Previous coronary surgery	
Percutaneous coronary intervention within the last 6 months	

Prognosis

Up to 25% of patients with NSTEMI progress to STEMI. Outcomes for acute coronary syndrome are presented in Table 1.16 on page 31.

Prior to hospital discharge, it is important to ensure that the risk factors for coronary artery disease have been addressed. In addition, patients should be on aspirin, a β-blocker and an ACE inhibitor. Patients should be advised on the need for risk factor modification and the appropriate amount of activity.

REFERENCES

(1) Steg PG, Goldberg RJ, Gore JM, et al. Baseline characteristics, management practices, and in-hospital outcomes of patients hospitalized with acute coronary syndromes in the Global Registry of Acute Coronary Events (GRACE). American Journal of Cardiology 2002; 90: 358–363.
(2) Theroux P, Ouimet H, McCans J, et al. Aspirin, heparin, or both to treat acute unstable angina. New England Journal of Medicine 1988; 319: 1105–1111.

ℹ FURTHER INFORMATION

Braunwald E, Antman EM, Beasley JW, et al. ACC/AHA guidelines for the management of patients with unstable angina and non-ST-segment elevation myocardial infarction: executive summary and recommendations: a report of the American College of Cardiology/American Heart Association Task Force on Practice Guidelines (Committee on the Management of Patients With Unstable Angina). Circulation 2000; 102: 1193–1209.

Braunwald E, Antman EM, Beasley JW, et al, Committee Members, Task Force Members. ACC/AHA guideline update for the management of patients with unstable angina and non-ST-segment elevation myocardial infarction—2002: summary article: a report of the American College of Cardiology/American Heart Association Task Force on Practice Guidelines (Committee on the Management of Patients With Unstable Angina). Circulation 2002; 106: 1893–1900.

ST-segment elevation myocardial infarction

Myocardial infarction was reclassified into NSTEMI and STEMI (p. 23) due to differences in pathogenesis and management. An important difference is the prompt thrombolytic therapy required for patients with STEMI.

Epidemiology

The epidemiology reflects that of chronic stable angina. In particular, for STEMI, the median age of presentation is 64 years, and it is 2.5 times more common in men.[1]

Pathology

Myocardial infarction is predominantly caused by coronary artery occlusion secondary to thrombosis around pre-existing coronary atherosclerotic plaque. The initiating stimulus is plaque instability leading to fissure or rupture, exposing the thrombogenic surfaces that incite a cascade of platelet activation and thrombin generation. Ultimately, this culminates in thrombus formation and vessel occlusion, occurring at the site of plaque instability or distal to it due to embolism. Other, more rare, causes are aortic dissection and coronary arteritis.

The extent of an infarct depends on the site of occlusion and the degree of collateral blood supply. Distal occlusions threaten smaller territories of myocardium, and a well-developed collateral blood supply from chronic coronary artery disease serves to limit the size of an infarct. An additional important influence in STEMI is the time to intervention (thrombolysis, percutaneous coronary intervention or surgery). Once the blood supply to an area of the heart is interrupted, irreversible cellular death commences within 20 minutes.

Scope of disease

The complications associated with myocardial infarction depend on the site and extent of infarction.

Arrhythmia

The borders of normal and ischaemic myocardium are zones of electrical instability. In addition, increased sympathetic activity (pain, distress) and sensitivity of injured myocardium to sympathetic stimulation predispose to cardiac arrhythmia. Complex ventricular arrhythmias are presumed to be the main cause of death prior to hospitalization. Ventricular fibrillation and ventricular tachycardia occur most commonly in the first 3 days following an infarct. New onset atrial flutter or fibrillation usually indicates a large area of infarct.

Infarction of myocardium carrying the conducting tissue gives rise to heart block (ranging from first-degree to complete heart block, depending on the extent of the infarct). More distal infarcts can give rise to left bundle branch or fascicle (hemi) blocks.

Myocardial rupture

The three sites of heart muscle rupture that produce characteristic clinical features are the left ventricular free wall (cardiac tamponade, circulatory shock and death), the septum (ventricular septal defect) and the papillary muscles of the left ventricle (acute mitral regurgitation, pulmonary oedema, circulatory shock).

Cardiac failure/circulatory shock

After a myocardial infarction, pump failure is usually caused by extensive infarction of the left ventricle; however, it may also arise from any of the complications detailed above. Progressive dysfunction can lead to circulatory shock, a very poor prognostic indicator. Extensive right coronary infarc-

Chronic stable angina

Acute coronary syndrome

Unstable angina/non ST segment elevation myocardial infarction

ST-segment elevation myocardial infarction

tions may result in right ventricular failure, although this is rarely clinically apparent (raised JVP, peripheral oedema without pulmonary oedema).

Late developments

Inflammation of the pericardium may give rise to pericarditis. Dressler's syndrome is thought to be an autoimmune reaction causing fever and recurrent chest discomfort; it is not always possible to differentiate between this and pericarditis.

Scar tissue eventually replaces the area of myocardial necrosis. If sufficiently extensive, this thin layer may develop into an aneurysm impairing myocardial performance.

Clinical features

Sudden onset of gripping chest pain, occurring at rest and lasting for more than 20 minutes, is the classical presentation. However, on history alone it cannot be differentiated from unstable angina, and serum cardiac markers are required to distinguish between the two. The diagnostic criteria for myocardial infarction are provided in Table 1.14.

On examination, the patient is usually in discomfort, distressed and sweating. There may be a resting tachycardia. It is important to ensure that all peripheral pulses are palpable as aortic dissection is a rare cause of myocardial infarction. The blood pressure may be low with cardiogenic shock. Other clinical indicators of poor tissue perfusion are slow capillary return, cold peripheries and cyanosis.

On auscultation, there may be the systolic murmur of mitral regurgitation or ventricular septal rupture. The heart sounds may be soft with pericardial effusion (pericarditis, tamponade from free wall rupture).

Initial investigations

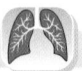

Serum cardiac markers and the ECG are the two fundamental investigations for the diagnosis and management of acute coronary syndrome.

Table 1.14	ACC/ESC definition of myocardial infarction*

1. Typical rise and fall of troponin or CK-MB with at least one of the following:
   a. ischaemic symptoms
   b. development of pathologic Q waves on ECG
   c. ECG changes indicative of ischaemia (ST elevation or depression)
   d. coronary artery intervention (e.g. coronary angioplasty)

or

2. Pathologic finding of an acute myocardial infarction

*Alpert JS, Thygesen K, Antman E, Bassand JP. Myocardial infarction redefined—a consensus document of The Joint European Society of Cardiology/American College of Cardiology Committee for the redefinition of myocardial infarction. Journal of the American College of Cardiology 2000; 36(3): 959–969.

Electrocardiogram

Myocardial ischaemia is diagnosed as ST segment depression and T wave inversion in the area affected by the coronary artery. This occurs with unstable angina and NSTEMI. Elevation of serum cardiac markers defines myocardial infarction. If the segment is depressed, it is considered NSTEMI and managed similarly to unstable angina (p. 25–26). On the other hand, if the ST segment is elevated (and serum cardiac markers raised) it is a STEMI (Fig. 1.17).

Arrhythmias and conduction blocks may also be revealed by the 12 lead ECG.

Serum cardiac markers

Currently, cardiac troponin is the gold standard for diagnosis of acute myocardial infarction. CK-MB is also useful, albeit as a less sensitive and specific marker. Troponin tends to be elevated for up to 7 days, whereas CK-MB tends to return to normal within 4 days. Within this time frame, therefore, troponin cannot reliably diagnose a re-infarction; CK-MB should be used for this purpose. Myoglobin is the first marker to rise and fall; however, myoglobin assays are

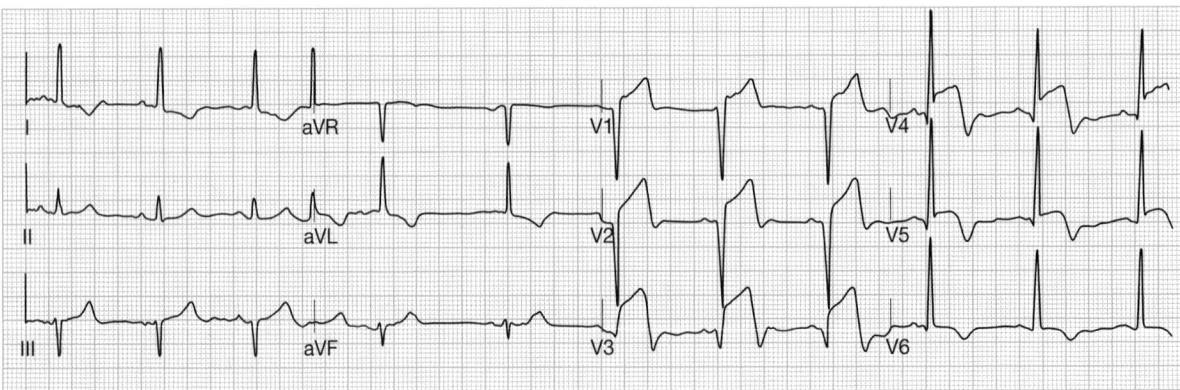

Fig. 1.17 Anterior ST segment elevation myocardial infarction (STEMI).

not commonly available in the UK. Figure 1.18 illustrates the rise and fall of the serum cardiac markers.

Full blood count
Haemoglobin estimation is useful to exclude anaemia, a potentially correctable condition that impairs myocardial oxygenation. The white cell count may be elevated from myocardial injury.

Urea and electrolytes
It is useful to document renal function, to monitor further deterioration from cardiogenic shock or drug therapy (ACE inhibitors).

Random plasma glucose
Serum glucose level may require treatment. It can be elevated as a result of diabetes or generally as a result of infarction.

Serum lipid profile
A serum lipid profile should be performed prior to discharge to assess the need for lipid-lowering therapy.

Group and save
Serum samples for group and save are generally taken on admission as bleeding complications can occur as a result of thrombolytic therapy.

Further investigations

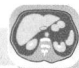

Further investigations are usually taken during the course of admission as time is of the essence in the initiation of thrombolysis.

Chest X-ray
A chest film can support a clinical diagnosis of pulmonary oedema, with the presence of widespread bilateral pulmonary infiltrates.

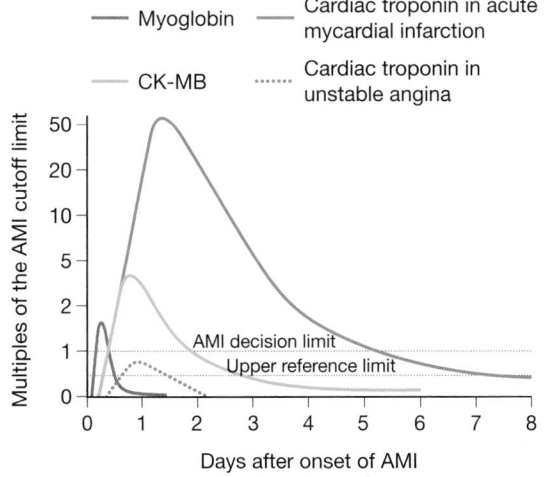

Fig. 1.18 Rise and fall of serum cardiac markers.

Transthoracic echocardiogram
An echocardiogram should be performed if there are any clinical features to suggest cardiac failure, or any mechanical complication (left ventricular free wall rupture, ischaemic ventricular septal defect and acute mitral regurgitation).

Coronary angiography
Coronary angiography is usually undertaken as an investigation prior to revascularization. It is indicated for high-risk patients, in the presence of ongoing ischaemia despite appropriate therapy, and for patients with previous percutaneous coronary intervention or coronary surgery.

Initial management

Oxygen
Supplementary oxygen should be provided to all patients to maintain peripheral oxygen saturations of more than 90%.

Nitrates
Immediate sublingual GTN should be administered, followed by intravenous infusion, to alleviate pain and promote coronary vasodilatation. It should not be used if the systolic pressure is below 90 mmHg or the heart rate is less than 50 bpm, and should be used with extreme caution in patients with suspected right ventricular infarction.

Opiate analgesia
If additional analgesia is required, intravenous morphine (or diamorphine) can be administered with an antiemetic (prochlorperazine).

Admission to coronary care unit
Where available, patients should be admitted to the coronary care unit for continuous monitoring by staff experienced in defibrillation and other aspects of advanced cardiac life support (ACLS).

Medical management

Antiplatelet therapy
Aspirin
Oral aspirin reduces the relative risk of death by 42% when used in conjunction with thrombolysis.[2] Aspirin should be administered in a dose of 160–325 mg to all patients on admission with suspected acute coronary syndrome.

Anti-ischaemic therapy
Thrombolysis
Fibrinolytic drugs such as streptokinase, recombinant tissue plasminogen activator (rTPA) and urokinase promote the conversion of plasminogen to plasmin, an enzyme that degrades fibrin and hence the thrombus. They should be administered to all patients within 12 hours of the onset

Chronic stable angina

Acute coronary syndrome

Unstable angina/non ST segment elevation myocardial infarction

ST-segment elevation myocardial infarction

Table 1.15	Absolute and relative contraindications to thrombolysis

Contraindications

Previous haemorrhagic stroke at any time; other strokes or cerebrovascular events within 1 year

Known intracranial neoplasm

Active internal bleeding (does not include menses)

Suspected aortic dissection

Cautions/relative contraindications

Severe uncontrolled hypertension on presentation (blood pressure >180/110 mmHg)

History of prior cerebrovascular accident or known intracerebral pathology not covered in contraindications

Current use of anticoagulants in therapeutic doses (INR ≥2–3); known bleeding diathesis

Recent trauma (within 2–4 weeks), including head trauma or traumatic or prolonged (>10 min) CPR or major surgery (<3 wk)

Non-compressible vascular punctures

Recent (within 2–4 weeks) internal bleeding

For streptokinase/anistreplase: prior exposure (especially within 5 days to 2 years) or prior allergic reaction

Pregnancy

Active peptic ulcer

History of chronic severe hypertension

INR, International Normalised Ratio; CPR, Cardiopulmonary resuscitation.

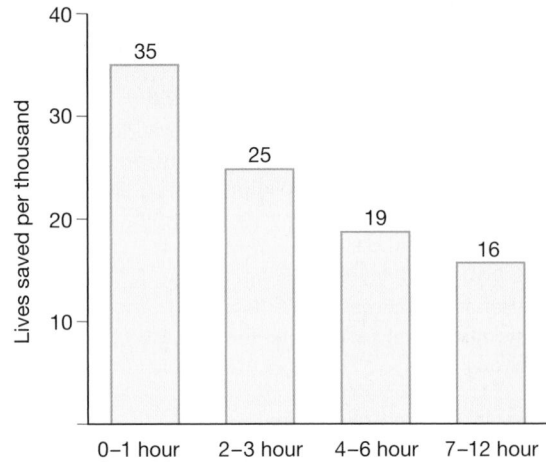

Fig. 1.19 Effect of time to initiate thrombolysis and survival. Source: Indications for fibrinolytic therapy in suspected acute myocardial infarction: collaborative overview of early mortality and major morbidity results from all randomised trials of more than 1000 patients. Fibrinolytic Therapy Trialists' (FTT) Collaborative Group. Lancet 1994; 343(8893): 311–322.

of chest pain, unless absolutely contraindicated (Table 1.15). The earlier fibrinolytic therapy is initiated, the more lives are saved (Fig. 1.19). The overall effect on survival is a 18% relative reduction in 35-day mortality; however, this is associated with an increase in the risk of intracranial haemorrhage (from 0.8% to 1.2%).[3]

β-Blocker

β-Blockers reduce myocardial oxygen demand by decreasing the heart rate, blood pressure and contractility, and should be administered in conjunction with thrombolysis to all patients without contraindications. The overall effects are a reduction in early mortality and in the size of infarct and rate of re-infarction. Adverse effects are hypotension and bradycardia.

ACE inhibitor

An ACE inhibitor should be prescribed to all patients following myocardial infarction. It is associated with a 7% relative reduction in mortality. The adverse effects are renal impairment (1.3%) and persistent hypotension (17.6%): both are approximately doubled compared to patients who do not receive ACE inhibitors.[4]

Anticoagulation therapy
Low molecular weight heparin

Low molecular weight heparin therapy is generally prescribed due to the increased risk of stroke and deep vein thrombosis.

Revascularization
Percutaneous coronary intervention

Percutaneous coronary intervention (PCI) is indicated as an alternative to thrombolysis for patients with absolute contraindications to thrombolytic therapy. In patients with cardiogenic shock, revascularization (PCI or surgery) improves late survival (but not 30-day mortality).[5]

Surgical management

The primary indications for coronary artery bypass surgery in the setting of acute myocardial infarction are to treat the mechanical complications (acute mitral regurgitation, ischaemic ventricular septal defect, left ventricular free wall rupture) and cardiogenic shock, and to revascularize patients with ongoing angina and coronary anatomy that is unsuitable for PCI. Urgent surgery in the setting of STEMI carries an increased risk of mortality and bleeding complications in view of the antiplatelet and anticoagulation therapy.

Prognosis

The average in-hospital mortality of STEMI is 7% (a significant proportion die before admission to hospital). Other outcome measures in comparison to unstable angina and NSTEMI are listed in Table 1.16.

Prior to discharge, it is important to ensure that predisposing risk factors to atherosclerosis have been corrected. In addition, patients should be on aspirin, a β-blocker and an ACE inhibitor. Patients should receive sufficient information regarding the importance of risk factor modification and recommended levels of activity.

Table 1.16	In-hospital outcomes for acute coronary syndrome*		
	Unstable angina	**NSTEMI**	**STEMI**
Death	3%	5%	7%
Cardiac failure	10%	18%	18%
Cardiogenic shock	2%	5%	7%
Reinfarction	N/A	2%	3%
Stroke	<1%	1%	2%
Major bleeding	2%	5%	5%
Acute renal failure	2%	6%	4%
Sustained VT/VF	2%	4%	10%
Atrial flutter/fibrillation	6%	12%	9%
Complete heart block	1%	2%	5%

* Adapted from Steg PG, Goldberg RJ, Gore JM, et al. Baseline characteristics, management practices, and in-hospital outcomes of patients hospitalized with acute coronary syndromes in the Global Registry of Acute Coronary Events (GRACE). American Journal of Cardiology 2002; 90(4): 358–363.

Patients should undergo risk stratification (exercise ECG) to screen for patient subsets that may benefit from revascularization.

FURTHER INFORMATION

Ryan TJ, Antman EM, Brooks NH, et al. 1999 update: ACC/AHA guidelines for the management of patients with acute myocardial infarction: executive summary and recommendations: a report of the American College of Cardiology/American Heart Association Task Force on Practice Guidelines (Committee on Management of Acute Myocardial Infarction). Circulation 1999; 100(9): 1016–1030.

REFERENCES

(1) Steg PG, Goldberg RJ, Gore JM, et al. Baseline characteristics, management practices, and in-hospital outcomes of patients hospitalized with acute coronary syndromes in the Global Registry of Acute Coronary Events (GRACE). American Journal of Cardiology 2002; 90(4): 358–363.
(2) Collaborative overview of randomised trials of antiplatelet therapy. Prevention of death, myocardial infarction, and stroke by prolonged antiplatelet therapy in various categories of patients. BMJ 1994; 308(6921): 81–106.
(3) Indications for fibrinolytic therapy in suspected acute myocardial infarction: collaborative overview of early mortality and major morbidity results from all randomised trials of more than 1000 patients. Fibrinolytic Therapy Trialists' (FTT) Collaborative Group. Lancet 1994; 343(8893): 311–322.
(4) Indications for ACE inhibitors in the early treatment of acute myocardial infarction: systematic overview of individual data from 100 000 patients in randomized trials. Circulation 1998; 97(22): 2202–2212.
(5) Hochman JS, Sleeper LA, Webb JG, et al. Early revascularization in acute myocardial infarction complicated by cardiogenic shock. New England Journal of Medicine 1999; 341(9): 625–634.

Heart failure

The degree of impairment to ventricular function is proportional to the site and extent of myocardial necrosis. In acute infarction, sudden loss of myocardial function is usually isolated to a specific territory and may produce features of isolated (left or right) ventricular failure.

Acute left ventricular failure

Left ventricular failure occurs in 10% of patients with acute myocardial infarctions: usually 40% or more of the heart muscle territory is infarcted before haemodynamic impairment occurs. The management of acute left ventricular failure is presented on page 60.

Acute right ventricular failure

Right ventricular impairment usually occurs in patients with acute inferior infarction; however, it is clinically apparent in less than 2%. Features of right ventricular failure are hypotension and raised venous pressures in the absence of pulmonary oedema. The diagnosis is best confirmed on transthoracic echocardiography.

In patients with clinically apparent right ventricular failure, the aims of management are to optimize cardiac output. This can involve invasive haemodynamic measurements, with central venous monitoring to optimize cardiac filling pressure. Pacing can increase cardiac output by optimizing heart rate (90–100 bpm). Further measures include pulmonary artery flotation, catheter insertion and introduction of inodilators (enoximone, milrinone) to augment ventricular contractility and reduce pulmonary pressures. Finally, right ventricular assist (p. 14) and heart transplantation (p. 71–72) are salvage options.

Arrhythmia and conduction abnormalities

In the border zone between normal and infarcted tissue, injured but viable cells are electrically unstable and constitute a potent source for arrhythmia.

Ventricular arrhythmia

Ventricular arrhythmias are common in the first 2 days after myocardial infarction. They range from ventricular premature beats to ventricular tachycardia to ventricular fibrillation. Ventricular premature beats alone require neither prophylaxis nor treatment.

The management of pulseless ventricular tachycardia is detailed on page 64. Otherwise, serum hypokalaemia should be corrected and treatment with lidocaine or amiodarone initiated. Any underlying cause should be carefully screened for and treated if successfully identified.

Ventricular fibrillation associated with poor left ventricular function carries an increased risk of in-hospital death.

Supraventricular arrhythmia

Atrial fibrillation occurs in approximately 15% of patients after myocardial infarction. It is associated with left

Chronic stable angina

Acute coronary syndrome

Unstable angina/non ST segment elevation myocardial infarction

ST-segment elevation myocardial infarction

ventricular failure and atrial infarction and carries a poor prognosis. Atrial flutter is less common. The management of both arrhythmias is covered on page 60.

Bradycardia and conduction blocks

Sinus bradycardia is common. It may be idiopathic or occur as a result of sinus node dysfunction or β-blocker therapy. In the absence of hypotension, treatment is not generally required. However, if the heart rate is below 40 bpm, atropine can be administered to raise the heart rate.

Conduction blocks occur in approximately 15% of patients. First-degree and Mobitz type I atrioventricular block do not require treatment. Mobitz type II and complete atrioventricular block will require temporary transvenous pacing. Failure of recovery to sinus rhythm indicates a requirement for the insertion of a permanent pacemaker (p. 12).

Myocardial rupture

Post-infarction heart muscle rupture usually leads to the following clinical syndromes related to the anatomical site of myocardial necrosis.

Ischaemic mitral regurgitation

Incompetence of the mitral valve may occur as a result of ischaemia and rupture of the chordae tendineae or papillary muscles and also as a consequence of impairment to the left ventricular free wall that anchors the papillary muscles. The severity of ischaemic mitral regurgitation ranges from transient and mild regurgitation from left ventricular free wall dysfunction, to acute torrential regurgitation and cardiogenic shock. Urgent or emergency mitral valve repair/replacement is the definitive procedure for patients with haemodynamically significant regurgitation.

Ischaemic ventricular septal defect

Myocardial necrosis from occlusion of the septal branches of the left anterior descending artery can result in the perforation of the ventricular septum, allowing free flow of blood from the left to the right ventricle. This rare complication usually occurs in the first week after myocardial infarction in approximately 2% and presents with a new onset systolic murmur in the lower left sternal border. Haemodynamic impairment can ensue in the subsequent hours to days depending on the size of perforation.

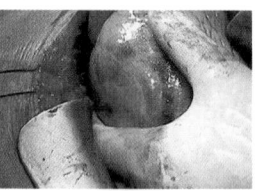

Fig. 1.20 Subacute left ventricular free wall rupture.

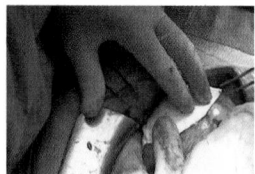

Fig. 1.21 Patch glue repair.

Management of acute heart failure is detailed on page 13–14. Haemodynamic impairment may require mechanical support such as an intra-aortic balloon pump. Currently, early surgery is advocated for clinically significant defects, with exclusion of the infarcted defect by pericardial patch sutured onto healthy heart muscle.

Left ventricular free wall rupture

Left ventricular free wall rupture occurs in approximately 5% and is usually fatal when a large 'blowout' rupture occurs. Subacute left ventricular free wall rupture becomes clinically apparent as pericardial tamponade. Left ventricular free wall rupture is managed surgically, with preoperative intra-aortic balloon pump support to augment left ventricular performance and reduce tension on the left ventricle. Emergency surgery is required to correct the defect (Fig. 1.20) and recent advances include the use of a patch that is simply glued onto the ventricular free wall (Fig. 1.21).[1]

Thromboembolism

Systemic emboli occur in approximately 5% of patients after myocardial infarction, usually as a result of mural thrombus in the akinetic infarcted segments. Emboli can manifest as stroke, mesenteric or renal infarction, and infarction of the digits.

Pericarditis

Pericarditis can occur as a result of localized inflammation from acute myocardial necrosis in approximately 10%, or occur as a result of an autoimmune response (Dressler's syndrome) that develops in the subsequent weeks or months in approximately 15%. Treatment of acute pericarditis is usually with high-dose aspirin or ibuprofen. Treatment of Dressler's syndrome may require corticosteroids.

REFERENCE

(1) Canovas SJ, Lim E, Dalmau MJ, et al. Midterm clinical and echocardiographic results with patch glue repair of left ventricular free wall rupture. Circulation 2003; 108 (Suppl 1): II237–240.

Heart valve disease

Infective endocarditis

Infective endocarditis results from microbial infection of the endothelial lining of the heart. Although not strictly synonymous, heart valve infection is the most common clinical manifestation of this disease.

Epidemiology

The incidence of infective endocarditis is approximately 4 per 100 000 and rises with age to 15 per 100 000 over the age of 50 years.[1] It is equally common in both sexes.

Pathology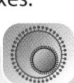

The most important predisposing factor is existing structural heart disease, such as heart valve disease, valve replacement and congenital heart disease. Intravenous drug abuse also predisposes to endocarditis, often resulting in right-sided heart valve infection. The majority (90%) of infections are due to streptococci, staphylococci and enterococci (Table 1.17).

Microorganisms can be introduced into the blood stream from dental procedures (streptococci), skin infections (staphylococci) and procedures on the gastrointestinal and urinary tract (enterococci). In a minority, the bacteraemia results in infection of the endothelium of the heart. Subsequent damage to heart valve surfaces produces platelet aggregation and fibrin deposition, culminating in friable vegetations that can harbour microorganisms and embolize. Infection of the heart valves can lead to perforation of the valve leaflets, rupture of papillary muscles and consequently aortic or mitral regurgitation. Extension of infection can erode into the fibrous skeleton of the heart, usually the aortic root, producing a paravalvular abscess.

Scope of disease

Cardiac

Acute heart failure and cardiogenic shock can result from free aortic or mitral regurgitation. Extension of infection can lead to fistula formation between great vessels and the heart, and within the chambers of the heart itself. Heart block can result from an aortic root abscess. Mycotic aortic aneurysm is a rare complication.

Embolic

Sterile or septic emboli from valve vegetations can lodge in the brain to cause stroke or cerebral abscesses. Other sites of emboli are the skin and mucous membranes (petechiae), the eye (retinal haemorrhages), the lung (septic emboli from right-sided endocarditis), the spleen (splenic infarcts), the kidney (renal infarcts) and rarely the coronary arteries (myocardial infarction).

Immunological

Immune complex mediated glomerulonephritis can occur as a result of endocarditis. In addition, the pathogeneses of arthralgia, arthritis and Osler's nodes are thought to be immune mediated. Rheumatoid factor may be (falsely) positive in the setting of endocarditis.

Clinical features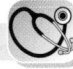

Infective endocarditis can be a difficult diagnosis as the presenting symptoms are of a non-specific flu-like illness. Fever, night sweats, rigors and malaise are typical. Patients may also present with embolic complications such as neurological deficits, abdominal pain (splenic infarcts) and immune mediated complications such as haematuria (glomerulonephritis) and arthralgia.

On examination, clubbing and splinter haemorrhages (more than five) may be evident. Osler's nodes (painful erythematous lesions on the pulps of the fingers) and

Table 1.17	Aetiological organisms of infective endocarditis
Culture-positive endocarditis	
Viridans streptococci	
Staphylococcus aureus	
Staphylococcus epidermidis	
Enterococcus faecalis	
Gram-negative bacilli	
Microaerophilic streptococcus	
Fungal species	
Culture-negative endocarditis	
Consider the effect of existing antibiotic usage	

'HACEK' organisms
   Haemophilus species
   Actinobacillus species
   Cardiobacterium hominis
   Eikenella species
   Kingella species	

Other organisms with fastidious culture requirements
   Coxiella species
   Chlamydia psittaci
   Fungal endocarditis	

Janeway lesions (small flat erythematous lesions from circulating immune complexes) are very rare. Petechiae may be visible on the skin, and pale conjunctiva may be suggestive of anaemia. A new murmur is a very important clinical finding and should be carefully auscultated for. Overt valve regurgitation and acute cardiac failure is rare. Abdominal examination may reveal splenomegaly.

The Duke diagnostic criteria (Table 1.18) are a useful adjunct to clinical assessment and investigations. The presence of two major, one major and three minor, or five minor criteria indicates infective endocarditis.

Initial investigations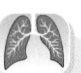

Three sets of blood cultures

Blood cultures are the key investigation for patients with suspected endocarditis. It is important to collect three sets of blood cultures before commencing antibiotic therapy, as the inability to isolate an organism impairs the ability to diagnose endocarditis and to identify a specific treatment regimen. The blood cultures should be collected over a 24-hour period, or over a 1–2-hour period if the patient is severely ill.

Full blood count

Anaemia and elevated white cell counts are the usual findings on a FBC.

Markers of inflammation

The non-specific markers of inflammation (erythrocyte sedimentation rate (ESR)/C-reactive protein (CRP) are usually raised but contribute little to the diagnostic process.

Urea and electrolytes

Glomerulonephritis can occur as a complication of endocarditis, although overt renal failure with elevated urea and creatinine is uncommon. Baseline estimation of renal function is essential as aminoglycosides are first-line therapy.

Urine dipstick

It is important to screen for blood and proteins in the urine that may indicate glomerulonephritis or renal infarct.

Transthoracic echocardiogram

This investigation forms part of the Duke criteria for the diagnosis of infective endocarditis. Echocardiographic features are oscillating masses on the valve (Fig. 1.22) or supporting structures or within regurgitant jets. Intracardiac fistulae, abscesses and mycotic aneurysms of the aortic root can also be detected.

Further investigations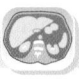

Serology

If blood cultures are negative, paired serology samples are collected to detect antibodies to *Coxiella burnetii*,

Table 1.18	Revised Duke criteria*

Major criteria

1. Positive blood culture
   a. typical microorganism for infective endocarditis from two separate blood cultures, *or*
   b. persistently positive blood culture of a microorganism consistent with infective endocarditis

2. Evidence of endocardial involvement
   a. positive echocardiogram for endocarditis (oscillating intracardiac mass, abscess or new partial dehiscence of prosthetic heart valve), *or*
   b. new valvular regurgitation

Minor criteria

a. Predisposition to infective endocarditis (structural heart disease, i.v. drug abuse)

b. Fever (more than 38°C)

c. Vascular phenomenon (emboli, septic pulmonary infarct, mycotic aneurysm, intracranial haemorrhage, conjunctival haemorrhage, Janeway lesions)

d. Immunologic phenomenon (glomerulonephritis, Osler's nodes, Roth spots, positive rheumatoid factor)

e. Microbiological evidence (positive blood culture not meeting major criteria, serological evidence of infection with organism consistent with endocarditis)

* Full details on pathological criteria and classification of diagnostic certainty (definite, possible and rejected endocarditis) can be found in Baddour LM, Wilson WR, Bayer ES, et al. Infective endocarditis: diagnosis, antimicrobial therapy, and management of complications: a statement for healthcare professionals from the Committee on Rheumatic Fever, Endocarditis, and Kawasaki Disease, Council on Cardiovascular Disease in the Young, and the Councils on Clinical Cardiology, Stroke, and Cardiovascular Surgery and Anesthesia, American Heart Association: endorsed by the Infectious Diseases Society of America. Circulation 2005; 111: 3167–3184.

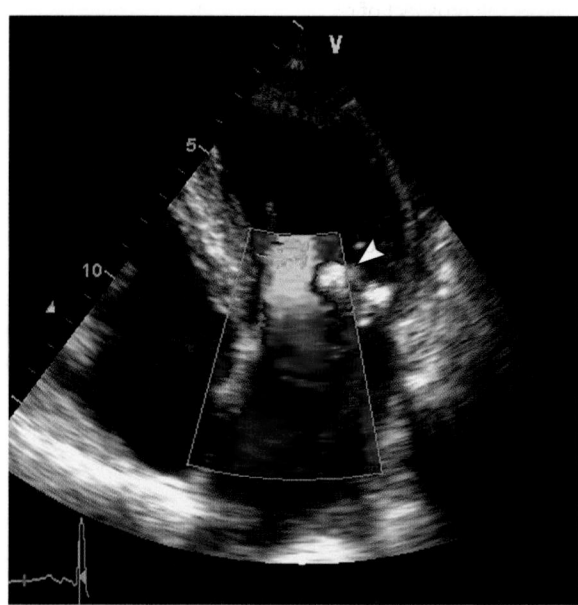

Fig. 1.22 Transthoracic echocardiogram. The echocardiogram shows the vegetation (arrow) on the anterior leaflet of the mitral valve, and valve destruction leading to severe mitral regurgitation (colour flow) from endocarditis.

Chlamydia psittaci, Mycoplasma, Bartonella and *Candida* (see Table 1.17).

Transoesophageal echocardiogram

Transoesophageal echocardiography is a more definitive investigation when transthoracic echocardiography is inadequate due to poor images, or negative despite strong clinical suspicion. It is the investigation of choice for suspected prosthetic heart valve endocarditis.

Medical management

Antibiotic therapy

Empirical antibiotic therapy should be initiated after collection of three sets of blood cultures in the acutely ill. In patients with native heart valves, intravenous benzylpenicillin plus gentamicin is the combination of choice. If there is a history of intravenous drug abuse, intravenous flucloxacillin should be added. For patients with prosthetic heart valves, vancomycin plus gentamicin is recommended.

Specific antibiotic therapy should be commenced as soon as the organism, antibiotic sensitivity and minimally effective concentrations of antibiotics are known.

Surgical management

Heart valve replacement

Haemodynamic instability is the primary indication for emergency heart valve replacement. This is usually undertaken in the setting of acute cardiac failure due to free aortic or mitral valve (Fig. 1.23) regurgitation unless the severity of comorbid conditions (severe cerebral damage) makes the prospect of recovery remote.

In patients who are haemodynamically stable, the indications for heart valve replacement are the development of complications such as aortic root abscess or intracardiac fistulae. Ideally the operation should take place when all evidence of the infection has subsided, as valve replacement involves the further prosthetic material in at a site of infection.

Surgery is also recommended for patients with evidence of valve dysfunction and persistent infection despite 7 days of antibiotics, and fungal endocarditis.

Approximately a third of patients will require surgery, and the operative mortality is similar to valve replacement procedures in the uncomplicated patient. Increased operative risk is proportional to extent of the infection, underlying health and immediate preoperative condition of the patient.

Prognosis

The overall in-hospital mortality is 15%,[2] and the 1- and 5-year survival is 76% and 58% respectively.[3] Most patients do not require valve replacement. In some, progressive valve dysfunction may continue with time and the indications for surgery are the same as patients with chronic valve disease.

i FURTHER INFORMATION

Baddour LM, Wilson WR, Bayer ES, et al. Infective endocarditis: diagnosis, antimicrobial therapy, and management of complications: a statement for healthcare professionals from the Committee on Rheumatic Fever, Endocarditis, and Kawasaki Disease, Council on Cardiovascular Disease in the Young, and the Councils on Clinical Cardiology, Stroke, and Cardiovascular Surgery and Anesthesia, American Heart Association: endorsed by the Infectious Diseases Society of America. Circulation 2005; 111: 3167–3184.

REFERENCES

(1) *Tak T, Reed KD, Haselby RC, McCauley CS Jr, Shukla SK. An update on the epidemiology, pathogenesis and management of infective endocarditis with emphasis on Staphylococcus aureus. WMJ 2002; 101: 24–33.*
(2) *Netzer RO, Zollinger E, Seiler C, Cerny A. Infective endocarditis: clinical spectrum, presentation and outcome. An analysis of 212 cases 1980–1995. Heart 2000; 84: 25–30.*
(3) *Netzer RO, Altwegg SC, Zollinger E, Tauber M, Carrel T, Seiler C. Infective endocarditis: determinants of long term outcome. Heart 2002; 88: 61–66.*

Rheumatic fever

Rheumatic fever is a delayed, non-suppurative connective tissue disease that develops after pharyngeal infection with group A β-haemolytic streptococci.

Epidemiology

Rheumatic fever is rare in developed countries following the introduction of antibiotic therapy for bacterial pharyngitis. It is still a significant worldwide problem, and was formerly the most common cause of childhood polyarthritis.

The prevalence of rheumatic fever is approximately 1 per 100 000 in developed countries and up to 2000 per 100 000 in developing countries. The peak age of onset is 6 years with the majority of cases developing between the ages of 4 and 15 years. Both sexes are equally affected.

Pathology

An abnormal humoral immune response develops to bacterial antigens which are cross-reactive with host antigens. A genetic predisposition has been found with an increased incidence of the MHC class II alleles HLA-DR. The inflammatory reaction generally involves connective tissue or collagen of the heart, joints and central nervous system. The basic structural change is fibrinoid necrosis, associated with the infiltration of mononuclear cells and histiocytes that form giant Aschoff's cells.

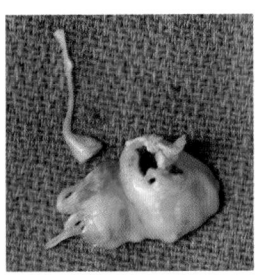

Fig. 1.23 Resected segment of anterior mitral valve leaflet.
Image courtesy of Mr Stephen Large, Cardiac Surgeon, Papworth Hospital, UK.

Rheumatic carditis is a pancarditis, affecting all the layers of the heart, although the predominant effect is scarring of the heart valves. The mitral and aortic valves are the most commonly affected. Polyarthritis is asymmetric and migratory involving the large joints of the knees, ankles, elbows and wrists. Chorea is usually a delayed manifestation, and multiple subcutaneous nodules can also occur.

Clinical features

Fever and arthralgia are non-specific initial symptoms of rheumatic fever. The development of complications such as chorea occurs approximately 3 months after the initial infection, and rheumatic heart disease (most commonly mitral regurgitation) develops 15 years after the initial attack. The diagnosis is established using the revised Jones criteria (Table 1.19).

Investigations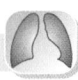

Full blood count
Mild anaemia may be present and the white cell count is usually elevated with acute infection.

Markers of inflammation
The CRP is almost always elevated with acute disease.

Electrocardiogram
A common finding is a prolonged PR interval.

Throat swab
Approximately 10% will have positive cultures on a throat swab.

Table 1.19	Revised Jones criteria (1992) for the diagnosis of rheumatic fever*
Major manifestations	
Carditis	
Polyarthritis	
Chorea	
Erythema marginatum	
Subcutaneous nodules	
Minor manifestations	
Fever	
Arthralgia	
Previous rheumatic fever or rheumatic heart disease	
Elevated ESR or CRP	
Prolonged PR interval	

Diagnosis is based on one major and two minor criteria plus supporting evidence of preceding group A streptococcal infection.
* Source: Dajani AS, Ayoub E, Bierman FZ, et al. Guidelines for the diagnosis of rheumatic fever: Jones criteria, updated 1992. Circulation 1993; 87: 302–307.

Management

Antibiotics
Prompt antibiotic therapy up to 9 days following the attack is effective in preventing the primary attack of rheumatic fever. Oral penicillin is the antibiotic of choice.

Analgesia
Non-steroidal anti-inflammatory agents are useful for the symptomatic treatment of arthritis.

Heart valve surgery
Eventually a proportion of patients will develop heart valve disease of sufficient severity to require heart valve surgery.

Prognosis

Prompt antibiotic therapy is effective in preventing the primary attack of rheumatic fever.

Aortic valve disease

Aortic stenosis

Aortic stenosis is narrowing of the aortic valve orifice. The site of narrowing is usually at the cusps or leaflets, but it can also occur proximal to the valve (subaortic stenosis) in the presence of a congenital membrane, or distal to the valve (supravalvular aortic stenosis) in Williams' syndrome. In conditions such as hypertrophic obstructive cardiomyopathy, aortic stenosis is mimicked with narrowing of the left ventricular outflow tract from gross septal hypertrophy.

The normal aortic valve area is 3–4 cm^2; narrowing to less than 1 cm^2 is regarded as severe stenosis, between 1 and 1.5 cm^2 as moderate, and between 1.5 and 3 cm^2 as mild. It is important to note that these are arbitrary values, and the degree of stenosis that a person can tolerate depends on body size (a small person will tolerate an aortic valve area of 1.5 cm^2 much better than a very large person).

RECENT ADVANCES
Increasingly, the aortic valve orifice area index is taken as a better measure of the severity of aortic valve stenosis and can be applied before and after valve replacement. It is calculated as the aortic valve orifice area divided by the body surface area. A 70 kg male has an aortic valve orifice area index of 2.2 and severe aortic stenosis is defined as an index of less than 0.6.

Epidemiology

Aortic stenosis is a common valve disease with an incidence that increases with age. The prevalence is approximately 3% of patients aged between 75 and 86 years.[1]

Pathology

The most common cause of aortic stenosis is termed degenerative (senile) calcific aortic stenosis. Unfortunately, this non-specific 'aetiology' can result from any degree of injury of the aortic valve as a pathophysiological response. It is thought that a congenitally bicuspid valve may predispose a person to aortic stenosis due to fibrosis and calcification that can potentially occur on the abnormal valve. A less common but more defined aetiology is rheumatic fever (Table 1.20).

Haemodynamic effects

The left ventricle adapts by increasing the force on contraction to generate higher pressures to overcome the narrowed aortic valve. This gradually leads to concentric hypertrophy. As heart muscle bulk increases, the compliance of the ventricle decreases. The inability of the ventricle to relax and fill completely gives rise to diastolic dysfunction. Eventually, the hypertrophy may not be able to keep up with the progression of disease and systolic heart failure sets in.

Natural history

Patients with aortic stenosis tend to be free of symptoms until late in the disease. Progression of aortic valve narrowing occurs at approximately 0.12 cm² per year, although this is variable depending on the aetiology (calcific faster than rheumatic). Following the onset of symptoms the mean life expectancy decreases to an average of 5 years with the onset of angina, 3 years with the onset of syncope, and 2 years with the onset of dyspnoea.[2]

Scope of disease

The increased heart muscle bulk and forceful systolic contractions lead to increased oxygen requirement: even in the presence of normal coronary arteries the supply may be inadequate, resulting in angina. Reduced cerebral perfusion on exercise can give rise to syncope as a symptom. Also, calcific debris from the valve has the potential to embolize and cause stroke. Sudden death is known to occur and may in part be due to ventricular arrhythmia.

Clinical features

Most patients are asymptomatic in the early stages of disease. Angina, syncope (on exertion) and dyspnoea are the three cardinal manifestations of symptomatic aortic stenosis.

Table 1.20	Causes of aortic stenosis
Calcific/degenerative aortic stenosis	
Congenitally bicuspid aortic valve	
Rheumatic fever	

Examination features depend on the severity of disease. The pulse may be low volume and slow rising with a narrow pulse pressure. The JVP is raised late in the disease when heart failure develops. A thrill may be palpable over the aortic area. On auscultation there is an ejection systolic murmur that is loudest in the aortic area and radiates into the carotids. It is the length not the intensity of the murmur that correlates with severity.

Initial investigations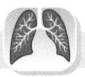

Electrocardiogram

There may be evidence of left ventricular hypertrophy and strain.

Chest X-ray

A chest film may be normal. The major features are post-stenotic dilatation of the aorta (Fig. 1.24) and calcification of the aortic valve. Evidence of left ventricular hypertrophy is subtle, and may be detected as rounding of the ventricular border. Cardiomegaly occurs late in the disease.

Transthoracic echocardiogram

A transthoracic echocardiogram is essential to confirm and grade the severity of stenosis. Severe aortic stenosis is defined as a valve orifice area of less than 1 cm², and in the presence of a normal cardiac output this corresponds to a pressure gradient of 50 mmHg (a pressure gradient of 100 mmHg or more is often considered critical aortic stenosis). It is important to note that the heart will not be able to generate high pressures when cardiac failure develops and therefore echocardiographic assessment of the severity of aortic stenosis requires the calculation of the aortic valve area and pressure gradient, and interpretation with the estimation of transvalvular flow.

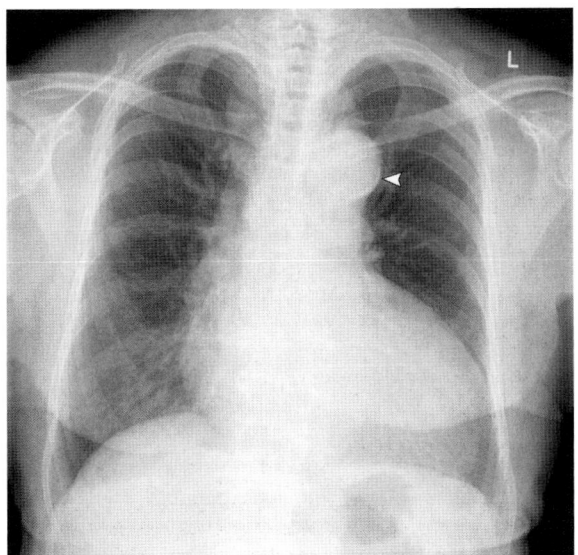

Fig. 1.24 A patient with aortic stenosis. The chest film shows left ventricular hypertrophy and calcification of the aortic arch (arrow).

Further investigations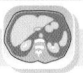

Left heart catheterization

Cardiac catherization is usually performed prior to cardiac surgery to assess the coronary arteries when concomitant ischaemic heart disease is suspected. It may also be performed when non-invasive assessment of the severity of aortic stenosis is inconclusive. Direct measurements of the aortic ventricular gradient can be obtained.

Initial management

Patient education

Patients should be informed of the importance of antibiotic prophylaxis for dental procedures. Patients with moderate to severe aortic stenosis should be advised to avoid competitive sports.

Medical management

There is no pharmacological therapy to treat aortic stenosis per se. Medical management consists of yearly clinical and echocardiographic assessment, and treatment of patients who are unsuitable to proceed to surgery.

Surveillance

Five-yearly clinical assessment and echocardiography is appropriate for asymptomatic patients with *mild* aortic stenosis, two-yearly assessment for asymptomatic patients with moderate aortic stenosis, and yearly assessment for patients with severe aortic stenosis.

Management of cardiac failure

In patients unsuitable for surgery in end stage aortic stenosis, digoxin, diuretics and the cautious use of ACE inhibitors may relieve symptoms of pulmonary oedema.

Surgical management

Surgery is indicated for patients with severe aortic stenosis and symptoms (angina, syncope, dyspnoea).

It is unusual for patients with echocardiographic evidence of severe aortic stenosis to remain asymptomatic for long periods of time. This subgroup should be followed up closely and referred for urgent surgery at the onset of symptoms.

Aortic valve replacement

The aortic valve may be replaced with a number of prostheses, however the decision is usually between a stented tissue (xenograft; Fig. 1.25) and a mechanical (Fig. 1.26) valve (Table 1.21). A tissue valve does not require anticoagulation and is the favoured prosthesis for the elderly (over 65), women of childbearing potential and patients who are involved in contact sports. The disadvantage of a tissue valve is its durability: the lifetime risk of revision operation is 28% and 12% in patients aged 65 and 75 at the time of implantation respectively[3].

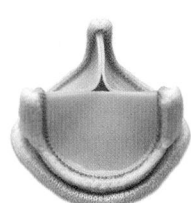
(a)

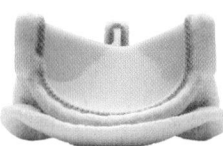
(b)

Fig. 1.25a,b Pericardial tissue aortic valve. Courtesy of Edwards Lifesciences, Irvine, California.

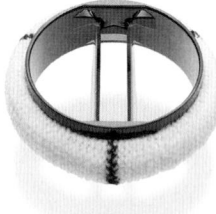
(a)

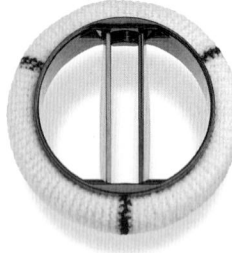
(b)

Fig. 1.26a,b Mechanical aortic valve Courtesy of ATS Medical Inc., Minneapolis, USA.

Table 1.21	Choice of aortic valve prosthesis
Tissue	
Animal valve	
Stented xenograft valve (porcine/bovine) Porcine/bovine aortic valve Pericardial valve (aortic valve made entirely from pericardium)	
Stentless xenograft valve Porcine aortic root Pericardial stentless valve	
Human	
Homograft (cadaveric donor)	
Autograft (use of the native pulmonary valve)	
Mechanical	

In this procedure a median sternotomy is performed, the pericardium is opened and cardiopulmonary bypass is established. The aorta is incised and the heart is stopped with cardioplegia solution via the aorta or direct cannulation into the coronary arteries. The native valve is excised and excess calcium is removed. The new valve is sutured into place and any air within the aorta is carefully removed before the access incision on the aorta is oversewn.

The risk of mortality with this procedure is approximately 2%. There is also a risk of stroke (air or debris embolism) and permanent pacemaker requirement (injury to the conduction system).

Prognosis

After tissue aortic valve replacement, the 5- and 10-year survival is approximately 78% and 55% respectively[3].

REFERENCES

(1) Lindroos M, Kupari M, Heikkila J, Tilvis R. Prevalence of aortic valve abnormalities in the elderly: an echocardiographic study of a random population sample. Journal of the American College of Cardiology 1993; 21: 1220–1225.

(2) Bonow RO, Carabello B, de Leon AC Jr, et al. ACC/AHA guidelines for the management of patients with valvular heart disease: a report of the American College of Cardiology/American Heart Association Task Force on Practice Guidelines (Committee on Management of Patients With Valvular Heart Disease). Journal of the American College of Cardiology 1998; 32: 1486–1588.

(3) Puvimanasinghe JPA, Steyerberg EW, Takkenberg JJM, Eijkemans MJC, van Herwerden LA, Bogers AJJC, Habbema JDF. Prognosis after aortic valve replacement with a bioprosthesis: predictions based on meta-analysis and microsimulation. Circulation 2001; 103: 1535–1541.

Aortic regurgitation

Competence of the aortic valve may be affected by any disease compromising the valve or the aortic root.

Epidemiology

Mild aortic regurgitation is common: the prevalence in a cohort of American Indians was 4.5% in patients less than 50 years old (4500 per 100 000), increasing with age to 16.4% patients aged between 70 to 79 years (16 400 per 100 000).[1] It is approximately one and a half times more common in women.

Pathology

Aortic regurgitation may arise from diseases affecting the valve leaflets, such as destruction from endocarditis, or valve mobility in degenerative calcific and rheumatic disease where the stiffened leaflets are unable to coapt (Table 1.22).

Dilatation of the aortic root also causes failure of the valve leaflet coaptation, and aortic dissection causes disruption of the structural support of the aortic valve.

Haemodynamic consequences

In acute severe aortic regurgitation (aortic dissection, endocarditis), the ventricle has a limited capacity to adapt to the sudden volume load. To increase cardiac output, heart rate increases and force of contraction increases with ventricular dilatation. However, in the unadapted ventricle, dilatation is limited and back pressure rapidly develops into pulmonary oedema.

Under chronic conditions, the ventricle adapts by dilatation and a combination of eccentric and concentric hypertrophy (combined volume and pressure overload). Increased compliance allows the ventricle to accommodate the excess volume load and eject a larger stroke volume. Left ventricular performance (ejection fraction) is usually normal and left ventricular systolic impairment is reversible in the early stages of the disease.

Table 1.22	Causes of aortic regurgitation
Diseases of the aortic valve	
Calcific degeneration	
Infective endocarditis	
Rheumatic fever	
Congenital bicuspid valve	
Diseases of the aortic root	

Dilatation
  Idiopathic (includes age related)
  Marfan's disease
Aortic dissection	

Other rare causes/associations	
Trauma	
Rheumatoid disease	
Systemic lupus erythematosus	
Ankylosing spondylitis	
Inflammatory bowel disease	

Natural history

The rate of progression to symptoms or left ventricular dysfunction is approximately 4% per year,[2] and following the onset of symptoms the mortality exceeds 10% per year. The severity of disease cannot be assessed by symptomatic status alone, as a proportion of patients with asymptomatic disease will have evidence of left ventricular dysfunction, a strong predictor of death.

Scope of disease

Progression of aortic regurgitation can lead to asymptomatic left ventricular dysfunction and, if left untreated, to congestive cardiac failure.

Clinical features

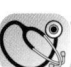

Symptoms of aortic regurgitation are dyspnoea and (less commonly) angina. On examination there may be a large volume (water hammer) pulse with a wide pulse pressure. The JVP is not usually raised unless congestive heart failure develops. The apex beat is displaced and has a thrusting quality. A diastolic murmur may be audible at the left sternal edge and accentuated with the patient's breath held on expiration. Increased flow may be audible across the aortic valve as a systolic murmur.

When assessing a patient with aortic valve disease, it is important to ascertain features of any disease that can cause aortic regurgitation (endocarditis, Marfan's syndrome), screen for complications (congestive cardiac failure), and quantify the severity of dyspnoea using the NYHA classification (p. 16) and angina using the CCS classification (p. 20).

Initial investigations

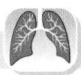

Electrocardiogram

There may be evidence of left ventricular hypertrophy and strain.

Chest X-ray

A chest film may be normal. The major features are dilatation of the ascending aorta and cardiomegaly.

Transthoracic echocardiogram

A transthoracic echocardiogram is essential to confirm the presence and grade the severity of aortic regurgitation and to assess left ventricular function. The degree of regurgitation is assessed semi-quantitatively (mild, moderate, severe) and left ventricular function is assessed by measuring ejection fraction and ventricular (end systolic, end diastolic) dimensions.

Further investigations

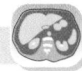

Left heart catheterization

Cardiac catheterization is usually performed prior to cardiac surgery to assess the coronary arteries when concomitant ischaemic heart disease is suspected.

Initial management

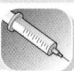

Patient education

It is important to stress the need for antibiotic prophylaxis during dental treatment.

Medical management

Medical management predominantly consists of yearly clinical and echocardiographic assessment. Vasodilator therapy is indicated for a small selected subgroup of patients.

Surveillance

Yearly clinical assessment and echocardiography is appropriate for asymptomatic patients with normal ejection fraction (more than 50%) and left ventricular dimensions (end systolic diameter less than 45 mm).

Vasodilator therapy

Vasodilator therapy is only suitable for patients with severe aortic regurgitation who are unsuitable for surgery or for severely symptomatic patients prior to surgery and asymptomatic patients with normal left ventricular function but enlarged left ventricular dimensions. Nifedipine and ACE inhibitors have been used in these circumstances.

Surgical management

Aortic valve replacement is indicated for patients with either:
1. symptoms (NYHA III/IV dyspnoea or CCS II–IV angina), *or*
2. left ventricular impairment, *either*
   a. ejection fraction less than 49%, *or*
   b. left ventricular end systolic diameter more than 55 mm, *or*
3. NYHA II dyspnoea and progressive left ventricular dilatation or declining ejection fraction.

Aortic valve replacement

The procedure for aortic valve replacement is detailed on page 38. Occasionally, when aortic valve regurgitation is associated with ascending aortic enlargement (aneurysm), replacement of the entire aortic root (aortic valve and proximal ascending aorta) is required (p. 38).

RECENT ADVANCES

Currently, the value of aortic valve repair is being evaluated for patients with aortic regurgitation secondary to aortic root enlargement.[3]

Prognosis

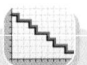

Following tissue aortic valve replacement, the 5- and 10-year survival is approximately 78% and 55% respectively.[4]

FURTHER INFORMATION

Bonow RO, Carabello B, de Leon AC Jr, et al. ACC/AHA guidelines for the management of patients with valvular heart disease: a report of the American College of Cardiology/ American Heart Association Task Force on Practice Guidelines (Committee on Management of Patients With Valvular Heart Disease). Journal of the American College of Cardiology 1998; 32: 1486–1588.

REFERENCES

(1) *Lebowitz NE, Bella JN, Roman MJ, et al. Prevalence and correlates of aortic regurgitation in American Indians: the Strong Heart Study. Journal of the American College of Cardiology 2000; 36: 461–467.*
(2) *Bonow RO, Carabello B, de Leon AC Jr, et al. ACC/AHA guidelines for the management of patients with valvular heart disease: a report of the American College of Cardiology/American Heart Association Task Force on Practice Guidelines (Committee on Management of Patients With Valvular Heart Disease). Journal of the American College of Cardiology 1998; 32: 1486–1588.*
(3) *David TE, Armstrong S, Ivanov J, Feindel CM, Omran A, Webb G. Results of aortic valve-sparing operations. Journal of Thoracic and Cardiovascular Surgery 2001; 122: 39–46.*
(4) *Puvimanasinghe JPA, Steyerberg EW, Takkenberg JJM, Eijkemans MJC, van Herwerden LA, Bogers AJJC, Habbema JDF. Prognosis after aortic valve replacement with a bioprosthesis: predictions based on meta-analysis and microsimulation. Circulation 2001; 103: 1535–1541.*

Mitral valve disease

Mitral regurgitation

Competence of the mitral valve may be compromised by disease affecting any component of the mitral apparatus from the annulus, leaflets, chordae and papillary muscles to the function of the left ventricle.

Epidemiology

In a population of American Indians, the overall prevalence of mitral regurgitation was 18% in patients less than 55 years old, increasing with age to 29% patients more than 75 years old.[1]

Pathology

The two most common aetiological factors that cause primary mitral regurgitation are myxomatous degeneration and ischaemic heart disease. Endocarditis and, in developed countries, rheumatic fever are less common. It is important to note that any cause of heart failure with accompanying ventricular dilatation can produce secondary (functional) mitral regurgitation.

Myxomatous degeneration, the most common cause of primary mitral regurgitation in developed countries, is due to defective fibroelastic tissue. In the early stage of disease it forms a distinct clinical entity (mitral valve prolapse or Barlow's syndrome). It results in annular dilatation and posterior leaflet prolapse. Elongated chordae are a common feature and sudden rupture can precipitate acute mitral regurgitation and pulmonary oedema.

Transient myocardial ischaemia can cause episodic and reversible mitral regurgitation (usually due to posterior papillary muscle ischaemia and dysfunction). Mitral regurgitation can also occur after myocardial infarction due to papillary muscle infarct and rupture.

Acute rheumatic fever can result in mitral annular dilatation, whilst the late effects are leaflet thickening chordal disease and commissural fusion with annular and leaflet calcification. Although mitral stenosis is a common end result, a fixed orifice can produce combined stenosis and regurgitation.

Acute endocarditis can result in bacterial destruction of the valve with leaflet perforation and chordal rupture leading to mitral incompetence.

Haemodynamic effects

As a result of mitral regurgitation, blood is ejected forwards into the aorta and backwards (regurgitant volume) into the left atrium (and pulmonary veins) simultaneously during each contraction. In acute severe mitral regurgitation, the heart does not have time to develop compensatory mechanisms and this often results in cardiogenic shock and pulmonary oedema.

Under more chronic conditions, the heart increases total stroke volume by eccentric hypertrophy and dilatation, initially detected on echocardiographic assessment as increased end diastolic volume and latterly as increased end systolic volume.

Ventricular contractility will appear hyperdynamic, but this is deceptive as the ventricle does not only eject into the aorta but also 'unloads' into the low-pressure pulmonary circuit. When the ejection fraction and contractility become 'normal' it often heralds the onset of moderate to severe ventricular impairment.

Scope of disease

Prolonged mitral regurgitation leads to compensatory dilatation of the left ventricle and atrium. With time, contractile dysfunction sets in and irreversible left ventricular impairment develops. Left atrial enlargement predisposes to atrial fibrillation, thrombus formation and stroke. Chronic back pressure into the pulmonary venous circulation eventually causes pulmonary hypertension, a poor prognostic sign.

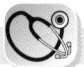

Clinical features

Clinical features of acute mitral regurgitation are presented on page 24. Dyspnoea is the primary symptom of chronic mitral valve regurgitation, however this tends to occur late in the disease. Patients may also present with features of complications such as palpitations (atrial fibrillation), stroke and haemoptysis (pulmonary hypertension).

On examination, the pulse may be irregular (atrial fibrillation), the JVP is not usually elevated (unless congestive heart failure has developed) and cardiomegaly may be evident by displacement of the apex beat (thrusting quality). On auscultation there is a soft first heart sound (failure of closure of the mitral valve) and pansystolic murmur that radiates into the axilla.

When assessing a patient with mitral valve disease, it is important to ascertain features of any disease that can cause mitral regurgitation (ischaemic heart disease, endocarditis), to screen for complications (atrial fibrillation) and to quantify the severity of dyspnoea using the NYHA classification.

Initial investigations

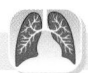

Electrocardiogram

A 12 lead ECG may confirm atrial fibrillation or reveal evidence of left ventricular hypertrophy or previous myocardial infarction.

Chest X-ray

A plain chest X-ray (Fig. 1.27) may reveal cardiomegaly, left atrial enlargement, calcification of the mitral annulus (rheumatic disease) and features of congestive cardiac failure.

Transthoracic echocardiogram

A transthoracic echocardiogram is an excellent investigation to quantify the extent and severity of mitral regurgitation, assess left ventricular function (ejection fraction, contractility) and measure left ventricular dimensions (end

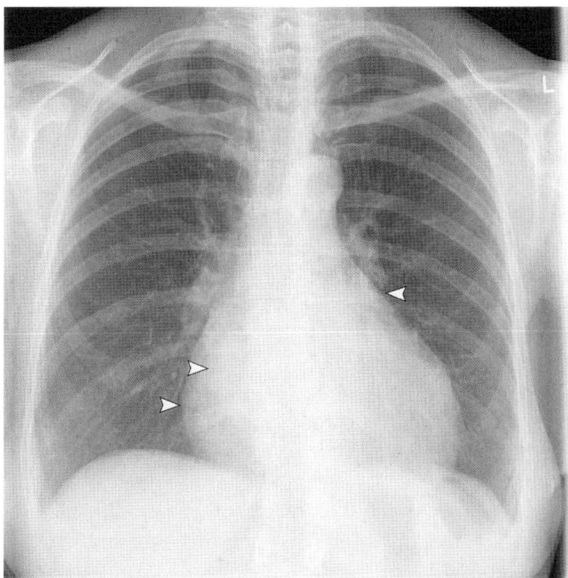

Fig. 1.27 Mitral regurgitation. The chest film illustrates cardiomegaly (left ventricular dilatation) and an enlarged left atrium (the two arrows indicate the double right heart border, and the single arrow points to the tented left heart border).

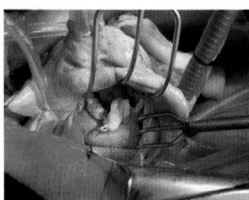

(a)

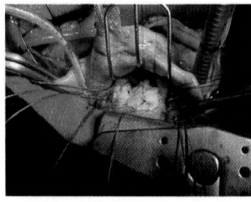

(b)

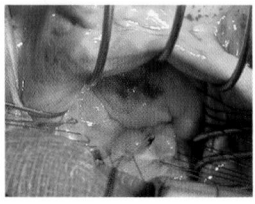

(c)

Fig. 1.29a–c Mitral valve repair. The prolapsing segment of the posterior mitral leaflet (a) is excised and the defect is closed (b), restoring the competency of the valve (c). Images courtesy of Mr Francis Wells, Consultant Cardiothoracic Surgeon, Papworth Hospital, Cambridge, UK.

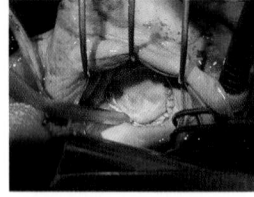

Fig. 1.30 Mitral valve repair. An annuloplasty ring is shown. Images courtesy of Mr Francis Wells, Consultant Cardiothoracic Surgeon, Papworth Hospital, Cambridge, UK.

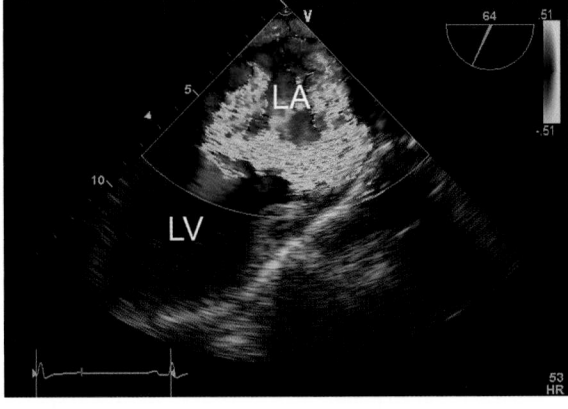

Fig. 1.28 Transoesophageal echocardiogram. The left ventricle is indicated (LV) and the colour flow illustrates the severe regurgitation across the mitral valve into the left atrium (LA).

systolic and end diastolic diameter). Figure 1.28 is an image from a transoesophageal echocardiogram.

Further investigations

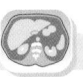

Further investigations to exclude aetiological factors should be guided according to clinical features (ischaemic heart disease, endocarditis).

Left heart catheterization

The utility of left heart catheterization and left ventricular angiography to diagnose and grade the severity of mitral regurgitation has largely been superseded by transthoracic echocardiography. Left heart catheterization should be performed in conjunction with coronary angiography in selected patients prior to valve surgery.

Initial management

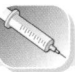

The following details the management of primary mitral regurgitation; the management of secondary (functional) mitral regurgitation is presented on page 35.

Patient education

Patients should be informed that the disease is stable in the majority of patients with mild mitral regurgitation, and only selected patients require surgery. It is important to stress the need for antibiotic prophylaxis during dental treatment.

Medical management

There is no generally accepted pharmacological therapy. Medical management consists of yearly clinical and echocardiographic assessment and management of atrial fibrillation.

Surveillance

Yearly clinical assessment and echocardiography is appropriate for asymptomatic patients with *mild to moderate*

mitral regurgitation who do not have evidence of left ventricular dysfunction or pulmonary hypertension on echocardiography.

Warfarin

Warfarin is recommended for patients in atrial fibrillation due to the increased risk of thromboembolism.

Surgical management

The decision for surgery rests on clinical features (dyspnoea) and echocardiographic assessment of ventricular function. Surgery is indicated for patients with *severe* mitral regurgitation with either:

1. NYHA II-IV dyspnoea, *or*
2. echocardiographic evidence of ventricular impairment:
   a. ejection fraction of less than 60%, *or*
   b. left ventricular end systolic diameter more than 50 mm.

> **RECENT ADVANCES**
>
> *As valve repair has become more established, many surgeons are considering mitral repair in patients with severe mitral regurgitation without symptoms, before the onset of left ventricular impairment, atrial fibrillation or pulmonary hypertension. The rationale is to correct the valve regurgitation before the onset of features that are associated with a poor outcome.*

Mitral valve repair

When at all possible, mitral valve repair is undertaken as the procedure of choice in mitral valve surgery. In this procedure, a median sternotomy is performed, the pericardium is opened and cardiopulmonary bypass is established. The heart is stopped with cardioplegia solution and access is usually gained into the left atrium directly by an incision posterior to the interatrial groove (lying posterior to the right atrium).

A repertoire of surgical techniques are employed to address individual defects of the mitral apparatus. These include resecting the prolapsing portion of the posterior leaflet (Fig. 1.29a–c), patch repair of perforations, chordal shortening, reconstruction of the chordae and suturing an annuloplasty ring to restore the size and shape of the annulus (Fig. 1.30). The incision over the left atrium is oversewn, and any residual air introduced into the heart is carefully removed before cardiopulmonary bypass is discontinued.

Postoperatively patients are managed on the intensive care unit and warfarin is often prescribed for 6 weeks.

Established benefits are prolonged survival through improved ventricular function and avoidance of long-term anticoagulation for patients in sinus rhythm. There is a risk of conversion to a valve replacement (approximately 5%).

Mitral valve replacement

When valve repair is not possible (multiple extensive valve lesions, the presence of severe calcification) valve replacement is undertaken.

Prognosis

The patient groups that undergo valve repair and valve replacement are different and therefore prognosis is presented according to surgical procedure.

Mitral valve repair

The overall 5- and 10-year survival rate is 83% and 68% respectively. Left ventricular function is the strongest predictor of long-term survival. Freedom from re-operation at 10 years is 93%, and freedom from thromboembolism at 10 years is approximately 68%.

Mitral valve replacement

The 5- and 10-year survival rate for mitral valve replacement is 69% and 52% respectively. Freedom from re-operation at 10 years is 80% and freedom from thromboembolism at 10 years is 70%.

_i_ FURTHER INFORMATION

Bonow RO, Carabello B, de Leon AC Jr, et al. ACC/AHA guidelines for the management of patients with valvular heart disease: a report of the American College of Cardiology/American Heart Association Task Force on Practice Guidelines (Committee on Management of Patients With Valvular Heart Disease). Journal of the American College of Cardiology 1998; 32: 1486–1588.

Wells FC, Shapiro LM. Mitral valve disease. Oxford: Butterworth-Heinemann, 1996.

REFERENCE

(1) _Jones EC, Devereux RB, Roman MJ, et al. Prevalence and correlates of mitral regurgitation in a population-based sample (the Strong Heart Study). American Journal of Cardiology 2001; 87: 298–304._

Mitral stenosis

Mitral stenosis refers to narrowing of the mitral valve orifice. Normally, this ranges from 4 to 5 cm^2, and symptomatic mitral stenosis usually occurs after the valve orifice area decreases to 2.5 cm^2. It is usually this amount of narrowing that corresponds to a pressure gradient developing across the mitral valve.

Epidemiology

The epidemiology reflects the prevalence of rheumatic fever, the predominant cause of mitral stenosis. This valve lesion can affect any age group; however, this becomes clinically apparent only after a latent period. Therefore symptomatic disease tends to present at a later age, usually after the age of 40. It is more common in women and in countries such as India where rheumatic fever prevails.

Pathology

Following rheumatic carditis, leaflet thickening or commissural or chordal fusion can occur, resulting in narrowing of the mitral apparatus.

Haemodynamic effects

When the aperture is reduced to half the normal orifice area, a pressure gradient develops and leads to left atrial enlargement and pulmonary hypertension. Eventually cardiac output may decrease as a result of the severe stenosis. The left ventricle is usually protected from the effects of mitral stenosis as the obstruction to flow occurs proximally.

Scope of disease

Left atrial dilatation predisposes to atrial fibrillation, thrombosis and stroke. Very rarely, severe left atrial enlargement may compress the oesophagus and cause dysphagia. Chronically elevated pulmonary venous pressures cause a reflex increase in pulmonary vascular resistance to protect the lungs, but this may lead to pulmonary hypertension.

Clinical features

Many patients remain asymptomatic as the disease progresses in severity. Dyspnoea is the principal feature, experienced initially on exercise as cardiac output is limited by the fixed narrowing of the mitral aperture. The onset of complications may give rise to haemoptysis (pulmonary hypertension), palpitations and stroke (atrial fibrillation).

On examination, characteristic mitral facies may be present (rare). The pulse may be of low volume and irregular in character (atrial fibrillation). The JVP may be elevated with raised pulmonary pressures and right heart failure. On auscultation, there is the classical opening snap (first heart sound) and a mid diastolic rumbling murmur. The Graham Steell murmur is a systolic murmur caused by pulmonary regurgitation, a result of pulmonary hypertension that accompanies severe mitral stenosis.

Initial investigations

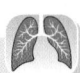

Electrocardiogram

ECG can confirm the presence of atrial fibrillation. Patients in sinus rhythm may have increased p-wave height and duration due to left atrial enlargement (p mitrale), and there may be evidence of right ventricular hypertrophy with chronic pulmonary hypertension.

Chest X-ray

Appearances on the standard chest film may be normal. The most characteristic feature is left atrial enlargement, evident as a double right heart shadow (Fig. 1.31), increased splaying of the carina and tenting of the left heart border. Features of congestive cardiac failure (p. 15) may also be evident.

Transthoracic echocardiogram

The transthoracic echocardiogram will readily diagnose mitral stenosis (Fig. 1.32) and estimate the size of the mitral orifice area. It is also a useful investigation to select suitable patients for balloon mitral valvuloplasty.

Further investigations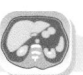

Left heart catheterization

Left ventricular angiography to diagnose mitral stenosis has largely been superseded by transthoracic echocardiography. This investigation is usually undertaken for coronary angiography in selected patients prior to surgery.

Initial management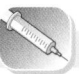

Patient education

It is important to stress the need for antibiotic prophylaxis during dental treatment.

Medical management

There is no generally accepted pharmacological therapy for mitral stenosis. Medical management consists of yearly clinical and echocardiographic assessment and management of atrial fibrillation and symptoms of congestive cardiac failure.

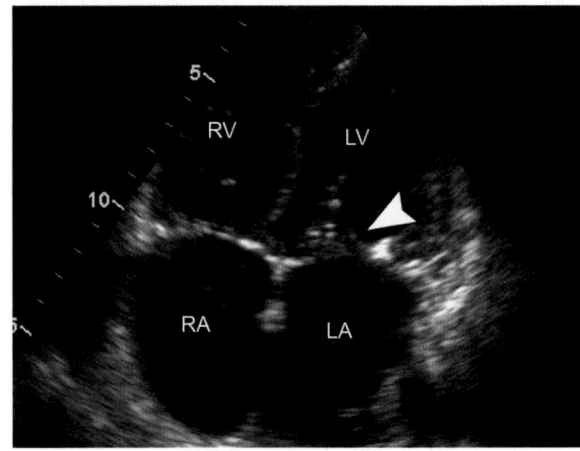

Fig. 1.32 Transthoracic echocardiogram. The four chambers are illustrated (LA, left atrium; LV, left ventricle; RA, right atrium; RV, right ventricle). The calcified and stenosed mitral valve is indicated by the arrow.

Surveillance

Yearly clinical assessment and echocardiography is appropriate for asymptomatic patients with *mild* mitral stenosis (mitral valve area more than 1.5 cm^2) who do not have evidence of pulmonary hypertension on echocardiography.

Warfarin

Warfarin is generally recommended for all patients in atrial fibrillation, and after the first thromboembolic event for patients in sinus rhythm.

Diuretics

A loop diuretic may be required for patients with symptoms and signs of pulmonary oedema.

Surgical management

Minimally invasive or surgical intervention is required for suitable candidates with symptoms (NYHA II–IV) and *moderate to severe* mitral stenosis (mitral valve area <1.5 cm^2).

In patients with symptomatic *mild* mitral stenosis (mitral valve area >1.5 cm^2), the following adverse prognostic features suggest the need for intervention:
1. elevated pulmonary artery pressures (>60 mmHg), *or*
2. elevated pulmonary artery wedge pressure (>25 mmHg), *or*
3. significant transmitral gradient (>15 mmHg).

Percutaneous balloon mitral commissurotomy

Dilatation of the mitral valve aperture can be performed percutaneously by cardiologists. This procedure may be performed for selected patients with favourable anatomy (pliable, non-calcified valve, minimal fusion of the chordae) and for those that have unacceptable risk for mitral valve surgery. It is not suitable for patients with left atrial thrombus (embolic risk) and patients with coexisting moderate to severe mitral regurgitation (there is the potential to worsen the degree of regurgitation).

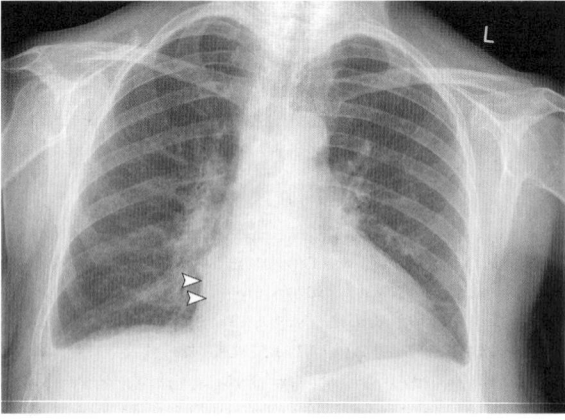

Fig. 1.31 Chest film of a patient with mitral stenosis. The arrows indicate the double right heart border from left atrial enlargement.

A balloon tipped catheter is introduced into the femoral artery and screened with fluoroscopy to confirm its position across the mitral valve. Inflation of the balloon causes mechanical disruption and widens the valve aperture.

The risk of mortality is 2%. Complications include severe mitral regurgitation (up to 10%), embolism and myocardial infarction.

Mitral valve repair

Open mitral valve repair has largely superseded closed mitral valvotomy due to the ability to directly inspect the severity of each lesion responsible for valve stenosis. In this procedure, a median sternotomy is performed, the pericardium is opened and cardiopulmonary bypass is established. The heart is stopped with cardioplegia solution and access is usually gained into the left atrium directly by an incision posterior to the interatrial groove that lies posterior to the right atrium. Fusion of the commissures is the most common valve lesion, and commissurotomy can be undertaken relatively easily. Extensive involvement of the chordae and papillary muscles or the presence of severe calcification usually suggests the need for valve replacement.

Postoperatively patients are managed on the intensive care unit and warfarin is often prescribed for 6 weeks in patients with sinus rhythm.

Mitral valve replacement

Early structural valve deterioration was a principal disadvantage of tissue valves in the mitral position, therefore mechanical valves were generally preferred unless pregnancy was anticipated or there were compelling contraindications to anticoagulation.

The access to the mitral valve is similar to that for valve repair. The importance of preservation of the subvalvar apparatus (chordae and papillary muscles) is established for the maintenance of normal ventricular function. Often the whole posterior leaflet is retained, with excision of the majority of the anterior leaflet. The prosthetic valve is then sutured into place. Closure is similar to that for valve repair.

Postoperatively patients are managed on the intensive care unit and warfarin is prescribed for life for all patients with a mechanical valve. As the valve is sutured in place, injuries can (rarely) occur to the conducting system (complete heart block), circumflex coronary artery (myocardial infarction) or coronary sinus (obstruction).

RECENT ADVANCES

New generation tissue valves in the mitral position (Fig. 1.33) have much better long-term durability leading to less stringent criteria for their use.

Prognosis

The 10-year survival for patients with mitral stenosis is 60%, however this decreases sharply to 15% following the onset of functionally limiting symptoms. The 5- and 10-year survival after mitral surgery is 75% and 56% respectively.[1]

 FURTHER INFORMATION

Bonow RO, Carabello B, de Leon AC Jr, et al. ACC/AHA guidelines for the management of patients with valvular heart disease: a report of the American College of Cardiology/ American Heart Association Task Force on Practice Guidelines (Committee on Management of Patients With Valvular Heart Disease). Journal of the American College of Cardiology 1998; 32: 1486–1588.

Wells FC, Shapiro LM. Mitral valve disease. Oxford: Butterworth-Heinemann, 1996.

REFERENCE

(1) *Hellgren L, Kvidal P, Horte LG, Krusemo UB, Stahle E. Survival after mitral valve replacement: rationale for surgery before occurrence of severe symptoms. Annals of Thoracic Surgery 2004; 78: 1241–1247.*

Tricuspid valve disease

Tricuspid regurgitation

Tricuspid regurgitation is rare. It is usually secondary to dilatation of the right ventricle and tricuspid annulus rather than intrinsic disease of the tricuspid valve.

Epidemiology

Tricuspid regurgitation is uncommon.

Pathology

Right ventricular and tricuspid annular dilatation causes functional tricuspid regurgitation and usually results from any cause of heart failure or pulmonary hypertension. Intrinsic valve disease may arise from rheumatic fever or infective endocarditis (usually as a result of intravenous drug abuse). Tricuspid regurgitation can also occur as a complication of carcinoid disease.

Clinical features

Tricuspid regurgitation is usually well tolerated (in the absence of pulmonary hypertension). Symptoms of right-sided heart failure predominate with peripheral oedema and ascites. On examination, peripheral oedema may be present, and jaundice can be caused by hepatic congestion. The pulse may be irregular from atrial fibrillation. Cannon waves are visible in the JVP due to unimpeded transmission of the pulse wave from right ventricular contraction. Right ventricular heave and a systolic murmur that is loudest in the 4th parasternal intercostal space may be present. The murmur is augmented by inspiration (Carvallo's sign).

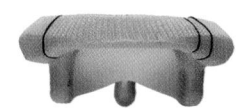

Fig. 1.33 Tissue (pericardial) mitral valve. Courtesy of Edwards Lifesciences, Irvine, California.

45

Investigations

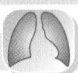

Electrocardiogram
The ECG is usually normal but may detect atrial fibrillation or evidence of right ventricular hypertrophy.

Chest X-ray
With functional tricuspid regurgitation, marked cardiomegaly may be evident on chest X-ray.

Transthoracic echocardiogram
Echocardiography will confirm the diagnosis, estimate the severity of regurgitation, assess pulmonary artery pressures and quantify right ventricular function.

Management

Tricuspid valve repair or replacement
The indications for the management of isolated tricuspid regurgitation are not well defined, as it is usually corrected in conjunction with mitral regurgitation. Tricuspid regurgitation in the absence of pulmonary hypertension is usually well tolerated and does not require surgical treatment. Tricuspid valve repair or replacement is usually considered in the setting of moderate to severe mitral valve regurgitation.

Prognosis

Patients with severe tricuspid regurgitation have a poor prognosis, and the prognosis worsens in the presence of pulmonary hypertension and right heart failure.

Tricuspid stenosis

Stenosis of the tricuspid valve is rare and is usually a result of rheumatic fever.

Epidemiology

Tricuspid stenosis is uncommon.

Pathology

The narrowed tricuspid valve orifice restricts the flow of blood to the right ventricle and limits cardiac output when severely narrowed. The back pressure of the rising right atrial pressure causes signs of isolated right heart failure, hepatomegaly, ascites and peripheral oedema.

Clinical features

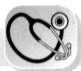

The main presenting complaint is dyspnoea on exertion due to a fixed cardiac output from restriction by the narrowed tricuspid valve. Abdominal distension and ankle swelling also arise from raised right atrial pressures. On examination peripheral oedema may be present and the JVP is elevated with large 'a' waves (forceful right atrial

contraction) that will be absent if atrial fibrillation occurs (loss of atrial contraction). The 'y' descent is prolonged due to the narrowed tricuspid orifice. A mid diastolic murmur may be audible. Abdominal examination may reveal hepatomegaly.

Investigations

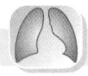

Electrocardiogram
ECG reveals large P waves (p pulmonale) and will confirm atrial fibrillation.

Chest X-ray
The chest X-ray may reveal a large right heart border.

Transthoracic echocardiogram
Echocardiography will confirm the diagnosis.

Management

Diuretics
Diuretic therapy and salt restriction may be required in fluid-overloaded patients to reduce the right atrial pressure.

Tricuspid valve replacement
Tricuspid valve replacement is not usually undertaken as an isolated procedure as concomitant mitral stenosis usually exists. It is rarely the isolated cause of severe symptoms.

Prognosis

The prognosis of patients with tricuspid stenosis is usually governed by coexistent mitral stenosis.

Pulmonary valve disease

Pulmonary stenosis is predominantly a congenital disease; survival into adulthood is common. Survival depends on the degree of stenosis and right ventricular function. Because of its rarity, it is not covered in any further detail, and the rest of this section concentrates on pulmonary regurgitation.

Pulmonary regurgitation

Epidemiology

Pulmonary regurgitation is rare and occurs secondary to pulmonary hypertension.

Pathology

Dilatation of the pulmonary valve ring from pulmonary hypertension or any other dilatation of the main pulmonary artery can result in pulmonary regurgitation. Other causes are infective endocarditis (usually from intravenous drug abuse) and carcinoid syndrome.

Clinical features

Pulmonary regurgitation is usually well tolerated unless it is complicated, or secondary to pulmonary hypertension when right ventricular failure ensues and symptoms of fatigue, peripheral oedema and abdominal distension (ascites) develop. On examination, a right ventricular heave may be palpable with a loud second heart sound (P2) if pulmonary hypertension is present. An early diastolic murmur (Graham Steell murmur) may be audible in the left 2nd to 4th intercostal space, resembling the murmur of aortic regurgitation.

Investigations
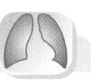

Electrocardiogram
An ECG may reveal right ventricular hypertrophy.

Chest X-ray
The pulmonary artery may be enlarged on the chest X-ray.

Transthoracic echocardiogram

Echocardiography confirms the diagnosis, estimates pulmonary artery pressures and quantifies right ventricular function.

Management

Expectant management
Unless intractable right ventricular failure occurs, pulmonary regurgitation is seldom severe enough to warrant valve replacement.

Prognosis

The majority of patients have mild disease and rarely require surgery.

SECTION 1.8   Cardiac tumours

Atrial myxoma

Epidemiology

The prevalence of primary tumours of the heart has been reported as 20 per 100 000 in autopsy series.[1]

Pathology

Secondary tumour metastasis to the heart is more common than primary cardiac tumours; the latter are rarities, of which the atrial myxoma is the most common variety. The majority arise in the left atrium and are usually solitary. A number of complications can arise, including pyrexia, embolism and obstruction to the mitral valve orifice.

Clinical features

When an atrial myxoma becomes symptomatic, patients may complain of dyspnoea, syncope (obstruction of the mitral valve orifice) or persistent unexplained pyrexia. Transient ischaemic attacks (TIA) or strokes can arise from tumour emboli. On examination, clubbing may be present and a tumour 'plop' may be audible on auscultation. Murmurs of mitral stenosis or regurgitation may coexist.

Investigations
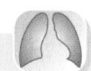

Echocardiogram
Echocardiography is the imaging modality of choice to confirm the diagnosis (Fig. 1.34).

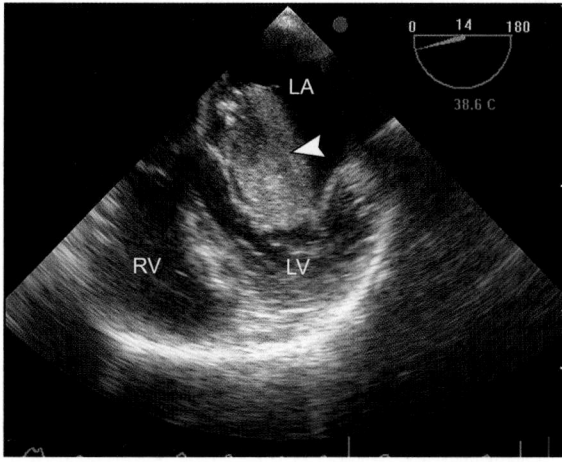

Fig. 1.34 The transoesophageal echocardiogram shows the left atrium (LA) and left ventricle (LV) and a large left atrial myxoma abutting onto the mitral valve (arrow).

Management

Surgical resection

For patients fit enough to withstand an operation, open heart surgery and resection is the treatment of choice.

Prognosis

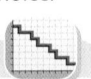

Complete cure is achieved in the majority; recurrence occurs in less than 5%.

REFERENCE

(1) *Reynen K. Frequency of primary tumors of the heart. American Journal of Cardiology 1996; 77: 107.*

SECTION 1.9 # Congenital heart disease

Atrial septal defect

Epidemiology

The foramen ovale remains patent in 26% of adults,[1] but the prevalence of atrial septal defects is approximately 30 per 100 000 births.[2] Atrial septal defect is more common in women than in men.

Pathology

Due to the anatomical valve-like construction, a foramen ovale may be patent but adopt a sealed position keeping both atria separate. Atrial septal defects are abnormal openings between the two atria. The ostium secundum defect is the most common site of an atrial septal defect, occurring at the foramen ovale. The ostium primum defect is situated close to the atrioventricular valves and may be associated with an atrioventricular septal defect (endocardial cushion defect). Least common is the sinus venosus defect that is situated high up in the atria and is associated with abnormal drainage of the pulmonary veins into the right atrium.

An atrial septal defect allows blood to divert from the left to the more compliant right atrium (left to right shunt) with a subsequent increase in pulmonary blood flow. Normally, the pulmonary circulation is able to accommodate the increase in blood flow; however, under chronic conditions, increased pulmonary resistance develops and eventually leads to irreversible pulmonary hypertension. The blood pressure in the pulmonary circulation can be high enough to reverse the flow of blood from the right atrium to the left atrium (Eisenmenger's syndrome).

Scope of disease

Under pathological conditions, blood (and emboli) may flow from the right to the left atrium and enter the systemic circulation. A patent foramen ovale is widely held to be an important cause of cryptogenic stroke, especially in young adults. Atrial septal defects also predispose patients to infective endocarditis.

RECENT ADVANCES

The patent foramen ovale is currently under investigation as a risk factor for migraine due to ischaemic stroke from paradoxical emboli.[3]

Clinical features

The clinical status and age of presentation depend on the size and position of the atrial septal defect. Small defects will cause no symptoms at all, whereas larger defects can give rise to shortness of breath, palpitations and fatigue. Clinical examination reveals a wide and fixed splitting of the second heart sound and a pulmonary flow murmur (increased flow) in some. The defect itself does not produce a murmur.

Investigations

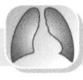

Electrocardiogram

An ECG will reveal a partial right bundle branch block with right axis deviation for an ostium secundum defect and left axis deviation for an ostium primum defect.

Chest X-ray

Chest X-ray may reveal cardiomegaly from right atrial enlargement with prominent pulmonary arteries from increased flow.

Echocardiography

Transthoracic echocardiography is sufficient to screen for an atrial septal defect, but transoesophageal imaging provides the best anatomical visualization. Cardiac catheterization to calculate pulmonary–systemic flow ratio is reserved as an investigation prior to intervention.

Management

Surveillance
Asymptomatic patients with small defects do not require intervention and should be kept under regular surveillance.

Surgical repair
Operation is advised for patients when pulmonary–systemic flow ratios reach 1.5:1.0, in the absence of complications such as pulmonary hypertension.

> **RECENT ADVANCES**
>
> *Percutaneous devices are currently being evaluated for the closure of anatomically favourable atrial septal defects (Fig. 1.35). The device is introduced via the femoral vein into the right atrium, across the defect and into the left atrium using fluoroscopy (Fig. 1.36a). It is then positioned across the defect, straddling the septum (Fig. 1.36d) and closing it.*

Prognosis

The natural history is associated with progressive disease and diminished exercise tolerance.[4]

REFERENCES

(1) *Meier B, Lock JE. Contemporary management of patent foramen ovale. Circulation 2003; 107: 5–9.*
(2) *Pradat P, Francannet C, Harris JA, Robert E. The epidemiology of cardiovascular defects, part I: a study based on data from three large registries of congenital malformations. Pediatric Cardiology 2003; 24: 195–221.*
(3) *Milhaud D, Bogousslavsky J, van Melle G, Liot P. Ischemic stroke and active migraine. Neurology 2001; 57: 1805–1811.*
(4) *Fredriksen PM, Veldtman G, Hechter S, et al. Aerobic capacity in adults with various congenital heart diseases. American Journal of Cardiology 2001; 87: 310–314.*

Ventricular septal defect

Epidemiology

The ventricular septal defect is the most common form of congenital heart disease with a prevalence of approximately 51 per 100 000 births.[1] Patients usually present in the few months after birth, or in early adulthood, depending on the size of the defect.

Pathology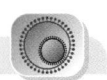

Defects occur most frequently in the membranous portion of the ventricular septum. The size of the defect may be

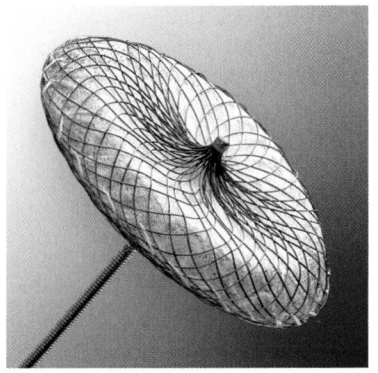

Fig. 1.35 Amplatzer® septal occluder.
Image courtesy of AGA Medical Corporation (Golden Valley, Minneapolis, USA). Copyright of the AGA Medical Corporation.

large in relation to the child at birth but, as the child grows, the size of the defect reduces proportionally.

Large ventricular septal defects allow blood to flow from the left to the right ventricle (left to right shunt), greatly increasing the flow in the pulmonary circulation. This may produce cardiac failure in the early months after birth. Significant defects are corrected in childhood, whilst less significant defects tend not to produce symptoms until early adult life. Increased pulmonary flow predisposes to pulmonary hypertension, and Eisenmenger's syndrome may also occur as a complication. Ventricular septal defects also predispose patients to endocarditis.

Clinical features

The uncomplicated ventricular septal defect is asymptomatic. When pulmonary hypertension develops, patients may present with shortness of breath, haemoptysis or syncope. On examination, the pulse pressure may be small, with evidence of right ventricular heave (right ventricular hypertrophy). A systolic thrill accompanied by pansystolic murmur may be evident. However, both are attenuated in the presence of pulmonary hypertension due to the reduced flow across the defect.

Investigations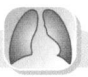

Electrocardiogram
The ECG is normal in patients with an uncomplicated defect. In the presence of pulmonary hypertension, both right and left ventricular hypertrophy may be evident.

Chest X-ray
Similarly, a chest X-ray is normal in patients with an uncomplicated defect, with evidence of cardiomegaly due to ventricular hypertrophy in patients with large defects.

Echocardiography
Echocardiography is a useful investigation to document the presence and estimate the size of a ventricular septal

49

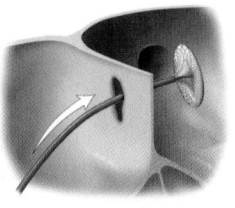

(a)

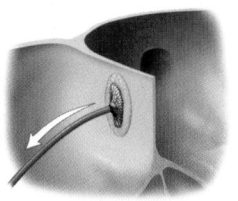

(b)

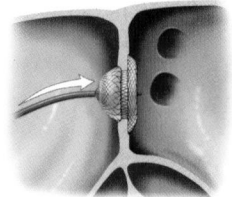

(c)

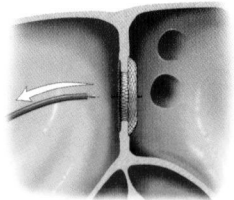

(d)

Fig. 1.36a–d Percutaneous closure of an atrial septal defect.
Images courtesy of AGA Medical Corporation (Golden Valley, Minneapolis, USA). Copyright of the AGA Medical Corporation.

defect. Patients with large symptomatic defects will need to progress to left heart catheterization to quantify the severity of the left to right shunt and measure pulmonary artery pressures.

Management

Surveillance
Asymptomatic patients with small defects do not require intervention and should be kept under regular surveillance.

Surgical repair
Operation is advised for symptomatic patients when pulmonary–systemic flow ratios reach 2.0:1.0.

Prognosis

Most affected children have a relatively normal lifespan if they have survived the first few years. Patients with small defects lead a normal life. However, patients with large uncorrected defects are at risk of death, usually between the ages of 20 and 40.

REFERENCE

(1) *Pradat P, Francannet C, Harris JA, Robert E. The epidemiology of cardiovascular defects, part I: a study based on data from three large registries of congenital malformations. Pediatric Cardiology 2003; 24: 195–221.*

Coarctation of the aorta

Coarctation of the aorta is narrowing of the aortic lumen—usually a discrete area of stenosis distal to the lumen of the left subclavian artery.

Epidemiology

Coarctation of the aorta occurs in approximately 11 per 100 000 births and is more common in males.[1]

Pathology

Although the most common site is just distal to the left subclavian artery, a spectrum of locations and lengths of stenosis may occur. The effects of the coarctation depend on the severity of the stenosis. As the heart pumps more forcefully to overcome the resistance from the narrowing, hypertension develops in the head and upper limb vessels. Collateral blood supply to the body and lower limbs includes the intercostal arteries that may dilate sufficiently to produce rib notching. Complications of coarctation include systemic hypertension, cardiac failure and predisposition to aortic dissection and endocarditis.

Clinical features

Most patients are asymptomatic and the coarctation is detected on routine clinical examination. Differential hypertension is confined to the upper limbs, with normal blood pressure in the lower limbs accompanied by radio-femoral delay. A systolic murmur is usually audible in the aortic area and is loudest posteriorly in the left 4th intercostal space. In addition, bruits may be audible over the intercostal arteries.

Investigations

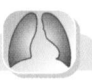

Electrocardiogram
The ECG is usually normal in the early years; however, later in life left ventricular hypertrophy develops.

Chest X-ray
The chest X-ray may reveal a prominent aortic knuckle and cardiomegaly from ventricular hypertrophy. Rib notching may be visible.

Computed tomography (CT)/magnetic resonance imaging (MRI)
The site of the coarctation may be visualized on echocardiography, but better anatomical definition is obtained from CT or MRI (Fig. 1.37) with the possibility of three-dimensional reconstruction (Fig. 1.38).

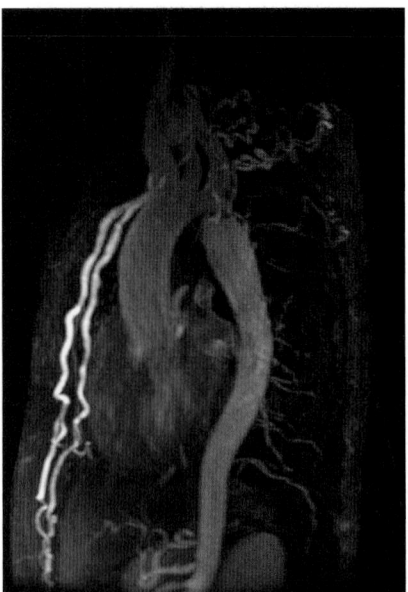

Fig. 1.37 Magnetic resonance angiogram (MRA) shows the coarctation with enlarged collateral flow from the internal thoracic arteries.
Image courtesy of Mr Sam Nashef, Consultant Cardiac Surgeon, Papworth Hospital, Cambridge, UK.

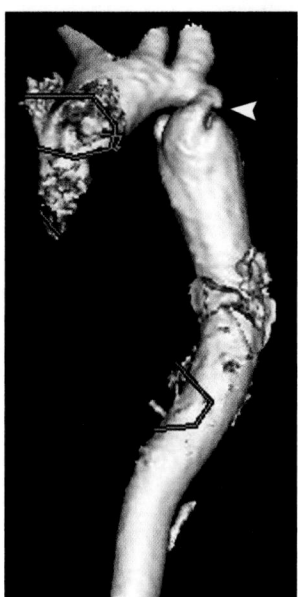

Management

Surgical correction is the preferred treatment unless the degree of stenosis is insignificant. Approximately 5% recur after corrective surgery.

Prognosis

The prognosis of patients with coarctation depends on the severity of the luminal stenosis. In the majority, hypertension develops by the age of 30 years.

REFERENCE

(1) Pradat P, Francannet C, Harris JA, Robert E. *The epidemiology of cardiovascular defects, part I: a study based on data from three large registries of congenital malformations. Pediatric Cardiology 2003; 24: 195–221.*

Fig. 1.38 A 3D MRA reconstruction of the aorta showing the coarctation (arrow).
Image courtesy of Mr Sam Nashef, Consultant Cardiac Surgeon, Papworth Hospital, Cambridge, UK.

SECTION 1.10   # Diseases of the myocardium

Myocarditis

Myocarditis refers to an inflammatory disease of the heart muscle. This occurs most commonly as a result of infection. The 1995 WHO classification defines inflammatory cardiomyopathy as myocarditis associated with impaired cardiac function.

Epidemiology

Although the proportion of patients with subclinical myocarditis during an acute viral infection is unknown, myocarditis of sufficient severity to produce heart failure is rare.

Pathology

Numerous viruses, bacteria and protozoa cause myocarditis; however, Coxsackie viruses are the most commonly identified agents. Myocardial injury can result from direct myocardial involvement, toxin production or immune mediated responses. Fulminant myocarditis can lead to overt cardiac failure and death. Other complications are atrial/ventricular arrhythmia, heart block and thromboembolism.

Clinical features

Patients may present with a flu-like illness progressing to fatigue and dyspnoea. Arrhythmias may give rise to palpitations, heart block is associated with syncope, and a proportion of patients will complain of chest pain.

On examination, a tachycardia and small volume pulse may be present. The blood pressure may be low, depending on the severity of haemodynamic impairment. Crepitations in the lung bases suggest pulmonary oedema.

Investigations

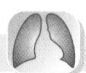

Full blood count and inflammatory markers
The white cell count is usually elevated along with the ESR or CRP.

Viral titres
Viral titres may identify an underlying infectious agent. Serum cardiac markers (p. 29) are elevated from myocardial inflammation.

Electrocardiogram
The ECG will detect conduction abnormalities that range from first-degree heart block to AV dissociation.

Chest X-ray
The chest X-ray may reveal cardiomegaly with pulmonary oedema if the course of events was sufficiently chronic, otherwise the heart will appear normal.

Echocardiogram

Echocardiography may demonstrate impaired left ventricular function.

Myocardial biopsy

Myocardial biopsy is required for confirmatory diagnosis, and this can be obtained histologically using Dallas criteria or with increased sensitivity by staining for upregulation of proteins associated with HLA.[1] The distinction is becoming increasingly relevant, as clinical trials are suggesting evidence for the use of immunosuppression in HLA-positive myocarditis.

Management

Immunomodulation

For patients with HLA-positive myocarditis, immuno-suppression is associated with improved left ventricular function on echocardiography and NYHA functional class, with no differences in death or heart transplantation.[2]

Supportive management

Treatment is otherwise supportive. A temporary pacemaker will be required for AV dissociation, and arrhythmias treated accordingly. Circulatory shock is managed in accordance with the severity of the acute heart failure (p. 13–14). Surgical support ranges from intra-aortic balloon pump to ventricular assist to heart transplantation.

Prognosis

The majority of patients will recover; however, the degree of improvement to ventricular function and performance status varies. Information on patient survival is limited due to small studies with varying diagnostic criteria and severity of disease.

REFERENCES

(1) Calabrese F, Thiene G. Myocarditis and inflammatory cardiomyopathy: microbiological and molecular biological aspects. Cardiovascular Research 2003; 60: 11–25.
(2) Wojnicz R, Nowalany-Kozielska E, Wojciechowska C, et al. Randomized, placebo-controlled study for immunosuppressive treatment of inflammatory dilated cardiomyopathy: two-year follow-up results. Circulation 2001; 104: 39–45.

Cardiomyopathies

Cardiomyopathies are defined as diseases of the myocardium associated with impaired cardiac function. The 1995 WHO classification classified the previously termed 'heart muscle diseases of unknown causes' by dominant pathophysiology as dilated, hypertrophic and restrictive cardiomyopathy.[1] The specific cardiomyopathies are heart muscle diseases associated with known cardiac or systemic disorders (Table 1.23). As our understanding of cardiomyopathy improves, the difference between the two main groups is starting to become indistinct.

Dilated cardiomyopathy

Dilated cardiomyopathy is a disease characterized by cardiac enlargement and impaired systolic function of one or both ventricles.

Epidemiology

The prevalence is 36 per 100 000 per year, and it is 2.5 times more common in males with an average age of presentation ranging from 20 to 50 years.[1]

Pathology

It is likely that dilated cardiomyopathy represents the end result of a variety of cytotoxic (chemotherapy), metabolic (thiamine deficiency, alcohol abuse), infectious (previous myocarditis) and familial disease that results in myocardial injury. Approximately 20% of patients will have an affected first-degree relative.

Clinical features

The clinical features are identical to those of congestive cardiac failure (p. 15). The diagnosis of idiopathic dilated cardiomyopathy is made after excluding established causes of cardiac failure.

Table 1.23	1995 WHO classification of cardiomyopathies*
Dilated cardiomyopathy	
Hypertrophic cardiomyopathy	
Restrictive cardiomyopathy	
Arrhythmogenic right ventricular cardiomyopathy (p. 63)	
Unclassified cardiomyopathy	
Specific cardiomyopathies	
Ischaemic cardiomyopathy	
Valvular cardiomyopathy	
Hypertensive cardiomyopathy	
Inflammatory cardiomyopathy	
Metabolic cardiomyopathy	
General system disease	
Muscular dystrophies	
Neuromuscular disorders	
Sensitivity and toxic reactions	
Peripartum cardiomyopathy	

* Report of the 1995 World Health Organization/International Society and Federation of Cardiology Task Force on the Definition and Classification of Cardiomyopathies. Circulation 1996; 93: 841–842.

Investigations

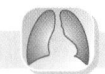

Investigations should proceed as for congestive cardiac failure (p. 16–17).

Echocardiography

Echocardiography is an excellent investigation that will reveal left-sided or four-chamber dilatation. Echocardiography can quantify the severity of ventricular impairment and exclude other causes of impaired cardiac function such as valvular heart disease and pericardial effusion.

Myocardial biopsy

Myocardial biopsy is usually performed in patients with unexplained cardiac failure and may reveal myocarditis in a proportion of patients.

Management

Supportive management

As dilated cardiomyopathy is a non-specific diagnosis, medical management is similar to chronic heart failure (p. 17–18). Heart transplantation may be required for suitable patients with end stage disease.

> **RECENT ADVANCES**
>
> *Surgical options currently being evaluated are ventricular restoration (excision of a portion of the left ventricular free wall to preserve the volume and pressure relations[2]) and mitral valve reconstruction (to improve clinical performance status by reducing the volume of secondary mitral regurgitation).[3]*

Prognosis

In general the prognosis is poor.

REFERENCES

(1) *Dec GW, Fuster V. Idiopathic dilated cardiomyopathy. New England Journal of Medicine 1994; 331: 1564–1575.*
(2) *Athanasuleas CL, Buckberg GD, Menicanti L, Gharib M. Optimizing ventricular shape in anterior restoration. Seminars in Thoracic and Cardiovascular Surgery 2001; 13: 459–467.*
(3) *Bolling SF. Mitral reconstruction in cardiomyopathy. Journal of Heart Valve Disease 2002; 11 (Suppl 1): S26–31.*

Hypertrophic cardiomyopathy

Hypertrophic cardiomyopathy is a disease characterized by left and/or right ventricular hypertrophy which is usually asymmetric and involves the ventricular septum.

Epidemiology

Echocardiographic population screening has identified the point prevalence of hypertrophic cardiomyopathy to be 170 per 100 000 in young adults.[1] It is equally common in both sexes.

Pathology

Hypertrophic cardiomyopathy results from mutation of genes that encode the protein components of the cardiac sarcomere; it is inherited as an autosomal dominant trait with variable penetrance. Myocardial hypertrophy increases the stiffness (reduced compliance) of the left ventricle and the interventricular septum, impairing diastolic filling of the ventricle.

A proportion develop obstruction of the left ventricular outflow tract, usually due to anterior displacement of the mitral valve during systole (systolic anterior motion); this also predisposes to mitral regurgitation. Less commonly (5%) septal hypertrophy causes obstruction due to muscular apposition in the mid cavity of the left ventricle. The obstruction is usually dynamic and occurs on exertion. Other complications of this condition are arrhythmia (atrial fibrillation), syncope and sudden death.

Clinical features

Many patients are asymptomatic, and most do not have evidence of outflow tract obstruction under resting conditions. Symptoms of angina, dyspnoea and syncope (similar to aortic stenosis) arise when left ventricular outflow tract obstruction occurs. On examination, classical findings are a steep upstroke of the pulse (forceful myocardial contraction), a systolic murmur of left ventricular outflow tract obstruction, or mitral regurgitation.

Investigations

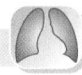

Electrocardiogram

The ECG is usually abnormal with non-specific ST and T wave abnormalities. Left ventricular hypertrophy may be evident.

Chest X-ray

Severe left ventricular hypertrophy may be evident on a chest X-ray as cardiomegaly.

Echocardiography

The definitive diagnosis is established on echocardiography with evidence of segmental (or diffuse) hypertrophy of the left ventricular free wall and asymmetric hypertrophy of the interventricular septum. A gradient of 30 mmHg or more across the left ventricular outflow tract indicates significant obstruction.

Management

Surveillance
Asymptomatic patients do not require treatment but should undergo regular surveillance.

β-Blockers
β-Blockers are recommended for symptomatic patients with evidence of outflow tract obstruction on exertion.

Septal myectomy
A minority with severe symptoms and extensive disease are referred for surgery. Ventricular septal myectomy (Morrow procedure) removes excess myocardium in the septum that obstructs the left ventricular outflow tract.

> **RECENT ADVANCES**
>
> *Current treatments under investigation are dual chamber pacing and percutaneous septal ablation by infusing alcohol into a septal artery inducing a controlled septal infarct.*

Prognosis

Hypertrophic cardiomyopathy is usually well tolerated and compatible with normal life expectancy.[2]

---

i FURTHER INFORMATION

American College of Cardiology/European Society of Cardiology clinical expert consensus document on hypertrophic cardiomyopathy. A report of the American College of Cardiology Foundation Task Force on Clinical Expert Consensus Documents and the European Society of Cardiology Committee for Practice Guidelines. Journal of the American College of Cardiology 2003; 42: 1687–1713.

REFERENCES

(1) *Maron BJ, Gardin JM, Flack JM, Gidding SS, Kurosaki TT, Bild DE. Prevalence of hypertrophic cardiomyopathy in a general population of young adults: echocardiographic analysis of 4111 subjects in the CARDIA Study. Circulation 1995; 92: 785–789.*
(2) *Maron BJ, Casey SA, Hauser RG, Aeppli DM. Clinical course of hypertrophic cardiomyopathy with survival to advanced age. Journal of the American College of Cardiology 2003; 42: 882–888.*

Restrictive cardiomyopathy

Restrictive cardiomyopathy is a disease characterized by restrictive filling and reduced diastolic volume of either or both ventricles with normal (or near normal) systolic function and wall thickness.

Epidemiology

Restrictive cardiomyopathy is the most rare of the three cardiomyopathies.

Pathology

Restrictive cardiomyopathy can result from a wide range of diseases such as infiltrative disease affecting the myocardium (amyloid, sarcoid), storage disorders (haemochromatosis, glycogen storage disease), endomyocardial fibrosis, carcinoid disease, and radiation and anthracycline toxicity. The main pathophysiological result is a stiff ventricle with impaired filling. Conduction abnormalities are associated with amyloidosis and sarcoidosis. Patients with no identifiable cause will be labelled as having idiopathic restrictive cardiomyopathy.

Clinical features

Patients with symptomatic disease present with dyspnoea on exertion as the cardiac chambers are unable to increase the stroke volume, and peripheral oedema. Chest pains may be experienced in the minority. On examination, clinical features are very similar to constrictive pericarditis, with peripheral oedema, elevated JVP and hepatomegaly. A distinguishing feature is a palpable apex beat in patients with restrictive cardiomyopathy.

Investigations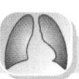

Electrocardiogram
The ECG usually reveals non-specific ST and T wave abnormalities and may detect atrial fibrillation, which is associated with amyloidosis and idiopathic restrictive cardiomyopathy.

Echocardiography
Echocardiography will reveal normal sized ventricles with impaired filling, normal or near normal systolic function, normal wall thickness and bi-atrial enlargement from raised diastolic pressures.

Determining the underlying cause
Further investigations should be directed at identifying any underlying cause.

Management

There is no specific management and treatment should be directed to any underlying cause.

Cardioversion
Cardioversion and maintenance of sinus rhythm is the aim in patients with atrial fibrillation to optimize cardiac output.

Pacing
Pacemakers are recommended for patients with conduction block.

Prognosis

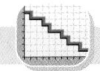

The prognosis of the disease is influenced by the underlying cause. For patients with idiopathic restrictive cardiomyopathy, the 1- and 5-year survival is approximately 95% and 64% respectively.[1]

REFERENCE

(1) Ammash NM, Seward JB, Bailey KR, Edwards WD, Tajik AJ. *Clinical profile and outcome of idiopathic restrictive cardiomyopathy.* Circulation 2000; 101: 2490–2496.

SECTION 1.11 Diseases of the pericardium

Advances in the understanding of pericardial disease have modified previous concepts and approaches to pericardial disease. It is currently recognized that the pericardium (to a variable extent) is involved in all disease states. Moreover, the causes of pericardial disease (Table 1.24) give rise to three main clinical syndromes: pericardial effusion and acute and constrictive pericarditis. These may coexist in any combination and can change from one predominant form of presentation to another.

Due to the broad spectrum of severity of disease, and the many different underlying causes, the general epidemiology of pericardial diseases has not been well documented and as such has been omitted from this section.

Table 1.24	Causes of pericardial disease
Infection	
Adenovirus	
Enterovirus	
Cytomegalovirus	
Herpes simplex virus	
Influenza virus	
HIV	
Bacterial infection (pyopericardium)	
Tuberculosis*	
Fungal infection	
Trauma	
Iatrogenic	
Cardiac surgery	
Radiation*	
Autoimmune	
Autoimmune pericarditis	
Post myocardial infarction	
Complication of systemic autoimmune disease	
Rheumatoid disease	
Systemic lupus erythematosus	
Scleroderma	
Sarcoidosis	
Rheumatic fever	
Metabolic disorders	
Renal failure	
Gout	
Neoplastic	
Lung cancer	
Breast cancer	
Haematological malignancy	
Idiopathic	
Idiopathic pericarditis is a diagnosis of exclusion	

* Conditions that tend to predispose to constrictive pericarditis as the primary presentation.

Pericardial effusion

The normal pericardium contains approximately 50 mL of clear fluid. A pericardial effusion refers to the accumulation of an abnormal amount of fluid in the pericardial cavity. Pericardial effusion is not a diagnosis but a manifestation of underlying disease.

Pathology

Haemoserous pericardial fluid is by far the most common constituent of a pericardial effusion; other fluids include pure blood (haemopericardium), pus (pyopericardium) and lymph (chylopericardium). The clinical effect of a pericardial effusion depends on the size, speed of accumulation and underlying state of the ventricle. With slowly progressive pericardial effusions, volumes of up to 2 litres can be accommodated. Normally, however, pericardial distension can accommodate up to 200 mL of fluid before intrapericardial pressure rapidly increases. When this occurs, intracardiac pressures become globally elevated, the diastolic relaxation of the ventricles becomes impaired, and this leads to a reduced stroke volume and eventually cardiogenic shock.

> ### ⚡ CLINICAL ALERT
>
> *Cardiac tamponade is the condition that arises from raised intrapericardial pressure of sufficient severity to impair haemodynamic performance of the heart. This usually occurs as a complication of pericardial effusion, but can also result from constrictive pericarditis. Tamponade can lead to cardiogenic shock, and its management is detailed on page 13.*

Clinical features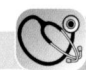

Although most pericardial effusions are small and asymptomatic, the range of presentation blends imperceptibly from an asymptomatic state to cardiogenic shock. Dyspnoea is the main presenting complaint, and this may be associated with tachypnoea. Depending on the underlying cause of the effusion, chest pain (acute pericarditis, myocardial infarction) may be associated. A detailed history should be directed to any underlying cause such as trauma, malignancy, connective tissue disease and renal failure.

On examination, peripheral oedema and ascites may be evident. Tachycardia is usually present and hypotension may result from poor cardiac output. A key finding is an elevated JVP, and a pericardial rub may be present due to pericarditis.

Investigations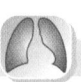

Full blood count
A full blood count may indicate anaemia if the cause is due to blood loss into the pericardial space.

Markers of inflammation
The ESR/CRP will be elevated with pericarditis and malignancy.

Serology
Paired sera should be requested for viral titres to identify a viral aetiology.

Serum cardiac markers
Serum cardiac markers may be elevated from pericarditis or myocardial infarction.

Electrocardiogram
The ECG will reveal a tachycardia with low voltage complexes due to pericardial effusion, and ST elevation from pericarditis and myocardial infarction (p. 28).

Chest X-ray
The chest film may reveal a globular cardiac silhouette (Fig. 1.39).

Transthoracic echocardiogram
An echocardiogram is the principal investigation that will confirm or exclude a pericardial effusion. The size of an effusion can be quantified and the presence of loculations identified (loculated effusions may not be adequately drained with percutaneous drainage). Raised intrapericardial pressures may cause collapse of the atria during diastole.

Management

Treatment should be directed to the underlying cause if possible.

Pericardiocentesis
Pericardiocentesis is required for tamponade, suspicion of purulent or neoplastic effusion and for patients who remain symptomatic despite one week of medical therapy.[1]

Drainage of pericardial effusion
Echocardiographic or fluoroscopic guided percutaneous drainage is best suited for anteriorly located, non-loculated, haemoserous effusions.

Surgical drainage (via a sternotomy or video assisted thoracoscopic approach) is usually required for traumatic, purulent and loculated effusions. As part of the surgical procedure a pericardial window is often created to allow any further fluid to drain into the pleural space.

Prognosis

The prognosis is related to the underlying cause with the poorest prognosis related to neoplastic disease and the best related to iatrogenic pericardial effusions. In patients with idiopathic pericardial effusions severe enough to warrant intervention, the long-term survival is similar to that of the general population.[2]

---

i **FURTHER INFORMATION**

Maisch B, Ristic AD. Practical aspects of the management of pericardial disease. Heart 2003; 89: 1096–1103.

REFERENCES

(1) *Maisch B, Ristic AD. Practical aspects of the management of pericardial disease. Heart 2003; 89: 1096–1103.*
(2) *Tsang TS, Barnes ME, Gersh BJ, Bailey KR, Seward JB. Outcomes of clinically significant idiopathic pericardial effusion requiring intervention. American Journal of Cardiology 2003; 91: 704–707.*

Acute pericarditis

Pericarditis is inflammation of the pericardium; it often exists subclinically in conjunction with many diseases.

Pathology

Pericarditis is an important prelude to a pericardial effusion and may lead to constrictive disease. The causes are listed on page 55.

Clinical features

Fever and chest pain is the main presentation of acute pericarditis; the pain is often described as a sharp pleuritic chest pain that may radiate to the back (trapezius ridge pain) and be relieved by sitting forwards. Patients with acute pericarditis complicated by effusion may also have the accompanying features listed.

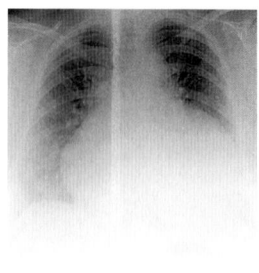
Fig. 1.39 This chest film shows a large pericardial effusion and a globular cardiac silhouette.

On examination, the presence of a pericardial rub often confirms the diagnosis of pericarditis (it is differentiated from a pleural rub by asking the patient to hold his/her breath).

The main differential diagnosis is myocardial infarction, which also presents with chest pain associated with ST segment elevation on the ECG; moreover, myocardial infarction itself can produce pericarditis. Features that would favour pericarditis over myocardial infarction are young age and ST segment configuration on ECG.

Investigations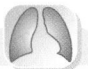

General investigations to determine the underlying aetiology should be performed as listed for pericardial effusion on page 55.

Electrocardiogram
ECG abnormalities characteristic of pericarditis are pan-ST segment elevation in a saddle configuration (Fig. 1.40).

Echocardiogram
Echocardiography is a useful screening tool for pericardial effusion.

Management

The management of complications such as pericardial effusion or tamponade is detailed on page 56.

Aspirin
High-dose aspirin (or ibuprofen) is the most commonly prescribed agent for patients with acute pericarditis.

Colchicine
Colchicine may be added in conjunction or as monotherapy.

Prognosis

Most cases will resolve with medical therapy with only a minority requiring intervention for complications.

i FURTHER INFORMATION

Spodick DH. Acute pericarditis: current concepts and practice. JAMA 2003; 289: 1150–1153.

Constrictive pericarditis

Constrictive pericarditis results from disease that causes thickening, scarring and calcification of the pericardium; it is the least common form of presentation of the pericardial diseases.

Pathology

The thickened and hardened pericardium impairs the diastolic relaxation of the heart, elevating the diastolic pressures in all four chambers and resulting in tamponade physiology. It is thought that constrictive pericarditis results as a complication of an initial episode of acute pericarditis.

Clinical features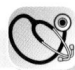

The presentation is similar to pericardial effusion with dyspnoea as the main symptom. Additional symptoms include atypical chest pains and peripheral oedema. A detailed history should also attempt to establish the underlying cause.

On examination, peripheral oedema and ascites may be present. A tachycardia may be accompanied by a low

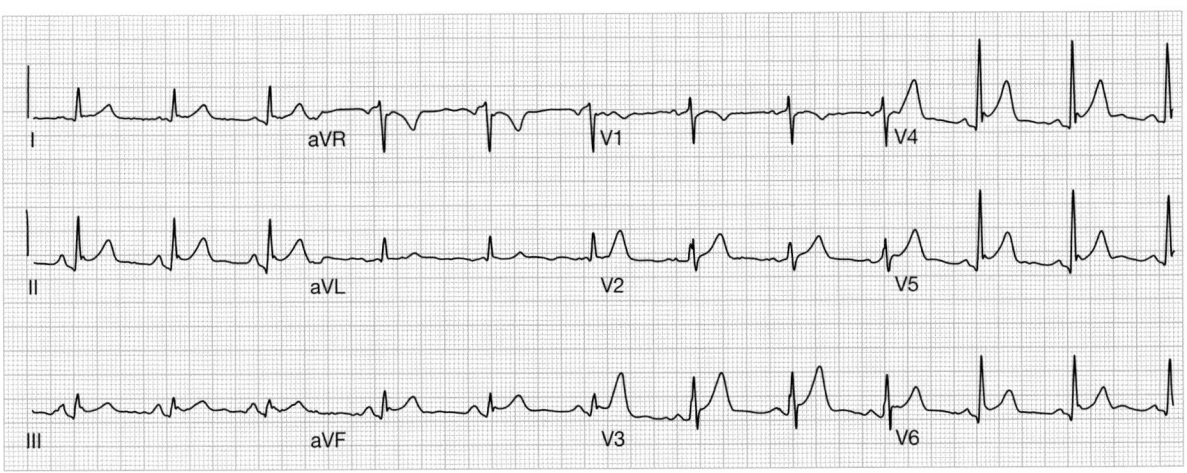

Fig. 1.40 ECG in pericarditis. This ECG shows the classic appearance of saddle-shaped ST segment elevation that is present uniformly in all leads.

volume pulse and hypotension. A key feature is Kussmaul's sign, when the elevated JVP increases on inspiration (normally, the JVP should decrease on inspiration as intrathoracic pressure becomes negative; with constrictive pericarditis, the negative intrathoracic pressure is not transmitted to the heart because of the thickened surrounding pericardium). The apex beat is not palpable and a pericardial rub may be present, depending on the presence of pericardial inflammation. Hepatomegaly may be present from hepatic congestion by raised right heart pressures.

Investigations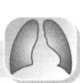

General investigations should proceed as for pericardial effusion.

Echocardiogram

The main distinguishing investigation is echocardiography, which will be able to identify the fluid of a pericardial effusion and the thickened peel of constrictive pericarditis.

CT/MRI

CT and MRI are often additional investigations to reveal the extent of the disease prior to surgical pericardiectomy.

Management

Pericardiectomy

Surgical excision of the pericardium is the definitive treatment for constrictive pericarditis. This is usually reserved for patients with NYHA class II or more, or patients with evidence of right heart failure. Pericardiectomy has a mortality rate of approximately 6% that is increased in patients with end stage or advanced underlying disease.

Prognosis

For patients who are well enough for surgery, the 5- and 10-year survival is 71% and 52% respectively.[1]

> ### *i* FURTHER INFORMATION
>
> Hoit BD. Management of effusive and constrictive pericardial heart disease. Circulation 2002; 105: 2939–2942.

> **REFERENCE**
>
> **(1)** *Ling LH, Oh JK, Schaff HV, Danielson GK, Mahoney DW, Seward JB, Tajik AJ. Constrictive pericarditis in the modern era: evolving clinical spectrum and impact on outcome after pericardiectomy. Circulation 1999; 100: 1380–1386.*

SECTION 1.12 · Arrhythmia

Supraventricular arrhythmias

The supraventricular arrhythmias are a family of abnormal rhythms that originate above the bifurcation of the bundle of His (i.e. in the atria, accessory electrical pathways and conduction tissue proximal to the bundle branches). A common feature is the conduction of electrical current to the bundle branches, producing narrow complex QRS intervals (with rates above 100/min). Because these arrhythmias are fast, they are known synonymously as the supraventricular tachycardias or tachyarrhythmias (SVT).

The types of supraventricular arrhythmia can be divided according to the tissue of origin: the atria (atrial fibrillation, atrial flutter), accessory pathways within the AV node (atrioventricular nodal re-entrant tachycardia) and accessory pathways that do not involve the AV node (atrioventricular re-entrant tachycardia, Wolff–Parkinson–White syndrome). These are listed in Table 1.25.

Table 1.25	Supraventricular arrhythmias/tachycardias*
Originating from the atria	
Atrial fibrillation	
Atrial flutter	
Multifocal atrial tachycardia	
Originating from accessory pathways	
Atrioventricular nodal re-entrant tachycardia (AVNRT)	
Atrioventricular re-entrant tachycardia (AVRT)	

*By definition, all arrhythmias that originate above the bundle branches are supraventricular arrhythmias; however, some books consider atrial fibrillation and atrial flutter to be separate from AVRT and AVNRT (which they regard as supraventricular tachycardias).

Atrial fibrillation

Epidemiology

The prevalence of atrial fibrillation is age related: it is present in 1% of patients under the age of 60, rising to 6% of patients over the age of 80.[1] It is 1.5 times more common in men.

Pathology

Atrial fibrillation is caused by haphazard conduction of electrical activity in atria that are enlarged or diseased. This results in irregular uncoordinated atrial contraction at a rate of 300–600/min, detected as a sawtooth baseline on the ECG. Some impulses are carried by the conduction tissue, producing irregularly timed QRS complexes and ventricular contraction.

Scope of disease

The atria contribute to 25% of the stroke volume, and the 'atrial kick' is lost with the onset of atrial fibrillation. In addition, the ventricles contract irregularly and often at a rapid rate. As ventricular filling is an important determinant of stroke volume, rapid and irregular ventricular contraction impairs the cardiac output. The severity of the haemodynamic compromise is dependent on the contractility of the ventricle. Patients with normal ventricles can tolerate atrial fibrillation and rapid ventricular rates without any appreciable haemodynamic consequence. However, if the ventricles are severely impaired, the onset of atrial fibrillation can result in circulatory shock.

Loss of atrial contraction predisposes to stasis and thrombus formation, greatly increasing the risk of stroke.

Clinical features

Atrial fibrillation is usually asymptomatic. Occasionally, patients may complain of palpitations, dyspnoea, fatigue or chest pains (atrial fibrillation can exacerbate angina) or present with the complication of stroke (p. 596). Patients may have a past medical history of ischaemic heart disease (angina, myocardial infarction) or hypertension (Table 1.26).

On examination, the pulse rate is irregularly irregular, both in rate and volume. The ventricular rate cannot be assessed from the pulse, as irregular ventricular contractions may not produce sufficient pulse pressure for all contractions to be detected. The ventricular rate is assessed by auscultating the apex: the discrepancy between apex and pulse rate is an indicator of rate control (the wider the discrepancy, the poorer the control). Evidence of underlying disease states that predispose to atrial fibrillation includes hypertension and the murmur of mitral valve disease.

On assessment, it is important to ascertain any acute precipitating factors (Table 1.27) and underlying risk factors and to assess the severity of disease (blood pressure, apex rate). Approximately a third will have no underlying cause: these are labelled as 'lone' atrial fibrillation.

Table 1.26	Underlying risk factors for atrial fibrillation	
Heart disease[a]		
Hypertensive heart disease	39%	
Ischaemic heart disease	17%	
Valvular heart disease	15%	
Heart failure (from any cause)	30%	
Other independent risks		
Increasing age	N/A	
Diabetes	11%	
Pulmonary disease[b]	11%	
Thyrotoxicosis[b]	3%	

[a] Proportions are not mutually exclusive and adapted from Benjamin EJ, Levy D, Vaziri SM, D'Agostino RB, Belanger AJ, Wolf PA. Independent risk factors for atrial fibrillation in a population-based cohort. The Framingham Heart Study. JAMA 1994; 271(11): 840–844.
[b] These conditions have been added to this list.

Table 1.27	Precipitating factors of atrial fibrillation
Hypoxia	
Excessive alcohol intake	
Pericarditis	
Myocardial infarction	
Pulmonary embolism	
Pneumonia	

Initial investigations

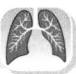

Urea and electrolytes
Chronic disturbances of electrolytes (hypokalaemia) may predispose to atrial fibrillation and have implications for therapy (hypokalaemia predisposes to digoxin toxicity).

Thyroid stimulating hormone
TSH is a useful screen for thyrotoxicosis and should be performed for all patients experiencing their first episode of atrial fibrillation.

Electrocardiogram
Atrial fibrillation is confirmed by the absence of p-waves, an irregular sawtooth baseline (Fig. 1.41) and an irregular ventricular rate. There may also be features of underlying

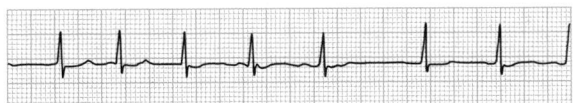

Fig. 1.41 ECG of atrial fibrillation. The irregularly irregular QRS complexes occur in the setting of a sawtooth baseline of uncoordinated atrial activity.

disease such as left ventricular hypertrophy (hypertension, heart valve disease) and previous myocardial infarction (abnormal Q waves).

Chest X-ray

A chest film is useful to screen for cardiomegaly, an indicator of underlying heart disease or congestive cardiac failure.

Transthoracic echocardiogram

Transthoracic echocardiography is able to measure the atrial size and screen for thrombus (sensitivity is low) and valvular heart disease. In addition, ventricular size and function can be quantified.

Further investigations

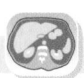

Holter monitoring

24-hour ECG monitoring may be required to monitor and diagnose paroxysmal atrial fibrillation in patients who have symptoms suggestive of atrial fibrillation but who remain in sinus rhythm on initial investigations.

Transoesophageal echocardiography

Transoesophageal echocardiography is indicated when there is a suggestion of left atrial thrombus on transthoracic imaging.

Electrophysiological studies

This investigation is not required for diagnosis; the main indications are to define the mechanism for atrial fibrillation in patients in whom curative catheter ablation is being considered.

Initial management

Address haemodynamic status

Although the majority of patients will not have clinically apparent haemodynamic compromise, it is important to identify and correct it if present.

Treat the precipitating cause

Identification and correction of an acute precipitating cause (e.g. oxygen for hypoxia) may correct atrial fibrillation.

Correct any underlying cause

Identification and correction of the underlying cause is an important aspect of patient management. The onset of atrial fibrillation in severe mitral regurgitation indicates the need for surgery.

Medical management

The foremost consideration in the management is the decision between rhythm or rate control. The aim of rhythm control is to achieve and sustain sinus rhythm, whereas the aim of rate control is to slow the ventricular rate and

prevent stroke by anticoagulation with warfarin. In patients over the age of 65, both treatments produced similar results for survival and risk of stroke.[2]

Rhythm control strategy
Pharmacological cardioversion

Amiodarone is a commonly used agent that can be given orally, in a decreasing loading dose over 2 weeks. An alternative agent is flecainide.

Electrical cardioversion

Synchronous DC cardioversion is usually undertaken following 4 weeks of anticoagulation with warfarin to reduce the risk of stroke. Alternatively, transoesophageal echocardiography may be used to screen for thrombus and pre-procedure anticoagulation undertaken only in patients with evidence of thrombus. DC cardioversion (p. 599) is successful in 95%, and the risk of stroke is 0.5% (increasing to 7% if pre-procedure anticoagulation was not undertaken). Post procedure, patients should continue anticoagulation therapy for 4 weeks.

Maintenance of sinus rhythm

Amiodarone, β-blockers or sotalol may be prescribed to maintain sinus rhythm.

Rate control strategy
Pharmacological rate control

Digoxin is a common agent used for rate control. Alternative agents are β-blockers and dihydropyridine calcium antagonists (verapamil and diltiazem).

Stroke prevention

Warfarin should be prescribed for patients at high risk of stroke to maintain an INR of 2.0–3.0; this subset of patients includes the elderly (age more than 75), patients with cardiac failure (or with an ejection fraction of less than 35%) or those with a history of hypertension. Low-risk patients, aged less than 60 years without any of the aforementioned risk factors, may receive 325 mg of aspirin daily instead.

Surgical management

The maze procedure

The maze procedure is currently under evaluation as a curative procedure for atrial fibrillation. The classic maze procedure requires cardiopulmonary bypass to perform multiple cuts on the atrial wall. The scarring resulting from the healing process of each incision acts as an insulator to electrical currents, and multiple cuts with a maze-like appearance prevent haphazard conduction of electrical activity. The atria are then reconstructed using sutures. More recently, radiofrequency probes have been developed that allow the creation of scar tissue by contact with the atria.

The maze procedure has a reported success rate of up to 80% in establishing and maintaining sinus rhythm, although this may take up to 8 weeks. Heart block is a common postoperative complication that resolves by 8 weeks.

RECENT ADVANCES

It has recently been discovered that the pulmonary vein ostia often harbour inciting foci that precipitate atrial fibrillation. Radiofrequency lesions that electrically isolate the region around the pulmonary veins are successful in eliminating atrial fibrillation in the short term, unfortunately the present recurrence rates are high.[3]

Prognosis

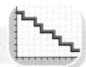

Atrial fibrillation is not a benign rhythm: approximately 15% of patients die within the first 30 days of diagnosis. The risk of death reduces thereafter: within the age group 55–74, the 1- and 5-year survival is approximately 82% and 60% respectively.[4] The annual incidence of stroke is 1.5% in patients aged between 50 and 59, and this increases to 23.5% in those aged between 80 and 89 years.[5]

REFERENCES

(1) *Fuster V, Ryden LE, Asinger RW, et al. ACC/AHA/ESC guidelines for the management of patients with atrial fibrillation: executive summary a report of the American College of Cardiology/American Heart Association Task Force on Practice Guidelines and the European Society of Cardiology Committee for Practice Guidelines and Policy Conferences (Committee to Develop Guidelines for the Management of Patients With Atrial Fibrillation) developed in collaboration with the North American Society of Pacing and Electrophysiology. Circulation 2001; 104: 2118–2150.*

(2) *The Atrial Fibrillation Follow-up Investigation of Rhythm Management (AFFIRM) Investigators. A comparison of rate control and rhythm control in patients with atrial fibrillation. New England Journal of Medicine 2002; 347: 1825–1833.*

(3) *Cappato R, Negroni S, Pecora D, et al. Prospective assessment of late conduction recurrence across radiofrequency lesions producing electrical disconnection at the pulmonary vein ostium in patients with atrial fibrillation. Circulation 2003; 108: 1599–1604.*

(4) *Benjamin EJ, Wolf PA, D'Agostino RB, Silbershatz H, Kannel WB, Levy D. Impact of atrial fibrillation on the risk of death: the Framingham Heart Study. Circulation 1998; 98: 946–952.*

(5) *Wolf PA, Abbott RD, Kannel WB. Atrial fibrillation as an independent risk factor for stroke: the Framingham Study. Stroke 1991; 22: 983–988.*

Atrial flutter

Atrial flutter is less common than atrial fibrillation and usually results from a re-entrant circuit within the right atrium. The rate of discharge of the atria is 250–350/min, but not all of the electrical activity is conducted to the ventricles—usually one out of every two or three beats (2:1 or 3:1 block). The causes of atrial flutter are similar to those of atrial fibrillation (p. 59), and a similar diagnostic workup should be employed. Synchronous DC cardioversion is usually the initial treatment of choice and is successful in the majority. If electrical cardioversion cannot be achieved, then pharmacological cardioversion using verapamil, diltiazem or amiodarone may be attempted. Maintenance

of sinus rhythm will require a β-blocker or amiodarone. Recurrent atrial flutter is an indication for electrophysiological studies to identify any inciting focus and to ablate it with radiofrequency waves. As the risk of stroke in patients with atrial flutter is low, routine anticoagulation is not required in the absence of other risk factors.

⚡ CLINICAL ALERT

Atrial flutter with 2:1 block can be difficult to diagnose on an ECG; the preceding non-conducted p wave is buried within the preceding QRS complex. Therefore, the ECG appears like sinus rhythm with an extremely regular rate of (classically) 150 bpm. The diagnosis can be confirmed using adenosine to transiently slow the heart rate.

Junctional arrhythmias

Currently, there is no uniformly accepted classification of junctional arrhythmias. They are commonly grouped together as 'paroxysmal supraventricular tachycardias (PSVT)'; however, the pathogenesis of these arrhythmias involves the ventricles as much as it involves the tissue 'above' the ventricles. In this section, the term junctional arrhythmia is used to encompass atrioventricular re-entrant tachycardia (AVRT) and atrioventricular nodal re-entrant tachycardia (AVNRT). The term PSVT refers to the narrow complex tachycardia that commonly results from this group of diseases.

Epidemiology

The incidence of PSVT has been estimated at 35 per 100 000 per year. It is twice as common in women than men before the age of 65, but three times as common in men thereafter.[1] AVNRT is approximately twice as common as AVRT.

Pathology

This group of arrhythmias is caused by an additional pathway of specialized conduction tissue that exists between the atrium and ventricle. Therefore, when normal electrical impulses are conduced from the atria to the atrioventricular node, they re-enter the atria via the accessory pathway, whilst simultaneous conduction to the rest of the bundle of His occurs. The result is the generation of an electrical circuit that is repeatedly cycled up into the atria and down into the bundle of His (and consequently the ventricles) generating a regular, narrow complex tachycardia.

Atrioventricular re-entrant arrhythmias are classified according to the site of the abnormal conducting tissue. If the specialized pathway exits within the atrioventricular node, the term atrioventricular nodal re-entrant tachycardia (AVNRT) is used; otherwise, if the specialized pathways are extranodal, it is termed atrioventricular re-entrant tachycardia (AVRT).

Scope of disease

Patients with accessory pathways are predisposed to PSVT, often a self-terminating narrow complex tachycardia. Sudden onset of PSVT can result in syncope; however, sustained haemodynamic compromise is uncommon because these arrhythmias are usually self-terminating in young patients with no other structural heart disease and normal ventricles.

Clinical features

This group of patients is asymptomatic until the onset of PSVT that results in palpitations and/or syncope.

Initial investigations

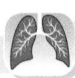

Electrocardiogram
A 12 lead ECG is sufficient to confirm the presence of a narrow complex regular tachycardia (Fig. 1.42). It is useful to compare with any previous ECG to screen for the appearance of a short PR interval that would suggest Wolff–Parkinson–White syndrome.

Further investigations

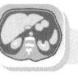

Electrophysiological studies
Once PSVT has been confirmed, formal electrophysiological studies should be arranged to map the site of the re-entrant pathway.

Initial management

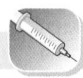

Vagal stimulation
The Valsalva manoeuvre and carotid sinus massage are two simple ways to increase vagal tone and slow atrioventricular conduction. Occasionally this is sufficient to interrupt the tachycardia circuit and restore sinus rhythm.

Medical management

Termination of PSVT
Adenosine
Termination of PSVT can be achieved with intravenous adenosine, a potent blocker of AV nodal conduction that lasts approximately 20 seconds. An alternative agent is intravenous verapamil.

DC cardioversion
If haemodynamic compromise is evident and PSVT is refractory to adenosine, then synchronous DC cardioversion should be undertaken.

Maintenance of sinus rhythm
Sotalol
Sotalol is often an effective first-line agent to prevent the recurrence of PSVT.

Catheter ablation
Radiofrequency ablation should be considered in all symptomatic patients. Initially, electrophysiological studies are performed with the primary aim of inducing a tachycardia to determine the mechanism of the arrhythmia. An ablation catheter is then positioned on a portion of the re-entry circuit that is critical for the maintenance of the tachycardia. Care is taken to ensure that this is not part of the normal cardiac conduction system. Radiofrequency energy is then delivered, rendering the small area of myocardium electrically inactive. The success rate has been reported to be 98%. Heart block is a complication that occurs in less than 1% of patients.

Prognosis

The clinical course of untreated PSVT is very variable; the reports in the literature on recurrence rates vary from 80% within a month to 20% at 2 years.[1]

REFERENCE

(1) Orejarena LA, Vidaillet H Jr, DeStefano F, Nordstrom DL, Vierkant RA, Smith PN, Hayes JJ. Paroxysmal supraventricular tachycardia in the general population. Journal of the American College of Cardiology 1998; 31: 150–157.

Wolff–Parkinson–White syndrome (WPW)

A subtype of AVRT may result from a defined abnormal pathway recognized as the 'bundle of Kent'. This results in a characteristic ECG appearance of pre-excitation, which is a short PR interval due to conduction of impulses from the atria (due to the bundle of Kent) and then the atrioventricular node, tachyarrhythmias and atrial fibrillation—a syndrome reported by Wolff, Parkinson and White. It is pre-excitation that distinguishes WPW as a subtype of AVRT,

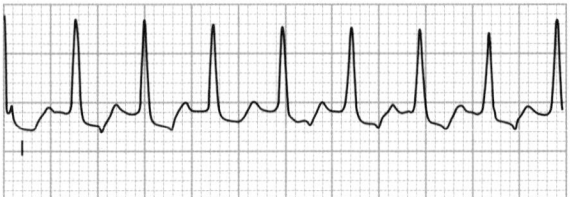

Fig. 1.42 ECG of supraventricular tachycardia.

although some regard them as separate entities. The clinical features of PSVT and its management are detailed on page 61–62. The ECG in WPW reveals a short PR interval and a slurred upstroke of the QS complex (Fig. 1.43).

The management of atrial fibrillation in WPW is different to that caused by other aetiologies. Digoxin and verapamil should be avoided as they slow the atrioventricular conduction and can precipitate uncontrolled ventricular activation via the accessory pathway. Cardioversion is the preferred treatment and sotalol or amiodarone may be used to prevent the recurrence of atrial fibrillation. In general, all patients should be referred for the consideration of radiofrequency catheter ablation, a curative procedure with a high overall success rate.

Ventricular arrhythmias

Ventricular tachycardia

Ventricular tachycardia is the occurrence of three or more consecutive premature ventricular complexes (p. 6). It is classified as monomorphic or polymorphic on the appearance of the QRS complex (Table 1.28).

Pathology

Monomorphic ventricular tachycardia and polymorphic ventricular tachycardia with normal baseline QT interval (during sinus rhythm) can result from acute myocardial infarction, existing ischaemic heart disease, ventricular aneurysms, heart valve disease, cardiomyopathies and arrhythmogenic right ventricular dysplasia. Ventricular tachycardia in the absence of structural heart disease is uncommon. Arrhythmogenic right ventricular dysplasia is a rare autosomal dominant condition characterized by fat or fibrous infiltration of the ventricles. It is more predominant, and can lead to right ventricular failure in addition to monomorphic ventricular tachycardia.

Polymorphic ventricular tachycardia with a prolonged baseline QT interval is known as torsade de pointes (twisting of the points). It is associated with hypokalaemia, hypomagnesaemia and antiarrhythmic drugs (quinidine, sotalol, amiodarone).

Scope of disease

The haemodynamic consequences depend on the underlying state of the ventricle and range from asymptomatic

Table 1.28 Classification and causes of ventricular tachycardia

Monomorphic ventricular tachycardia
Acute myocardial infarction
Ischaemic heart disease
Ventricular aneurysm
Heart valve disease
Cardiomyopathies
Arrhythmogenic right ventricular dysplasia
Polymorphic ventricular tachycardia with normal baseline QT interval
Causes are the same as monomorphic ventricular tachycardia
Polymorphic ventricular tachycardia with prolonged baseline QT interval (torsade de pointes)
Hypokalaemia
Hypomagnesaemia
Antiarrhythmic drugs (quinidine, sotalol, amiodarone)

Atrial fibrillation

Atrial flutter

Wolff–Parkinson–White syndrome (WPW)

Ventricular tachycardia

status to cardiac arrest and death. Torsade de pointes can precipitate ventricular fibrillation.

Clinical features

The clinical features associated with ventricular tachycardia depend on the rate and duration of the arrhythmia as well as the underlying function of the heart. The presenting symptoms are varied and range from palpitations to collapse. It is important to screen for symptoms such as angina, suggesting underlying ischaemic heart disease, or dyspnoea from heart valve disease or cardiomyopathy.

Initial investigations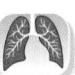

Urea and electrolytes, serum magnesium
Low potassium or magnesium levels can predispose to ventricular tachycardia.

Electrocardiogram
A 12 lead ECG will allow classification into monomorphic or polymorphic ventricular tachycardia (Fig. 1.44). In addition, previous ECGs (if available) should be used to determine the duration of the baseline QT interval.

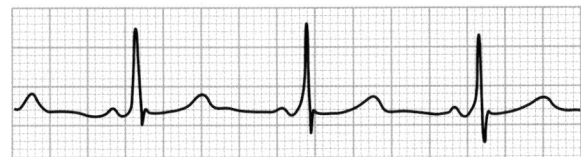
Fig. 1.43 ECG of Wolff–Parkinson–White syndrome.

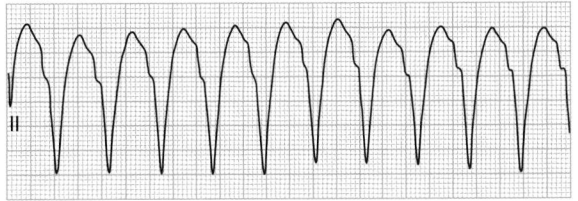
Fig. 1.44 ECG of monomorphic ventricular tachycardia.

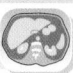

Further investigations

Serum cardiac markers
Serum cardiac markers should be requested for patients with a history of chest pain to screen for myocardial infarction.

Transthoracic echocardiography
Echocardiography is indicated for patients with clinical features suggestive of cardiac failure or murmurs associated with heart valve disease.

Electrophysiological studies
Electrophysiological studies should be performed for patients with recurrent, symptomatic ventricular tachycardia. Catheter ablation is indicated for bundle branch re-entry ventricular tachycardia and may be suitable in selected patients with scar-related ventricular tachycardia.

Initial management

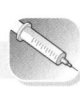

Resuscitation
Basic and advanced life support algorithms should be followed, and resuscitative efforts should commence immediately if haemodynamic comprise is evident.

> **CLINICAL ALERT**
>
> *Pulseless ventricular tachycardia is life threatening and is treated as ventricular fibrillation. Defibrillation should be initiated immediately.*

Admission to CCU
Where available, patients should be admitted to the coronary care unit for continuous monitoring by staff experienced in defibrillation and other aspects of advanced cardiac life support (ACLS).

Identify and correct the underlying cause
Low serum potassium or magnesium levels should be corrected. The management of ischaemic and valvular heart disease is presented on pages 21 and 36.

Medical management

Lidocaine
Lidocaine is currently the second-line treatment for patients with sustained ventricular tachycardia and stable haemodynamic status.

Amiodarone
For patients with ventricular tachycardia, amiodarone is a good first-line agent.

DC cardioversion
For patients with haemodynamic instability, DC cardioversion should be employed.

Implantable cardioverter defibrillator
Implantable cardioverter defibrillators are indicated for patients who experienced an episode of cardiac arrest, patients with spontaneous sustained ventricular tachycardia in association with structural heart disease not amenable to surgical correction, and those with haemodynamically significant sustained ventricular tachycardia when drug therapy is ineffective or not tolerated.

Surgical management

Surgical management of patients with ventricular tachycardia is confined to the correction of predisposing factors such as ischaemic heart disease, valvular heart disease and excision of ventricular aneurysms.

Prognosis

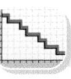

The prognosis of patients experiencing a first episode of ventricular tachycardia depends on underlying cause.

SECTION 1.13   Diseases of the thoracic aorta

Thoracic aortic aneurysm

Epidemiology

The prevalence of asymptomatic thoracic aortic aneurysm has been reported as 463 per 100 000 in a population post mortem study.[1] It is more common in men than in women.

Pathology

Atherosclerosis (degenerative aneurysms) has been implicated as the most common cause for dilatation of the thoracic aorta. Another important cause is annulo-aortic ectasia with cystic medial degeneration, a condition that occurs in patients with Marfan's syndrome (p. 923). Rare causes are syphilis, chronic dissection and chronic transection. The natural history of thoracic aortic aneurysms is progressive enlargement that can lead to aortic regurgitation, aortic rupture or aortic dissection.

Clinical features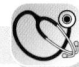

In the majority, thoracic aneurysms are asymptomatic. Patients may complain of non-specific chest pain that radiates to the back, and occasionally hoarseness of voice due to tension on the recurrent laryngeal nerve. On examination, a pulsatile mass may (rarely) be detected in the root of the neck.

Investigations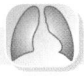

Chest X-ray

The dilated thoracic aorta may be evident on the chest film (Fig. 1.45).

CT/MRI chest

The anatomy is best delineated by CT or MRI (Fig. 1.46).

Management

Treatment of hypertension

Patients with small aneurysms should be kept under surveillance. Hypertension should be treated if present (p. 70).

Replacement of the ascending aorta

Resection and replacement of the aneurysm (Fig. 1.47a–c) is indicated when the aortic index (ratio of the diameter of the aneurysm and body surface area) approaches 1.5 (4.8 cm in an average adult) or 1.3 (4.3 cm in the average adult) in patients with Marfan's syndrome due to the increased risk of rupture.

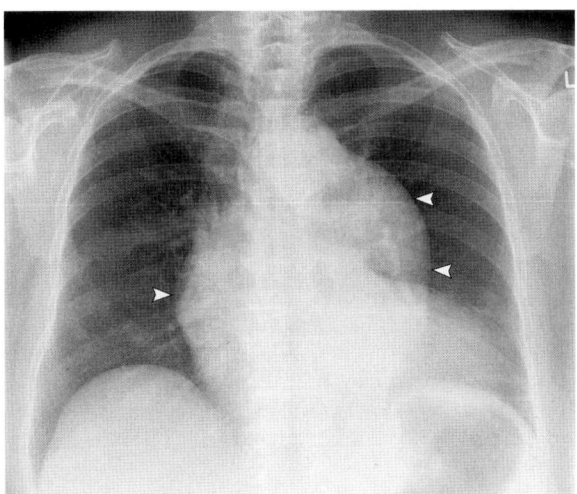

Fig. 1.45 Chest film of a thoracic aneurysm. The arrows demarcate the left lateral border of the aneurysm.

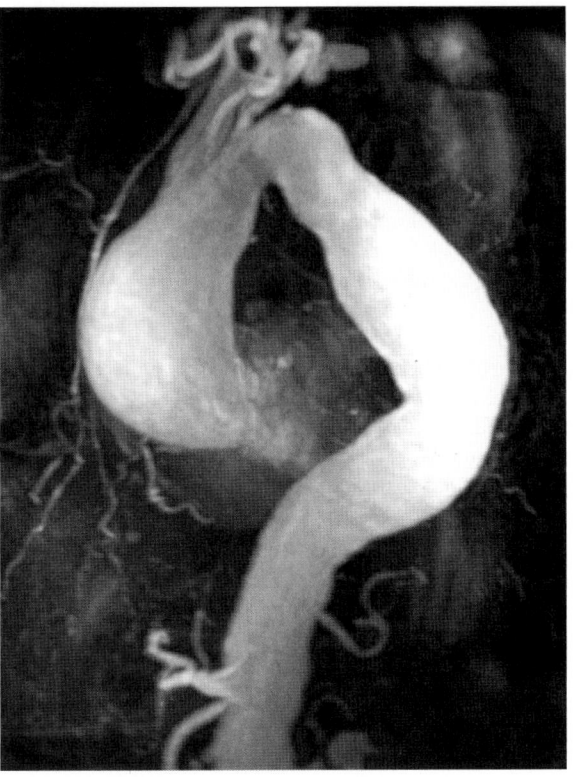

Fig. 1.46 Three-dimensional reconstructed MRI.

Prognosis

In a post mortem study, the incidence of aortic rupture as a cause of death in the general population due to previously asymptomatic thoracic aortic aneurysm has been reported to be 1 per 100 000, and that of dissection as 3 per 100 000.[1] Operative mortality depends on the experience of the centre and in general is less than 10%. The 5-year survival free of any complications has been reported to be 79%.[2]

REFERENCES

(1) Svensjo S, Bengtsson H, Bergqvist D. Thoracic and thoracoabdominal aortic aneurysm and dissection: an investigation based on autopsy. British Journal of Surgery 1996; 83: 68–71.
(2) Ergin MA, Spielvogel D, Apaydin A, Lansman SL, McCullough JN, Galla JD, Griepp RB. Surgical treatment of the dilated ascending aorta: when and how? Annals of Thoracic Surgery 1999; 67: 1834–1839; discussion 1853–1856.

Thoracic aortic dissection

Acute aortic dissection is a surgical emergency characterized by the sudden separation of the intima and media of the aorta. Often, blood leaves the normal aortic lumen,

Thoracic aortic aneurysm

Thoracic aortic dissection

65

travels into a discrete entry point, and dissects the intima from the media to produce a false channel.

Epidemiology

The incidence of aortic dissection has been reported as 2.9 per 100 000 per year.[1] The mean age of presentation is 63 years. The condition is 2 times more common in men.[2]

Pathology

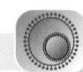

Increased shear stresses (hypertension) and any mechanism that weakens the aortic media (connective tissue disease) will predispose to dissection; the risk factors are detailed in Table 1.29. Dissection, by separating the intima from the media, can shear off blood vessels from the aortic lumen, rendering the vascular territory ischaemic. It may proceed in an antegrade (away from the heart) or retrograde (towards the heart) fashion. Most life-threatening complications occur in the ascending aorta: if the carotid arteries are involved, stroke ensues; if the coronary arteries are involved, myocardial infarction occurs. In addition, aortic dissection can shear the entire aortic valve, leading to free aortic regurgitation. When blood extravasates into the pericardial space, tamponade and death is the usual result.

In view of the gravity of the complications involving the ascending aorta, aortic dissections are classified according to proximal aortic involvement (Stanford classification). Any dissection involving the ascending aorta is classified as type A, and any dissection not involving the ascending aorta is classified as type B (Fig. 1.48).

Clinical features

Pain is the most common presenting complaint (95%) and may be experienced in the chest, back or abdomen (mesenteric infarction).[2] It is often described as the worst pain ever experienced and is an important differential diagnosis of patients with myocardial infarction (due to dissection that involves the coronary arteries). Syncope, stroke, acute limb ischaemia and paraplegia at presentation are less common.

Although hypertension is a risk factor in the majority, less than 50% will have a systolic blood pressure over 150 mmHg at presentation.[2] Other examination findings may include the murmur of aortic regurgitation (32%), with pulse deficits present in only 15%.

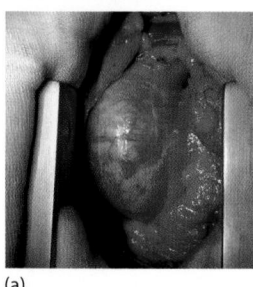

(a)

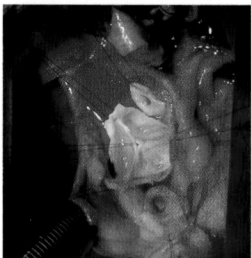

(b)

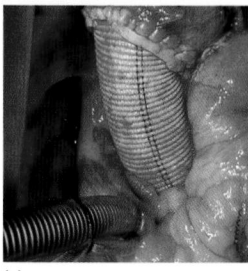

(c)

Fig. 1.47a–c Resection and repair of a thoracic aneurysm. The dilated ascending thoracic aneurysm is visible. It is excised and reconstructed with a polytetrafluoroethylene (PTFE) graft. Image courtesy of Mr Francis Wells, Consultant Cardiothoracic Surgeon, Papworth Hospital, Cambridge, UK.

Table 1.29	Risk factors of aortic dissection
Hypertension	
Connective tissue disease (Marfan's, Ehlers–Danlos syndrome)	
Coarctation of the aorta	
Arteritis	
Trauma (deceleration injury)	
Iatrogenic (cardiac surgery, catheter intervention of the aorta)	

Type A   Type B

Fig. 1.48 Stanford classification of aortic dissection.

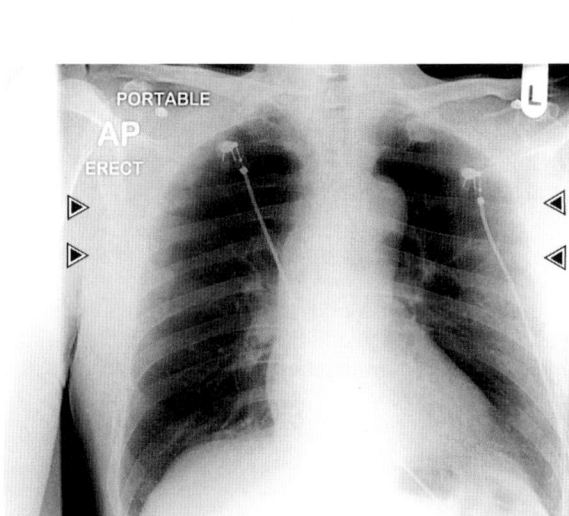

Fig. 1.49 Chest film of aortic dissection. The abnormal aortic contour is a subtle feature.

Investigations

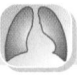

Electrocardiogram
Non-specific ST segment or T wave abnormalities and left ventricular hypertrophy are the most common abnormalities. The ECG is normal in a third of patients.

Chest X-ray
The CXR is abnormal in 87%, with a widened mediastinum and abnormal aortic contour being the most commonly reported abnormalities (Fig. 1.49).

CT chest

CT of the chest will confirm the diagnosis, the extent of a dissection and the type of dissection (Fig. 1.50).

Transoesophageal echocardiogram

An alternative imaging modality is transoesophageal echocardiography.

Management

Type A dissection

Blood pressure control with labetalol (to achieve a target systolic pressure of 110 mmHg) and emergency surgery is required for all patients with a confirmed diagnosis of a type A aortic dissection (within the last 14 days). Operation involves resection and replacement of the ascending aorta (and aortic arch if required) with an interposition graft (Fig. 1.51). The aortic valve may need to be replaced and coronary artery bypass grafts performed, depending on the extent of the dissection.

Type B dissection

In patients with type B dissection, the management is conservative. The indications for surgery are persisting pain, rapidly expanding aorta or the presence of periaortic or mediastinal haematoma (impending rupture). An alternative treatment is endovascular stenting with percutaneous fenestrations to perfuse the side branches of the aorta.

Prognosis

The mortality of untreated type A dissections is approximately 1% per hour in the first 24 hours, peaking with an overall in-hospital mortality of 58%. Surgery is associated with an in-hospital mortality of 26%.[2] For medically treated type B dissections the in-hospital mortality is 11%, compared to 31% in those who underwent surgery.[2]

REFERENCES

(1) Meszaros I, Morocz J, Szlavi J, Schmidt J, Tornoci L, Nagy L, Szep L. Epidemiology and clinicopathology of aortic dissection. Chest 2000; 117: 1271–1278.
(2) Hagan PG, Nienaber CA, Isselbacher EM, et al. The International Registry of Acute Aortic Dissection (IRAD): new insights into an old disease. JAMA 2000; 283: 897–903.

Thoracic aortic aneurysm

Thoracic aortic dissection

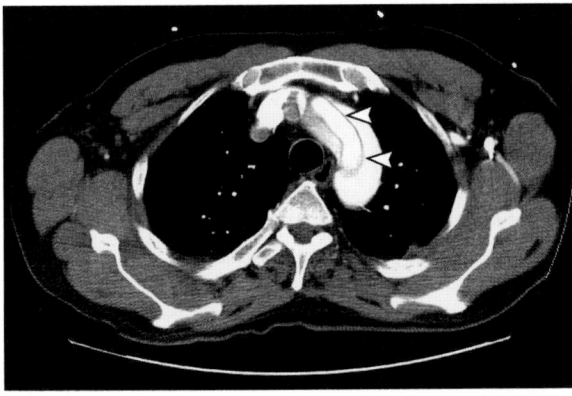

(a)

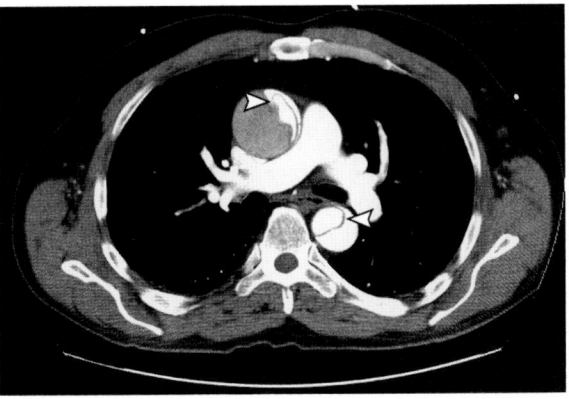

(b)

Fig. 1.50 a,b CT of aortic dissection. (a) The dissection flap in the aortic arch. (b) There is proximal and distal extension with a double-barrelled aorta. Contrast is seen in the true lumen proximally and in both lumina distally.

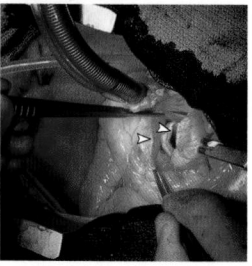

(a)

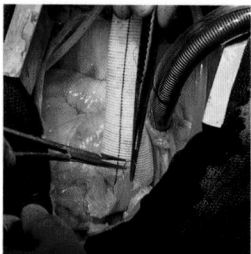

(b)

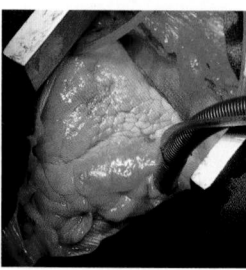

(c)

Fig. 1.51a–c Repair of aortic dissection. The true and false lumen (two arrows) can be seen in (a). The aorta is excised and a PTFE interposition graft sutured in place (b) to repair the dissection (c). Images courtesy of Mr Stephen Large, Consultant Cardiac Surgeon, Papworth Hospital, Cambridge, UK.

SECTION 1.14 Systemic hypertension

Hypertension is a very common disease. The morbidity and mortality associated with hypertension are mainly due to its contribution as a major risk factor for coronary artery disease and stroke.

Epidemiology

Hypertension is a very common disease in developed countries and is a growing problem in developing countries. The overall prevalence in Europe is 44 000 per 100 000 (that is 44% of the entire population) and both sexes are affected equally. The prevalence increases with age from 27% in 35–44-year-olds to 78% in those aged between 65 and 74 years.[1]

Pathology

An underlying cause (Table 1.30) is established in less than 10% and most patients will be classified with essential hypertension. Pathological changes associated with chronic sustained hypertension are hyaline and hyperplastic arteriolosclerosis.

Scope of disease

Hypertension is a major risk factor for atherosclerosis. Complications involve the eye (hypertensive and arterio-sclerotic retinopathy), heart (coronary heart disease, heart failure), brain (stroke) and kidney (nephrosclerosis and hypertensive renal disease).

Clinical features

Uncomplicated essential hypertension is asymptomatic and is identified during the course of routine physical examination. Patients with secondary hypertension, however, may complain of symptoms from the underlying disorder. A detailed drug history should reveal any offending drug that can cause hypertension.

In addition to establishing the diagnosis of hypertension (sustained rise in blood pressure above 140/90 mmHg on three or more readings, each at least a week apart), a detailed clinical assessment will also screen for any evidence of complications and attempt to ascertain any underlying cause (Table 1.30).

General investigations

The aim of general investigations in hypertension is to screen for secondary causes and complications and to evaluate concomitant risk factors for atherosclerosis.

Table 1.30	Causes of hypertension
Renal	
Renal parenchymal diseases (glomerulonephritis)	
Renal artery stenosis	
Chronic pyelonephritis	
Polycystic kidney disease	
Connective tissue disease (systemic sclerosis)	
Diabetic nephropathy	
Endocrine	

Adrenal
    Conn's syndrome
    Phaeochromocytoma	

Cushing's syndrome	
Acromegaly	
Drugs	
Glucocorticoids (corticosteroids)	
Mineralocorticoids (liquorice)	
Monoamine oxidase inhibitors and tyramine	
Sympathomimetic agents (salbutamol)	
Cardiovascular	
Coarctation of the aorta	

Urinalysis

Urine strip testing may reveal blood and protein, suggestive of renal disease. Urine microscopy is necessary to confirm the presence of red blood cells and also casts.

Urea and electrolytes

Urea and creatinine may be elevated with renal failure, and low serum potassium levels in untreated patients may be due to Conn's syndrome (p. 427).

Blood glucose

Plasma glucose is performed to screen for diabetes (p. 442) as it is associated with atherosclerosis, renal vascular disease and nephropathy. All of these may contribute to hypertension. Moreover, causes of secondary hypertension such as Cushing's syndrome, acromegaly and phaeochromocytoma are associated with hyperglycaemia.

Serum cholesterol

Serum cholesterol screening should be performed as it is an additional risk factor for atherosclerosis and may require treatment for the prevention of cerebrovascular and ischaemic heart disease.

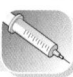

Electrocardiogram

A 12 lead ECG is required as a baseline investigation and to screen for left ventricular hypertrophy, a complication of hypertension.

Specific investigations

Specific investigations are usually tailored to suspected secondary causes. Details of each screening test are provided for phaeochromocytoma (p. 431), Cushing's syndrome (p. 422), Conn's syndrome (p. 427), coarctation of the aorta (p. 50) and renal artery stenosis (p. 734).

Renal ultrasound

Renal ultrasound is a good screening investigation for hypertensive patients when the suspected underlying cause is renal disease. It is best at detecting structural disorders such as polycystic kidney disease and renal artery stenosis.

Initial management

Apart from blood pressure lowering, an important aspect of the management of hypertension encompasses modification of cardiovascular risk.

Lifestyle and risk factor modification

Weight loss towards ideal weight, regular exercise, limiting alcohol consumption, reduced salt intake and increased fruit and vegetable intake have been proven in clinical trials to reduce blood pressure and may obviate the need for pharmacological therapy for hypertension. This advice should be offered to all patients and is best supplemented with written information.

Aspirin

Aspirin reduces major cardiovascular events in hypertensive patients and should be prescribed for primary preven-

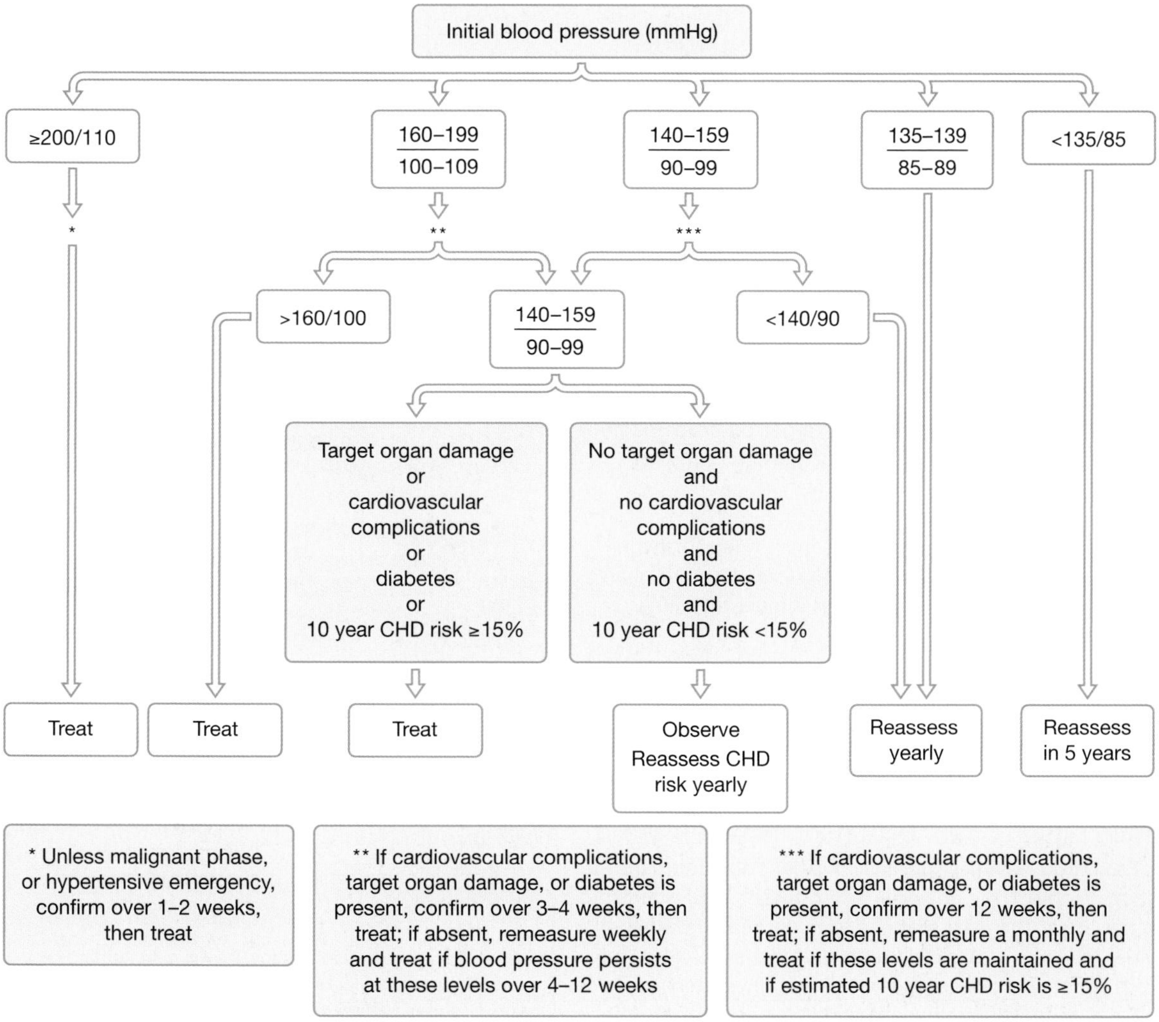

Initial blood pressure (mmHg)

≥200/110 | 160–199 / 100–109 | 140–159 / 90–99 | 135–139 / 85–89 | <135/85

* | ** | ***

>160/100 | 140–159 / 90–99 | <140/90

Target organ damage or cardiovascular complications or diabetes or 10 year CHD risk ≥15%

No target organ damage and no cardiovascular complications and no diabetes and 10 year CHD risk <15%

Treat | Treat | Treat | Observe / Reassess CHD risk yearly | Reassess yearly | Reassess in 5 years

* Unless malignant phase, or hypertensive emergency, confirm over 1–2 weeks, then treat

** If cardiovascular complications, target organ damage, or diabetes is present, confirm over 3–4 weeks, then treat; if absent, remeasure weekly and treat if blood pressure persists at these levels over 4–12 weeks

*** If cardiovascular complications, target organ damage, or diabetes is present, confirm over 12 weeks, then treat; if absent, remeasure a monthly and treat if these levels are maintained and if estimated 10 year CHD risk is ≥15%

Fig. 1.52 Initiation of drug therapy for hypertension.
From Ramsay LE, Williams B, Johnston GD, et al. British Hypertension Society guidelines for hypertension management 1999: summary. BMJ 1999; 319: 630–635.

Table 1.31 Choice of drug therapy for hypertension

Class of drug	Indication		Contraindications	
	Compelling	*Possible*	*Possible*	*Compelling*
α-Blockers	Prostatism	Dyslipidaemia	Postural hypotension	Urinary incontinence
ACE inhibitors	Heart failure Left ventricular dysfunction Type I diabetic nephropathy	Chronic renal disease[a] Type II diabetic nephropathy	Renal impairment[a] Peripheral vascular disease[b]	Pregnancy Renovascular disease
Angiotensin II receptor antagonists	Cough induced by ACE inhibitor[c]	Heart failure Intolerance of other antihypertensive drugs	Peripheral vascular disease[b]	Pregnancy Renovascular disease
β-Blockers	Myocardial infarction Angina	Heart failure[d]	Heart failure[d] Dyslipidaemia Peripheral vascular disease	Asthma or chronic obstructive pulmonary disease Heart block
Calcium antagonists (dihydropyridine)	Isolated systolic hypertension in elderly patients	Angina Elderly patients	—	—
Calcium antagonists (rate limiting)	Angina	Myocardial infarction	Combination with β-blockade	Heart block Heart failure
Thiazides	Elderly patients	—	Dyslipidaemia	Gout

[a] Angiotensin-converting enzyme (ACE) inhibitors may be beneficial in chronic renal failure but should be used with caution. Close supervision and specialist advice are needed when there is established and significant renal impairment.
[b] Caution with ACE inhibitors and angiotensin II receptor antagonists in peripheral vascular disease because of association with renovascular disease.
[c] If ACE inhibitor indicated.
[d] β-Blockers may worsen heart failure, but in specialist hands may be used to treat heart failure.

tion in patients aged 50 or more with satisfactory control of blood pressure and those with target organ damage, diabetes or a 10-year coronary risk of more than 15%.

Statin
Cholesterol lowering therapy is recommended for hypertensive patients when serum cholesterol is more than 5.0 mmol/L and 10-year coronary risk is more than 30%.

Medical management

Antihypertensive medication
Guidelines for the decision to initiate pharmacological therapy were produced by the British Hypertension Society in 1999 and are shown in Figure 1.52.

Each drug class has specific indications and contraindications (Table 1.31); however, when these circumstances do not apply, the drug that has been backed by the most evidence is the thiazide diuretic, and this should be the initial agent of choice for the treatment of hypertension.[2]

Each drug should be allowed 4 weeks before the response is assessed. The dose of each drug (except thiazide diuretics) should be increased accordingly if satisfactory control (less than 140/85 mmHg) is not achieved.

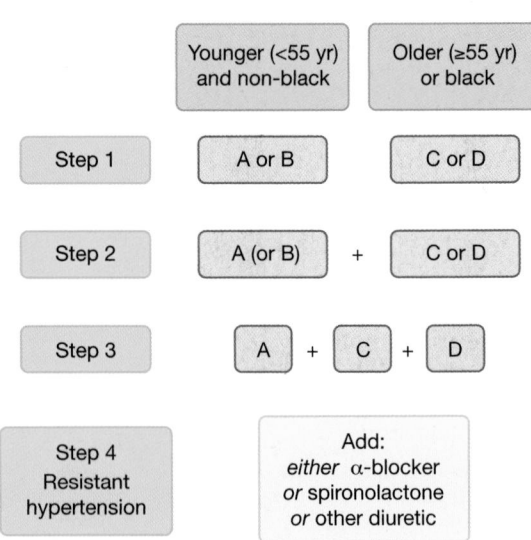

Guidelines for combination therapy. A, ACE inhibitor or angiotensin receptor blocker; B, β-blocker; C, calcium channel blocker; D, diuretic (thiazide).

Fig. 1.53 From Brown MJ, Cruickshank JK, Dominiczak AF, et al. Better blood pressure control: how to combine drugs. Journal of Human Hypertension 2003; 17: 81–86.

If the first drug is well tolerated but the response is small, substitution with another drug is appropriate when hypertension is mild and uncomplicated. However, in severe or complicated hypertension it is safer to add drugs stepwise until blood pressure control is attained. Drug combinations are best tailored to the individual, with guidance from Figure 1.53.

Prognosis

Death from hypertension relates primarily to the increased risk of ischaemic heart disease and stroke. The risk of premature death increases with blood pressure and age. Each 20 mmHg increase in systolic (or 10 mmHg increase in diastolic) pressure increases the risk of death by coronary heart disease or stroke approximately 2-fold in patients aged 40–69 years, and approximately 1.5-fold in patients aged 70–89 years.[3]

REFERENCES

(1) *Wolf-Maier K, Cooper RS, Banegas JR, et al. Hypertension prevalence and blood pressure levels in 6 European countries, Canada, and the United States. JAMA 2003; 289: 2363–2369.*
(2) *The ALLHAT Officers and Coordinators for the ALLHAT Collaborative Research Group. Major outcomes in high-risk hypertensive patients randomized to angiotensin-converting enzyme inhibitor or calcium channel blocker vs diuretic: the Antihypertensive and Lipid-Lowering treatment to prevent Heart Attack Trial (ALLHAT). JAMA 2002; 288: 2981–2997.*
(3) *Lewington S, Clarke R, Qizilbash N, Peto R, Collins R. Age-specific relevance of usual blood pressure to vascular mortality: a meta-analysis of individual data for one million adults in 61 prospective studies. Lancet 2002; 360: 1903–1913.*

SECTION 1.15   Heart transplantation

Indications

Cardiac transplantation is the only established surgical treatment of advanced heart failure and is reserved for patients with irreversible cardiac disease, unacceptable quality of life and high risk of mortality despite optimum medical therapy.

Patient preparation

Appropriate candidate selection by precise risk stratification and exclusion of patients with unacceptable operative risk, irreversible end organ failure or active malignancy is performed as part of a stringent and comprehensive preoperative workup. Donor organs are matched principally on ABO blood compatibility, followed by height and weight.

Procedure

The recipient operation is undertaken through a median sternotomy, and cardiopulmonary bypass is employed. The superior and inferior vena cava are cannulated separately to divert the flow of blood to the bypass machine and back into the aorta. On arrival of the donor organ, the heart is explanted by excising into the right atrium and cutting along the circumference of the atria, leaving the bases of both atria in the chest. The aorta and pulmonary artery

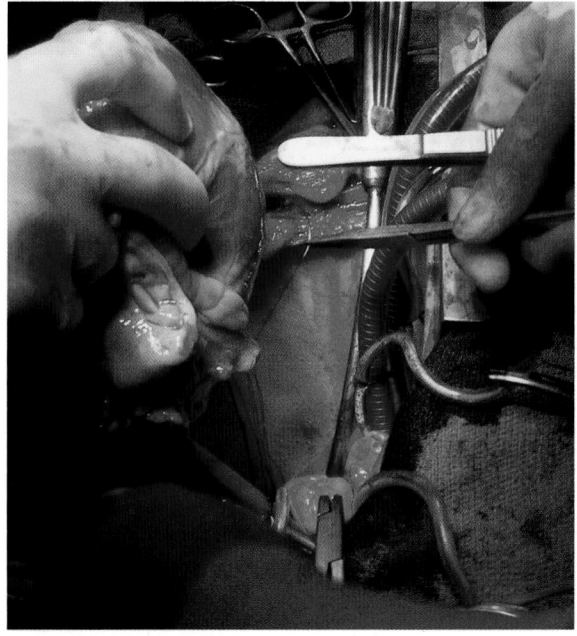

Fig. 1.54 Heart transplantation
Image courtesy of Mr David Jenkins, Consultant Cardiac Surgeon, Papworth Hospital, Cambridge, UK.

are sectioned and the heart is lifted out of the chest. The donor heart is sutured (Fig. 1.54) to the left atrial cuff, then the right atrial cuff and the procedure is completed by performing an end to end anastomosis with the pulmonary artery and aorta.

Complications

Long-term complications of heart transplantation are rejection, predisposition to infection (from immunosuppression), diabetes, hypercholesterolaemia and graft arteriosclerosis.

Post procedure care

Postoperatively, transplant patients are managed on the intensive care unit. Immunosuppression commences from in theatre and standard triple therapy consists of ciclosporin, azathioprine and prednisolone.

Prognosis

After heart transplantation the 1- and 5-year survival is approximately 80% and 70% respectively.[1]

 FURTHER INFORMATION

Selection and treatment of candidates for heart transplantation. A statement for health professionals from the Committee on Heart Failure and Cardiac Transplantation of the Council on Clinical Cardiology, American Heart Association. Circulation 1995; 92: 3593–3612.

REFERENCE

(1) Taylor DO, Edwards LB, Boucek MM, Trulock EP, Keck BM, Hertz MI. The Registry of the International Society for Heart and Lung Transplantation: twenty-first official adult heart transplant report—2004. Journal of Heart and Lung Transplantation 2004; 23: 796–803.

Diseases of the peripheral vascular system

Introduction

Applied basic science of the peripheral vascular system

Anatomy

The distal aorta divides at the level of L2 into the common iliac arteries. The internal iliac artery branches off to supply the pelvic organs 5–8 cm distal to the bifurcation, whilst the common iliac carries on as the external iliac artery. The external iliac becomes the common femoral artery as it passes beneath the inguinal ligament. The profunda femoris artery branches off from the common femoral 5–10 cm below the inguinal ligament supplying the thigh muscles. The common femoral then becomes the superficial femoral artery down to the popliteal area behind the knee. The popliteal artery divides into three branches: the anterior tibial artery, the posterior tibial artery and the peroneal artery. The anterior tibial becomes the dorsalis pedis artery in the foot.

Atherosclerotic disease often manifests due to stenosis or occlusion secondary to thrombosis or emboli. This often occurs at branch points where the calibre of the artery changes, and in the subsartorial canal in the lower thigh. Localized symptomatic stenoses often occur in the iliac (20%), femoral (40%) and distal (20%) arteries. In 20% of patients disease can be found at all of these levels.

The long saphenous vein begins as the continuation of the dorsal venous arch and continues approximately 2 fingerbreadths anterior and superior to the medial malleolus, up the medial aspect of the leg to one hand's breadth posterior to the patella, ending in the saphenofemoral junction approximately 3 cm inferolateral to the pubic tubercle. The anatomical landmarks of the long saphenous vein are important as it is a commonly harvested conduit for vascular and cardiac surgery. In extreme circulatory shock, the consistency of the location in relation to the medial malleolus makes it the venous conduit of choice when emergency access is required (saphenous cutdown).

The short saphenous vein begins posterior to the lateral malleolus, ascending lateral to the tendo calcaneus, progresses to the posterior aspect of the mid calf and terminates in the popliteal vein. Incompetence and varicosities of the short saphenous system are not controlled with a tourniquet applied to the thigh, which is the basis of the Trendelenburg test. Numerous perforating veins are present in the short saphenous system in the ankle, distal calf and knee.

Physiology
Endothelium

Endothelial cells line all vascular tissue and represent a non-thrombogenic biocompatible barrier between blood and extravascular tissue. They allow and facilitate passage of molecules and blood gases to and from blood and tissue. The endothelium together acts as a potent endocrine organ and carefully mediates vascular homeostasis.

Prostacyclin (PGI_2) is produced by the endothelium and inhibits platelet aggregation and formation of platelet derived growth factors. In combination with nitric oxide, it inhibits procoagulants such as thrombin and thromboxane A_2. Heparin sulphate and thrombomodulin also act to reduce the procoagulant effect of thrombin. In addition, the negatively charged vessel wall acts to repel the negatively charged platelets, further inhibiting aggregation.

Dysfunction of the endothelium leads to vasoconstriction, platelet and leukocyte activation, cellular proliferation, pro-oxidation, thrombosis, procoagulation, vascular inflammation and ultimately atherosclerosis.

Venous system

At rest, the pressure in the venous system at the foot is equal to the column of standing blood that extends from the heart to the foot. The presence of one-way valves and the muscular activity of the calf muscles act to pump the blood back to the heart. When the valves become incompetent the pressure exerted on the veins causes dilatation and tortuosity (i.e. veins become varicose); as the system of valves is lost, venous pressure increases. Eventually, the increased venous pressure limits the outflow of blood from the leg and results in tissue hypoxia predisposing to venous ulceration.

Symptoms of peripheral vascular disease

Arterial disease

Blood flow through the arterial system may be reduced gradually or suddenly, in either large or small vessels. This leads to a range of potential presenting symptoms.

Claudication

Claudication is muscle pain that occurs with exercise. It is often cramping in nature and relieved by rest. Once recovered, the patient is able to exercise again for a similar duration before the cramp recurs. It is caused by chronic stenosis or occlusion in the artery feeding the muscle group: for example, calf pain on walking due to superficial femoral artery occlusion.

Rest pain

Pain occurring at rest reflects more severe ischaemia, either chronic or acute. The distal parts of the limb and foot are most affected, unlike claudication which involves the muscle groups in the calf and thigh. Typically rest pain is aggravated by elevation of the limb. Foot pain is therefore worse at night. The patient may wake to hang the foot out of the bed, or get up and walk around until the foot recovers. The pain is severe and often requires strong analgesics to control it.

Colour changes of the limb

Acute arterial occlusion leads to a pale 'white' leg because the vessels in the skin contain little blood. These vessels then dilate and fill slowly with de-oxygenated blood producing a 'mottled blue' discolouration. If the occlusion is acute on chronic there will be some collateral supply: the colour change may not be so dramatic and may recover to normal.

In chronic ischaemia the foot will become pale when elevated but is often red when dependent due to reactive hyperaemia. These colour changes form the basis of Buerger's test for chronic severe ischaemia.

Sensory motor symptoms

With severe ischaemia patients may describe numbness of the foot or toes. Loss of motor function with weakness or paralysis is seen in severe acute ischaemia.

Change in temperature

The ischaemic limb fails to maintain a normal temperature and becomes cold. Patients may take to wearing thick socks and wrapping the feet in blankets. This does help to warm the limb to some extent and can occasionally be misleading.

Venous disease

Pain

The pain associated with venous insufficiency is often an ache on standing that gets worse as the day progresses. Distended varicose veins may be a focus of pain and tenderness. Inflamed thrombosed veins (thrombophlebitis) are acutely painful, red and tender.

Swelling

Oedema from the ankle extending up the leg is a common symptom in patients with worsening venous insufficiency.

Examination of the peripheral vascular system

Arterial system

The vascular examination involves looking for signs of ischaemia, listening for bruits and feeling for pulses.

Upper limbs

The hands should be inspected looking for anaemia (this can worsen symptoms of claudication) and tendon xanthoma (associated with hypercholesterolaemia). The radial pulse is obtained, noting the rhythm, rate and strength. An irregularly irregular pulse from atrial fibrillation is an important indicator of the source of emboli. The ulnar and brachial pulses should be palpated simultaneously in both arms. Compare the blood pressure in both arms. Feel the radial pulse with the arm elevated and abducted to assess subclavian artery compression at the thoracic outlet. A bruit in the supraclavicular fossa may also be heard during this manoeuvre with subclavian stenosis.

The supply to the palmar arch of the hand via the ulnar and radial arteries can be assessed by Allen's test. The radial and ulnar arteries are occluded at the wrist and the patient elevates the hand and opens and closes the fist. The palm becomes blanched and the pressure on the ulnar artery is released. The flow from the ulnar artery results in colour returning quickly to the palm. The procedure is repeated, releasing the radial artery. Both arteries should fill the palmar arch.

Head and neck

Pallor of the conjunctiva may suggest anaemia, and xanthelasma or arcus senilis is associated with hyperlipidaemia. The carotid pulse is palpable in front of the sternomastoid muscle in the anterior triangle of the neck. A bruit may be due to carotid stenosis (subtotal stenosis or occluded carotid arteries do not have bruits). Bilateral bruits of similar nature may be transmitted from aortic stenosis.

Abdomen

The epigastrium is palpated to screen for an aortic aneurysm, which is usually noticeable as an expansile swelling. A pulsatile mass in the iliac fossa may represent an iliac aneurysm. An abdominal bruit may arise from the abdominal aorta, iliac arteries, renal or mesenteric arterial stenoses.

Lower limbs

The feet are examined for discolouration, ulcers, gangrene and deformities. With peripheral vascular disease, the foot and leg are cold. Capillary refill is assessed in the toes. The femoral, popliteal, posterior tibial and dorsalis pedis pulses are palpated and compared between the two limbs. Pulses distal to the site of disease are weak or absent.

Auscultation is performed along the course of all major arteries to screen for bruits. Buerger's test is the angle at which the leg is elevated before it becomes white. Normally, the legs can be raised to 90 degrees without any discolouration. Buerger's test is the angle at which the leg is elevated before it becomes white, however the dependent hyperaemia that occurs when the leg is lower is usually a more important sign.

Venous system
Lower limb
The lower limb is inspected for skin changes and oedema. Brown staining can occur from haemosiderin deposition with venous insufficiency. Other features of venous insufficiency include the red, flaky, itchy patches that can arise from venous eczema. Purple tender plaques of inflamed skin and subcutaneous tissues can arise from lipodermatosclerosis (Fig. 1.55), or white scars of healed previous ulcers, 'atrophie blanche', may be observed (Fig. 1.56). Open non-healed ulceration commonly occurs in the gaiter area of the leg (p. 95–96).

The patient should also be examined standing, to assess the distribution of any varicose or distended veins (Fig. 1.57). The varicose veins should be palpable along their course and the tap test can be performed to assess their distribution and connection to the saphenous systems. The saphenofemoral and saphenopopliteal junctions are palpated and an impulse is elicited with coughing in an incompetent system. The level of major venous incom-

petence can be assessed with the Trendelenburg test in which the leg veins are emptied and a tourniquet is applied to the mid thigh. Control of the varicose veins in the lower leg implies insufficiency at the saphenofemoral junction. The location of insufficiency can be more accurately identified with a hand-held Doppler, listening for reflux in the long and short saphenous systems.

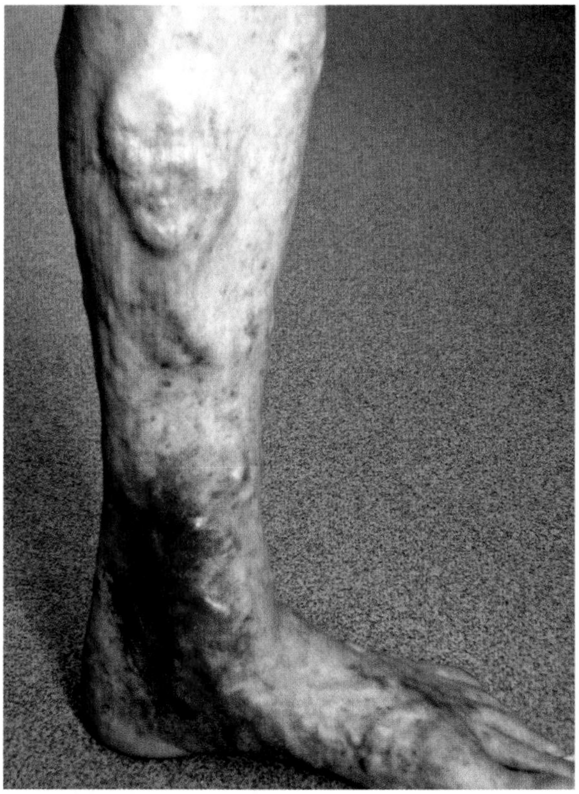

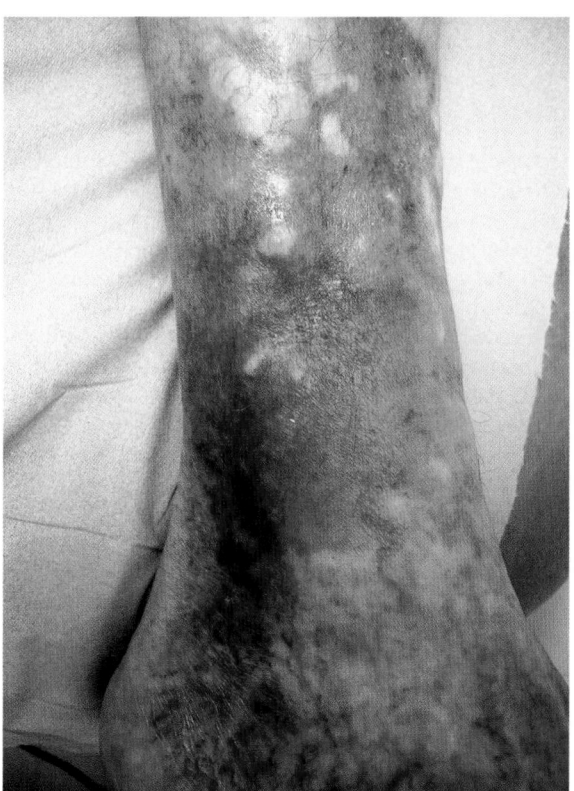

Fig. 1.56 Atrophie blanche.

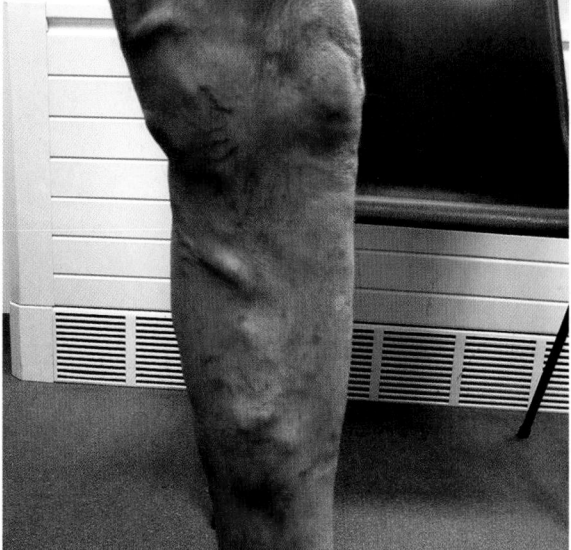

Fig. 1.57 Varicose veins.

Applied basic science
of the peripheral
vascular system

Symptoms of peripheral
vascular disease

**Examination of the
peripheral vascular
system**

Fig. 1.55 Lipodermatosclerosis.

Investigations for peripheral vascular disease

Ankle brachial pressure index

The ankle brachial pressure index (ABPI) is the ratio of the systolic blood pressure in the ankle as compared to the arm (which is used as the reference value). Using a hand-held Doppler, an arterial signal from the dorsalis pedis, posterior tibial and peroneal arteries at the ankle can normally be heard. A blood pressure cuff can be used to occlude the arteries in the lower calf and the pressure at which the arterial signal is lost is the ankle systolic pressure (Fig. 1.58). The highest pressure from the three ankle arteries should be used to calculate the ABPI.

In the absence of any stenosis or occlusions in the lower limb arteries this pressure should be equal to or greater than the systolic pressure in the arm. The ABPI is normally more than 1.0. It decreases with increasing severity of peripheral arterial disease. Patients with mild to moderate claudication often have an ABPI of 0.7–0.9. Patients with rest pain often have an ABPI of less than 0.5. Some classifications place more emphasis on the absolute ankle pressure rather than the ratio, and an ankle pressure of less than 50 mmHg is used to indicate critical ischaemia (p. 79).

There are a few situations in which the ABPI may be difficult or misleading. If the calf arteries are heavily calcified (as in diabetes) the ABPI may be falsely elevated, as the pressure cuff fails to occlude the rigid calcified arteries. Patients with painful ulceration in the calf may not tolerate a tight cuff on the leg, and a toe pressure can be used in these situations. Measurement of toe pressure is usually undertaken with specialized equipment in a vascular laboratory.

Colour duplex ultrasound

Most ultrasound scanners produce an ultrasound image and are able to detect the Doppler shift effect due to flowing blood. This is added into the image as a colour signal that is related to the velocity of the blood flow. Arterial and venous flow can therefore be mapped and quantified using colour duplex ultrasound—a very useful, non-invasive technique for investigating both arterial and venous disease (Fig. 1.59).

Arterial duplex is particularly useful for easily accessible vessels such as the carotid artery and the lower limb vessels. For more diffuse and complex disease, particularly involving deeper arteries such as the iliac and aorta, formal angiography may be required.

In venous disease, duplex ultrasound has become the gold standard investigation, and contrast venography is now rarely used.

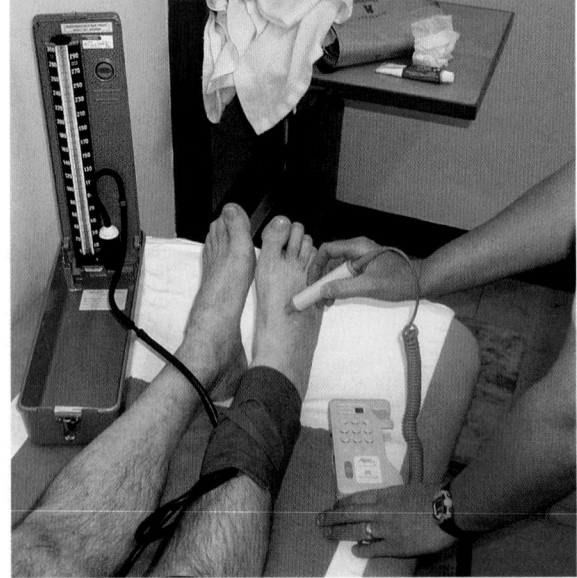

Fig. 1.58 Ankle pressure measurements.

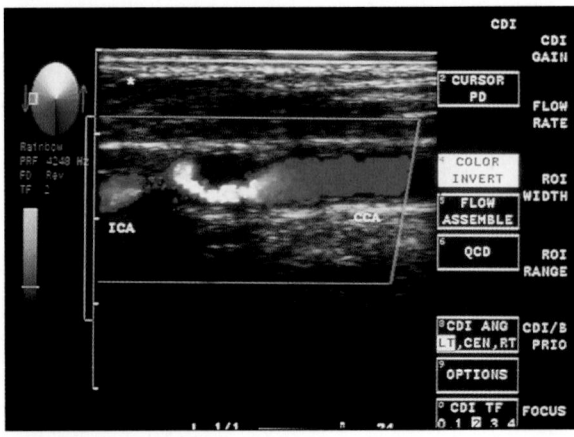

Fig. 1.59 Carotid duplex scan.

Digital subtraction angiography (DSA)

The arterial tree can be imaged by the use of contrast injected into the arteries and imaged on conventional X-ray. The image is processed by subtracting the background of bones and soft tissues, leaving a clear view of the arteries alone. In most cases a catheter is inserted over a wire into the arterial system via the common femoral artery in the groin under local anaesthetic. If the femoral arteries are blocked, the brachial or axillary artery in the arm may be used. Contrast is injected via the catheter and outlines the lumen of the artery to provide an accurate map of any stenoses or occlusions (Fig. 1.60). By carefully placing the catheter in the area of interest, excellent images of most arterial territories can be obtained.

DSA is an invasive technique. Its complications include bleeding from the arterial puncture site, occasionally leading to haematoma and less commonly false aneurysm formation. Damage to the femoral artery can lead to occlusion, dissection, thrombosis and embolism. The presence of the catheter itself in the artery being studied may also cause local thrombosis, embolism, dissection or perforation. The use of contrast may lead to anaphylactic reactions and renal impairment. In general, the major complication rate after diagnostic DSA is only 2%.

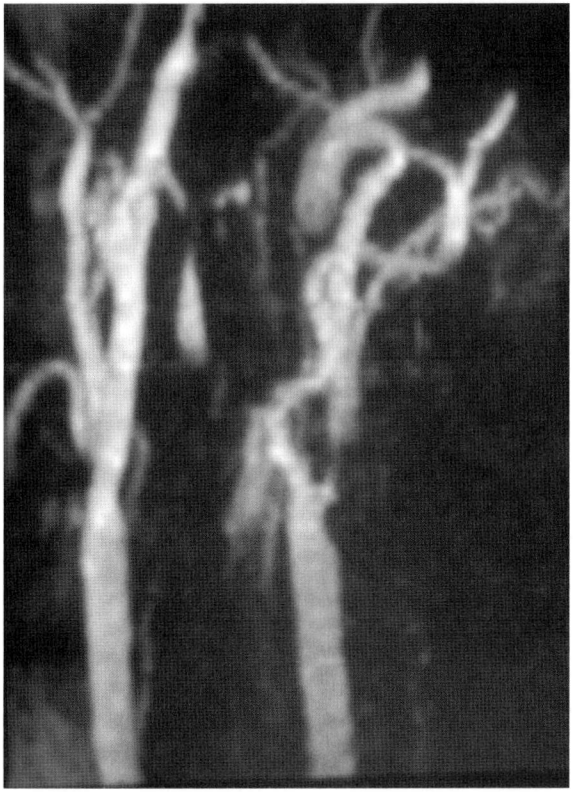

Fig. 1.61 Magnetic resonance angiogram of the carotid arteries.

Ankle brachial pressure index

Colour duplex ultrasound

Digital subtraction angiography (DSA)

Magnetic resonance angiography (MRA)

Computed tomographic angiography

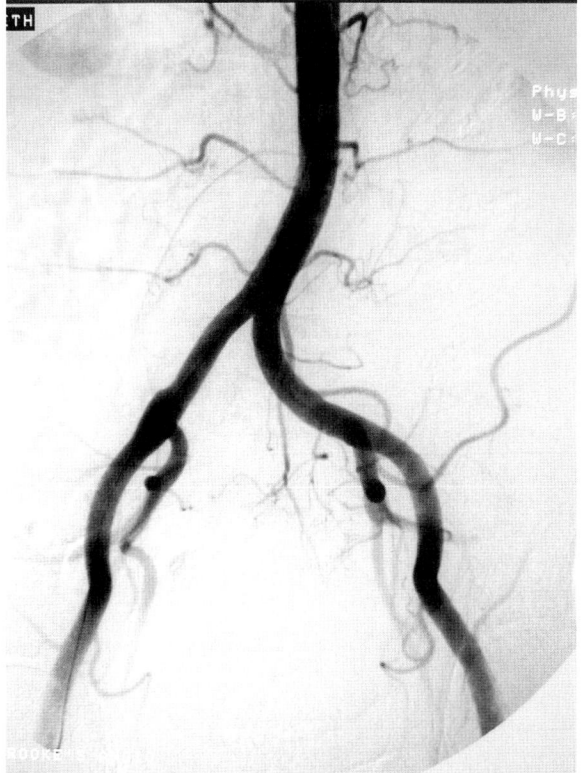

Fig. 1.60 Digital subtraction angiogram. This investigation shows the aorta, iliac and femoral arteries.

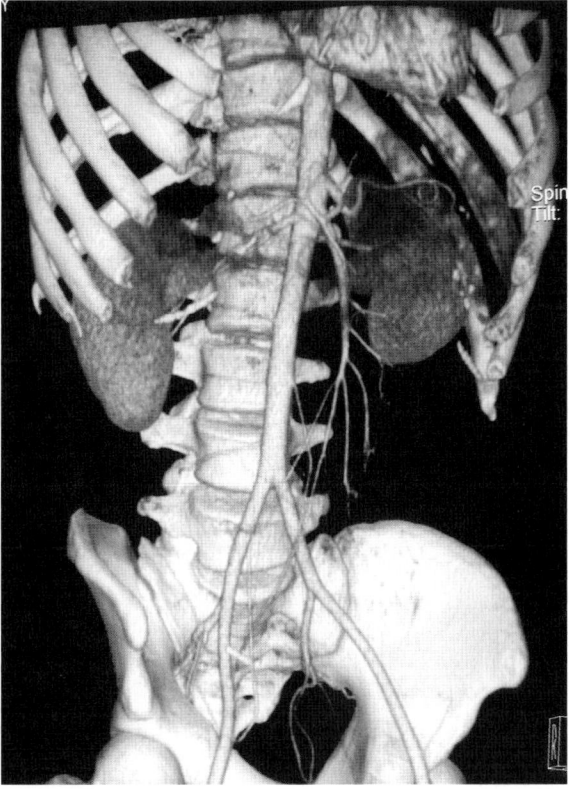

Fig. 1.62 CT angiography. Three-dimensional CT reconstruction of the aorta and iliac arteries.

Magnetic resonance angiography (MRA)

Magnetic resonance imaging (MRI) can be used to study blood flow. Intravenous contrast injected via the brachial veins is used to improve image quality, and with modern MRI machines and appropriate processing of the data excellent images of the arterial tree can be obtained (Fig. 1.61). MRA is less invasive than DSA; the contrast load is significantly less and X-ray exposure is avoided. However, in many countries, the cost and unavailability of MRI (especially for out of hours imaging) may limit the extent to which MRA is used.

Computed tomographic angiography

As with MRI, modern helical or spiral CT scanners can be used to study arteries and veins (Fig. 1.62). Intravenous contrast is used to enhance the images, therefore the procedure is less invasive than DSA.

SECTION 1.18 — Peripheral arterial disease

Acute limb ischaemia

Acute limb ischaemia occurs when there is a sudden reduction in blood supply to a large proportion of the limb. There is a spectrum of presentation but the most common is within 24–48 hours with a threatened limb requiring urgent revascularization.

Epidemiology

Acute limb ischaemia is a common surgical emergency, often in elderly patients (mean age 75) with significant cardiac comorbidity. Men and women are equally affected. Acute limb ischaemia is five times more common in the lower limb compared to the upper limb.

Pathology

The two major pathological processes leading to acute limb ischaemia are thrombosis in situ and embolism. Thrombosis in situ has now become a more common cause of acute limb ischaemia, accounting for 60% of patients with acute limb ischaemia. Two decades ago, embolism secondary to rheumatic atrial fibrillation was more common.

Thrombosis in situ refers to the acute occlusion of a major limb artery by thrombosis in a vessel with pre-existing disease. The patient with established atherosclerosis in the limb suffers an acute major deterioration.

The majority of emboli to the limb originate in the heart (90%). Other sources include the aorta (5%). Emboli often lodge at branch points of peripheral arteries where the vessel diameter decreases, but the eventual site is determined by the size of the embolus. Smaller emboli tend to lodge more distally. Common sites include the femoral artery (75%) and the popliteal artery (15%); large emboli may lodge in the aorto-iliac junction (aorto-iliac saddle embolus in 10%). The arteries in the leg may be free of disease.

Other less common causes of acute limb ischaemia are trauma, dissection, non-occlusive limb ischaemia (low flow states such as cardiogenic shock) and venous gangrene due to extensive venous occlusion combined with compartment syndrome (Table 1.32).

Scope of disease

Unresolved acute limb ischaemia threatens limb viability with the development of gangrene, systemic sepsis and even death. Muscle necrosis releases myoglobin into the circulation which will precipitate in the renal tubules and cause acute renal failure. Pain control can be difficult since severe ischaemia induces a severe unremitting pain.

Clinical features

Patients with acute limb ischaemia present with a painful, pulseless, paralyzed leg (Table 1.33). It is important to

Table 1.32	Causes of acute limb ischaemia
Thrombosis in situ	
Embolism (from the heart and aorta)	
Trauma	
Dissection	
Non-occlusive limb ischaemia (cardiogenic shock)	
Venous gangrene	

Table 1.33	Clinical features of acute limb ischaemia
Pale	
Painful	
Perishing cold	
Pulseless	
Paraesthesia	
Paralysis	

ascertain if the patient has severe existing atherosclerosis (smokers, diabetics, patients with existing claudication) as he/she is more likely to have suffered from thrombosis in situ. Alternatively, patients with a history of cardiac disease (atrial fibrillation, recent myocardial infarction, known ventricular aneurysm) are more likely to have suffered an arterial embolus.

On examination, the limb is pale and cold. Palpation of pulses in both lower limbs is important. Patients with existing atherosclerotic disease (arteriopaths) with thrombosis in situ may have few lower limb pulses. Patients with a unilateral embolus usually have good distal pulses in the non-affected leg. Neurosensory deficit with loss of sensation and movement indicates a more severe level of ischaemia. Calf muscle tenderness may indicate the development of muscle swelling and compartment syndrome. A prominent swelling behind the knee (pulsatile or not) may indicate a popliteal aneurysm as the underlying cause, and the abdomen should also be examined for the presence of an aortic aneurysm which may have been the source for an embolus.

Initial investigations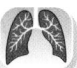

Full blood count
Polycythaemia and thrombocythaemia both predispose to thrombosis.

Coagulation screen
A baseline coagulation screen is important, as anticoagulant agents are often required.

Urea and electrolytes
Impaired renal function with rising serum creatinine and elevated serum potassium can result from acute limb ischaemia.

Glucose
Serum glucose is performed to screen for diabetes.

Electrocardiogram
An ECG is important to confirm the rhythm and screen for atrial fibrillation. New Q waves may indicate a recent myocardial infarction.

Chest X-ray
A chest film may reveal an enlarged heart (cardiac failure, left ventricular aneurysm) or a dilated thoracic aorta (source of emboli).

Ankle Doppler pressures
Listen for an arterial signal over the dorsalis pedis, posterior tibial and peroneal arteries. The presence of one arterial signal is a good sign. If possible, the pressure is measured using the Doppler signal. The absence of any arterial signals usually indicates severe ischaemia requiring urgent revascularization. Venous signals may become difficult to hear when limbs become non-viable.

Further investigations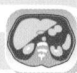

Arteriogram
Imaging of the arterial tree is required to make a precise diagnosis. The urgency is dictated by the condition of the limb. In most severe cases an emergency arteriogram (DSA, CT or MRA) is required. If the clinical diagnosis is highly suggestive of an embolus, an embolectomy may be performed without an arteriogram.

Initial management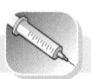

Intravenous fluids
It is important to establish venous access and to commence maintenance fluids as patients should initially be kept nil by mouth.

Analgesia
Analgesia is administered and intravenous opiates may be required in patients with severe ischaemic pain.

Intravenous unfractionated heparin
A 5000 unit bolus of unfractionated heparin is administered to inhibit clot propagation and prevent further deterioration. For patients with mild symptoms due to distal occlusion, heparin alone may be sufficient treatment (Table 1.34).

Forced alkaline diuresis
Early intravenous fluids and furosemide administered to patients with renal impairment may limit the renal injury from myoglobinuria.

Medical management

Revascularization is required for patients with viable limbs. The decision for the optimum treatment usually lies between thrombolysis and surgery.

Thrombolysis
Local catheter-directed thrombolysis can be used to treat acute limb ischaemia. The characteristics of patients most suitable for this technique are listed in Table 1.35.

Under angiographic control, a narrow-bore catheter is placed within the clot. A bolus of the lytic agent is administered into the clot and an infusion commenced. The patient is monitored in the high-dependency unit or a vascular ward for bleeding or failure of treatment and deterioration

Table 1.34	Management options for acute limb ischaemia
Heparin alone	
Intra-arterial thrombolysis	
Embolectomy	
Surgical bypass	
Amputation	

Table 1.35	Indications and contraindications for intra-arterial thrombolysis
Indication	**Contraindication**
Short history of ischaemia (<7 days)	Chronic ischaemia
Viable limb with time for lysis to occur	Threatened limb (early resolution required)
No bleeding risk (no cerebrovascular accident or gastrointestinal bleed)	Bleeding risk
Young age	Age more than 75
Short occlusion on angiography	Long occlusion, poor run-off

of the condition. Further angiographic images are obtained to confirm successful lysis of the clot. Lysis commonly takes 8–12 hours but may take up to 48 hours.

Although thrombolysis may reduce the need for a surgical procedure in the majority, more patients subsequently develop recurrent ischaemia or require amputation compared to patients undergoing surgery.[1,2]

Surgical management

Embolectomy

Surgical embolectomy is performed by a cutdown onto the vessel containing the embolus (common femoral, popliteal or brachial) under local or general anaesthetic. An arteriotomy is made and a balloon embolectomy catheter is introduced into the vessel and advanced distal to the embolus. The balloon is then inflated and the clot is extracted by pulling back on the catheter. The arteriotomy is closed and flow restored to the limb.

Bypass surgery

For patients with thrombosed diseased arteries, balloon embolectomy is less successful and a formal surgical bypass procedure is preferred (p. 82–83).

Fasciotomy

If compartment syndrome is present or suspected, a fasciotomy can be performed at the end of the procedure (Fig. 1.63).

Amputation

Amputation is the most appropriate management option for patients with non-viable limbs.

Prognosis

In-hospital outcomes are poor: the amputation rate is up to 30% and there is an overall mortality rate of 25%. Many patients are high risk as they have cardiac comorbidity and widespread atherosclerosis.

i FURTHER INFORMATION

Callum K, Bradbury A. Acute limb ischaemia. ABC of arterial and venous disease. BMJ 2000; 320: 764–767.

REFERENCES

(1) *Weaver FA, Comerota AJ, Youngblood M, Froehlich J, Hosking JD, Papanicolaou G. Surgical revascularization versus thrombolysis for nonembolic lower extremity native artery occlusions: results of a prospective randomized trial. The STILE Investigators. Surgery versus Thrombolysis for Ischemia of the Lower Extremity. Journal of Vascular Surgery 1996; 24: 513–521; discussion 521–523.*
(2) *Korn P, Khilnani NM, Fellers JC, Lee TY, Winchester PA, Bush HL, Kent KC. Thrombolysis for native arterial occlusions of the lower extremities: clinical outcome and cost. Journal of Vascular Surgery 2001; 33: 1148–1157.*

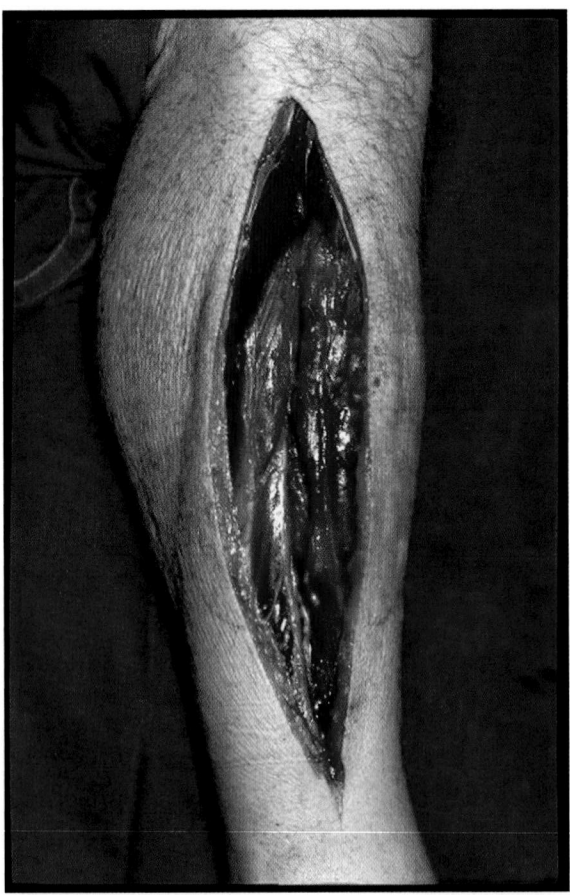

Fig. 1.63 Medial fasciotomy.

Chronic limb ischaemia

Chronic limb ischaemia refers (usually) to gradual onset ischaemic symptoms (Table 1.36) in the limbs of more than 14 days.

Table 1.36	Fontaine classification of chronic lower limb ischaemia
I	Asymptomatic
IIa	Mild claudication
IIb	Moderate/severe claudication
III	Ischaemic rest pain
IV	Ulceration or gangrene

Epidemiology

Intermittent claudication is common and affects up to 10% of patients over the age of 65 years. More severe critical limb ischaemia (Table 1.37) occurs in up to 30 per 100 000 per year. The incidence increases with age; it is initially more common in men but there is equal incidence by the age of 80 years.

Table 1.37	Definition of chronic critical leg ischaemia

Chronic critical leg ischemia is defined as either:

1. more than 2 weeks of recurrent foot pain at rest that requires regular use of analgesics, or
2. a non-healing wound or gangrene of the foot or toes that is associated with ankle systolic pressure of 50 mmHg or less or a toe systolic pressure of 30 mmHg or less

Pathology

The most common cause of limb ischaemia is stenosis of the blood vessels due to atherosclerosis. The risk factors include increasing age, male sex, smoking, diabetes, hypertension and hypercholesterolaemia (p. 460). With time, non-flow-limiting disease progresses to subcritical then critical stenosis, finally leading to occlusion. Multilevel disease is often responsible for more severe ischaemia. Over a third of patients are diabetic.

Scope of disease

Skin breakdown with severe ischaemia leads to painful non-healing ulceration. More extensive necrosis leads to gangrenous change. This may remain localized but can be associated with superadded infection, extension of the gangrene and septicaemia (Fig. 1.64). As patients often have widespread atherosclerosis, concomitant coronary and cerebrovascular disease is common.

Clinical features

Depending on the duration and severity of the disease, the symptoms of chronic limb ischaemia may include claudication, rest pain, ulceration and gangrene.

Claudication is lower limb pain that occurs with exercise and is relieved by rest. It commonly affects the calf muscles due to femoral and popliteal artery disease. Symptoms in the thigh and buttock suggest more proximal disease of the aorto-iliac segment. It is important to note the claudication distance as it is a simple measure of disease progression.

The classical history of shortening claudication distance progressing to rest pain at night is uncommon as many elderly patients do not walk fast or far enough to develop claudication. Therefore the first presentation of chronic lower limb ischaemia in the elderly may be rest pain or ulceration of relatively short duration.

A detailed history also includes the risk factors for atherosclerosis and complications of atherosclerosis (angina, myocardial infarction, cerebrovascular accident, transient ischaemic attack). Patients with few or none of the risk factors or atypical symptoms may have other causes of leg pain such as nerve entrapment, hip or knee arthritis, or cauda equina stenosis.

On examination, the leg may be pale with loss of hairs. There may be evidence of gangrene (Fig. 1.64) or ulcers on the pressure points such as the soles of the feet. Capillary refill time may be prolonged. Palpation of the leg pulses is important and will characterize the distribution of the disease. In diabetics with foot ulceration and ischaemia, the extent of the neuropathy can be assessed by sensory testing.

Initial investigations

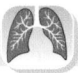

Full blood count
Anaemia will aggravate claudication symptoms.

Lipid profile
Hypercholesterolaemia is an important modifiable risk factor.

Urea and electrolytes
Elevated serum creatinine can result from coexisting renovascular disease (p. 734).

Ankle brachial pressure index
The ankle brachial pressure index (ABPI) can confirm the presence of peripheral vascular disease and assess its severity (p. 76).

Further investigations

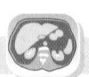

Treadmill test
If the ABPI is normal (more than 1.0) at rest but claudication is suspected, a repeat ABPI after exercise is performed. Patients with less severe stenosis may develop an abnormal ABPI only after exercise as the vessel calibre is sufficient

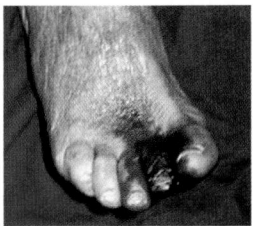

Fig. 1.64 Chronic limb ischaemia with distal gangrene.

81

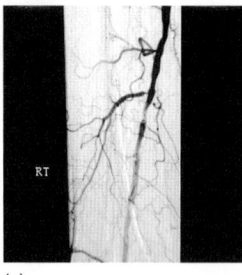

(a)

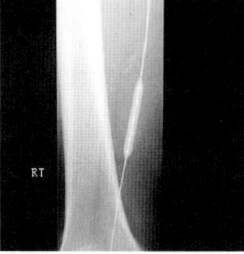

(b)

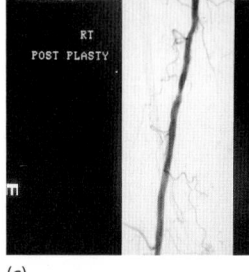

(c)

Fig. 1.65 Percutaneous balloon angioplasty. This series of images shows (a) multiple stenoses in the femoral artery, a fully inflated angioplasty balloon (b), and the post angioplasty result (c).

to provide normal flows at rest but cannot accommodate higher flows on exercise compared to the upper limb arteries.

Colour duplex ultrasound

Localized disease in patients with claudication is often effectively imaged with colour duplex ultrasound. The information provided may indicate whether the underlying disease is likely to be suitable for angioplasty.

Angiography

Patients with critical ischaemia often have widespread multilevel disease that is better imaged with digital subtraction angiogram (see Fig. 1.65a), CT or MR angiography.

Initial management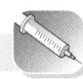

Exercise

An exercise programme (preferably supervised) can help patients to increase their walking distance.

Risk factor modification

Patients with claudication due to relatively mild peripheral vascular disease benefit from an initial period of exercise and risk factor modification. Patients should be encouraged and assisted to stop smoking as walking distance and mortality are both improved. Statin treatment reduces cardiovascular events by up to 33%.

Antiplatelet therapy

All patients with confirmed peripheral vascular disease will benefit from an antiplatelet agent to reduce thromboembolic events such as myocardial infarction, stroke and death.[1] Low-dose aspirin (75 mg) is well tolerated, and clopidogrel may be a suitable alternative.

RECENT ADVANCES

Combined antiplatelet treatments (aspirin and clopidogrel) are being evaluated but no evidence for their superiority yet exists.

Medical management

Pentoxifylline

Pentoxifylline may be helpful in rare patients who do not respond to exercise therapy or who cannot exercise. Definitive supportive evidence for the use of pentoxifylline is lacking.

 CLINICAL ALERT

In critical limb ischaemia there is no time available for the above medical measures to take effect. Antiplatelet agents and analgesia are useful whilst planning urgent angioplasty or surgical revascularization to salvage the limb.

Surgical management

Angioplasty and stenting

In general, angioplasty is more suited to patients with focal short arterial lesions in the larger proximal vessels of the limb. In high-risk patients, angioplasty may be attempted for more diffuse disease down into the popliteal and calf vessels.

Access to the arterial lumen is usually achieved via the femoral artery. A needle is inserted under local anaesthesia, then a wire is threaded through the needle and the needle is removed. The wire is then manipulated across the narrowed or occluded segment of artery under X-ray control. Once the wire is in position, a catheter with a balloon can be passed over the wire into position (Seldinger technique). As each balloon will inflate to a predetermined size, the artery can be 'stretched' in a controlled fashion to re-establish the normal lumen diameter by selecting the appropriate balloon (Fig. 1.65a–c). The underlying atherosclerotic plaque is split and remoulded within the adventitia.

There is a risk of embolism and thrombosis resulting from this process. The wall may re-stenose due to elastic recoil and spasm in the adventitia. Insertion of an expandable, inert metal stent can be used to overcome these problems. Stenting is commonly used in the iliac arteries but is less successful in the smaller femoral, popliteal and calf arteries.

Other complications of angioplasty are vessel rupture, dissection, bleeding from the puncture site and contrast induced renal impairment. Serious complications occur in approximately 5%.

RECENT ADVANCES

Trials of drug eluting stents, as used in the coronary arteries, are ongoing in the femoral arteries. If successful, there may be an increased role for stenting in the femoral arteries in the future.

Surgical bypass/endarterectomy

A bypass procedure is the most common open surgical procedure carried out in the lower limb for ischaemia, requiring a general or regional anaesthetic. Patient fitness is a key factor in deciding on the risks of surgery, and preoperative preparation is vitally important to optimize the patient's cardiac, respiratory, and renal function.

The name given to each procedure describes where the bypass starts and finishes: for example, axillo-femoral, aorto-femoral, ilio-femoral, femoro-popliteal, and femoro-crural bypass. Artificial Dacron or PTFE conduits are used to bypass larger arteries above the groin. Below the groin, best results in the smaller femoral and popliteal are achieved using the patient's own long saphenous vein as a conduit (Fig. 1.66).

An important principle underlying bypass operations is the exposure and control of the inflow and outflow artery above and below the diseased segments. The arteries can then be clamped, opened and the conduit sewn on to both

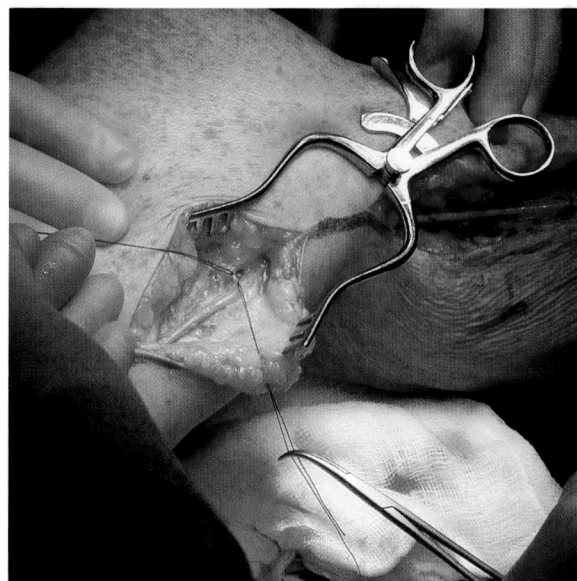
Fig. 1.66 Femoropopliteal bypass using long saphenous vein.

ends. When the clamps are released, blood flows through the conduit, bypassing the diseased segment to supply blood to the distal vessel. Occasionally, if the diseased section is short, an endarterectomy can be performed which involves coring out the atheroma.

Complications after surgery include thrombosis leading to graft occlusion, bleeding and infection (more common with artificial grafts). Patients with vascular disease frequently have comorbid conditions and are therefore prone to a wide number of systemic postoperative problems such as angina, myocardial infarction, arrhythmia, chest infection, deep vein thrombosis, pulmonary embolism, renal failure, coagulopathy and bowel ischaemia. A high level of postoperative monitoring and early intervention is required to minimize the risk and limit the effects of these complications.

Prognosis

In general, the symptoms of claudication stabilize in 80%; 20% progress to more severe ischaemia. Only 4% of claudicants undergo an amputation; however, their 5- and 10-year survival probability is 70% and 50% respectively. The excess mortality is largely due to cardiovascular causes such as myocardial infarction and stroke. Patients with critical limb ischaemia have a 75% survival probability and a 29% amputation rate at 1 year despite intervention.

i FURTHER INFORMATION

Beard JD Chronic lower limb ischaemia. ABC of arterial and venous disease. BMJ 2000: 320; 854–857.

Shearman CP Management of intermittent claudication. British Journal of Surgery 2002: 89; 529–531.

Audit Committee of the Vascular Surgical Society of Great Britain and Ireland. Recommendations for the management of chronic critical lower limb ischaemia. European Journal of Vascular and Endovascular Surgery 1996; 12: 131–135.

REFERENCE

(1) *Collaborative overview of randomised trials of antiplatelet therapy. Prevention of death, myocardial infarction, and stroke by prolonged antiplatelet therapy in various categories of patients. BMJ 1994; 308: 81–106.*

SECTION 1.19 Carotid artery disease

Epidemiology

The prevalence of asymptomatic carotid disease has been estimated to be 6400 per 100 000 in patients aged 50–79 years.[1] It is more common in men than in women and the prevalence increases with age.

Pathology

Atherosclerosis is the main aetiological agent of carotid artery disease. The build-up of atherosclerotic plaque leads to narrowing of the carotid lumen. The resulting transient ischaemic attacks (TIA) and strokes are a result of plaque emboli.

Clinical features

Many patients with carotid stenosis are asymptomatic; in those with symptoms, transient ischaemic attacks and anterior circulation strokes are the main manifestations. On examination a bruit may be auscultated; however, patients with subtotal stenosis and occluded carotid vessels do not have sufficient blood flow to generate a bruit. Overall, the sensitivity and specificity of carotid auscultation for the detection of important (70–99%) stenosis was 56% and 91% respectively.[2] Therefore, the presence of a bruit is useful to rule in the diagnosis, but the absence of a bruit cannot reliably rule out important stenoses.

Investigations

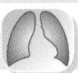

High-resolution Doppler ultrasonography

Doppler assessment is the investigation of choice for patients with carotid disease. Colour flow assessment measures flow velocity to confirm the diagnosis and quantify the degree of stenosis. The stenosis is defined as moderate if it is between 50% and 70%, and severe if more than 70% stenosed.

Magnetic resonance angiography

Magnetic resonance angiography (p. 77) is excellent in detecting severe (70–99%) stenosis, but performs less well in discriminating above and below the 70% threshold, which is important for surgical decision making.[3]

Cerebral angiography

In general, carotid ultrasound is sufficient to guide the management for most patients. Cerebral angiography (Fig. 1.67) is usually reserved to evaluate the carotid anatomy of patients with neurological events without severe stenosis on Doppler ultrasound, when more extensive disease is suspected (e.g. brachiocephalic trunk), and when the anatomy is unclear on Doppler ultrasound imaging. Although cerebral angiography is the gold standard, it is an invasive procedure with complications that include TIA (4%), stroke (1%), and contrast allergy.

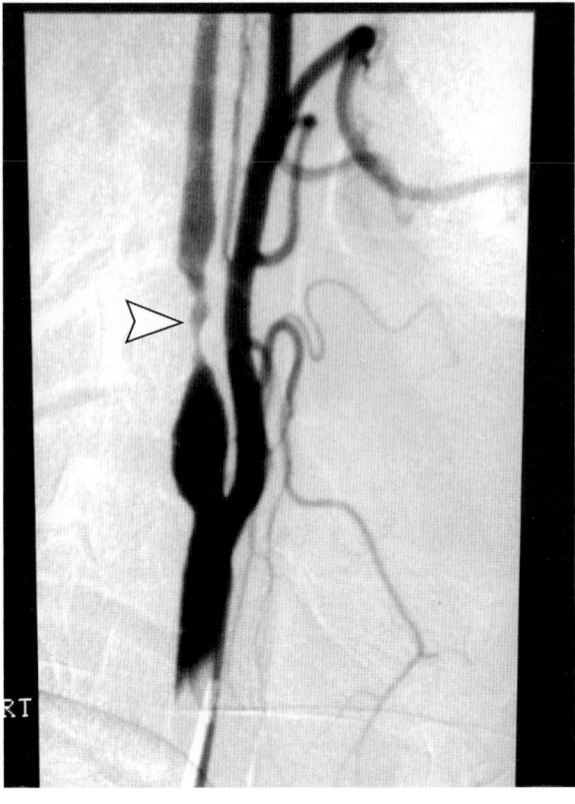

Fig. 1.67 Carotid angiography. This image shows a stenosis of the internal carotid artery (arrow).

> **RECENT ADVANCES**
>
> *The utility of spiral CT angiography is currently being investigated for determining the degree of carotid stenosis.*

Management

Risk factor modification

Carotid arterial disease is a classic manifestation of widespread atherosclerotic disease, and the first step in management should be risk factor modification (Table 1.38).

Antiplatelet therapy

Antiplatelet therapy should be prescribed to reduce further stroke and transient ischaemic attacks.[4] Symptomatic patients should be prescribed between 150 and 300 mg, reduced to 75 mg after 1 year. Asymptomatic patients should be prescribed 75 mg once daily. Clopidogrel is of proven benefit in those whom aspirin is contraindicated. Anticoagulants have no benefits over antiplatelet therapy and should not be prescribed unless indicated for other reasons.

Table 1.38	Targets for risk factor modification	
Risk factor	**Target**	**Comment**
Hypertension	≤140/90	ACE inhibitors reduce the risk of stroke and decrease vessel intima/media thickness. Aim for blood pressure ≤130/85
Diabetes mellitus	Fasting blood glucose of <7 mmol/L	
Hypercholesterolaemia	LDL <2.6 mmol/L	Diet consisting of less than 30% fat, 7% saturated, and 200 mg of cholesterol. Statins may cause plaque regression
Smoking	Cessation	Nicotine patches, smoking cessation clinics
Alcohol use	Eliminate excessive use	Excess alcohol consumption is associated with increased all-cause mortality
Physical activity	30–60 minutes exercise 3 times a week	

Carotid endarterectomy

The indications for carotid endarterectomy and selection of best management regimen are presented in Table 1.39 and Figure 1.68.

For patients with symptomatic disease and severe stenosis (more than 70%), carotid endarterectomy reduces the risk of ipsilateral stroke (relative risk reduction of 65%) and improves survival.[5–7] In symptomatic patients with moderate stenosis (50–69%) the evidence is less clear. In the ECST trial[6] no benefit was identified, whereas in NASCET[5] there was an absolute risk reduction of 6.5% in stroke in the surgical treatment arm at 5 years. The patients that benefited most in this subgroup were male, aged less than 75, with recent stroke (less than 3 months), hemispheric symptoms, no intracranial stenosis and absence of microvascular ischaemia. Symptomatic patients with mild stenosis (<50%) do not benefit from surgery compared to medical therapy alone.

For patients with asymptomatic carotid stenosis, the risk of ipsilateral stroke with stenosis of more than 50% is up to 3% per year, and if the stenosis ranges from 60% to 99% the risk of stroke is approximately 5% per year. The results of surgery in this group of patients are less clear-cut, with approximately 50% relative risk reductions in the risk of stroke with some trials[8,9] and no benefit in others.[10]

Carotid endarterectomy can be performed under general or local anaesthesia. The patient is positioned

Table 1.39	Recommendations for carotid endarterectomy

Symptomatic carotid stenosis

Patients with severe stenosis (70–99%) should undergo carotid endarterectomy

Patients with moderate stenosis (50–69%) should be considered on a case by case basis for carotid endarterectomy based on patient fitness, risk factors, and experience of surgeons

Patients with mild stenosis (less than 50%) in general should be managed with risk factor modification. Carotid endarterectomy is not recommended for patients with mild stenosis

Asymptomatic carotid stenosis

Patients with more than 60% stenosis should be considered for carotid endarterectomy if an experienced surgeon is available, and taking into account patient fitness and risk factors

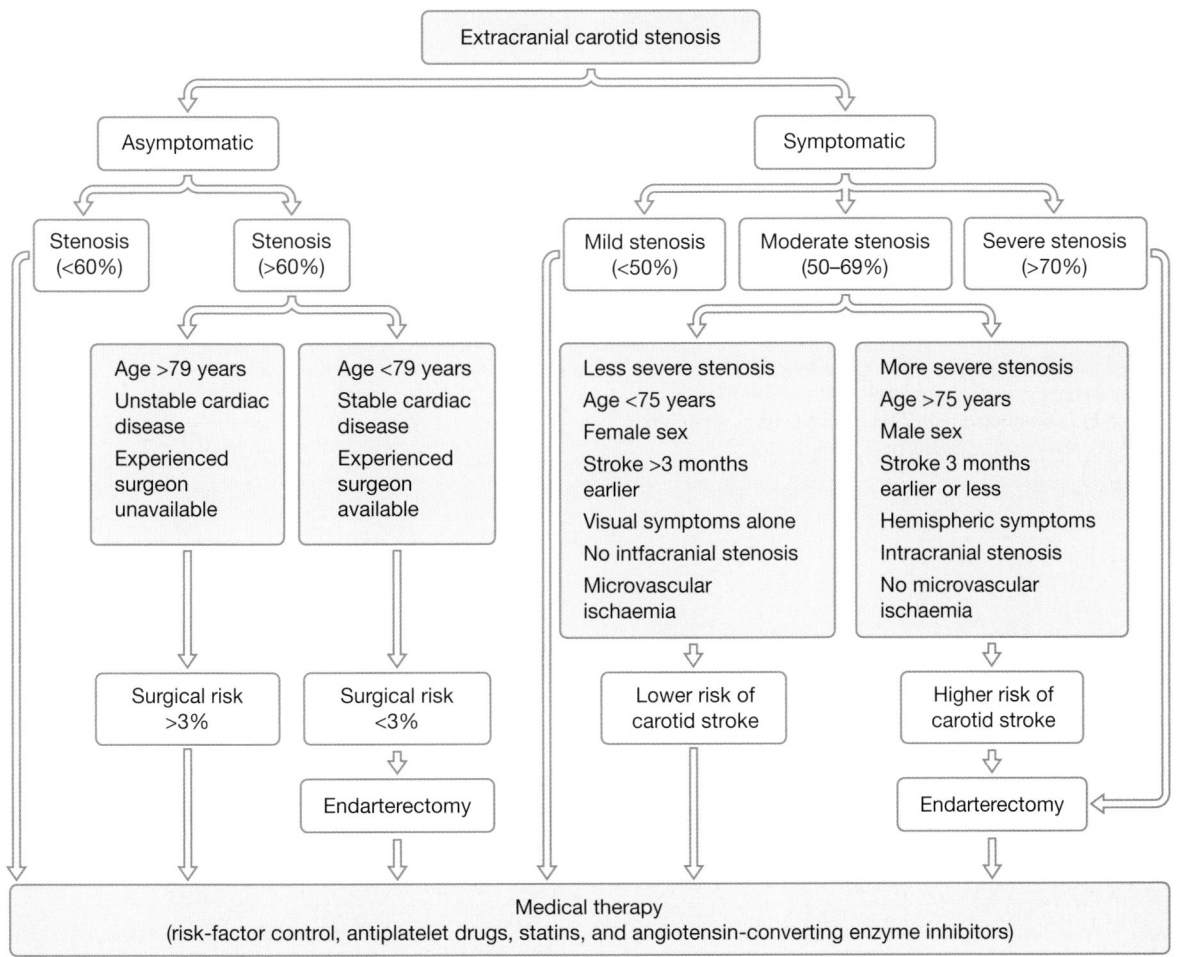

Fig. 1.68 Treatment algorithm for patients with carotid stenosis.
Sacco RL. Extracranial carotid stenosis. New England Journal of Medicine 2001; 345: 1113–1118.

supine with the neck extended and turned away from the affected side. A longitudinal incision is made on the medial border of the sternocleidomastoid muscle, and the carotid artery identified posterior to the muscle. The carotid sinus nerve is anaesthetized to prevent excessive fluctuations in blood pressure. Heparin is administered and a longitudinal arteriotomy performed. A shunt may be used to preserve the blood supply to the brain. The plane between the plaque and artery wall is developed and the full extent of the plaque removed. A vein patch or prosthetic patch can be sutured to prevent stenosis of a small-calibre carotid artery.

Postoperatively, the risk of death is small and the risk of stroke is 3% or less.

Carotid artery stenting

Advances in endovascular techniques have made carotid artery stenting a viable option for treating carotid artery disease. Randomized trials of surgical coronary endarterectomy have demonstrated that medical treatment is inferior to carotid stenting in symptomatic patients with more than 50% stenosis and asymptomatic patients with more than 70% stenosis. Compared to carotid endarterectomy, both techniques reduce the risk of stroke, but restenosis is more common in the endovascular treatment group (14% vs 4%) at 3 years.[11]

Prognosis

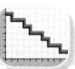

The prognosis of patients depends on the presence of symptoms, severity of stenoses and the chosen management strategy, as discussed above.

i FURTHER INFORMATION

Biller J, Feinberg WM, Castaldo JE, et al. Guidelines for carotid endarterectomy: a statement for healthcare professionals from a special writing group of the Stroke Council, American Heart Association. Circulation 1998; 97: 501–509.

REFERENCES

(1) *Mineva PP, Manchev IC, Hadjiev DI. Prevalence and outcome of asymptomatic carotid stenosis: a population-based ultrasonographic study. European Journal of Neurology 2002; 9: 383–388.*
(2) *Magyar MT, Nam EM, Csiba L, Ritter MA, Ringelstein EB, Droste DW. Carotid artery auscultation—anachronism or useful screening procedure? Neurological Research 2002; 24: 705–708.*
(3) *Westwood ME, Kelly S, Berry E, et al. Use of magnetic resonance angiography to select candidates with recently symptomatic carotid stenosis for surgery: systematic review. BMJ 2002; 324: 198–201.*
(4) *Jackson MR, Clagett GP. Antithrombotic therapy in peripheral arterial occlusive disease. Chest 2001; 119: 283S–299S.*
(5) *Beneficial effect of carotid endarterectomy in symptomatic patients with high-grade carotid stenosis. North American Symptomatic Carotid Endarterectomy Trial Collaborators. New England Journal of Medicine 1991; 325: 445–453.*
(6) *MRC European Carotid Surgery Trial: interim results for symptomatic patients with severe (70–99%) or with mild (0–29%) carotid stenosis. European Carotid Surgery Trialists' Collaborative Group. Lancet 1991; 337: 1235–1243.*
(7) *Mayberg MR, Wilson SE, Yatsu F, et al. Carotid endarterectomy and prevention of cerebral ischemia in symptomatic carotid stenosis. Veterans Affairs Cooperative Studies Program 309 Trialist Group. JAMA 1991; 266: 3289–3294.*
(8) *Endarterectomy for asymptomatic carotid artery stenosis. Executive Committee for the Asymptomatic Carotid Atherosclerosis Study. JAMA 1995; 273: 1421–1428.*
(9) *Hobson RW, Weiss DG, Fields WS, Goldstone J, Moore WS, Towne JB, Wright CB, Veterans Affairs Cooperative Study Group. Efficacy of carotid endarterectomy for asymptomatic carotid stenosis. New England Journal of Medicine 1993; 328: 221–227.*
(10) *Carotid surgery versus medical therapy in asymptomatic carotid stenosis. The CASANOVA Study Group. Stroke 1991; 22: 1229–1235.*
(11) *Endovascular versus surgical treatment in patients with carotid stenosis in the Carotid and Vertebral Artery Transluminal Angioplasty Study (CAVATAS): a randomised trial. Lancet 2001; 357: 1729–1737.*

SECTION 1.20 # Visceral ischaemia

Epidemiology

Chronic visceral ischaemia is uncommon, accounting for 5% of all intestinal ischaemic events.[1] It is uncommon in the young: the incidence increases with age.

Pathology

Atherosclerotic disease of the aorta may lead to narrowing of the orifices of the visceral arteries. The coeliac axis, superior and inferior mesenteric arteries supply blood to the gastrointestinal tract through many branch vessels. Only acute occlusion of the superior mesenteric artery leads to small bowel infarction due to the rich collateral supply. Approximately a quarter of such occlusions result from systemic embolization (usually in association with atrial fibrillation).

Chronic visceral artery ischaemia (mesenteric angina) is the result of progressive atherosclerotic disease of the major visceral vessels. Ingestion of food activates the sympathetic nervous system and the increased blood requirements lead to 'mesenteric angina'. Abdominal pain is the lone presenting symptom in 75% of patients, usually representing a superior mesenteric artery lesion.

Clinical features

Patients with acute visceral ischaemia as a result of systemic embolization or venous thrombosis present with an acute abdomen.

Patients with chronic visceral ischaemia usually present with severe central dull abdominal pain after food that lasts for several hours. It is often associated with marked weight loss and may present in a similar manner to gastrointestinal malignancy. However, it is the fear of eating and precipitating abdominal pain rather than loss of appetite that is the discriminating factor. Involvement of the inferior mesenteric artery often leads to food-associated diarrhoea and rectal bleeding. On examination, the presence of an abdominal bruit is a specific but insensitive physical sign.

Investigations
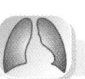

Full blood count, markers of inflammation
In patients with acute visceral ischaemia, the white cell count (neutrophilia), CRP and ESR may be elevated.

Arterial blood gas
In acute ischaemia, the venous bicarbonate is low and arterial blood gas analysis will show a metabolic acidosis as a result of lactic acid being released into the circulation from cell death. Lactate dehydrogenase is usually raised.

Mesenteric angiography
Mesenteric angiography remains the gold standard investigation for the diagnosis of chronic visceral ischaemia.

Management

Surgical embolectomy/bowel resection
Acute visceral ischaemia is treated by surgical embolectomy or more often surgical resection if there is an infarcted segment of bowel that does not recover.

Revascularization
Revascularization in chronic ischaemia can be performed by balloon angioplasty, venous bypass grafting or side to side anastomosis between the ileocolic and right colic arteries. Treatment with balloon angioplasty is associated with a 70% incidence of restenosis.

Prognosis

Untreated acute ischaemia carries a high mortality rate. In general, surgical treatment of arterial embolism improves outcome whereas the mortality rate following surgery for arterial thrombosis and non-occlusive ischaemia remains poor.[2]

REFERENCES

(1) Sreenarasimhaiah J. Chronic mesenteric ischemia. Best Practice & Research Clinical Gastroenterology 2005; 19: 283–295.
(2) Schoots IG, Koffeman GI, Legemate DA, Levi M, van Gulik TM. Systematic review of survival after acute mesenteric ischaemia according to disease aetiology. British Journal of Surgery 2004; 91: 17–27.

Abdominal aortic aneurysm

Epidemiology

The prevalence of abdominal aortic aneurysms (AAA) is 4.9% (4900 per 100 000) in men aged 65–74 years.[1] Although AAA is four times more common in men, AAAs that occur in women are three times more likely to rupture.[2] There is marked geographical variation, and the higher prevalence in the Western world is associated with atherosclerosis. Familial clustering occurs: up to 19% of patients with an AAA will have first-degree relatives with an aneurysm.[3]

Pathology

An arterial aneurysm is a permanent increase in arterial diameter to greater than 50% of the normal (Table 1.40). The risk factors for the development of abdominal aortic aneurysms are smoking, hypertension, atherosclerosis and connective tissue disorders. Recent clinical and experimental studies are now challenging the long-held belief that AAA results primarily as a complication of atherosclerosis.[4]

Table 1.40	Classification of aneurysms
Congenital or acquired	
True or false aneurysm	
A true aneurysm consists of all three layers of the vessel wall	
A false aneurysm consists of only part of the vessel wall	
Aetiology	
Atherosclerotic	
Ischaemic	
Hypertensive	
Infective (syphilis)	
Traumatic	
Inflammatory	
Connective tissue disorder	
Site	
Infrarenal	
Juxtarenal	
Suprarenal	
Thoracic	
Shape	
Fusiform	
Saccular	
Dissecting	

The inflammatory theory of aortic aneurysm formation suggests that chronic inflammation leads to smooth muscle cell depletion and an imbalance in proteolytic enzymes, causing degradation of matrix proteins that weakens the aorta.[5] The inflammatory milieu within the vessel wall further contributes to aneurysm formation by promoting increased levels of metalloproteinase, a group of enzymes known to degrade extracellular matrix of the arterial wall.[6]

Mechanical factors such as high blood pressure and the shape of the aorta are also pertinent, but hypertension alone is only a weak risk factor for aneurysm formation (3%); when associated with concomitant systemic vascular disease, the risk of aortic aneurysm rises dramatically (18%).[7] High blood pressure is also an independent risk factor for aneurysm rupture.[2] According to Laplace's law, at a given pressure, wall tension is proportional to the radius. Therefore, as aneurysms dilate, the wall tension and risk of rupture increase. Other risk factors for rupture include smoking, female sex and low FEV_1.

Scope of disease

Rupture is the most dramatic complication of abdominal aneurysms; the majority of patients do not arrive at hospital in time for treatment. Other complications include distal thromboembolism, compression on adjacent viscera and fistula formation.

Clinical features

Approximately 75% of AAAs are asymptomatic and detected on routine examination or investigation of unrelated disease. Clinical symptoms usually arise from impending or established complications.

Abdominal pain

The diagnosis of a ruptured abdominal aneurysm should be considered in any patient with hypotension and vague abdominal pain. The severity of the symptoms varies with the size and site of the leak. Intraperitoneal leaks are rapidly fatal, and a minority with small retroperitoneal (contained) leaks may present with the classical triad of hypotension, abdominal or back pain, and a pulsatile abdominal mass. Periaortic tissue may tamponade a small leak with hypertension as a response to slow volume loss. Large amounts of blood loss lead to hypovolaemic shock with hypotension, tachycardia, peripheral vasoconstriction and depressed consciousness.

Isolated abdominal pain is typically related to stretching of the aortic wall or compression of nearby structures. Continuous abdominal pain is often regarded as a symptom of potential rupture, but evidence to support this is limited.

Embolization

Propagation of thrombus or atheroma can give rise to a variety of thromboembolic complications ranging from acute limb ischaemia to multiple areas of distal infarction (trash foot).

Fistula

Fistula formation is a rare complication that occurs from abnormal connection of the inflamed aorta to the gastrointestinal tract. The presenting symptom of aorto-enteric fistula is massive gastrointestinal bleeding. It rarely occurs as a primary symptom and can occur as a complication after aortic aneurysm surgery.

Examination

On examination there may be hypertension. The abdominal examination is unreliable for the presence and estimation of the size of abdominal aortic aneurysms. The lower limbs should be examined for evidence of embolic complications.

Initial investigations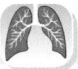

Abdominal ultrasound

Abdominal ultrasound is the investigation of choice for non-emergency imaging of the abdominal aorta. It can identify the presence of an aneurysm, measure the diameter, assess the disease extent (involvement of the iliac arteries) and screen for complications (mural thrombus). Ultrasound is not useful to assess the presence of a leak or the proximal

extent of the aneurysm and in general underestimates the true diameter of the aneurysm.

CT abdomen

For emergency or painful aneurysms, CT of the abdomen is the investigation of choice (Fig. 1.69). It provides all of the information that an ultrasound does, but in addition is able to accurately visualize the proximal extent and the relationship of the aneurysm to the renal arteries, information that is important for surgery and to assess the anatomical suitability for stent insertion. If required, three-dimensional images can be obtained (Fig. 1.70).

Surgical management

The main aim of surgery for aortic aneurysm is the prevention of rupture and other complications. Aneurysm diameter is the strongest independent predictor of rupture and hence the most important guide to management.

Expectant management

In general there are no benefits in operating on aneurysms that are less than 5.5 cm. Early surgery is more costly and not associated with any survival benefit.[8] The 8-year mortality in patients under observation compared to surgery was 1.0% vs 5.9%.[9]

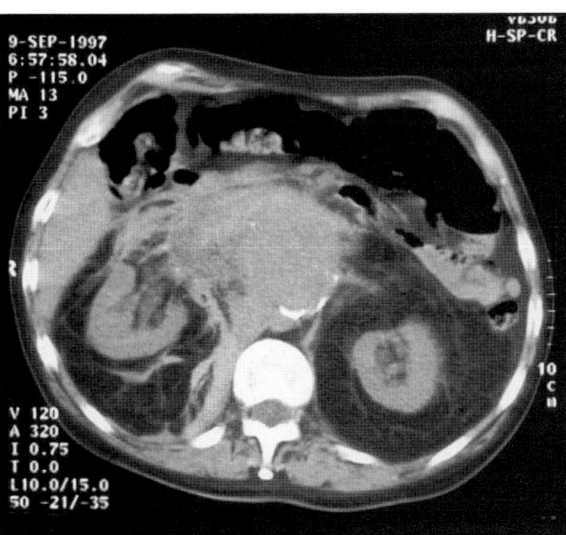

Fig. 1.69 CT abdomen. This CT shows a ruptured aortic aneurysm.

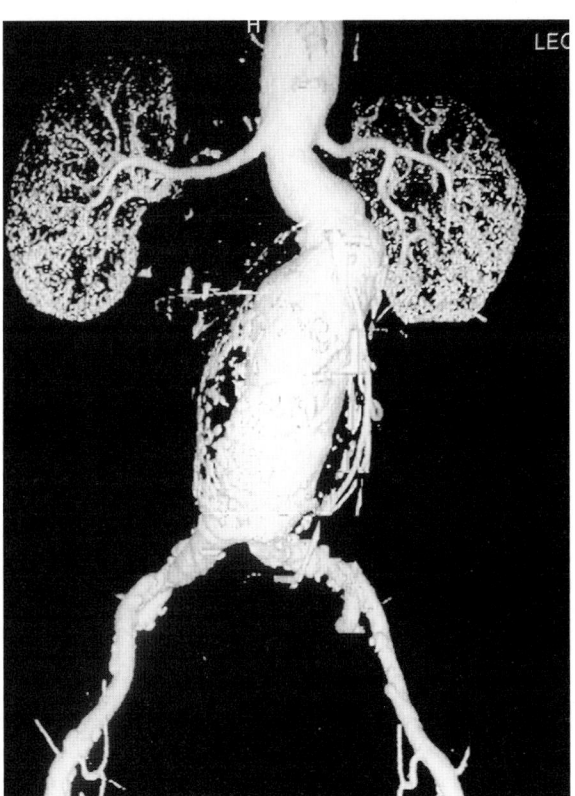

Fig. 1.70 Spiral CT of the aorta, reconstructed to provide a three-dimensional image of the abdominal aneurysm.

Elective operative repair

It is generally accepted that patients with aneurysms greater than 5.5 cm should undergo elective surgery despite the lack of direct evidence, as the risk of rupture increases with aneurysm diameter.

A midline laparotomy incision is performed and the bowel is reflected away to expose the abdominal aorta. The aneurysm and iliac arteries are dissected free of adhesions (Fig. 1.71). Heparin is administered and a cross clamp is applied to the aortic neck and the iliac arteries. The aneurysm sac is opened, mural thrombus is removed and the lumbar arteries (and inferior mesenteric artery) are oversewn. A Dacron tube graft is sewn to the proximal and distal ends within the native aortic lumen. A Dacron trouser graft is used if the iliac arteries are involved in the disease process (Fig. 1.72). The aneurysm sac is closed over the top of the graft to prevent adhesion, infection and fistula formation.

Emergency operative repair

The mortality of untreated ruptured aortic aneurysm is 100%, and many patients are unfit for operative intervention. Age over 80 years, altered consciousness, haemoglobin less than 8 g/dL, systolic pressure less than 80 mmHg, cardiac arrest and severe cardiorespiratory disease are independent predictors of death in the emergency setting.[10]

Leak from a ruptured aneurysm causes physiological reflex contraction of the abdominal wall to maintain high intra-abdominal pressure. This is reversed with anaesthesia, causing a sudden drop in blood pressure. Therefore rapid sequence induction is used and the operation begun immediately. A laparotomy incision is made and a cross clamp is applied on the aorta above the coeliac artery through the lesser omentum. Once control is achieved, dissection of the infrarenal aorta is performed. An initial supracoeliac clamp is applied (high above the aneurysm neck) as haematoma obscures the dissection. When the aneurysm is identified a second cross clamp is placed at the neck of the aneurysm and the supracoeliac clamp removed. The remainder of the operation carries on as described for the elective repair.

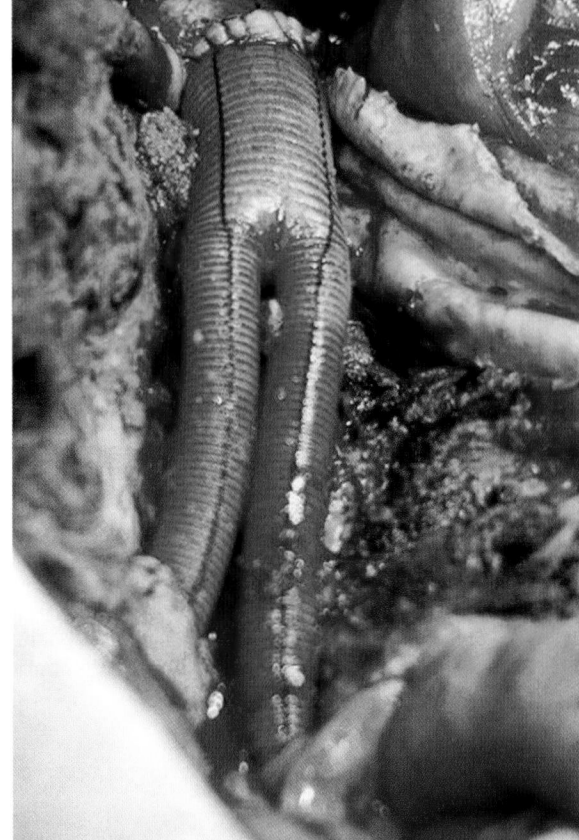

Fig. 1.72 Replacement of the abdominal aorta with a trouser graft.

Complications of emergency surgery include a mortality rate of 46%. In addition there is a risk of postoperative coagulopathy, myocardial infarction, renal failure and ischaemic colitis.

RECENT ADVANCES

Endovascular repair can be performed by employing a stent graft (Fig. 1.73a) to the aneurysm via the femoral artery (Fig. 1.73b). There is no need for an abdominal incision, the aorta is not cross clamped, postoperative cardiorespiratory function is better, and renal failure and hospital stay are reduced.[11]

To be eligible for endovascular aortic repair the aneurysm neck must be infrarenal, at least 1.5 cm in length, with less than 45 degree angulation, and less than 3.0 cm in diameter. The iliac arteries must also be large enough to allow the passage of the stent.

Currently data on the long-term durability of stent grafts are unavailable. Deployment of the stent graft does not inevitably change the natural course of expansion and the stent graft can migrate leading to endoleak and possible rupture. The rupture rate in patients with an endovascular stent is estimated at 3% and re-intervention occurs at approximately 10% per year. Surgical intervention for failed stent grafts carries a significant morbidity and mortality.

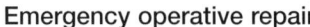

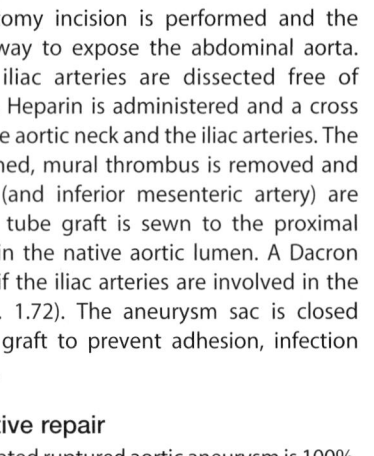

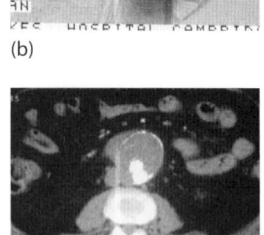

(a)

(b)

(c)

Fig. 1.73a–c Stenting of the abdominal aorta. (a) Aortic stents, (b) endovascular insertion and (c) post procedure CT result.

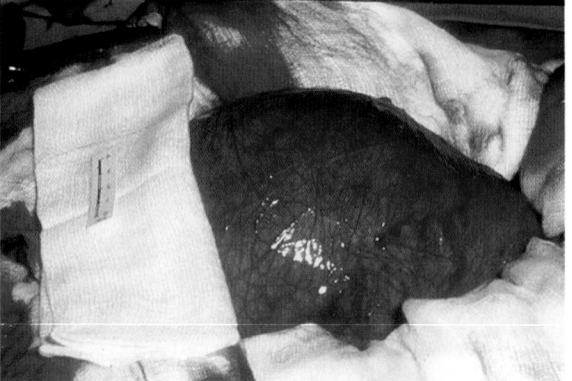

Fig. 1.71 Operative photo of an abdominal aneurysm.

Prognosis

The 1-year incidence of rupture is 9.4% for unoperated aneurysms 5.5–5.9 cm, rising to 32.5% for aneurysms with a diameter of 7.0 cm or more.[12] The mortality risk of open elective surgery is approximately 6%, that of stent grafting 2–3%, and emergency surgery is associated with a mortality risk of approximately 50%.

REFERENCES

(1) Ashton HA, Buxton MJ, Day NE, et al. The Multicentre Aneurysm Screening Study (MASS) into the effect of abdominal aortic aneurysm screening on mortality in men: a randomised controlled trial. Lancet 2002; 360: 1531–1539.

(2) Brown LC, Powell JT. Risk factors for aneurysm rupture in patients kept under ultrasound surveillance. UK Small Aneurysm Trial Participants. Annals of Surgery 1999; 230: 289–296; discussion 296–297.

(3) van Vlijmen-van Keulen CJ, Pals G, Rauwerda JA. Familial abdominal aortic aneurysm: a systematic review of a genetic background. European Journal of Vascular and Endovascular Surgery 2002; 24: 105–116.

(4) Shah PK. Inflammation, metalloproteinases, and increased proteolysis: an emerging pathophysiological paradigm in aortic aneurysm. Circulation 1997; 96: 2115–2117.

(5) Walton LJ, Franklin IJ, Bayston T, Brown LC, Greenhalgh RM, Taylor GW, Powell JT. Inhibition of prostaglandin E2 synthesis in abdominal aortic aneurysms: implications for smooth muscle cell viability, inflammatory processes, and the expansion of abdominal aortic aneurysms. Circulation 1999; 100: 48–54.

(6) McMillan WD, Tamarina NA, Cipollone M, Johnson DA, Parker MA, Pearce WH. Size matters: the relationship between MMP-9 expression and aortic diameter. Circulation 1997; 96: 2228–2232.

(7) MacSweeney ST, O'Meara M, Alexander C, O'Malley MK, Powell JT, Greenhalgh RM. High prevalence of unsuspected abdominal aortic aneurysm in patients with confirmed symptomatic peripheral or cerebral arterial disease. British Journal of Surgery 1993; 80: 582–584.

(8) The United Kingdom Small Aneurysm Trial Participants. Long-term outcomes of immediate repair compared with surveillance of small abdominal aortic aneurysms. New England Journal of Medicine 2002; 346: 1445–1452.

(9) Lederle FA, Wilson SE, Johnson GR, et al, the Aneurysm Detection and Management Veterans Affairs Cooperative Study Group. Immediate repair compared with surveillance of small abdominal aortic aneurysms. New England Journal of Medicine 2002; 346: 1437–1444.

(10) Chen JC, Hildebrand HD, Salvian AJ, Taylor DC, Strandberg S, Myckatyn TM, Hsiang YN. Predictors of death in nonruptured and ruptured abdominal aortic aneurysms. Journal of Vascular Surgery 1996; 24: 614–620; discussion 621–623.

(11) Yusuf SW, Hopkinson BR. Endovascular repair of aortic aneurysm. British Journal of Surgery 1995; 82: 289–291.

(12) Lederle FA, Johnson GR, Wilson SE, et al, for the Veterans Affairs Cooperative Study #417 Investigators. Rupture rate of large abdominal aortic aneurysms in patients refusing or unfit for elective repair. JAMA 2002; 287: 2968–2972.

Varicose veins

Venous ulceration

Peripheral venous insufficiency

Return flow from the lower limbs is caused by the calf muscle pump action, venomotor tone and cardiac output maintaining a gradient across the venous system. Abnormality or dysfunction of any of these mechanisms leads to venous hypertension and ultimately venous insufficiency manifesting as varicose veins or venous ulceration.

Varicose veins

The WHO defines varicose veins as saccular dilatations of veins, often being tortuous. Varicose veins can be classified as trunk varicosities, reticular varicosities or telangiectasia (thread veins). Although the majority of varicose veins are primary (due to inherent weakness of the wall of the veins), it is important to recognize secondary causes as they are managed differently.

Epidemiology

Varicose veins occur in approximately 17% of males and 31% of females between the ages of 35 and 70 years. The prevalence increases with age. Varicose veins are more common in women and in developed countries.

Pathology

Venous return is dependent on venous valve integrity. Varicose veins are the manifestation of venous reflux and vein dilatation that develop due to imbalance between hydrostatic (gravitational) and hydrodynamic (muscle pump) forces within the limbs. The risk factors for the development of venous insufficiency can be primary or secondary (Table 1.41).

In primary disease, there is an inherent weakness within the walls of the vein, causing dilatation and widening of the space between valve cusps. As the valve becomes incompetent, hydrostatic forces increase and lead to peripheral pooling, standing columns of blood within the veins and the development of varicosities. A genetic predisposition in the development and severity of varicosities can be identified in up to 70% of patients.

Secondary causes are damage to the venous walls (deep venous thrombosis), outflow obstruction (pelvic tumours) and, rarely, congenital absence of venous valves.

Scope of disease

The sizes of the veins are unrelated to the extent or severity of complications (Table 1.42).

Clinical features

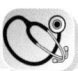

The majority of patients with varicose veins are asymptomatic. Of symptomatic patients, men often attend complaining of itch whilst females usually present with heaviness, tension and aching. It is important to take a careful history as up to a third of patients' symptoms can be attributed to other problems. It is vital to ascertain whether the patient has had varicose vein surgery in the past and/or suffered a deep venous thrombosis or thrombophlebitis. These conditions make varicose vein surgery more difficult

Table 1.42	Complications of varicose veins and venous hypertension
Complications of varicose veins	
Bleeding	
Ulceration	
Thrombophlebitis	
Complications of venous hypertension	
Pigmentation	
Lipodermatosclerosis	
Oedema	
Eczema	

and increase the likelihood of deep venous insufficiency for which treatment is markedly different.

Examination should focus on the distribution of disease, particularly whether the long (Fig. 1.74), short or both saphenous veins are involved. The presence of complications should also be noted (Table 1.42). The skin changes associated with venous insufficiency have been described on page 75. The American College of Phlebology has designed an objective standardized classification system

Table 1.41	Risk factors for the development of venous insufficiency
Primary	
Age	
Female sex	
Contraceptive pill use	
Prolonged standing	
Obesity	
Positive family history	
Secondary	
Deep venous valvular insufficiency	
Incompetent perforating veins	
Venous outflow obstruction (pelvic tumours)	
Congenital abnormalities	
Arteriovenous malformation	

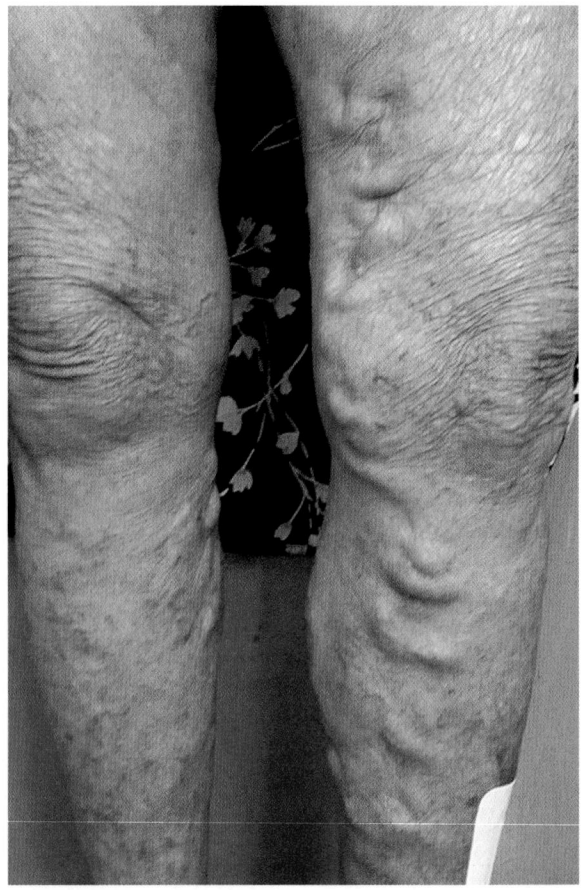

Fig. 1.74 Varicose veins.

known as CEAP to allow treatment comparisons and documentation of progress (Table 1.43).

Clinical techniques to determine reflux such as the tourniquet and Perthes test have been superseded by the use of hand-held Doppler (Fig. 1.75). For completeness, the two traditional examination techniques are described.

The tourniquet test is performed by laying the patient flat and emptying the superficial veins in the leg. A tourniquet is applied and the patient is instructed to stand (Fig. 1.76a). Absence of varicosities implies control of the site of reflux proximal to the tourniquet and implies a positive test (Fig. 1.76b). Perthes test is performed by repeating the tourniquet test but allowing some blood into the leg. The patient stands up and down on tiptoes and emptying of the veins implies that the muscle pump is functioning.

Initial investigations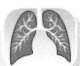

Hand-held Doppler evaluation
The tip of the Doppler probe is applied to the sapheno-femoral junction and the calf is squeezed or varicosities are tapped with the fingertips. A single swoosh implies a competent valve and a double swoosh indicates an incompetent valve. The procedure is repeated at the sapheno-popliteal junction.

Further investigations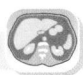

Duplex Doppler evaluation
Duplex evaluation provides real time images with physiological data on blood flow which can be amalgamated to determine luminal and parietal diameter, compressibility, echogenicity, flow direction, and valve leaflet function of the vessel.

Colour duplex should be performed in all patients who have recurrent disease, skin changes, or a history of deep venous thrombosis (DVT) or thrombophlebitis. Patients presenting with venous flaring or telangiectasia should also have colour duplex as up to a third will have superficial venous insufficiency.

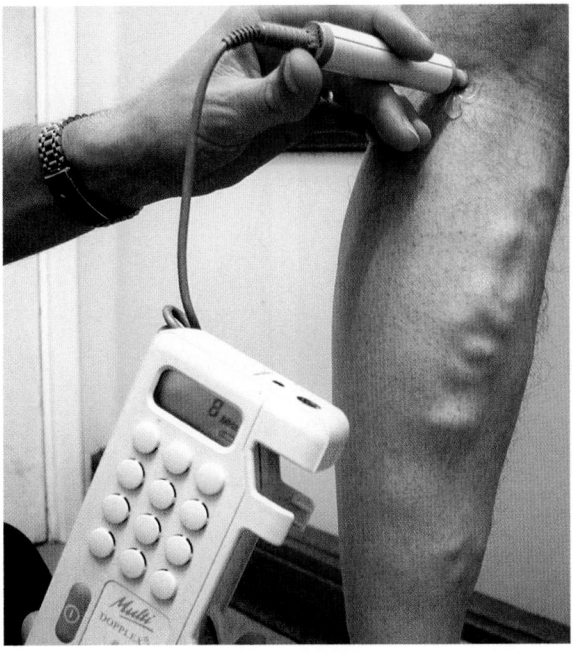

Fig. 1.75 Hand-held Doppler to assess for venous insufficiency.

Photoplethysmography
Patients noted to have both superficial and deep venous reflux should undergo functional testing to determine the relative contribution of each system to reflux. Photoplethysmography works on the premise that infrared light is absorbed in varying degrees based on the volume of haemoglobin present within the limbs, and measures venous refilling time as well as the efficiency of the calf muscle pump.

Initial management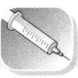

Exercise
There is an exponential rise in the prevalence of venous disease as the amount of daily movement is reduced,

Varicose veins

Venous ulceration

Table 1.43	CEAP classification of varicose veins		
C (Clinical findings)	**E (Etiology)**	**A (Anatomy)**	**P (Pathophysiology)**
C0—no disease	c—Congenital	s—Superficial	r—Reflux
C1—telangiectasia	p—Primary	d—Deep	o—Obstruction
C2—varicose veins	s—Secondary	p—Perforating	r, o—Both
C3—oedema			
C4—skin changes/no ulcer			
C5—skin changes/healed ulcer			
C6—skin changes/active ulcer			
Add 'a' for asymptomatic or 's' for symptomatic			

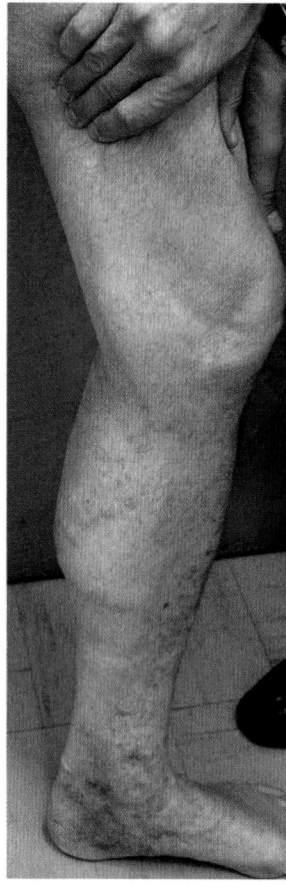
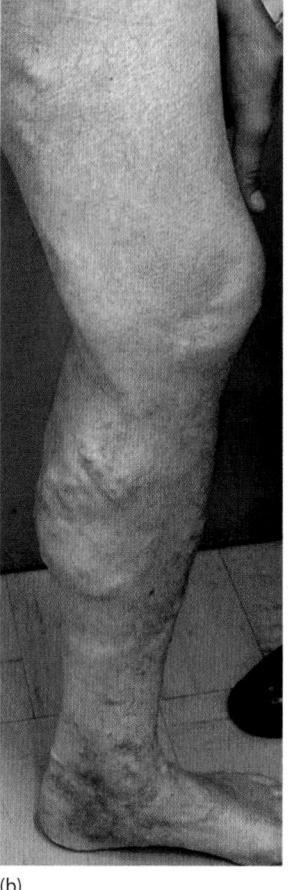

(a)   (b)

Fig. 1.76 Tourniquet test. (a) Hand pressure is used instead of a tourniquet for clarity, which shows control of the varicose veins. (b) When the hand is lifted, the veins are visible.

therefore exercises that emphasize ankle flexion are encouraged. Activation of the musculo-venous pump provides periods of lowered venous pressure and improves function of the calf muscle pump.

Elevation

Raising the feet above the level of the heart for 15–30 minutes per day reduces symptoms and oedema.

Compression hosiery

Compression reduces the diameter of the veins, increases the blood flow velocity and lymphatic flow and reduces oedema. It is the first-line therapy in patients who are unwilling or unfit for surgery, or if there is a possibility that the symptoms are not from venous disease. Response to compression stockings usually indicates that surgery will be beneficial

Elastic compression comes in four classes based on the pressure exerted at the ankle (Table 1.44). The pressure is reduced further up the leg to create a gradient to encourage venous flow. Elastic therapy may reduce the severity of symptoms and halt progression of disease but poorly fitting stockings can lead to a 'tourniquet effect', creating an opposite gradient and worsening the reflux.

Inelastic compression is more effective in augmenting venous pumping, as the semi-rigid compression ensures that the muscular pump directs blood towards the heart, rather than a circle of pumping blood in and around muscles which can occur with elastic hosiery; however, compliance is more difficult.

Laser therapy

Laser therapy is increasingly used for the treatment of telangiectasia and venous flaring. Laser and light therapy produce foci of high-intensity heat which potentially cause less inflammation and chemical irritation as the target tissue absorbs different wavelengths of light compared to surrounding structures. To date these methods are unsuitable for coloured skin.

Surgical management

High tie strip and avulsions

Surgery is indicated in patients with skin changes, venous ulceration and intractable pain. The decision for surgical treatment is less straightforward for patients with symptomatic trunk varices with no skin changes as it is impossible to determine which of these patients go on to develop ulceration.

High tie strip and avulsions is the preferred operation for long saphenous reflux. A short oblique incision 2 cm below and lateral to the pubic tubercle is made along the groin crease. The five specific tributaries are identified and ligated: the superficial inferior epigastric, deep external pudendal, superficial external pudendal, superficial circumflex iliac vein and the anteromedial and posterolateral thigh veins. A stripper is placed down the distal part of the disconnected saphenous vein to as far down as 5 cm

Table 1.44	Grades of compression hosiery	
Class	**Pressure (approximate)**	**Indications**
I	15–25 mmHg	Aching, swelling, telangiectasias, reticular veins
II	25–35 mmHg	Symptomatic varicose veins, CVI, post-ulcer
III	35–45 mmHg	CVI, post-ulcer, lymphoedema
IV	> 45 mmHg	CVI, post-ulcer, lymphoedema

CVI, chronic venous insufficiency.

below the knee and a ligature placed proximally. An oblique 1.5 cm incision is made at the tip of the stripper and the distal vein ligated and divided. The stripper is then pulled down, stripping the saphenous vein from groin to knee. Stab avulsion incisions are made for the remaining varicosities and pulled out using a hook and artery forceps. At the completion of the operation a crepe bandage should be applied firmly from ankle to mid thigh in order to aid haemostasis and minimize postoperative bruising.

For short saphenous reflux a 3–5 cm incision is made in the popliteal fossa targetted to the sapheno-popliteal junction using a hand-held Doppler. The vein is disconnected at the junction using a similar technique to that above, with or without avulsions. The deep fascial layer should be closed with care to avoid the potential of popliteal hernia developing. Extreme attention must be paid not to damage the nearby sural nerve.

Complications of surgery include saphenous or sural nerve neuralgia (10%), postoperative bruising (90%), wound infection (2%), and transient lymphocele (2%). Recurrence is 20–30% at 10 years from surgical therapy. The most common cause is failure to identify and ligate all the saphenous vein tributaries. In the past many surgeons would tie and ligate the saphenous vein in isolation without stripping. This method has a high rate of recurrence secondary to venous recanalization.

Sclerotherapy

Intravenous injection of sclerosants (such as sodium tetradecyl sulphate) causes venous fibrosis and obliteration. This method of treatment is usually reserved for residual varicosities after surgery. Its use as first-line treatment lost favour due to high recurrence rates, skin staining and the risk of ulceration and deep venous thrombosis. An important principle in successful sclerotherapy is the prevention of exposure of the sclerosant to normal vessels.

RECENT ADVANCES

Radiofrequency endovenous occlusion is a technique that uses radiofrequency energy delivered through an endovenous electrode (Fig. 1.77). Heat dissipates within the lumen of the vessel leading to vein shrinkage and occlusion by contraction of venous collagen. Vein occlusion rates are reported as high as 97% at 1 week, 95% at 6 weeks, and 92% at 1 year. The major complication of this technique is the creation of venous thrombus (1%). Other side effects include phlebitis (6%), skin burn (3%) and temporary paraesthesia (18%). Endovenous laser therapy (EVLT) is a laser version that works in a very similar manner.

Prognosis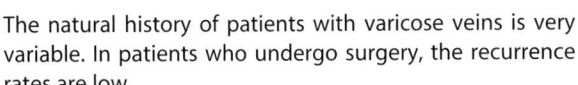

The natural history of patients with varicose veins is very variable. In patients who undergo surgery, the recurrence rates are low.

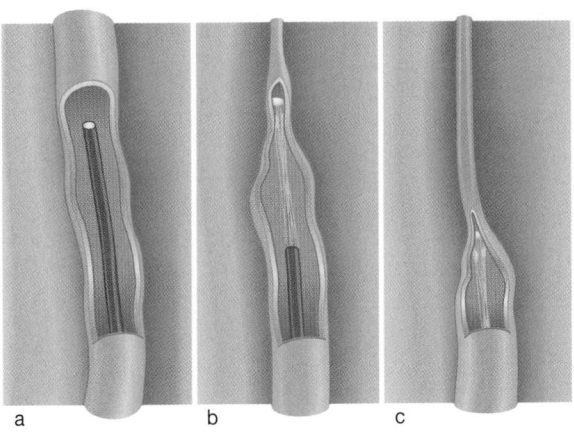

a   b   c

Fig. 1.77 Radiofrequency endovenous occlusion. (a) The catheter is inserted; (b) the vein is warmed and collapses; (c) the catheter is slowly withdrawn, closing the vein.

Venous ulceration

Epidemiology

Leg ulceration is common, affecting 1% of all adults and 3.6% of adults over 65 years. Venous ulcers are the most common cause of leg ulceration (Table 1.45).

Pathology

Venous insufficiency is the underlying cause of venous ulceration that is often precipitated by injury. Approximately 40% of cases are associated with insufficiency of the superficial system of leg veins. Any pathology leading to dysfunction of the calf muscle pump (outflow obstruction, neuromuscular disorders) predisposes to venous insufficiency and the development of ulceration.

In chronic venous hypertension, the microcirculation in the skin and subcutaneous tissues of the lower leg becomes deranged. The capillaries are abnormal and leak fibrinogen, leading to a pericapillary fibrin cuff. This may act as a barrier to oxygen diffusion according to the theory of Browse and Burnand. The trapping of activated leukocytes may also cause tissue damage. These deficiencies in the microcirculation lead to skin damage and ultimately ulceration.

Clinical features

It is important to determine the duration of ulceration, the character of any exudate, whether it is recurrent, and if it is painful. A careful history should note risk factors for ulceration, particularly previous deep vein thrombosis (30–50%), diabetes mellitus, trauma, varicose veins, immobility and rheumatoid arthritis.

Venous ulcers vary in size and location, but are most common in the gaiter area, which is the distal medial aspect of the lower limb (Fig. 1.78) surrounded by telangiectasia

95

Table 1.45	Causes of lower limb ulceration
Venous disease	
Arterial disease	
Mixed arteriovenous	
Trauma	
Neuropathic	
Malignant	
Lymphoedema	
Vasculitis	
Osteomyelitis	
Diabetes	
Pyoderma gangrenosum	
Vasculitis	

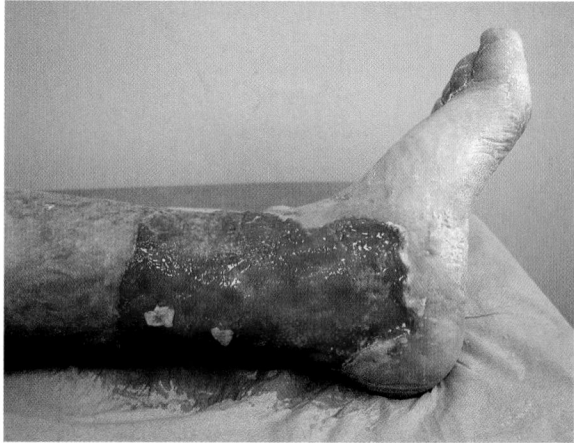

Fig. 1.79 Large venous ulcer with a granulating base.

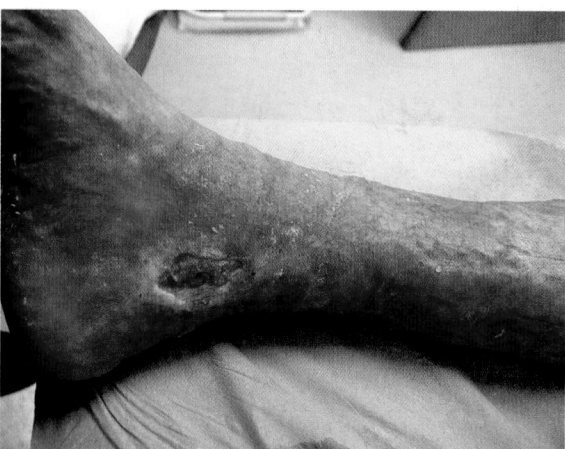

Fig. 1.78 Venous ulcer.

(corona phlebectatica). Pain is not a major feature unless they are infected or there is coexistent ischaemia.

On examination, venous ulcers are well-circumscribed, irregularly shaped, partial thickness ulcers with gently sloping edges. The ulcer is often surrounded by erythematous and hyperpigmented skin. An elevated overlapping edge can result from associated squamous cell carcinoma (Marjolin's ulcer).

The colour of the base is a useful indicator of the state of healing. A red and velvety base indicates a well-healing uninfected ulcer (Fig. 1.79); a white and fibrous base indicates a chronic and non-progressive ulcer; and a yellow and offensive base is usually indicative of infection.

Careful inspection for varicose veins should be made and it is also important to assess the arterial supply to the lower limb (ulcers are less likely to heal in the presence of ischaemia). In the presence of normal pinprick sensation, a normal ABPI indicates that the aetiology of the ulcer will be venous in 95% of patients.

Initial investigations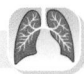

Full blood count
The white cell count may be elevated in the presence of infection.

Random blood glucose
Random blood glucose is estimated as a screening test for diabetes.

Wound swab
A wound swab should be performed to isolate any bacteria.

Further investigations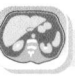

Serum autoantibodies
In patients with a history of joint disorders, autoantibodies should be performed to screen for connective tissue and rheumatoid disease.

Duplex ultrasound
A duplex ultrasound is performed to evaluate the presence of the superficial (60%) and deep venous insufficiency.

Plain X-ray
A plain film X-ray of the underlying bone should be performed in diabetics to exclude osteomyelitis.

Initial management

Lifestyle modification
Patients are advised to reduce weight, avoid smoking, and exercise regularly. When seated, patients should elevate their legs if possible.

General ulcer care
In general only culture-positive ulcers should be treated with antibiotics as clinical diagnosis of infection is unreli-

able. Washing the ulcer with saline is an excellent method for wound cleansing, and patients should be taught this to do at home. Liquid paraffin with silver sulfadiazine should be applied to the ulcer with a light dressing for ulcers associated with substantial exudation. The skin of the lower leg should be kept moist with simple aqueous cream, and topical corticosteroids may be applied to any surrounding eczema.

Compression hosiery

Compression hosiery improves venous flow, reduces reflux and increases ejection of the calf muscle pump. Initially, compression bandaging (except in those with concomitant arterial disease) should be applied and this should be done by an experienced practitioner.

Once the ulcer has healed or is healing well, class II (30 mmHg) or III (40 mmHg) calf length compression stockings should be used instead of compression bandages. Intermittent pneumatic compression should be reserved for those patients who fail to respond to this regimen. In general 70% of venous ulcers heal with compression hosiery treatment by 6 months, although this varies with the initial size of the ulcer.

Surgical management

Varicose vein surgery

Surgery is associated with a better rate of ulcer healing in patients with long or short saphenous incompetence and a normal deep system. Patients with evidence of extensive deep reflux should remain on compression therapy.

Prognosis

The recurrence rate of venous ulceration is 19% in patients who remain on long-term compression hosiery and 40% otherwise.

Varicose veins

Venous ulceration

Diseases of the respiratory system

2

Eric Lim, Mitra Shahidi, Michael Polkey, Peter Goldstraw

SECTION 2.1 | **Introduction**

Applied basic sciences of the respiratory system

Anatomy

The trachea

The trachea starts at the cricoid cartilage and descends slightly to the right of the midline. It bifurcates into the left and right bronchi at the carina, which is at the level of the manubriosternal angle of Louis. It is 10–12 cm long and consists of a series of U-shaped cartilages joined by fibrous tissue and muscle. The site of a tracheostomy is usually over the 2nd to 4th cartilage.

The bronchi

The right main bronchus is wider, shorter and more vertical, providing an easier passage of aspiration. It divides into the upper lobe and intermediate bronchi. The intermediate bronchus subdivides into the middle and lower lobe bronchi. The left main bronchus divides into the upper lobe bronchus (that divides into the upper division and lingula bronchus) and lower lobe bronchus.

Each lobar bronchus divides further to form segmental and subsegmental bronchi; the bronchopulmonary segments are shown in Figure 2.1. The terminal bronchioles divide within an acinus into smaller respiratory bronchioles with alveoli arising from the surface, each bronchiole supplying around 200 alveoli.

The alveoli

There are approximately 300 million alveoli in each lung. They are lined by type I pneumocytes, which provide the thin barrier for gas exchange. Type I pneumocytes are derived from type II pneumocytes, the principal source of surfactant. The interstitium is the lung parenchyma that includes the space between the epithelial and endothelial basement membranes, the target site of inflammation and fibrosis for the pulmonary parenchymal lung disorders. Diseases of the interstitium impair diffusion and gas exchange, and the severity is reflected by the degree of reduction in diffusing capacity.

The lungs

The right lung is divided into upper, middle and lower lobes, the left into upper (lingula) and lower lobes. Blood is supplied for gas exchange by the pulmonary arteries; the bronchial tree is supplied by the bronchial arteries, which are small branches directly from the descending aorta. The nerve supply is from the vagus and sympathetic trunk.

The pleura

This is a layer of fibrous connective tissue covered by a single layer of mesothelial cells which lines the inside of the chest wall (parietal pleura) and reflects back to cover the surface of the lungs (visceral pleura). The visceral and parietal pleurae are in close apposition with some lubricating fluid in between, so the pleural cavity is only a potential space

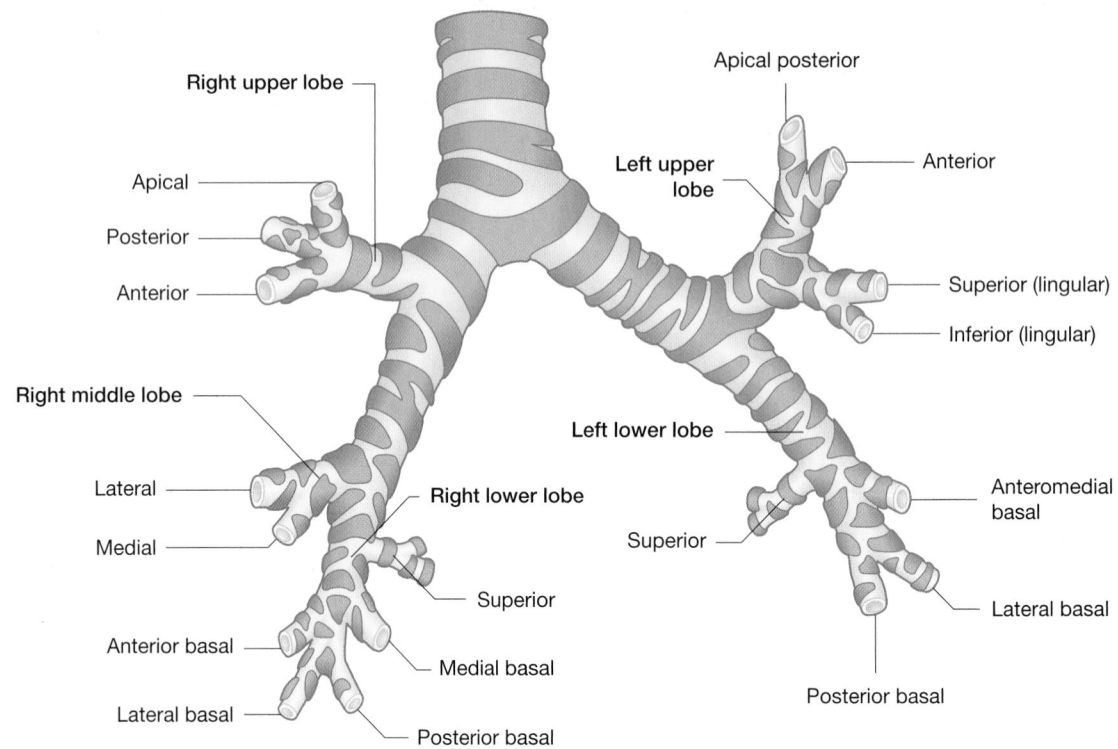

Fig. 2.1 The lobes and segments of the lungs.

until it becomes filled with air (pneumothorax) or fluid (pleural effusion). Normally, 5–10 litres of pleural fluid are produced and absorbed each day, with only 5 mL present in the pleural space at any time.

The mediastinum

The mediastinum is the area between the mediastinal pleura, bounded anteriorly by the sternum, posteriorly by the spine, inferiorly by the diaphragm and superiorly by the thoracic inlet. The anatomical classification of Shields divides the mediastinum into anterior, middle (visceral) and posterior (paravertebral sulci) compartments (p. 172).

The blood supply of the lungs

The lung has a dual blood supply via the pulmonary arteries and the bronchial circulation (bronchial arteries that originate directly from the aorta). Hence, emboli rarely cause pulmonary infarction unless they are small and impact in the terminal arterioles where the vascular territory is predominantly supplied via the pulmonary arteries.

The pulmonary artery accompanies the dividing bronchioles. The arterioles accompanying the respiratory bronchioles are thin-walled for efficient gas exchange. The pulmonary venules drain the periphery of the lobules and pass along the septa to drain centrally into the pulmonary veins. The bronchial veins drain into the pulmonary veins.

Physiology

Breathing

Inspiration is an active process achieved by contraction of the diaphragm and external intercostals that increases the thoracic volume, generating negative pressure to cause air to flow from the environment into the chest (through the airways). Accessory muscles that assist this procedure include the sternocleidomastoid, anterior serrati and the scalene muscles. In quiet breathing, elastic recoil of the diaphragm and intercostal muscles are sufficient to produce expiration.

Unilateral paralysis of the diaphragm may cause reasonably few symptoms in patients with normal lung function; however, patients may experience dyspnoea on exertion or when abdominal pressure rises (bath or swimming pool). Bilateral paralysis is usually asymptomatic at rest, but can lead to dyspnoea on exercise or when lying flat. The use of the accessory muscles at rest is usually seen in patients with obstructive lung disease (severe COPD, acute asthma).

The dynamic compliance of the lung is defined as the change in volume per unit change in transpulmonary pressure. It is a measure of how much the volume will increase (in litres) for each unit decrease in pressure (usually in cm of water). Normal compliance ranges from 0.1 to 0.2 L/cmH$_2$O. Diseases that cause destruction of lung tissue tend to result in increased compliance (COPD) and diseases that cause inflammation, fibrosis (IPF) or restricted thoracic expansion (kyphosis) result in a reduced lung compliance.

The work of breathing is divided into three components: compliance work, tissue resistance work (this is the work required to overcome the viscosity of the lung and chest wall structures) and airways resistance work. As compliance falls or airway resistance increases (COPD, asthma), the work of breathing increases. This results in greater oxygen consumption. If consumption is not matched by increased ventilation for gas exchange (severe pulmonary disease), or if the situation is not reversed with medication (e.g. bronchodilators with acute severe asthma), respiratory failure ensues and mechanical ventilation will be required to maintain life.

Ventilation and perfusion relationships

Alveolar ventilation is the total volume of new air entering the alveoli each minute (respiratory rate per minute multiplied by tidal volume minus dead space volume). During quiet respiration, the tidal volume (p. 102) is sufficient only to reach the terminal bronchioles. Only a very small amount actually reaches the alveoli directly, the remaining distance is achieved by diffusion. This is due to the dead space volume, which is the volume of air in the respiratory passages that do not take part in ventilation. After a period of prolonged mechanical ventilation, a tracheostomy is sometimes used to reduce the dead space volume (from mid trachea to the oropharynx) to improve alveolar ventilation and assist in weaning.

Normally, in the vast majority of the lung, ventilation and perfusion is well matched. In diffuse lung disease, the overall ventilation and perfusion may be matched; however, there will be wide variation in the matching of ventilation with perfusion. In areas of ventilation and perfusion mismatch, carbon dioxide levels are usually held within normal limits because it is carried in solution and therefore high levels can be lowered by mixing with blood from areas of well-matched ventilation and perfusion. Oxygen, however, is carried principally by haemoglobin, therefore normal lung tissue can only compensate for low levels in areas of poor ventilation and perfusion up to the point where haemoglobin is fully saturated. As disease progresses, a point will be reached where no further compensation can occur and oxygen levels will decrease.

Pulmonary embolism is an example in which gross ventilation and perfusion mismatch can occur, leading to hypoxaemia. Carbon dioxide levels are usually within normal limits for the reasons given above, and may be lower than normal due to hyperventilation in an attempt to compensate for low oxygen levels.

Symptoms of respiratory disease

Cough

Cough is a reflex explosive expiration that prevents aspiration and promotes the removal of secretions and foreign particles from the lung. It is a common symptom of respiratory disease described on page 111. Cough may be productive of clear, discoloured or frankly purulent sputum. Haemoptysis is coughing up of blood and is detailed on page 114.

Dyspnoea

The causes of shortness of breath are varied, and may be due to respiratory, cardiac, neuromuscular, haematological or metabolic causes. Dyspnoea is covered in detail on page 113.

Wheeze

A wheeze is a continuous expiratory high-pitched whistling sound of air flowing through narrowed airways. It is a common symptom of obstructive respiratory diseases such as asthma or COPD.

Stridor

Stridor is a monophonic inspiratory wheeze-like sound heard with upper airways obstruction. Acute stridor, such as in anaphylactic reactions, can lead to rapid respiratory arrest due to complete closure of the inflamed cords.

Chest pain

Respiratory disease may be associated with pleuritic chest pain that is worse on inspiration.

Examination of the respiratory system

For the respiratory examination, patients should be positioned at 45 degrees and undressed from the waist up.

Inspection

General inspection reveals a lot of information. The conscious level of the patient is immediately apparent, as is any shortness of breath at rest. The respiratory rate can be counted from the end of the bed. The effort required to breathe should be noted: patients with obstructive airways disease may have pursed lip breathing, prolonged exhalation and use of accessory muscles. Inspection of the chest from the end of the bed will detect any deformities such as kyphosis or a barrel-shaped chest. Scars may require closer scrutiny. Symmetry of lung expansion may be noted. Finally, it is important to examine the surroundings of the patient, and any sputum pots.

Inspection then progresses to the hands. Finger clubbing may be noted; this is a drumstick appearance of the tips of the fingers with loss of the angle between the nailbed and the nail. Asterixis is a flapping tremor of the hands due to carbon dioxide retention.

The mucous membranes of the lips should be examined for cyanosis, a blue discolouration of the skin due to deoxygenated haemoglobin (low oxygen levels). Central cyanosis is a sign of hypoxia but peripheral cyanosis (bluish discolouration of the fingers) can occur with normal oxygen levels in the presence of peripheral vasoconstriction (cold weather, low blood pressure).

Palpation

The position of the trachea is palpated in the suprasternal notch. Deviation from the midline suggests mediastinal shift that can occur by a large pleural effusion pushing it across the midline or collapse of a lobe pulling it towards the side of the disorder.

The supraclavicular fossae should be palpated for enlarged lymph nodes. Expansion of the upper chest is assessed by placing the hands on the upper anterior chest either side of the sternum and asking the patient to take a deep breath. Expansion of the lower chest is assessed by placing both hands around the lateral walls of the chest.

Percussion

Percussion of the chest can detect whether there is hyper-resonance such as with a pneumothorax, or dullness such as with an effusion ('stony dull') or consolidation. Percussion should be performed comparing the same area on the right as the left and working down the chest back and forth across both sides.

Auscultation

As with percussion, the right and left sides of the chest should be compared at the same levels. Normal sounds are described as vesicular. If breath sounds are absent or reduced this may be a sign of pneumothorax, effusion or a collapsed area of lung. Bronchial breathing is a continuous (wind-like) breath sound with no gap between inspiration and expiration, and is suggestive of consolidation. This type of sound is normally audible when the stethoscope is placed over the trachea.

Vocal resonance is the relative loudness of speech. The stethoscope is placed on the chest and the patient is asked to say '99'. If the sound is louder compared with the unaffected side, vocal resonance is increased (consolidation). If the sound is dampened down compared with the unaffected side, vocal resonance is decreased (pleural effusion).

Additional sounds include crepitations, which are crackly sounds that can occur on inspiration or expiration; they may be indicative of sputum or fibrotic lung disease. Wheezing is usually a sign of narrowed airways and may indicate asthma. A pleural rub is a sound like feet crunching on snow, usually caused by inflamed pleura.

SECTION 2.2

Investigations for respiratory disease

Arterial blood gases

Arterial blood is usually sampled from the radial brachial or femoral artery using a pre-heparinized syringe. The sample is analyzed and the partial pressures of oxygen (PO_2) and carbon dioxide (PCO_2) and the hydrogen ion concentrations (H^+) are determined. From these values, the bicarbonate concentration, base excess and oxygen saturations are calculated. Apart from blood gas estimation, disorders of acid–base balance will also be revealed (Table 2.1).

Pulmonary function tests

Three important types of test are used in standard lung function laboratories. These are spirometric indices, plethysmographic lung volumes and carbon monoxide gas transfer. They can be used to aid diagnosis, assess disease severity, monitor progression of the disease and/or treatment response, as a screening tool, and for operative risk assessment and planning for lung resection.

Spirometry

Patients are asked to inhale maximally and breathe out through the spirometer as hard and as fast as they can, continuing until all the breath has been exhaled.

The volume expired in the first second of this manoeuvre is the FEV_1 (forced expired volume in one second), a measure of how quickly the lungs can be emptied. The forced vital capacity (FVC) is the total volume of air exhaled during the manoeuvre, which arbitrarily is conventionally measured at 6 seconds (Fig. 2.2). In patients with severe airflow limitation the slow vital capacity may be significantly

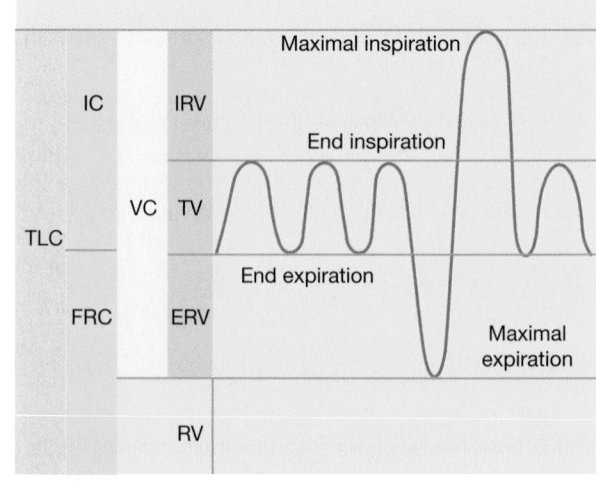

Fig. 2.2 Schematic illustration of lung volumes.

Table 2.1	Acid–base disturbances				
	H^+	Po_2	Pco_2	HCO_3	Examples
Respiratory acidosis					
Acute (uncompensated)	↑	↓	↑	N	Exacerbation of COPD
Chronic (compensated)	N	↓	↑	↑	Motor neuron disease
Metabolic acidosis					
Acute (uncompensated)	↑	N	N	↓	Diabetic ketoacidosis
Chronic (compensated)	N	↑	↓	↓	Chronic renal failure
Respiratory alkalosis					
Acute (uncompensated)	↓	↑	↓	N	Acute hyperventilation
Chronic (compensated)	N	↑	↓	↓	Chronic hyperventilation
Metabolic alkalosis					
Acute (uncompensated)	↓	N	↑	↑	Acute severe vomiting
Chronic (compensated)	N	↓	↑	↑	Chronic vomiting (anorexia nervosa)

greater than the FVC. The FEV_1/FVC ratio gives a clinically useful index of airflow limitation. Ratios of less than 70% indicate an obstructive lung defect (Table 2.2). Patients with restrictive lung defects have normal or raised FEV_1/FVC ratio with reduced FVC.

Forced expiratory flow between 25% and 75% of FVC ($FEF_{25-75\%}$) is the average expired flow over the middle part of the FVC manoeuvre and is a more sensitive measure of small airways narrowing. Peak expiratory flow rate is the maximal expiratory flow rate achieved measured in litres per second, and is considered to not reflect the large airways.

Static lung volumes

Whole body plethysmography is used to measure residual volume (RV), functional residual capacity (FRC) and total lung capacity (TLC) (Figure 2.2, Table 2.3). Two types of plethysmographs may be constructed but the most commonly used is a constant volume box. Changes in lung volume moving from one lung volume to another are inferred, using Boyle's law from changes in pressure. In addition, dynamic lung volumes can also be assessed using flow volume loops (Fig. 2.3).

Diffusing capacity (transfer factor)

Carbon monoxide is used to measure the diffusing capacity of the lung (TL_{co}); the older term DL_{co} is still used in North America. Carbon monoxide is similar to oxygen in molecular weight and solubility and has a high affinity for haemoglobin. The amount inspired is known and the amount expired is measured; the difference is used to calculate the diffusing capacity of the lung, a measure of the surface area and nature of the air–blood interface. Therefore it has to be taken in context with alveolar ventilation (Va).

The TL_{co} divided by the alveolar volume (Va) gives rise to the transfer coefficient (K_{co}), and further correction for haemoglobin concentration gives the K_{coc} (transfer coefficient, corrected for haemoglobin).

Any disease process that involves the lung parenchyma rather than or in addition to the airways may bring about a decrease in the TL_{co}, e.g. emphysema or interstitial lung disease. Gas transfer measurements are influenced by anaemia/polycythaemia and so should be corrected for haemoglobin.

Bronchial challenge tests

This test involves provoking bronchospasm by inhalation of an irritant such as methacholine or histamine. The allergen is inhaled at increasing concentrations and the FEV_1 is measured. The concentration at which the FEV_1 falls by 20% is called the provocation concentration (PC_{20}). A PC_{20} of less than 8 mg/mL is indicative of bronchial hyperresponsiveness.

Walk tests

The 6-minute walk test and shuttle walk test measure exercise capacity. During the 6-minute walk, patients are asked to walk at their own pace and the distance covered in 6 minutes is measured.

The shuttle walk test involves the patient walking between two posts at an increasing pace, determined by audio signals from a cassette. The level at which the patient is unable to keep up with the paced signals determines his or her level of breathlessness.

Cardiopulmonary exercise testing

Cardiopulmonary exercise testing provides a global assessment of the integrative exercise responses involving the pulmonary, cardiovascular, neurological and skeletal muscle

103

Table 2.2 Pulmonary function tests results with disease

Disease	FEV$_1$	FVC	FEV$_1$/FVC	TLC	TL$_{CO}$	K$_{CO}$
Emphysema	↓↓	↓/N	<70%	↑	↓	↓/N
COPD	↓↓	↓/N	<70%	↑	N	N
Asthma (during exacerbation)	↓	N/↓	<70%	N	N	N/↑
Lung fibrosis	↓	↓↓	>80%	↓	↓	N
Neuromuscular disease/obesity/scoliosis	↓	↓	>80%	↓	N	N/↑
Pneumonectomy	↓↓	↓↓	>80%	↓↓	↓↓	N

Table 2.3 Measurements of static lung volumes

Measurement	Derivation
Tidal volume (V$_T$)	The amount of air in the lungs between normal resting inspiration and expiration
Inspiratory reserve volume (IRV)	The volume of air in the lung from end inspiration to maximal inspiration
Expiratory reserve volume (ERV)	The volume of air in the lung from end expiration to maximal expiration
Residual volume (RV)	The volume of air left in the lungs after maximal expiration (this cannot be measured directly)
Total lung capacity (TLC)	The total volume of air in the lungs at maximal inspiration (this cannot be measured directly)
Inspiratory capacity (IC)	The volume measured from resting end expiration to maximal inspiration TLC – FRC
Functional residual capacity (FRC)	The volume of air in the lungs at resting end expiration, i.e. RV + ERV
Vital capacity (VC)	The volume of air from maximal inspiration to maximal expiration (IRV + TV + ERV)

systems. The indications are undiagnosed exercise intolerance, exercise related symptoms, and the objective determination of functional capacity and impairment.

During this test the patients exercise up to the limits of their breathlessness on the treadmill or a cycle ergometer. Maximum oxygen consumption (Vo$_2$ max), carbon dioxide output (Vco$_2$), minute ventilation, 12 lead ECG, blood pressure, pulse oximetry, and occasionally arterial blood gases are documented during exercise.

Respiratory muscle tests

The strength of the respiratory muscles, in particular the diaphragm, can be measured through voluntary manoeuvres and stimulation of the phrenic nerve externally. These tests may be indicated to screen for respiratory muscle dysfunction in patients with unexplained breathlessness, apparently small lungs on chest X-ray in the absence of lung disease (i.e. bilateral diaphragm paralysis) and for patients with suspected global neurological disease.

Diagnostic imaging

Chest X-ray (CXR)

This is probably the most essential investigation when assessing a patient with respiratory disease. Ideally the film is taken in a postero-anterior (PA) projection (the X-rays pass through the patient from back to front and the X-ray plate is placed in front of the chest) in full inspiration with the patient upright.

When looking at the film a system should be employed which ensures that all elements of the X-ray are examined. One method is to look at the lung fields first, then the mediastinal and hilar structures and the heart, next looking at the inner surface of the chest wall for pleural abnormalities, the diaphragms, the bony structures and finally any abnormalities in extra-thoracic structures such as the breast.

When examining the lung fields, it is useful to screen for abnormalities (opacities) in the upper, middle and lower zones, comparing left with right lung fields (Fig. 2.4). The mediastinal borders pass through the medial aspect of each clavicle and merge on the right with the right heart border and on the left with the aortic arch and left heart border. The hilar shadows consist of the pulmonary arteries and branches, and normal lymph nodes are not visible. The size and position of the heart is described on page 1–2.

The diaphragmatic surfaces should be smooth and clearly visible from one costophrenic angle to the other. When examining the clavicle, ribs and spine there should not be any evidence of abnormal lucencies or bony prominences.

Computed tomography (CT)

With CT scanning, cross-sectional images delineate mediastinal and hilar structures clearly and provide detailed

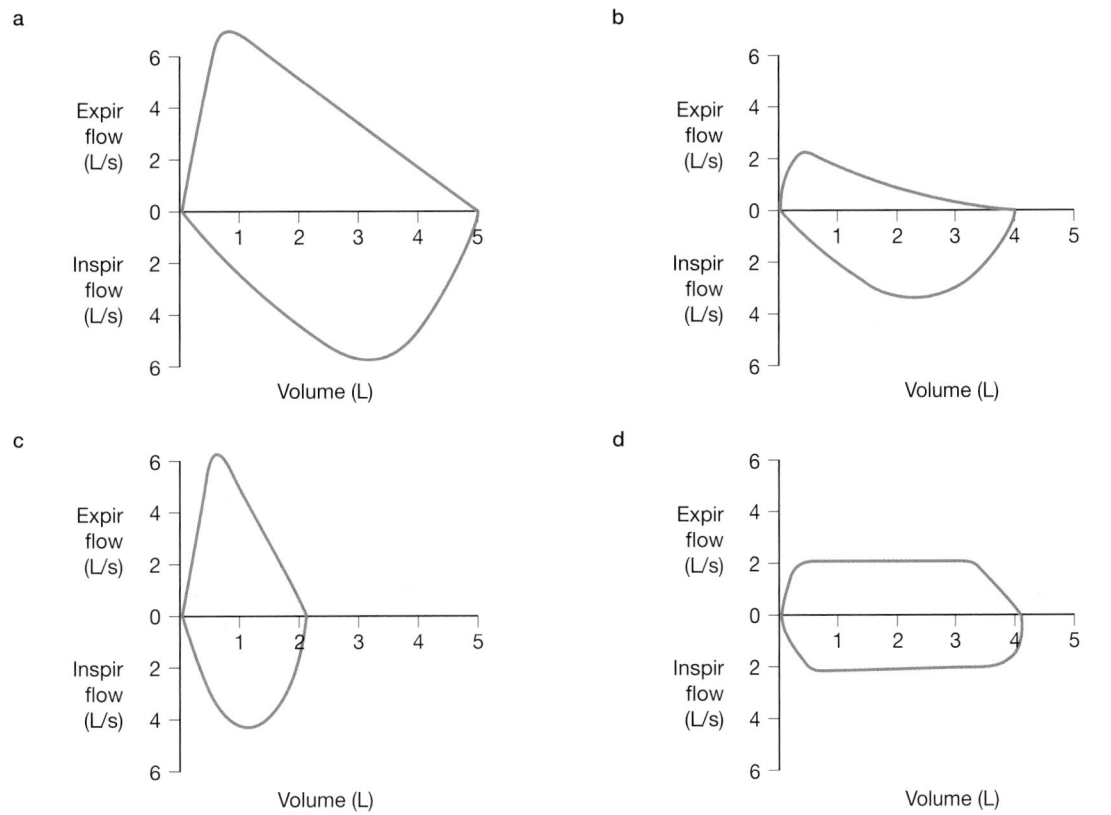

Fig. 2.3 Pulmonary flow volume loops. (a) Normal. (b) Obstructive. (c) Restrictive. (d) Fixed.

information on the lung parenchyma. Masses can be visualized accurately and their relation to adjacent structures clearly defined (Figs 2.5 and 2.6).

CT can be conventional, high-resolution or spiral. Conventional CT is useful for characterizing masses, pleural disease or structures in the mediastinum. High-resolution CT (HRCT) enables resolution of smaller structures and gives images comparable to macroscopic pathology specimens. This is useful for looking more closely at the lung parenchyma in conditions such as diffuse parenchymal lung disorders

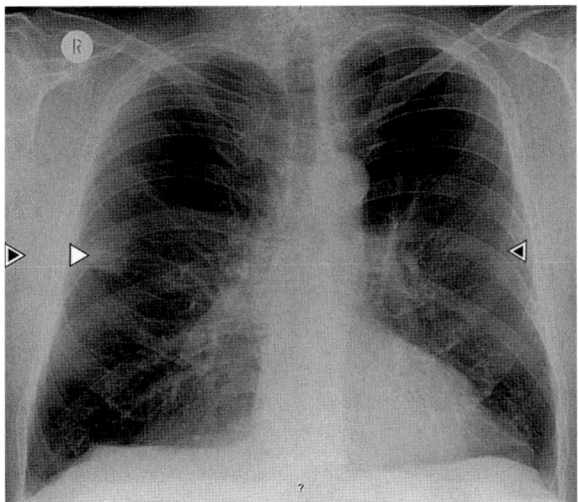

Fig. 2.4 This plain chest film reveals a mass in the right middle zone.
Image courtesy of Mr Michael Dusmet, Consultant Thoracic Surgeon, Royal Brompton Hospital, London, UK.

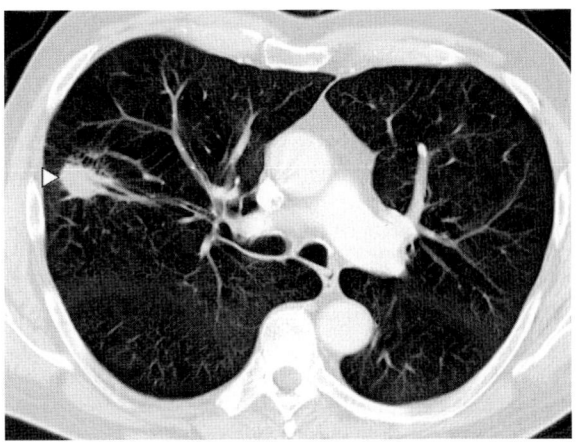

Fig. 2.5 The CT thorax confirms a mass in the right upper lobe.
Image courtesy of Mr Michael Dusmet, Consultant Thoracic Surgeon, Royal Brompton Hospital, London, UK.

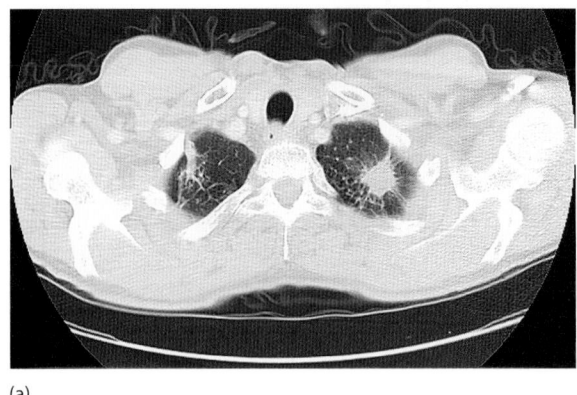
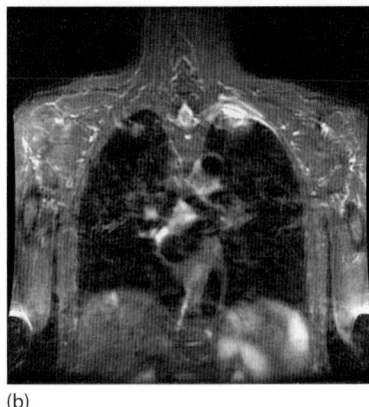

(a)   (b)

Fig. 2.6 CT and MRI of the thorax. The CT scan (a) identifies a left upper lobe (superior sulcus). Pancoast tumour and confirmation of invasion into the brachial plexus can be seen with the MRI (b).

(p. 140), bronchiectasis and emphysema. Spiral CT takes continuous images in a spiral fashion in one breath hold and so has the advantage of being quicker, which may of necessity be a consideration in patients who are breathless at rest. Images can be reconstructed to provide the same information as conventional or high-resolution CT. Contrast enhanced CT can also be used to visualize the pulmonary arteries and has now become the investigation of choice for suspected pulmonary embolism.

Ultrasound scan (USS)

Ultrasound of the chest can be useful in detecting pleural fluid, estimating the thickness of abnormal pleura, and pinpointing the best site to insert an intercostal drain or obtain pleural biopsies. Ultrasound can also determine the presence of loculations within pleural effusions.

Positron emission tomography (PET) scan

PET scanning is achieved by injection of a glucose analogue tagged to a fluorine-18 isotope, [18]fluorodeoxyglucose. Metabolically active tissue (neoplasms, infections) exhibits an increased rate of glucose metabolism and this is detected by a gamma camera as a PET avid area (Fig. 2.7). Current uses of PET scanning include the evaluation of malignancy in focal lung lesions. PET scanning has an overall sensitivity of 97% and specificity of 78% to diagnose cancer.[1] False positive results can be obtained with inflammatory conditions such as tuberculosis and benign tumours.

Ventilation/perfusion scan (V/Q)

This is a nuclear medicine scan that images ventilation ($\dot{V}$) and perfusion ($\dot{Q}$) of the lungs separately, mainly in the diagnosis of pulmonary embolism. The scans can then be looked at together to see if there is any $\dot{V}/\dot{Q}$ mismatch, suggesting a pulmonary embolus. If there is underlying lung disease the scans may be difficult to interpret and this limits the use of this investigation.

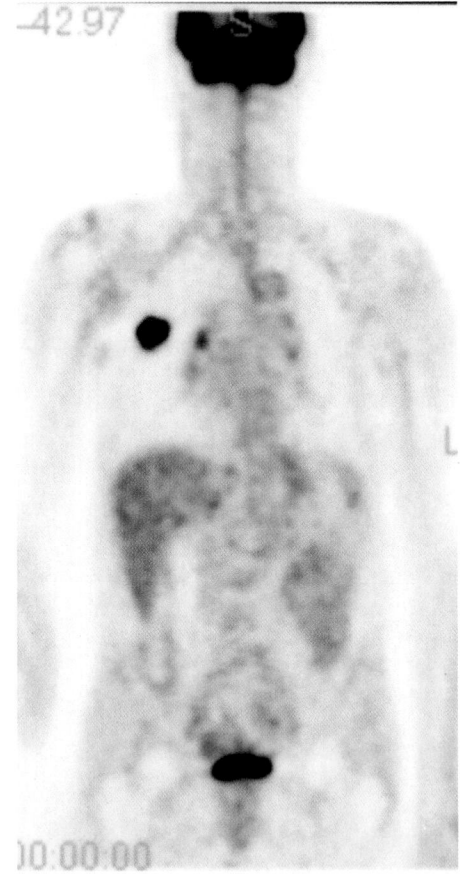

Fig. 2.7 PET scan. The mass identified in Figures 2.4 and 2.5 is PET positive.
Image courtesy of Mr Michael Dusmet, Consultant Thoracic Surgeon, Royal Brompton Hospital, London, UK.

Conventional pulmonary angiography

Conventional pulmonary angiography is performed by injecting contrast into the pulmonary arteries under fluoroscopic (X-ray) control to delineate the pulmonary arteries. This investigation is now reserved for patients with suspected massive pulmonary embolism as, in addition, intra-arterial thrombolysis or mechanical clot disruption can be performed. Pulmonary angiography may be indicated in patients with massive haemoptysis to find the offending vessel with a view to embolization.

REFERENCE

(1) *Gould MK, Maclean CC, Kuschner WG, Rydzak CE, Owens DK. Accuracy of positron emission tomography for diagnosis of pulmonary nodules and mass lesions: a meta-analysis. JAMA 2001; 285: 914–924.*

SECTION 2.3 **Diagnostic procedures**

Bronchoscopy

Flexible and rigid bronchoscopy are two different methods of gaining access to and visualizing the airways.

Flexible bronchoscopy

Indications

A flexible fibreoptic bronchoscope can be used to examine the bronchial tree and vocal cords (to exclude a recurrent laryngeal nerve palsy) prior to surgery. It can also be used for the diagnosis of endobronchial lesions. Additional techniques such as endobronchial biopsy can be performed to obtain specimens of endobronchial lung tumours or to sample abnormal respiratory epithelium. Bronchial brushings may increase the diagnostic yield.

Bronchial washings may be used to obtain cytology in cases of suspected malignancy and are also useful in the diagnosis of suspected infections, notably tuberculosis and *Pneumocystis carinii*. Bronchial lavage and cell counts may be useful for the differential diagnosis of parenchymal lung disease (transbronchial biopsies can be performed to diagnose parenchymal lung disease). In addition, transbronchial lymph node aspiration may be performed to stage lung cancer. Fibreoptic bronchoscopy also allows for the aspiration of pus and impacted secretions and retrieval of selected foreign bodies.

Patient preparation

Informed consent is obtained and patients should be fasted for 4 hours prior to the procedure (in case of any complications that may arise requiring general anaesthesia). Oxygen saturation monitoring is required and resuscitation/ anaesthetic facilities are essential.

Procedure

Intravenous sedation is normally offered. The choice of drug varies with the operator but a typical sedative could be midazolam. Topical lidocaine is sprayed into the nasal passage and sufficient time allowed for anaesthesia. The fibreoptic scope is introduced into the nose and further lidocaine administered through the side arm of the scope to progressively anaesthetize the hypopharynx, larynx and vocal cords. Progressing from the trachea, the entire tracheobronchial tree should be readily visualized.

Complications

Major complications are few, occurring in 1.7%. These include mortality (0.1%), respiratory arrest, pneumonia and airway obstruction. Minor complications include vasovagal reactions, fever, cardiac arrhythmias, bleeding, nausea and vomiting, and aphonia in 6.5%.[1] Supplemental procedures such as transbronchial biopsy carry additional risks of pneumothorax (10%).

Post procedure care

Post procedure, patients are observed for up to 4 hours before returning to a ward or being discharged home.

Rigid bronchoscopy

Indications

A wider range of therapeutic procedures can be performed with rigid bronchoscopy, however general anaesthesia is required. The range of indications includes massive haemoptysis, airway obstruction, and local therapy for tumours that invade the airways and strictures (e.g. stenting).

Patient preparation

Informed consent is required. Patients should be fasted overnight as general anaesthesia is required.

Procedure

After general anaesthesia is administered, the patient is ventilated with a high inspired concentration of oxygen. The eyes are taped and the neck extended. The rigid bronchoscope is introduced under direct vision through the mouth (taking care not to injure the gums or teeth), past the epiglottis and vocal cords and into the trachea. Intermittent jet ventilation (through the bronchoscope) is required to maintain gas exchange during the procedure.

The entire tracheobronchial tree can be visualized and a wide variety of diagnostic and therapeutic procedures undertaken.

Complications

Injuries to the lips, gums and teeth can occur but pharyngeal lacerations are rare. Bleeding can occur from trauma to the airway during this procedure but major haemorrhage is rare and is usually associated with biopsies of vascular tumours. Barotrauma from jet ventilation can produce surgical emphysema and/or pneumothorax.

Post procedure care

Patients are recovered on a high-dependency unit for 4 hours, and a chest X-ray is usually performed to screen for complications.

> **REFERENCE**
>
> (1) Pereira W Jr, Kovnat DM, Snider GL. *A prospective cooperative study of complications following flexible fiberoptic bronchoscopy. Chest 1978; 73: 813–816.*

Pleural biopsy

Indications

The main indication for a pleural biopsy is to provide samples for histopathology, usually as part of a diagnostic workup for a pleural effusion of unknown cause (p. 165). Coagulation abnormality (bleeding) and positive pressure ventilation (risk of pneumothorax by inadvertent lung biopsy) are relative contraindications to this procedure.

Patient preparation

Informed consent is required. The positioning, preparation of the patient and local anaesthetic administration is exactly the same as that for a thoracocentesis (p. 109).

After the local anaesthetic is infiltrated, a small skin incision is made and the syringe with the fitted Abrams needle is introduced into the same puncture hole. Aspiration of the needle is performed to confirm the position in the pleural space and the cutting trocar is then rotated into the closed position to obtain a pleural biopsy. Multiple biopsies are taken and the samples should be placed in formalin. Unless tuberculosis (TB) can be excluded on clinical grounds it is good practice to send specimens for TB culture.

Complications

A small pneumothorax is the most common complication (few require treatment). Other complications include bleeding, vasovagal reaction (bradycardia, hypotension) and pain.

Post procedure care

A chest X-ray is obtained after the procedure to screen for pneumothorax.

> **RECENT ADVANCES**
>
> *Blind pleural biopsy has largely been superseded by CT-guided pleural biopsy as specific areas of abnormalities can be identified.*

Cervical mediastinoscopy

Indications

Cervical mediastinoscopy is undertaken as a diagnostic procedure to obtain tissue samples from mediastinal masses (p. 153) and mediastinal lymph nodes (paratracheal, subcarinal) for the diagnosis of benign disorders (sarcoidosis) and staging of malignant disease (p. 152–153).

Patient preparation

Informed consent is required. Patients should be starved appropriately for general anaesthesia.

Procedure

Under general anaesthesia, a small sandbag is placed between the patient's shoulder blades and the neck is extended. A 2–3 cm transverse cervical incision is performed and a combination of diathermy and sharp dissection proceeds along the midline to the pretracheal fascia. A finger is introduced deep to the pretracheal fascia and along the anterior trachea. A cervical mediastinoscope (often with video-assisted visualization) is introduced to examine any mediastinal masses or to obtain lymph node biopsies. After ensuring haemostasis, the wound is closed in layers.

Complications

Complications occur in approximately 2%.[1] They include major bleeding, tracheal rupture, recurrent laryngeal nerve palsy and perforation of the oesophagus. Other less severe complications are wound infection, haematoma and pneumothorax.

Post procedure care

Patients are recovered on the high-dependency unit for 4 hours prior to returning to the ward. A chest X-ray is usually performed to screen for pneumothorax.

> **REFERENCE**
>
> (1) Luke WP, Pearson FG, Todd TR, Patterson GA, Cooper JD. *Prospective evaluation of mediastinoscopy for assessment of carcinoma of the lung. Journal of Thoracic and Cardiovascular Surgery 1986; 91: 53–56.*

Open lung biopsy

Indications

An open lung biopsy is usually performed to obtain histopathological specimens to assist in the diagnosis of parenchymal lung disease after less invasive methods have failed to provide a diagnosis.

Patient preparation

Informed consent is required. Patients should be fasted appropriately for a general anaesthetic. Preoperative investigations should include a CT thorax to determine the target biopsy site. Full lung function tests should be performed to assess the pulmonary reserve and determine the best approach (thoracotomy or video-assisted thoracoscopy—VATS).

Procedure

In patients with relatively well-preserved lung function (able to tolerate single lung ventilation) and the absence of pleural adhesions, the VATS approach may be employed. Under general anaesthesia, patients are positioned in a lateral position. An initial incision (2–3 cm) is usually performed in the midaxillary line and the VATS camera introduced to examine the pleural space and lung surfaces. The second and third portholes are usually made under direct vision in an inverted triangle to allow the entry of a grasper and a lung stapler. The target sections of lung are identified (usually along a fissure) and removed with an endoscopic lung stapler.

In patients with poor lung function who would not tolerate single lung ventilation, a mini-thoracotomy is undertaken, the appropriate section of lung identified and stapled or clamped, incised, and repaired in two layers (horizontal mattress, followed by a running layer of vertical mattress sutures). A single drain is usually left at the apex of the pleural cavity (with either approach).

Complications

Significant mortality is associated with this procedure, and is usually reflective of the poor general health of patients requiring open lung biopsy. It ranges from 12% to 54% depending on indication and urgency.[1,2]

Post procedure care

Postoperatively, patients are recovered on the high-dependency or intensive care unit depending on general health. The chest drain is usually removed 24 hours after any air leak has ceased.

REFERENCES

(1) *Temes RT, Joste NE, Qualls CR, Allen NL, Crowell RE, Dox HA, Wernly JA. Lung biopsy: is it necessary? Journal of Thoracic and Cardiovascular Surgery 1999; 118: 1097–1100.*
(2) *Satterfield JR Jr, McLaughlin JS. Open lung biopsy in diagnosing pulmonary infiltrates in immunosuppressed patients. Annals of Thoracic Surgery 1979; 28: 359–362.*

Thoracocentesis

Insertion of an intercostal chest drain

SECTION 2.4 Therapeutic procedures

Thoracocentesis

Indications

The indications for thoracocentesis are diagnostic aspiration of pleural fluid in the investigation for a pleural effusion of unknown cause (p. 164) and also to relieve the symptoms of a pleural effusion. Occasionally, it is used for the aspiration of a pneumothorax (p. 169). Abnormal coagulation is a relative contraindication.

Patient preparation

Patients are seated on the edge of a bed, leaning comfortably on a pillow placed on a bedside table of appropriate height. A chest X-ray or CT scan (if performed) should be examined to guide the level and site of entry. Alternatively, the procedure can be performed under ultrasound guidance.

Procedure

The operator should be gowned and gloved, the skin prepared with antiseptic solution and draped. A syringe with 10 mL 1% lidocaine is required and the site of the subsequent biopsy should be entered, while sustaining gentle aspiration. The point of entry should be lateral to the paraspinal muscles and inferior to the scapula for aspiration of pleural effusion, or the second intercostal space in the midclavicular line for aspiration of a pneumothorax. A small amount of lidocaine (1–2 mL) should be infiltrated into the skin at the point of entry (to create a wheal) before advancing into the pleural space. When the pleural space has been entered, there is a flash of pleural fluid (or air with a pneumothorax) with release of the tension on the syringe. The syringe is withdrawn until no pleural fluid or air is aspirated and the lidocaine infiltrated at this point.

Once the needle has been removed from the patient, and the anaesthetic given time to work, the patient is asked to take a deep breath and slow exhalation (asked to say 'Eeeeeee') while a 14 G cannula is introduced into the pleural space through the same puncture site as the local anaesthetic. Once the flash of pleural fluid or air is seen, a three-way tap is attached (it is important that the patient continues to exhale whilst a three-way tap is attached to minimize the risk of a pneumothorax).

A 50 mL syringe is then attached to the three-way tap and the pleural fluid or air is aspirated.

Complications

Complications include a pneumothorax (often a small pneumothorax manifests by the loss of the pleural fluid meniscus), bleeding and rarely infection of the pleural space (empyema).

Post procedure care

A chest X-ray is performed to assess the size of or screen for a pneumothorax, to assess the amount of remaining fluid and to check for re-expansion of the lung.

Insertion of an intercostal chest drain

Intercostal chest tube drainage with an underwater seal is a simple and effective method to eliminate air or fluid in the pleural space.

 CLINICAL ALERT

Emergency decompression of tension pneumothorax is undertaken by a wide-bore cannula in the second intercostal space (midclavicular line) of the affected side.

Indications

The main indications for chest drain insertion are moderate to large spontaneous pneumothoraces, symptomatic pleural effusions or haemothorax (traumatic or spontaneous).

Relative contraindications are abnormal coagulation status and suspected pleural adhesions (specialist expertise is required).

Patient preparation

The patient is positioned lying with the shoulder elevated and undressed to the waist with the arm abducted at 90 degrees. The arm may be held behind the head, but this often results in a slow downward drift as the patient becomes tired or experiences pain. Absorbent pads are placed under the patient to prevent soiling of the clothes or bed.

Procedure

The triangle (or, more correctly, quadrangle) of safety is bounded posteriorly by the posterior axillary line, anteriorly by the lateral border of pectoralis major, and overlies the 3rd to 5th intercostal spaces (Fig. 2.8). Usually the 4th intercostal space is chosen just anterior to the midaxillary line.

The surgical field is prepared with antiseptic solution and the patient is draped. Approximately 2 mL of 1% lidocaine is then injected to create a transverse wheal to demarcate the length and position of the skin incision. The tip of the scalpel blade is used to make a skin incision large enough to comfortably admit the index finger.

Blunt dissection with Roberts forceps can usually proceed painlessly through the subcutaneous fat up to deep fascia without any lidocaine. Once the deep fascia is reached, the intercostal space becomes distinctive. Further lidocaine (8 mL) is used to create a field block by injecting multiple intercostal nerves. The needle is advanced to identify the rib immediately superior to the chosen intercostal space

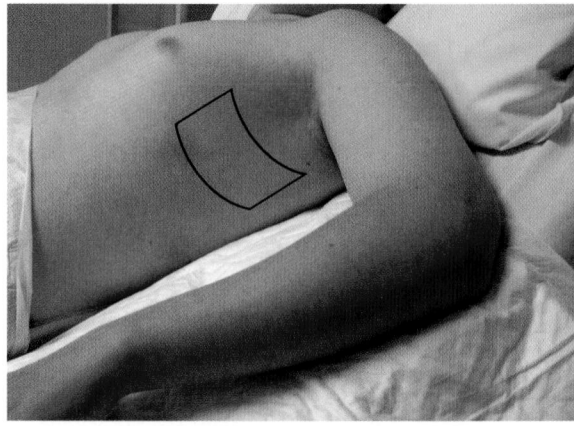

Fig. 2.8 Positioning for chest drain insertion.

and 'walked' down the rib until soft tissue is felt. The needle is then angled 45 degrees upwards and the syringe aspirated to ensure that the tip does not lie within the vessels of the neurovascular bundle before injecting 2–3 mL of 1% lidocaine. Using the same method, a further 2 mL is injected in the targeted intercostal space to block the intercostal nerve anteriorly and also in the intercostal nerve of the space above and below the targeted intercostal space.

After leaving adequate time for the intercostal block to work, the Roberts clamp is then used with gentle but firm pressure, spreading the intercostal muscles apart and dissecting superiorly starting at the lower margin of the intercostal space (to avoid the neurovascular bundle). The Roberts clamp should enter the pleural cavity easily once the deep fascia and muscle layer has been negotiated. A gush of air or fluid is normally experienced at this point. The jaw of the Roberts is opened to dilate the puncture site, and then followed by the index finger to dilate a track into the pleural space. This is an important step. The tip of the finger will detect any adherent lung tissue, and the track is dilated in the process to comfortably admit a 28 F chest drain. If this manoeuvre is not performed satisfactorily, it can become difficult to find the tract for the chest drain as the tissues retract to seal the path made by the Roberts clamp.

Once it has been ascertained that there is no lung tissue adherent to the chest wall, a 28 F drain is introduced into the pleural space without a trocar. The drain is advanced continuously until a change in resistance is felt as the tip abuts the pleural apex or base of the diaphragm. Occasionally, pain is experienced in the neck and shoulder as the tip of the drain impinges on the apex. Withdrawal of the drain by an inch ensures a perfectly apical position and alleviation of pain. At this point, make a mental note of the distance marker at skin level.

Once the drain is sited, it is attached to an underwater seal. Entry into the thoracic cavity is suggested by fogging of the tube, a respiratory swing and bubbling of the fluid level on coughing. The drain is then fixed with a suture.

Complications

Major complications are rare and include perforation of the lung and haemorrhage (laceration to the intercostal artery).

Post procedure care

It is standard practice to obtain a post chest drain insertion film to ensure that the drain lies within the thoracic cavity, evaluate the position of the drain, ensure re-expansion of the lung and screen for complications (such as a new effusion from intrathoracic bleeding).

SECTION 2.5 Manifestations of respiratory disease

Cough

Cough is a reflex explosive expiration that prevents aspiration and promotes the removal of secretions and foreign particles from the lung.

History

The onset of a cough may be acute or chronic (usually defined as a cough that has persisted for more than 3 weeks) (Table 2.4). Sudden onset of unrelenting violent coughing can be due to an inhaled foreign body.

Cough that is continuously productive of purulent sputum is suggestive of chronic bronchitis and bronchiectasis. Expectorated bloodstained sputum tends to be a complaint of patients with bronchogenic carcinoma, pulmonary embolism and tuberculosis.

Smoking alone may cause a chronic cough; however, a long smoking history should alert the clinician to bronchogenic carcinoma and chronic bronchitis as underlying causes, especially if there is a change in the character of the cough.

Episodic (or even seasonal) wheezing with shortness of breath is common with asthma. This should be differentiated from the monophonic wheeze, which is suggestive of intraluminal obstruction from foreign bodies or tumour.

Most of the respiratory causes of coughing tend to be accompanied by shortness of breath, but sudden onset of dyspnoea may result from aspiration or pulmonary embolism. Shortness of breath that is worse on recumbency is suggestive of pulmonary oedema; however, asthma may also be worse at night. Weight loss can be a prominent feature with lung tumours and tuberculosis.

Associated pleuritic chest pain may be experienced with pulmonary emboli and pneumonia; unrelenting chest pain is more suggestive of bone involvement from lung cancer. Associated symptoms of gastro-oesophageal reflux disease may indicate aspiration of refluxed material. Frequent clearing of the throat due to nasal discharge or a history of allergy with rhinitis may result in postnasal drip and precipitate coughing.

Examination

The presence of pyrexia usually indicates an infective aetiology; the temperature may also be raised with pulmonary embolism.

The chest may be barrel-shaped with chronic obstructive pulmonary disease. These patients, as well as those with lung cancer or tuberculosis, may appear cachectic. Clubbing is associated with bronchial carcinoma, fibrotic lung disease and bronchiectasis. The supraclavicular nodes may be palpable with respiratory tract infections, tuberculosis and lung cancer.

On auscultation, coarse crepitations are a feature of bronchiectasis and pulmonary oedema. Widespread wheezing is suggestive of asthma, and a fixed inspiratory wheeze may be heard with bronchial luminal obstruction.

Investigations

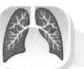

Investigations are not required for all patients that present with a cough, and should be reserved for patients in whom

Table 2.4	Causes of a cough
Acute	
Inhaled foreign body	
Respiratory tract infection	
Pulmonary embolism (bloodstained sputum)	
Chronic	
Productive	
Chronic obstructive pulmonary disease (mucoid/purulent)	
Bronchiectasis (purulent)	
Pulmonary oedema (pink, frothy)	
Lung cancer (bloodstained)	
TB (bloodstained)	
Non-productive	
Asthma	
Postnasal drip	
Gastro-oesophageal reflux	
Drugs (ACE inhibitors)	
Sarcoidosis	

the underlying aetiology is not clear after initial clinical assessment, patients with suspected chest infections or if a serious underlying disorder is suspected.

Sputum cultures

If a productive cough is present, sputum should be sent for cultures in an attempt to isolate any bacterial cause. If tuberculosis is suspected, Ziehl–Neelsen staining and specific culture on Löwenstein–Jensen media is required.

Full blood count

A raised white cell count is a non-specific indicator of infection.

Chest X-ray

A chest film is most useful in patients in whom pneumonia, lung cancer or cardiac failure is suspected.

Respiratory function tests

Formal respiratory function tests are usually reserved for patients with suspected airway obstruction (asthma, chronic bronchitis and bronchiectasis).

Dyspnoea

Dyspnoea is the uncomfortable awareness of breathing.

History

As many cardiac or respiratory diseases produce dyspnoea, it is useful to classify the causes by speed of onset (Table 2.5). An obvious precipitating factor may be evident, such as trauma (fractured ribs, pneumothorax) or aspiration of a foreign body. Position is important as dyspnoea on recumbency relieved by sitting upright can be caused by cardiac failure.

Dyspnoea may be seasonal (asthma induced by pollen) or perennial (house dust mite faecal proteins), depending on the precipitating allergen. A history of severe allergy should lead to the consideration of anaphylaxis.

Dyspnoea associated with productive cough may be due to chest infection. Concomitant haemoptysis may result from chest infection (especially tuberculosis), pulmonary embolism or tumour. Wheezing may result from asthma or aspiration of a foreign body.

Examination

Cyanosis reflects hypoxia and is an indicator of severe underlying disease, and decreased consciousness is usually an indication of a life-threatening situation. The respiratory rate is used as an approximate estimate of severity (very low or very high). An elevated temperature may occur with infection or pulmonary embolism.

Clubbing is associated with bronchial carcinoma, suppurative lung disease, idiopathic pulmonary fibrosis and cyanotic heart disease. A change in rate or regularity of the pulse may indicate an arrhythmia as a precipi-

Table 2.5	Causes of dyspnoea
Sudden (seconds–minutes)	
Pneumothorax	
Pulmonary oedema	
Pulmonary embolism	
Aspiration	
Anaphylaxis	
Anxiety	
Chest trauma	
Acute (hours–days)	
Asthma	
Respiratory tract infection	
Lung tumours	
Pleural effusion	
Metabolic acidosis	
Chronic (months–years)	
Chronic obstructive pulmonary disease	
Cardiac failure	
Fibrosing alveolitis	
Anaemia	
Valvular heart disease	
Chest wall deformities	
Neuromuscular disorders	
Cystic fibrosis	
Pulmonary hypertension	

tating factor (usually in pre-existing heart or lung disease).

Acute elevation of the JVP suggests tension pneumothorax, pulmonary embolism or tricuspid regurgitation (prominent v waves). Chronic elevation results from congestive heart failure or any chronic lung disease with right heart failure (cor pulmonale).

On palpation, the trachea deviates away from the side of a tension pneumothorax, pleural effusion and any large mass. It deviates to the side of a collapsed segment, which can result from obstruction of the bronchial lumen from tumour or foreign bodies. Chest wall movement on inspiration may be reduced on the side of an area of consolidation (infection), pneumothorax and effusion, or bilaterally with chronic obstructive pulmonary disease.

The area overlying consolidation, effusion or collapse is dull to percussion. Hyperresonance is often described on the affected side of a pneumothorax; however, a 'relative dullness' of the unaffected side is the usual finding.

Auscultation may reveal murmurs associated with valvular heart disease. The presence of a third heart sound or a displaced apex beat is consistent with cardiac failure, and quiet heart sounds may be secondary to chest hyperexpansion from chronic obstructive pulmonary disease.

Localized reduction in the intensity of breath sounds occurs over areas with consolidation or collapse of the lung; however, it may be reduced generally with asthma and COPD. Wheezing may be appreciated in a localized area following intraluminal airway obstruction from inhaled foreign body or tumour. Generalized wheezing usually occurs with asthma. When a history of pre-existing asthma is not evident, then consider anaphylaxis. Localized crepitations may be auscultated over areas of pulmonary consolidation. Extensive bilateral crepitations occur with idiopathic pulmonary fibrosis (fine inspiratory), pulmonary oedema and bronchopneumonia.

Investigations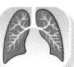

Full blood count
Anaemia may be the primary cause or an exacerbating factor of underlying disease. Polycythaemia may be seen in chronic lung disease. An elevated white cell count usually indicates infection, but it can also occur with other conditions such as pulmonary embolism, or after steroid usage.

Serum cardiac markers
Cardiac troponin is elevated with myocardial infarction (acute left ventricular failure).

Arterial blood gases
Arterial blood gases are useful to quantify the severity of the disease and subtype of respiratory failure. Normal levels of oxygenation, however, are not useful to exclude respiratory or cardiac disease. Low levels of bicarbonate indicate metabolic acidosis and should lead to investigation of the underlying cause, such as diabetic ketoacidosis. An alkalosis (high pH) with low $P\text{CO}_2$ and high $P\text{O}_2$ points to hyperventilation. CO_2 retention may result from chronic lung disease (type II respiratory failure) or may indicate the need for ventilation (especially with coexisting hypoxia) in asthmatics.

ECG
Arrhythmias are readily appreciated on the ECG. Atrial fibrillation or supraventricular tachycardia may precipitate dyspnoea in patients with pre-existing heart or lung disease. However, an arrhythmia may be a manifestation of the underlying cause, such as myocardial infarction, pulmonary embolism and hypoxia. ST segment elevation occurs with myocardial infarction and are also a non-specific finding in pulmonary embolism. Right bundle branch block may occur in the presence of long-standing lung disease.

Pulse oximetry
Although a low saturation *per se* is not discriminatory, acute severe impairment of oxygen saturation is associated with pulmonary embolus and pneumothorax. Post exercise desaturation occurs with parenchymal lung disease.

Peak expiratory flow rate
Reduced peak expiratory flow may indicate asthma or chronic obstructive pulmonary disease.

Chest X-ray
Hyperinflation of the lungs (if the hemidiaphragm is below the seventh rib anteriorly or the twelfth rib posteriorly) is a feature of emphysema and may also result from asthma. Areas of consolidation are seen on a plain film; however, radiographic changes of a chest infection may take a few days to develop. The presence of cardiac failure is appreciated by cardiomegaly, upper lobe diversion of the pulmonary veins, bilateral pleural effusions, Kerley B lines (1–2 cm horizontal lines in the periphery of the lung fields) and patchy pulmonary oedema. A pneumothorax may be diagnosed by identifying the line of the pleura and the absence of lung markings beyond it (but beware of giant lung bullae that have a similar appearance but entirely different management). Bronchial carcinoma may present as a hilar mass, peripheral opacity, or collapse and consolidation of the lung due to airways obstruction.

Haemoptysis

Haemoptysis is the expectoration of blood or bloodstained sputum.

History

Sudden onset of haemoptysis can occur with pulmonary embolism and acute respiratory tract infections; the remaining conditions listed in Table 2.6 pursue chronic recurrent courses. Although the amount of blood expectorated is not very useful as a discriminating feature, small amounts of blood sufficient to stain the sputum pink are characteristic of pulmonary oedema.

Acute onset of cough with haemoptysis may occur with respiratory tract infections and pulmonary embolism. Associated sputum production may be purulent and long-

Table 2.6	Causes of haemoptysis
Respiratory	
Bronchial carcinoma	
Pneumonia	
TB	
Chronic bronchitis	
Bronchiectasis	
Pulmonary oedema	
Goodpasture's syndrome	
Wegener's granulomatosis	
Vascular	
Pulmonary embolism	
Pulmonary hypertension—mitral stenosis	
Hereditary haemorrhagic telangiectasia	
Systemic	
Coagulation disorders	

standing with chronic bronchitis and bronchiectasis. Blood-stained sputum would suggest infection, pulmonary embolism (sudden onset dyspnoea), lung cancer (smoking, weight loss), tuberculosis or mitral stenosis.

Enquiry should be undertaken about other sites of bleeding: haemoptysis and haematuria may be due to systemic disease such as Goodpasture's syndrome. Epistaxis and haemoptysis occur together with Wegener's granulomatosis and hereditary haemorrhagic telangiectasia. Epistaxis per se may occasionally be confused with haemoptysis when expectorated sputum is mixed with blood originating from the nasal passages. A careful history is taken to identify any coagulation disorder or anticoagulant drug use.

Examination

Cachexia is a prominent feature of cancer, tuberculosis and chronic lung disease. Loss of the nasal bridge and saddling of the nose may be apparent in patients with Wegener's granulomatosis. The presence of clubbing is associated with bronchial carcinoma, chronic bronchitis and bronchiectasis. The malar flush characteristic of mitral facies may be present with mitral stenosis. Small dilated blood vessels present on the mucous membranes are features of hereditary haemorrhagic telangiectasia. The JVP may be elevated with a large pulmonary embolus or accompanying congestive cardiac failure secondary to mitral stenosis. The chest may be hyperexpanded with decreased inspiratory movement in chronic bronchitis.

The presence of an irregularly irregular heartbeat of atrial fibrillation is associated with mitral stenosis (and usually anticoagulant therapy). Supraclavicular lymphadenopathy may be present with pulmonary infections or carcinoma.

Localized crepitations and bronchial breathing may be audible with lobar pneumonia. Generalized coarse crepitations are suggestive of bronchiectasis, pulmonary oedema and chronic bronchitis. Breath sounds tend to be decreased in intensity with chronic bronchitis. Patients with bronchial carcinoma may present with a number of clinical features from the primary tumour, such as wheezing due to large airway obstruction, pulmonary collapse, pleural effusion or superior vena cava obstruction.

Investigations

Sputum analysis
Sputum should be collected for microscopy, culture and cytology. Infective organisms may be isolated or cytological features of malignancy may be present. When tuberculosis is suspected, serial cultures should be taken from sputum, urine, bronchial washings or lung biopsy specimens during bronchoscopy. Polymerase chain reaction amplification techniques may also be performed on smear-positive cultured specimens to provide a more rapid diagnosis and to assess drug resistance.

ECG
Sinus tachycardia may be noted with violent coughing, anxiety and blood loss. S1Q3T3 is indicative of right heart strain with pulmonary embolism, although non-specific ST abnormalities are very much more common.

Full blood count
Anaemia can result from chronic haemoptysis, but acute bleeding will not be associated with an immediate change in the blood count. An elevated white cell count may be due to infection or bleeding alone.

Urea and electrolytes
The presence of impaired renal function with deranged urea and creatinine estimations may be due to glomerulonephritis from Goodpasture's syndrome or Wegener's granulomatosis. However, prerenal failure may also be precipitated by acute blood loss and volume depletion.

Coagulation screen
A coagulation screen is performed to identify any abnormality that may lead to spontaneous haemorrhage.

Chest X-ray
Bilateral patchy areas of consolidation may be seen on a chest film with bronchopneumonia and pulmonary oedema. Opacification of an entire lobe suggests lobar pneumonia, although pulmonary emboli may have a similar appearance due to the wedge-shaped shadowing of a pulmonary infarct. Recurrent fluffy shadowing may be seen with Goodpasture's syndrome and Wegener's granulomatosis, due to repeated intra-alveolar haemorrhage. Areas of ground glass opacity may indicate the site of bleeding.

Features of tuberculosis (p. 123), bronchial carcinoma (p. 111), pulmonary hypertension (p. 161) and mitral stenosis (p. 44) may be evident.

CT thorax
A CT of the thorax may occasionally identify the source of bleeding.

Bronchoscopy
Flexible bronchoscopy is indicated in all patients with haemoptysis of unknown cause. Rigid bronchoscopy may be required to locate the site of major bleeding. In addition, biopsies of the bleeding site may be sampled for pathological analysis. Multiple arterio-venous malformations will be visible with hereditary haemorrhagic telangiectasia.

Diseases of the upper respiratory tract

The common cold (coryza)

The common cold is caused by an upper respiratory viral infection that can also involve the sinuses, ears and bronchial airways.

Epidemiology

Cold is common: on average adults suffer 2–3 colds per year and children around 6–10. Colds can occur at any time but there is an increased incidence during autumn and winter months in temperate climates.

Pathology

There are over 100 different viruses that cause the common cold. Rhinoviruses account for approximately half; other viruses include coronavirus, respiratory syncytial virus (RSV), adenovirus, parainfluenza, influenza, enteroviruses and the newly discovered metapneumovirus.[1]

The viruses are transported to the nose and eyes by contaminated hands from contact, or directly through coughs and sneezes. From there the virus infects the upper respiratory airways. Inflammatory mediators (histamine, kinins, interleukins, prostaglandins) are responsible for the classical symptoms. Inflammation also increases the permeability of blood vessels and mucous gland secretion, activating the sneeze and cough reflexes and stimulating pain nerve fibres.

The highest concentration of viral load in nasal secretions is in the first 3 days, when the infected person is most contagious; antibody production usually starts after 2 weeks, reaching a maximum at 4 weeks. This helps to prevent repeat infections by the same virus but does not protect against other viruses. Since there are over a hundred different types of cold virus, over the period of a lifetime one could have a few infections each year, each caused by a different virus.

The cold may be complicated by acute bacterial sinusitis and otitis media. Patients with pre-existing lung disease (asthma, COPD) may experience exacerbations.

Clinical features

The symptoms of a common cold are sneezing, runny nose, nasal obstruction, sore throat, cough, hoarseness, headache, fever and general malaise. The incubation period is 8–12 hours. The time from the beginning of the infection to the peak of symptoms is typically 36–72 hours, and a cold usually lasts from 2 days to 2 weeks. Approximately 25% do not develop any symptoms.

Investigations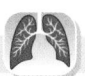

No investigations are required for uncomplicated cases.

Management

Symptomatic relief
Paracetamol, cough suppressants and decongestants may help to relieve the symptoms, but no treatment can cure the illness or speed its resolution.

Preventative measures
Infected patients should be advised to keep their hands out of their eyes and noses, and to wash their hands regularly (to reduce the viral load on the skin of the hands and fingers). Contact with known cold sufferers, especially during the first 3 days of their illness, should be avoided.

Prognosis

The majority of patients recover without any complications. In the minority (children and elderly) the prognosis is specific to the complication developed (e.g. bronchiolitis, pneumonia).

REFERENCE

(1) *Williams JV, Harris PA, Tollefson SJ, et al. Human metapneumovirus and lower respiratory tract disease in otherwise healthy infants and children. New England Journal of Medicine 2004; 350: 443–450.*

Allergic rhinitis

Allergic rhinitis is characterized by nasal itching, sneezing, watery rhinorrhoea and nasal obstruction after inhaled allergen exposure due to IgE mediated inflammation of the nasal membranes.

Epidemiology

Approximately 24% (24 000 per 100 000) of the population suffers with rhinitis, of which allergic rhinitis makes up the majority.[1]

Pathology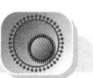

In atopic individuals, exposure to an aeroallergen incites an IgE mediated immediate hypersensitivity reaction resulting

115

in chemotaxis, release of cytokines and chemokines, and activation of mast cells, eosinophils, T cells and epithelial cells, which in turn release a host of mediators including histamine. The result is mucosal inflammation, oedema and reduced sinus drainage.

Common triggers include house dust mite (faeces), domestic pets, flower or grass pollen and occupational exposures (e.g. latex).

Scope of disease

Headaches, nasal blockage, difficulty sleeping and coughing (postnasal drip) can also occur.

Clinical features

Depending on the inciting allergen, rhinitis can be seasonal (pollen) or perennial (house dust mite). The symptoms are rhinorrhoea (usually a watery discharge), sneezing which is paroxysmal, itching, nasal blockage and conjunctivitis (Table 2.7). Additional symptoms include headache, cough and impaired smell. Generally symptoms are reversible (spontaneously or with medication) and are worse during the day compared to the night.

Examination of the nose is usually unremarkable but occasionally may reveal pale or bluish oedematous mucosa with a watery discharge.

Initial investigations

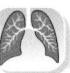

No investigations are generally required, as the diagnosis is usually evident from the history.

Further investigations

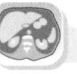

Specific investigations are only required when symptoms remain uncontrolled despite allergen avoidance and medication.

Skin prick testing

Skin prick testing is performed by introducing a small amount of diluted antigen into the epidermis of the forearm and measuring the maximum diameter of the inflammatory ('wheal') response. Over 90% of patients who test positive react to one of the four most common allergens: grass pollen, house dust mite (faeces), *Aspergillus fumigatus* and domestic pets with which the patient is in regular contact. Whilst not diagnostic, the sensitivity of this test makes the diagnosis of allergic rhinitis very unlikely if negative.

Radioallergosorbent tests

Radioallergosorbent tests (RASTs) measure serum levels of allergen-specific IgE. This is a useful test for specific allergens that are not tested on the skin prick test.

Initial management

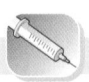

Allergen avoidance

Allergen avoidance is usually successful for specific triggers such as a domestic pet or occupational exposure.

Medical management

The current approach of stepped care management of allergic rhinitis may be disrupted by the widespread availability of antihistamines and nasal corticosteroids over the counter, i.e. pharmacists may already have placed patients on the treatment ladder.

Mild to moderate symptoms

An oral antihistamine or nasal corticosteroid should be prescribed. For patients with seasonal allergy, the medication should ideally be commenced 2–3 weeks before the season commences and continued for several months. Patients with perennial symptoms may require long-term therapy.

Severe symptoms

Nasal corticosteroids and topical cromoglycate in conjunction with oral antihistamine can be prescribed for patients with more severe symptoms.

If symptoms persist or are disabling despite initial treatment, further options include a short course of oral corticosteroids or immunotherapy (this involves desensitizing the patient by administering increasing amounts of the allergen subcutaneously over the course of a few months).

Prognosis

Good symptom control is usually achieved in the majority of patients with allergen avoidance and stepped care therapy.

Table 2.7	Assessment of severity of allergic rhinitis
Mild	Symptoms that do not interfere with daily activities and/or sleep
Moderate	Symptoms that disturb daily activities and/or sleep
Severe	Symptoms that are so pronounced that the patient cannot function properly during the day and/or cannot sleep without treatment

> ***i*** **FURTHER INFORMATION**

van Cauwenberge P, Bachert C, Passalacqua G, et al. Consensus statement on the treatment of allergic rhinitis. European Academy of Allergology and Clinical Immunology. Allergy 2000; 55: 116–134.

REFERENCE

(1) Sibbald B, Rink E. *Epidemiology of seasonal and perennial rhinitis: clinical presentation and medical history. Thorax* 1991; 46: 895–901.

Obstructive sleep apnoea/hypopnoea syndrome

The obstructive sleep apnoea syndrome is a condition in which unwanted daytime sleepiness results from recurrent episodes of upper airway obstruction during sleep. Obstructive sleep apnoea is present when the patient has had more than 5 episodes of apnoea per hour that each last at least 10 seconds (i.e. an apnoea hypopnoea index (AHI) of more than 5).[1]

Epidemiology

The prevalence of obstructive sleep apnoea is critically dependent on the disease definition, age, sex and body mass index (BMI) of the population studied. In a US-based population study, using an AHI of 5 or more, the obstructive sleep apnoea/hypopnoea syndrome was estimated to be present in 24% of men (24 000 per 100 000) and 9% of women (9 000 per 100 000).[2] Using the stricter criteria of AHI 5 or more and daytime sleepiness, more recent epidemiological studies estimate the prevalence to be approximately 4% (4000 per 100 000) in men and 2% (2000 per 100 000) in women.[1]

Pathology

In susceptible individuals, complete or partial collapse of the pharyngeal airway brings about apnoea or hypopnoea during sleep. Consequently, oxygen saturation drops and arousal occurs briefly, allowing a few deep breaths to be taken. Sleep is resumed and the cycle repeats (up to 60 to 100 times an hour). The patient may awake feeling unrefreshed and suffer with daytime somnolence.

The primary defect is a small and collapsible airway; contributing factors include a small jaw, large tonsils and increased soft tissues of the oropharynx (obesity). Population risk factors for this condition are increasing age, male sex and obesity.[3]

Scope of disease

Obstructive sleep apnoea syndrome is a relatively new diagnosis, and morbidity related to this disease is still being studied. Epidemiological studies have reported a causal relationship between obstructive sleep apnoea and hypertension; current studies are evaluating the benefits of treatment on hypertension.[3] Other complications are impaired cognitive function, altered mood and personality, ventilatory failure and an increased risk of road traffic accidents.

Clinical features

The cardinal symptoms are excessive daytime somnolence, snoring and mood changes. Additional symptoms that may be noticed by the partner are apnoea, choking during sleep and poor concentration. Less common features are nocturia and erectile dysfunction.

On examination the patient is often obese (BMI >30 kg/m^2) with a small mandible, crowded oropharynx, hypertension and a large neck size (more than 42 cm). Nasal patency and the size of the tongue and uvula should be assessed.

Clinical assessment should also include the Epworth score to quantify the severity of daytime somnolence (Table 2.8). Patients should also be screened for coexisting diseases such as COPD, hypothyroidism, Marfan's syndrome and acromegaly.

Initial investigations

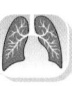

No initial investigations are required to diagnose obstructive sleep apnoea.

Further investigations

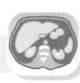

Sleep studies

Sleep studies are indicated for unwanted daytime somnolence (Epworth Score greater than 10), snoring associated with hypertension or cardiovascular disease, or when uvulopalatoplasty is considered for snoring.

The patient is attached to pulse oximetry and abdomen and ribcage movement monitors as well as airflow monitors (through the nose and mouth). If there is doubt as to the diagnosis of obstructive sleep apnoea, or if narcolepsy or restless legs syndrome is being considered, full polysomnography is performed. During sleep, an EEG is also recorded, and the pattern of rapid eye movements (REM) may suggest narcolepsy or periodic leg movement syndrome (arousals in association with limb movement).

Initial management

Weight loss

Currently weight loss is the only intervention strategy associated with improved outcome.[3] Other measures include avoiding alcohol at night, elevation of the foot of the bed, and positional therapy to stop the patient lying on his or her back (e.g. a tennis ball sewn into the pyjama jacket).

Medical management

Nasal continuous positive airway pressure ventilation (CPAP)

The indications for CPAP are an apnoea – hypopnoea index (AHI) > 15 events/hour accompanied by excessive daytime

117

Table 2.8	The Epworth sleepiness scale*

How likely are you to doze off or fall asleep in the following situations, in contrast to feeling just tired?
This refers to your usual way of life in recent times. Even if you have not done some of these things recently, try to work out how they would have affected you.
Use the following scale to choose the most appropriate number for each situation:
0: would *never* doze
1: *slight* chance of dozing
2: *moderate* chance of dozing
3: *high* chance of dozing

Activity	Chance of dozing
Sitting and reading	_____
Watching TV	_____
Sitting inactive in a public place (meeting, theatre, etc.)	_____
As a passenger in a car for 1 hour without a break	_____
Lying down in the afternoon when circumstances permit	_____
Sitting and talking to someone	_____
Sitting quietly after lunch without alcohol	_____
In a car, while stopped for a few minutes in traffic	_____
Total	_____

Each question is answered with a number from 0 (not at all likely to fall asleep) to 3 (very likely to fall asleep). This yields a total score of 0 (minimum) to 24 (maximum).

*Johns MW. A new method for measuring daytime sleepiness: the Epworth sleepiness scale. Sleep 1991; 14: 540–545.

sleepiness, impaired cognition, mood disorders, insomnia or documented cardiovascular disease (including hypertension, ischaemic heart disease and stroke).[4]

A CPAP mask is worn over the nose (or nose and mouth) and a ventilator blows air continuously at a fixed pressure (usually around 10 cm of water). This keeps the airway open during sleep and prevents desaturation and arousal. Problems with CPAP include nasal bridge pressure sores, claustrophobia, nasal congestion, sneezing and disrupted sleep. Many adjustments are usually required to optimize treatment (minimize air leaks), and it may be some time before patients and their carers are able to cope and use it successfully.

Mandibular advancement splints

A mandibular advancement splint is an option for patients with mild obstructive sleep apnoea or those intolerant of CPAP (it is not as effective as CPAP for patients with severe disease). The splint is a personalized device made by an orthodontist which pulls the mandible forward, keeping the airway open during sleep.

Surgical management

Uvulopalatopharyngoplasty

Uvulopalatopharyngoplasty may be an option for highly selected patients; at present results are no better than with the use of a mandibular splint.[5] Laser uvulopalatoplasty reduced the level of snoring in mild obstructive sleep apnoea, but improvements to the apnoea hypopnoea index and symptoms are minor compared to no treatment.[6]

Tracheostomy

Tracheostomy is seldom required, and is used only as a last resort in the treatment of obstructive sleep apnoea.

Prognosis

Patients are expected to have a normal life expectancy, currently treatment aims are intended to minimize behavioural and cardiovascular morbidity.

i FURTHER INFORMATION

Stradling JR, Davies RJO. Sleep 1: Obstructive sleep apnoea/hypopnoea syndrome: definitions, epidemiology, and natural history. Thorax 2004; 59: 73–78.

Fogel RB, Malhotra A, White DP. Sleep 2: Pathophysiology of obstructive sleep apnoea/hypopnoea syndrome. Thorax 2004; 59: 159–163.

REFERENCES

(1) *Stradling JR, Davies RJO. Sleep 1: Obstructive sleep apnoea/hypopnoea syndrome: definitions, epidemiology, and natural history. Thorax 2004; 59: 73–78.*
(2) *Young T, Palta M, Dempsey J, Skatrud J, Weber S, Badr S. The occurrence of sleep-disordered breathing among middle-aged adults. New England Journal of Medicine 1993; 328: 1230–1235.*
(3) *Young T, Peppard PE, Gottlieb DJ. Epidemiology of obstructive sleep apnea: a population health perspective. American Journal of Respiratory and Critical Care Medicine 2002; 165: 1217–1239.*
(4) *Loube DI, Gay PC, Strohl KP, Pack AI, White DP, Collop NA. Indications for positive airway pressure treatment of adult obstructive sleep apnea patients: a consensus statement. Chest 1999; 115: 863–866.*
(5) *Walker-Engstrom M-L, Tegelberg A, Wilhelmsson B, Ringqvist I. 4-Year follow-up of treatment with dental appliance or uvulopalatopharyngoplasty in patients with obstructive sleep apnea: a randomized study. Chest 2002; 121: 739–746.*
(6) *Ferguson KA, Heighway K, Ruby RRF. A randomized trial of laser-assisted uvulopalatoplasty in the treatment of mild obstructive sleep apnea. American Journal of Respiratory and Critical Care Medicine 2003; 167: 15–19.*

SECTION 2.7   Pulmonary infections

Community acquired pneumonia

In the community, pneumonia is defined as symptoms of an acute lower respiratory tract illness (cough and at least one other lower respiratory tract symptom) with new focal chest signs on examination and at least one systemic feature (either a symptom complex of sweating, fevers, shivers, aches and pains and/or temperature of 38°C or more) and no other explanation for the illness.[1]

In hospital, community acquired pneumonia is defined as symptoms and signs consistent with an acute lower respiratory tract infection associated with new radiographic shadowing for which there is no other explanation (e.g. not pulmonary oedema or infarction).[1]

Epidemiology

The incidence of community acquired pneumonia ranges from 110 (Canada) to 400 (USA) per 100 000 per year depending on geography.[2,3] There is a bimodal age distribution, with the young and elderly most affected.

Pathology

Pneumonia tends to cause intra-alveolar exudation that results in consolidation (solidification) of lung parenchyma. This is visible on a chest X-ray (after a certain period of time) either as patchy shadowing involving more than one lobe (bronchopneumonia) or uniformly involving an entire lobe (lobar pneumonia). The causative pathogens are listed in Table 2.9.

Scope of the disease

With severe infection, tissue destruction and necrosis can occur, giving rise to a lung abscess. Sterile pleural effusions can occur; however, extension of infection into the pleural space results in an empyema. Organization of the exudate can convert the affected areas into solid fibrous tissue. Dissemination of infection can result in bacteraemia with or without endocarditis, cerebral abscesses, meningitis and arthritis.

Clinical features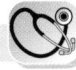

The symptoms of pneumonia are a productive cough, sweating, fevers, shivers, aches and pains and a temperature of 38°C or more. It is not possible to determine the aetiological organism on the history alone; however, certain organisms have specific predisposing risk factors and a classical presentation (Table 2.10).

On examination, the patient may be breathless, tachycardic, hypotensive or confused. Signs of consolidation are reduced expansion, dullness to percussion, quiet breath sounds, bronchial breathing and increased vocal resonance. In addition scattered crepitations may be audible.

Table 2.9   Causative pathogens of community acquired pneumonia

	UK (5 studies, n = 1137)		Rest of Europe (23 studies, n = 6026)		Australia and New Zealand (3 studies, n = 453)		North America (4 studies, n = 1306)	
	Mean (%)	95% CI	Mean (%)	95% CI	Mean (%)	95% CI	Mean (%)	95% CI
Streptococcus pneumoniae	39	36.1–41.8	19.4	18.4–20.4	38.4	33.9–42.9	11.3	9.5–13.0
Haemophilus influenzae	5.2	4.0–6.6	3.9	3.4–4.4	9.5	7–12.6	6.3	5.0–7.7
Legionella spp.	3.6	2.6–4.9	5.1	4.6–5.7	7.5	5.3–10.3	4.8	3.7–6.0
Moraxella catarrhalis	1.9	0.6–4.3	1.2	1.0–1.5	3.1	1.4–6.1	1.2	0.5–2.5
Staphylococcus aureus	1.9	1.2–2.9	0.8	0.5–1.1	2.9	1.5–4.9	3.8	2.9–5.0
Gram-negative enteric bacilli	1	0.5–1.7	3.3	2.8–3.7	4.6	2.9–7	5.3	4.1–6.6
Mycoplasma pneumoniae	10.8	9.0–12.6	6	5.4–6.6	14.6	11.3–17.8	4.1	3.1–5.3
Chlamydia pneumoniae	13.1	9.1–17.2	6.3	5.5–7.3	3.1	1.4–6.1	5.9	4.3–7.8
Chlamydia psittaci	2.6	1.7–3.6	1.4	1.1–1.8	1.4	0.5–3.2	0.1	0–0.7
Coxiella burnetii	1.2	0.7–2.1	0.9	0.6–1.1	0	0–3.4	2.3	1.5–3.7
All viruses	12.8	10.8–14.7	9.5	8.6–10.3	10.6	7.8–13.4	8.9	7.4–10.6
Influenza A and B	10.7	8.9–12.5	5.3	4.6–6.1	6.4	4.3–9.1	5.9	4.5–7.6
Mixed	14.2	12.2–16.3	6.3	5.5–7.1	19.6	16–23.3	8.5	7.0–10.3
Other	2	1.3–3	2	1.7–2.4	4	2.4–6.2	8.0	6.6–9.7
None	30.8	28.1–33.5	50.7	49.5–52.0	31.6	27.3–35.8	40.7	38.1–43.4

CI, confidence interval.

Table 2.10   Classical presentations of selected organisms

Organism	Season	Risk factors	Clinical features
Streptococcus pneumoniae	Winter	Increasing age, comorbidity, overcrowded settings (men's shelters, prisons)	Acute onset, high fever, pleuritic chest pains, rusty sputum, herpes labialis
Staphylococcus aureus	Winter	Prior viral (especially influenza) infection, hospital/ICU admission	
Mycoplasma pneumoniae	Winter, every 3–4 year cycle	Young, prior antibiotics	
Legionella spp.	September to October	Young, smokers, travel to the Mediterranean, infected water sources in buildings	Diarrhoea, neurological symptoms, severe infection, multisystem involvement (abnormal LFTs, elevated creatine kinase)
Chlamydia pneumoniae	N/A	Epidemics in closed communities	Long duration of symptoms, headache
Chlamydia psittaci	N/A	Birds as pets (including parrots, poultry, ducks)	
Coxiella burnetii	April to June	Male sex, animal exposure (sheep)	Dry cough, high fever
Influenza virus	Winter		

When assessing patients with pneumonia, it is important also to determine the severity of disease using the CRB-65 score that can help determine the need for hospital admission (Table 2.11). The indications for ICU admission are persisting hypoxia with P_aO_2 <8 kPa despite maximal oxygen administration, progressive hypercapnia, severe acidosis (pH <7.26), shock or depressed consciousness.

General investigations

Full blood count

An elevated white cell count is the usual finding; however, a white cell count at either extreme (less than 4 or more than 20×10^9 per litre) is indicative of severe infection.

Table 2.11	CRB-65 score for severity assessment in community acquired pneumonia
Confusion	
Respiratory rate ≥30	
Blood pressure (SBP <90 mmHg or DBP ≤60 mmHg)	
Age ≥65	
Each feature scores 1 point	
0	Likely suitable for home treatment
1 or 2	Consider hospital treatment
3 or more	Manage in hospital as severe pneumonia

C-reactive protein

In pneumonia, the CRP is usually elevated above 100 (75% of patients). It is a relatively more sensitive indicator of pneumonia than pyrexia or elevated white cell count.

Urea and electrolytes

Elevated urea is an indicator of disease severity. Renal impairment may be evident with severe infection.

Liver profile

Organisms such as *Legionella* are associated with abnormal liver profile.

Chest X-ray

Lobar consolidation appears as an opaque lobe and is virtually diagnostic of lobar pneumonia (Fig. 2.9). Patchy consolidation may occur with bronchopneumonia (but also with heart failure and pulmonary embolism). Parapneumonic pleural effusions may occur, and less commonly may indicate the development of an empyema (Fig. 2.10).

Cavitation may be evident with a single air–fluid level, and is associated with *S. aureus, Klebsiella, Mycobacterium tuberculosis* and anaerobic bacteria.

Radiological resolution often lags behind clinical symptoms, therefore it is not a useful investigation to document evidence of improvement but may be useful in screening for complications.

Blood and sputum cultures

Blood cultures are a highly specific investigation for the diagnosis of pneumonia; bacteraemia is also a marker of disease severity. Sputum should be sent for microscopy, culture and sensitivities prior to the initiation of antibiotic therapy.

Urinalysis

Detection of *Legionella* and pneumococcal antigen in the urine is a specific investigation for *Legionella* and pneumococcal pneumonia.

Further investigations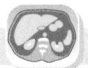

Arterial blood gases

Arterial blood gases are required for patients with oxygen saturations less than 92% to screen for respiratory failure and to guide the need for oxygen therapy.

Serology

Serological tests are indicated in severe pneumonia, in the presence of an epidemic, and if patients are unresponsive to β-lactam antibiotics. Respiratory serological tests usually comprise antibody tests for the atypical pathogens (*M. pneumoniae, Chlamydia spp., Coxiella burnetii*), influenza A virus, influenza B virus, adenovirus, respiratory syncytial virus, and *L. pneumophila*.

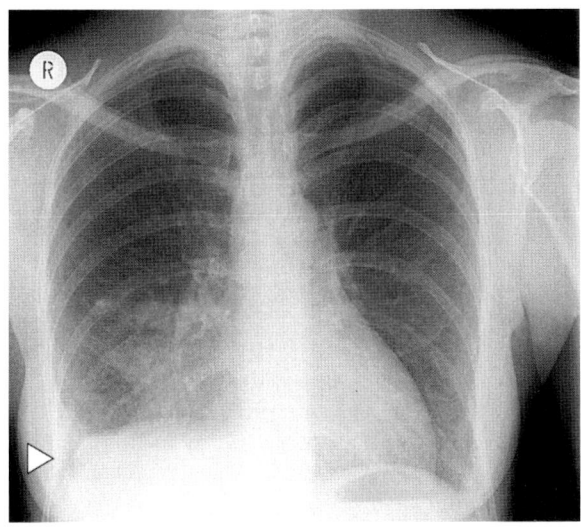

Fig. 2.9 Chest X-ray of right lower lobe pneumonia.

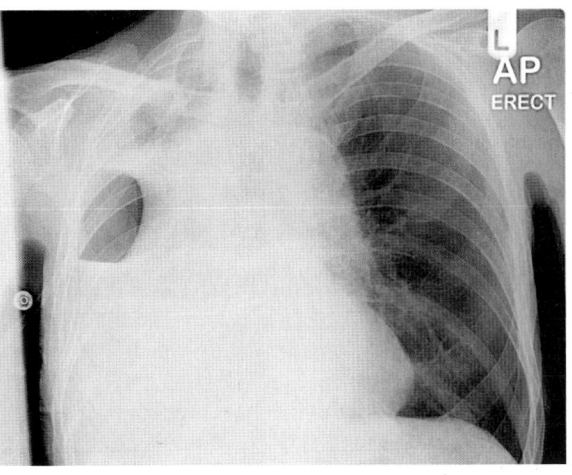

Fig. 2.10 Chest X-ray of a right empyema. Multiple air–fluid levels are visible in the right chest due to the development of an empyema.

Initial management

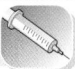

Oxygen
Supplemental oxygen should be given to maintain S_aO_2 >92% and PO_2 >8 kPa.

Fluid replacement
Intravenous fluids are required in patients who are dehydrated.

Nutritional supplementation
Nutritional support may be necessary for patients with prolonged illness either prior to admission or during the course of admission.

Medical management

Non-severe pneumonia
In the community, the empirical antibiotic of choice for non-severe community acquired pneumonia is high-dose *amoxicillin* (500 mg to 1 g tds). In patients who are allergic to penicillin, a macrolide (*erythromycin* or *clarithromycin*) should be prescribed. The recommended duration of treatment is 7 days.

For patients admitted to hospital, in general, combination therapy with *amoxicillin and a macrolide* is required (20% will be infected with β-lactam resistant organisms such as *Legionella*, *Mycoplasma* or *Chlamydia*). The oral route is preferred unless there is evidence of impaired consciousness, loss of swallowing reflex or malabsorption. The recommended duration of treatment is 7 days.

Severe pneumonia
For patients with severe pneumonia, a broad-spectrum β-lactamase stable antibiotic *(co-amoxiclav)* or a cephalosporin (cefuroxime, cefotaxime) is prescribed in conjunction with a macrolide (*erythromycin* or *clarithromycin*). The intravenous route is preferred for patients with severe pneumonia. The recommended duration of treatment is 10 days, but atypical pathogens may require a longer course of antibiotics. Advice from the local microbiologist should be sought and the possibility of infection with methicillin resistant *S. aureus* or *Pneumocystis carinii* pneumonia should be considered.

Surgical management

Decortication of empyema
Surgical intervention is usually only required for complications such as a lung abscess and empyema that develop despite medical therapy.

Prognosis

The mortality for pneumonia treated in the community (not severe enough to warrant hospital admission) is less than 1%. However, mortality is as high as 15% for hospital treated pneumonia[4] and up to 58% if admission to ICU is required.[5]

i FURTHER INFORMATION

British Thoracic Society Guidelines on the management of community acquired pneumonia. Thorax 2001; 56(Suppl 4): ii–64.

British Thoracic Society Pneumonia Guidelines Committee. BTS guidelines for the management of community acquired pneumonia in adults: 2004 update. www.brit-thoracic.org.uk/guidelines

REFERENCES

(1) *British Thoracic Society Guidelines for the management of community acquired pneumonia in adults. Thorax 2001; 56(Suppl 4): IV1–64.*
(2) *Marrie TJ. Epidemiology of community-acquired pneumonia in the elderly. Seminars in Respiratory Infections 1990; 5: 260–268.*
(3) *Lave JR, Fine MJ, Sankey SS, Hanusa BH, Weissfeld LA, Kapoor WN. Hospitalized pneumonia. Outcomes, treatment patterns, and costs in urban and rural areas. Journal of General Internal Medicine 1996; 11: 415–421.*
(4) *Lim WS, Macfarlane JT, Boswell TC, Harrison TG, Rose D, Leinonen M, Saikku P. Study of community acquired pneumonia aetiology (SCAPA) in adults admitted to hospital: implications for management guidelines. Thorax 2001; 56: 296–301.*
(5) *The aetiology, management and outcome of severe community-acquired pneumonia on the intensive care unit. The British Thoracic Society Research Committee and The Public Health Laboratory Service. Respiratory Medicine 1992; 86: 7–13.*

Tuberculosis

Tuberculosis (TB) is a bacterial infection caused by *Mycobacterium tuberculosis*. It can affect any organ but the most common site is the lung. *Infection* occurs after patients have been exposed to the organism, but this does not always lead to disease. Thus infection can be asymptomatic, or minimally symptomatic and self-limiting. When clinical manifestations of active tuberculosis become apparent this is called *disease* (rather than infection). This distinction is important as many can be infected but not suffer with active tuberculosis.

Epidemiology

Tuberculosis is the most common infectious disease in the world: 2 billion people are currently infected. The global incidence was 137 per 100 000 in the year 2000, with the highest incidence in Africa.[1] Tuberculosis is more common in men, and the peak age of infection is 15–34 years. The increase in tuberculosis has been attributed to poverty, neglect of the disease and collapse of the health infrastructure in developing countries where the disease is rife. The HIV epidemic also contributes: currently 12% of new cases of tuberculosis are associated with HIV.[1]

Pathology

Mycobacterium tuberculosis infection occurs through droplet transmission; the organism is inhaled into the lungs where it causes a type IV immune response. Tissues show granulomatous inflammation with caseous necrosis (usually in the lower aspects of the upper lobe, or upper aspects of the lower lobe). The tubercle bacilli travel to the regional lymph nodes and occasionally to the rest of the body via blood and lymph.

Primary tuberculosis is usually contained and, when resolved, often leaves a calcified scar in the periphery of the lung (Ghon focus). The Ghon focus together with mediastinal lymphadenopathy is known as the primary complex. Post primary tuberculosis includes tuberculous bronchopneumonia and fibrocaseous tuberculosis. Secondary tuberculosis can be caused by reactivation of the organism many years later in any site of the body (classically located at the lung apices).

Scope of disease

Pulmonary tuberculosis accounts for 62% of all cases. Extra-pulmonary disease occurs in 29% and is more common in children. Pulmonary and lymph node tuberculosis occur in 9%. A summary of the multisystem manifestations is presented in Table 2.12.

Clinical features

Primary tuberculosis is usually asymptomatic. Secondary tuberculosis presents with nonspecific symptoms such as fever, drenching night sweats, anorexia, weight loss and malaise. Eventually, in the majority, a productive cough with bloodstained sputum develops. Extensive disease can lead to dyspnoea and ARDS. Organ-specific clinical features are presented in Table 2.12.

Few abnormalities are detected on examination of patients with pulmonary tuberculosis. There may be cachexia, clubbing, and occasionally bronchial breathing; scattered crepitations may be audible over localized areas of consolidation.

Initial investigations

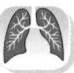

Full blood count
The white cell count may be raised, and a normochromic normocytic anaemia may be present.

Liver profile
The liver profile may be deranged, with a low serum albumin. Antituberculous drugs can cause hepatotoxicity; therefore it is important to document baseline liver function tests.

Community acquired pneumonia

Tuberculosis

Table 2.12	Clinical features of tuberculosis	
Location	**Effects**	**Clinical features**
Lungs	Invasion of pulmonary vessels, cavitation, miliary spread, fibrosis, bronchiectasis	Cough, sputum, haemoptysis, shortness of breath
Pleura	Effusion; if untreated, calcification can occur, causing restrictive lung defect	Dyspnoea Type II respiratory failure
Lymph nodes	Cold abscess, ulceration, scarring	Painless fluctuant swellings (cervical, supraclavicular, axillary, inguinal nodes)
Pericardium	Pericardial effusion, leading to scarring and restrictive pericarditis	Dyspnoea, pericardial rub
Central nervous system	Tuberculous abscess, obstructive hydrocephalus, meningitis	Neurological deficits, headache, papilloedema (obstructive hydrocephalus), coma
Renal	Pyonephritis, abscess, scarring, renal failure	Flank pain, frequency, nocturia, haematuria, sterile pyuria
Abdominal	Obstruction, psoas abscess	Abdominal pain, mass, pain on hip flexion (psoas abscess)
Bone/spine	Bony deformities, nerve root compression, vertebral collapse	Back pain, nerve root pain
Eye	Phlyctenular conjunctivitis	Visual impairment/blindness
Reproductive organs	Infection, scarring	Infertility, abdominal, testicular pain, swelling
Skin	Erythema nodosum, lupus vulgaris	Painful skin nodules

Urea and electrolytes

Assessment of renal function is important prior to commencing ethambutol as dose adjustments are required if renal impairment is present.

Chest X-ray

In primary disease, the Ghon focus appears as an area of consolidation, usually in the periphery of the mid or upper zones. Consolidation may be accompanied by visible mediastinal lymphadenopathy (primary complex).

Multiple small areas of consolidation are the usual CXR appearance of secondary tuberculosis (Fig. 2.11). Areas of fibrosis and calcification may also be seen. Pleural effusions are common and may lead to pleural thickening. New lesions and cavity formation suggest active disease.

Microbiological specimens

Three early morning sputum specimens should be sent for microscopy and culture. Pleural fluid and any other pus specimen that is possible to obtain should also be sent for examination.

Ziehl–Neelsen or auramine stain is used to identify mycobacteria, which show up as acid- and alcohol-fast bacilli (AFBs) on light microscopy. Identification is positive in only 25% of those infected and therefore treatment should not be withheld whilst waiting for culture results in patients with suspected tuberculosis.

Tuberculin testing

The Mantoux test is performed by injecting a small amount of tuberculin (purified protein derivative of *Mycobacterium tuberculosis*) into the skin. A positive reaction to the tuberculin indicates either infection (it does not necessarily indicate active disease) or prior BCG vaccination. False negative readings can occur in extensive disease (miliary tuberculosis) and HIV coinfection.

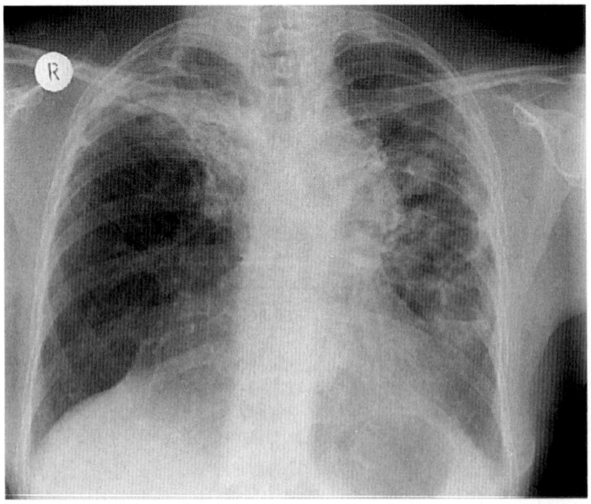

Further investigations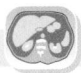

Bronchoscopy

Bronchoscopy and bronchoalveolar washings are performed to obtain specimens for microbiology in patients who are unable to produce sputum, when there is suspicion of active disease despite negative sputum cultures, or if lung cancer is a differential diagnosis. For patients with miliary tuberculosis, transbronchial biopsies are obtained for microbiology and histology.

Liver biopsy

Liver biopsies are usually obtained when miliary tuberculosis is suspected.

Lymph node excision biopsy

When lymph node tuberculosis is suspected, accessible nodes can be aspirated for pus or excised for microbiology and histology. This is a particularly useful investigation to screen for alternative diagnoses (e.g. lymphoma) in patients who have not responded to initial antituberculosis therapy.

Site-specific investigations

Depending on the site of extrapulmonary disease, specific investigations may be required such as lumbar puncture for suspected meningeal tuberculosis and plain X-ray or isotope bone scans for suspected bone involvement.

HIV test

Where appropriate, patients under the age of 50 years should be offered a HIV test as 12% of patients with tuberculosis are HIV positive.

Initial management

Isolation

Patients with pulmonary tuberculosis are considered infectious if acid-fast bacilli have been identified in sputum specimens (smear positive). Isolation in a negative pressure room is required for 2 weeks whilst treatment is commenced or until the sputum microscopy is smear negative on three successive examinations. Extrapulmonary disease is not considered to be infectious even if it is smear positive.

Patient education

Patients should be informed that tuberculosis is only infectious if it is smear-positive pulmonary disease, and that after 2 weeks on compliant treatment they are no longer infectious. Compliance with medication is a very important issue with tuberculosis treatment because resistance develops if treatment is undertaken with less than three drugs in the initial phase.

Fig. 2.11 Chest X-ray of a patient with widespread tuberculosis.

Medical management

Antituberculous therapy

As bacteriological cultures can take up to 8 weeks and false negative results can occur, patients are treated on clinical suspicion before culture results are obtained. The drugs used as first-line treatment of tuberculosis are rifampicin, isoniazid and pyrazinamide (Table 2.13). Ethambutol is added when the sensitivities are unknown. (Patients should be warned that if their sight deteriorates, they should stop ethambutol immediately and contact the medical team.) Pyridoxine is prescribed in malnourished patients to reduce the risk of isoniazid-induced peripheral neuropathy.

Hepatotoxicity is a known complication of isoniazid, rifampicin and pyrazinamide (Table 2.14). Liver function tests are done before starting treatment and usually again at the end of the initial phase of treatment, or if any signs or symptoms of liver disease develop such as itching (pruritus) or jaundice. If the decision is made to withdraw treatment because of deranged LFTs, the drugs should then be reintroduced individually (isoniazid first, then rifampicin, and pyrazinamide) to identify the offending drug and exclude it.

Directly observed therapy (DOT) is a treatment regimen in which patients are given high-dose medication three times a week and are observed taking their medicine to confirm compliance. This is as effective as daily treatment and can be initiated from the start or when poor compliance is suspected. Tuberculosis specialist nurses play a very important role by visiting (non-DOT) patients to ensure compliance (tablet counting) and to check that treatment is taken correctly.

Notification

The Centre for Communicable Diseases must be notified of patients with confirmed or suspected tuberculosis.

Contact tracing and screening

Contact tracing is an important aspect of the control of tuberculosis infection. All close (family and household) contacts should be screened with a chest film and a Mantoux test. Screening new immigrants and contacts is a time-consuming but important aspect of tuberculosis control.

Prevention

Vaccination with the Bacille Calmette–Guerin (BCG) is only recommended in all children in high-risk areas (where vaccination is undertaken in neonates) and Heaf-negative health-care workers.

Community acquired pneumonia

Tuberculosis

Table 2.13	Selection and duration of drug treatment of tuberculosis	
Complications	**Initial phase**	**Continuation phase**
None (fully sensitive organism)	2 months: rifampicin isoniazid pyrazinamide	4 months: rifampicin isoniazid
Sensitivity unknown	2 months: As above, but add ethambutol	4 months: As above
Multidrug resistance (isoniazid and rifampicin resistance)	2 months: 5 or more sensitive drugs from the list above	22 months: 5 or more sensitive drugs
Miliary TB, or TB meningitis	2 months: As above	10 months: As above
TB pericarditis	2 months: As above, but add prednisolone	4 months: As above, but add prednisolone

Table 2.14	Adverse effects of antituberculous medication	
Drug	**Adverse effect**	**Management**
Rifampicin	Pink urine, tears, secretions	None
Rifampicin, isoniazid and pyrazinamide	Hepatotoxicity	Withhold medication until liver function tests improve
Ethambutol	Optic neuritis	Stop medication, ophthalmic referral
Pyrazinamide	Joint pains	NSAIDs

Nausea, rash and hepatotoxicity are complications of rifampicin, isoniazid and pyrazinamide.

Prognosis

Of patients infected with tuberculosis, 10–15% will develop active disease. The prognosis is related to the severity of disease at presentation and the extent of extrapulmonary disease.

REFERENCE

(1) *Corbett EL, Watt CJ, Walker N, Maher D, Williams BG, Raviglione MC, Dye C. The growing burden of tuberculosis: global trends and interactions with the HIV epidemic. Archives of Internal Medicine 2003; 163: 1009–1021.*

i **FURTHER INFORMATION**

BTS Guidelines for the chemotherapy and management of tuberculosis in the United Kingdom: recommendations 1998. Thorax 1998; 53: 536–548.

Blumberg HM, Burman WJ, Chaisson RE, et al. American Thoracic Society/Centers for Disease Control and Prevention/ Infectious Diseases Society of America: treatment of tuberculosis. American Journal of Respiratory and Critical Care Medicine 2003; 167: 603–662.

World Health Organization. Treatment of tuberculosis: guidelines for national programmes. Geneva: World Health Organization, 2003.

SECTION 2.8 Diseases of the airways

Asthma

Asthma is a chronic inflammatory disorder with symptoms associated with widespread but variable airflow obstruction and an increase in airway response to a wide variety of stimuli. Airways obstruction is often reversible, either spontaneously or with treatment.[1]

Epidemiology

The prevalence of asthma is very variable. Depending on geography, the range extends from 1.6% to 36.8% (36 800 per 100 000),[2] with the highest prevalence in the United Kingdom, Australia and North America, and the lowest in Eastern Europe, China and India. The age of onset is bimodal: more cases of extrinsic asthma occur in childhood and more cases of intrinsic asthma occur in later life. Both sexes are affected equally.

Pathology

Current evidence points to bronchial inflammation as the cause of the hyper-responsiveness. The bronchi in asthmatic patients show damaged epithelium with a persistent inflammatory cell infiltrate. In extrinsic (allergic) asthma, the cause of the inflammation is usually an aeroallergen. The cause in intrinsic asthma is less clear. There is increased sputum production and this can form plugs that can cause localized blockages of the airways.

Histologically there is oedema, hyperaemia and an inflammatory cell infiltrate in particular with eosinophils, lymphocytes and mast cells in the bronchial walls. The submucosal glands are enlarged and there may be increased numbers of goblet cells. Patchy necrosis and shedding of epithelial cells is seen, and the basement membrane is thickened. There is also hyperplasia and hypertrophy of the smooth muscle in the bronchial wall. The cycles of chronic inflammation and repair ultimately lead to 'airway remodelling', which is thought to be the cause of the irreversible airflow obstruction seen in some asthmatic patients. On post mortem examination, hyper-inflation and sputum plugging is often evident.

The determinants for asthma are both genetic and environmental. Asthma is more frequent in patients with atopy; established environmental triggers include chest infection, house dust mite (faeces), smoking, exercise, drugs (e.g. NSAIDs), air pollution, emotion/stress and occupational exposure to dusts (e.g. flour) or chemicals (e.g. isocyanate).

Scope of disease

Patients experience acute severe asthma attacks that may be severe enough to cause death.

Clinical features

The classical symptoms of asthma are episodic wheezing, breathlessness and cough. In addition patients may complain of chest tightness. The hallmark characteristics of asthma are intermittent symptoms that are worse at night and provoked by established triggers (allergens, infection, cold air, exercise). It is important to document the frequency and severity of attacks, known or suspected precipitants and a family history of asthma or atopy.

Examination may be normal during symptom-free periods. During an acute attack, there may be widespread wheezing (a silent chest may indicate life-threatening asthma), tachypnoea, tachycardia, prolonged expiration with the use of accessory muscles for breathing and a hyperinflated chest.

When assessing a patient with acute asthma (p. 130), it is important to assess the severity of the attack (Table 2.15) and determine if hospital or intensive care admission is required (Tables 2.16, 2.17).

For patients with a known history of asthma, it is important to ensure that the patient is on the correct step of the treatment ladder by assessing the frequency and severity of asthma attacks and reviewing the daily peak expiratory flow (PEF) diary. In addition, compliance with medication and the degree of successful allergen avoidance should be documented.

Table 2.15	Assessment of severity of acute asthma
Moderate exacerbation	
Increasing symptoms	
PEF >50–75% best or predicted	
No features of acute severe asthma	
Acute severe asthma	
Any one of:	
PEF 33–50% best or predicted	
Respiratory rate more than 25/min	
Heart rate more than 110 bpm	
Inability to complete sentences in one breath	
Life-threatening asthma	
Any one of the following in a patient with severe asthma:	
PEF <33% best or predicted	
Respiratory rate >25/min	
Heart rate >110 bpm	
Inability to complete sentences in one breath	
Near fatal asthma	
Raised P_aCO_2 and/or requiring mechanical ventilation with raised inflation pressures	

Table 2.16	Criteria for hospital admission in asthma
Life-threatening features	
Feature of acute severe asthma present after initial treatment	
Previous near fatal asthma	

Table 2.17	Criteria for admission to intensive care in asthma
Indications for admission to intensive care facilities or a high-dependency unit include patients requiring ventilatory support and those with severe acute or life-threatening asthma who are failing to respond to therapy as evidenced by:	
Deteriorating PEF	
Persisting or worsening hypoxia	
Hypercapnia	
Arterial blood gas analysis showing fall in pH or rising H^+ concentration	
Exhaustion, feeble respiration	
Drowsiness, confusion	
Coma or respiratory arrest	

Not all patients admitted to ICU need ventilation, but those with worsening hypoxia or hypercapnia, drowsiness or unconsciousness and those who have had a respiratory arrest require intermittent positive pressure ventilation. Intubation in such patients is very difficult and ideally should be performed by an anaesthetist or ICU consultant.

Initial investigations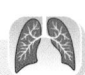

Asthma is a clinical diagnosis (there is no confirmatory investigation). In some cases, the clinical diagnosis can be supported by suggestive changes in lung function tests.

Peak expiratory flow rate

Assessments of airway calibre (PEF and FEV_1) may be normal between attacks or if patients are well controlled on treatment. The presence of marked diurnal variation is highly suggestive of asthma. The absence of variation, however, cannot be used to exclude asthma as a diagnosis. Patients may be required to document their PEF readings (diary) and return for assessment before the diagnosis of asthma can be established, as it is important to document objective evidence of asthma prior to commencing treatment.

Further investigations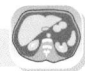

Pulmonary function testing

Formal lung function testing may be used as an alternative to identify and document variable airflow limitation. It is a useful investigation if other diagnoses (such as COPD in older patients) or a coexisting condition are suspected. Airflow reversibility is defined as a 15% or more increase in FEV_1 following therapy (inhalation of a short-acting β-agonist or a 14-day steroid trial) or a 15% or more decrease in FEV_1 after 6 minutes of exercise.

Methacholine or histamine challenge

If the diagnosis of asthma is still in doubt because of an atypical history or borderline changes on the PEF diary recordings, a methacholine or histamine challenge can be performed. This involves getting the patient to inhale increasing concentrations of methacholine or histamine and measuring the percentage drop in FEV_1 from baseline. The result is expressed as the provocation concentration that causes a 20% fall in the FEV_1 (PC 20). The lower the concentration required, the more hyper-responsive the airways and greater the likelihood of asthma. Increased bronchial responsiveness is also common in the general population without asthma, but failure to demonstrate bronchial responsiveness should prompt the search for an alternative diagnosis.

Initial management

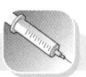

Patient education
Self-management is an essential and continuous aspect of asthma care. Self-monitoring of PEF on a twice-daily basis should be encouraged, and patients taught to maintain 90% of their best ever reading (in the mornings) with medication. In addition, patients and parents are informed about how to deal with attacks effectively and when to seek assistance. Inhaler technique should be taught and assessed regularly to ensure that the most effective inhaler device is used.

Avoiding precipitating factors
Avoiding known triggers may reduce the severity of existing disease. The clinical efficacy of measures that reduce house dust mite exposure is still under evaluation. Patients, parents and partners should be advised to stop smoking.

Medical management

The pharmacological management of patients with non-acute asthma involves increasing (and decreasing) treatment in a stepwise fashion, guided by the patient's symptoms and use of relieving bronchodilator. The aims of pharmacological management are the control of symptoms, prevention of exacerbations and the achievement of best possible physical activity and pulmonary function with minimal side effects.

Step 1. Mild intermittent asthma (short-acting bronchodilator)
Inhaled bronchodilators in the form of β_2-agonists such as salbutamol or terbutaline are the preferred starting point for treatment of mild intermittent asthma as they work quickly and have few side effects. Oral and parenteral formulations have a higher risk of systemic adrenergic adverse effects such as tachycardia, tremor and hypokalaemia.

Step 2. Regular preventer therapy (standard dose inhaled steroid)
Although preventers are not used for the treatment of acute attacks, regular use of a preventer is very important in maintaining long-term disease control. Inhaled steroids such as beclometasone, budesonide, fluticasone and mometasone are effective. Serious adverse effects of corticosteroids are seldom seen in patients using inhaled steroids at doses such as beclomethasone 200–800 µg daily.

Step 3. Add-on therapy
A. Long-acting β-agonist (LABA)
Long-acting inhaled β_2-agonists such as salmeterol and formoterol are the first choices in this step. Unlike their short-acting counterparts (which only work for 3–5 hours), the duration of action is up to 12 hours, and they are particularly suitable for nocturnal asthma. There is some debate over their anti-inflammatory effects, but they have a proven clinical role in improving lung function and symptoms. In recent years the combination of steroids and LABAs in a single inhaler has been produced.

B. Increase inhaled steroid dose
If there is benefit from a long-acting β-agonist, but with an inadequate response, the dose of inhaled steroid should be increased (e.g. beclometasone to 800 µg daily). Alternatively, if there is no response to the long-acting β-agonist, it should be stopped and the steroid dose increased.

C. Leukotriene receptor antagonists
At this stage, if there is no response to a long-acting β-agonist then leukotriene receptor antagonists should be introduced in conjunction with an increased inhaled steroid dose. Montelukast and zafirlukast (only available as tablets) act by blocking cysteinyl leukotrienes implicated in the allergic inflammatory process and improve lung function and symptoms and decrease exacerbations. Their main side effects are abdominal pain, headache and diarrhoea.

D. Methylxanthines
A methylxanthine may be prescribed instead of a leukotriene receptor antagonist. Both theophylline and aminophylline improve lung function and reduce symptoms. They are usually given as modified-release tablets, which are particularly suitable for nocturnal asthma. Care must be taken when prescribing methylxanthines: they have a narrow therapeutic window (10–20 µg/L) and interact with a number of other medications. Toxic side effects include tachycardia, nausea and headache.

E. Slow-release β2-agonist tablets
Modified-release tablets of salbutamol improve lung function and symptoms, and may be prescribed as part of a trial of therapy.

Step 4. Persistent poor control
A. Further increase in inhaled steroids
The dose of inhaled beclometasone may be increased to 2000 mg per day in adults.

B. Addition of a fourth drug
A sequential therapeutic trial of a leukotriene receptor antagonist, methylxanthine or an oral β_2-agonist, which was not added in step 3, should now be introduced.

Step 5. Addition of continuous or frequent oral steroids

Prednisolone is prescribed at this step for continuous or frequent use.

Stepping down

Regular review of treatment is important so that it can be stepped down as well as up, where appropriate. If a drug is not bringing about any benefit it should be stopped, thus ensuring patients are not over treated.

RECENT ADVANCES

Recent trials of administration of a recombinant human anti-IgE monoclonal antibody omalizumab that forms complexes with free IgE to block its interaction with mast cells and basophils have demonstrated improved symptoms and lung function in some patients with severe allergic asthma.[3]

Prognosis

In general, asthma is not a progressive disorder. Of patients diagnosed with childhood asthma, attacks in the majority (73%) will abate without returning in adult life.[4] The survival of patients with asthma (and without other concomitant lung disease) is no different from that of the general population.[5]

i FURTHER INFORMATION

British guideline on the management of asthma. Thorax 2003; 58(Suppl 1):i1–94.

REFERENCES

(1) *International consensus report on diagnosis and treatment of asthma. National Heart, Lung, and Blood Institute, National Institutes of Health. Bethesda, Maryland 20892. Publication no. 92-3091, March 1992. European Respiratory Journal 1992; 5: 601–641.*
(2) *Worldwide variation in prevalence of symptoms of asthma, allergic rhinoconjunctivitis, and atopic eczema: ISAAC. The International Study of Asthma and Allergies in Childhood (ISAAC) Steering Committee. Lancet 1998; 351: 1225–1232.*
(3) *Busse W, Corren J, Lanier BQ, et al. Omalizumab, anti-IgE recombinant humanized monoclonal antibody, for the treatment of severe allergic asthma. Journal of Allergy and Clinical Immunology 2001; 108: 184–190.*
(4) *Sears MR, Greene JM, Willan AR, et al. A longitudinal, population-based, cohort study of childhood asthma followed to adulthood. New England Journal of Medicine 2003; 349: 1414–1422.*
(5) *Silverstein MD, Reed CE, O'Connell EJ, Melton LJ, O'Fallon WM, Yunginger JW. Long-term survival of a cohort of community residents with asthma. New England Journal of Medicine 1994; 331: 1537–1541.*

Acute severe asthma

The majority of patients with acute severe asthma attacks who arrive in hospital have developed symptoms over 6 hours or more. Many deaths are preventable but delay can be fatal. The aims in the management of acute severe asthma are recognition of disease severity (p. 127) and prompt treatment.

Initial investigations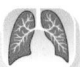

PEF

This is a mandatory investigation to assess the severity of asthma (Table 2.15).

Pulse oximetry

Oxygen saturations can be estimated non-invasively with pulse oximetry. The aim of oxygen therapy is to maintain oxygen saturations greater than 92%.

Arterial blood gases

These should be assessed in patients with oxygen saturations less than 92% or with any life-threatening features of asthma (Table 2.16). The aim is to classify the severity of the asthma.

Further investigations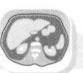

Further investigations are usually directed to identify any precipitating cause or alternative diagnosis. Treatment should not be withheld while these investigations are performed.

Chest X-ray

The indications for a chest radiograph are clinical features to suggest pneumothorax, pneumonia, life-threatening asthma, failure to respond to treatment, and (if safe) prior to the commencement of ventilation. Figure 2.12 is a chest

Asthma

Chronic obstructive pulmonary disease

Cystic fibrosis

Bronchiectasis

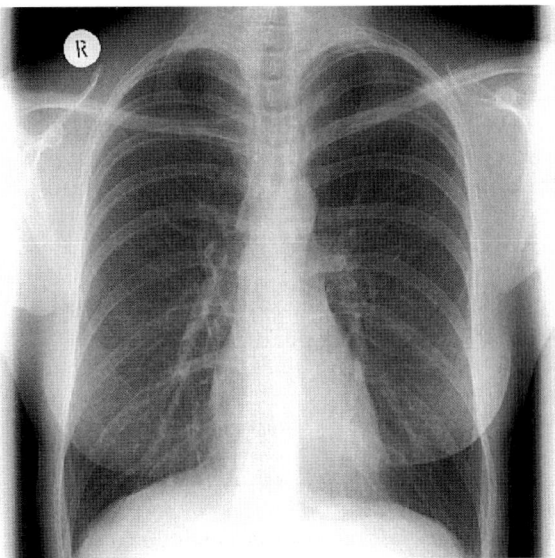

Fig. 2.12 Chest X-ray of a patient with acute severe asthma.

X-ray of a patient with acute severe asthma. The lungs are hyperexpanded with flattening of the diaphragms, and there is no suggestion of pneumothorax or pneumonia.

Sputum and blood cultures

Microbiological specimens should be collected prior to commencing antibiotics in cases of infective exacerbation of asthma.

Initial management

Oxygen

Patients should be sat upright to optimize breathing. Oxygen (40% or greater) should be administered via a Hudson face mask.

Treat precipitating cause

Attempts should be made to identify and correct any precipitating cause.

Risk assessment

If life-threatening features are present, discuss the patient with a senior clinician and the ICU team.

Medical management

High-dose inhaled β_2-agonist

Oxygen driven nebulized salbutamol is the preferred drug and route of administration, although administration of a β_2-agonist can also be achieved with a metered dose inhaler and appropriately sized spacer if a nebulizer is not available. Intravenous β_2-agonists are reserved for patients who cannot reliably use the inhaled formulations.

Steroid therapy

Oral prednisolone or intravenous hydrocortisone should be administered in all cases of acute severe asthma. Oral prednisolone should be continued for 5 days or until recovery.

Ipratropium bromide

Nebulized ipratropium bromide should be added to β_2-agonist treatment for patients with acute severe or life-threatening features, or in those with a poor initial response to a β_2-agonist alone.

Magnesium

Intravenous magnesium should be administered to patients who have not responded well to initial nebulizer therapy or those who have life-threatening features.

RECENT ADVANCES

The use of routine antibiotic therapy is controversial, as viral infections are the most common cause of infective exacerbation of asthma.[1] Current British guidelines do not support their routine prescription.[2]

Prognosis

In-hospital mortality is rare; most deaths from acute severe asthma occur as a result of respiratory arrest prior to hospital admission.[3,4]

FURTHER INFORMATION

British guideline on the management of asthma. Thorax 2003; 58(Suppl 1):i1–94.

REFERENCES

(1) Graham V, Lasserson T, Rowe BH. Antibiotics for acute asthma. Cochrane Database Systematic Review 2001: CD002741.
(2) British guideline on the management of asthma. Thorax 2003; 58(Suppl 1):i1–94.
(3) Burr ML, Davies BH, Hoare A, et al. A confidential inquiry into asthma deaths in Wales. Thorax 1999; 54: 985–989.
(4) Bucknall CE, Slack R, Godley CC, Mackay TW, Wright SC. Scottish Confidential Inquiry into Asthma Deaths (SCIAD), 1994–6. Thorax 1999; 54: 978–984.

Chronic obstructive pulmonary disease

Chronic obstructive pulmonary disease (COPD) is a disease characterized by airflow limitation that is not fully reversible. The airflow limitation is usually both progressive and associated with an abnormal inflammatory response of the lungs to noxious particles or gases.[1]

Previous distinctions between chronic bronchitis and emphysema, and definitions of chronic obstructive airways disease, chronic airflow limitation and chronic asthma are no longer applied.

Epidemiology

COPD is common: the world prevalence is estimated to be 830 per 100 000 with an approximately equal sex distribution. By country, the prevalence ranges from 4% to 10% in Europe and North America depending on disease definition and diagnostic criteria (symptoms, physician diagnosis or spirometry).[2]

Pathology

The risk factors for COPD are genetic and environmental (often an interaction of the two). Cigarette smoking is the single most important cause (the risk of disease increases with the number of cigarettes smoked); however, only 18% of smokers develop clinically significant COPD.[3] Other known environmental risk factors are heavy exposure to pollution, wood smoke and occupational dusts or chemicals (e.g. cadmium). A rare hereditary deficiency of

(α_1-antitrypsin) is the best characterized genetic predisposing factor to COPD.

COPD is characterized by chronic inflammation in the airways, lung parenchyma and pulmonary vasculature. Activated inflammatory cells release a variety of mediators that can also damage the lung. In addition there appears to be an imbalance between the destructive effects of protease and protective effects of anti-protease activity. Smoking stimulates the release and accumulation of elastase from neutrophils and macrophages. The oxidants in cigarette smoke also inhibit α_1-antitrypsin (an anti-protease).

The overall effects are ciliary dysfunction with mucus hypersecretion (chronic cough), repeated cycles of injury and repair to the bronchial wall leading to scar tissue formation and luminal narrowing (airflow limitation, reduced FEV_1), alveolar destruction leading to pulmonary hyperinflation (increased residual volume) and thickening of the intima of the pulmonary vasculature (impaired diffusing capacity).

Scope of disease

Chronic cough and sputum production may precede the development of airflow limitation by many years. Long-standing disease can result in right heart failure from pulmonary hypertension (from hypoxaemia).

Clinical features

The symptoms of COPD are cough, sputum production and dyspnoea in patients with a long history of smoking (or exposure to another risk factor). Spirometric evidence of airflow obstruction is required for confirmatory diagnosis (Table 2.3).

On examination, patients may be barrel chested, breathless at rest and cyanosed. Pursed lip breathing, the use of accessory muscles of respiration and in-drawing of the lower ribs on inspiration (due to a flattened diaphragm) may be evident. Asterixis (flapping tremor) can result from carbon dioxide retention and this may be accompanied by tachycardia and a bounding pulse. Percussion is hyper-resonant obliterating the cardiac and hepatic dullness. On auscultation there may be expiratory wheezing but breath sounds are usually diminished.

Initial investigations

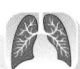

Spirometry

The presence of airflow obstruction is suggested by an FEV_1/FVC ratio of less than 70%, and the severity of COPD is defined, arbitrarily, on the degree of impairment of FEV_1 as mild (FEV_1 more than 50% predicted), moderate (FEV_1 between 30% and 50% predicted) and severe (FEV_1 less than 30% predicted). Bronchodilator reversibility testing is helpful to predict response to treatment. A positive response is considered to be an increase in FEV_1 by 200 mL or 15% of baseline, although non-responders often benefit from the prescription of bronchodilators, presumably by reducing dynamic hyperinflation. If a marked response is seen, the diagnosis of chronic asthma should be considered.

Other measurements of static lung volumes show an increased functional residual capacity, residual volume

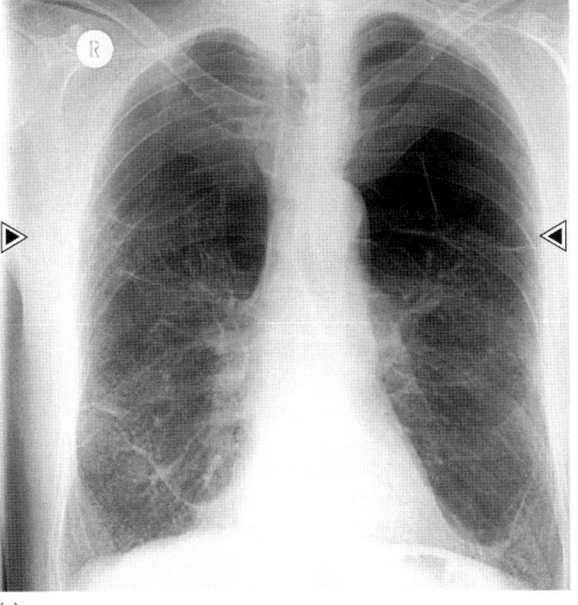

(a)

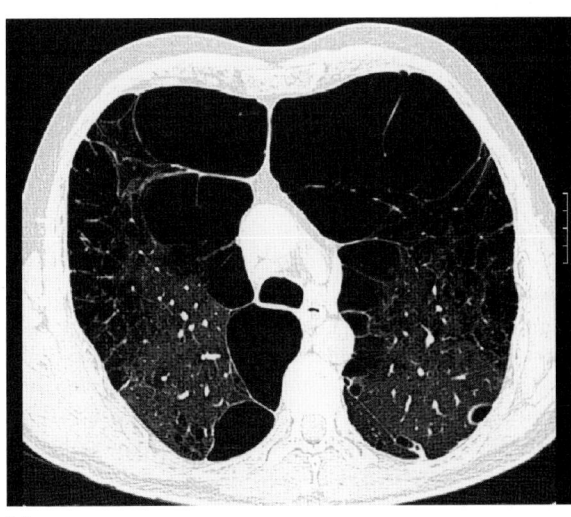

(b)

Fig. 2.13a, b Chest x-ray and CT thorax of a patient with severe bullous emphysema. The chest X-ray (a) shows hyperinflated lungs with loss of lung markings in the upper zones due to large bullae, which are evident on the CT thorax (b).

and total lung capacity. Diffusing capacity is impaired with severe disease.

Further investigations

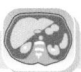

For patients with moderate to severe disease as assessed by spirometry, further investigations may be helpful.

Chest X-ray

Often the lungs appear hyperinflated with flattened diaphragms. However, a chest film is seldom diagnostic unless large bullae are present (Fig. 2.13a). It is more useful as a means to exclude other pathology.

CT Thorax

A CT thorax (Fig. 2.13b) is not usually required unless surgical treatment is contemplated or initial investigations suggest other pathology (such as bronchiectasis).

Alpha-1-antitrypsin levels

Screening for α_1-antitrypsin deficiency is indicated in young patients (below 45 years) and those with a positive family history.

Arterial blood gases

Since domiciliary oxygen is of proven benefit, arterial blood gas estimation is important in patients with resting Sao_2 <94% or clinical features of respiratory or right heart failure.

> **RECENT ADVANCES**
>
> Trials of oral steroids (typically prednisolone 30 mg daily for 2 weeks) are no longer recommended as the results fail to predict the response to inhaled corticosteroids.

Initial management

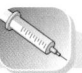

Risk factor modification

Smoking cessation is the single most import determinant of outcome. It should be encouraged and the patient should be helped to obtain appropriate information and nicotine replacement therapy or amfebutamone. This does not restore lung function but reduces the rate of further decline (Fig. 2.14).

Pulmonary rehabilitation

Pulmonary rehabilitation involves multidisciplinary management and addresses a wide range of issues such as exercise training, nutritional assessment/advice, counselling (for depression) and general patient education about COPD. The benefits to the patients are reduced hospital admission and improved exercise tolerance.[4]

Influenza vaccination

Influenza vaccination is recommended to all patients with COPD.

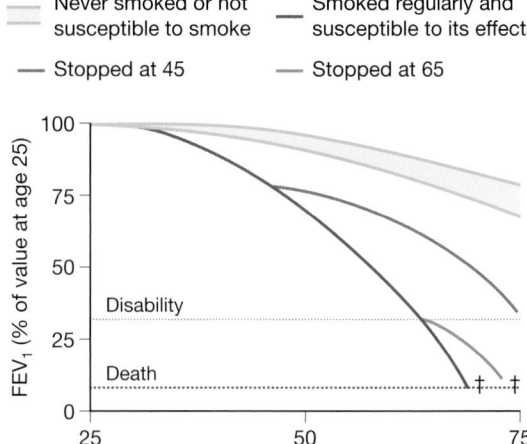

Fig. 2.14 Annual FEV_1 with age, smoking and cessation. From Fletcher C, Peto R. The natural history of chronic airflow obstruction. BMJ 1977; 1:1645–1648.

Medical management

The aims of pharmacological management are to prevent and control symptoms, reduce the frequency of exacerbations, and improve symptomatic status and exercise tolerance. However, none of the medications appears effective in arresting the progressive long-term decline in lung function. A stepwise approach may be employed and tailored according to disease severity and response to treatment.

Mild disease—short-acting bronchodilator

An inhaled short-acting bronchodilator (either a β_2-agonist or anticholinergic agent) is prescribed to be used as required.

Moderate disease—regular single or combination bronchodilator therapy

Regular use of a short-acting bronchodilator is recommended. Patients who are still poorly controlled should receive combination therapy with a β_2-agonist and anticholinergic drug. Combination therapy produces greater and more sustained improvements to FEV_1 than either agent alone.

Moderate to severe disease—combination bronchodilator therapy and corticosteroids

Inhaled combination LABA + corticosteroids should be given when the FEV_1 is <50% of predicted, or if frequent exacerbations occur (more than two per year). Corticosteroid should be stopped if no discernible benefit is evident after 4–6 weeks; those who do not respond can be given a trial of tiotropium.

Long-term oxygen therapy

Continuous nocturnal oxygen therapy improves survival[5] and should be prescribed for patients with respiratory failure (Po_2 <7.3 kPa or S_aO_2 <88%) or if Po_2 is less than 8 kPa with coexistent pulmonary hypertension, cardiac failure or polycythaemia. The aim is to increase the Po_2 to 8 kPa or S_aO_2 to 90% or more.

Domiciliary non-invasive ventilatory support is helpful for COPD patients with recurrent acidotic ventilatory failure.

Surgical management

Lung volume reduction surgery

Selected patients may benefit from lung volume reduction surgery. This subset includes patients with moderate to severe COPD, heterogeneous disease (usually predominantly upper lobe disease), with FEV_1 and carbon monoxide diffusing capacity more than 20% predicted[6] and without undue steroid dependence.

Lung volume reduction surgery involves resection of the non-functioning diseased lung to improve chest wall to lung volume matching. Access can be obtained thorough a thoracotomy, video assisted thoracoscopy or median sternotomy. The diseased lung tissue (usually the upper third of each upper lobe) is resected by a stapling device and 2–3 chest drains are left in the pleural cavity.

The patients who undergo this procedure are usually in poor health, and this surgery carries risks of mortality (approximately 8% at 90 days) and morbidity (postoperative respiratory failure, prolonged air leak, empyema).

Results are improved FEV_1, exercise capacity and quality of life.[7,8] However, there is no evidence at present to suggest any difference in survival.

> **RECENT ADVANCES**
>
> *Bronchoscopic lung volume reduction by therapeutic pulmonary segment atelectasis using a one-way valve implanted in terminal bronchioles is currently being evaluated as a potential treatment option with promising results.*[9]

Prognosis

The 5-year survival of patients with COPD ranges from 30% to 60%, depending on severity of disease (FEV_1, Po_2, Pco_2), age and comorbidity.[10] Low body mass index is an independent risk factor for mortality, an association that is strongest in subjects with severe COPD.[11]

i FURTHER INFORMATION

Pauwels RA, Buist AS, Calverley PM, Jenkins CR, Hurd SS. Global strategy for the diagnosis, management, and prevention of chronic obstructive pulmonary disease. NHLBI/WHO Global Initiative for Chronic Obstructive Lung Disease (GOLD) Workshop summary. American Journal of Respiratory and Critical Care Medicine 2001; 163: 1256–1276.

REFERENCES

(1) *Pauwels RA, Buist AS, Calverley PM, Jenkins CR, Hurd SS. Global strategy for the diagnosis, management, and prevention of chronic obstructive pulmonary disease. NHLBI/WHO Global Initiative for Chronic Obstructive Lung Disease (GOLD) Workshop summary. American Journal of Respiratory and Critical Care Medicine 2001; 163: 1256–1276.*

(2) *Halbert RJ, Isonaka S, George D, Iqbal A. Interpreting COPD prevalence estimates: what is the true burden of disease? Chest 2003; 123: 1684–1692.*

(3) *Tashkin DP, Clark VA, Coulson AH, et al. The UCLA population studies of chronic obstructive respiratory disease. VIII. Effects of smoking cessation on lung function: a prospective study of a free-living population. American Review of Respiratory Disease 1984; 130: 707–715.*

(4) *Berry MJ, Rejeski WJ, Adair NE, Zaccaro D. Exercise rehabilitation and chronic obstructive pulmonary disease stage. American Journal of Respiratory and Critical Care Medicine 1999; 160: 1248–1253.*

(5) *Continuous or nocturnal oxygen therapy in hypoxemic chronic obstructive lung disease: a clinical trial. Nocturnal Oxygen Therapy Trial Group. Annals of Internal Medicine 1980; 93: 391–398.*

(6) *National Emphysema Treatment Trial Research Group. Patients at high risk of death after lung-volume-reduction surgery. New England Journal of Medicine 2001; 345: 1075–1083.*

(7) *Geddes D, Davies M, Koyama H, et al. Effect of lung-volume-reduction surgery in patients with severe emphysema. New England Journal of Medicine 2000; 343: 239–245.*

(8) *National Emphysema Treatment Trial Research Group. A randomized trial comparing lung-volume-reduction surgery with medical therapy for severe emphysema. New England Journal of Medicine 2003; 348: 2059–2073.*

(9) *Toma TP, Hopkinson NS, Hillier J, et al. Bronchoscopic volume reduction with valve implants in patients with severe emphysema. Lancet 2003; 361: 931–933.*

(10) *Nishimura K, Tsukino M. Clinical course and prognosis of patients with chronic obstructive pulmonary disease. Current Opinion in Pulmonary Medicine 2000; 6: 127–132.*

(11) *Landbo C, Prescott E, Lange P, Vestbo J, Almdal TP. Prognostic value of nutritional status in chronic obstructive pulmonary disease. American Journal of Respiratory and Critical Care Medicine 1999; 160: 1856–1861.*

Asthma

Chronic obstructive pulmonary disease

Cystic fibrosis

Bronchiectasis

Acute exacerbation of COPD

Clinical features

Increased breathlessness is the main symptom of an exacerbation. It may be accompanied by wheezing, chest tightness, increasing volume/purulence of sputum and fever. The most common causes of an exacerbation are infection (viral and bacterial) and air pollution.[1]

Enquiry into the baseline exercise tolerance, current treatment regimen, social circumstances and previous hospital admissions is important when assessing the need for hospital (Table 2.18) or ICU (Table 2.19) admission.

Examination findings tend to be similar to those listed on page 131. However, in acute exacerbations it is important to exclude pneumonia, pulmonary embolism and cardiac failure as coexistent causes for the presumed 'acute exacerbation'.

Table 2.18	Indications for hospital admission in COPD
Marked increase in intensity of symptoms, such as sudden development of resting dyspnoea	
Severe background COPD	
Onset of new physical signs (e.g. cyanosis, peripheral oedema)	
Failure of exacerbation to respond to initial medical management	
Significant comorbidities	
Newly occurring arrhythmias	
Diagnostic uncertainty	
Older age	
Insufficient home support	

Table 2.19	Indications for ICU admission
Severe dyspnoea that responds inadequately to initial emergency therapy	
Confusion, lethargy, coma	
Persistent or worsening hypoxaemia (P_aO_2 <6.7 kPa, 50 mmHg), or severe/worsening hypercapnia (P_aCO_2 >9.3 kPa, 70 mmHg), or severe/worsening respiratory acidosis (pH <7.30) despite supplemental oxygen and NIPPV	

RECENT ADVANCES

The role of bacterial infection as a cause for acute exacerbation is controversial[2] as bacterial colonization occurs in a third of patients with stable COPD.[1] Therefore, the value of positive sputum cultures in the diagnosis and antibiotics in the treatment of acute exacerbation for a presumed bacterial cause should be carefully evaluated.

Investigations

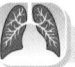

Peak expiratory flow rate/spirometry

It is difficult for ill patients to perform spirometry; however, PEFR less than 100 L/min or FEV$_1$ less than 1 L indicates severe disease.

Full blood count

Anaemia can worsen the symptoms of COPD, and polycythaemia can result from chronic hypoxia. The white count alone is not a very discriminatory investigation for infection, especially if steroids have been given.

Arterial blood gases

Screening for features of respiratory failure (P_O_2 <8.0 kPa or P_{CO_2} >7.0 kPa on room air) is an important investigation on admission. Life-threatening features (P_O_2 <6.7 kPa, P_{CO_2} >9.3 kPa or pH <7.3) require senior clinician and ITU involvement. Acidosis (pH <7.35) indicates a recent deterioration. Hypercapnia without acidosis is a feature of advanced disease but indicates that enough time has elapsed to allow balancing of the acidosis by bicarbonate retention (i.e. at least 3 days).

Chest X-ray

A chest film is useful to screen for alternative diagnoses (such as lobar pneumonia, cardiac failure, pneumothorax) that may mimic an acute exacerbation.

Sputum cultures

Purulent sputum alone is an indication for antibiotic treatment. The most commonly isolated organisms are *Streptococcus pneumoniae*, *Haemophilus influenzae* and *Moraxella catarrhalis*.

Initial management

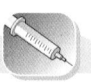

Oxygen therapy

Oxygen therapy is the cornerstone for the management of acute exacerbations. It is important to maintain P_O_2 >8 kPa and oxygen saturations >90%. Once oxygen is started, it is important to check the P_{CO_2} levels approximately 30 minutes later to ensure that satisfactory oxygenation has not precipitated carbon dioxide retention.

Medical management

Bronchodilator therapy

A β$_2$-agonist and an anticholinergic are usually given together, at 4–6-hourly intervals, by nebulizer. The role of aminophylline in this setting is controversial, and if used, will require close monitoring of levels to minimize systemic toxicity.

Corticosteroids

High-dose prednisolone (40 mg) is recommended for 5–10 days and has been shown to shorten recovery time (by 1–2 days) and improve FEV$_1$ (approximately 100 mL).[3]

Antibiotics

Antibiotics are only effective with worsening dyspnoea, increased sputum volume and purulence. The choice of antibiotic depends on local sensitivities and the results of the previous sputum cultures.

Ventilation

The aims of ventilatory support are to relieve symptoms and to decrease morbidity and mortality. Ventilation can be undertaken non-invasively (not requiring endotracheal intubation) or invasively (e.g. mechanical ventilation).

The indications for non-invasive positive pressure ventilation (NIPPV) are provided in Table 2.20. In acute severe exacerbation of COPD, the use of NIPPV decreases the rate of endotracheal intubation (by 28%), hospital stay (by approximately 5 days) and in-hospital mortality (by 10%).[4,5] Where the pH (1 hour) after nebulized β-agonist is between

7.25 and 7.35 the patient may be safely managed on a general ward but patients with pH <7.25 require HDU or ICU admission.

Invasive mechanical ventilation is usually required for patients with impending respiratory arrest, impairment of consciousness or life-threatening acid–base abnormalities despite medical therapy (p. 136) (Table 2.21). Making a decision on whether the patient is likely to benefit from endotracheal ventilation is an important part of the management of COPD and depends on the patient's premorbid lung function and level of disability, where known.

Prognosis

The overall in-hospital mortality for acute exacerbation of COPD is 8%, and the overall 1-year survival is 77%, decreasing to 65% if ITU admission for respiratory failure was required.[6]

REFERENCES

(1) White AJ, Gompertz S, Stockley RA. Chronic obstructive pulmonary disease. 6: The aetiology of exacerbations of chronic obstructive pulmonary disease. Thorax 2003; 58: 73–80.
(2) Pauwels RA, Buist AS, Calverley PM, Jenkins CR, Hurd SS. Global strategy for the diagnosis, management, and prevention of chronic obstructive pulmonary disease. NHLBI/WHO Global Initiative for Chronic Obstructive Lung Disease (GOLD) Workshop summary. American Journal of Respiratory and Critical Care Medicine 2001; 163: 1256–1276.
(3) Niewoehner DE, Erbland ML, Deupree RH, et al. Effect of systemic glucocorticoids on exacerbations of chronic obstructive pulmonary disease. Department of Veterans Affairs Cooperative Study Group. New England Journal of Medicine 1999; 340: 1941–1947.
(4) Keenan SP, Sinuff T, Cook DJ, Hill NS. Which patients with acute exacerbation of chronic obstructive pulmonary disease benefit from noninvasive positive-pressure ventilation?: a systematic review of the literature. Annals of Internal Medicine 2003; 138: 861–870.
(5) Lightowler JV, Wedzicha JA, Elliott MW, Ram FSF. Non-invasive positive pressure ventilation to treat respiratory failure resulting from exacerbations of chronic obstructive pulmonary disease: Cochrane systematic review and meta-analysis. BMJ 2003; 326: 185–189.
(6) Groenewegen KH, Schols AMWJ, Wouters EFM. Mortality and mortality-related factors after hospitalization for acute exacerbation of COPD. Chest 2003; 124: 459–467.

Cystic fibrosis

Cystic fibrosis is a genetic disease caused by the inheritance of a defective autosomal recessive gene that results in abnormal ion transport of the epithelia.

Epidemiology

The prevalence of cystic fibrosis is approximately 33 per 100 000 in North America and Europe, with a carrier frequency (of the genetic defect) of 1 in 25. It is more common in Caucasians; the prevalence is markedly lower in continents such as Asia and Africa. It has an equal sex incidence and usually presents before the age of 18.

Pathology

The cystic fibrosis gene is located on the long arm of chromosome 7 and encodes for a gene-protein product, the cystic fibrosis transmembrane conductance regulator (CFTR). The CFTR functions both as a cyclic AMP regulated chloride channel, and as a regulator of other ion channels. The most common mutation is the delta F508 (ΔF_{508}) mutation that leads to intracellular degradation of the CFTR protein and impaired ion transport.

The effects of impaired ion transport vary according to the type of epithelium: some are volume-absorbing (airways and intestinal epithelia), others are salt- but not volume-absorbing (sweat ducts), others are secretory (pancreas). In the lung the defect causes dehydration of the mucus layer in the airways leading to defective mucociliary action with accumulation of viscid secretions that obstruct the airways and predispose to recurrent pulmonary infections. In addition the neutrophil responses are exaggerated, leading to damage of the lung tissue, bronchiectasis and lung abscesses. On the skin, the inability to reabsorb chloride results in high chloride content of the sweat, a test used to diagnose cystic fibrosis.

Scope of disease

The multisystem manifestations of cystic fibrosis are presented in Table 2.22.

Table 2.20	Indications and contraindications for non-invasive ventilation in COPD	
Selection criteria (at least two should be present)	**Exclusion criteria (any may be present)**
Moderate to severe dyspnoea with use of accessory muscles and paradoxical abdominal motion	Respiratory arrest
Moderate to severe acidosis (pH 7.25–7.35) and hypercapnia (P_aCO_2 6.0–8.0 kPa, 45–60 mmHg)	Cardiovascular instability (hypotension, arrhythmias, myocardial infarction)
Respiratory frequency >25 breaths/min	Somnolence, impaired mental status, uncooperative patient
	High aspiration risk; viscous or copious secretions
	Recent facial or gastro-oesophageal surgery
	Craniofacial trauma, fixed nasopharyngeal abnormalities

Table 2.21	Indications for invasive mechanical ventilation
Severe dyspnoea with use of accessory muscles and paradoxical abdominal motion
Respiratory frequency >35 breaths/min
Life-threatening hypoxaemia (P_aO_2 <5.3 kPa, 40 mmHg or P_aO_2/F_iO_2 <200 mmHg)
Respiratory arrest
Somnolence, impaired mental status
Cardiovascular complications (hypotension, shock, heart failure)
Other complications (metabolic abnormalities, sepsis, pneumonia, pulmonary embolism, barotrauma, massive pleural effusion)
NIPPV failure (or exclusion criteria, see Table 2.20)

Table 2.22	Multisystem manifestation of cystic fibrosis	
Location	**Effect**	**Clinical features**
Lungs	Bronchiectasis, airflow obstruction, allergic bronchopulmonary aspergillosis	Cough, purulent sputum, respiratory failure, pneumothorax, haemoptysis
Hepatobiliary system	Exocrine and endocrine pancreatic failure, biliary cirrhosis, gallstones	Steatorrhoea, malnutrition, diabetes mellitus, liver failure, portal hypertension, cholecystitis
Reproductive system	Obstruction of the vas deferens	Male infertility
Gastrointestinal	Gastro-oesophageal reflux, intestinal obstruction, pseudomembranous colitis, rectal prolapse	Abdominal pain, diarrhoea
Skin	Vasculitis	Palpable purpuric rash
Musculoskeletal	Osteoporosis, joint disease	Kyphosis, fractures, arthritis
Nose	Nasal polyps	Recurrent sinusitis

Clinical features

The symptoms of cystic fibrosis are chronic productive cough (with purulent thick tenacious sputum), wheezing (airways obstruction), dyspnoea and decreasing exercise tolerance. In addition, adult patients may present with any of the multisystem manifestations listed in Table 2.22 such as pancreatitis, steatorrhoea, chronic sinusitis or infertility.

On examination, patients are often thin and short and look prepubertal. Clubbing (Fig. 2.15), cyanosis and halitosis may be present. On auscultation coarse crackles and wheezing are usually audible (most often in the upper zones).

Initial investigations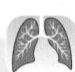

Chest X-ray
Radiological findings are ill-defined consolidation (opacities) mainly in the upper lobes with cavitation (nodular cystic lesions), bronchial wall thickening, hyperinflation, areas of subsegmental atelectasis and bronchiectatic cysts. These features are visible in Figure 2.16.

Sweat test
There are over 1000 different mutations, and routine genetic testing for cystic fibrosis is not practical (at present). Measuring the amount of chloride in sweat is the

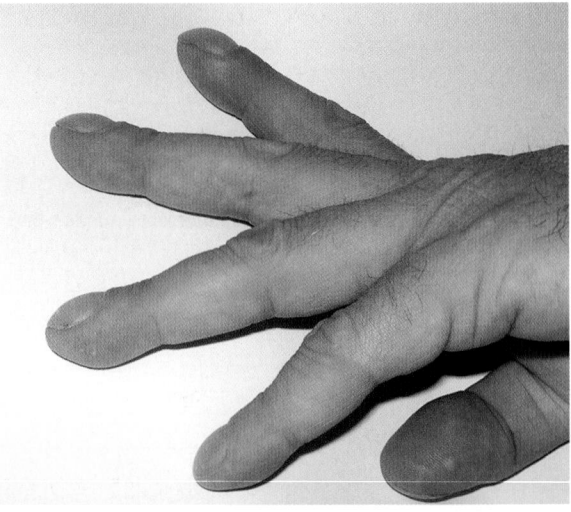
Fig. 2.15 Clubbing.

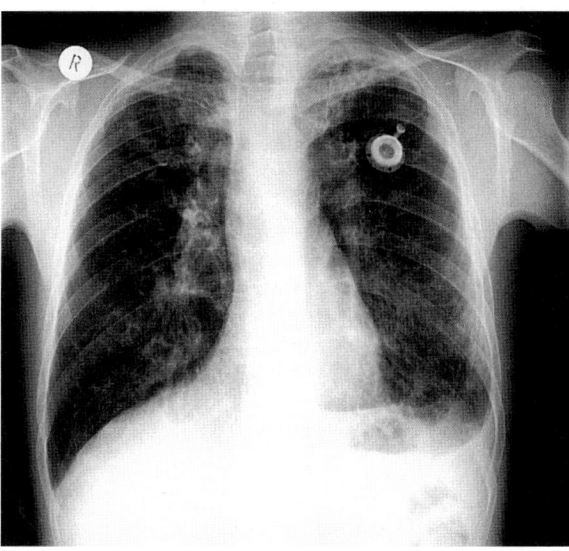

Fig. 2.16 Chest X-ray of cystic fibrosis. The artefact is a Port-a-Cath (a subcutaneous reservoir for intravenous access).

diagnostic test of choice. Normal levels are usually less than 40 mM; cystic fibrosis is diagnosed (in 90%) with sweat chloride levels higher than 60 mM. For patients with borderline sweat chloride values, CFTR mutation testing should be performed. Measurement of nasal potential differences may be performed in some centres for diagnostic purposes.

Further investigations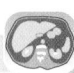

Lung function tests
Lung function testing reveals a pattern of airflow obstruction (FEV_1/FVC less than 70%). With disease progression FEV_1 decreases whilst FRC and RV increase. Eventually, a mixed severe obstructive and restrictive defect is observed.

Lung function is an important prognostic predictor for patients with cystic fibrosis, and is also an indicator of the efficacy of treatment.

Genetic studies
CFTR mutation testing should be performed to diagnose cystic fibrosis in patients with borderline sweat chloride values.

Sputum cultures
Sputum cultures are performed every 3 months to screen for colonizing organisms and detect new infections.

Other screening investigations
Screening for diabetes (random plasma glucose) and liver cirrhosis (liver function tests) is usually performed annually.

Initial management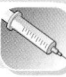

Referral for specialist care
The management of cystic fibrosis should be confined to specialist centres and multidisciplinary teams. Patient education and psychological support (including genetic counselling) is required for these young patients to help them cope with their chronic illness.

Physiotherapy
Airways clearance is an important aspect of the management of patients with cystic fibrosis; percussion and postural draining is the standard technique employed.

Nutritional support
A high-fat, high-calorie diet with liberal salt intake is recommended, with vitamin (A, D, E, K) supplementation and microencapsulated pancreatic enzymes (to normalize digestion). Weight and BMI are closely monitored throughout the course of this disease.

Medical management

Chronic suppressive antibiotic therapy
Long-term aerosolized tobramycin is recommended for patients with chronic *Pseudomonas* infection, as the treatment of pulmonary exacerbations often does not eradicate the lung infection. The decision to treat specific colonizing organisms varies from centre to centre; increasingly, however, the use of azithromycin in patients chronically infected with *Pseudomonas* has been associated with modest improvement of lung function and weight gain.[1] In general, oral or intravenous antibiotics are usually reserved for the treatment of acute severe exacerbations.

Bronchodilator therapy
Most patients demonstrate a degree of bronchial hyperreactivity and therefore experience improved pulmonary function with short- and long-acting bronchodilators.[2]

Mucolytic agents
Recombinant human DNAase decreases sputum viscosity by catalyzing cellular DNA into smaller fragments. It may be suitable for patients with chronic productive cough with moderate to severe obstructive airways disease, with subjective response (after several months) as the main indicator to continue treatment.

Surgical management

Lung transplantation
The indications for lung transplantation (p. 163) for patients with cystic fibrosis are FEV_1 <30% predicted, P_aCO_2 >6.7 kPa, P_aO_2 <7.3 kPa or young patients with rapid deterioration.[3]

137

RECENT ADVANCES

Gene therapy is currently being developed to deliver the CFTR protein using viral vectors. At present, clinical use is limited by inadequate uptake and the induction of airway inflammation.[4]

Prognosis

Cystic fibrosis is a relentlessly progressive disease. Due to advances in management, the life expectancy of patients born in the 1990s is estimated to be over 40 years.[5]

i **FURTHER INFORMATION**

Yankaskas JR, Marshall BC, Sufian B, Simon RH, Rodman D. Cystic fibrosis adult care: consensus conference report. Chest 2004; 125: 1S–39.

REFERENCES

(1) *Wolter J, Seeney S, Bell S, Bowler S, Masel P, McCormack J. Effect of long term treatment with azithromycin on disease parameters in cystic fibrosis: a randomised trial. Thorax 2002; 57: 212–216.*
(2) *Hordvik NL, Sammut PH, Judy CG, Colombo JL. Effects of standard and high doses of salmeterol on lung function of hospitalized patients with cystic fibrosis. Pediatric Pulmonology 1999; 27: 43–53.*
(3) *International guidelines for the selection of lung transplant candidates. The American Society for Transplant Physicians (ASTP)/ American Thoracic Society (ATS)/European Respiratory Society (ERS)/ International Society for Heart and Lung Transplantation(ISHLT). American Journal of Respiratory and Critical Care Medicine 1998; 158: 335–339.*
(4) *Kennedy MJ. Current status of gene therapy for cystic fibrosis pulmonary disease. American Journal of Respiratory and Critical Care Medicine 2002; 1: 349–360.*
(5) *Elborn JS, Shale DJ, Britton JR. Cystic fibrosis: current survival and population estimates to the year 2000. Thorax 1991; 46: 881–885.*

Bronchiectasis

Bronchiectasis is the permanent dilatation of bronchi and bronchioles caused by destruction of the muscle and supporting elastic tissue, resulting from (or associated with) chronic necrotizing infections.

Epidemiology

Bronchiectasis is uncommon and its global epidemiology is not well reported. In Finland, the overall incidence is 3.98 per 100 000 per year, with a bimodal distribution: 0.49 per 100 000 per year in the young (0–14 years) and 10.4 per 100 000 per year in the elderly (over the age of 65).[1]

Pathology

Bronchiectasis itself is not a primary disorder but occurs as a complication of other diseases (Table 2.23). The pathogenesis is due to two related processes, distal airways obstruction and persistent chronic infection. Chronic infection (as a primary event or distal to an obstructed airway) damages the bronchial walls, leading to weakness and dilatation (usually visible on chest X-ray and CT scan). Conversely, chronic infection can cause obstructive secretions, inflammation, fibrosis and scarring of the airways, leading to obstruction. Eventually fibrosis and scarring develops. Bronchial wall thickening as a result is thought to be an important determinant in the development and progression of an obstructive lung defect on pulmonary function testing.[2]

Scope of disease

Depending on the aetiology, bronchiectasis may be localized to a lobe (foreign body obstruction) or diffuse and involving both lungs (primary ciliary dyskinesia). Recurrent lower respiratory tract infection is a common complication, a third of patients have sinusitis, and amyloidosis may complicate chronic cases. Male patients with cilial disorders may have associated infertility.

Table 2.23	Causes of bronchiectasis
Bronchial obstruction	
Foreign bodies	
Tumours	
Mucus impaction	
Infection	
Pneumonia (bacterial or viral)	
Whooping cough	
Tuberculosis	
Allergic bronchopulmonary aspergillosis (excessive immune response)	
Congenital	
Primary ciliary dyskinesia (Kartagener's syndrome—bronchiectasis, sinusitis, situs inversus)	
Primary immune deficiency	
Cystic fibrosis	
Toxic inhalation or aspiration	
Chlorine	
Heroin overdose	
Other systemic diseases	
Rheumatoid disease	
SLE	
Inflammatory bowel disease	
Acquired immune deficiency (cancer, post transplant)	
Young syndrome (secondary ciliary dyskinesia)	

Clinical features

Cough and chronic (daily) purulent sputum production are the two main symptoms of bronchiectasis. The absence of a smoking history makes the diagnosis much more likely, and is an important differentiating feature from COPD (the two may coexist in smokers). Dyspnoea, wheezing, haemoptysis (especially during infective exacerbations), malaise and fatigue can also result. It is important also to screen for any of the causes listed in Table 2.23 which would further support the diagnosis.

On examination the patient may be cachetic with clubbing and halitosis. On auscultation coarse crepitation and wheezing may be audible (either localized or widespread depending on the extent of the disease).

Initial investigations

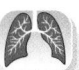

Chest X-ray

Radiographic imaging and anatomical visualization of dilated bronchi confirms the diagnosis of bronchiectasis. The chest film may be abnormal with linear atelectasis or tramlines (visible thickened bronchial walls), ring-like shadows (bronchial walls end on) or focal areas of consolidation.

CT Thorax

High-resolution CT is currently the imaging modality of choice, clarifying the plain film findings and providing a detailed map of disease. Pathological dilatation of the bronchial lumen is defined as a width of more than 1.5 times the size of an adjacent blood vessel. Cystic dilatations, thickened bronchial walls, mucus plugs and lymphadenopathy may also be visible.

Further investigations

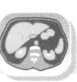

Lung function tests

Spirometry often reveals an obstructive defect (FEV_1 / FVC ratio <70%). Assessment for bronchodilator reversibility (p. 102–103), present in 20–40%,[3,4] is an important adjunct that assists medical management.

Sputum microscopy and culture

This is performed to determine the type and antibiotic sensitivities of colonizing pathogens and provides useful information during subsequent admissions for infective exacerbations.

Specific investigations for an underlying cause

Guided by the history and clinical features, specific investigations may be required to screen for foreign body (bronchoscopy), allergic aspergillosis (skin allergen testing, IgE and RAST to aspergillus), primary ciliary dyskinesia (nasal mucociliary clearance test) and congenital immunodeficiencies (immunoglobulin levels).

Initial management

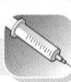

The aims are to interrupt the cycle of infection and inflammation. Conventional therapy usually involves physiotherapy and intermittent antibiotic therapy for exacerbations.

Physiotherapy and mucus clearance

Exercise is encouraged, and patients are taught postural drainage and mucus clearance techniques such as active cycles of breathing (ACBT).

Hydration

Maintaining adequate systemic hydration is important for patients with thick and viscous sputum; in addition, nebulized saline may be required.

Medical management

Bronchodilator therapy

Bronchodilator therapy improves pulmonary function in patients with reversible airflow obstruction.

Antibiotics

Antibiotic prescription is usually reserved for acute infective exacerbation, although nebulized aminoglycosides may be useful for a subgroup of patients with advanced disease. The evidence for long-term antibiotic therapy is limited; although there is a significant response, there are no differences in the frequency of subsequent exacerbations or in lung function.[5]

Management of exacerbations

Exacerbation of bronchiectasis is suggested by a combination of increasing cough or sputum production, worsening dyspnoea, reducing exercise tolerance, pyrexia, increased wheezing, reduced pulmonary function or new X-ray changes. Common pathogens responsible for infective exacerbation are *H. influenzae* (amoxicillin), *M. catarrhalis* and *P. aeruginosa* (ciprofloxacin). Antibiotic prescription in this setting should be pathogen specific and sensitivities may be known from previous sputum cultures.

Surgical management

The role of surgery in bronchiectasis is limited. The main indications are removal of the offending stimulus (foreign body), management of complications (haemoptysis) and, in selected patients, excision of the bronchiectatic segments of lung.

Lung resection

Lung resection for bronchiectasis may be an option for patients with localized disease that is amenable to resection. The indications are progressive disease despite medical therapy, massive haemoptysis and the development of a lung abscess.[6] Details of lung resection are provided on page 153.

Prognosis

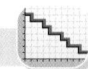

Bronchiectasis tends to be a relatively stable disease. The decline in pulmonary function is similar to the general population in non-smoking patients, and more accelerated in smokers. Spontaneous improvements compared to the time of diagnosis occur in a third. Survival is related to the severity of pulmonary function impairment and the presence of right heart failure.[7]

i FURTHER INFORMATION

Barker AF. Bronchiectasis. New England Journal of Medicine 2002; 346: 1383–1393.

REFERENCES

(1) Saynajakangas O, Keistinen T, Tuuponen T, Kivela SL. Evaluation of the incidence and age distribution of bronchiectasis from the Finnish hospital discharge register. Central European Journal of Public Health 1998; 6: 235–237.

(2) Sheehan RE, Wells AU, Copley SJ, et al. A comparison of serial computed tomography and functional change in bronchiectasis. European Respiratory Journal 2002; 20: 581–587.

(3) Murphy MB, Reen DJ, Fitzgerald MX. Atopy, immunological changes, and respiratory function in bronchiectasis. Thorax 1984; 39: 179–184.

(4) Hassan JA, Saadiah S, Roslan H, Zainudin BM. Bronchodilator response to inhaled beta-2 agonist and anticholinergic drugs in patients with bronchiectasis. Respirology 1999; 4: 423–426.

(5) Evans DJ, Bara AI, Greenstone M. Prolonged antibiotics for purulent bronchiectasis. Cochrane Database Systematic Reviews 2003: CD001392.

(6) Agasthian T, Deschamps C, Trastek VF, Allen MS, Pairolero PC. Surgical management of bronchiectasis. Annals of Thoracic Surgery 1996; 62: 976–978; discussion 979–980.

(7) Ellis DA, Thornley PE, Wightman AJ, Walker M, Chalmers J, Crofton JW. Present outlook in bronchiectasis: clinical and social study and review of factors influencing prognosis. Thorax 1981; 36: 659–664.

SECTION 2.9 Diffuse parenchymal lung disease

Many acute and chronic lung disorders with variable degrees of pulmonary inflammation and fibrosis are collectively referred to as diffuse parenchymal lung diseases or interstitial lung diseases.

The interstitium is the lung parenchyma that includes the space between the epithelial and endothelial basement membranes and is the target site of injury for this group of disorders. However, the extent of inflammation and fibrosis involves not only the interstitium but also the airspaces, airways and vessels, along with their epithelial and endothelial linings, hence the preferred term, diffuse parenchymal lung disease.

In 2001, international consensus on the nomenclature of diffuse parenchymal lung diseases was based on known causes (e.g. associated with collagen vascular disease) and unknown causes (idiopathic interstitial pneumonia, granulomatous diffuse parenchymal lung disorders and other forms), as summarized in Figure 2.17.[1] This section covers the more common of the diffuse parenchymal lung disorders: sarcoidosis, idiopathic pulmonary fibrosis, Goodpasture's disease, radiation-induced lung injury and eosinophilic pneumonia.

It is important to note that disorders such as COPD and pulmonary hypertension are also considered diffuse parenchymal lung disease but are often excluded from this classification.

REFERENCE

(1) American Thoracic Society/European Respiratory Society International Multidisciplinary Consensus Classification of the Idiopathic Interstitial Pneumonias. This joint statement of the American Thoracic Society (ATS), and the European Respiratory Society (ERS) was adopted by the ATS board of directors, June 2001 and by the ERS Executive Committee, une 2001. American Journal of Respiratory and Critical Care Medicine 2002; 165: 277–304.

Sarcoidosis

Sarcoidosis is a systemic granulomatous disease that primarily affects the lungs and lymphatic (lymphoreticular) systems of the body.[1]

Epidemiology

There are few population-based studies on sarcoidosis. In a US population cohort, the incidence of sarcoidosis was 6.1 per 100 000 person-years,[2] with an approximately equal sex distribution. The peak incidence in males was 30–39 years old and in females 40–49 years old.

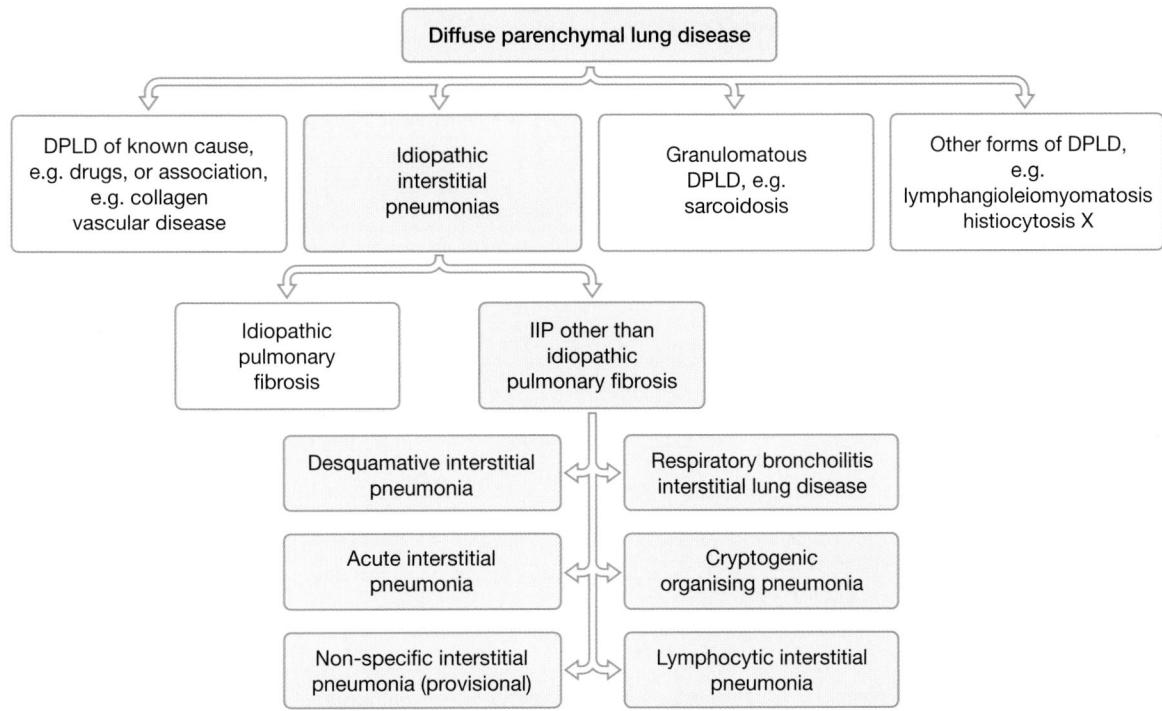

Fig. 2.17 Classification of diffuse parenchymal lung disorders.
From the American Thoracic Society/European Respiratory Society International Multidisciplinary Consensus Classification of the Idiopathic Interstitial Pneumonias. This joint statement of the American Thoracic Society (ATS), and the European Respiratory Society (ERS) was adopted by the ATS board of directors, June 2001 and by the ERS Executive Committee, June 2001. American Journal of Respiratory and Critical Care Medicine 2002; 165: 277–304.

Pathology

Although the exact cause of sarcoidosis is unknown, the risk factors are genetic and environmental. Numerous human leukocyte antigens (HLAs) have been associated with increased (A1, B8, DR3) or decreased (B12, DR4) risk of sarcoidosis and may influence disease expression. Implicated environmental exposures include infection and dusts (talc, aluminium, zirconium).

The characteristic lesion is due to a non-caseating granulomatous inflammatory process. In the lung, the granulomas are predominantly in the interstitium around bronchioles, pulmonary venules and the pleura. With ongoing disease, pulmonary fibrosis develops (honeycomb lung).

Scope of disease

Sarcoidosis is a multisystem disorder that can potentially affect all organs of the body (Table 2.24).

Clinical features

The nonspecific constitutional manifestations of sarcoidosis are low-grade fever, fatigue, malaise and weight loss.

Respiratory symptoms are dyspnoea, dry cough and chest pain. Two-thirds of patients with pulmonary sarcoidosis are asymptomatic and diagnosed on routine chest X-ray or blood tests. Less common manifestations include Löfgren's syndrome (erythema nodosum, polyarthritis, bilateral hilar lymphadenopathy and uveitis) and Mikulicz's syndrome (bilateral swelling of the lacrimal and parotid glands (uveoparotitis) with fever). Other important but rare regional/systemic manifestations are cardiac sarcoid, which may cause rhythm disturbances, and neuro sarcoid which carries a poor prognosis.

Few patients have palpable lymph nodes on examination. Clubbing is rare. On auscultation of the lungs, there may be wheezing or scattered crepitations. It is also important to screen for the clinical features of multisystem disease listed in Table 2.24.

Initial investigations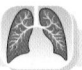

Apart from the diagnosis of sarcoidosis, the aims of initial investigations are also to screen for systemic involvement.

Full blood count
Anaemia, leukopenia and thrombocytopenia may be present.

Table 2.24	Extrapulmonary manifestations of sarcoidosis	
Location	**Effects**	**Clinical features**
Heart	Infiltration	Arrhythmia, heart block, restrictive cardiomyopathy
Peripheral nervous system	Infiltration	Cranial (Bell's palsy), peripheral neuropathy
Central nervous system	Infiltration, space-occupying lesions	Aseptic meningitis, hydrocephalus, seizures, personality changes
Musculoskeletal	Infiltration	Arthralgia, polyarthritis, myopathy
Liver	Infiltration	Hepatomegaly, jaundice, cirrhosis, portal hypertension
Haematological	Infiltration	Splenomegaly, anaemia, leukopenia, thrombocytopenia, lymphadenopathy
Ocular	Infiltration	Anterior uveitis, optic neuritis
Skin	Infiltration	Erythema nodosum, lupus pernio, alopecia
Nose and sinuses	Infiltration	Congestion, sinus pains, 'saddle' nose deformity
Salivary glands	Infiltration	Parotitis, enlargement
Endocrine	Dysregulated calcitriol production (macrophages and granulomas), pituitary infiltration	Hypercalcaemia, diabetes insipidus
Kidneys	Interstitial nephritis, space-occupying lesions	Renal failure

Urea and electrolytes

Rarely, interstitial nephritis can occur. However, renal failure is more commonly due to hypercalcaemia.

Liver profile

Deranged liver profile is common due to hepatic infiltration.

Serum calcium

Hypercalcaemia occurs in approximately 10% of patients.

Serum angiotensin converting enzyme

Serum levels of angiotensin converting enzyme may be elevated. If so, these are a useful way of monitoring treatment.

Chest X-ray

The chest film is abnormal in more than 90%: bilateral hilar lymphadenopathy, with or without interstitial infiltrates, is the most common feature (Fig. 2.18a). The severity

Table 2.25	Chest X-ray staging of sarcoidosis
Stage 0	Normal
Stage 1	Bilateral hilar lymphadenopathy
Stage 2	Bilateral hilar lymphadenopathy and interstitial infiltrates
Stage 3	Interstitial infiltrates only
Stage 4	Fibrocystic interstitial lung disease

of pulmonary involvement can be evaluated on the radiological features listed in Table 2.25.

Pulmonary function testing

Patients with sarcoidosis have diffuse parenchymal lung disease. This is reflected by a restrictive defect (reduced FEV_1 and FVC) and reduced carbon monoxide diffusing capacity (DL_{CO}).

Further investigations

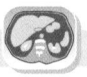

CT Thorax

The CT thorax is a useful investigation for patients with atypical chest X-ray findings or normal CXR and clinical suspicion of disease. In addition, a CT scan is an excellent investigation prior to transbronchial or surgical lymph node biopsy. The common features on CT are bilateral mediastinal lymphadenopathy and pulmonary infiltrates (Fig. 2.18b). In advanced disease fibrosis and bronchiectasis may be seen.

Bronchoscopy and transbronchial biopsies

On bronchoscopy, the mucosa of the airways can be nodular, oedematous and hypervascular. Endobronchial biopsies can be taken from the affected airways, and transbronchial lung biopsies should also be taken.

Surgical biopsy

When transbronchial biopsies have been unsuccessful, or if the lymph nodes are not accessible to transbronchial

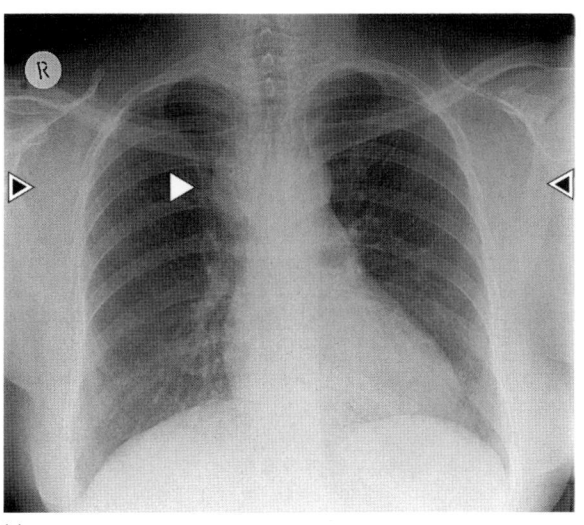

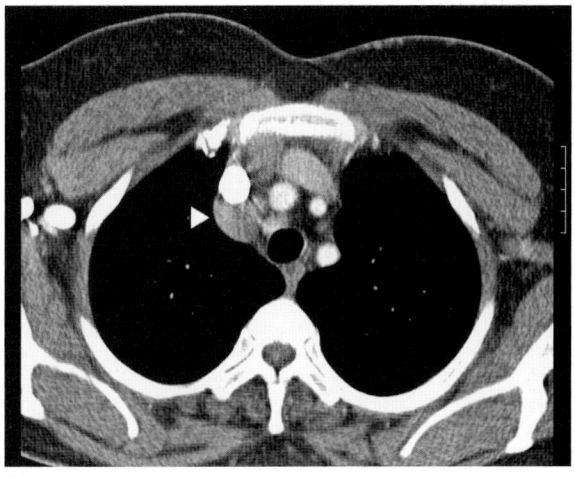

(a)   (b)

Fig. 2.18a, b Chest X-ray and CT thorax of a patient with sarcoidosis. The white arrow illustrates right hilar lymphadenopathy on the chest film (a), the CT thorax (b) reveals the enlarged lymph node seen in (a).

biopsy, mediastinoscopy and lymph node biopsies (p. 124) will usually provide sufficient tissue for histopathological analysis.

Additional investigations

Specific investigations may be required based on individual organ involvement. Routine ophthalmic investigation is recommended for all patients diagnosed with sarcoidosis. If a diagnosis of TB is also being considered, a Mantoux test should be performed. Elevated serum angiotensin converting enzyme (ACE) levels are a poor indicator of disease due to the lack of specificity.

Medical management

Corticosteroids

Patients with mild disease (skin lesions, uveitis, cough) do not require systemic treatment. Oral corticosteroids are indicated for patients with symptomatic systematic disease.[1] The starting dose of prednisolone is often 20–40 mg per day, but higher doses may be required for cardiac and neurological sarcoidosis. Treatment usually results in relief of respiratory symptoms and improvements in radiographic appearance and pulmonary function.[3]

Other cytotoxic agents

Alternative cytotoxic agents have been used to treat sarcoidosis, but the evidence supporting their use is limited. The two most commonly used agents are methotrexate and azathioprine. Other agents that have been used are cyclophosphamide, chlorambucil and ciclosporin.

Surgical management

Lung transplantation

Lung transplantation is an option for selected patients with end stage disease.[4] However, there are no current guidelines on the stage of disease in which optimum benefit from lung transplantation would be derived.

Prognosis

Sarcoidosis is a relapsing and remitting condition. Symptoms resolve spontaneously in approximately 50% by 6 months[3] with recurrences at a later date. Data on survival have not been well documented in the literature; however, higher stage on CXR and extrathoracic involvement are poor prognostic indicators.[5]

ι FURTHER INFORMATION

Statement on sarcoidosis. Joint Statement of the American Thoracic Society (ATS), the European Respiratory Society (ERS) and the World Association of Sarcoidosis and Other Granulomatous Disorders (WASOG) adopted by the ATS Board of Directors and by the ERS Executive Committee, February 1999. American Journal of Respiratory and Critical Care Medicine 1999; 160: 736–755.

REFERENCES

(1) *Statement on sarcoidosis. Joint Statement of the American Thoracic Society (ATS), the European Respiratory Society (ERS) and the World Association of Sarcoidosis and Other Granulomatous Disorders (WASOG) adopted by the ATS Board of Directors and by the ERS Executive Committee, February 1999. American Journal of Respiratory and Critical Care Medicine 1999; 160: 736–755.*

(2) *Henke CE, Henke G, Elveback LR, Beard CM, Ballard DJ, Kurland LT. The epidemiology of sarcoidosis in Rochester, Minnesota: a population-based study of incidence and survival. American Journal of Epidemiology 1986; 123: 840–845.*

(3) *Gibson GJ, Prescott RJ, Muers MF, Middleton WG, Mitchell DN, Connolly CK, Harrison BD. British Thoracic Society Sarcoidosis study: effects of long term corticosteroid treatment. Thorax 1996; 51: 238–247.*

(4) *Shorr AF, Helman DL, Davies DB, Nathan SD. Sarcoidosis, race, and short-term outcomes following lung transplantation. Chest 2004; 125: 990–996.*

(5) *Reich JM. Mortality of intrathoracic sarcoidosis in referral vs population-based settings: influence of stage, ethnicity, and corticosteroid therapy. Chest 2002; 121: 32–39.*

Idiopathic pulmonary fibrosis

Idiopathic pulmonary fibrosis (IPF, cryptogenic fibrosing alveolitis) is a diffuse pulmonary parenchymal disease belonging to the idiopathic interstitial pneumonia group (p. 141).

Idiopathic pulmonary fibrosis is a distinctive type of chronic fibrosing interstitial pneumonia of unknown cause, limited to the lung and associated with a histological pattern of 'usual interstitial pneumonia (UIP)'.[1]

Epidemiology

The prevalence of idiopathic pulmonary fibrosis ranges from 3 to 20 per 100 000, with the highest prevalences in countries such as Mexico and Finland.[2] It is more common in males with a mean age at diagnosis of 66 years.[1]

Pathology

Within the idiopathic interstitial pneumonias (p. 141), idiopathic pulmonary fibrosis is the most common subtype. Whilst little is known of the underlying cause, reported risk factors include smoking, drugs (antidepressants), chronic aspiration, environmental exposures (metal and wood dusts) and infection (Epstein–Barr virus, influenza, cytomegalovirus, hepatitis C). Genetic predisposition has also been regarded as a risk factor.

Alveolar wall injury, interstitial oedema and accumulation of chronic inflammatory cells are thought to be the starting points. Persistence of the injurious agent results in fibroblast proliferation and subsequent lung fibrosis. The histological subtype of this fibrotic process is 'usual interstitial pneumonia', a heterogeneous appearance with alternating areas of normal lung, interstitial inflammation, fibrosis and honeycomb change.

Scope of disease

Respiratory failure and death can result from advanced disease. Right ventricular failure can occur with pulmonary hypertension secondary to hypoxia. In addition, lung carcinoma has been identified with increased frequency in patients with idiopathic pulmonary fibrosis.

Clinical features

A gradual progressive dyspnoea and a dry cough are the two main symptoms of idiopathic pulmonary fibrosis. Dyspnoea is usually the most prominent and disabling symptom.

On examination, finger clubbing may be present (50%). Cyanosis and peripheral oedema (from right heart failure) are usually indicators of late stage disease. On auscultation, bibasal, dry, end-inspiratory ('Velcro' sounding) crackles are usually present; these may be audible in the upper zones with advanced disease.

Extrapulmonary involvement does not occur; fever, joint pains or eye symptoms should prompt the search of another diagnosis such as connective tissue disease or sarcoidosis. It is important that clinical assessment is undertaken to exclude other causes of pulmonary fibrosis such as extrinsic allergic alveolitis, pneumoconiosis, sarcoid and systemic sclerosis.

Initial investigations

Chest X-ray

Nearly all patients will have an abnormal CXR at presentation (however, a normal CXR does not exclude the diagnosis). Bibasal, asymmetrical reticular shadowing is the characteristic feature (Fig. 2.19a). Lung volumes appear small unless there is coexistent COPD.

CT Thorax

The precision of a high-resolution CT scan (HRCT) allows for earlier diagnosis of idiopathic pulmonary fibrosis, helps narrow the differential diagnosis and can identify associated emphysema. Classical findings are patchy peripheral, subpleural, bibasal reticular abnormalities with limited ground glass opacity (Fig. 2.19b). Traction bronchiectasis and honeycombing (Fig. 2.19b) may be seen with severe disease.

Usually, a confident diagnosis of idiopathic pulmonary fibrosis can be made in only two-thirds of patients.

Pulmonary function tests

Lung function tests will reveal a restrictive defect (reduced vital capacity and total lung capacity). The carbon monoxide transfer factor (TL_{CO}) is usually reduced and may precede abnormalities in the lung volumes. FEV_1 and FVC are also reduced but their ratio (FEV_1/FVC) is maintained.

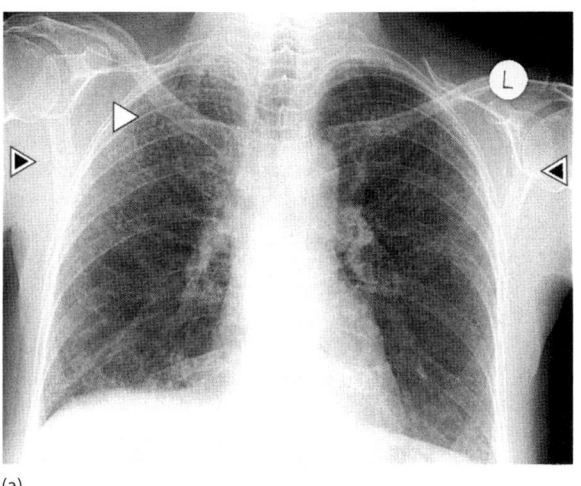
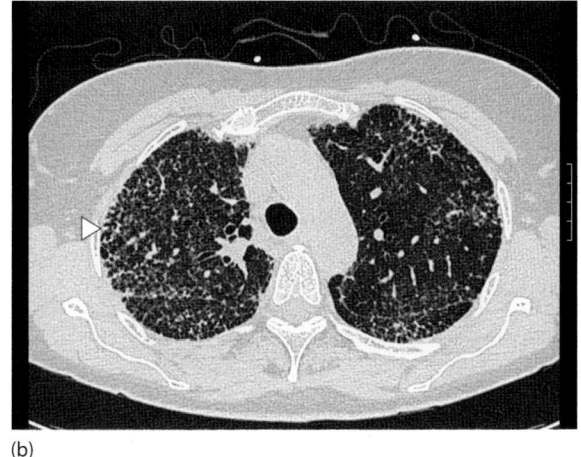

(a)   (b)

Fig. 2.19a, b X-ray and CT thorax of a patient with idiopathic pulmonary fibrosis. On the chest film (a) the arrows indicate reticular shadowing which corresponds to the honeycomb appearance as highlighted on the CT (b).

Further investigations
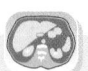

Bronchoscopy and bronchoalveolar lavage (BAL)
The use of bronchoalveolar lavage in the diagnosis and monitoring of disease progression in idiopathic pulmonary fibrosis is limited to specialist centres. The presence of neutrophilia in the lavage fluid increases the likelihood of an underlying fibrotic process.

Surgical lung biopsy
Surgical lung biopsy is recommended for patients who are likely to tolerate the procedure when the diagnosis is in doubt or there is no response to treatment. Lung biopsy (p. 108–109) provides the best tissue samples to diagnose idiopathic pulmonary fibrosis, to document the extent and stage of disease, and to differentiate it from the other idiopathic interstitial pneumonias.

Medical management

At present there is no evidence that any treatment improves the survival or quality of life in patients with idiopathic pulmonary fibrosis.[1]

Immunosuppression regimen
Current recommended treatment is combination immuno-suppression therapy using corticosteroid (prednisolone) with either azathioprine or cyclophosphamide for an indefinite period. Recent reports suggest that carbocysteine can be usefully added to this regime.

After a minimum of 6 months, patients are re-evaluated. If their clinical condition is stable or improved, the therapy is continued. If their clinical condition is worse, therapy should be stopped or changed (e.g. prednisolone with a different cytotoxic agent).

Surgical management

Lung transplantation
Lung transplantation should be considered for patients with symptomatic progressive disease that fails to improve with steroids or immunosuppressive therapy, or when pulmonary function becomes severely limited (FVC <60% predicted, corrected diffusing capacity <50% predicted).[3]

Prognosis

The progression of idiopathic pulmonary fibrosis is relentless, often in an insidious manner. Spontaneous remission does not occur. The 5-year survival is approximately 40% (ranging from 30% to 50%),[1] with respiratory failure as the most frequent cause of death.

FURTHER INFORMATION

American Thoracic Society. Idiopathic pulmonary fibrosis: diagnosis and treatment. International consensus statement. American Thoracic Society (ATS), and the European Respiratory Society (ERS). American Journal of Respiratory and Critical Care Medicine 2000; 161: 646–664.

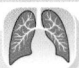

REFERENCES

(1) *American Thoracic Society. Idiopathic pulmonary fibrosis: diagnosis and treatment. International consensus statement. American Thoracic Society (ATS), and the European Respiratory Society (ERS). American Journal of Respiratory and Critical Care Medicine 2000; 161: 646–664.*
(2) *Hodgson U, Laitinen T, Tukiainen P. Nationwide prevalence of sporadic and familial idiopathic pulmonary fibrosis: evidence of founder effect among multiplex families in Finland. Thorax 2002; 57: 338–342.*
(3) *International guidelines for the selection of lung transplant candidates. The American Society for Transplant Physicians (ASTP)/ American Thoracic Society (ATS)/European Respiratory Society (ERS)/International Society for Heart and Lung Transplantation (ISHLT). American Journal of Respiratory and Critical Care Medicine 1998; 158: 335–339.*

Goodpasture's disease

Goodpasture's disease is a small vessel vasculitis affecting the lung and kidney (p. 721) which causes inflammatory destruction of the arterioles, venules and alveolar capillaries in the interstitial compartment. Goodpasture's syndrome is characterized by pulmonary haemorrhage, rapidly progressive glomerulonephritis and anti-basement membrane antibodies (Goodpasture's antigen).

Epidemiology

Goodpasture's disease is rare: the incidence has been reported to be 0.1 per 100 000 per year in European populations and even less in people of Asian and Afro-Caribbean origin. There is a bimodal age distribution that peaks between the ages of 18 and 35 and 50 and 65. There is an equal sex incidence.[1]

Pathology

The histology of this autoimmune disease shows focal necrosis of the alveolar walls with extensive intra-alveolar haemorrhage, haemosiderin-laden macrophages (not seen acutely), fibrous thickening of the septa, hypertrophy of the septal lining and linear immunofluorescence. Fibrosis, obstructive or restrictive lung defects, massive (occasionally fatal) haemoptysis, respiratory failure and a rapidly progressive glomerulonephritis are potential complications.

Clinical features

Symptoms often start with an upper respiratory tract infection, followed by haemoptysis. Approximately a third have significant haemorrhage without any haemoptysis. Other symptoms include shortness of breath, cough, low-grade fever, and general malaise that evolves over days to weeks.

Initial investigations

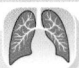

Full blood count
The haemoglobin falls with continued bleeding. The white cell and platelet counts can be slightly raised. However, if the platelet count is low this suggests that the haemorrhage may be due to another diagnosis such as idiopathic thrombocytopenic purpura or thrombotic thrombocytopenic purpura.

Clotting
A clotting screen should be performed to screen for abnormalities.

Urea and electrolytes
If renal disease is also present, the renal function will be abnormal and progress rapidly if untreated. In the early stages of coexistent renal disease, the renal function may actually be normal and so should be monitored regularly.

Urinalysis
If the kidneys are also involved, there will be proteinuria, haematuria and red blood cell casts in the urine.

Chest X-ray
This shows patchy or diffuse bilateral fluffy infiltrates. There is relative sparing of the upper lobes.

Lung function tests
Sequential increase in the transfer factor (K_{co}) is seen, as more haemoglobin is available in the alveoli to absorb the carbon monoxide.

Further investigations

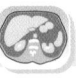

Bronchoscopy
Urgent bronchoscopy is usually performed for patients with haemoptysis although there will be no endobronchial lesion in this condition. Blood may be visible, however, and bronchoscopy provides an opportunity to remove blood from the airways. Bronchoalveolar lavage fluid may reveal haemosiderin-laden macrophages.

Renal biopsy
A renal biopsy is usually required to confirm the diagnosis (linear immunofluorescence) and assess the severity of renal disease.

Anti-GBM antibodies
Antibodies directed against the basement membrane of the lung and kidney can be found in over 90% of patients with Goodpasture's disease.

Management

Initial management consists of resuscitation by ensuring airway patency and adequate oxygenation. Intravenous access should be obtained in patients with haemoptysis, and an urgent bronchoscopy arranged. The subsequent management of the disease is detailed on page 721.

Prognosis

Pulmonary complications usually resolve without any impact on long-term respiratory function. Further information on renal function is provided on page 721.

REFERENCE

(1) Turner AN. *Goodpasture's disease. Nephrology, Dialysis, Transplantation* 2001; 16(Suppl 6): 52–54.

Radiation-induced lung injury

Radiation-induced lung injury is usually a complication of therapeutic irradiation for thoracic malignancy.

Epidemiology

The frequency of this complication depends on the disease definition and the radiation dose. Radiographically, it may occur in 13–100% of patients, depending on the radiation dose. Clinically symptomatic radiation-induced lung injury may be evident in up to 34%.[1]

Pathology

Within 24 hours of irradiation, sloughing of the alveoli or lining cells and accumulation of fibrin and inflammatory cells within the intra-alveolar spaces are visible on histology. This either resolves or undergoes organization to leave fibrosis and loss of lung volume over a period of 3–6 months. The hallmarks of fibrosis are intimal thickening, obliterative vasculitis, sclerosis and loss of airspaces.

There are three recognized phases of radiation-induced lung injury. The initial latency period occurs immediately after exposure, where inflammatory events are sub-clinical. This is followed by the acute phase 4–6 weeks later, when symptoms become apparent and CXR changes occur (radiation pneumonitis). The chronic phase lasts up to 2 years, and it is during this period that pulmonary fibrosis develops. Some patients may develop pulmonary fibrosis without ever having experienced pneumonitis. The disease process usually stabilizes after 2 years.

In patients with a large volume of irradiated lung, pulmonary hypertension and right heart failure can develop.

Clinical features

Shortness of breath, cough, low-grade fever and occasional haemoptysis may occur. As pulmonary fibrosis develops, exercise tolerance decreases to the point where patients with severe disease may become oxygen dependent.

Examination is usually unremarkable; radiation injury to the overlying skin may be present, with the occasional crepitation or pleural rub on auscultation.

Investigations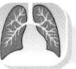

Chest X-ray
CXR changes can pre-date symptoms by 2 weeks. Initial findings are a diffuse haziness within the irradiated area that develops into fluffy infiltrates with clearly defined borders that do not conform to an anatomical pattern. These changes will be fully reversible, partially reversible, or develop into an area of fibrosis (6–9 months later) with linear reticular shadowing. Contraction associated with fibrosis can cause mediastinal shift and tenting of the diaphragm.

CT Thorax
High-resolution CT will clearly delineate the plain film findings. The infiltrates usually have a ground glass appearance with increased attenuation with radiation pneumonitis and chronic soft tissue changes consistent with radiation fibrosis.

Lung function tests
Depending on the severity of injury, lung function tests may reveal impaired diffusing capacity with decreased TL_{CO}. If fibrosis is present, a restrictive defect usually develops (reduced FVC with normal FEV_1/FVC ratio).

Management

Corticosteroid therapy
Most cases are mild and do not require treatment. High-dose corticosteroid therapy is the treatment of choice for patients with moderate to severe disease. A dose of 100 mg of prednisolone is prescribed for several weeks and tailed off gradually. The response rate has been reported to be 80%.[1] However, the treatment of radiation pneumonitis does not guarantee prevention of subsequent fibrosis.

> **RECENT ADVANCES**
>
> *A recent trial reported that pentoxifylline reduced the higher degrees of lung injury (detected radiologically) and improved diffusing capacity and lung perfusion in patients receiving thoracic irradiation (compared to placebo).*[2]

Prognosis

The prognosis is variable and relates primarily to the severity of the initial injury and volume of lung irradiated.

i FURTHER INFORMATION

Movsas B, Raffin TA, Epstein AH, Link CJ Jr. Pulmonary radiation injury. Chest 1997; 111: 1061–1076.

REFERENCES

(1) *Movsas B, Raffin TA, Epstein AH, Link CJ Jr. Pulmonary radiation injury. Chest 1997; 111: 1061–1076.*
(2) *Ozturk B, Egehan I, Atavci S, Kitapci M. Pentoxifylline in prevention of radiation-induced lung toxicity in patients with breast and lung cancer: a double-blind randomized trial. International Journal of Radiation Oncology, Biology, Physics 2004; 58: 213–219.*

Eosinophilic pneumonia

The term eosinophilic pneumonia encompasses a variety of disorders, characterized by eosinophilic pulmonary infiltrates and peripheral blood eosinophilia.

Epidemiology

All eosinophilic pneumonias are rare.

Pathology

Acute eosinophilic pneumonia
The cause of acute eosinophilic pneumonia is unknown. It tends to present in young patients, and histopathology shows diffuse alveolar damage, hyaline membranes, and marked numbers of interstitial and alveolar eosinophils.

Chronic eosinophilic pneumonia
The cause of chronic eosinophilic pneumonia is also unknown. It tends to present in middle-aged (50 years) women with a concomitant history of asthma. Histopathology shows interstitial and alveolar eosinophils and histiocytes including multinucleated giant cells.

Allergic bronchopulmonary aspergillosis
Allergic bronchopulmonary aspergillosis is due to a type I hypersensitivity reaction to airway colonization with *Aspergillus fumigatus*, usually in patients with asthma or cystic fibrosis.

Churg–Strauss syndrome
Churg–Strauss syndrome is the pulmonary manifestation of a systemic vasculitis, characterized by asthma, peripheral eosinophilia and palpable purpura (vasculitis), usually presenting in middle age. Other organs includ-ing the heart (coronary occlusion, pericardial effusion) may be affected.

Clinical features

Most patients tend to present with fever, dry cough and shortness of breath. Night sweats, wheeze and chest pain can also occur with chronic eosinophilic pneumonia. Associated symptoms of arthralgia, pericarditis, purpura, rhinitis and sinusitis would suggest Churg–Strauss syndrome.

Asthma predisposes to the development of eosinophilic pneumonia, but repeated episodes of bronchial obstruction, fever, malaise, brown mucus plugs and haemoptysis may herald allergic bronchopulmonary aspergillosis.

On examination, scattered crepitations are the most common finding.

Investigations

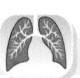

Full blood count
Peripheral blood eosinophilia is the usual finding, but eosinophil counts may be normal with acute eosinophilic pneumonia.

Chest X-ray
Often CXR reveals fluffy interstitial infiltrates. The appearance of a 'photographic negative' of pulmonary oedema is the classic finding with chronic eosinophilic pneumonia. In allergic bronchopulmonary aspergillosis, changing perihilar shadowing may be present. With disease progression, fibrosis, proximal bronchiectasis and cavitation can occur.

Other investigations
Bronchoscopy and bronchoalveolar lavage (revealing a high eosinophil count) may be required if initial investigations fail to provide a firm diagnosis. *Aspergillus* skin tests and precipitins will be positive with allergic bronchopulmonary aspergillosis, and a raised ESR with positive p-ANCA and rheumatoid factor would suggest Churg–Strauss syndrome. Modestly raised levels of IgE are consistent with acute bronchopulmonary aspergillosis but very high levels suggest parasitic infection.

Management

In general, most patients will benefit from a course of corticosteroids. Antifungal therapy (e.g. itraconazole) may be required for patients with allergic bronchopulmonary aspergillosis as an adjunctive therapy.

Prognosis

The prognosis is generally good if the disease is recognized and treated early. Relapse can occur with chronic eosinophilic pneumonia.

SECTION 2.10 Neoplastic disease

Benign lung tumours

Benign tumours of the lung are rare and usually present incidentally on a chest film as a solitary pulmonary nodule (p. 152).

Epidemiology

As benign tumours encompass a variety of disorders, there is limited information on the epidemiology of this disease as a group.

Pathology

Benign lung tumours include hamartomas, clear cell tumours, papillomas, fibromas, leiomyomas, chondromas and haemangiomas.

Clinical features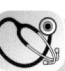

Benign tumours of the lung are usually asymptomatic. Occasionally, if the tumour obstructs an airway, distal pneumonitis (and bronchiectasis) can occur, resulting in the patient presenting with a persistent productive cough.

Investigations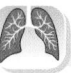

Investigation should proceed as detailed on page 151–152 for the solitary pulmonary nodule.

Management

Expectant management
In general, uncomplicated benign tumours do not require treatment.

Surgical resection
Surgical resection by simple excision is curative and is reserved for patients in whom the diagnosis of malignancy cannot confidently be excluded (p. 153) or as part of a procedure to address complications such as distal lobar bronchiectasis.

Prognosis

A normal life expectancy is usual.

Neuroendocrine tumours

Primary neuroendocrine tumours of the lung constitute an important family of lung tumours that range from typical carcinoid to small-cell lung cancer.

Epidemiology

Small-cell lung cancer is the histopathological tumour type in approximately 20% of lung cancer patients, whilst typical carcinoid, atypical carcinoids and large cell neuroendocrine tumours constitute approximately 2%.

Pathology

The malignant potential is specific to cell type (Table 2.26). Typical carcinoids are low-grade malignancies, atypical carcinoids are intermediate-grade malignancies, and large cell neuroendocrine and small-cell lung cancers are high-grade malignancies (80% have evidence of metastasis at presentation).

Neuroendocrine tumours can present anywhere in the tracheobronchial tree. When localized to an airway, they may manifest as a persistent monophonic inspiratory wheeze or with distal obstructive pneumonitis. Carcinoid

Table 2.26	Characteristics of pulmonary neuroendocrine tumours		
Type	**Malignant potential**	**5-year survival**	**10-year survival**
Typical carcinoid	Low grade	87%	87%
Atypical carcinoid	Intermediate grade	56%	35%
Large cell neuroendocrine tumour	High grade	27%	9%
Small cell lung cancer	High grade	9%	5%

syndrome is rare with primary neuroendocrine tumours of the lung.

Clinical features

With central tumours, patients may present with a persistent inspiratory wheeze (due to endobronchial obstruction) that may have been misdiagnosed as asthma, a persistent cough due to obstructive pneumonitis or haemoptysis. Peripheral tumours can be asymptomatic and may only be detected on routine chest films.

Investigations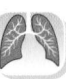

The diagnostic workup of patients and staging investigations are detailed on page 151–152.

Management

Surgical resection
Complete surgical resection is the treatment of choice for patients with neuroendocrine tumours. The extent of resection depends on tumour type. Lung-conserving surgery (segmentectomy, bronchotomy and reimplantation of the distal airways) is suitable for patients with typical carcinoid tumours. Formal anatomical lung resection (lobectomy or pneumonectomy) is appropriate for suitable patients with atypical carcinoid and large cell neuroendocrine tumours.

Radiotherapy
Patients with small-cell lung cancers are classified as having limited stage disease (Veterans Administration Lung Cancer Study Group) when disease is confined to the ipsilateral hemithorax within a singe radiation port (i.e. field of radiation). Treatment for patients in this stage comprises combination radiotherapy and chemotherapy or surgical resection for patients with very limited (T1–2, N0) disease. Prophylactic cranial irradiation is offered to all patients in complete remission due to improved disease-free survival and reduction in subsequent cerebral metastasis.[1]

Patients with small-cell lung cancers and metastatic disease are classified as having extensive stage disease; platinum-based chemotherapy is the treatment of choice for patients in this stage.[2] Prophylactic cranial irradiation is also offered to all patients in complete remission.

Prognosis

The prognosis of patients with neuroendocrine tumours is specific to cell type (Table 2.26).[3]

> ### *i* FURTHER INFORMATION
>
> Simon GR, Wagner H. Small cell lung cancer. Chest 2003; 123(90010): 259S–271.

REFERENCES

(1) Auperin A, Arriagada R, Pignon JP, et al. Prophylactic cranial irradiation for patients with small-cell lung cancer in complete remission. Prophylactic Cranial Irradiation Overview Collaborative Group. New England Journal of Medicine 1999; 341(7): 476–484.
(2) Pujol JL, Carestia L, Daures JP. Is there a case for cisplatin in the treatment of small-cell lung cancer? A meta-analysis of randomized trials of a cisplatin-containing regimen versus a regimen without this alkylating agent. British Journal of Cancer 2000; 83(1): 8–15.
(3) Travis WD, Rush W, Flieder DB, et al. Survival analysis of 200 pulmonary neuroendocrine tumors with clarification of criteria for atypical carcinoid and its separation from typical carcinoid. American Journal of Surgical Pathology 1998; 22(8): 934–944.

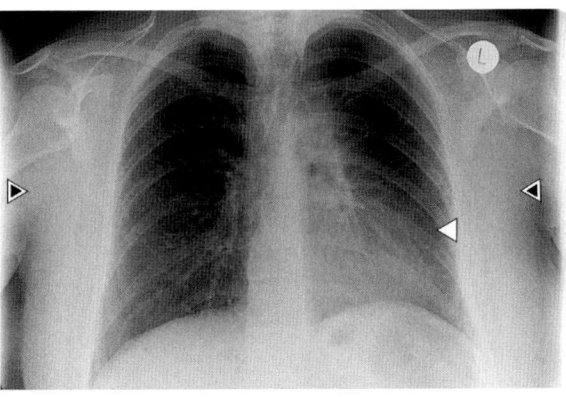

(a)

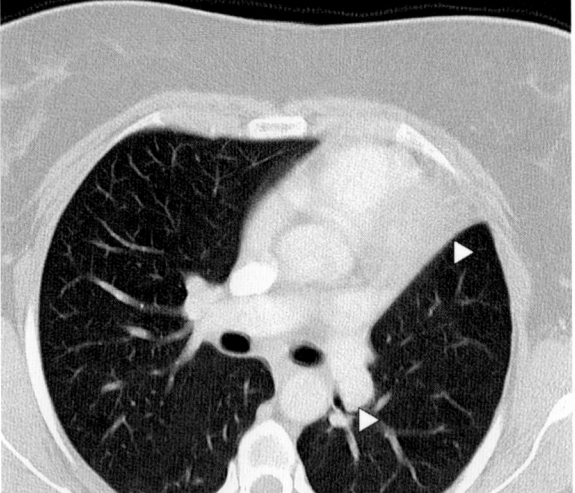

(b)

Fig. 2.20a, b Chest X-ray and CT of a patient with a carcinoid tumour. The chest X-ray (a) illustrates an endobronchial carcinoid, not directly visible but obstructing the lingula bronchus, causing lingula collapse and obscuring the left heart border. The corresponding CT scan (b) reveals the collapsed lingula (top arrow) and the endobronchial tumour (bottom arrow).

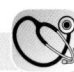

Non-small-cell lung cancer

Lung cancer is the leading cause of cancer death worldwide and cigarette smoking is the primary cause.

Epidemiology

The incidence of lung cancer is highest at 69.6 and 59.1 per 100 000 in North America and Europe respectively.[1] It is approximately twice as common in men and the median age range at diagnosis is 65–70 years.[2]

Pathology

Cigarette smoking is the primary cause of lung cancer, and the risk increases with the number of cigarettes smoked. However, not all smokers develop lung cancer. By the age of 75, the cumulative risk is 15.9% and 9.5% in male and female lifelong smokers respectively.[3]

The main histological subtypes of invasive malignant epithelial lung cancers are squamous cell carcinoma, small-cell carcinoma, adenocarcinoma and large cell carcinoma. Clinically, it is usual to consider small-cell (p. 149) and non-small-cell types, because of the differences in management.

Scope of disease

Local disease

The local effect of lung cancer depends on the site and size of the tumour. Cancers located close to or within the bronchial lumen can lead to obstruction of the distal airway or blood in the airway from the ulcerative surface of the tumour or invasion into a local blood vessel.

Tumours situated at the apex of the lung (Pancoast tumours) can produce Horner's syndrome and invade the brachial plexus. Obstruction of the superior vena cava (compressive effects or direct invasion) can lead to superior vena cava syndrome. Invasion of the phrenic nerve can lead to diaphragmatic paralysis, and invasion into the recurrent laryngeal nerve will result in voice hoarseness. Invasion into the chest wall, vertebral bodies or ribs can cause chest pain.

Metastatic disease

Specific symptoms can occur at the sites of metastasis including the brain, bones, liver and adrenal glands.

Paraneoplastic disease

Clubbing and hypertrophic pulmonary osteoarthropathy can occur as a result of underlying lung cancer. Ectopic hormone production includes parathyroid hormone (hypercalcaemia) and ACTH (Cushing's syndrome). Paraneoplastic neurological manifestations include Lambert–Eaton myasthenic syndrome (p. 630). Acanthosis nigricans and dermatomyositis are among the known cutaneous manifestations.

Clinical features

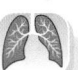

Cough, wheeze, dyspnoea and fever can occur as a result of obstruction to the bronchial lumen and sputum production from distal obstructive pneumonitis. However, many patients are lifelong smokers and differentiating the symptoms from underlying chronic obstructive pulmonary disease may be difficult. The combination of haemoptysis and weight loss is a suggestive feature of lung cancer.

Chest pain can occur with chest wall invasion or bony metastasis. New onset Horner's syndrome or hoarseness of voice suggests invasion of the sympathetic chain or recurrent laryngeal nerve respectively.

On examination, clubbing or hypertrophic pulmonary osteoarthropathy may be present. The small muscles of the hand may be wasted with localized invasion of the first thoracic nerve. Facial oedema with fixed engorgement of the head and neck veins are prominent features of superior vena cava syndrome. In addition features of chronic obstructive pulmonary disease may be present (p. 132).

Supraclavicular lymphadenopathy can result from nodal metastasis. Chest wall invasion may be evident, and areas of localized tenderness can result from bony metastasis. On percussion and auscultation, lobar consolidation or collapse may be detected with tumours obstructing the bronchial lumen. Pleural effusions may also be present. Abdominal examination may reveal hepatomegaly indicative of extensive liver metastasis.

A detailed clinical assessment includes evaluation of the functional status of the patient (exercise tolerance), severity of any underlying comorbidity, evidence of any distal metastasis and screening for any paraneoplastic effects.

Initial investigations

The initial investigations are to screen for evidence of lung cancer, to define the anatomical site and size, and to acquire (histopathological) confirmation of the type of lesion.

Full blood count

Abnormalities on full blood count are usually non-specific. Anaemia may be present. A leukoerythroblastic blood film is occasionally seen.

Liver profile

Elevated transaminases may occur with liver metastasis, and raised alkaline phosphatase from bony metastasis.

Serum calcium

Serum calcium levels may be raised from bony metastasis or ectopic parathyroid or parathyroid releasing hormone production.

Sputum cytology

Microscopic examination of sputum cytology is a simple and very specific method to diagnose lung cancer. Negative sputum cytology does not exclude lung cancer, as this test has an intermediate sensitivity that decreases with increasingly peripheral tumours.

Chest X-ray

A postero-anterior (PA) and lateral chest film may reveal a lung mass, hilar lymphadenopathy or effects of the tumour mass (Fig. 2.21a). Central cavitating lesions are characteristic of squamous cell carcinoma. Obstruction of a bronchus can cause collapse or consolidation of the distal lung parenchyma. A pleural effusion may be present, and an elevated hemidiaphragm on the side of the tumour may imply invasion of the phrenic nerve. Bony metastasis may be evident as lytic lesions in the vertebrae or ribs.

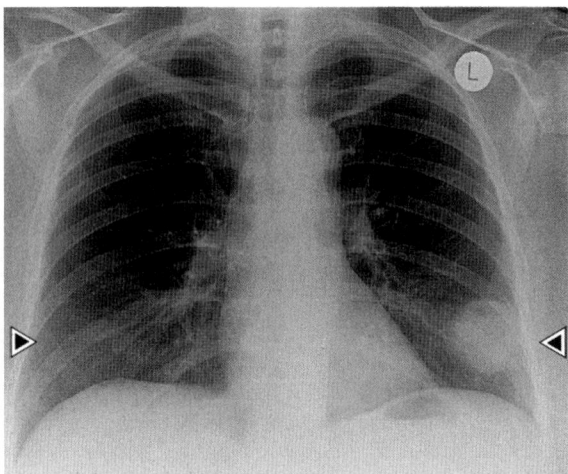

(a)

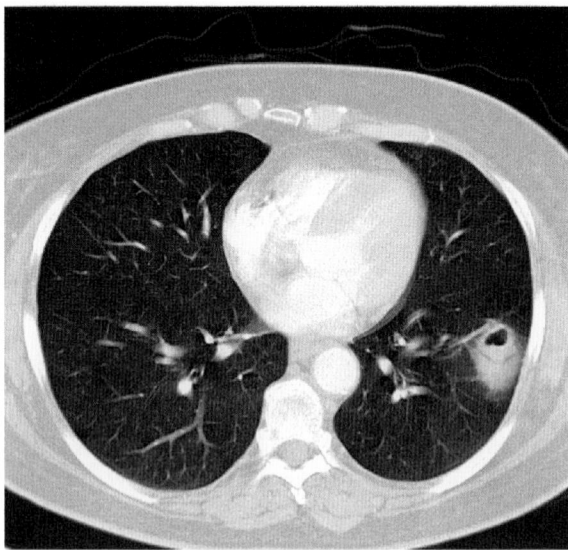

(b)

Fig. 2.21a, b Chest X-ray and CT thorax of left lower lobe non-small-cell lung cancer. The chest film (a) reveals a peripheral cavitating mass, confirmed on CT thorax (b), with no evidence of distant disease.

CT Thorax

A CT scan of the chest will accurately delineate the site and extent of a tumour mass. In addition, chest CT can also detect enlarged mediastinal lymph nodes (Fig. 2.21b) that may warrant further staging investigations. The anatomical resolution facilitates the assessment of direct pleural, chest wall, vertebral or mediastinal invasion. If required, transthoracic needle aspiration can be undertaken with CT guidance for histopathological confirmation of the tumour.

Flexible bronchoscopy

For centrally located tumours, flexible bronchoscopy permits visualization and biopsy of an endobronchial tumour. In addition bronchial washings and brush cytology specimens can be taken.

RECENT ADVANCES

PET scanning is currently being evaluated as a non-invasive method to diagnose lung cancer (Fig. 2.7).

---

i **FURTHER INVESTIGATIONS**

Having acquired a histopathological diagnosis confirming lung cancer, the next step is to stage the patient to decide the best treatment option.

▶▶▶ **TNM staging of lung cancer**

T—Tumour

T1   A tumour that is 3.0 cm or less in greatest dimension, surrounded by lung or visceral pleura, and without evidence of invasion proximal to a lobar bronchus at bronchoscopy

T2   A tumour more than 3.0 cm in greatest dimension, or a tumour of any size that either invades the visceral pleura or has associated atelectasis or obstructive pneumonitis extending to the hilar region. At bronchoscopy, the proximal extent of demonstrable tumour must be within a lobar bronchus or at least 2.0 cm distal to the carina. Any associated atelectasis or obstructive pneumonitis must involve less than an entire lung

T3   A tumour of any size with direct extension into the chest wall (including superior sulcus tumours), diaphragm, or the mediastinal pleura or pericardium without involving the heart, great vessels, trachea, oesophagus or vertebral body, or a tumour in the main bronchus within 2 cm of the carina without involving the carina, or associated atelectasis or obstructive pneumonitis of entire lung

T4   A tumour of any size with invasion of the mediastinum or involving heart, great vessels, trachea, oesophagus, vertebral body or carina or presence of malignant pleural or pericardial effusion, or with satellite tumour nodules within the ipsilateral, primary tumour lobe of the lung

TNM staging of lung cancer—cont'd

N—Nodes

N0   No demonstrable metastasis to regional lymph nodes

N1   Metastasis to lymph nodes in the peribronchial or the ipsilateral hilar region, or both, including direct extension

N2   Metastasis to ipsilateral mediastinal lymph nodes and subcarinal lymph nodes

N3   Metastasis to contralateral mediastinal lymph nodes, contralateral hilar lymph nodes, ipsilateral or contralateral scalene or supraclavicular lymph nodes

M—Distant metastasis

M0   No (known) distant metastasis

M1   Distant metastasis present

Stage

Stage			
Stage 0	Carcinoma in situ		
Stage IA	T1–N0–M0		
Stage IB	T2–N0–M0		
Stage IIA	T1–N1–M0		
Stage IIB	T2–N1–M0		
	T3–N0–M0		
Stage IIIA	T3–N1–M0		
	T1–N2–M0	T2–N2–M0	T3–N2–M0
Stage IIIB	T4–N0–M0	T4–N1–M0	T4–N2–M0
	T1–N3–M0	T2–N3–M0	T3–N3–M0
	T4–N3–M0		
Stage IV	Any T	Any N	M1

Staging CT head/abdomen

A staging abdominal CT scan is usually performed to detect liver or adrenal metastasis. In patients with neurological symptoms or signs, a staging CT of the head should be performed to detect cerebral metastasis.

Bone scan

A technetium-99m (^{99m}Tc) labelled phosphate bone scan (Fig. 2.7) should be performed in patients with symptoms of chest pain, localized bony tenderness, raised serum alkaline phosphatase or raised serum calcium.

Mediastinoscopy

Cervical mediastinoscopy and lymph node biopsy is performed if enlarged mediastinal lymph nodes (more than 2 cm in the short axis) are evident on the staging CT scan. The aim is to screen for ipsilateral mediastinal nodal metastasis (N2) that may be indicative of inoperable disease (stage IIIA).

Initial management

Surgery is the only curative management option for patients with non-small-cell lung cancer. Prior to the consideration of surgery, it is necessary to evaluate pulmonary function and any concomitant disease that may increase the risk of operative mortality. This is usually undertaken by a multi-disciplinary team.

Patients with stage I/II disease, good lung function and permissive operative risk should undergo lung resection. Patients with stage III disease, poor lung function or high operative risk should be referred to a specialist thoracic centre for further evaluation as selected patients may be eligible for surgery. These options should be discussed with the patient.

Surgical management

Pulmonary resection

The patient is anaesthetized and a double lumen endotracheal tube is positioned to allow single lung ventilation. The patient is positioned in a lateral position, and a posterolateral thoracotomy is performed (Fig. 2.22a). A systematic nodal dissection is undertaken to evaluate any lymph node metastases. Then an anatomical resection is performed of the lung or lobe depending on the size and position of the tumour and the presence of N1 disease. For a lobectomy, the lung fissures are dissected and separated (Fig. 2.22b), the pulmonary artery branches supplying the lobe are ligated (Fig. 2.22c), then the corresponding pulmonary veins, and finally the lobar bronchus is transected and the lobe delivered. The bronchus is oversewn (Fig. 2.22d) and chest drains are inserted before a layered closure is performed (Fig. 2.22e) for the thoracotomy incision.

The mortality associated with a lobectomy and pneumonectomy is approximately 3%[4] and 6% respectively. Other postoperative complications are bleeding, wound infection and prolonged air leak.

After surgery, all patients should receive regular postoperative surveillance for recurrence. This usually consists of regular clinical assessment and screening chest films on an annual basis. If there is any suspicion of recurrence, the patient needs to undergo full diagnostic evaluation as detailed in the earlier part of this section.

Medical management

Completely resected stage I to IIB non-small-cell lung cancer

In general, completely resected lung cancers in stage I to IIB do not require further treatment. Currently, the role of adjuvant therapy is being investigated.

Unresectable stage III non-small-cell lung cancer

Thoracic irradiation and a platinum-based combination chemotherapy regimen should be offered to patients with unresectable stage III disease.[5] The effect of chemotherapy is small, improving median survival from 11.4 to 13.2 months.[6]

Unresectable stage IV non-small-cell lung cancer

A two-drug combination chemotherapy regimen should be offered to patients with good performance status.[5] Patients with poor performance status should be offered palliative care. Apart from pain control and psychological support, palliative care encompasses active measures such as irradiation for local symptom control and airway stenting for selected patients with bronchial obstruction.

Prognosis

The prognosis of patients with non-small-cell lung cancer depends on stage. The overall 5-year survival is 61% and 38% for patients with pathological stage IA and IB respectively.[7]

REFERENCES

(1) Parkin DM, Pisani P, Ferlay J. Global cancer statistics. CA: A Cancer Journal for Clinicians 1999; 49(1): 33–64.
(2) Bilello KS, Murin S, Matthay RA. Epidemiology, etiology, and prevention of lung cancer. Clinics in Chest Medicine 2002; 23(1): 1–25.
(3) Peto R, Darby S, Deo H, Silcocks P, Whitley E, Doll R. Smoking, smoking cessation, and lung cancer in the UK since 1950: combination of national statistics with two case-control studies. BMJ 2000; 321(7257): 323–329.
(4) Treasure T, Utley M, Bailey A. Assessment of whether in-hospital mortality for lobectomy is a useful standard for the quality of lung cancer surgery: retrospective study. BMJ 2003; 327(7406): 73–70.
(5) Pfister DG, Johnson DH, Azzoli CG, et al. American Society of Clinical Oncology treatment of unresectable non-small-cell lung cancer guideline: Update 2003. Journal of Clinical Oncology 2004; 22(2): 330–353.
(6) Sause W, Kolesar P, Taylor S IV, et al. Final results of phase III trial in regionally advanced unresectable non-small cell lung cancer: Radiation Therapy Oncology Group, Eastern Cooperative Oncology Group, and Southwest Oncology Group. Chest 2000; 117(2): 358–364.
(7) Fry WA, Phillips JL, Menck HR. Ten-year survey of lung cancer treatment and survival in hospitals in the United States: a national cancer data base report. Cancer 1999; 86(9): 1867–1876.

Secondary lung tumours

Secondary lung tumours are metastatic deposits from cancers that originate outside the lung.

Epidemiology

Secondary lung tumours are more common than primary lung cancer, although the exact frequency is difficult to quantify. The epidemiological characteristics of patients with secondary lung tumours reflect those of the primary cancer.

Pathology

Tumours with a predisposition to metastasize to the lung are osteosarcomas, germ cell tumours, colorectal carci-

nomas, renal carcinomas, melanomas, breast and thyroid cancers. The frequency with each is related to the frequency of the primary tumour.

Clinical features

Secondary lung tumours are usually silent and detected on routine surveillance chest X-rays of patients with treated cancer (Fig. 2.23a). Occasionally, pulmonary metastasis may produce symptoms of pleuritic pain, cough or haemoptysis. Extensive pulmonary metastases can lead to progressive dyspnoea.

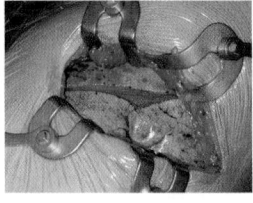

(a)

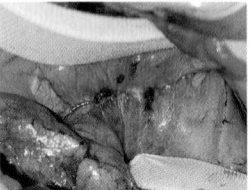

(b)

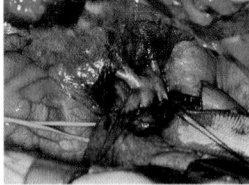

(c)

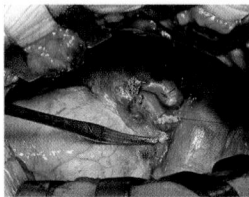

(d)

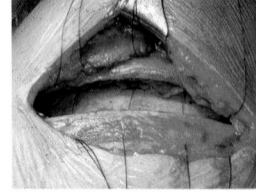

(e)

Fig. 2.22 Left lower lobectomy.

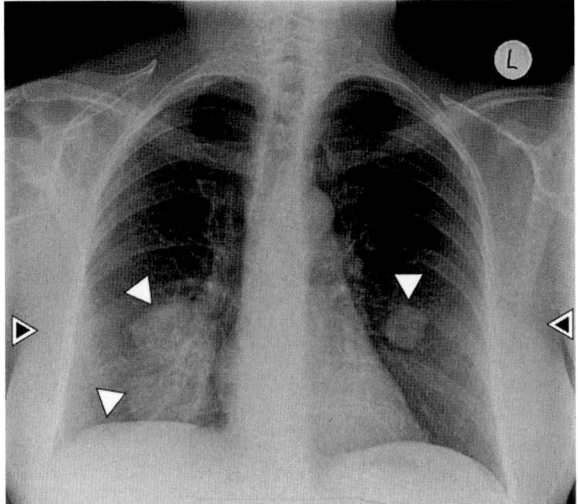

(a)

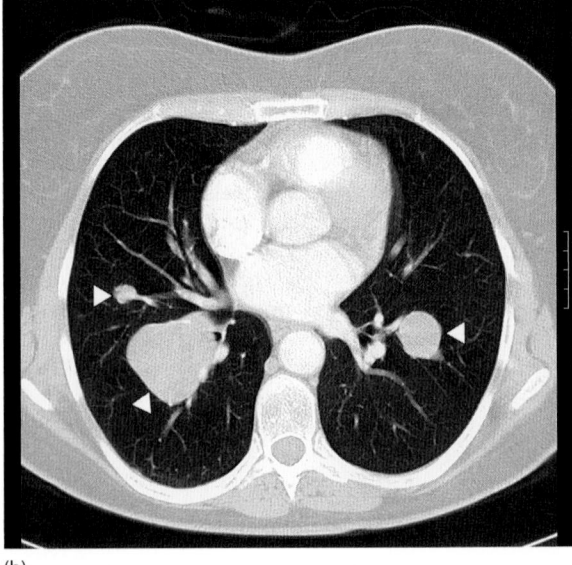

(b)

Fig. 2.23 Chest X-ray and CT thorax of a patient with secondary lung tumours.

Investigations

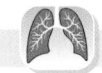

In the majority of patients, the onset of pulmonary metastasis indicates end stage disease and no further investigations would be appropriate. In a highly selected subset of patients (detailed below), a CT scan of the chest (Fig. 2.23b) and further staging investigations may be indicated if surgical resection is considered.

Management

Palliative care
In the majority of patients, palliative care is appropriate for this stage of disease.

Chemotherapy
Chemotherapy may be suitable for patients with subgroups of chemo-responsive tumours (e.g. breast cancer).

Pulmonary metastasectomy
In patients with limited pulmonary metastases, in whom the primary tumour is controlled (no evidence of local recurrence) with no evidence of extrapulmonary metastases and who are able to tolerate lung resection, pulmonary metastasectomy can be considered. Pulmonary metastasectomy is performed via a thoracotomy (or median sternotomy for simultaneous bilateral procedures) and precision diathermy excision of CT-identifiable and any other palpable tumour deposits.

Prognosis

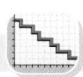

The operative mortality of pulmonary metastasectomy is 1%, and the 5- and 10-year survival is 36% and 26% respectively.[1] Approximately 50% of tumours will recur at a median time interval of 10 months.

REFERENCE

(1) Pastorino U, Buyse M, Friedel G, et al. Long-term results of lung metastasectomy: Prognostic analyses based on 5206 cases. Journal of Thoracic and Cardiovascular Surgery 1997; 113(1): 37–49.

Silicosis

Coal-worker's
pneumoconiosis

Asbestosis

Occupational lung disease

Pneumoconioses

Pneumoconioses are inflammatory lung conditions caused by the inhalation of mineral dusts. The most common types are coal dust, asbestos and silica.

With all pneumoconiosis, there is usually a lag period of up to 30 years from exposure until symptoms arise. The proposed pathogenesis begins with an inflammatory reaction after dust inhalation. Inhaled dust is trapped in the mucous blanket and most are removed by ciliary movement, however, some particles travel to alveolar duct bifurcations where they impact and are engulfed by macrophages, inciting a further inflammatory response with fibroblast proliferation and collagen deposition. Fibrosis can be nodular (silicosis) or diffuse (asbestosis). Silica and asbestos are more reactive than coal dust and can cause fibrosis at lower concentrations.

In most developed countries, state compensation is available for all patients with pneumoconioses.

Silicosis

Epidemiology

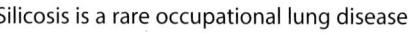

Silicosis is a rare occupational lung disease.

Pathology

Silicosis is caused by the inhalation of crystalline silica found in trades such as mining, quarrying, masonry, sandblasting and glass making. The pathologies of acute and chronic silicosis are different. In acute silicosis, there is interstitial inflammation with accumulation of protein-rich fluid in the alveolar spaces. In chronic silicosis, nodules form from dust-laden macrophages with a whorled appearance due to collagen fibre deposition. The centres of these nodules fibrose and enlargement continues at the periphery due to inflammation, even after cessation of exposure.

Clinical features

The mildest form is simple silicosis; these patients are usually asymptomatic. Acute silicosis develops after inhalation of high levels of silica dust, presenting with shortness of breath, cough, cyanosis and fulminant respiratory failure. With chronic silicosis, there is a latent period which is inversely proportional to the length of exposure. Initial symptoms are shortness of breath and cough; respiratory failure may ensue.

Investigations

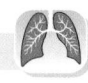

Chest X-ray
In simple silicosis, small nodules are seen in the upper zones that increase in size and number with disease progression.

As the disease progresses to the chronic form, fibrosis occurs causing the upper lobes to contract; the lower zones may become emphysematous. Hilar nodal eggshell calcification is sometimes seen and occasionally the nodules can contain small calcified areas.

The plain film in acute silicosis usually shows extensive ground glass shadowing, starting in the bases and progressing to large opacities in the mid zones. Nodules are not typical.

Pulmonary function tests

Initially the results are normal, but later in the disease a restrictive defect with a low gas transfer and reduced lung volumes occurs.

Rheumatoid and anti-nuclear factor

Rheumatoid disease may develop in patients with advancing fibrosis, giving rise to rheumatoid and anti-nuclear factors.

Management

The management is largely symptomatic, in conjunction with efforts to stop further occupational exposure.

Prognosis

Simple silicosis has a very good prognosis, but continued exposure to silica can cause disease progression to chronic silicosis and respiratory failure. Acute silicosis has a poor prognosis and is almost invariably fatal within 2 years.

Coal-worker's pneumoconiosis

Epidemiology

Coal-worker's pneumoconiosis is present in approximately 2% of miners.

Pathology

The extent of disease caused by exposure to coal dust varies in severity. Asymptomatic anthracosis is due to accumulation of carbon pigment without a cellular reaction, and is common in urban dwellers and smokers as well as coal miners. In simple coal-worker's pneumoconiosis, coal macules form within the lung and develop into nodules. With progressive massive fibrosis, extensive fibrosis develops with pulmonary nodules that coalesce over years. Central necrosis and melanoptysis (black sputum) can occur. Centrilobular emphysema can occur in non-smokers; if the patient has smoked as well, the impact on lung function is multiplicative rather than additive.

Caplan's syndrome is the coexistence of rheumatoid arthritis with any of the pneumoconioses, although it is usually thought of in conjunction with coal-worker's pneumoconiosis. Serum rheumatoid factor is often present and rheumatoid nodules may be seen elsewhere in the body.

Investigations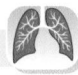

Chest X-ray

Discrete nodules are the main abnormality in simple coal-worker's pneumoconiosis. Massive pulmonary fibrosis with homogeneous shadowing may be seen, usually in the upper zones. Occasionally, large opacities may necrose and cavitate.

Pulmonary function tests

Lung function remains preserved unless progressive massive fibrosis occurs; a restrictive defect is then seen with loss of lung volume and a reduced TL_{CO}. If centrilobular emphysema occurs, an obstructive defect may also be seen.

Management

Supportive management

Management consists of supportive measures, and smoking cessation should be encouraged.

Prognosis

The prognosis of simple coal-worker's pneumoconiosis is comparatively good; however, the onset of progressive massive fibrosis leads to respiratory failure and eventually death.

Asbestosis

Epidemiology

The epidemiology of asbestos-related lung disease is detailed on page 170.

Pathology

Asbestosis is lung fibrosis caused by prolonged exposure to asbestos dust, a mineral fibre of silicate origin. Occupations classically associated with asbestos exposure are shipbuilding, construction, plumbing and welding. There are three types of asbestos fibres: crocidolite (blue), amosite (brown), and chrysotile (white). Chrysotile is thought to be the most pathogenic. Histologically, asbestos bodies may be seen; these originate from asbestos fibres coated with brown phagocyte ferritin consequent upon being engulfed by macrophages. Asbestos exposure also causes benign pleural plaques, pleural effusion and mesothelioma, and greatly increases the risk of lung cancer, especially in smokers.

Clinical features

Shortness of breath and a productive cough are the usual non-specific symptoms. Patients may also present with symptoms of a mesothelioma (p. 153) or lung cancer (p. 170). On examination clubbing may be seen and crepitations may be heard in the bases.

Investigations

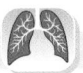

Chest X-ray

Initially linear opacities are seen in the lower zones progressing to fibrotic changes in the costophrenic and cardiophrenic angles. Fibrosis begins in the lower lobes subpleurally and progresses proximally. Calcified pleural plaques may be seen on the diaphragmatic or lateral pleural surfaces (Fig. 2.24a). Pleural thickening or effusions can occur, but should not be assumed to be benign. Fibrosis that occurs in the absence of pleural plaques is unlikely to be due to asbestos exposure.

CT Thorax

The findings on CT are peripheral septal lines, bronchiolar thickening, honeycombing of the lung, pleural thickening and plaques (Fig. 2.24b). The density of parenchymal abnormalities correlates well with the severity of symptoms.

Pulmonary function tests

A restrictive defect occurs with reduced gas transfer ($T_{L_{CO}}$).

Management

Supportive management

The management is essentially supportive. Occupational exposure should stop. In the UK, mesothelioma and asbestosis are recognized as industrially related. Patients or their estate are entitled to compensation from the state and may also resort to the law to sue their former employers.

Prognosis

The prognosis is variable and can range from stable disease with mild symptoms to progressive deterioration and respiratory failure. Usually, disease progression slows over a period of a decade after cessation of exposure. Lung cancer is the commonest cause of death in patients with asbestosis.

Silicosis

Coal-worker's pneumoconiosis

Asbestosis

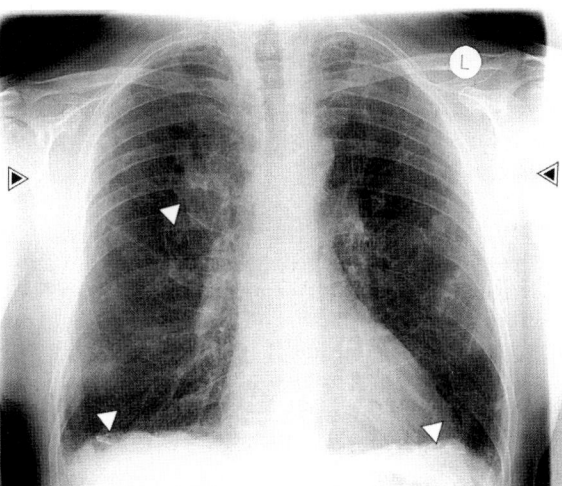

(a)

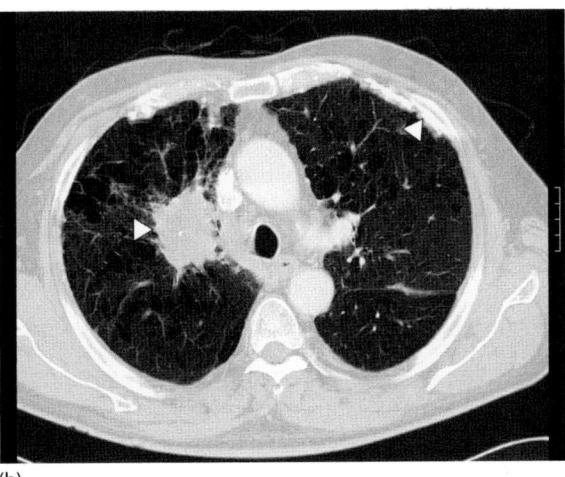

(b)

Fig. 2.24 Chest X-ray and CT thorax of asbestosis. Multiple pleural plaques can be seen on the plain film (a). The CT thorax details the plaques and also reveals emphysema and a central right-sided non-small-cell lung cancer from long-term smoking.

Pulmonary vascular disease

Pulmonary embolism

Pulmonary embolism (PE) usually refers to the lodging of venous emboli in the pulmonary arterial circulation.

Epidemiology

The incidence of pulmonary embolism is approximately 65 per 100 000 per year,[1] increasing with age. Pulmonary embolism is more common in men than in women.[2]

Pathology

Approximately 70% of pulmonary embolisms are associated with emboli from deep vein thrombosis (usually clinically undetectable). The major risk factors for venous thrombo-embolism are surgery, cardiac disease, lower limb immobility and cancer. More than 80% of patients who present with pulmonary embolism will have one or more of the risk factors listed in Table 2.27.

Scope of disease

The effects of a pulmonary embolus depend on its size. Small emboli tend to cause pulmonary infarcts (haemoptysis, pleuritic chest pain), medium-sized emboli can produce dyspnoea from ventilation/perfusion mismatch, and large emboli can give rise to right ventricular failure and cardiogenic shock from obstruction of a major pulmonary artery.

Clinical features

The most common symptoms are dyspnoea, pleuritic chest pain, cough and haemoptysis. Approximately 60% present with pulmonary haemorrhage (haemoptysis, pleuritic chest pain), 25% present with isolated dyspnoea, and a minority present with circulatory collapse. Loss of consciousness and central chest pains can be caused by a large embolus (or small to medium-sized embolus in patients with poor cardiopulmonary reserve).

On examination the most common clinical findings are tachypnoea, tachycardia and, occasionally, evidence of deep vein thrombosis. Individually the symptoms and signs are non-specific and therefore the clinical diagnosis of pulmonary embolus can be difficult. Diagnostic sensitivity can be improved, however, by the combination of dyspnoea and tachypnoea (respiratory rate >20 per minute), which is absent in only 10% of patients with pulmonary embolism. Only 3% have neither dyspnoea nor tachypnoea.

Two other factors influence diagnostic probability: the possibility that another diagnosis is unlikely (on clinical assessment and laboratory investigations) and the presence of a major risk factor. The clinical probability of pulmonary embolus is low, intermediate or high depending if no, one or both factors are present. It is important that low molecular weight heparin should be initiated for patients in the intermediate and high probability categories before diagnostic imaging is performed.

Initial investigations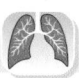

D-dimer assay

D-dimer assays have high sensitivity (but low specificities), therefore a negative test is helpful to rule out the diagnosis of a pulmonary embolism. This investigation need not be performed in patients with a high clinical probability of pulmonary embolus, as a negative result will still require confirmation with further imaging.

Arterial blood gases

A low Po_2 with a low Pco_2 are the usual findings, due to ventilation/perfusion mismatch and hyperventilation. A normal Po_2 level does not exclude the diagnosis of a pulmonary embolus.

Electrocardiogram

Tachycardia and non-specific ST segment and T wave abnormalities are usually the most common findings (50%). Features of right heart strain (S1 Q3 T3, right axis deviation and a dominant R wave in V1) are rare (less than 6%) and usually indicate massive emboli. Atrial fibrillation occurs in approximately 4%.

Chest X-ray

The CXR (Fig. 2.25a) often appears normal, but subtle non-specific features such as segmental collapse, raised hemi-diaphragm and a pleural effusion are present in more than half of patients. Classic features of pulmonary embolism, such as a wedge-shaped pleural-based opacity due to pulmonary infarction and hypovascularity, are rare. A chest film is useful to exclude other diseases that may present with similar features such as cardiac failure, pneumonia and pneumothorax.

Further investigations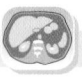

CT Pulmonary angiography

CT pulmonary angiography is currently the imaging modality of choice for the detection of suspected non-massive

Table 2.27	Risk factors for venous thromboembolism

Major risk factors (relative risk 5–20)
Surgery
Major abdominal/pelvic surgery

Hip/knee replacement

Postoperative intensive care

Obstetrics
Late pregnancy

Caesarean section

Puerperium

Lower limb problems
Fracture

Varicose veins

Malignancy
Abdominal/pelvic

Advanced/metastatic

Reduced mobility
Hospitalization

Institutional care

Miscellaneous
Previous proven venous thromboembolism

Minor risk factors (relative risk 2–4)
Cardiovascular
Congenital heart disease

Congestive cardiac failure

Hypertension

Superficial venous thrombosis

Indwelling central vein catheter

Oestrogens
Oral contraceptive

Hormone replacement therapy

Miscellaneous
COPD

Neurological disability

Occult malignancy

Thrombotic disorders

Long-distance sedentary travel

Obesity

Surgery
    Orthopaedic (hip and knee surgery)
    Abdominal and pelvic surgery

Cardiac disease
    Acute myocardial infarction
    Congestive cardiac failure

Lower limb immobility
    Limb fractures
    Stroke/spinal injury

Malignancy
    Metastatic cancer
    Breast, uterine, stomach, pancreatic cancer

Pregnancy

From British Thoracic Society guidelines for the management of suspected acute pulmonary embolism. Thorax 2003; 58 Suppl 1: 470–483.

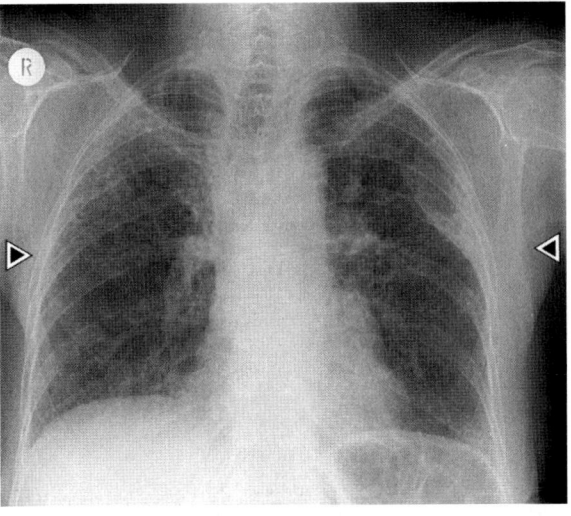

(a)

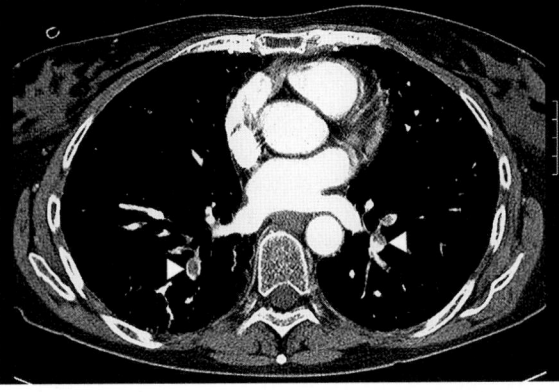

(b)

Fig. 2.25 Chest X-ray and CT thorax of a patient with pulmonary embolus. (a) CXR of a patient with idiopathic pulmonary fibrosis (note the reticular shadowing) with sudden onset increased dyspnoea. (b) CT pulmonary angiography confirms the new pulmonary embolus as a filling defect (arrow).

pulmonary embolism (Fig. 2.25b). This technique is fast and non-invasive.

Isotope lung scan (V̇/Q̇ scan)
Isotope lung scanning can only confirm or refute a diagnosis of pulmonary embolism in a minority of patients with pulmonary embolism. It is not recommended in the presence of an abnormal chest film or chronic cardiorespiratory disease (due to difficulties in interpreting the results of the V̇/Q̇ scan). An indeterminate scan needs to be confirmed by further imaging.

Conventional pulmonary angiography
Pulmonary angiography is indicated (Fig. 2.25b) in the presence of cardiovascular collapse or hypotension and when other investigations have failed to give a firm diagnosis. Access to the pulmonary artery facilitates intraarterial thrombolysis or clot fragmentation.

Other imaging strategies

Transthoracic/transoesophageal echocardiography can detect indirect evidence of massive pulmonary emboli (right heart failure, raised pulmonary artery pressure). Doppler ultrasound of the leg veins can be performed in patients with clinical evidence of a deep vein thrombosis. In the presence of deep vein thrombus, respiratory symptoms are usually attributed to pulmonary embolism. A negative scan, however, has limited value.

Initial management

Oxygen

High-flow oxygen should be administered to all patients who are hypoxic on peripheral oxygen saturations.

Analgesia

Analgesia should be administered for patients with pleuritic chest pain, but opiates should be avoided in patients with incipient cardiovascular collapse (due to the vasodilatory effects).

Low molecular weight heparin

Low molecular weight heparin should be commenced on the clinical suspicion of a pulmonary embolus. Intravenous unfractionated heparin is preferred where rapid anticoagulation is required for massive emboli. Heparin is continued until adequate maintenance of anticoagulation with warfarin (INR 2.0–3.0) is achieved.

Medical management

Warfarin

Warfarin is continued for 4–6 weeks in patients with temporary risk factors for venous thromboembolism, 3–6 months for patients with a first idiopathic embolism, and as long-term therapy in patients with thrombotic disorders, recurrent emboli or persisting risk factors.

Thrombolysis

The main indication for thrombolytic therapy is cardiovascular collapse in patients with acute massive embolism, although evidence for reduced mortality is lacking. Intravenous thrombolytics may be administered to patients who are at imminent risk of cardiac arrest.

Surgical management

Pulmonary embolectomy

Pulmonary embolectomy is usually reserved for patients with acute massive embolus when thrombolytic therapy fails or is contraindicated. A median sternotomy is performed, the pericardium is opened and cardiopulmonary bypass is instituted. The pulmonary artery is incised and emboli are removed under direct vision using suction catheters and forceps.

Inferior vena cava filter

Patients who develop recurrent emboli on warfarin, or who have contraindications to anticoagulation, may benefit from the insertion of an inferior vena cava filter.

Prognosis

The overall in-hospital mortality rate for pulmonary embolism is 22%; however, mortality varies with presentation. The mortality rate in haemodynamically stable patients is 8% and this increases to 25% in patients presenting with cardiogenic shock. Recurrent thromboembolism occurs in 17% and a proportion of patients will progress to develop chronic thromboembolic pulmonary hypertension (see p. 161).

i **FURTHER INFORMATION**

Suspected acute pulmonary embolism: a practical approach. British Thoracic Society, Standards of Care Committee. Thorax 1997; 52(Suppl 4): S1–24.

British Thoracic Society guidelines for the management of suspected acute pulmonary embolism. Thorax 2003; 58: 470–483.

REFERENCES

(1) *British Thoracic Society guidelines for the management of suspected acute pulmonary embolism. Thorax 2003; 58: 470–483.*
(2) *Heit JA, Silverstein MD, Mohr DN, Petterson TM, Lohse CM, O'Fallon WM, Melton LJ III. The epidemiology of venous thromboembolism in the community. Thrombosis and Haemostasis 2001; 86: 452–463.*

Pulmonary hypertension

The normal mean pulmonary artery pressure is approximately 15 mmHg, and pulmonary hypertension is usually considered to be present when this is elevated above 25 mmHg at rest or 30 mmHg on exercise. It is classified as primary (cause unknown) or secondary (known underlying cause).

Epidemiology

The incidence of primary pulmonary hypertension is approximately 5 per 100 000 per year.[1] The mean age at diagnosis is 36 years, and it is approximately twice as common in women as in men.[2] The epidemiology of secondary pulmonary hypertension reflects that of the underlying disease.

Pathology

The pathophysiological mechanisms that lead to pulmonary hypertension can be a combination of elevated left atrial

Table 2.28	WHO diagnostic classification of pulmonary hypertension

Pulmonary arterial hypertension

Primary pulmonary hypertension
Sporadic disorder
Familial disorder

Related conditions
Collagen vascular disease
Congenital systemic-to-pulmonary shunt
Portal hypertension
Human immunodeficiency virus infection
Drugs and toxins
Anorectic agents (appetite suppressants)
Others

Persistent pulmonary hypertension of the newborn

Others

Pulmonary venous hypertension

Left-sided atrial or ventricular heart disease

Left-sided valvular heart disease

Extrinsic compression of central pulmonary veins
Fibrosing mediastinitis
Adenopathy and/or tumours

Pulmonary veno-occlusive disease

Others

Pulmonary hypertension associated with disorders of the respiratory system and/or hypoxaemia

Chronic obstructive pulmonary disease

Interstitial lung disease

Sleep-disordered breathing

Alveolar hypoventilation disorders

Chronic exposure to high altitudes

Neonatal lung disease

Alveolar–capillary dysplasia

Others

Pulmonary hypertension resulting from chronic thrombotic and/or embolic disease

Thromboembolic obstruction of proximal pulmonary arteries

Obstruction of distal pulmonary arteries
Pulmonary embolism (thrombus, tumour, ova and/or parasites, foreign material)
In situ thrombosis
Sickle cell disease

Pulmonary hypertension resulting from disorders directly affecting the pulmonary vasculature

Inflammatory conditions
Schistosomiasis
Sarcoidosis
Others

Pulmonary capillary haemangiomatosis

From Runo JR, Loyd JE. Primary pulmonary hypertension. Lancet 2003; 361: 1533–1544.

hypertension are listed within the WHO classification in Table 2.28.

Clinical features

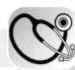

Pulmonary hypertension is usually clinically silent until right ventricular failure supervenes and shortness of breath develops. Most other symptoms are non-specific and can include palpitations, syncope and chest pain. It is important to screen for evidence of underlying disease that may result in secondary pulmonary hypertension (Table 2.28). On examination the blood pressure is normal unless severe right failure develops when hypotension and tachycardia may be present at rest. The JVP will be elevated with right ventricular failure, and cannon waves of tricuspid regurgitation may be evident. On palpation there may be a right ventricular heave and auscultation may reveal a loud and widely split P2. Hepatomegaly, ascites and peripheral oedema indicate severe right ventricular impairment.

Initial investigations

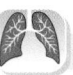

Electrocardiogram
An ECG will reveal right axis deviation and a tall R wave in V1 from right ventricular hypertrophy. An enlarged P wave may be attributable to right atrial enlargement.

Chest X-ray
A chest film may reveal cardiomegaly due to right ventricular hypertrophy. The right pulmonary artery may be visibly enlarged (more than 16 mm), with decreased peripheral lung markings.

Transthoracic echocardiogram
Transthoracic echocardiography can confirm the presence of right ventricular enlargement and quantify the pulmonary artery pressure.

Right heart catheterization
Pulmonary artery catheterization may be required to confirm the diagnosis and/or assess the severity of pulmonary hypertension. A selective pulmonary vasodilator test is usually performed to assess the response of the pulmonary vascular resistance.

Further investigations

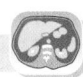

Further investigations such as magnetic resonance imaging may be required to assess the distribution of disease prior to surgery (Fig. 2.26) or to ascertain any evidence for an underlying cause.

Management

Supportive management
The management of primary pulmonary hypertension includes diuretics for symptomatic peripheral oedema,

pressure (poor left ventricular function, left-sided heart valve disease), elevated pulmonary vascular resistance (from hypoxia or hypercarbia) or chronic obstruction (thrombo-embolic disease). The causes of secondary pulmonary

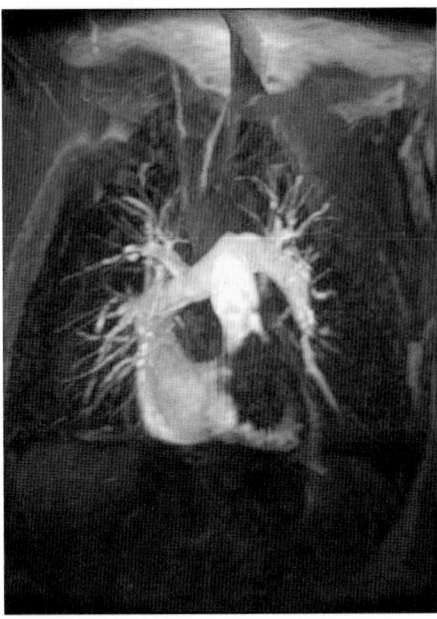

Fig. 2.26 Magnetic resonance angiography. This MRA shows the short 'tails' of the pulmonary artery that are abruptly cut off due to the presence of thromboembolic disease.
Image courtesy of Mr David Jenkins, Consultant Cardiac Surgeon, Papworth Hospital, Cambridge, UK.

oxygen supplementation for hypoxaemia at rest, and anti-coagulation (warfarin) for the prevention of in situ thrombosis.

Vasodilator therapy

Vasodilator therapy (calcium channel blockers) may be appropriate for patients in whom there is documented evidence of reduced pulmonary vascular resistance in response to an acute vasodilator test on right heart catheterization. In severely symptomatic patients that do not respond to vasodilators, a trial of continuous prosta-cyclin PGI_2 (epoprostenol) a modern oral analogue may be initiated.

Lung transplantation

Lung transplantation or heart–lung transplantation (for patients with cor pulmonale) is reserved for younger (<60 years) patients with end stage disease.

The management of patients with secondary pulmonary hypertension should be directed to the underlying cause.

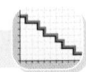

RECENT ADVANCES

Pulmonary endarterectomy is a relatively new surgical technique for selected patients with chronic thromboembolic pulmonary hypertension. The pulmonary artery is approached via median sternotomy on full cardiopulmonary bypass and a fibrothrombotic layer is removed (Fig. 2.27), relieving the obstructive effects.

Prognosis

The prognosis of primary pulmonary hypertension is poor. The 1- and 3-year survival has been reported as 64% and 48% respectively.[2]

REFERENCES

(1) *Galie N, Manes A, Uguccioni L, Serafini F, De Rosa M, Branzi A, Magnani B. Primary pulmonary hypertension: insights into pathogenesis from epidemiology. Chest 1998; 114: 184S–194.*
(2) *Gaine SP, Rubin LJ. Primary pulmonary hypertension. Lancet 1998; 352: 719–725.*

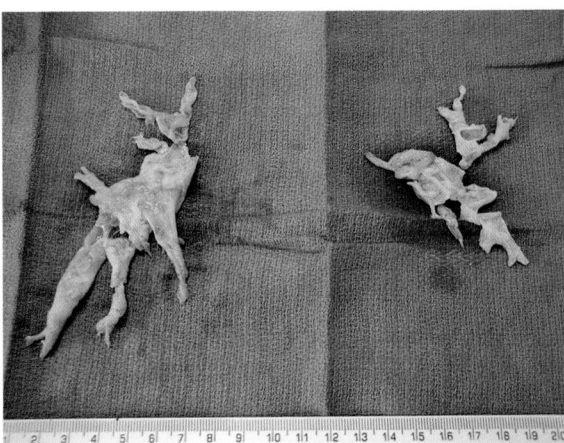

Fig. 2.27 The removed cast of the pulmonary arteries corresponding to the image in Figure 2.26.
Image courtesy of Mr David Jenkins, Consultant Cardiac Surgeon, Papworth Hospital, Cambridge, UK.

SECTION 2.13   Lung transplantation

Lung transplantation is becoming established therapy for the treatment of patients with end stage respiratory disease and declining lung function despite optimum therapy.

Indications

Generally, patients to be considered for lung transplantation should have chronic lung disease with limited life expectancy with no further medical or surgical therapy available. Chronic obstructive pulmonary disease, idiopathic pulmonary fibrosis, cystic fibrosis and primary pulmonary hypertension make up 85.6% of the indications for lung transplants worldwide.[1]

Patient preparation

All patients undergo formal medical and psychological assessment prior to consideration for transplantation (Table 2.29). Current contraindications are other end organ failure (although patients with specific combinations of end organ failure may be eligible for dual organ transplantation, e.g. heart–lung transplant), active malignancy, HIV or hepatitis B/C infection.

Procedure

Different approaches are undertaken depending on the need for single or double lung transplantation and the current practice of the lung transplant centre.

Unilateral lung transplantation (Fig. 2.28) is undertaken through a postero-lateral thoracotomy; a double lumen ventilation tube is required to selectively ventilate the non-transplant side. A pneumonectomy is performed and the donor main bronchus anastomosed end to end, followed by the donor to recipient pulmonary artery, and donor left atrial cuff (containing the pulmonary veins) to the recipient left atrium.

Bilateral lung transplantation can be undertaken through bilateral thoracotomies, median sternotomy or a clamshell incision (bilateral thoracotomies that meet via a horizontal incision through the sternum). In addition, cardiopulmonary bypass is utilized by some centres to perform the operation.

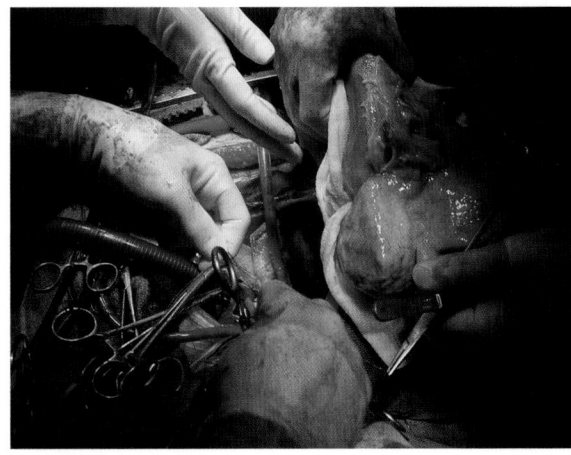

Fig. 2.28 Lung transplantation. A donor lung is being implanted into the recipient's chest.
Image courtesy of Mr Stephen Large, Consultant Cardiac Surgeon, Papworth Hospital, Cambridge, UK.

Table 2.29	Common lung diseases and selection criteria for lung transplantation
Disease	**Selection criteria**
Non-bronchiectatic chronic obstructive pulmonary disease	FEV_1 <25% predicted P_aco_2 >7.3 kPa
Cystic fibrosis	FEV_1 <30% predicted P_aco_2 >6.7 kPa P_ao_2 <7.3 kPa Or young patients with rapid deterioration
Idiopathic pulmonary fibrosis	Symptomatic progressive disease that fails to improve with steroids or immunosuppressive therapy When pulmonary function becomes abnormal (FVC <60% predicted, corrected diffusing capacity <50% predicted)
Pulmonary hypertension	Symptomatic (NYHA III/IV) and progressive disease despite optimum medical/surgical treatment Cardiac index <2 L/min/m², right atrial pressure >15 mmHg and mean pulmonary pressure >55 mmHg

Complications

The mortality at 3 months is approximately 17%, mainly due to rejection or cytomegalovirus infection.[1] Other postoperative complications are the development of rejection, infection, bronchiolitis obliterans, hypertension, renal impairment (from immunosuppressive drugs), diabetes (from steroids) and hyperlipidaemia.

Post procedure care

Postoperatively, transplant patients are managed on the intensive care unit. Standard triple therapy for immunosuppression consists of ciclosporin, azathioprine and prednisolone. Long-term complications of lung transplantation are rejection (manifests with declining FEV₁), predisposition to infection (from immunosuppression), diabetes and hypercholesterolaemia.

Prognosis

The 1- and 5-year survival after lung transplantation is 73% and 45% respectively.[1]

i FURTHER INFORMATION

International guidelines for the selection of lung transplant candidates. The American Society for Transplant Physicians (ASTP)/American Thoracic Society (ATS)/European Respiratory Society (ERS)/International Society for Heart and Lung Transplantation (ISHLT). American Journal of Respiratory and Critical Care Medicine 1998; 158: 335–339.

REFERENCE

(1) *Trulock EP, Edwards LB, Taylor DO, Boucek MM, Mohacsi PJ, Keck BM, Hertz MI. The Registry of the International Society for Heart and Lung Transplantation: Twentieth Official adult lung and heart-lung transplant report—2003. Journal of Heart and Lung Transplantation 2003; 22: 625–635.*

SECTION 2.14 # Diseases of the pleura

Pleural effusions

A pleural effusion is the accumulation of fluid in the pleural space. It is not a diagnosis but a manifestation of an underlying disease process. Although there are many causes, the most common are heart failure, pneumonia and cancer.

Epidemiology

Pleural effusions are common. The epidemiology is specific to the underlying cause.

Pathology

Pleural effusions are classified by pathophysiology into transudates and exudates. Transudate results from an imbalance between hydrostatic and oncotic pressure while an exudate results when pleural or local capillary permeability is altered. The causes for a transudative and exudative pleural effusion are provided in Tables 2.30 and 2.31 respectively.

A pleural fluid protein content of less than 25 g/L or more than 35 g/L normally differentiates between transudate and exudate; if the protein concentration lies between 25 and 35 g/L, then Light's criteria will be required to distinguish the two (Table 2.32).

Scope of disease

Gradual fluid accumulation and progressive dyspnoea is the usual manifestation of pleural effusion.

Clinical features

Shortness of breath is the principal complaint of patients with pleural effusions. The degree of fluid sufficient to cause dyspnoea varies according to the underlying state of the lungs. An otherwise healthy individual may tolerate up to several litres of fluid before experiencing dyspnoea on exertion. On examination the trachea may be deviated away from the (very large) effusion; there may be decreased expansion on the affected side, dullness to percussion and absent breath sounds.

Table 2.30	Causes of a transudative pleural effusion

Cardiac
    Cardiac failure*
    Mitral stenosis
    Constrictive pericarditis	

Pulmonary Pulmonary embolism	
Hepatic Liver cirrhosis*	
Renal Nephrotic syndrome	

General
    Hypoalbuminaemia*
    Superior vena cava obstruction	

* Common causes	

Table 2.31	Causes of an exudative pleural effusion
Malignancy*	
Lung	
Mesothelioma	
Breast	
Genito-urinary tract	
Gastrointestinal tract	
Pulmonary	
Pneumonia*	
Pulmonary infarction	
Autoimmune	
Rheumatoid disease	
SLE	
Drugs	
Amiodarone	
Phenytoin	
Methotrexate	
Others	
Pancreatitis	
Haemothorax	
Chylothorax	
* Common causes	

Table 2.32	Light's criteria to distinguish between an exudative and a transudative pleural effusion
The diagnosis (of an exudate) is based on one or more of the following three:	
Ratio of pleural fluid protein level to serum protein level >0.5	
Ratio of pleural fluid lactate dehydrogenase (LDH) level to serum LDH level >0.6	
Pleural fluid LDH level more than 2/3 the upper limit of normal for serum LDH	
Light's criteria have an overall sensitivity of 98% and specificity of 83%. From Light RW. Clinical practice. Pleural effusion. New England Journal of Medicine 2002; 346: 1971–1977.	

It is important to take a detailed drug history and also screen for symptoms and signs of the underlying diseases mentioned in Tables 2.30 and 2.31. A history of coagulation disorder is also pertinent as thoracocentesis may be required when the cause is unknown.

Initial investigations

Serum albumin and lactate dehydrogenase (LDH)
These two investigations are usually required to provide comparison with the results of pleural fluid analyses.

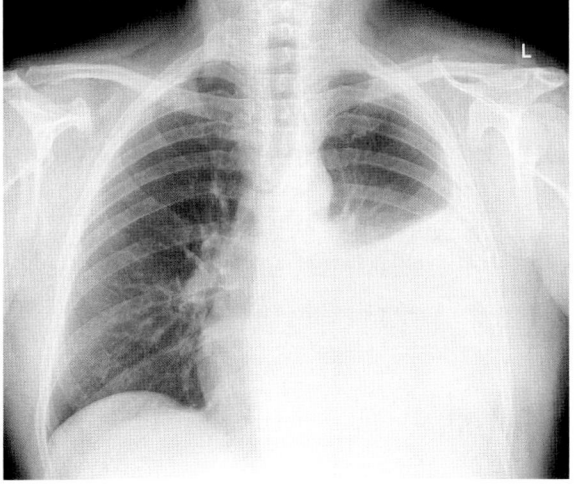

Fig. 2.29 Chest film of a left pleural effusion.

Chest X-ray
Postero-anterior and lateral films should be performed. An accumulation of approximately 200 mL of fluid is required before it is detectable on the PA chest film (blunting of the costophrenic angle); 500 mL would obscure the hemi-diaphragm (Fig. 2.29). On a lateral film, 50 mL of fluid is generally detectable.[1]

Pleural fluid aspiration (thoracocentesis)
The indication for pleural fluid aspiration (p. 109) is for clinically significant effusions with no known cause. Aspiration should not be undertaken in patients with bilateral effusions with clinical features suggestive of a transudative effusion (unless there are atypical features or the patient fails to respond to therapy).[2] Ultrasound-guided aspiration is recommended for small or loculated effusions.

The pleural fluid should be inspected and sent for microbiology (bacterial and TB cultures), cytology (successful in identifying 60% of malignant effusions) and clinical chemistry analysis (protein, LDH, pH, glucose, differential cell count; Table 2.33). Additional investigations are requested on clinical suspicion of pancreatitis (pleural fluid amylase), haemothorax (pleural fluid haematocrit) or chylothorax (pleural fluid lipid and chylomicrons level; Fig. 2.30).

Bloody effusions can result from trauma, malignancy, tuberculosis or pulmonary infarction (pulmonary embolus). A cloudy or turbid appearance would suggest infection (empyema) or chylothorax (lymph in the pleural space, Fig. 2.30).

Further investigations

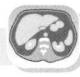

CT Thorax
CT of the thorax is a useful investigation when initial investigations fail to determine the underlying cause. It is also useful to help differentiate between benign and malignant disease (such as mesothelioma). Pleural biopsies can be taken with CT guidance.

165

Table 2.33	Results and interpretation of pleural fluid analyses	
Test	**Result**	**Underlying diagnosis**
Glucose	Less than 3.3 mmol/L	Consider infection, tuberculosis, rheumatoid disease, malignancy
pH	Less than 7.2	Consider infection, the need for chest tube drainage, rheumatoid disease, malignancy
Differential cell count	Lymphocytosis	Consider malignancy and tuberculosis
Additional investigations when indicated		
Amylase	More than the serum upper limit of normal	Pancreatitis
Haematocrit	More than 50% of serum haematocrit	Haemothorax
Triglycerides	More than 1.24 mmol/L	Chylothorax

Percutaneous pleural biopsies

Percutaneous pleural biopsies are usually performed to obtain tissue samples for suspected malignant disease of the pleura. There is an approximate 10% risk of pneumothorax, 2% risk of haemothorax (less than 1% risk of death from haemorrhage) and 40% risk of needle tract invasion if the underlying diagnosis is mesothelioma (hence the requirement for needle site irradiation).[2]

Medical management

Drainage of effusion

In patients with transudative effusions (and in some cases of exudative effusion), treatment of the underlying cause can result in the resolution of effusion. In patients with dyspnoea from accumulating fluid, percutaneous pleural aspiration, narrow bore pigtail catheter or formal chest tube drainage may be required for symptomatic relief in conjunction with treatment of the underlying cause. It is important not to remove more than 1 litre per hour to minimize the risk of re-expansion pulmonary oedema.

Chemical pleurodesis (for malignant effusions)

There is an extremely high recurrence rate after drainage of a malignant effusion. Once drainage has been achieved and lung re-expansion confirmed on chest X-ray, a chemical sclerosant (talc, tetracycline, bleomycin) may be instilled to promote an inflammatory reaction and pleurodesis.

Surgical management

Surgical management is largely confined to diagnosis or the treatment of malignant effusions (occasionally surgical biopsies can assist in the diagnosis of an underlying cause after initial investigations have failed to identify a diagnosis).

Surgical pleurodesis

A video-assisted thoracoscopic (VATS) approach is usually employed. With the patient in a lateral position, a VATS camera is introduced into the pleural cavity. The fluid is drained and sent for cytology, and the lung and pleural surfaces are carefully inspected. Biopsies are taken of any suspicious nodules. Only after histopathological confirmation of malignancy has been obtained is pleurodesis undertaken. The lung must fully expand (otherwise a pleuroperitoneal shunt may be used instead) for a successful pleurodesis; talc is usually the preferred sclerosant. Pleurectomy is rarely performed.

Pleuro-peritoneal shunt

For patients in whom the lung is trapped by tumour deposits, failure of contact with the chest wall will result in unsuccessful pleurodesis. In such cases a pleuro-peritoneal shunt is placed from the pleural into the abdominal cavity. A small one-way pump is situated subcutaneously for patients to ensure continuous drainage of the pleural space.

Long-term pleural drain

A long-term pleural drain is usually reserved for patients who are not fit for surgery, or for patients with terminal illness where repeated hospitalizations can be avoided.

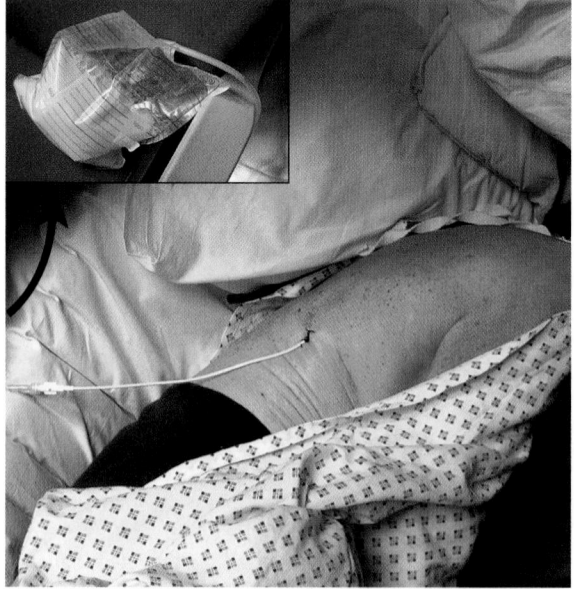

Fig. 2.30 Chylothorax.

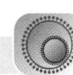

Prognosis

The prognosis is related to the underlying cause.

 FURTHER INFORMATION

Maskell NA, Butland RJA. BTS guidelines for the investigation of a unilateral pleural effusion in adults. Thorax 2003; 58(Suppl 2): 8ii–17.

Antunes G, Neville E, Duffy J, Ali N. BTS guidelines for the management of malignant pleural effusions. Thorax 2003; 58(Suppl 2): 29ii–38.

REFERENCES

(1) *Blackmore CC, Black WC, Dallas RV, Crow HC. Pleural fluid volume estimation: a chest radiograph prediction rule. Academic Radiology 1996; 3: 103–109.*
(2) *Maskell NA, Butland RJA. BTS guidelines for the investigation of a unilateral pleural effusion in adults. Thorax 2003; 58(Suppl 2): 8ii–17.*

Pneumothorax

A pneumothorax is defined as the entry of air into the pleural space; it is classified as spontaneous when there is no evidence of any precipitating cause (Table 2.34).

Epidemiology

The overall incidence of pneumothorax is 16.8 per 100 000 per year.[1] There is a biphasic age distribution: the initial peak at 15–34 years is followed by one at over 55 years, corresponding to the incidence of primary and secondary pneumothoraces respectively. Pneumothorax is 2.5 times more common in males than in females and does not exhibit seasonal variation.

Table 2.34	Classification of pneumothoraces
Spontaneous	**Acquired**
Primary	**Traumatic**
Apical blebs	**Iatrogenic**
Secondary	Central line insertion
Chronic obstructive pulmonary disease	Pleural aspiration
Pneumonia	Barotrauma (ventilation)
Lung cancer	
Asthma	
Pulmonary fibrosis	
Cystic fibrosis	

Pathology

Pneumothoraces are categorized as primary when there is no evidence of underlying lung disease. Despite this nomenclature, subpleural bullae are found in the majority during video-assisted thoracoscopy (VATS), and 'primary' pneumothoraces are often attributed to rupture of these bullae. Secondary pneumothoraces occur as a complication of pre-existing lung disease, most commonly chronic obstructive pulmonary disease. Acquired causes of pneumothoraces are traumatic and iatrogenic (central line insertion, pleural aspiration, barotrauma from ventilation).

Scope of disease

Progression to tension pneumothorax is an uncommon but potential complication. The increasing amount of air accumulating in the pleural space leads to mediastinal shift, reducing venous return to the heart and resulting in circulatory shock.

> **CLINICAL ALERT**
>
> *A tension pneumothorax is diagnosed by severe dyspnoea, cyanosis, tachycardia, tracheal deviation (away from the affected site) and absent breath sounds. It is treated initially by a large bore (14 G) cannula introduced into the pleura via the second intercostal space in the midclavicular line. A gush of air confirms the diagnosis. A chest X-ray should be performed prior to insertion of an intercostal chest drain.*

Clinical features

Sudden onset ipsilateral pleuritic chest pain and dyspnoea are the most common symptoms. The degree of dyspnoea depends on the size of pneumothorax and presence of underlying lung disease.[2] Most episodes of spontaneous pneumothoraces occur at rest and symptoms tend to settle within 24 hours even without resolution of the pneumothorax.[3]

Clinical examination may reveal tachycardia, tracheal deviation (away from the side of the pneumothorax), decreased expansion, vocal resonance and air entry on the affected side. Although hyper-resonance of the affected side is often reported, relative dullness of the unaffected side is often better appreciated. Features of underlying disease resulting in secondary pneumothoraces may be evident on clinical examination.

In addition to the aforementioned clinical features, tension pneumothorax is characterized by severe dyspnoea, tachycardia and hypotension. Treatment should be instituted immediately on clinical diagnosis.

Initial investigation

Chest X-ray

The diagnosis of pneumothorax is suggested by the history and examination and confirmed by a standard chest film. The thin pleural edge will be visible as a faint line with loss

167

of lung markings distal to it (Fig. 2.31a). A chest film on expiration will accentuate any pneumothorax that is difficult to diagnose on a standard view. It is inappropriate to request a chest film to diagnose a tension pneumothorax as this can result in an unacceptable delay in treatment.

Medical management

The principal aims for the management of pneumothoraces are lung re-expansion and prevention of recurrence (Fig.

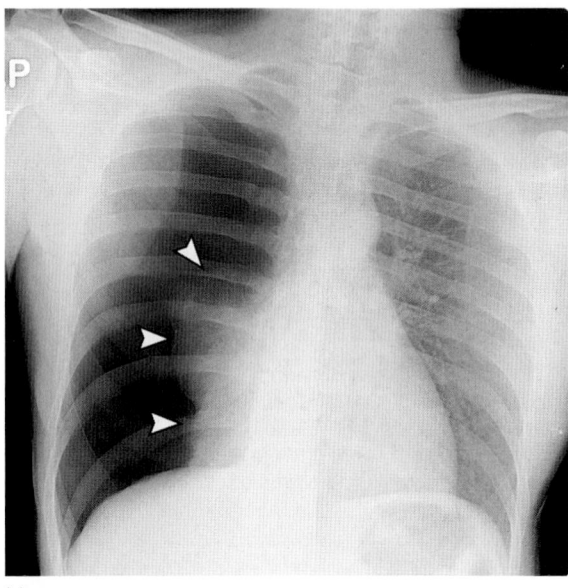

(a)

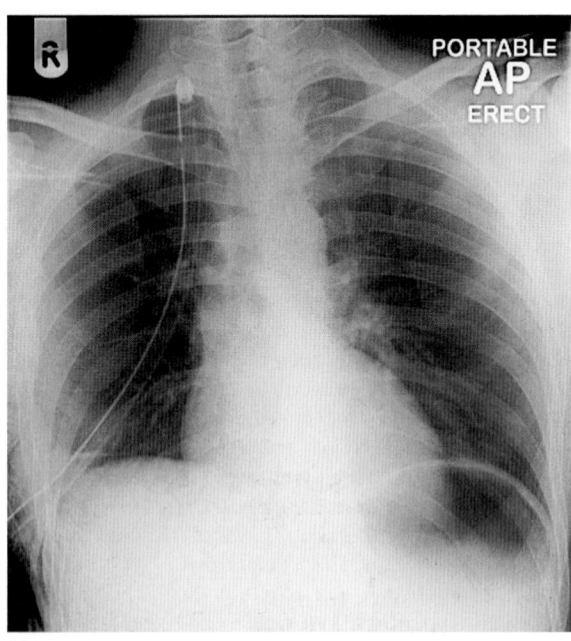

(b)

Fig. 2.31 Chest X-ray of a right pneumothorax. The plain film shows a complete right pneumothorax, with the pleural edge indicated (a), and complete re-expansion with a right chest drain (b).

2.32). Estimation of the size of a pneumothorax is useful to direct further treatment. However, visual estimation of size as a percentage is imprecise, and sophisticated nomograms are cumbersome to use. The American College of Chest Physicians has defined a small pneumothorax to be less than 3 cm and a large pneumothorax to be more than 3 cm when measuring from the apex of the lung to the top of the thoracic cavity (apex to cupola distance).

Lung re-expansion

Observation

A period of observation in the emergency department with a repeat chest film in 6–12 hours prior to discharge is appropriate for patients with a small pneumothorax who are clinically stable and have no underlying lung disease. The rate of resolution is approximately 1% per day. Patients may be discharged with clear follow-up instructions if there

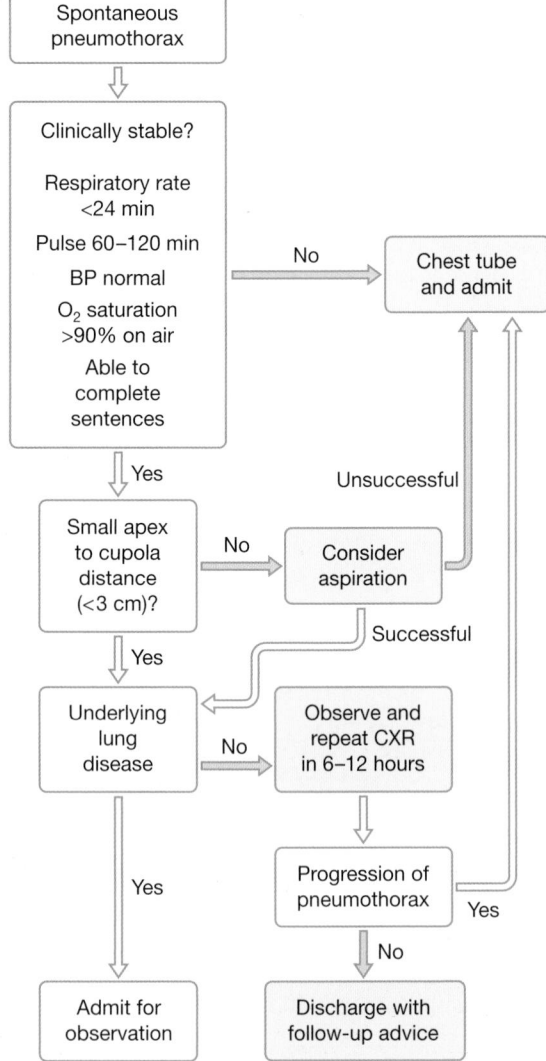

Fig. 2.32 Management of spontaneous pneumothorax.

is no evidence of progression. All patients with underlying lung disease should be admitted for inpatient observation.

Simple aspiration

Simple aspiration is recommended by the British Thoracic Society for the treatment of moderate to large pneumothoraces in clinically stable patients. The use of this technique is controversial and it has an overall success rate of 55%. Occasionally, multiple aspirations may be required. When compared to chest tube insertion as first line treatment, simple aspiration results in more patients having a subsequent air leak at 10 days.[4]

Chest tube insertion

The insertion of an intercostal chest tube is indicated for patients who are unstable, or when simple aspiration fails, or in the presence of a large pneumothorax. The size of the tube should be 28 F and it should be directed as high into the apex of the thoracic cavity as possible. Initially, 7.5 cm H_2O or 0.75 kPa of suction should be applied. A repeat chest film should be performed to assess the position of the drain and confirm full re-expansion of the lung (Fig. 2.31b). Suction should continue until any air leak has resolved. Once the patient has been taken off suction, a repeat chest film should be taken after 12–24 hours to confirm full re-expansion of the lung before the chest tube is removed. After 5 days, if there is a persistent air leak, surgical intervention should be considered.

Prevention of recurrence

Unless a persistent air leak occurs or occupational requirements demand (divers, pilots), measures to prevent recurrence of pneumothorax are usually reserved for the second episode.

Pleurodesis

Chemical pleurodesis can be achieved with talc, tetracycline, or bleomycin. This form of therapy is suitable for patients who are at high risk for surgery. In the absence of contraindications, however, surgical therapy is preferred due to lower recurrence rates.

Surgical management

The main aims for surgical intervention are to address the air leak and prevent recurrence. The indications for surgical intervention are provided in Table 2.35. Surgeons and patients differ in their preference to the approach (minimal access or open thoracotomy) for pleurodesis.

Bullectomy and pleurodesis (video-assisted thoracoscopic (VATS) approach)

Two to three thoracoscopic ports are introduced into a laterally positioned patient (Fig. 2.33a). The entire lung is examined for bullae and the apex (the most common site) is carefully scrutinized (Fig. 2.33b). Offending bullae are stapled and excised (Fig. 2.33c, d), then either pleural abrasion, apical pleurectomy (Fig. 2.33e) or talc insufflation is performed to prevent recurrence. One or two apical drains are positioned, the lung re-inflated under direct vision and the remaining port sites sutured. The recurrence rate following VATS pleurectomy has been reported as 6.7% after 15 months.[5]

Bullectomy and pleurodesis (open thoracotomy approach)

Bullectomy and pleurectomy via a thoracotomy is the preferred approach for patients with previous thoracic surgery (due to adhesions). Axillary mini-thoracotomy or limited posterolateral thoracotomy is used. The lung is collapsed and complete parietal pleurectomy can be performed by peeling the pleura from the chest wall. The recurrence rate is less than 1% at 4 years.

Overall, the in-hospital recurrence rate is 2.5% and persistent air leak (more than 5 days) occurs in 3%.

Prognosis

A third of pneumothoraces treated by lung expansion alone will recur. The aforementioned recurrence rates are dependent on the type of procedure and the approach used (Table 2.36).

i FURTHER INFORMATION

Baumann M, Strange C, Heffner JE, et al. Management of spontaneous pneumothorax. An American College of Chest Physicians Delphi consensus statement. Chest 2001; 119: 590–602.

Miller AC, Harvey JE. Guidelines for the management of spontaneous pneumothorax. BMJ 1999; 307: 114–116.

Table 2.35	Indications for surgical therapy

First episode of spontaneous pneumothorax for:
     Persistent air leak (>5 days)
     Secondary pneumothorax
     Occupational requirement (pilots, divers)
     Previous contralateral pneumonectomy	

Recurrent pneumothoraces (2 or more episodes)	

Table 2.36	Recurrence rates (mean interval of 45 months) according to management
Observation only	36%
Chest tube only	35%
Tetracycline pleurodesis	9%
Surgery	0%

From Alfageme I, Monreno L, Huertas C, et al. Spontaneous pneumothorax: long term results with tetracycline pleurodesis. Chest 1994; 106: 347–350.

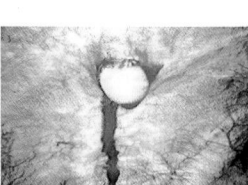

(a)

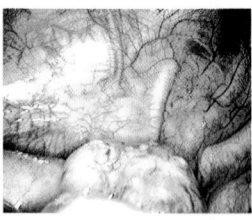

(b)

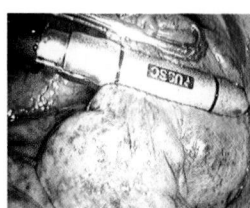

(c)

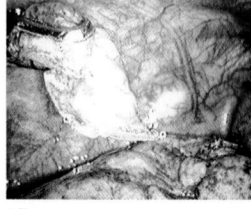

(d)

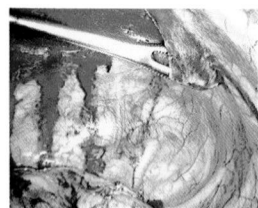

(e)

Fig. 2.33 VATS bullectomy and pleurectomy. Images courtesy of Mr Andrew Ritchie, Consultant Cardiothoracic Surgeon, Papworth Hospital, Cambridge, UK.

REFERENCES

(1) *Gupta D, Hansell D, Nichols T, Duong T, Ayres JG, Strachan D. Epidemiology of pneumothorax in England. Thorax 2000; 55: 666–671.*
(2) *Seremetis MG. The management of spontaneous pneumothorax. Chest 1970; 57: 65–68.*
(3) *Sahn SA, Heffner JE. Spontaneous pneumothorax. New England Journal of Medicine 2000; 342(12): 868–873.*
(4) *Andrivet P, Djedaini K, Teboul JL, et al. Spontaneous pneumothorax: comparison of thoracic drainage vs immediate or delayed needle aspiration. Chest 1995; 108: 335–339.*
(5) *Waller, Forty J, Morritt GN. Video assisted thoracoscopic surgery versus thoracotomy for spontaneous pneumothorax. Annals of Thoracic Surgery 1994; 58: 372–377.*

Pleural mesothelioma

Mesothelioma is a tumour of the mesothelial lining of the pleural, pericardial and peritoneal cavities.

Epidemiology

Pleural mesothelioma is currently uncommon, with an incidence of 8 per 100 000 per year in the United Kingdom.[1] However, asbestos use was widespread in Europe until the 1980s and, due to an approximate 40-year latent period between exposure and presentation, it has been projected that the peak incidence is likely to occur around 2020, individuals born between 1945 and 1950 being at greatest risk.[2] Pleural mesothelioma is more common in men than in women.

Pathology

Asbestos is the primary aetiological exposure that results in the development of mesothelioma. Any evidence of exposure is relevant, as no threshold exposure exists for the risk of mesothelioma. The four histopathological subtypes are epithelioid, sarcomatoid, biphasic (epithelioid and sarcomatoid) and desmoplastic.

Clinical features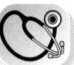

The presentation of malignant pleural mesothelioma is often insidious and non-specific. Progressive dyspnoea and/or dull and diffuse chest pain are the two most common symptoms. The pain may radiate to shoulder, arm, chest wall or abdomen and may occasionally be pleuritic. Systemic symptoms of malignancy include anorexia, weight loss and pyrexia. A detailed occupational history is the key to determine any evidence of asbestos exposure.

On examination, clubbing may be present. Chest examination may reveal features exactly like those of a pleural effusion (p. 164). In advanced disease, cachexia, chest wall mass, hepatomegaly or ascites may be present.

Investigations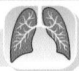

Chest X-ray

The plain film appearances may be similar to a pleural effusion, but the abnormal area may be composed in part or entirely of tumour, or isolated pleural thickening. Other evidence of asbestos exposure may be present such as pleural plaques (nodular or irregular pleural shadowing) that may extend to the mediastinal aspect, pleural calcifications or pulmonary fibrosis—asbestosis (Fig. 2.24).

CT Thorax

A CT scan may have been part of the diagnostic workup for a pleural effusion of unknown cause. Features of mesothelioma are the presence of discrete pleural masses. Multiloculated effusions may be present and a think pleural rind in more established disease. In addition, CT-guided biopsy of a pleural nodule can provide valuable tissue samples for histopathological analysis. The CT scan is also an excellent staging investigation that can assess the extent of local invasion and regional lymphadenopathy. The UICC (IMIG) staging of pleural mesothelioma is provided below.

▸▸▸ Staging of malignant pleural mesothelioma	
T—Primary tumour	
T1	Tumour involves ipsilateral parietal pleura, with or without focal involvement of the visceral pleura
T1a	Tumour involves ipsilateral parietal (mediastinal, diaphragmatic) pleura. No involvement of the visceral pleura
T1b	Tumour involves ipsilateral parietal (mediastinal, diaphragmatic) pleura, with focal involvement of the visceral pleura
T2	Tumour involves any of the ipsilateral pleural surfaces with at least one of the following:
	Confluent visceral pleural tumour (including fissure)
	Invasion of diaphragmatic muscle
	Invasion of lung parenchyma
T3*	Tumour involves any of the ipsilateral pleural surfaces with at least one of the following:
	Invasion of the endothoracic fascia
	Invasion into mediastinal fat
	Solitary focus of tumour invading the soft tissues of the chest wall
	Non-transmural involvement of the pericardium
T4**	Tumour involves any of the ipsilateral pleural surfaces with at least one of the following:
	Diffuse or multifocal invasion of soft tissues of the chest wall
	Any involvement of rib
	Invasion through the diaphragm to the peritoneum

Staging of malignant pleural mesothelioma—cont'd

Invasion of any mediastinal organ(s)

Direct extension to the contralateral pleura

Invasion into the spine

Extension to the internal surface of the pericardium

Pericardial effusion with positive cytology

Invasion of the myocardium

Invasion of the brachial plexus

T3*   Describes locally advanced potentially resectable tumour

T4**   Describes locally advanced technically unresectable tumour

N—Regional lymph nodes

N1   Metastases in the ipsilateral bronchopulmonary and/or hilar lymph node(s).

N2   Metastases in the subcarinal lymph node(s) and/or the ipsilateral internal mammary or mediastinal lymph node(s).

M—Distant metastasis

M0   No distant metastasis

M1   Distant metastasis

Stage

Stage			
Stage I	T1	N0	M0
Stage IA	T1a	N0	M0
Stage IB	T1b	N0	M0
Stage II	T2	N0	M0
Stage III	T1, T2	N1	M0
	T1, T2	N2	M0
	T3	N0, N1, N2	M0
Stage IV	T4	Any N	M0
	Any T	N3	M0
	Any T	Any N	M1

Pathological diagnosis

Pleural aspiration cytology (p. 165) and percutaneous pleural biopsies (p. 166) have poor sensitivity, therefore a negative test cannot confidently rule out disease. However, confirmatory histopathological diagnosis is essential, and if necessary a surgical biopsy should be undertaken.

Management

As with all other tumours, confirmatory histopathological diagnosis and staging are fundamental to the management of patients with malignant pleural mesothelioma.

Patient education

Patients should be informed that the prognosis is poor despite a current trimodality approach of surgery (where appropriate), radiotherapy and chemotherapy. Financial compensation is usually provided for industry-related mesothelioma, and advice on how to make a claim is important.

Surgery

The efficacy of radical surgery has not been evaluated in the setting of a randomized trial. Surgery for stage I/II disease should be confined to patients with a favourable histological subtype (epithelioid) and centres with specialist expertise in pleural mesothelioma. Extrapleural pneumonectomy (resection of the lung, viscera, parietal pleura, pericardium, and ipsilateral diaphragm) has a mortality rate of approximately 30% in inexperienced and less than 5% in experienced centres.[3] Video-assisted thoracoscopic (VATS) decortication and pleurodesis is also an option for the palliative management of symptomatic pleural effusions, although it remains controversial as a definitive management strategy.

Radiotherapy

Pleural mesothelioma is a relatively radioresistant disease. The role of radiotherapy is confined to palliation (of chest pain), prophylactic (along needle aspiration, biopsy and surgical incision, and chest drain sites) and postoperative adjuvant therapy that may reduce recurrence in selected patients.[4]

Chemotherapy

Pleural mesothelioma is also a relatively chemoresistant disease. Initial single agent chemotherapy regimens have failed to produce response rates above 30%.[5] Pemetrexed, a potent inhibitor of proteins required for DNA synthesis, prolongs median survival from 9 to 12 months.[6] Gemcitabine in combination with cisplatin has also resulted in objective response rates and improved quality of life.[7]

RECENT ADVANCES

The results of biological therapy with imatinib (platelet derived growth factor inhibitor) and gefitinib (epidermal growth factor receptor blocker) have not yet yielded convincing responses.[8]

Prognosis

The prognosis of pleural mesothelioma is related to stage. In general, the prognosis is very poor with a median survival of less than one year.[9]

i FURTHER INFORMATION

Statement on malignant mesothelioma in the United Kingdom. Thorax 2001; 56: 250–265.

REFERENCES

(1) *Montanaro F, Bray F, Gennaro V, et al. Pleural mesothelioma incidence in Europe: evidence of some deceleration in the increasing trends. Cancer Causes and Control 2003; 14: 791–803.*
(2) *Peto J, Decarli A, La Vecchia C, Levi F, Negri E. The European mesothelioma epidemic. British Journal of Cancer 1999; 79: 666–672.*
(3) *van Ruth S, Baas P, Zoetmulder FAN. Surgical treatment of malignant pleural mesothelioma: a review. Chest 2003; 123: 551–561.*
(4) *Rusch V, Rosenzweig K, Venkatraman E, et al. A phase II trial of surgical resection and adjuvant high-dose hemithoracic radiation for malignant pleural mesothelioma. Journal of Thoracic and Cardiovascular Surgery 2001; 122: 788–795.*
(5) *Tomek S, Manegold C, Senan S. Chemotherapy for malignant pleural mesothelioma. Indications and limitations of radiotherapy in malignant pleural mesothelioma. Current Opinion in Oncology 2003; 15: 148–156.*
(6) *Vogelzang NJ, Rusthoven JJ, Symanowski J, et al. Phase III study of pemetrexed in combination with cisplatin versus cisplatin alone in patients with malignant pleural mesothelioma. Journal of Clinical Oncology 2003; 21: 2636–2644.*
(7) *Nowak AK, Byrne MJ, Williamson R, et al. A multicentre phase II study of cisplatin and gemcitabine for malignant mesothelioma. British Journal of Cancer 2002; 87: 491–496.*
(8) *Robinson BW, Lake RA. Advances in malignant mesothelioma. New England Journal of Medicine 2005; 353: 1591–1603.*
(9) *Herndon J, Green M, Chahinian A, Corson J, Suzuki Y, Vogelzang N. Factors predictive of survival among 337 patients with mesothelioma treated between 1984 and 1994 by the Cancer and Leukemia Group B. Chest 1998; 113: 723–731.*

SECTION 2.15 | Diseases of the mediastinum

The mediastinum is the area between the mediastinal pleura, bounded anteriorly by the sternum, posteriorly by the spine, inferiorly by the diaphragm and superiorly by the thoracic inlet. In this section we use the anatomical classification of Shields that divides the mediastinum into anterior, middle (visceral) and posterior (paravertebral sulci) compartments, as demonstrated in Figure 2.34.

Mediastinal tumours

Epidemiology

Mediastinal tumours are uncommon, and patient characteristics are related to the underlying cause (Table 2.37).

Pathology

Anterior compartment

In adults, thymic tumours (thymoma, rarely thymic carcinoma) are usually the most common cause. Germ cell

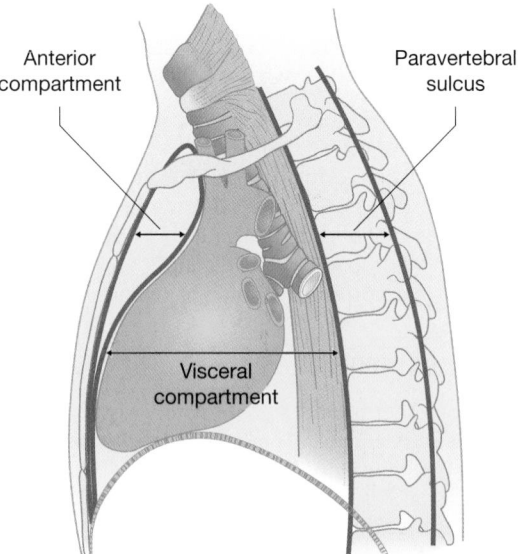

Fig. 2.34 Shields' three-compartment model of the mediastinum. From Dresler CM. Anatomy and classification. In: Pearson FG (ed) Thoracic surgery. New York: Churchill Livingstone, 1995, p. 1326.

Table 2.37	Mediastinal tumours and other masses	
Anterior	**Middle (visceral)**	**Posterior (paravertebral sulci)**
Thymic tumours	Lymphomas	Neurogenic tumours
Germ cell tumours	Foregut cysts	Meningoceles
Lymphomas	Pericardial cysts	Foregut cysts (enteric)
Goitre (substernal)		
Ascending aortic aneurysm	Left ventricular aneurysm	Descending aortic aneurysm
Sternal tumours	Pulmonary artery aneurysm	Diaphragmatic hernias
	Enlarged lymph nodes	Oesophageal tumours

tumours include metastasis from seminomas, teratomas and embryonal carcinomas. Primary germ cell tumours of the mediastinum are rare. Mediastinal lymphoma can be of the Hodgkin's or non-Hodgkin's type.

Middle (visceral compartment)
Pericardial cysts are characteristically located at the right costophrenic angle and usually appear contiguous with the right hemidiaphragm. Bronchogenic cysts are usually located adjacent to the bronchial tree.

Posterior (paravertebral sulci)
Neurogenic tumours (schwannomas, neurofibromas) are the most common posterior compartment tumour in the adult, presenting as round circumscribed masses on chest X-ray.

Clinical features

In the majority, mediastinal tumours present as asymptomatic masses on chest X-ray. Occasionally, mediastinal masses may present with compressive effects such as cough, stridor or dyspnoea, dysphagia from oesophageal compression, and hoarseness from compression of the recurrent laryngeal nerve.

Patients may also have symptoms or signs of the underlying disease such as myasthenia with thymoma, hyperthyroidism from a substernal goitre or a previous history of malignancy (lymphoma, seminoma).

Investigations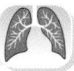

Serum tumour markers
Beta human chorionic gonadotrophin (β-hCG) and α-fetoprotein may be elevated in non-seminomatous germ cell tumours. Anti-acetylcholinesterase antibodies may be elevated with thymoma.

Chest X-ray
Both PA (Fig. 2.35) and lateral chest films are required. The lateral film may be able to locate the mediastinal compartment and narrow the differential diagnosis.

CT Thorax
A contrast enhanced CT scan of the thorax (Fig. 2.36) can accurately delineate the position and extent of the mediastinal mass. CT-guided biopsy may be undertaken if features suggest that surgical treatment is not likely to be required (e.g. lymphoma).

Surgical biopsy
Confirmatory histopathological diagnosis of the tumour type is required for management. This may necessitate surgical biopsy when the diagnosis remains indeterminate after initial investigations. Depending on the location of the tumour, tissue can be obtained by mediastinoscopy, anterior mediastinotomy or video-assisted thoracoscopy.

Management

The management of thymoma is surgical excision and that of lymphoma and is covered on page 153. With regard to the other underlying aetiologies, readers are advised to consult more specialized reference books.

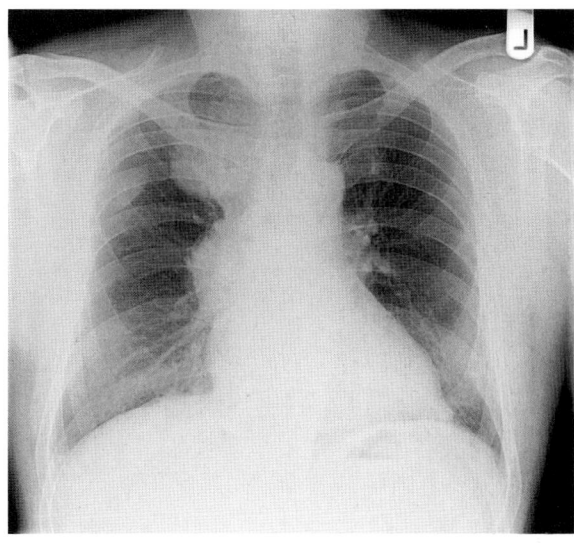

Fig. 2.35 Chest X-ray of thymoma. A well-circumscribed mass can be seen in the upper right mediastinum.

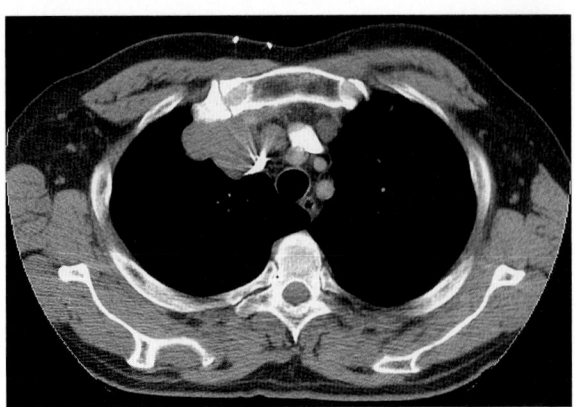

Fig. 2.36 CT of thymoma. CT of the same patient as in Figure 2.35 reveals an anterior mediastinal mass corresponding to CXR findings.

 FURTHER INFORMATION

Pearson FG, Cooper JD, Deslaurier J, Ginsberg RJ, Hiebert CA, Patterson GA, Urschel HC. Thoracic surgery, 2nd edn. New York: Churchill Livingstone, 2002.

Diseases of the ear, nose and throat

3

Jeevendra Kanagalingam, Azhar Shaida

Afflictions of the ear, nose and throat are very common. Approximately 15% of patients in the United Kingdom have consulted general practitioners for ear, nose or throat (ENT) symptoms. A significant number of emergency room attendances too are for ENT emergencies such as nosebleeds and foreign bodies in the ears, nose and throat.

ENT has grown rapidly as a specialty and this has led to the development of subspecialties within this field. Otology is concerned with the surgical management of ear diseases, encompassing skull base surgery or otoneurosurgery where tumours of the lateral skull base or cerebello-pontine angle are excised. Audiological medicine has grown as a medical counterpart to otology. Rhinology is concerned with the management of nasal conditions, closely allied to clinical allergy and immunology (allergic rhinitis makes up a significant portion of the workload).

ENT cancers are managed within the subspecialty of head and neck surgery. Due to their complex nature, the treatment of head and neck malignancies is managed by multidisciplinary teams comprising ENT, plastic and maxillo-facial surgeons, oncologists, radiologists, pathologists, speech therapists and dieticians.

The ear

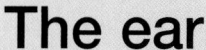

SECTION 3.1 | **Introduction**

Applied basic sciences of the ear

The ear is a complex sensory end organ that is responsible for hearing and balance. It is divided into the external, middle and inner ear. All three parts are important in the perception of sound, but only the inner ear plays a part in the maintenance of balance.

The pinna and external auditory canal

The pinna or auricle is made up of elastic fibrocartilage and thin skin which is closely adherent to the perichondrium. The lateral surface is thrown into several prominences and depressions which help the pinna function as a receptacle of sound waves (Fig. 3.1).

The external auditory canal slopes forwards and downwards for approximately 2.5 cm in the adult towards the

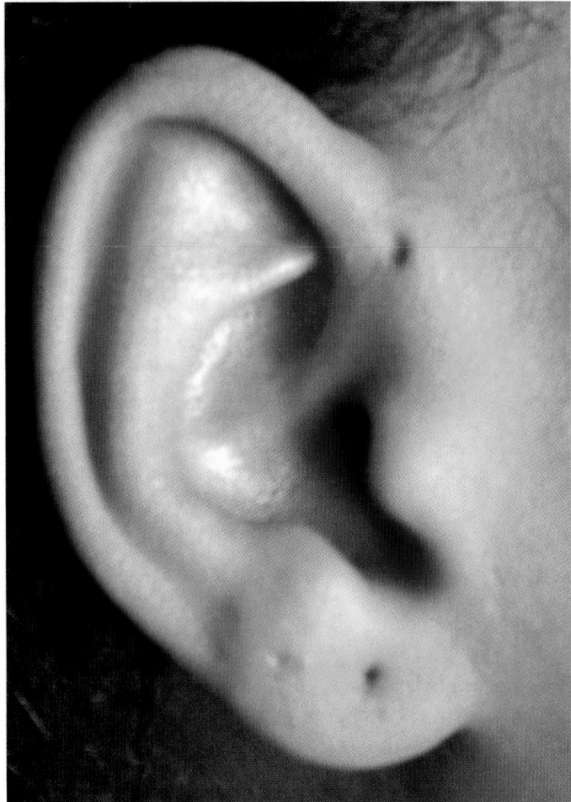

Fig. 3.1 The external ear functions as a receptacle of sound. This pinna exhibits a pre-auricular sinus which predisposes a patient to recurrent infections and abscesses. Note the scar on this patient from previous incision and drainage of an abscess.

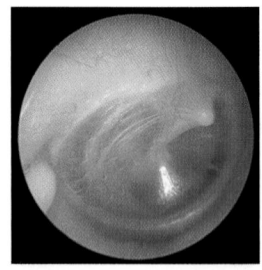

(a)

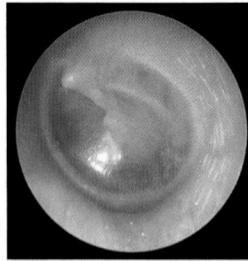

(b)

Fig. 3.2 The normal tympanic membrane may be divided into the upper pars flaccida and a lower and larger pars tensa for the right (a) and left (b) eardrum.

this space and connect the tympanic membrane to the cochlea of the inner ear through a small oval window. These bones are known as the ossicular chain and enable the mechanical amplification of sound waves arriving at the tympanic membrane and their subsequent transmission into the cochlea (see Fig. 3.3). Middle ear mechanics magnify the amplitude of sound waves arriving at the eardrum by 22 times.

The middle ear space is kept ventilated by the eustachian tube which passes antero-medially and inferiorly towards the post-nasal space or nasopharynx, where it opens on the lateral nasopharyngeal wall. In childhood, this tube is wider, shorter and more horizontal in position than in adulthood. This anatomical fact and the presence of adenoidal tissue in the post-nasal space may explain the prevalence of otitis media with effusion or 'glue ear' in childhood, when ventilation of the middle ear is poor.

The middle ear communicates posteriorly with a system of air-filled sinuses which fill the mastoid process of the petrous temporal bone. Suppuration of the middle ear may therefore spread posteriorly and produce an osteomyelitis of this process, a condition known as acute mastoiditis.

The inner ear

The inner ear can be conveniently divided into the cochlea and the labyrinth. The cochlea is responsible for hearing and the vestibular labyrinth is important for balance.

The cochlea is a coiled or helical neuroepithelial structure which is partitioned into two compartments by a membrane. Sound waves transmitted into the cochlea by the ossicular chain set up a waveform along this membrane. Specialized cells known as hair cells detect the perturbation of this membrane and send action potentials along nerve fibres of the auditory nerve. These impulses pass the brainstem to reach the auditory cortex where sound is perceived.

The vestibular labyrinth consists of three semicircular canals which lie at right angles to each other, and two vestibular 'sacs' known as the utricle and saccule. The canals contain a specialized fluid, perilymph, and a specialized neuroepithelial structure within the dilated ends of the canals. Movements of fluid within these canals due to circular motion of the head are detected. Impulses from the canals tell the brain that the head is rotating. The saccule and utricle detect linear movement in the vertical and horizontal planes respectively.

Symptoms of ear disease

Earache

Earache or otalgia is often felt as a throbbing pain deep in the ear. It may also be felt behind or in front of the ear, and may radiate towards the jaw, throat or neck. It may be very severe, as in otitis externa, or fairly mild and described as 'discomfort' in eustachian tube dysfunction.

The ear receives sensory innervation from cranial nerves V, VII, IX and X and from dorsal rami of C2 and C3. Pathology outside the ear, in the distribution of any of these nerves,

eardrum or tympanic membrane. The canal is cartilaginous in its outer third and bony in its inner two thirds. The skin overlying the outer cartilaginous portion is hair-bearing and contains sebaceous and ceruminous glands. The latter are modified sweat glands. Secretions of both these glands mix to form wax. Wax contains fatty acids, amino acids, lysozymes and immunoglobulins, which make it bactericidal, fungicidal and antiseptic. It serves a useful purpose and is not problematic unless it is pushed deeper into the ear canal by attempts to clean the canal.

The skin of the ear canal does not mature directly towards the surface. Instead, lateral migration of the epidermis occurs with shedding of squamous epithelial cells or keratin towards the surface opening of the canal. This is also true of the superficial or epidermal layer of the tympanic membrane, which is contiguous with the epidermal layer of the ear canal.

The middle ear

The tympanic membrane has three layers and is approximately 1 cm^2 in surface area. It can be divided into an upper flaccid section (pars flaccida) and a lower tense section (pars tensa) (see Fig. 3.2). The tympanic membrane separates the ear canal from an air-filled middle ear space. Three small bones (the malleus, incus and stapes) straddle

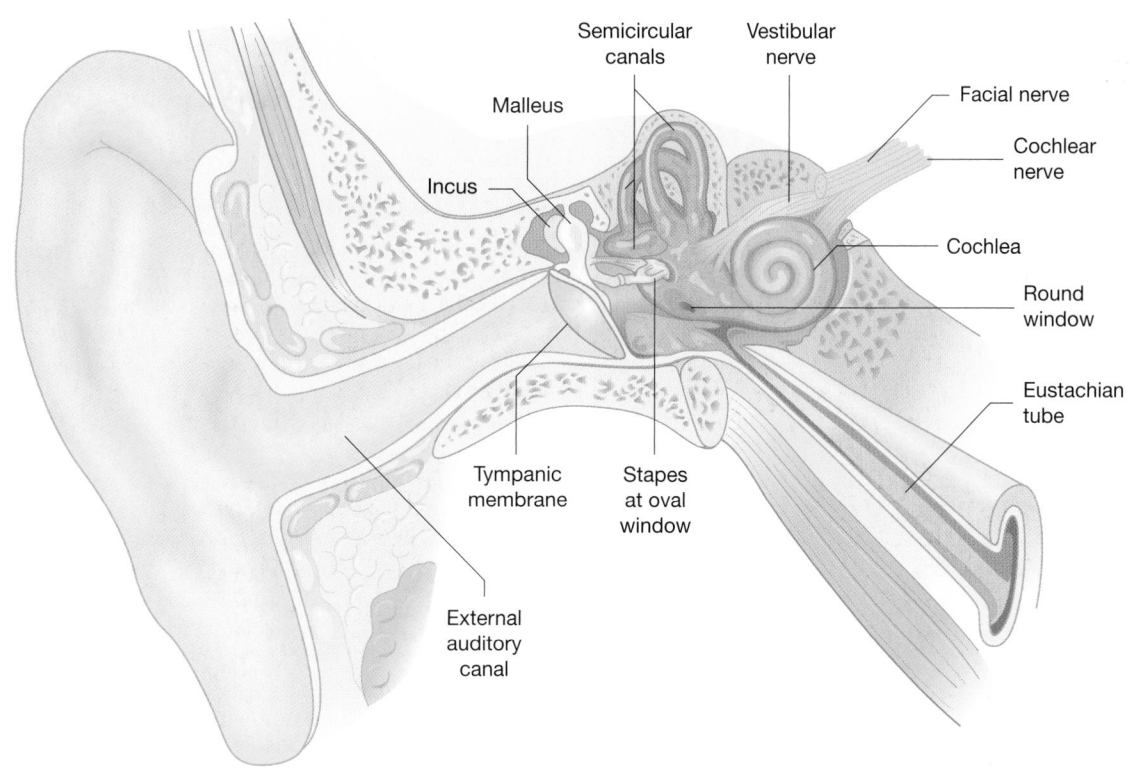

Semicircular canals
Vestibular nerve
Malleus
Incus
Facial nerve
Cochlear nerve
Cochlea
Round window
Eustachian tube
Tympanic membrane
Stapes at oval window
External auditory canal

Fig. 3.3 A diagrammatic representation of the external, middle and inner ear.

may produce earache; this is called *referred otalgia*. Common causes of referred otalgia include acute tonsillitis, dental infections, tumours of the pharynx and larynx, jaw joint problems and cervical spine pathology.

Deafness

Deafness is the perception of hearing loss. If hearing loss is due to damage to the external or middle ear, it is often termed conductive hearing loss. Damage to the sensory end organ, i.e. the cochlea, or to neural pathways results in sensorineural hearing loss. To the patient, both forms of hearing loss can be equally debilitating. Speech discrimination is said to be worse in the sensorineural variety. Age-related symmetrical sensorineural hearing loss is described as presbyacusis. In cases where outer hair cell loss is predominant, high-tone loss occurs with preservation of speech discrimination (sensory presbyacusis). When auditory nerve fibres start to fail, hearing loss is equal across all thresholds with significant impairment of speech discrimination (neural presbyacusis).

It is important to elicit from the patient whether hearing loss is bilateral or unilateral. Unilateral cases often have a specific underlying cause. The mode of onset of deafness is also important, as is any progression, fluctuation or improvement in hearing. Finally, it is important to ask if hearing loss is worse in group conversation. Patients with sensorineural hearing loss are particularly disabled in crowds. Paradoxically, in a condition called otosclerosis where there is conductive loss, hearing is better when there is environmental noise, a phenomenon known as paracusis Willisii.

Discharge

Discharge or otorrhoea is usually mucopurulent in nature. Infections of the ear canal (otitis externa) often produce scanty creamy discharge which contains keratinous debris. Middle ear suppuration often produces copious discharge which is offensive in the presence of cholesteatoma (p. 191). Bloody or serosanguinous discharge may result from trauma, severe infections or tumours (Fig. 3.4). Trauma may also result in 'gin-clear' watery otorrhoea which is, in fact, cerebrospinal fluid leaking through a skull-base fracture.

Tinnitus

Tinnitus is the perception of noise in the head. Patients may describe a single sound or a spectrum. Most commonly these sounds are described as 'ringing' or 'hissing' sounds. A distinction should be made between subjective and objective tinnitus, which the examiner may hear. Pulsatile or unilateral tinnitus usually suggests organic pathology that requires further investigation. For the most part, tinnitus has no underlying cause and most patients 'get used' to it, a process known as habituation.

177

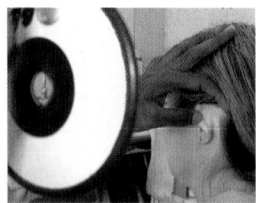

Fig. 3.6 Examination of the post-aural skin may reveal, as in this case, a scar from previous surgery.

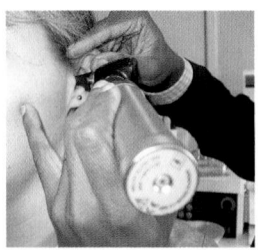

Fig. 3.7 The correct way of holding the auroscope and pinna. The little finger rests on the patient's cheek, so that the auroscope moves with the patient.

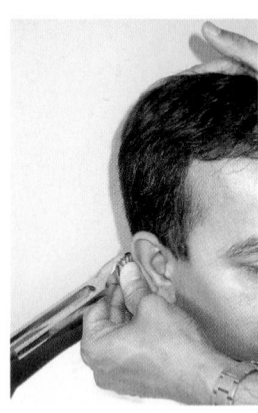

Fig. 3.8 Rinne's test. A 512 Hz tuning fork is placed on the mastoid process with counterpressure on the opposite side of the head. Once no sound is heard, it is held two inches from the external auditory meatus in the coronal plane.

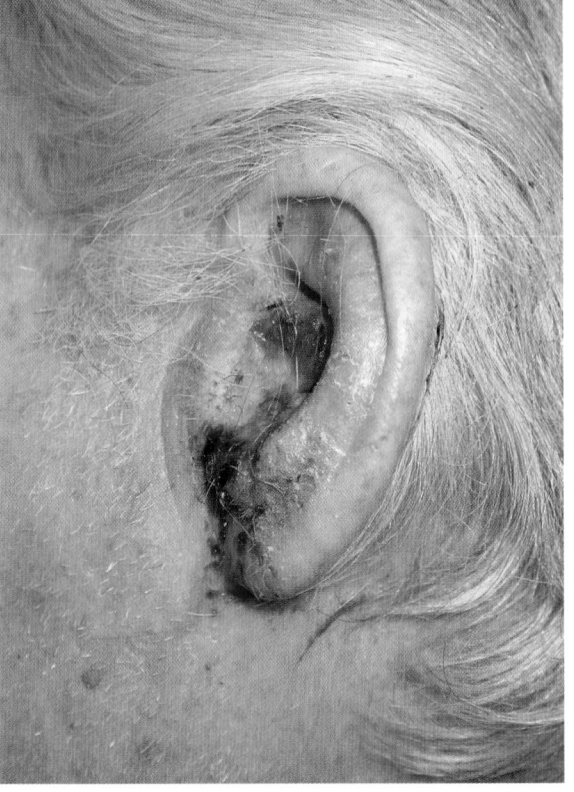

Fig. 3.4 Bloody discharge from squamous cell carcinoma of the external auditory canal.

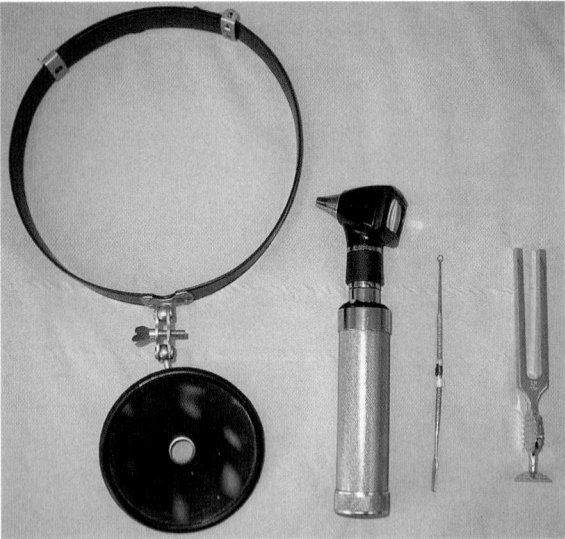

Fig. 3.5 Basic instruments needed for examining the ear are (from left to right) a head-mirror, an auroscope (or otoscope), a Jobson-Horne probe and a 512 Hz tuning fork

Vertigo

Vertigo is the illusion of movement which is often rotatory in nature. It is vital to distinguish this from 'dizziness' or 'light-headedness' which is often unrelated to ear disease.

When severe, vertigo may be associated with nausea and vomiting. This symptom is often due to disorders of the peripheral vestibular sensory end organ (i.e. semicircular canals, saccule or utricle) or central vestibular pathways.

Examination of the ear

Examination of the ear requires a head-mirror and light source, an auroscope (or otoscope) with disposable speculae, a Jobson-Horne probe for wax removal or dry-mopping the ear canal, and a 512 Hz tuning fork (Fig. 3.5).

Inspection

Examination of the pinna should begin with bending the pinna forward and inspecting the post-aural area for surgical scars or inflammatory swellings (Fig. 3.6). The folds of the pinna and the skin of the conchal bowl may then be examined. In protruding or bat ears, the antihelical fold is often absent or poorly formed. The skin of the conchal bowl may be inflamed with exfoliation in otitis externa. Crusting in the external meatus alludes to an on-going discharge from the ear.

In the pre-auricular or pre-tragal area, sinuses or auricular appendages may be noticed.

Otoscopy

The auroscope allows for examination of the ear canal and tympanic membrane. In some patients, wax in the outer third of the ear canal or purulent discharge should be removed beforehand. This can often be easily done with the looped end of the Jobson-Horne probe or a wisp of cotton wool rolled on to the other end of the same probe.

The auroscope should be held in the left hand when examining the left ear and in the right hand when examining the right ear. The handle of the auroscope should be gripped like a pen between the thumb and index, middle and ring fingers. The little finger should be extended to rest on the patient's cheek (Fig. 3.7). This will ensure that the auroscope when inserted will move with the patient should the patient turn his or her head suddenly. The largest speculum that will fit comfortably into the ear canal should be chosen.

The ear canal should be straightened before the auroscope is inserted. In the adult, this is best done by gently pulling the pinna gently backwards and upwards. In the infant, the pinna need only be pulled backwards to straighten the ear canal.

The best otoscopists develop a set routine when examining the ear with an auroscope. The canal is inspected first, then the tympanic membrane, paying close attention to the translucency of the eardrum and features such as the lateral process and handle of the malleus, and the light reflex. The upper portion of the eardrum, or pars flaccida, is then carefully examined as this is where cholesteatoma is frequently seen.

Some auroscopes have a pneumatic bulb attached. This allows for a puff of air to be blown towards the eardrum to check its mobility. An alternative is to get the patient to perform a Valsalva manoeuvre or swallow (Toynbee's manoeuvre).

Tuning fork tests

These are simple tests that may be performed in the clinic. They are useful in making the distinction between conductive and sensorineural hearing loss, and giving an objective sense as to which ear is the better hearing ear. A 512 Hz tuning fork must be used as lower frequencies tend to cause significant vibration that is detected by the patient's vibrotactile sensory end organs.

Rinne's test

Rinne's test determines whether sound is best heard by air conduction (AC) through the ear canal or by bone conduction (BC) from the mastoid process located behind the ear to the bony labyrinth. The tuning fork is struck and its base placed on the mastoid process (Fig. 3.8). The patient is asked to indicate when he or she can no longer hear a sound. At this point, the tuning fork is held two inches from the external auditory meatus with both prongs in the coronal plane. If the patient hears a tone, AC is better than BC and the test is positive. If BC is better than AC the test is negative.

A positive test suggests either normal hearing or sensorineural hearing loss. A negative test suggests conductive hearing loss. The situation is complicated in the case of unilateral sensorineural hearing loss where the inter-aural hearing thresholds are significantly different (i.e. more than 40 dB). In patients with profound unilateral sensorineural hearing loss, or a unilateral 'dead' ear, BC across to the contralateral unaffected ear is better than AC in the bad ear. The patient detects the sound when conducted by bone, not realizing that it is in fact the good ear which is helping him or her to do so. Rinne's test is therefore negative. A negative Rinne's test in sensorineural deafness is termed a false negative Rinne's test. To distinguish between false and true negative Rinne's tests, it is crucial to 'mask' the contralateral ear and repeat the test. The concept of masking is complex and beyond the scope of this text.

Weber's test

In this test, the tuning fork is struck and the base placed on the top or vertex of the skull (Fig. 3.9). The patient is asked where the sound is heard. Placing the tuning fork on the forehead reduces its sensitivity and placing it on the upper incisors increases its sensitivity.

In unilateral or asymmetrical conductive hearing loss, the tone is heard loudest in the affected (or worse hearing) ear. In unilateral or asymmetrical sensorineural hearing loss, the tone localizes to the unaffected (or better hearing) ear. In normal hearing, or symmetrical hearing loss, the sound is heard centrally (Fig. 3.10).

Applied basic sciences of the ear

Symptoms of ear disease

Examination of the ear

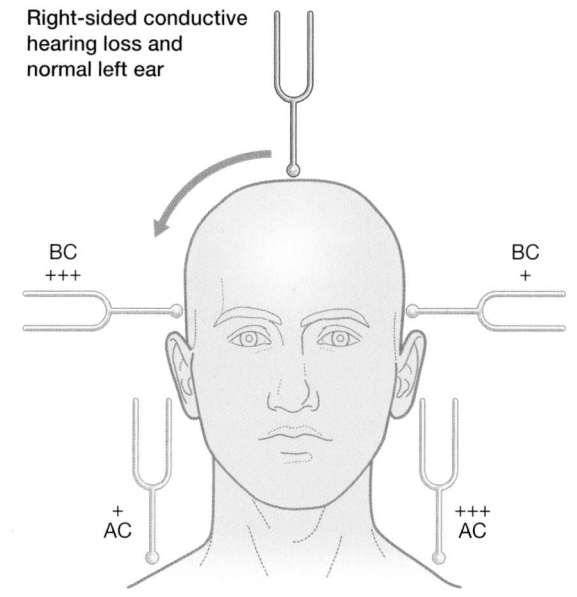

Right-sided conductive hearing loss and normal left ear

BC +++   BC +

+ AC   +++ AC

Right Rinne: negative (BC>AC)
(a)   Weber: lateralizes to ear with conductive loss

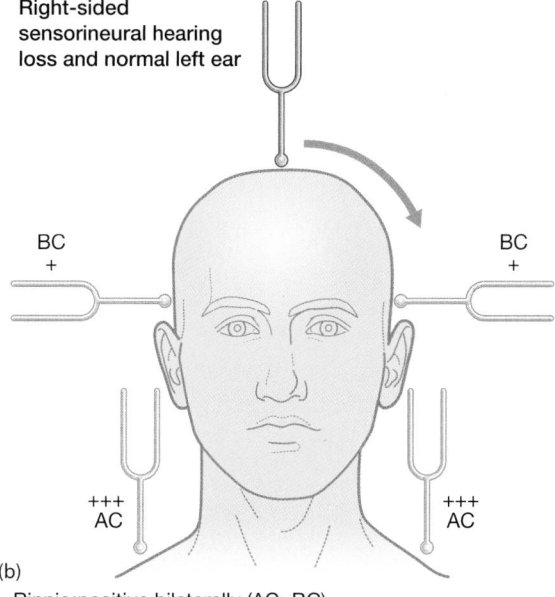

Right-sided sensorineural hearing loss and normal left ear

BC +   BC +

+++ AC   +++ AC

(b)
Rinnie: positive bilaterally (AC>BC)
Weber: lateralizes to the ear with greater cochlear function

BC: hearing via ear canal and middle ear
BC: direct transmission to the inner ear via the mastoid process + subjective loudness

= Weber test   = Rinnie test

Fig. 3.10 Tuning fork test in (a) unilateral conductive hearing loss, (b) unilateral sensorineural hearing loss.

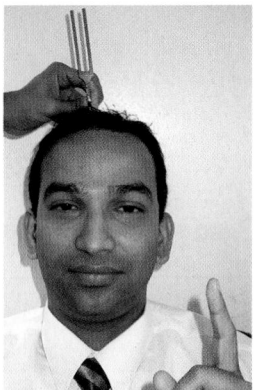

Fig. 3.9 Weber's test. A 512 Hz tuning fork is placed on the vertex of the skull.

179

Investigations for ear disease

Pure-tone audiogram

The most commonly performed hearing test is pure-tone audiometry. This is a subjective hearing test in which the patient is presented with a series of pure tones in each ear sequentially. The patient sits in a soundproof room wearing headphones, and responds by pressing a button every time he or she hears a tone (Fig. 3.11). The quietest sound that is heard is recorded as the hearing threshold for that frequency.

International symbols depicting right and left ears are used to record the hearing level on a decibel hearing level (dB HL) scale. By convention, the frequencies tested are 1, 2, 4, 8 kHz, then 250 and 500 Hz (Fig. 3.12).

In young children, play audiometry or visual reinforced audiometry is used to obtain reliable hearing thresholds. These tests require a degree of cooperation and concentration on the part of the child.

Tympanometry

Tympanometry is a test of middle ear compliance. It is also known as impedance audiometry. This test measures the stiffness of the eardrum and estimates middle ear pressure and the volume of the external canal (Fig. 3.13). It is useful in detecting middle ear effusions in glue ear, underventilation of the middle ear space in eustachian

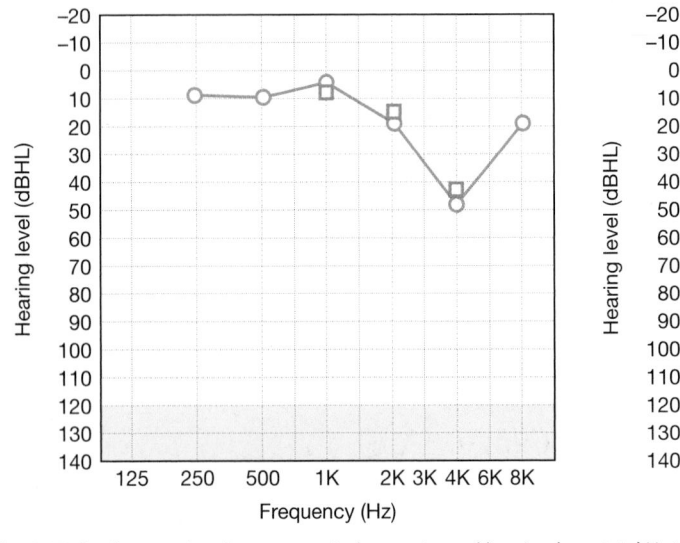

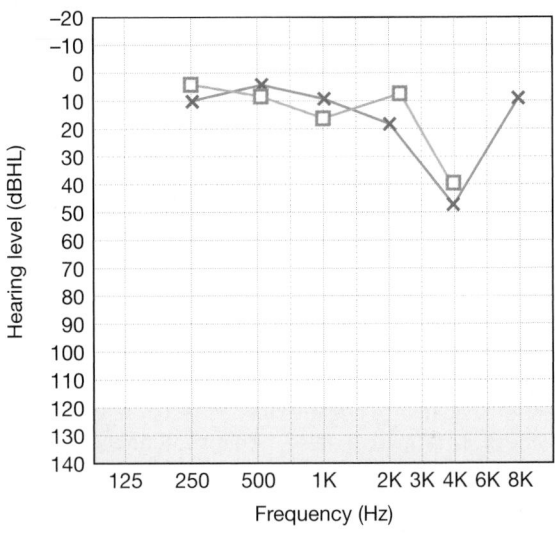

Fig. 3.12 Audiogram showing symmetrical sensorineural hearing loss at 4 kHz to 45 dB, which is characteristic of noise-induced hearing loss.

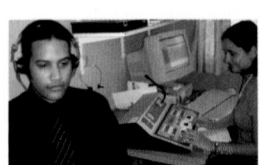

Fig. 3.11 For a pure-tone audiogram, the patient usually sits in a soundproof room.

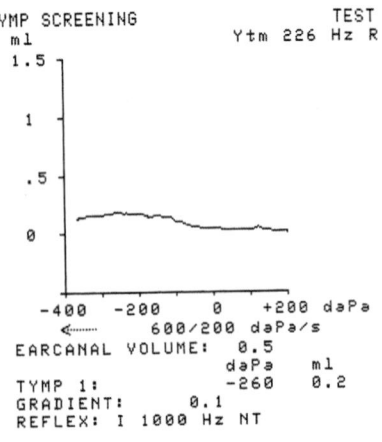

(a)

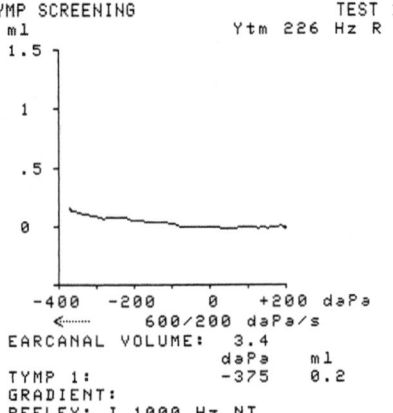

(b)

Fig. 3.13 Tympanogram. Tracing (a) is obtained from an ear with a middle ear effusion and is therefore flat. Tracing (b) shows an increased ear canal volume of 3.4 cm³, which is seen in eardrum perforations, i.e. the tympanogram measures both ear canal and middle ear volumes.

tube dysfunction, and small perforations that are not seen on otoscopy.

Electrical response audiometry

Electrical response audiometry is a useful objective measure of hearing. A sound, usually a series of clicks, is presented to the ear, and electrodes placed along the auditory pathway detect the electrical responses that occur. In electrocochleography (ECochG), a fine needle is inserted through the eardrum to rest on the promontory or basal turn of the cochlea. Here it detects any electrical activity in the cochlea. Electrodes placed elsewhere on the head may detect electrical activity in the brainstem or auditory cortex. These responses are termed brainstem evoked responses or cortical evoked responses, respectively.

Vestibular testing

Vestibular testing involves a range of tests that measure peripheral and central vestibular function. The most common test employed is caloric testing. In this test, irrigation of the ear canal with cold and warm water creates convection currents in the lateral semicircular canals. This in turn causes nystagmus (rhythmic involuntary

oscillations of the eyes), which eventually settles. The loss of this reflex, or canal paresis, points to peripheral vestibular failure.

Diagnostic imaging

In common otological practice, the use of plain X-rays has been superseded by computed tomography (CT) and magnetic resonance imaging (MRI).

CT scan

High-resolution CT scanning of the petrous temporal bone is able to identify the ossicles and detect bony erosion of the middle ear as a result of inflammatory or neoplastic conditions. It is, unfortunately, less effective in distinguishing soft tissue lesions such as cholesteatoma from simple fluid or pus (Fig. 3.14).

MRI scan

MRI scanning allows for better soft tissue definition and reliably distinguishes soft tissue lesions from fluid or secretions. In the skull base, MRI scanning identifies lesions as small as 2 mm in the cerebello-pontine angle and has become a useful tool for the diagnosis of tumours of this region, including vestibular schwannomas (Fig. 3.15).

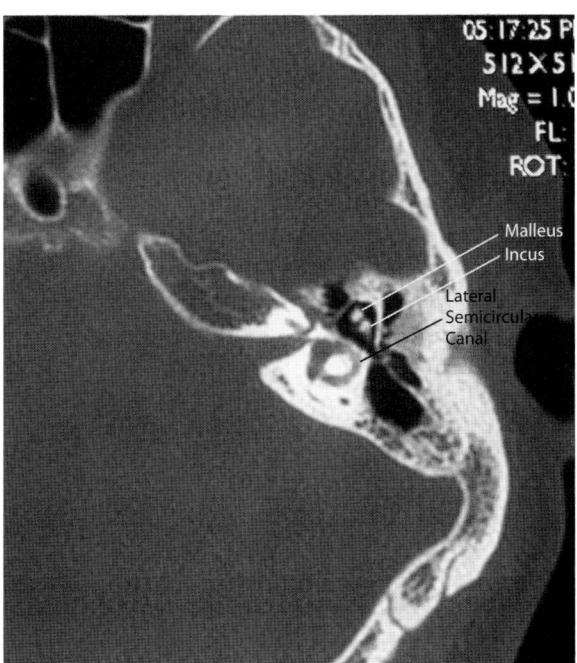

Fig. 3.14 A normal CT scan of the left temporal bone. This axial slice passes through the malleus and the incus. The articulation of these two ossicles is often described as the ice cream (malleus) sitting on the cone (incus).

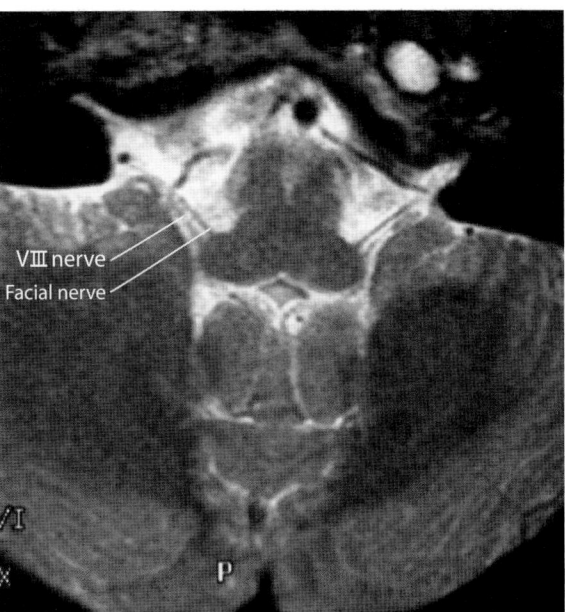

Fig. 3.15 A T_2-weighted MRI scan of the cerebello-pontine angle. Cranial nerves VII (Facial) and VIII are clearly seen.

Manifestations of ear disease

Sensorineural hearing loss

Sensorineural hearing loss (SNHL) is deafness due to disease affecting the inner ear ('sensory') or the central nervous pathways involved in auditory function ('neural'). It is defined as loss of 30 dB in three continuous frequencies. The external and middle ear are normal.

SNHL encompasses a large variety of pathological conditions. The causes may be classified as congenital or acquired (see Table 3.1). Idiopathic sudden onset SNHL is an important entity that deserves special mention. It is an otological emergency that requires prompt recognition and urgent treatment.

Pathology

Congenital SNHL

Genetic causes account for the overwhelming majority of cases of congenital SNHL: 80% of these genetic conditions are transmitted by autosomal recessive inheritance, 15% follow an autosomal dominant pattern, and the remainder are X-linked. The hereditary forms of deafness may be syndromic in nature. Markers of genetic hearing loss now exist (e.g. connexin 26), allowing for early recognition and hopefully genetic therapy in the future.

Non-genetic congenital SNHL is due to infections acquired in utero.

Acquired SNHL

Infection

Meningitis accounts for 90% of acquired SNHL in children. It is estimated that between 8% and 12% of children suffer SNHL following meningitis. In a quarter, the loss is profound. It is important to assess these children fairly quickly following recovery. Cochlear implantation may be feasible but must be undertaken before the irreversible changes of cochleosclerosis occur.

Postnatally, mumps and measles may affect the cochlea and cause SNHL. In adults, a variety of viruses may cause damage to the cochlea. These viral infections are often insidious with SNHL occurring suddenly. Bacterial toxins from middle ear suppuration or frank suppurative labyrinthitis may cause irreversible SNHL. One ototoxic protozoal infection worthy of mention is toxoplasmosis.

Trauma

Head injuries may be severe enough to cause cochlea concussion. This is reversible SNHL. Transverse fractures of the petrous temporal bone which pass through the bony labyrinth will cause irreversible severe to profound SNHL.

Table 3.1	Causes of sensorineural hearing loss
Congenital	
Genetic	
Non-syndromic	
Syndromic, e.g. Alport's, Usher's, Pendred's and	
Waardenburg's	
In utero infection	
Rubella	
Cytomegalovirus	
Toxoplasmosis	
Congenital syphilis	
Acquired	
Infection	
Meningitis	
Mumps	
Measles	
Toxoplasmosis	
Trauma	
Head injuries (cochlea concussion—reversible)	
Temporal bone fractures (often irreversible)	
Noise-induced hearing loss	
Degenerative	
Ageing (degeneration of the outer hair cells and auditory	
nerve fibres)	
Idiopathic	
Probably an unproven 'viral' cochleitis	
Tumours	
Vestibular schwannoma (asymmetric hearing loss)	
Ototoxic drugs	
Aspirin	
Loop diuretics	
Aminoglycoside antibiotics	
Platinum-based chemotherapy	
Haematological	

Noise-induced hearing loss

Noise-induced hearing loss is SNHL secondary to loud noise exposure. Commonly, this is due to occupational exposure to machinery, but recreational pursuits such as shooting and nightclubbing increasingly account for more cases. Exposure to more than 85 dB noise for more than 8 hours a day is deemed hazardous.

Initially, there is a temporary threshold shift which is accompanied by subjective tinnitus. No microscopic damage is seen in the cochlea. Eventually, the outer hair cells are damaged and a permanent threshold shift is noted with little to no tinnitus. Classically, audiometric measures show a steep dip in thresholds at 4–6 kHz.

Degenerative SNHL

Ageing results in degeneration of the outer hair cells and auditory nerve fibres. This causes a symmetrical SNHL which is described as presbyacusis. In cases where outer hair cell loss is predominant, high-tone loss occurs with preservation of speech discrimination (sensory presbyacusis). When auditory nerve fibres start to fail, hearing loss is equal across all thresholds with significant impairment of speech discrimination (neural presbyacusis).

Idiopathic sudden onset SNHL

The incidence of idiopathic sudden onset sensorineural hearing loss has been estimated at 6 per 100 000 per year. It can affect any age group and either sex. No cause is known, but there is reason to attribute this condition to a viral cochleitis.

Tumours

Tumours of the internal auditory meatus where the facial (VII) and vestibulocochlear (VIII) nerves enter the petrous temporal bone may cause asymmetrical SNHL. Losses in the low frequencies are more specific for these lesions. Vestibular schwannomas (or acoustic neuromas), which are benign entities, are the most common tumours encountered. Advances in imaging of this area with MRI allow detection of tumours as small as 2 mm (see Fig. 3.16). All patients with significant asymmetrical SNHL should be referred for this scan.

Ototoxic drugs

Several drugs may cause SNHL. Those commonly encountered which are worthy of mention are aspirin, loop diuretics

and aminoglycoside antibiotics. Some chemotherapeutic agents, particularly platinum-based compounds, may also affect hearing.

Haematological causes

Hypercoagulopathies and hyperlipidaemia may cause sudden sensorineural hearing loss. It is postulated that microemboli in the blood supply to the labyrinth can cause irreversible ischaemic damage to the cochlea.

Clinical features

Adults present with a history of muffled or reduced hearing. Characteristically, difficulties are experienced in noisy environments where there is a lot of background sound. Patients with presbyacusis often present at the behest of their relatives. They often have little difficulty with one-to-one conversation but find conversing in crowds problematic.

Hearing loss may be preceded by symptoms of an upper respiratory tract infection, and it is important to rule out causes of conductive hearing loss such as otitis media with effusion (p. 190). A past medical and drug history is important to screen for known precipitating factors.

Tinnitus often accompanies SNHL. It is important to elicit the nature of any tinnitus. Pulsatile tinnitus may be a manifestation of a vascular lesion in the middle ear.

Otoscopy is usually normal and tuning fork tests (see p. 179) will confirm sensorineural deafness.

> ⚡ **CLINICAL ALERT**
>
> Sudden onset sensorineural hearing loss should be considered an otological emergency.

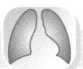

Investigations

Audiogram

Pure-tone audiometry should be performed to establish the diagnosis and estimate the severity of the hearing loss. This should be performed urgently in idiopathic sudden onset SNHL. In addition, the audiogram is also used to monitor disease progression and the response to treatment.

Speech audiometry

This is a more subjective test of hearing and assesses the patient's ability at speech discrimination. In neural-type SNHL, speech discrimination scores tend to be worse than expected.

MRI

MRI of the internal auditory meatus and posterior cranial fossa is performed to identify cochlear anomalies which may be part of a congenital syndrome. In idiopathic sudden onset SNHL, it should be performed to exclude an acoustic neuroma (also known as vestibular schwannoma), which is a rare cause of sudden onset sensorineural hearing loss.

Sensorineural hearing loss

Vertigo

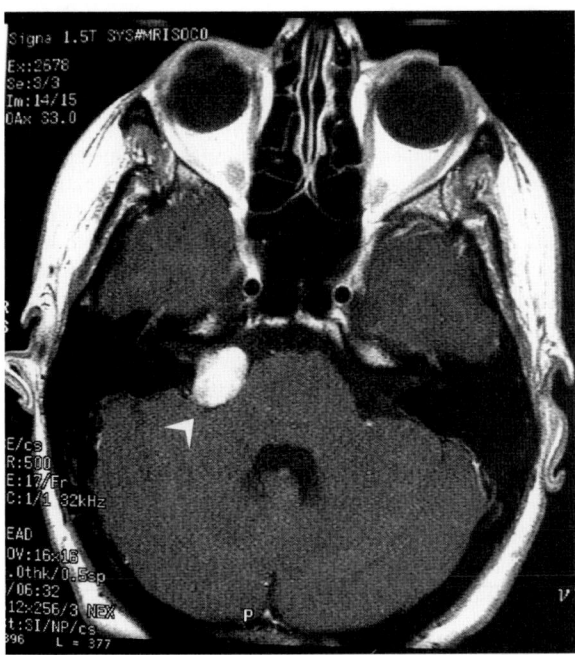

Fig. 3.16 Post-contrast T₁-weighted MRI scan of the internal auditory meatus demonstrating a right cerebello-pontine angle acoustic neuroma (arrow).

Management

Idiopathic sudden onset SNHL

There are various treatment options for this condition. Immunomodulation with high-dose steroids is of proven efficacy. Approximately 78% of patients with moderate hearing loss recover their hearing when high-dose steroids (prednisolone 60–80 mg) are administered within 10 days compared to 38% when steroids are not used.[1] In patients who cannot tolerate steroids, intratympanic injection of steroids to the round window of the cochlea is an option.

Other treatment options include inhalation of carbogen (a mixture of 95% oxygen and 5% carbon dioxide), oral betahistine to improve cochlear perfusion, antivirals and aspirin.

Other SNHL

There is little that can be done in other irreversible causes of SNHL. Aiding the ear with a hearing aid is the only option. In profound deafness where hearing aids offer little benefit, cochlear implantation is an alternative.

Hearing rehabilitation has much to offer those with impaired hearing. Clinicians should always work closely with other allied health-care professionals to optimize the care of these patients.

Prognosis

In idiopathic sudden onset SNHL, the prognosis for recovery of hearing is related to the severity of hearing loss. Patients with profound hearing loss (more than 90 dB) are unlikely to recover their hearing. Patients with mild hearing loss usually recover spontaneously with or without treatment. Prompt steroid administration is an important aspect that improves the prognosis of patients with moderate hearing loss.

REFERENCE

(1) Wilson WR, Byl FM, Laird N. *The efficacy of steroids in the treatment of idiopathic sudden hearing loss. A double-blind clinical study. Archives of Otolaryngology* 1980; 106: 772–776.

Vertigo

Vertigo is an illusion of movement. In its most typical form it is rotatory and likened to the sensation obtained after spinning around on a swivel chair.

Vertigo may be confused with other symptoms that patients may report as 'dizziness'. Vertigo is a consequence of peripheral (labyrinth) or central (neural connections) vestibular pathology. Light-headedness, blackouts (syncope, or pre-syncope) and incoordination are commonly confused with vertigo and the causes are almost always non-vestibular.

Epidemiology

Of all patients presenting with dizziness, only a third will have symptoms classified as true vertigo. In the United Kingdom, true vertigo accounts for 1070 consultations per 100 000 patients per year. The prevalence of vertigo increases with age. It is rare in children, but the symptom must always be taken seriously and thoroughly investigated.

Pathology

Any peripheral or central insult to the vestibular system may cause vertigo. Peripheral vestibular failure is often unilateral and irreversible. Although the contralateral labyrinth often compensates adequately, compensation takes time and requires the patient to resume daily activities. This often leaves patients with some disequilibrium after vertiginous symptoms have waned.

The commonest causes of vertigo are vestibular neuronitis, benign paroxysmal positional vertigo (BPPV) and Ménière's disease. Vestibular neuronitis is due to isolated degeneration of the vestibular nerve or its connections. BPPV is due to the presence of particles or 'sand' in the semicircular canals (canaliths). It is postulated that these break off from the otoliths within the utricle. Not surprisingly, there is often a history of a head injury in these patients.

Ménière's disease is due to endolymphatic hydrops. The increased pressure in the endolymphatic system causes the episodic triad of tinnitus, vertigo and fluctuating hearing loss. As the disease progresses, hearing loss becomes permanent and worsens. Vertigo eventually 'burns out'.

Clinical features

Patients often have difficulty describing their symptoms, and it is important to take a structured and precise history without the use of leading questions.

Acute vestibular failure may present dramatically with sudden onset of vertigo accompanied by intense nausea or vomiting. The patient struggles to get on to his/her feet and is usually moribund. This attack often settles in hours but may recur. There is often an association with tinnitus and deafness.

Episodes of true vertigo usually settle spontaneously but leave the patient with disequilibrium and a loss of confidence. The clinical features distinguishing between the three common causes of vertigo are summarized in Table 3.2.

A good history and thorough neuro-otological examination is more important than any investigation. Examine the cranial nerves, in particular funduscopy for papilloedema or optic atrophy (cranial nerve II), eye movements (III, IV, and VI), corneal reflex (V), and facial movement (VII). Nystagmus is common in acute vertigo. Check cerebellar function (past pointing, dysdiadochokinesia). Testing vibration sense (a 128 Hz tuning fork on the ankle) is useful to screen for peripheral neuropathy. Otoscopy is unlikely to be abnormal without hearing loss, pain or discharge.

Table 3.2	Common causes of vertigo		
Condition	**Clinical features**	**Tinnitus**	**Hearing**
Benign paroxysmal positional vertigo (BPPV)	Vertigo associated with head turning or rolling over in bed. Often accompanied by nausea and vomiting. Resolves over days but is followed by dysequilibrium. There may be a history of a head injury	None	Not affected
Ménière's disease	Triad of vertigo, tinnitus and hearing loss often associated with a pressure sensation in the affected ear. Attacks last between 1 and 24 hours but are often followed by persistent dysequilibrium	Present and often increases in severity over years	Hearing loss initially fluctuates with normal hearing between attacks. Permanent hearing loss eventually occurs
Vestibular neuronitis	Recurrent attacks of vertigo lasting hours or even days. Followed by dysequilibrium, while central compensation occurs. A preceding viral illness is common	None	Not affected

The Dix–Hallpike manoeuvre is a useful clinical test for BPPV. Sit the patient on the examining bench, then lay her down quickly with her head turned to one side (Fig. 3.17). Rotatory nystagmus observed after a short latency is a positive test for the dependent ear.

Initial investigations

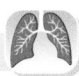

Investigations are not required in patients without any central symptoms or hearing loss.

Further investigations

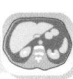

Audiogram
In the presence of hearing loss, a pure-tone audiogram is indicated to quantify the range and severity of the loss.

Balance tests
Tests of vestibular function such as caloric testing, electronystagmography (ENG) and rotation tests are available in specialist units. These are useful when there is diagnostic doubt.

Imaging
A contrast-enhanced MRI scan of the brain and internal auditory meatus is indicated when a central cause is suspected.

Initial management

Labyrinthine sedatives
In the acute setting, supportive treatment is all that is necessary. The patient should be given a labyrinthine sedative such as prochlorperazine or cinnarizine. Sublingual preparations are ideal when patients are vomiting. Antiemetic treatment should not be prolonged as this may cause extrapyramidal side effects or delay vestibular compensation.

In Ménière's disease, betahistine (a histamine analogue that improves labyrinthine perfusion), a low-salt and low-caffeine diet, and a diuretic are said to be of prophylactic benefit. There is little evidence, however, to support their use.

Intravenous rehydration
In severe cases, admission to hospital for intravenous rehydration may be necessary.

Vestibular rehabilitation
In BPPV, a canalith repositioning manoeuvre known as the Epley manoeuvre produces good results and a series of head and neck exercises—the Cawthorne–Cooksey exercises—helps vestibular rehabilitation.

Surgical management

Surgical procedures
Most surgical approaches to vertigo have focused on Ménière's disease. Strategies that have been adopted include endolymphatic sac decompression, vestibular neurectomy and chemical labyrinthectomy with intratympanic gentamicin.

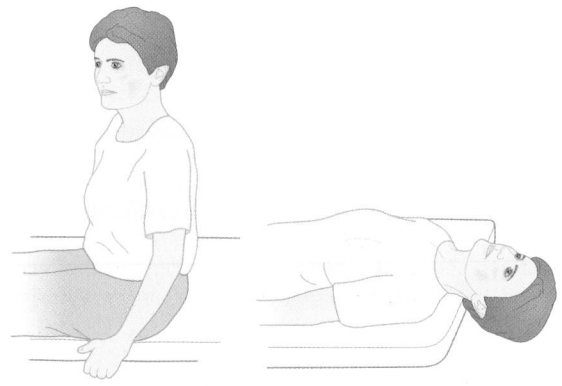

Fig. 3.17 Dix–Hallpike manoeuvre.

The use of intratympanic gentamicin yields highly favourable results and is gaining popularity. The drug is delivered into the middle ear cleft and is absorbed into the vestibule. A recent meta-analysis of this strategy concluded that complete resolution of vertigo occurred in 74.7% of patients, and complete or substantial control was achieved in 92.7%. Hearing level and word recognition were not adversely affected.

Prognosis

The symptoms of vertigo resolve spontaneously by 2 months in 50% of patients with vestibular neuronitis.

i FURTHER INFORMATION

Kanagalingam J, Hajioff D, Bennett S. Vertigo. [Review.] BMJ 2005; 330(7490): 523.

Cohen-Kerem R, Kisilevsky V, Einarson TR, Kozer E, Koren G, Rutka JA. Intratympanic gentamicin for Meniere's disease: a meta-analysis. [Review.] Laryngoscope 2004; 114(12): 2085–2091.

Hilton M, Pinder D. The Epley (canalith repositioning) manoeuvre for benign paroxysmal positional vertigo. [Review.] Cochrane Database of Systematic Reviews 2004;(2): CD003162.

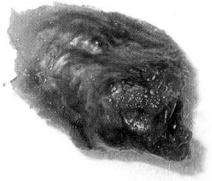

Fig. 3.18 A solid wax plug forming a 'cast' of the ear canal.

SECTION 3.4 | Diseases of the ear

Impacted wax

Impaction of wax deep in the external auditory canal is a common primary care problem.

Epidemiology

The incidence of wax impaction is 2–6% among the general population but rises to 25–28% among 'institutionalized' adults.

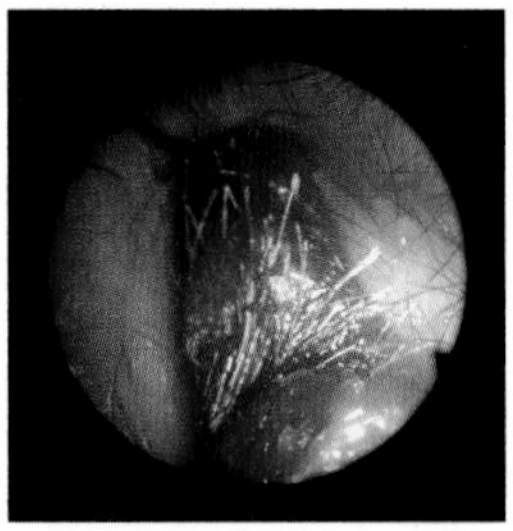

Pathology

Wax is only produced by the outer third of the ear canal. It poses no problems unless it is pushed deeper into the meatus (usually by attempts to rid the ear of it). Once wax falls deep into the ear canal, spontaneous extrusion fails to occur. Repeated attempts to clear the ear canal contribute further to impaction until a solid wax plug is formed (Fig. 3.18).

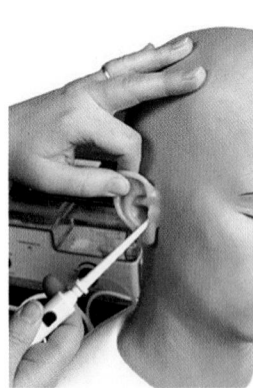

Fig. 3.19 Wax impaction of the external auditory canal.

Scope of disease

Plugs may form a nidus for recurrent intractable outer ear infections (otitis externa). Damage to the tympanic membrane as a consequence of wax impaction is rare. However, aggressive or improper syringing of the ear to clear wax can cause eardrum perforations.

Clinical features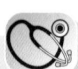

Wax impaction typically causes mild conductive hearing loss. The patient often reports a sense of 'blockage'. Occasionally, mild irritation of the ear canal may produce discomfort. If the wax plug becomes wet following swimming or bathing, symptoms may be exacerbated. Rarely, stimulation of glossopharyngeal or vagal afferents by the wax plug may produce symptoms in the throat.

On otoscopy, a wax plug is clearly visible (Fig. 3.19). The tympanic membrane is often completely obscured by this plug.

Initial investigations

No investigation is generally required, as the diagnosis is established under direct vision.

Initial management

Wax softeners

The first line treatment for wax impaction is the use of a suitable softener or ceruminolytic. A large variety of softeners are available from pharmacies without a doctor's prescription. Some of these contain hydrogen peroxide, which may irritate an inflamed or infected ear canal. Olive oil or sodium bicarbonate drops are popular, effective and inexpensive. Hard wax plugs often respond best to the effervescent sodium bicarbonate drops. Softeners should be used for a week before further assessment.

Surgical management

Syringing

In some circumstances, wax has to be physically removed. This can be achieved by syringing water into the ear canal. The water used should be warmed to body temperature so as not to precipitate vertigo (p. 185). The stream of water should be directed towards the posterior canal wall, to flush wax plugs out (Fig. 3.20).

Syringing should not be attempted in patients with previous ear conditions or surgery, in patients with only one hearing ear, or in patients with active ear infection.

Fig. 3.20 Syringing with water at body temperature flushes out wax plugs.

Microsuction

If syringing is contraindicated or unsuccessful, referral to an ENT specialist is necessary. Removal of wax can then be undertaken with the help of an operating microscope and vacuum suction in the clinic.

Prognosis

Wax plugs in the ear canal usually cause few complications and are effectively treated with simple ear wax softeners.

i FURTHER INFORMATION

Burton MJ, Dorée CJ. Ear drops for the removal of ear wax (Cochrane Review). The Cochrane Library, Issue 4, 2003.

Foreign bodies

Foreign bodies inserted into the ear, or live insects that enter the ear canal, are a common problem encountered in the emergency department.

Epidemiology

Amongst children, the curious toddler is usually predisposed to insert small objects such as beads into the ear. It is rare for older children to present with this complaint. Children with learning difficulties occasionally present having inserted a large number or variety of objects. A significant number of adults present with infective complications of foreign bodies, although the history of inserting a foreign body is seldom volunteered for fear of embarrassment.

Pathology

It is important to consider the underlying reason for the insertion of a foreign object. In children, there is often an underlying conductive hearing loss such as glue ear, and the child inserts objects simply to try to 'clear a blockage'. In adults, eczema or a fungal otitis externa may cause intense itching and drive patients to insert cotton buds, matchsticks or hairpins into the ear canal.

A distinction must be made between organic and inorganic foreign bodies. Organic foreign bodies such as peas swell when water is introduce into the ear canal. Syringing is unlikely to be successful in removing them. Inorganic foreign bodies such as beads lend themselves to syringing but can be difficult to remove if they lie deep in the ear canal.

Scope of disease

Inert, inorganic foreign bodies cause few problems in the ear canal. Indeed, some patients may present with such foreign bodies many years after their initial insertion. Organic foreign bodies are more likely to cause severe ear canal infections. Often, treatment with topical antibiotics is unsuccessful until the foreign body is identified and removed. Lithium button batteries may leak corrosive alkali that erodes the ear canal skin and bone.

Clinical features

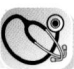

Patients often report a history of foreign body insertion into the ear canal. In a minority, a history is not volunteered and the patient presents with intractable infections. When a live insect has entered the ear canal, a highly distressed patient often presents with objective tinnitus.

Otoscopy often reveals the foreign body or insect. Occasionally, an infection may produce pus or squamous debris which obscures the foreign body.

Initial investigations

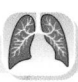

No investigation is generally required as the foreign body is diagnosed by direct vision.

Initial management

Syringing

Syringing is reserved for inorganic foreign bodies that do not completely occlude the ear canal. Organic foreign bodies will swell on contact with water, making removal difficult.

Surgical management

Microsuction

Removal of most foreign bodies, with the particular exception of lithium button batteries, need not be done urgently. Live insects should be killed first by instilling warm olive oil into the ear canal to drown the insect.

In most cases, removal under the operating microscope is possible with vacuum suction, wax hooks or fine 'crocodile' forceps. The choice of instrument is important as there is a risk of pushing foreign bodies deeper into the ear canal. In young children, general anaesthesia may be necessary to allow for removal.

Prognosis

In the majority, the foreign body is removed without any residual complications.

Acute otitis media

Acute otitis media or acute suppurative otitis media is an infection of the middle ear space characterized by pus in the middle ear.

Epidemiology

Acute otitis media is common in children, particularly after an upper respiratory tract infection. Incidence in the first year of life approaches 50 000 per 100 000, and remains high for the first 5 years of life. The incidence is marginally higher in boys, and episodes are more frequent in winter when upper respiratory tract infections are more common.

Recurrent episodes of acute otitis media occur in a minority of children. The risk of recurrent acute otitis media is highest in children who attend a nursery and have multiple siblings, allergies or parents who smoke.

Pathology

Upper respiratory tract infections cause hyperaemia and oedema of the respiratory mucosa of the middle ear and eustachian tube. An exudate forms in the middle ear space and negative middle ear pressures develop. This sucks an infected bolus of mucus from the nasopharynx into the middle ear via the eustachian tube. The most common causative organisms are *Streptococcus pneumoniae* and *Haemophilus influenzae*, which are nasopharyngeal commensals.

A purulent effusion develops and increases middle ear pressures. This increases pressure on the eardrum and produces rapidly escalating pain. In a third of cases, the bulging tympanic membrane then ruptures.

Scope of disease

Recurrent episodes of acute otitis media that result in repeated rupture of the tympanic membrane may produce a permanent perforation of the pars tensa. Although it does not usually lead to impaired hearing, it leaves the ear prone to chronic suppurative otitis media. Recurrent acute otitis media may produce hyaline degeneration of the collagen in tympanic membranes (tympanosclerosis). Calcification and ossification may then occur, leaving a white chalk-like plaque on the eardrum. This may affect the sound-conducting properties of the middle ear.

Mastoiditis is a rare consequence of untreated acute otitis media (p. 189). The facial nerve passes through a bony canal along the medial wall of the middle ear space. In some instances, this bony canal is dehiscent and acute otitis media results in inflammation of the facial nerve producing a facial palsy.

Clinical features

Children with acute otitis media usually present with severe ear pain. They may be irritable, tug at the ear, and have disturbed sleep. Fever is common and may be the only sign. As the eardrum bulges, pain reaches a crescendo. If the eardrum then ruptures, pus is seen at the external auditory meatus and the symptoms resolve quickly. Associated symptoms of an upper respiratory tract infection may be present with rhinorrhoea, coughing and vomiting.

Otoscopy is difficult in irritable and distressed children. Often it is only possible to obtain a glimpse of the eardrum. The eardrum will appear hyperaemic, bulging and featureless. If the eardrum has ruptured, there will be pus in the ear canal and this is occasionally misdiagnosed as otitis externa.

Initial management

Analgesia

Good analgesia is critical as the child will suffer significant earache. It is important to give the child a good dose at bedtime as pain is often worst at night. Non-steroidal anti-inflammatory drugs (NSAIDs) delivered per rectum often provide better analgesia in a vomiting child than paracetamol. The child should be kept well hydrated and in a well-humidified room.

Medical management

Antibiotic therapy

Whilst there may be clinical improvement or rapid resolution of symptoms with antibiotics, this is at a risk of increased vomiting, diarrhoea and rashes. A recent meta-analysis of six trials concluded that children under two with bilateral acute otitis media, and children with both acute otitis media and otorrhoea (ear discharge) benefit most from antibiotics.[1] In these groups, 4 children need to be treated to prevent an extended course of disease in one.

When antibiotics are indicated, amoxicillin is sufficient unless there is a high prevalence of β-lactamase microbes, when co-amoxiclav is a suitable first line agent. In cases of recurrent acute otitis media, daily low-dose antibiotics for 6–12 weeks may help break the cycle of re-infection.

Surgical management

Myringotomy and drainage

Patients who develop complications such as a facial nerve palsy or acute mastoiditis (without a subperiosteal abscess) require urgent myringotomy (incision of the eardrum) to drain the middle ear space. A ventilation tube or grommet may be inserted to ensure good middle ear ventilation. Routine myringotomy and drainage of pus from the middle ear in patients without complications is practised in the United States, but is not common in the United Kingdom.

Recurrent acute otitis media that has failed long-term low-dose antibiotic prophylaxis can be effectively treated with grommet insertion.

Prognosis

The outlook after a single episode of acute otitis media is excellent. In most cases, spontaneous resolution occurs regardless of whether the eardrum ruptures or antibiotics are prescribed. Surgery for the development of facial palsy as a complication has a favourable outcome, usually with complete resolution of facial weakness.

In all cases, there is a residual effusion in the middle ear that clears within 3 months. Children who suffer recurrent acute otitis media are prone to complications and may suffer tympanosclerosis (Fig. 3.21) or middle ear adhesions that affect hearing in the long term.

> **REFERENCES**
>
> (1) Rovers MM, Glasziou P, Appelman CL et al. *Antibiotics for acute otitis media: a meta-analysis with individual patient data.* Lancet 2006; 368: 1429–35.

Mastoiditis

Mastoiditis is infection of the mastoid air cells, often as a complication of untreated acute otitis media or chronic suppurative otitis media. Acute mastoiditis is rare in the age of antibiotics; however, masked mastoiditis is common.

Epidemiology

In Europe, the annual incidence of mastoiditis is 4 per 100 000 per year. Under half of all cases occur in infants.

Pathology

Infection of the middle ear invariably involves the mucosa of the mastoid air cells. Bacterial isolates from mastoiditis mirror those from cases of acute otitis media; however, pneumococci and β-haemolytic streptococci are more common. Infection extends into the bone of the mastoid process and destroys the bony trabeculae. A single cavity of infected pus is formed (so-called 'coalescent mastoiditis') and this may breach the cortex of the mastoid process to form a subperiosteal abscess.

Scope of disease

Life-threatening complications can occur if left untreated. Mastoid infection can spread to the brain, resulting in meningitis or cerebral abscess. Infection of the cerebral venous sinuses may lead to thrombosis.

Facial nerve involvement can result in facial paralysis, especially with tuberculous mastoiditis. A subperiosteal abscess may also track into the sheath of the sternocleidomastoid muscle and produce a neck abscess.

The inner ear is also at risk: purulent labyrinthitis may cause irreversible sensorineural hearing loss and damage the vestibular apparatus, thus affecting balance.

Clinical features

Otalgia (predominantly retro-auricular) and fever are the main features of acute mastoiditis. On examination, a retro-auricular swelling with protrusion of the pinna is seen and the mastoid process is tender to touch (Fig. 3.22).

Otoscopy is normal in approximately two-thirds. In a third, the eardrum may be injected, dull and bulging. Occasionally, there is gross oedema of the posterior canal wall and the tympanic membrane cannot be seen.

In addition to the features of mastoiditis, clinical features of meningitis (p. 616) or a cerebral abscess (p. 620) can occur due to intracranial extension of mastoiditis.

When antibiotics are used to treat acute otitis media suboptimally, 'masked' mastoiditis may develop. The classical picture is that of recurrent attacks of acute otitis media in which the ear does not return to normal between attacks. There is also earache behind the ear during attacks.

Initial investigations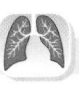

Investigations are not required for patients without any features of complications.

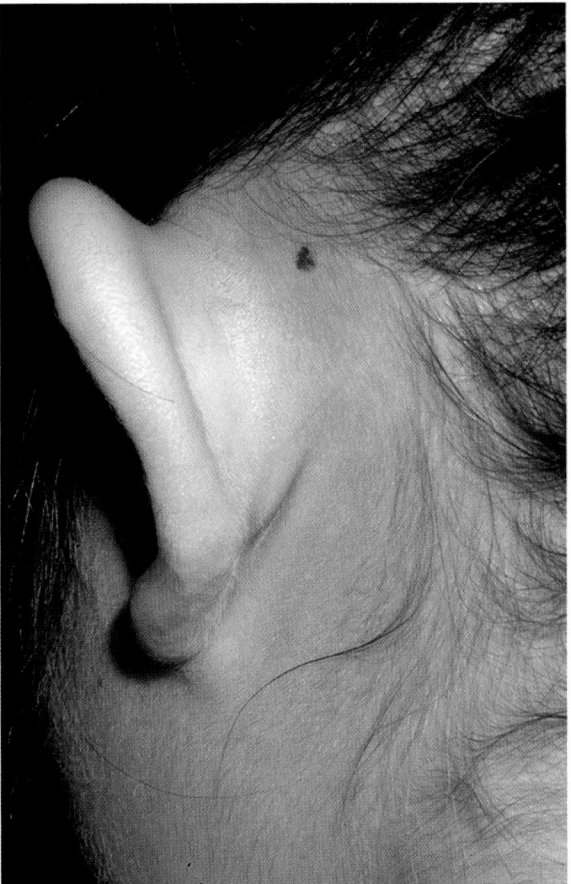

Fig. 3.22 Post-aural swelling. At presentation the eardrum was perforated, allowing drainage of mucopus from the middle ear.

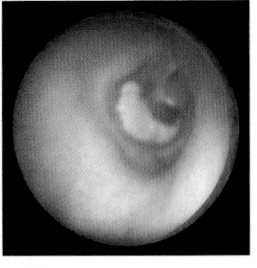

Fig. 3.21 Tympanosclerosis. Hyaline degeneration within the layers of the eardrum produces the white plaque. If tympanosclerosis is extensive, conductive hearing loss may occur.

Further investigations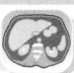

CT of the head

If there are clinical signs of intracranial infection, or failure to respond to 24 hours of intravenous antibiotics, a CT scan of the temporal bones and brain should be obtained. In infants, this may necessitate general anaesthesia.

Medical management

Antibiotics

All cases of mastoiditis require admission and treatment with intravenous antibiotics. A broad-spectrum antibiotic with good anaerobic cover is best.

Surgical management

Myringotomy

Myringotomy, with or without grommet insertion, may be used as an initial measure. This allows mucopus in the middle ear to drain and effectively ventilates the middle ear and mastoid air cell system.

Simple or cortical mastoidectomy

All cases of mastoiditis with a subperiosteal abscess warrant urgent drainage. This is achieved by removing the cortex of the bone of the mastoid process.

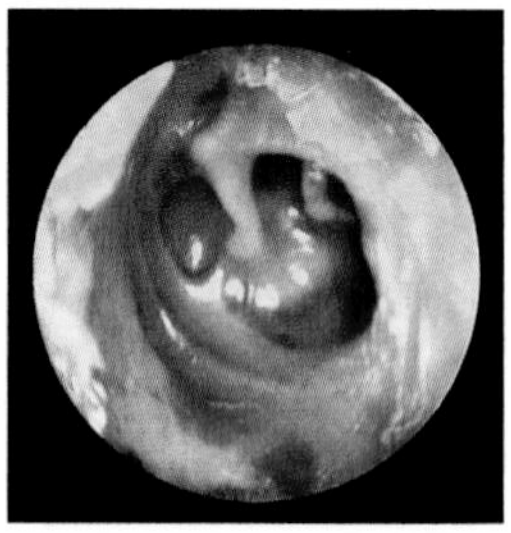

Prognosis

The majority of patients with early disease experience resolution with antibiotics. In patients who require surgical drainage, results are often excellent with complete recovery of hearing. Recurrent mastoiditis in cases following surgical drainage is rare.

Fig. 3.23 Retraction pockets of the pars tensa of the left eardrum. Here the drum is draped over the ossicles.

Otitis media with effusion

Otitis media with effusion (OME), better known as 'glue ear', is characterized by the presence of sterile, thick and tenacious fluid in the middle ear space. It is considered chronic if the fluid is present for more than 12 weeks.

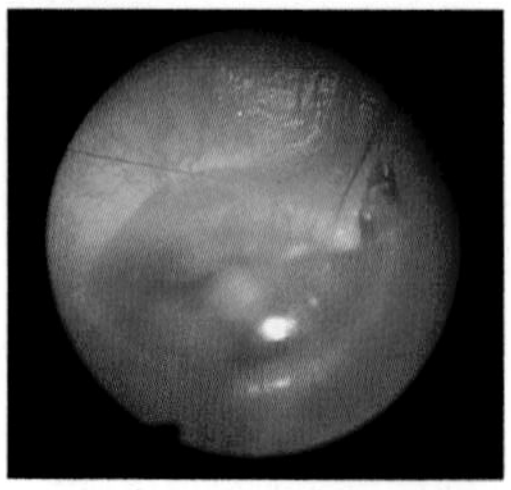

Epidemiology

Otitis media with effusion is very common in Western countries. Between the ages of 18 months and 6 years, the prevalence of chronic middle ear effusions is 20 000 per 100 000 in the UK. The prevalence decreases with age to 6000 per 100 000 at 8 years of age and 2000 per 100 000 by the age of 12. Otitis media with effusion is rare in adults.

Pathology

The pathogenesis of otitis media with effusion is incompletely understood. In children, the most popular theory is underventilation of the middle ear space (due to poor eustachian tube function) with negative middle ear pressure allowing a transudate to form. Adenoidal hypertrophy may worsen eustachian tube function and predispose to chronic middle ear effusions. Other contributing factors include exposure to other children, allergy, impaired immune defences and unresolved acute otitis media. The pathogenesis in adults is probably different: predisposing factors include post-nasal tumours, radiation of the head and neck, barotrauma and AIDS.

In addition to the accumulation of thick fluid in the middle ear, metaplasia occurs in the respiratory mucosa of the middle ear and mastoid air cells. Cuboidal mucosa is replaced by pseudostratified mucus-secreting mucosa, rich with goblet cells. Ciliary function appears to be less effective. The effusion contains all types of inflammatory cells, and bacteria are isolated in approximately 20% of patients.

Scope of disease

Complications associated with chronic middle ear effusions are uncommon. They include thinning and collapse of the eardrum into the middle ear (atelectasis), retraction pockets of the drum (Fig. 3.23), erosion of ossicles and recurrent acute otitis media (p. 188).

Undiagnosed hearing loss in children with otitis media with effusion may result in impairment of speech, language and cognitive development, and behavioural difficulties. The child may appear uninterested in his or her environment and is described as a 'silent child'.

Clinical features

Children with otitis media with effusion suffer hearing loss that may be covert or manifest. Parents may report that they are inattentive or repetitively question instructions. Perceptive teachers may pick up this inattention in the classroom.

Otalgia is often less dramatic. The child may pull at his or her ear, or occasionally insert foreign bodies into the ear.

On otoscopy, the eardrum appears featureless, dull and immobile. Often, prominent radial vessels are noted (Fig. 3.24). Occasionally, air bubbles in the middle ear may be seen through the eardrum.

 CLINICAL ALERT

Unilateral otitis media with effusion in an adult may be an early feature of nasopharyngeal carcinoma (see p. 225).

Fig. 3.24 Otitis media with effusion or 'glue ear' in the left ear.

Initial investigations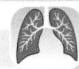

Audiometry

Audiometry often reveals a mild conductive hearing loss in excess of 20 dB, which is more significant in the low tones.

Tympanometry

Tympanometry is an easy and effective way of demonstrating middle ear effusions (see Fig. 3.13a).

Initial management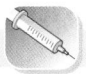

Patient education

There is no evidence to substantiate the use of antibiotics, decongestants, mucolytics, antihistamines or steroids in the treatment of glue ear. Any resolution of glue with these drugs appears to be short-lived.

In children under 3 years of age with persistent bilateral effusions, thresholds better than 25 dB and no obvious consequence for development, there are strong grounds for the adoption of a watchful waiting approach, and reassurance is required for the parents. In children over 3 years of age, or in those with adverse development consequences or losses of more than 25 dB, referral to a specialist is necessary.

Auto-inflation of the eustachian tube

Auto-inflation of the eustachian tube with an Otovent balloon has been shown to produce short-term improvement in older children who are able to use this device.

Surgical management

Insertion of ventilation tubes

Surgical treatment of bilateral effusions comprises the insertion of ventilation tubes or grommets (Figs 3.25 and 3.26).

Adenoidectomy

In children with gross upper airway obstruction, adenoidectomy to improve eustachian tube function or possibly remove a sump of infection is advisable.

Prognosis

The outcome following treatment of glue ear is good. Unfortunately, half of all those treated with ventilation tubes will require re-insertion. Speech or developmental delay often corrects itself quickly.

> *i* **FURTHER INFORMATION**
>
> Diagnosis and management of childhood otitis media in primary care: A national clinical guideline. Scottish Intercollegiate Guideline Network. www.sign.ac.uk

Chronic suppurative otitis media

Chronic suppurative otitis media (CSOM) is characterized by a chronic discharging middle ear cleft. By implication, there is a defect in the eardrum, either a perforation or a 'retraction pocket' which allows mucopurulent discharge to leak into the ear canal. This discharge may be persistent or episodic (active chronic suppurative otitis media) or cease altogether, leaving a stable 'burnt out' condition (inactive chronic suppurative otitis media).

A simple (but inaccurate) subdivision is into cases with or without cholesteatoma. A cholesteatoma is the term given to a 'skin bag' of keratinizing squamous epithelium in the middle ear. It contains osteolytic enzymes that can erode bone. This is therefore a destructive entity and has earned its description as 'unsafe' chronic suppurative otitis

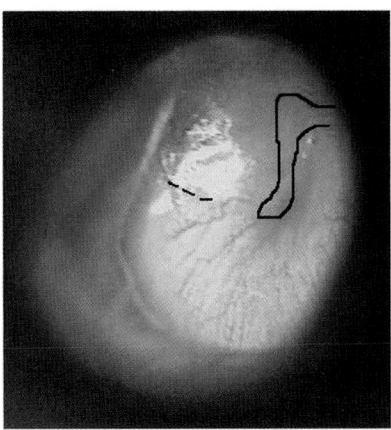

(a)

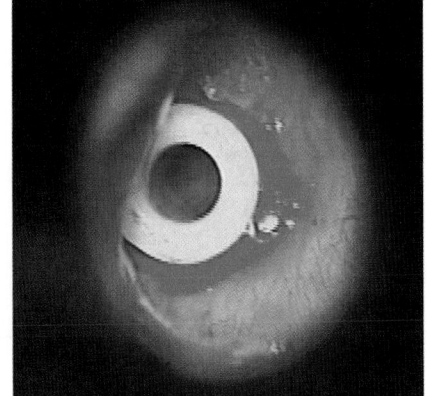

(b)

Fig. 3.25 Grommet insertion. (a) An otoscopic view of the left eardrum showing dilated radial vessels in keeping with OME. The malleus is outlined for orientation. A radial 'myringotomy' is made (dotted line) and the grommet inserted (b).

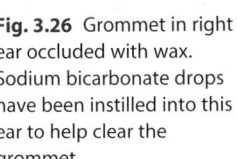

Fig. 3.26 Grommet in right ear occluded with wax. Sodium bicarbonate drops have been instilled into this ear to help clear the grommet.

media. A more accurate international classification system is presented in Table 3.3.

Epidemiology

The overall prevalence in the United Kingdom of healed, inactive and active otitis media is 12 000, 2600 and 1500 per 100 000 respectively. In practice, half of all active cases are associated with cholesteatoma. Despite improvements in health care, the incidence has not lessened in recent years. There is, however, a clear association between lower socio-economic status and the prevalence of this condition. The prevalence is high amongst indigenous peoples, such as the Maoris in New Zealand. It has an equal incidence in both sexes.

Pathology

The aetiology of chronic suppurative otitis media is multi-factorial. There is an important role for bacterial infection, previous otitis media, upper respiratory tract infection, eustachian tube dysfunction, autoimmunity, allergy, genetics and environmental factors.

There are a number of theories for the pathogenesis of a cholesteatoma. A cholesteatoma may form from negative middle ear pressures (creating a narrow-necked attic retraction pocket), or squamous epithelium may invade the middle ear following perforation of the eardrum, or there may be squamous metaplasia of the middle ear mucosa in response to otitis media with effusion.

Bacteria are isolated from the middle ear in all patients with active suppurative otitis media and up to 50% of patients with inactive chronic suppurative otitis media. Although a variety of organisms may be isolated, the Gram-negative 'bowel-type' flora predominates. There is no difference in the pathogens seen in patients with or without cholesteatoma.

Scope of disease

The subdivision of chronic suppurative otitis media into 'safe' or 'unsafe' due to the presence of a cholesteatoma is misleading as complications can occur in all varieties. As with all cases of middle ear suppuration, spread of infection to the inner ear, facial nerve canal, brain and cerebral venous sinuses may occur. Spread of infection to the labyrinth may cause suppurative labyrinthitis, whilst spread to the cochlea can produce sensorineural deafness (in addition to any conductive loss). Facial palsy is common in patients with a dehiscent facial canal and, occasionally, recurrent meningitis results from (unrecognized) chronic suppurative otitis media.

Cholesteatoma has the propensity to erode bone, and erosion of the ossicles will cause conductive hearing loss. Erosion into the semicircular canals of the labyrinth may create a 'perilymph fistula' resulting in severe vertigo.

Clinical features

Patients with chronic suppurative otitis media often (but not invariably) present with a discharging ear. The effluent is often mucoid and described as foul or offensive. In some cases, the discharge is minimal but otological symptoms predominate (hearing loss, aural fullness, tinnitus or episodic vertigo). Pain is unusual.

On otoscopy, the ear canal will be full of mucopus in patients with active disease. Simple dry-mopping will fail to clear the discharge. Suction clearance under the microscope allows visualization of any defect in the eardrum. Perforations may vary in size from pinhole defects to complete loss of the pars tensa (subtotal perforations). They may be centrally located or marginal. The middle ear mucosa may be dry and healthy in inactive cases or moist and oedematous. In severe cases, a polyp may arise from middle ear mucosa and protrude through the defect in the eardrum. Persistent discharge may cause granulation tissue to form in the deep portion of the external ear canal.

Cholesteatoma may be visible in some cases, but often its presence has to be inferred from other clinical features such as erosion of the bony attic with the presence of offensive squamous epithelial debris.

Clinical testing with a tuning fork will reveal a hearing loss that is often purely conductive in nature. In cases

Table 3.3	Classification of chronic suppurative otitis media
Subtype	**Features**
Healed otitis media	Eardrum is intact, but scarred, thickened or tympanosclerotic. Classically, a healed perforation appears as a 'transparent scar'. There is no discharge. Any hearing loss is due to disruption or fixation of the ossicles
Active mucosal chronic otitis media ('wet perforation')	Permanent defect in the pars tensa of the eardrum, with oedematous middle ear. There is a discharge of mucus or mucopus. Granulation tissue or polyps may develop
Inactive mucosal chronic otitis media ('dry perforation'; see Fig. 3.27)	Permanent defect in the pars tensa of the eardrum, with normal middle ear mucosa. No discharge
Active squamous epithelial chronic otitis media ('cholesteatoma'; see Fig. 3.28)	In addition to active mucosal disease, there is a squamous epithelium lined pocket filled with epithelial cells and debris. The defect is often in the pars flaccida. Discharge is characteristically offensive
Inactive squamous epithelial chronic otitis media ('retraction pocket')	A 'retraction pocket' is present in the eardrum. There is no accumulation of epithelial cells or debris, and no discharge. Middle ear mucosa is normal

where chronic suppuration has been untreated, the patient may have a superadded sensorineural loss.

Features of complications or coexistent upper respiratory tract infections may also be present. A frequent association is with chronic infective rhinosinusitis.

Initial investigations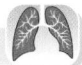

Microbiological swab
A swab of the discharge should be sent for microscopy and culture in an attempt to isolate an organism.

Initial management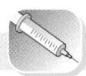

Oral antibiotics
A swab for bacteriological analysis should precede treatment with topical and oral antibiotics in primary care. Antibiotic treatment may occasionally render a discharging ear inactive.

Patient education
Patients should be warned against allowing water to enter their ears. This entails abstaining from swimming and the use of cotton wool balls, smeared with petroleum jelly, placed in the ears when bathing or showering. A variety of watertight ear plugs may be used.

Surgical management

Suction clearance
In ENT clinics, suction clearance of mucopus and examination for any perforations, retraction pockets, polyps, granu-

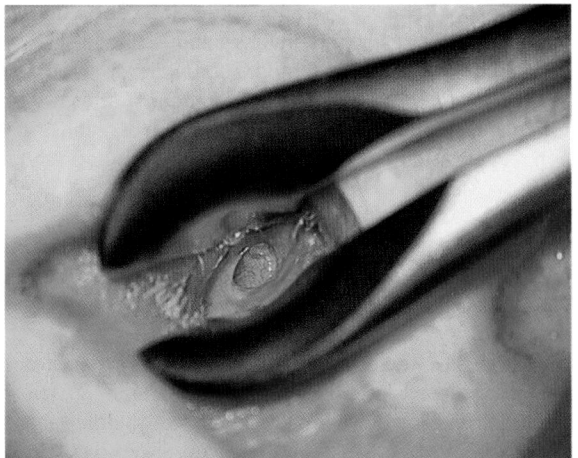

Fig. 3.27 A dry perforation of the right eardrum seen through an aural speculum prior to surgical repair (myringoplasty).

lations and cholesteatoma may be performed. Any dry perforations (Fig. 3.27) or stable retraction pockets may simply be observed in clinic with regular follow-up.

Combination treatment
Polyps and granulation tissue often respond to a steroid, antibacterial and antifungal ointment (e.g. Tri-Adcortyl, which contains triamcinolone, gramicidin, neomycin and nystatin). Gentle chemical cauterization with silver nitrate is sometimes undertaken.

Middle ear surgery
In active cases with cholesteatoma (Fig. 3.28) or persistently wet perforations, surgery is necessary.

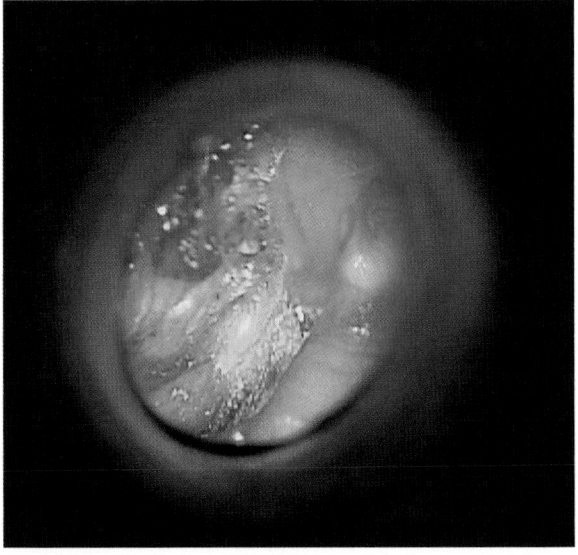

(a)

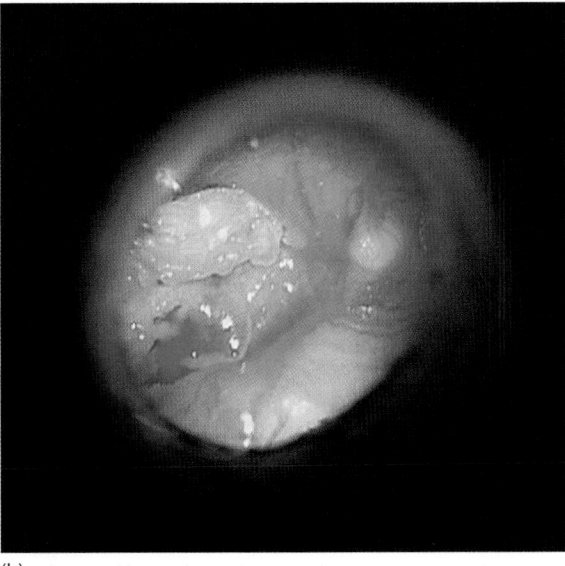

(b)

Fig. 3.28a, b A right ear posterior superior quadrant cholesteatoma. Often the cholesteatoma is obscured by a small piece of wax (a), removed to reveal the underlying keratin of cholesteatoma (b).

Myringoplasty is an operation to repair a perforation of the eardrum. Usually this involves harvesting fascia or perichondrium from the temporalis muscle or tragus of the ear respectively to graft the perforation. In cases where ossicular disruption has occurred, some form of reconstruction may be attempted (tympanoplasty or ossiculoplasty).

Mastoid exploration

When cholesteatoma is present, it is necessary to explore the middle ear and mastoid cavity to rid the ear of disease. Various surgical approaches to achieve this have been described.

Historically, the mastoid cavity is approached from behind the ear (post-aural approach) and the posterior canal wall is 'taken down'. The ossicles of the middle ear are often affected by disease and have to be removed. In a radical mastoidectomy, all the ossicles are removed and the eustachian tube orifice left exposed. In a modified radical mastoidectomy, some ossicles are left or only partially removed, and the middle ear is sealed.

This operation leaves the patient with a large defect in the posterior ear canal wall that communicates with the surgically created mastoid cavity. This has lifelong implications in terms of continuing ENT care for the patient, as regular microscopic suction clearance of wax and debris from the ear canal and 'mastoid bowl' is necessary.

RECENT ADVANCES

Combined approach tympanoplasty is an operation that approaches the middle ear and mastoid without disrupting the posterior canal wall. Although this operation leaves the patient with a normal external ear canal, it does not allow recurrent or residual cholesteatoma to be easily visualized in clinic. This approach, therefore, necessitates a 'second look' procedure to ensure that the middle ear is free of disease.

Prognosis

Frequently, simple medical treatment and, thereafter, adequate water precautions will render chronic suppurative otitis media inactive.

Otitis externa

Infection of the ear canal skin or external ear is known as otitis externa. The middle ear space is free from involvement.

Epidemiology

Otitis externa is a common presenting complaint. It usually occurs in younger age groups and equally in both sexes.

Pathology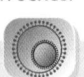

Otitis externa is often caused by a bacterial infection of the ear canal skin by staphylococci and *Pseudomonas* species.

Fungal otitis externa (*Candida* and *Aspergillus*) is frequently seen following long-term and ineffective treatment of simple bacterial otitis externa with topical antibiotic drops.

Predisposing factors to external ear infection are underlying skin conditions such as eczema, mild abrasions (inflicted with a cotton bud or fingernail) which permit infection with bacteria or fungi, and warm moist conditions such as those encountered on sun, sand and sea holidays. Otitis externa may also result from a middle ear infection discharging through a perforated eardrum into the ear canal.

Scope of disease

Otitis externa may spread to the pinna and cause an intense perichondritis. If this is left unchecked, destruction of cartilage may result in significant disfigurement of the pinna. Infrequently, infection may spread to the face and produce facial cellulitis.

In diabetic or other immunocompromised patients, otitis externa may spread and cause a skull base osteomyelitis ('malignant' otitis externa). Typically, patients complain of a severe headache and exhibit cranial nerve palsies. Cranial nerve VI may be affected, leading to lateral rectus palsy (Gradenigo's syndrome). Alternatively, the facial and last four cranial nerves may be affected.

Clinical features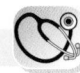

Typically, an episode of otitis externa begins with itching or irritation of the ears which builds up to severe pain. Itching is often severe in fungal cases. The patient may report a discharge or simply a moist ear canal. As the infection progresses, the ear canal becomes blocked and a mild conductive hearing loss develops.

On examination, the pinna and tragus are tender on gentle movement. The external meatus and pinna may be inflamed with evidence of a discharge (Fig. 3.29). A reactive post-aural lymph node may cause post-aural tenderness

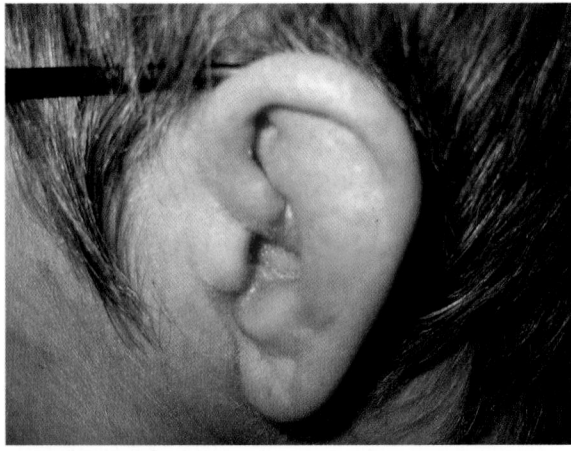

Fig. 3.29 Otitis externa of the ear with creamy discharge and inflamed ear canal skin.

over the mastoid process which can mimic acute mastoiditis. Otoscopy may be painful or simply impossible due to the pain. If the ear canal is swollen, the tympanic membrane may be obscured (Fig. 3.30). The canal skin is usually thickened and inflamed, and there is a scanty, creamy discharge. There are no mucous glands in the ear canal and therefore discharge is classically not mucoid. In fungal infections, hyphae or spores may be seen, aiding diagnosis.

Initial investigations

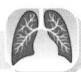

Ear swab

A swab for microbiological analysis should always be taken, as the results may guide further antibiotic therapy if there is no response to initial empirical treatment.

Initial management

Analgesia

It is important to provide patients with adequate analgesia as the pain from otitis externa may be severe. A non-steroidal anti-inflammatory drug (NSAID) is often necessary.

Antibiotics

There is a range of topical antibiotic drops available. Most of these preparations are combined with steroids. Aminoglycoside drops, such as gentamicin and framycetin, should only be used with caution in patients with eardrum perforations due to the increased risk of ototoxicity.

Topical antibiotic treatment should be used for one week before further assessment. There is little evidence to support the use of oral antibiotics in uncomplicated otitis externa.

Surgical management

Aural toilet

In severe cases of otitis externa, where there is a considerable amount of debris or discharge in the ear canal, dry-mopping or suction clearance using an operating microscope is necessary. This is known as aural toilet. In cases where the ear canal is severely oedematous, a wick soaked in ichthammol and glycerin or an otowick (Fig. 3.31) should be inserted. This allows for a quick resolution to the infection and should be removed after 2–3 days.

Petrosectomy

In cases of malignant otitis externa that fail to respond to medical treatment, surgical debridement of osteomyelitic bone is vital. This usually involves extensive skull base surgery to remove parts of the petrous temporal bone.

Prognosis

The prognosis of uncomplicated otitis externa is good. However, if the predisposing factors are not addressed, e.g. eczema or cotton bud abuse, the risk of developing recurrent or chronic infections is high. Malignant otitis externa has a 50% mortality rate.

Otitis externa

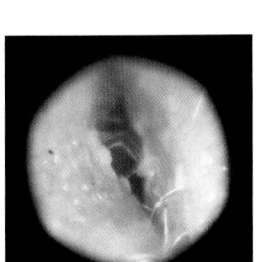

Fig. 3.30 Otoscopic view of otitis externa. Oedema of the ear canal obscures the tympanic membrane.

SECTION 3.5   Hearing aids

Hearing aids are small devices which selectively amplify sounds. They are ideal for conductive hearing losses where the inner ear is intact and functioning normally. In general, patients with chronic but stable middle ear diseases or otosclerosis derive more benefit from aids than patients with sensorineural hearing loss.

A hearing aid consists of a microphone which picks up sound, an amplifier which makes the sound louder, a receiver which transmits sound into the ear canal, and a mould which sits snugly in the conchal bowl and outer ear canal. The amplifier processes sound in a variety of ways. Hearing aids with linear processing systems amplify input sound by a set ratio. Non-linear processing systems are more sophisticated and the ratio of amplification varies according to input sound intensity and frequency.

Conventional hearing aids convert incoming sound into a continuously varying electrical signal. This is known as analogue signal processing. Recently, digital hearing aids have been introduced. This simply means that input sound is converted into a series of electronic impulses which can have one of two (binary) values: 0 or 1. This digital information may be manipulated in a variety of ways, which gives these aids more flexibility.

The common limitation of hearing aids is the amplification of background noise. This noise is often low-frequency and therefore poses a problem for people with good low-frequency but poor high-frequency hearing (e.g. presbyacusis). Some patients with sensorineural hearing loss are exquisitely sensitive to loud noise (a phenomenon known as 'recruiting'). This makes it difficult for them to derive optimum benefit from hearing aids.

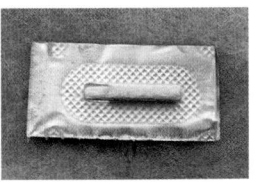

Fig. 3.31 An otowick keeps an oedematous ear canal patent, allowing topical antibiotic drops to penetrate deep into the ear canal.

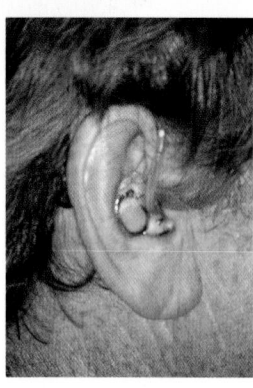

Fig. 3.32 Behind-the-ear hearing aid. The aid is connected to the mould which sits in the ear canal.

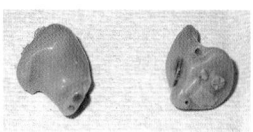

Fig. 3.33 In-the-ear (ITE) aids are cosmetically more acceptable, but less powerful.

Behind-the-ear hearing aid

Behind-the-ear hearing aids are the most commonly used type. They are powerful and rest behind the ear. Some people find them cosmetically displeasing. Figure 3.32 shows a new digital behind-the-ear hearing aid. Adjusting the setting of the aid requires some manual dexterity and may be a challenge for the arthritic elderly patient.

Body-worn hearing aid

Body-worn aids are powerful aids which are suitable for patients with severe to profound hearing loss with poor manipulative skills.

In-the-ear or in-the-canal hearing aids

These aids are more cosmetically acceptable and sit within the ear canal. They are expensive and not suitable for people with significant hearing losses. Figure 3.33 shows typical in-the-ear devices.

Bone-anchored hearing aids

Bone-anchored hearing aids are fixed by means of a titanium abutment onto the skull. This titanium screw is fitted surgically and undergoes 'osseointegration'. The aid is clipped onto the titanium screw and sound vibration is transmitted to the cochlea through bone. Bone-anchored hearing aids are suitable for patients with congenital external ear deformities (pinna or canal atresia) or discharging ears.

The nose

SECTION 3.6   Introduction

Applied basic sciences of the nose

The external nose

The shape of the external nose displays rich ethnic and racial diversity. In Figure 3.34, the different parts of the nose are named. The skeleton of the nose is made up of paired nasal bones in the upper part, and two paired cartilages in the lower part (Fig. 3.35). The skeleton of the nose gives it its shape, and there are several muscles attached to the nose that allow for movement and flaring of the nostrils.

The nasal cavity

The cavity of the nose extends from the nostrils towards the posterior nasal aperture or choanae. The floor of the nasal cavity runs directly backwards in a horizontal direction (Fig. 3.36). This is often forgotten when attempts are made to pack the nose to arrest bleeding. The nasal cavity is divided into two parts by the midline nasal septum.

The lateral wall of the nose has three projecting shelves of bone which are covered by highly vascular erectile tissue. These structures are called turbinates; they serve to warm and humidify inhaled air. Below each turbinate is a cleft or meatus. The sinuses and the nasolacrimal duct drain into the meati.

The nasal cavity is lined by two types of epithelium, olfactory and respiratory. Olfactory epithelium occupies the superior part of the nasal cavity and detects odours. It is non-ciliated and comprises bipolar cells. The axons of these cells combine to form olfactory nerve fibres that pass through the cribriform plate of the skull towards the brain. The respiratory epithelium is pseudostratified ciliated columnar epithelium, which is similar to the mucosa of the trachea and bronchus. Its submucosa contains mucus-secreting glands.

The nasal septum

The nasal septum is a wall that partitions the nasal cavity into two equal halves. It is made up of two bones posteriorly: the vomer of the sphenoid and the perpendicular plate of the ethmoid. Anteriorly it is made up of hyaline cartilage (quadrilateral cartilage).

The paranasal sinuses

The sinuses are bony cavities within the skull that communicate with the nasal cavity. They are formed as diverticula from the nasal cavity and therefore share the respiratory epithelial lining of the nose. The sinuses consist of paired frontal, maxillary and sphenoid sinuses. There is a labyrinth of small sinuses between the eyes called the ethmoid sinuses; these are divided into an anterior and posterior group.

All sinuses except the frontal sinuses are present at birth. The frontal sinuses start to develop from the age of 6 onwards. In children the ethmoid sinuses are the largest, but as the facial skeleton matures the maxillary sinuses attain the greatest size.

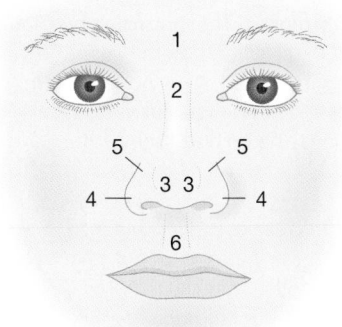
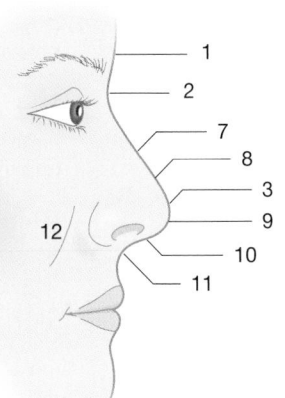

Fig. 3.34 Surface anatomy of the frontal and lateral views of the nose. 1, Glabella; 2, nasion; 3, tip-defining points; 4, alar side-wall; 5, supra-alar crease; 6, philtrum; 7, rhinion (osseocartilaginous junction); 8, supratip; 9, infratip lobule; 10, columella; 11, columella–labial angle or junction; 12, alar-facial groove or junction.

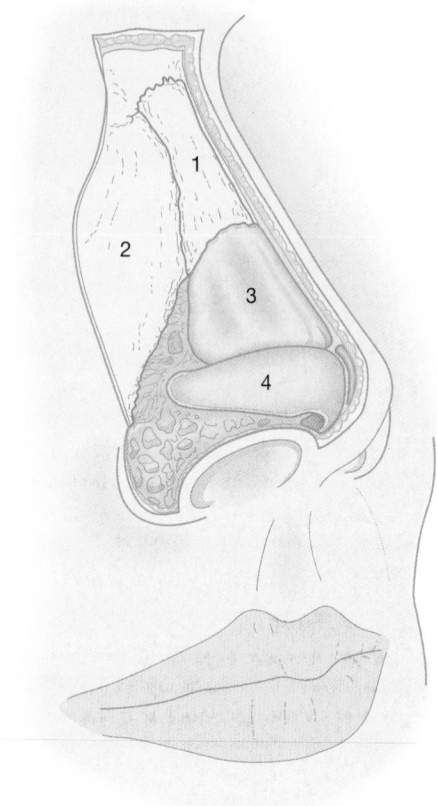

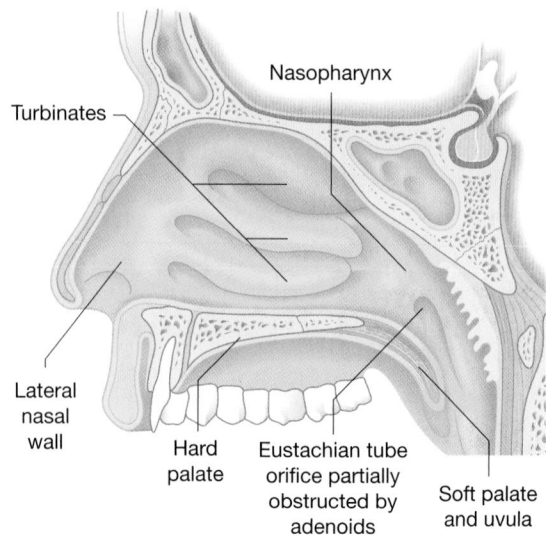

Fig. 3.36 The nasal cavity and lateral wall of nose.

Fig. 3.35 The nasal skeleton is made up of the nasal bones (1), ascending process of the maxilla (2), upper lateral cartilages (3) and the lower lateral cartilages (4).

The ethmoid sinuses lie adjacent to the orbit and are separated by a thin plate of bone called the lamina papyracea. This is a weak barrier to infection spreading from the sinuses into the orbit (orbital cellulitis). The skull base lies just superior to the ethmoid sinuses and this must be borne in mind when operating on these sinuses. The sphenoid sinus lies anterior to the pituitary gland; and allows for surgical access to the gland for excision (i.e. transsphenoidal hypophysectomy).

The nasopharynx

The nasopharynx is the uppermost part of the pharynx that opens anteriorly into the nasal cavity. In the young child it contains the adenoids, comprised of lymphoid tissue. As the child matures, the adenoids involute. The eustachian tubes open into the lateral wall of the nasopharynx. Adenoidal hypertrophy may obstruct the orifices of the eustachian tubes and impair eustachian tube function and middle ear ventilation.

Blood supply

The nose and sinuses have a rich blood supply. They are supplied by both the internal and external carotid arteries. Crudely, the internal carotid artery is said to supply the nasal cavity above the level of the middle turbinate and the external carotid to supply the nose below this level.

In the front part of the nose, the nasal mucosa of the anterior septum receives a rich supply by a plexus of vessels that anastomose in this area. The plexus is called *Kiesselbach's plexus*, and the area is often described as *Little's area*. Most nosebleeds, particularly in children, originate from this area.

Symptoms of diseases of the nose

All patients with nasal symptoms should be asked about precipitating or exacerbating factors and seasonal variation. This may identify patients with allergy-related conditions. Unilateral nasal symptoms, particularly unilateral discharge, should raise concerns about a foreign body or sinonasal tumour.

Nasal congestion or blockage

Persistent unilateral nasal congestion may due to anatomical deformity such as a deviated septum, a foreign body, a large antrochoanal polyp or a sinonasal tumour. Rhinitis produces bilateral symptoms. The normal physiological nasal cycle means that nasal airway patency varies between right and left nasal cavities every 4–12 hours. A primitive nasal reflex also causes the nasal airway to decongest in the upper nasal cavity when lying on one's side.

Rhinorrhoea

Nasal discharge may be clear or mucopurulent. To assess severity, it is useful to ask patients about the need to carry tissues. Beware of the 'gin-clear' nasal discharge, which may indicate a leak of cerebrospinal fluid into the nose, either spontaneously or due to pathology of the skull base.

Post-nasal drip

Post-nasal drip is a constant flow of mucus from the nasal cavity and paranasal sinuses into the nasopharynx. It may cause throat irritation and a chronic cough with resultant laryngitis.

Sneezing or itching

Sneezing is a reflex response to nasal irritation. It occurs commonly when irritative substances are inhaled (pepper) or in disease states such as the common cold. Persistent bouts of sneezing or nasal itching with lacrimation are the hallmark of allergic rhinitis, which may be seasonal or perennial.

Anosmia or hyposmia

Loss of smell may be complete (anosmia) or partial (hyposmia). This loss may be conductive if thickened nasal mucosa or nasal deformity prevents odours from reaching the olfactory neuroepithelium in the vault of the nose. Fractures of the skull base may shear the olfactory nerves as they pass through the cribriform plate and cause 'sensory' anosmia. More commonly, these nerves are destroyed by neuropathic 'cold' viruses, leaving patients anosmic following a bad cold.

Cacosmia

Cacosmia refers to a bad smell sensed by the patient. This is due to malodorous infected mucus retained in the sinuses.

Sinofacial pain

Pain on the forehead, between the eyes and over the cheek may be caused by sinus inflammation. Characteristically, this pain increases with stooping, atmospheric pressure changes on descent in an aircraft, and nose blowing. The differential diagnosis of facial pain includes neurological entities such as cluster headaches, migraine and trigeminal neuralgia.

Examination of the nose

Examination of the nose requires a head-mirror with light source, a Thudicum's nasal speculum, a Lacks oral speculum and a range of fibreoptic endoscopes or Hopkin's rods (Fig. 3.37).

Inspection

Examination should begin with a careful examination of the external nose. This is particularly important in patients requesting cosmetic nasal surgery or rhinoplasty. Start by looking at the nose from the front, paying attention to the 'facial aesthetic lines' that run from the eyebrow, along the side of the nose, towards the edge of the nostrils. Any deformity of this smooth curved line may be in the upper, middle or lower third of the nose. The nose is then viewed from above, below and the sides to assess its profile, projection and tip appearance. The skin is then assessed

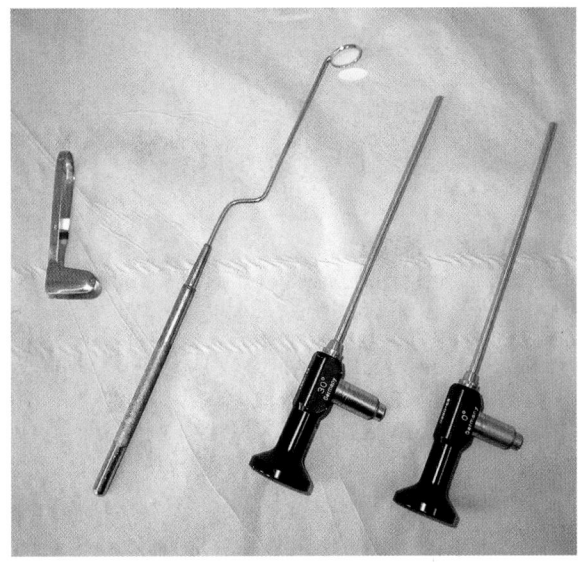
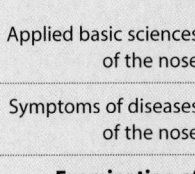

Fig. 3.37 Instruments for examining the nose (from left to right): Thudicum's speculum, post-nasal mirror and rigid fibreoptic scopes.

Applied basic sciences
of the nose

Symptoms of diseases
of the nose

**Examination of
the nose**

for thickness and scars. Running a finger along the nose allows the examiner to further appreciate deformities of the nasal skeleton.

Rhinoscopy

Rhinoscopy is examination of the internal nasal cavity. Begin with assessing nasal patency by holding a cold speculum against the nostrils and observing the misting pattern. In children, a wisp of cotton wool may be held against the nostril to detect airflow.

Examination of the anterior nasal cavity (anterior rhinoscopy) is performed with a Thudicum's nasal speculum. An appropriately sized speculum is inserted just into the nostrils and offers a good view of the anterior nasal septum, inferior and middle turbinates (Fig. 3.38). The rest of the nasal cavity is best examined with a fibreoptic endoscope. The rigid scopes vary in diameter between 2.7 and 4.0 mm and may have an angled view ranging from 30 to 120 degrees. In patients with a deviated nasal septum, rigid nasendoscopy may be impossible and a lubricated flexible scope may prove useful.

Children often fear anterior rhinoscopy with a pair of Thudicum's. Some clinicians simply lift the nasal tip with a thumb to obtain a good view. Alternatively an otoscope can be used.

Before the advent of fibreoptics, the post-nasal space was examined with a post-nasal space mirror. This mirror is warmed and introduced into the oropharynx facing upwards, whilst the tongue is depressed. In experienced hands and cooperative patients, this method offers a good view of the adenoids, eustachian tube cushions and any other post-nasal mass.

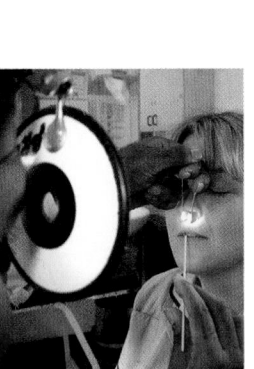

Fig. 3.38 Anterior rhinoscopy. The speculum is held in the non-dominant left hand leaving the right hand free to use other instruments.

Investigations for nose disease

Rhinomanometry

Rhinomanometry is an objective measure of nasal airway resistance. By measuring nasal airflow and pressure at the nostrils, nasal airway resistance may be calculated. Acoustic rhinomanometry uses sound waves to give a topographical picture of the nasal airway. These tools are largely research tools; they give an accurate objective measure of nasal airway narrowing due to mucosal thickening or septal deformity.

Smell tests

The University of Pennsylvania Smell Identification Test (UPSIT) is a simple 'scratch and sniff' card test of 40 questions. Patients are given four options to choose from to identify the odour. They are forced to guess if they are unable to detect a smell. This test usefully identifies malingerers, who score 0/40. Truly anosmic patients, who are forced to guess, will get some answers right by pure chance!

A simple modification of this test is the nez du vin test which is used by professional wine tasters. Patients have to identify six different odours.

Immunological investigations

Skin-prick testing

Skin-prick testing is a quick and inexpensive test for identifying allergies in clinic. The active components of most airborne allergens are isolated and mixed with glycerin. Droplets of these solutions are then placed on the volar aspect of the forearm and the skin is pricked with a lancet through the droplets. One of these solutions is histamine, which acts as a positive control; the other is normal saline, which is a negative control (Fig. 3.39).

A positive result is one where a wheal develops measuring more than 3 mm in diameter than that produced by normal saline. Tests where a wheal does not develop in response to histamine (positive control) cannot be interpreted. This commonly occurs in patients taking oral antihistamine. Finally, significant wheals developing to the negative control raises the possibility of dermatographism or a related dermatological condition.

Radio-allergo-sorbent test (RAST)

The RAST is a simple blood test that detects the level of circulating specific IgE in a patient's serum. A sample of serum is taken and mixed with the various antigens. Specific IgEs then bind to the related antigen and form a complex. This antigen–antibody complex may then be detected by adding radiolabelled anti-IgE antibodies.

Both skin-prick testing and RAST fail to identify some patients with allergic rhinitis. This is explained by the concept of 'local' allergy in which there is no systemic manifestation of the allergy in the form of circulating or dermal IgE. These patients are sometimes referred to as non-atopic allergic rhinitis sufferers.

Investigations of mucociliary clearance

The cilia of the respiratory epithelium of the nose beat rhythmically to sweep surface mucus back to the pharynx. This mucociliary clearance may be deficient or absent in a variety of conditions such as cystic fibrosis, where mucus is thick and tenacious, or primary ciliary dyskinesia (PCD) where ciliary function is impaired. A simple way of testing this is the saccharin test. A fragment of saccharin is placed on the anterior end of the inferior turbinate. In normal subjects, saccharin is tasted within 20 minutes as mucociliary clearance transports the saccharin to the pharynx. Alternatively, a brush biopsy of the turbinates may harvest some ciliated epithelium. The ciliary action may be observed with phase contrast microscopy.

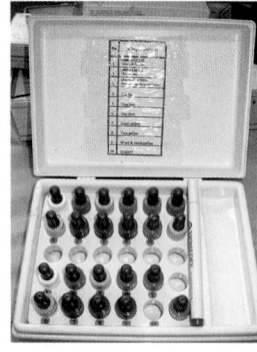

Fig. 3.39 A standard skin prick testing kit for common aero-allergens.

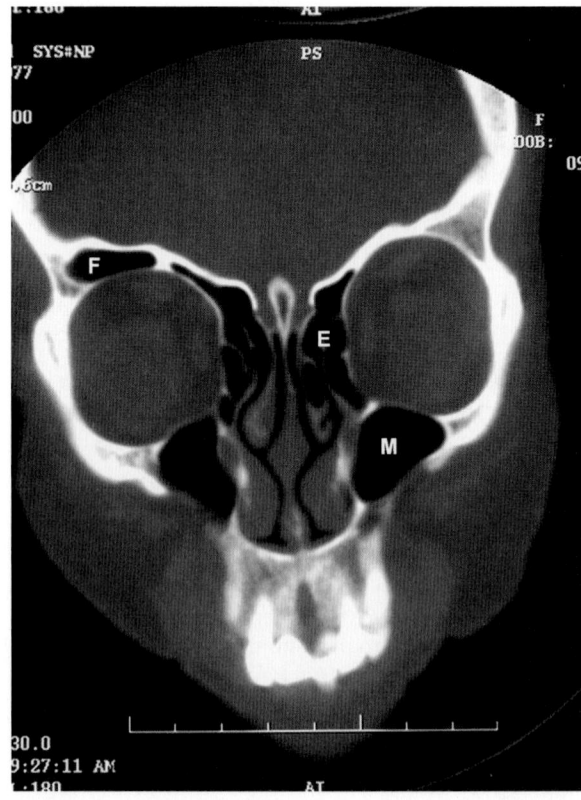

Fig. 3.40 A normal CT scan of the paranasal sinuses: E, ethmoidal; F, frontal; M, maxillary.

Diagnostic imaging

Plain X-rays

Plain sinus X-rays are of limited value in the modern practice of rhinology. They may help to identify foreign bodies, fractures or fluid levels in the sinuses, but are of limited value in the management of chronic rhinosinusitis.

CT scan

Coronal reconstruction of the axial images through the paranasal sinuses give excellent anatomical information about the paranasal sinuses, skull base and orbits (Fig. 3.40) and have replaced direct coronal sequences. CT provides better bony detail than MRI.

MRI scan

MRI is useful in distinguishing soft tissue from retained sinus secretions and the intracranial involvement of sinonasal tumours.

SECTION 3.8   Manifestations of nose disease

Epistaxis

Nosebleeds, or epistaxis, can range from a trivial to a life-threatening complaint.

Epidemiology

Epistaxis is extremely common, particularly in children and the elderly.

Pathology

In children, bleeding is almost always from the mucosa lining the anterior nasal septum (Little's area). In the elderly, posterior nosebleeds may occur. These can be very severe and impossible to control.

Allergic rhinitis in children causes itching and encourages nose-picking, leading to epistaxis. Juvenile angiofibroma is a rare, highly vascular post-nasal tumour that affects young boys, usually causing recurrent heavy nosebleeds. Occasionally, such tumours are mistaken for adenoidal tissue and the unfortunate child is subjected to a catastrophic 'adenoidectomy'.

Hypertension does not cause epistaxis but may increase the severity of a nosebleed. Moreover, most patients with hypertension may be taking antiplatelet agents such as aspirin.

Scope of disease

The severity of a nosebleed should never be underestimated as it may be life threatening.

Clinical features

Anterior nosebleeds often start unilaterally and suddenly. All the blood that is lost is visible. Posterior nose bleeds often result in blood entering the oral cavity and oropharynx. A significant amount of blood is ingested and the apparent blood loss may not reflect the true loss. Eventually, the patient may vomit and the severity of the haemorrhage comes to light.

Patients are often highly anxious when they suffer a severe nosebleed. This anxiety causes a tachycardia and raises blood pressure, contributing to further blood loss. If bleeding does not stop or is not controlled, hypovolaemia and shock ensue.

The overwhelming majority of nosebleeds are idiopathic in nature. In a minority, there are specific local or systemic causes. Every attempt should be made to identify treatable causes of epistaxis (Table 3.4) to minimize recurrence.

Table 3.4	Predisposing factors of epistaxis
Local	**Systemic**
Traumatic, e.g. fractures, foreign bodies, nose-picking	Drugs (clopidogrel, aspirin, warfarin)
Inflammatory, e.g. rhinitis	Haematological disease (haemophilia, acute leukaemias)
Neoplastic, e.g. tumours of the nose, sinuses or nasopharynx	Familial disease (hereditary haemorrhagic telangiectasia or Osler–Weber–Rendu syndrome)
Environmental, e.g. high altitude, air-conditioning	Raised venous pressure, e.g. whooping cough or bronchopneumonia
Endocrine, e.g. menstruation	
Iatrogenic, e.g. nasal surgery, topical nasal steroids	

Initial investigations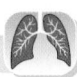

No investigation is required for young patients with mild nosebleed.

Further investigations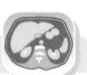

Investigations are appropriate for patients with severe recurrent nosebleeds.

Full blood count

Anaemia may be present with severe recurrent nosebleeds. The haemoglobin concentration may not drop until approximately 24 hours after bleeding.

Coagulation screen

It is important to identify any existing coagulopathies that may worsen the bleeding.

Group and crossmatch

Patients with severe bleeding will require blood transfusion.

Initial management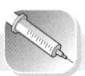

Resuscitation

In cases of severe epistaxis, always secure the airway and ensure adequate ventilation before addressing circulatory collapse. Resuscitation with crystalloid, colloid or blood may be necessary. In the elderly, careful fluid balance with the help of central venous pressure monitoring is important.

Correct coagulopathy

Nosebleeds due to haematological causes or anticoagulation are difficult to arrest until the underlying aberration in clotting is corrected. This may involve a platelet transfusion in thrombocytopenia and antiplatelet anticoagulation, or fresh frozen plasma (FFP) in warfarin overdose. In significant haemorrhage due to other causes, consumption coagulopathy ensues and must be addressed.

Control of haemorrhage

Mild anterior nosebleeds, particularly in children, may be controlled by pinching the nasal tip and thereby applying direct pressure to Little's area. Sucking on ice or placing ice over the nose or on the back of the neck encourages vasoconstriction. Inserting tissues into the nostril is seldom helpful.

Cauterization of the bleeding vessels by application of silver nitrate ($AgNO_3$) or electrocautery is an effective method of arresting haemorrhage (Fig. 3.41). Topical anaesthesia is necessary. Posterior bleeding points may be treated by endoscopic-assisted cautery.

Nasal packing

When bleeding is torrential, and no single bleeding point is obvious, the nasal cavity should be packed. There are a variety of nasal packs available. Traditionally, ribbon gauze impregnated with bismuth iodoform paraffin paste (BIPP)

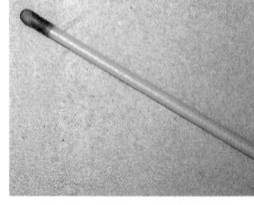

Fig. 3.41 Silver nitrate applicator.

was used to pack the nasal cavity. This ribbon gauze is layered into the nose from the floor to the vault (Fig. 3.42). This required experience on the part of the clinician and a very tolerant patient. The newer nasal 'tampons', e.g. Merocel packs, are much easier to insert. On contact with fluid, they expand and fill the nasal cavity.

For posterior nasal bleeds, a post-nasal balloon catheter is used to provide sufficient tamponade posteriorly. A urinary Foley catheter is often used although it is not licensed for this purpose. In noses with severe septal deformity, nasal packing may not be effective until the deformity is corrected. For this reason, submucous resection of the septum (SMR) is often performed to improve the efficacy of nasal packing.

Nasal packing is usually left in situ for 24 hours and this alone is sufficient to treat a nosebleed. Whilst packs are in, hypoventilation and hypoxia may occur, particularly in the elderly. Myocardial ischaemia following nasal packing is a recognized complication.

Surgical management

Artery ligation

When bleeding continues after pack removal, it is often necessary to ligate the feeding blood vessels. The nasal mucosa below the level of the middle turbinate receives its blood supply from the external carotid artery via the maxillary and then sphenopalatine branches. Before endoscopes were available, the maxillary artery had to be ligated via a transantral approach. A sublabial incision was

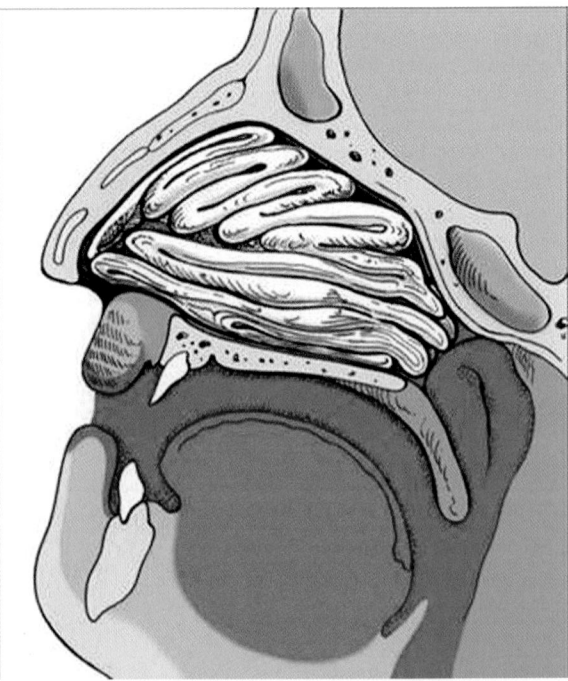

Fig. 3.42 A BIPP-impregnated ribbon gauze is layered into the nose from the floor to the vault, extending antero-posteriorly.

necessary and both the anterior and posterior wall of the maxillary sinus had to be drilled away. Today, endoscopic surgery allows the ENT surgeon to identify and clip the sphenopalatine artery as it passes through the lateral wall of the nose (Fig. 3.43).

The nasal mucosa of the upper half of the nose is supplied by the anterior and posterior ethmoidal arteries. These are branches of the ophthalmic artery, which is a branch of the internal carotid artery. These vessels are disrupted following significant nasal fractures and account for intractable nosebleeds. The anterior ethmoidal artery is usually the larger and therefore more commonly the culprit. Ligation requires an external approach, exposing the artery as it passes through the medial orbital wall.

The nose has a rich collateral blood supply and occasionally vessels need to be ligated bilaterally. Rarely, the external carotid artery must be exposed and ligated in the neck.

Intra-arterial embolization

In some cases, bleeding is due to abnormal blood vessels or an unusual feeding vessel. Angiography and intra-arterial embolization may be useful.

Coagulating laser therapy

In hereditary haemorrhagic telangiectasia, the troublesome telangiectasia may be 'spot-welded' by KTP or Argon laser. This effectively seals these blood vessels. Patients often require multiple treatments with the argon laser throughout their lives.

Prognosis

In most patients, bleeding stops with conservative measures; only a very small proportion require additional measures such as surgery.

> *i* **FURTHER INFORMATION**
>
> Pashen D, Stevens M. Management of epistaxis in general practice. Australian Family Physician 2002; 31(8): 717–721.

Adenoidal hypertrophy

Nasal polyps

Rhinosinusitis

Nasal trauma

SECTION 3.9 # Diseases of the nose

Nasal symptoms are the most common reason for adult referrals to ENT clinics in the United Kingdom. The nose is not only important for breathing, but is functionally important for smell and taste. The paranasal sinuses are important resonators of the voice, and the external appearance of the nose is key to the perception of beauty.

Diseases of the nose and paranasal sinuses may be a manifestation of systemic disease. Indeed the close association of nasal conditions with lung diseases, such as the co-existence of rhinitis and asthma, has earned the nose the appropriate title of 'window to the lung'.

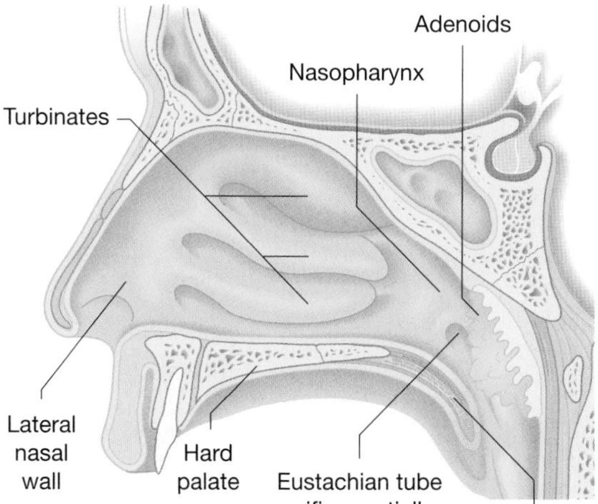

Adenoidal hypertrophy

Adenoidal tissue is lymphoid tissue situated on the postero-superior wall of the nasopharynx (Fig. 3.44). It does not have a capsule and is aggregated in vertical ridges that abut the eustachian cushions laterally. Adenoids, like tonsils, are part of Waldeyer's ring and are hypertrophic in early childhood.

Epidemiology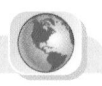

Adenoidal hypertrophy is virtually universal in children between the ages of 3 and 7.

Pathology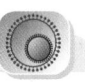

Hypertrophy of the adenoids may be physiological or a response to recurrent infection. Whilst adenoidal hypertrophy is extremely common, it is the relative size of the adenoids to the nasopharynx that leads to symptoms. Large adenoids cause problems when they obstruct the choanae and hinder normal nasal breathing.

Turbinates

Nasopharynx

Adenoids

Lateral nasal wall

Hard palate

Eustachian tube orifice partially obstructed by adenoids

Soft palate and uvula

Fig. 3.44 The adenoids lie on the ceiling and posterior wall of the nasopharynx, and may obstruct the choanae or eustachian tube orifices.

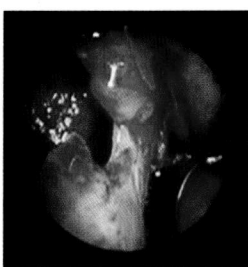

Fig. 3.43 An endoscopic view of the sphenopalatine artery as it passes through the lateral wall of the nose (left). This vessel may be diathermied or clipped, as in this case, to stem bleeding from the lower nasal cavity. Here a large opening has been made into the maxillary sinus on the left (a middle meatal antrostomy).

203

Scope of disease

It is hypothesized that the proximity of enlarged adenoids to the eustachian tube orifices prevents normal ventilation of the middle ears, predisposing to acute middle ear infections and glue ear (p. 190). Severe disease can lead to failure to thrive: the effort of breathing expends energy and feeding is poor as the child has to mouth-breathe through each meal. Adenoidal hypertrophy may be severe enough to cause obstructive sleep apnoea with an inherent risk of right heart failure (cor pulmonale).

Clinical features

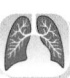

Adenoidal hypertrophy causes nasal congestion and mouth breathing. These children are described as 'always having a cold'. They often snore at night and occasionally suffer from obstructive sleep apnoea. Hyponasal speech may be noted, with some children being referred to speech therapists before an otolaryngologist is consulted. Children with severe disease may present with failure to thrive.

On inspection, purulent thick nasal secretions may be present in patients with adenoidal hypertrophy (the main differential diagnosis is allergic rhinitis). Classical 'adenoidal facies' (open-mouthed posture, narrow upper alveolus, hypoplastic maxilla and high-arched palate) is seldom seen and often correlates poorly with adenoidal size.

Examination of the post-nasal space with a mirror or fibreoptic scope is the most accurate method of assessing adenoidal size. Unfortunately, this is rarely tolerated by children less than 5 years old.

Initial investigations

Lateral soft tissue X-ray

A lateral soft tissue X-ray of the post-nasal space is a useful alternative to fibreoptic endoscopy.

Surgical management

Adenoidectomy

There are no absolute indications for adenoidectomy, and the risks of surgery must be weighed against the expected benefits. Adenoidectomy relieves chronic nasal obstruction and is indicated with tonsillectomy in children with proven obstructive sleep apnoea (OSA). Snoring is not an indication for adenoidectomy in the absence of OSA. In children with recurrent glue ear (otitis media with effusion) after initial treatment with grommets, there is evidence to suggest that adenoidectomy will improve eustachian tube function and middle ear ventilation. Finally, there is growing evidence to show that children enjoy a better general health status, with fewer respiratory tract infections, and fewer symptoms of chronic sinusitis following adenoidectomy.

Adenoidectomy is achieved by curettage (Fig. 3.45) of the adenoidal pad or electrocautery. The adenoidal tissue in the post-nasal space is removed intra-orally (Fig. 3.46).

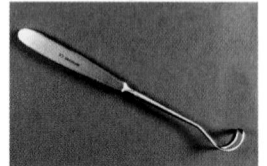

Fig. 3.45 Adenoidectomy curette.

Complete removal is important as tags of remnant adenoidal tissue can cause primary or reactionary haemorrhage. Haemostasis is ensured by packing the nasopharynx. There is a risk of haemorrhage in the first 12 hours following surgery, and in some patients velopharyngeal incompetence may result in hypernasal speech (rhinolalia aperta) in the long term.

Prognosis

The majority of patients with adenoidal hypertrophy do not require surgery. The adenoids begin to recede in size from the age of 7 and the nasopharynx enlarges around them. Adenoidectomy therefore simply expedites nature's course.

Nasal polyps

Polyps of the sinonasal mucosa are a common cause of intractable nasal obstruction. This is a distinct entity and may not be associated with an allergy. Swollen inferior turbinates are often mistaken for nasal polyps as they may be dramatically enlarged and occlude the nares.

Epidemiology

The prevalence of nasal polyps is between 0.2% and 4.3% of the population. Incidence appears to rise with age, and there is a clear male predominance (2–4-fold increase). At autopsy, up to 42% of individuals have evidence of nasal polyposis. There is a higher prevalence of nasal polyps in patients with aspirin sensitivity (36%), cystic fibrosis (20%) and asthma (10%). Amongst patients with polyps, 45% are asthmatic. The association of asthma, aspirin sensitivity and nasal polyps was described by Widal, but is now widely known as *Samter's triad*.

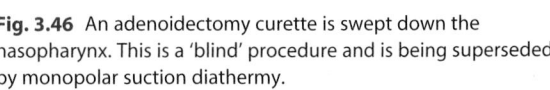

Fig. 3.46 An adenoidectomy curette is swept down the nasopharynx. This is a 'blind' procedure and is being superseded by monopolar suction diathermy.

Pathology

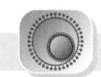

The factors that initiate polyp formation are unknown. However, increasing oedema of the connective tissue stroma of the nasal mucosa eventually causes herniation through the basement membrane to form a nasal polyp. This stroma contains a variety of inflammatory mediators and cells, with eosinophils predominating. The epithelium of the polyp remains respiratory, with an increase in the goblet cell population. There are often areas of squamous metaplasia.

Polyps appear to arise from the middle meatus and lining of the ethmoid sinuses. They are frequently found in the maxillary antrum. A distinct entity is the large antrochoanal polyp which arises in the maxillary antrum, protrudes into the nasal cavity through the middle meatus and then passes posteriorly towards the choana.

There is no evidence to link general allergy to nasal polyposis. Indeed, skin-prick testing does not show a higher incidence of atopy in polyp patients, and the incidence of polyps in allergic patients is no higher than in normal controls (1.5% vs 1%). The incidence of polyposis is higher in non-allergic asthmatics (12%) than in atopic asthmatics (5%).

There is, however, evidence of 'local' allergy in the nasal mucosa with mast cell degranulation, raised IgE levels and eosinophilia. Recent research has suggested a role for fungi in the pathogenesis of polyps. The ubiquitous nature of fungal spores in the paranasal sinuses of all individuals makes proving causation immensely difficult.

Scope of disease

Nasal polyps predispose individuals to chronic rhinosinusitis and infective exacerbations. Indeed, any of the complications of sinusitis may be seen in these patients. Gross nasal polyposis may cause facial deformity, with widening of the nasal bridge and even displacement of the globes.

Clinical features

Nasal polyps may be asymptomatic but characteristically cause nasal obstruction. The patient may also complain of a post-nasal drip, rhinorrhoea and hyponasal speech. There is a profound loss of smell and therefore reduced taste. Symptoms of sinusitis, such as facial pressure and headache, may occur but are not as common as one might expect.

In severe cases, nasal polyps may protrude from the patient's nostrils and prove an embarrassment. Polyps are insensate and therefore amenable to removal using snares in the clinic. A unilateral nasal polyp and a history of bleeding should raise the suspicion of malignancy and warrants urgent biopsy.

Initial investigations

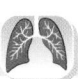

Skin-prick testing/RAST

Few investigations are mandatory, but the exclusion of allergy by skin-prick testing or RAST is advisable.

Peak expiratory flow

Assessment of peak expiratory flow rates (PEFR) will identify mild asthmatics who may have no overt respiratory symptoms.

Sweat test

All children with nasal polyposis should have a sweat test to exclude cystic fibrosis (p. 136).

Further investigations

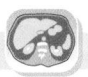

CT of the paranasal sinuses

For patients in whom medical management has failed, CT scanning provides important anatomical information for endoscopic sinus surgery and polypectomy. Simple plain sinus radiographs are of no value.

Medical management

Nasal topical steroids

All patients should have a trial of optimal medical therapy before surgical polypectomy is contemplated. Nasal steroid drops instilled in the head-dependent position offer better drug delivery to the sinonasal mucosa than sprays.

Oral steroids

In severe cases, a short course of oral steroids (e.g. prednisolone at 1 mg/kg body weight daily for 5 days) will offer spontaneous short-term benefit.

> **RECENT ADVANCES**
>
> *There is some evidence that leukotriene receptor antagonists (e.g. montelukast, zafirlukast) may be beneficial in reducing congestion in aspirin-sensitive asthmatics with nasal polyps.*

Surgical management

Endoscopic polypectomy

When medical measures have failed, surgical endoscopic polypectomy is indicated. This is often combined with sinus surgery to lay open the paranasal sinuses. The purpose of surgery is to allow topical steroids to access the sinonasal mucosa. It is an adjunct to medical treatment and not an alternative.

Powered instrumentation in the form of a suction debrider with its own irrigation system has allowed surgeons to perform polypectomy swiftly, effectively and safely.

Caldwell–Luc procedure

Occasionally, complete removal of large antrochoanal polyps arising from the maxillary sinus is not possible endoscopically. A fenestration is made in the front wall of the maxillary sinus through a sublabial incision. This was, in fact, a common procedure before the advent of endoscopes and is known as the Caldwell–Luc procedure.

Prognosis

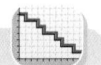

Polyps invariably recur to some extent: 5–10% of sufferers have severe intractable disease that necessitates repeated surgery. Overall, 60% of those undergoing polypectomy will have a repeat procedure in the first 5 years following surgery.

Rhinosinusitis

The respiratory epithelium lining the nose is confluent with the mucosa of the paranasal sinuses. Inflammation of the nasal mucosa, or rhinitis, is often associated with some degree of sinus inflammation, or sinusitis. The two entities are therefore not distinct but are part of a clinical spectrum which is correctly referred to as rhinosinusitis.

Epidemiology

Rhinosinusitis affects 1 in 6 people, and 1 in 4 adolescents. It is extremely common and accounts for an increasing number of consultations with general practitioners in the United Kingdom. Allergic rhinitis is now the commonest immunological disorder and the commonest chronic disorder in man. It is estimated that chronic sinusitis has a prevalence of 15% in most urban communities.

Table 3.5	Common causes or categories of rhinitis
Infective	
Viral (adenoviruses)	
Bacterial (*Streptococcus pneumoniae*)	
Fungal (*Aspergillus*)	
Allergic	
Seasonal or intermittent (tree or grass pollen allergy)	
Perennial or persistent (house dust mite allergy)	
Atrophic rhinitis	
This is due to any condition that causes persistent drying of the nose	
Inflammatory	
Wegener's granulomatosis	
Sarcoidosis	
Occupational	
Occupational exposure to irritants such as aerosols may cause severe rhinitis	
Pregnancy	
Rhinitis of pregnancy may be a consequence of hormonal changes although rapid resolution soon after delivery throws this theory into doubt	
Drug-induced	
Many antihypertensive agents cause nasal stuffiness	
Vasoconstricting agents that are used for the short-term relief of nasal congestion can themselves cause a severe rebound phenomenon (rhinitis medicamentosa)	

Pathology

Rhinitis may be caused by infection, allergy or a variety of other factors. Table 3.5 lists some of the common causes. The immunological response to the allergens, for example, generates inflammatory mediators such as histamine, kinins, prostaglandins and leukotrienes. Some of these mediators cause 'early phase' symptoms such as itching, sneezing and rhinorrhoea, whilst others cause 'late phase' symptoms such as nasal blockage. Mast cell degranulation has a pivotal role in the early phase response, whilst eosinophils are the key players in the late response.

Oedema of the nasal mucosa not only produces nasal congestion but also causes obstruction of the normal sinus openings or ostia into the nasal cavity. Mucociliary clearance may also be inhibited, resulting in stasis of nasal secretions and then infection. This leads to chronic rhinosinusitis.

Asthma frequently coexists with rhinitis: up to 80% of patients with asthma also have rhinitis. Rhinitis appears first in 45% of asthmatics with a 'lead' time of up to 2 years. This relationship is important to recognize as treating rhinitis in asthmatics improves pulmonary function.

Scope of disease

Complications that arise from untreated or uncontrolled rhinosinusitis are rare. The most serious complications are caused by infective rhinosinusitis. They are local and acute, and are divided into orbital, intracranial and bony complications.

Orbital complications

Infection from the ethmoid air cells may spread into the soft tissues of the orbit. This is more common in children, 50% of patients being under 6 years of age. This complication often begins as a cellulitis of the periorbital tissue. The patient develops a unilateral painful eye with erythema of the lids and periorbital skin. An abscess may then develop and there is often proptosis (outward displacement of the globe) and ptosis (closure) of the eye (Fig. 3.47).

Increased intraorbital pressure leads to compression of the optic nerve and neuropathy, often manifesting as deteriorating colour vision or a relative afferent pupillary defect. This is a warning sign for impending permanent visual loss and necessitates urgent drainage of the abscess.

A serious sequela of orbital cellulitis is cavernous sinus thrombosis; this complication has a 10–27% mortality rate.

Intracranial complications

Intracranial abscesses may be extradural, subdural or intracerebral. Subdural abscesses are by far the most common. Other intracranial complications of rhinosinusitis are meningitis, encephalitis, cavernous sinus and superior sagittal thrombosis.

Bony complications

The frontal bone is diploic and has a narrow cavity. This cavity is prone to infection spreading from the frontal sinus, which may progress to osteomyelitis. This condition presents

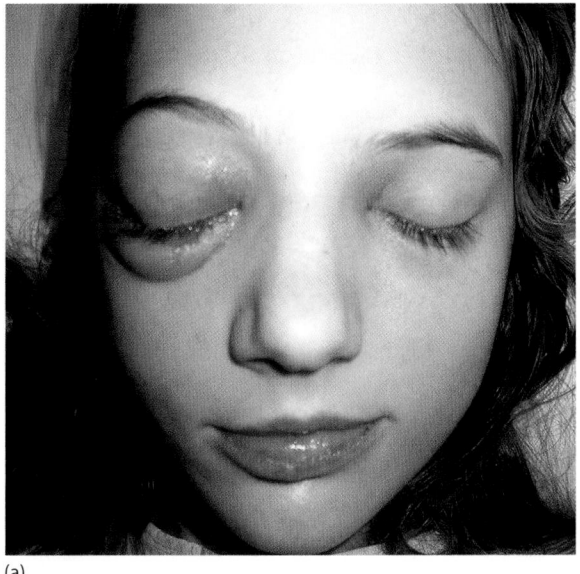

(a)

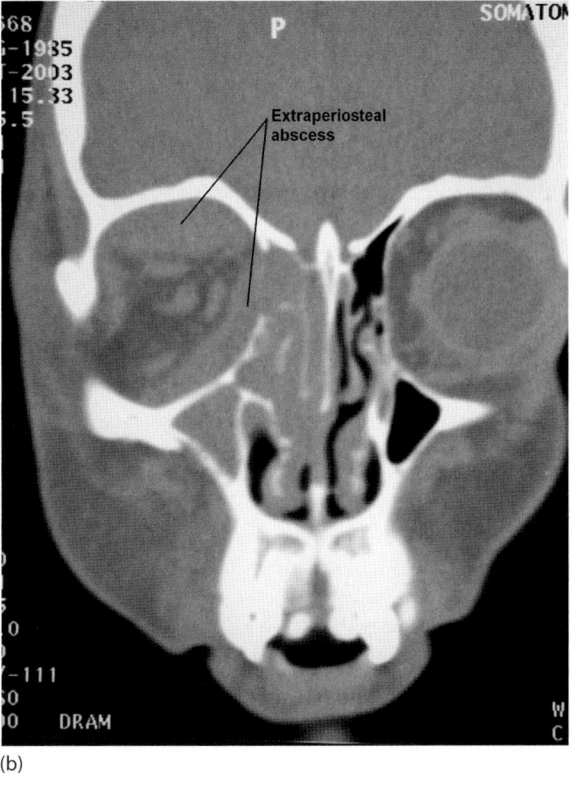

Extraperiosteal abscess

(b)

Fig. 3.47a, b Orbital cellulitis. (a) Patient with a right orbital abscess. (b) Direct coronal CT scan of her sinuses shows a dehiscent lamina papyracea and an abscess within the bony orbit but outside the orbital periosteum.

as a fluctuant swelling over the forehead. Treatment is by surgical debridement and long-term antibiotics.

Clinical features

Clinically, rhinitis is defined by the presence of two of the three cardinal symptoms (nasal discharge, blockage, sneezing/itching) for at least an hour on most days. Patients with allergic rhinitis will have more in the way of sneezing and itching of the nose and eyes. Nasal blockage may be very uncomfortable and disrupt sleep. These patients will be constantly mouth-breathing.

Nasal discharge or rhinorrhoea may be clear, yellow or green in nature. The colour of the discharge does not reliably predict the likelihood of infection. A thick 'peanut-butter' secretion, however, is suggestive of allergic fungal rhinosinusitis. Patients often carry tissues or a handkerchief with them. Eliciting this when taking a history is often a useful way of establishing the severity of any rhinorrhoea.

Nasal oedema often causes a 'conductive' olfactory loss. Patients may report having no sense of smell (anosmia), although more often their sense of smell is poor (hyposmia).

When inflammation of the sinuses or sinusitis develops, patients report facial pain or headache that worsens with stooping. Fever, halitosis, cacosmia (an offensive smell), cough or fatigue may also be reported. If these symptoms have been present for more than 12 weeks, the condition is often labelled 'chronic rhinosinusitis'.

Examination may identify mucopus, polyps or simply congested and oedematous nasal mucosa (Fig. 3.48).

Initial investigations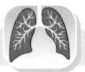

Anterior rhinoscopy

In the primary care setting, anterior rhinoscopy (p.199) may reveal gross nasal polyps, mucopus or simply hypertrophic inferior turbinates.

Further investigations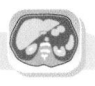

Nasal endoscopy

Further examination of the nose can be undertaken by ENT specialists using rigid nasal endoscopy.

Skin-prick testing

This is a quick way of demonstrating allergies. An alternative would be radio-allergo-sorbent testing (RAST), which detects specific type E immunoglobulins (IgE).

CT of the paranasal sinuses

When endoscopic surgery is contemplated or complications of rhinosinusitis have occurred, CT scanning of the sinuses and/or brain is useful. Direct coronal scans are most useful to the surgeon in planning endoscopic surgery, and contrast-

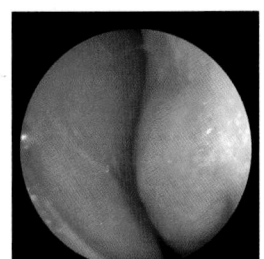

(a)

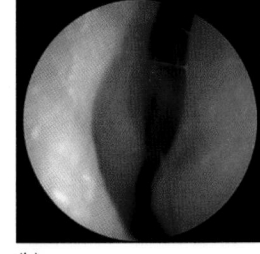

(b)

Fig. 3.48a, b Intranasal images of a 'rhinitic' nose. In both images the septum is on the left. In (a) there is gross inferior turbinate hypertrophy obstruction, and in (b) there are mucus 'strings' traversing the nasal cavity (string sign).

207

enhanced scans are mandatory to rule out intracranial sepsis.

Medical management

Anti-inflammatory and immunomodulation therapy

The use of allergen avoidance, antihistamines, mast cell stabilizing agents and steroids in the management of allergic rhinitis is detailed on page 116.

Antibiotics

Antibiotic therapy is indicated in the presence of infection. Nasal swabs are of little value as multiple organisms are often cultured. Antibiotic therapy should continue for at least 10 days to ensure complete bactericidal effect. Penicillin-type antibiotics are often sufficient. Macrolides are said to have an anti-inflammatory effect on the nasal mucosa, and are often prescribed in long courses.

Antifungals

In invasive fungal sinusitis, early treatment with antifungals is important. In rhinocerebral mucormycosis, which is seen in immunocompromised patients, early treatment with amphotericin significantly alters the prognosis.

Surgical management

Reduction of inferior turbinates

When optimum medical treatment has failed to improve nasal congestion or symptoms of sinusitis such as facial pain or headache, surgery is indicated. A simple procedure that improves the nasal airway is reduction of the inferior turbinates. These are often severely hypertrophic in long-standing untreated rhinitis, and fail to shrink with topical treatment.

Surgical reduction is most commonly done by sub-mucous diathermy, although laser and radiofrequency ablation and trimming are also widely practised. The results of this procedure are excellent initially, but only 60% of patients have continuing benefit at 1 year.

Functional endoscopic sinus surgery

When sinus symptoms predominate, endoscopic sinus surgery may be undertaken to widen the natural drainage channels of the sinuses into the nasal cavity. Functional endoscopic sinus surgery is minimally invasive surgery performed using rigid fibreoptic scopes intranasally. It seeks to open or remove structural obstructions to the normal channels of sinus drainage.

This procedure has a higher satisfaction rate than previous methods such as antral washouts and intranasal or external ethmoidectomies. The 5-year satisfaction rates are typically between 85% and 95%. Although functional endoscopic sinus surgery is minimally invasive, extensive sinus dissection runs the risk of creating CSF leaks and damaging orbital contents or the optic nerve.

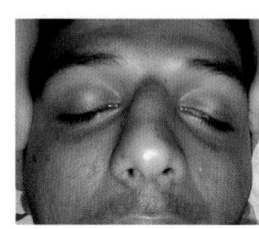
(a)
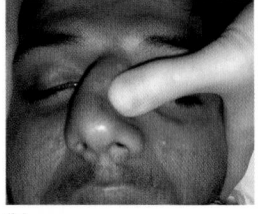
(b)
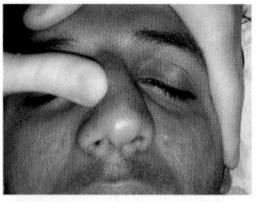
(c)
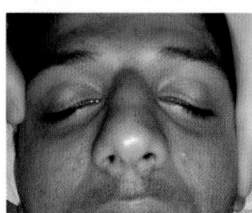
(d)
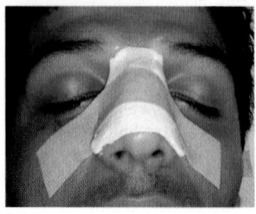
(e)

Fig. 3.49a–e Reduction of nasal fracture performed under general anaesthesia.

A recent innovation is the use of image guidance systems which help the surgeon navigate through the paranasal sinuses.

Prognosis

The symptoms of most patients with allergic rhinitis can be controlled with simple medication. Non-allergic or idiopathic rhinitis is less responsive to antihistamine treatment but responds well to nasal steroids.

ℹ FURTHER INFORMATION

British Society for Allergy and Clinical Immunology. Rhinitis management guidelines, 3rd edn. London: Dunitz, 2000.

Nasal trauma

Epidemiology

Nasal trauma is common. In the United Kingdom, approximately 500 000 cases of facial injury occur each year, of which 125 000 are due to assault. Assault accounts for an increasing proportion of nasal injuries, as the use of seatbelts and improved road safety have reduced the contribution of facial injuries from road-traffic accidents. In 60% of assaults resulting in facial injury, alcohol has been consumed by either assailant or victim.

Pathology

Nasal trauma causes both soft tissue and bony damage. The skin overlying the nose may be contused and lacerated. Trauma from sharp objects, such as broken pint glasses, may totally deglove the nose. The nasal bones may be fractured and displaced, and the nasal septum may be similarly fractured or dislocated.

High-velocity injuries to the nose may cause extensive naso-frontoethmoid fractures. There may be associated zygomatic fractures and damage to the orbits. In all cases of severe trauma, brain and cervical spine injuries must be excluded.

Scope of disease

Septal haematoma

Shearing of blood vessels deep to the perichondrium of the septal cartilage may result in the development of a sub-perichondral septal haematoma. Unless drained urgently, the haematoma may devitalize the septal cartilage as it receives its blood supply from the perichondrium. Cartilage necrosis from an untreated septal haematoma may leave a patient with a depressed nasal dorsum or saddle-shaped nose.

Cerebrospinal fluid leak

Fractures of the base of the skull may cause a CSF leak, resulting in clear rhinorrhoea, often described as 'gin-clear'. A CSF leak leaves a patient at risk of ascending infection from the nose, causing meningitis.

Clinical features

Virtually all significant trauma to the nose causes epistaxis (p. 201). In most cases this is transient and self-limiting. Later, bruising over the nose and around the eyes develops. Swelling and tenderness in the acute situation often makes assessment difficult. In mild cases with no immediate complications, assessment may be deferred for 5–7 days to allow the swelling and bruising to settle.

Nasal obstruction is universal, and initially bilateral. When the nasal mucosal oedema settles, symptoms lateralize to the side of anatomical obstruction. In some cases there are subconjunctival ecchymoses. Naso-frontoethmoid fractures may cause diplopia due to telecanthus and epiphora (tearing) due to disruption of the nasolacrimal ducts.

Associated mid-face fractures may cause noticeable deformity and airway obstruction as the mid-face falls backwards. Orbital 'blow-out' fractures may cause diplopia on upgaze as a result of inferior rectus entrapment by an orbital floor fracture.

Septal fractures may be obvious. Mild trauma causes vertical fractures of the septum whereas more severe trauma may cause a C-shaped septal fracture. This has implications for the ease of subsequent reduction.

Ocular movement, dental occlusion and the integrity of the infra-orbital nerve should be tested. Photography is useful to aid documentation and for medicolegal reasons.

Initial investigations
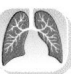

Routine investigations are not required for patients with mild injuries and no other clinical features of underlying complications.

Further investigations
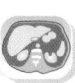

X-ray of the nasal bones

X-rays of the nasal bones are inaccurate (missing up to 50% of clinically evident fractures) and financially inefficient. Plain films are performed when there is a suspicion of foreign bodies (glass or shrapnel), or for medicolegal purposes.

CSF testing

Fluid from patients with clear rhinorrhoea should be tested with a dipstick for glucose; high levels of glucose suggest CSF. Confirmation may be obtained by sending a sample for a β_2-transferrin assay.

CT of the head

If there is significant trauma, a high-resolution CT scan should be performed to identify any fracture of the base of the skull and orbits.

Initial management
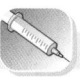

Airway management

It is imperative to secure the airway if it is obstructed by a displaced mid-face fracture. Epistaxis that continues despite simple measures may require immediate packing. If bleeding settles to allow further assessment, the nasal airway may then be examined, principally to exclude a septal haematoma.

Surgical management

Drainage of septal haematoma

Septal haematoma requires urgent drainage before the septal cartilage is devitalized.

Repair of CSF leaks

A significant proportion of CSF leaks close spontaneously, but a small number require surgical repair. There is much controversy about the need for prophylactic antibiotics in treating CSF leaks. Bed rest is clearly desirable and some clinicians advocate a lumbar drain to keep CSF pressures low.

Reduction of nasal fractures

Simple nasal fractures may be reduced under local or general anaesthesia. This involves disimpaction of the fractured bony fragments by accentuating the deviation, then realignment. Simple digital pressure will achieve this in most cases (Fig. 3.49a–d). In depressed fractures, elevators may be used to raise any bony fragments. Septal fractures may be reduced using special forceps. Fixation of reduced fractures is achieved by the application of a plaster of Paris splint (Fig. 3.49e).

Manipulation of nasal fractures has a poor outcome: some 40% of patients will have residual deformity. This can be addressed electively by rhinoplasty or septorhinoplasty. Some centres adopt a more pro-active management of nasal fractures, advocating septoplasty, osteotomies and surgery on the nasal tip cartilages following injury. This produces a lower rate of residual deformity.

Prognosis
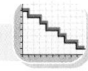

The prognosis of patients with nasal trauma relates to the underlying severity of injury.

i **FURTHER INFORMATION**

Staffel JG. Optimising treatment of nasal fractures. Laryngoscope 2002; 112(10): 1709–1719.

The throat

SECTION 3.10 Introduction

Applied basic sciences of the throat

The 'throat' is a lay term that usually refers to the pharynx and larynx. The pharynx may be divided into the nasopharynx, oropharynx and hypopharynx. The nasopharynx is often considered a part of the nose, as is the case in this text.

Anatomy

The pharynx and larynx in the human are intimately related. Inhaled air passes through the oropharynx into the larynx whilst ingested food is directed from the oropharynx into the hypopharynx. The pharynx and larynx are aptly called the upper aerodigestive tract (UADT), which emphasizes the union of these two passages. This means that man, unlike lower mammals, cannot breathe and swallow simultaneously.

Pharynx

The pharynx is a single muscular tube which opens anteriorly into the nasal and oral cavities (Fig. 3.50). The nasopharynx is separated from the oropharynx by the soft palate, which acts like a 'trap door'. The oropharynx extends from the anterior faucial pillar posteriorly towards the posterior pharyngeal wall, and then inferiorly toward the larynx. The larynx invaginates into the pharynx anteriorly, and this portion of the pharynx is termed the hypopharynx. The hypopharynx commences at the level of the upper border of the hyoid bone and extends to the lower level of the cricoid cartilage.

Oropharynx

The oropharynx is the anterior communication of the pharynx into the oral cavity. The anterior faucial pillar is made up of the palatoglossus muscle whilst the posterior pillar is made up of the palatopharyngeus. The palatine tonsils are sandwiched between these pillars and form a continuous ring of lymphoid tissue called Waldeyer's ring (Fig. 3.51). The adenoids and lingual tonsils form the other parts of this ring.

The lateral and posterior walls of the oropharynx are made up of the muscular fibres of the superior and middle constrictors. The walls of the nasopharynx, by contrast, do not contain muscle but comprise the fibrous buccopharyn-geal membrane. This fibro-muscular tube lies over the alar fascia, which allows it to move with ease. The alar fascia extends from the skull base to the level of the second thoracic vertebra (T2).

The space lateral to the naso- and oropharynx is termed the parapharyngeal space. The space between the posterior pharyngeal wall and the so-called alar fascia, which extends through the neck to the level of the second thoracic vertebra, is termed the retropharyngeal space. The space contained behind the alar fascia and anterior to the prevertebral fascia is called the 'danger space' and extends to the level of the diaphragm (Fig. 3.52). Finally, the space behind the prevertebral fascia which extends along the entire length of the vertebral column is the prevertebral space. An abscess may form in any of these deep neck spaces and require surgical drainage.

Hypopharynx

The hypopharynx is the continuation of the oropharynx below the level of the hyoid bone or floor of the valleculae.

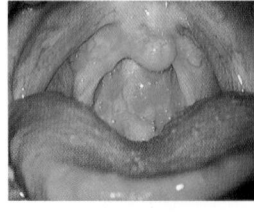

Fig. 3.51 The palatine tonsil is sandwiched between the muscular faucial pillars.

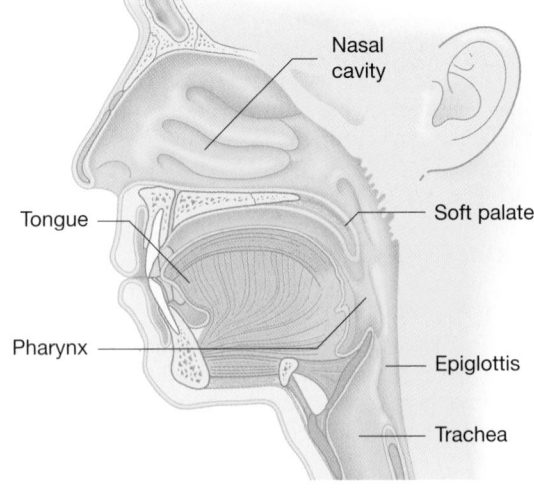

Fig. 3.50 Sagittal section of head and neck. The pharynx opens anteriorly into the nose and oral cavity. The soft palate is a 'trapdoor' between the upper nasopharynx and the lower oropharynx.

Nasal cavity

Tongue

Soft palate

Pharynx

Epiglottis

Trachea

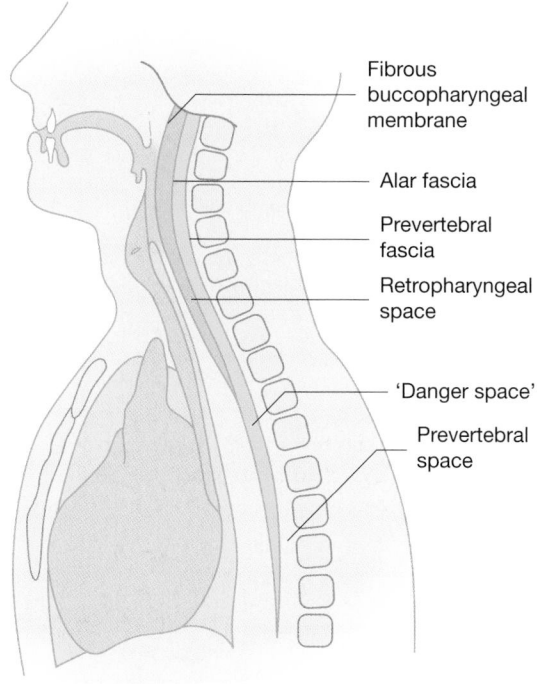

Fig. 3.52 The deep neck spaces extend into the mediastinum. This explains how abscesses in the neck may track and cause fatal mediastinal abscesses.

framework, and the signet ring-shaped cricoid cartilage lies inferiorly and is the only complete ring of cartilage in the upper airway. The entire laryngeal apparatus is suspended from the hyoid bone by strap muscles and the thyrohyoid membrane.

The three paired cartilages of the larynx are the large pyramidal arytenoids and the smaller corniculate and cuneiforms. The latter two are insignificant and lie within the aryepiglottic folds. The arytenoids sit on the posterior lamina of the cricoid cartilage and form a synovial cricoarytenoid joint. This allows both arytenoids to glide laterally and rotate on the cricoid. The arytenoid cartilages have vocal processes anteriorly that form the posterior third of the true vocal folds. Vocal ligaments pass anteriorly from the vocal processes to meet in the midline just behind the apex of the thyroid cartilage. The vocal ligaments form the remaining anterior two-thirds of the true vocal folds. Movement of the arytenoids away from the midline and lateral rotation of the vocal processes cause abduction of the true vocal folds and opening of the glottis. Movement of the arytenoids towards the midline and medial rotation of the vocal processes cause adduction of the true vocal folds and closing of the glottis (Fig. 3.55).

The larynx may be subdivided into the supraglottis, glottis and subglottis. The supraglottis extends superiorly from the level of the true vocal folds. The glottis encompasses the true vocal folds, the floor of the laryngeal ventricle and the region 1 cm below the upper surface of the folds. The subglottis extends inferiorly from the glottis to the level of the first tracheal ring. In the adult, the glottis is the narrowest portion of the upper airway, but in the infant it is the subglottis (Fig. 3.56).

The arytenoid cartilages move by virtue of small intrinsic laryngeal muscles. The posterior cricoarytenoid is the only muscle that abducts the vocal folds. The lateral cricoarytenoid, the interarytenoid and the oblique interarytenoid muscles bring about adduction. The vocalis muscle runs within the vocal folds and increases tension whilst shortening the folds. The cricothyroid muscle, which is an extrinsic muscle, tenses and lengthens the vocal folds by approximating the cricoid and thyroid cartilages anteriorly.

The vocal folds have a mucosal layer and underlying lamina propria over the vocal ligament. The lamina propria has several layers, but the superficial layer is the most important and is termed Reinke's space. This gelatinous layer allows a standing mucosal wave to develop as air passes across the adducted vocal folds.

The larynx is covered by pseudostratified ciliated columnar epithelium except at three sites where there is non-keratinizing squamous epithelium. These sites are the true vocal folds, the edge of the aryepiglottic folds, and the laryngeal surface of the epiglottis. The vocal folds are made up of three histologically distinct layers in cross-section: the cover (squamous epithelium), the intermediate layer (superficial layer of the lamina propria) and the deep layer (remainder of the lamina propria and the vocalis muscle).

Applied basic sciences of the throat

Symptoms of throat disease

Examination of the throat

It surrounds the laryngeal apparatus laterally and posteriorly. Inferiorly, the hypopharynx communicates with the cervical oesophagus.

The hypopharynx forms lateral passages for food and fluid to pass. These passages are called pyriform sinuses and are separated from the larynx medially by the aryepiglottic folds. As the name suggests, this fold connects the epiglottis anteriorly to the arytenoid cartilages, which rest on the cricoid cartilage posteriorly (Fig. 3.53).

Behind the arytenoid cartilages and the posterior lamina of the cricoid cartilage is the postcricoid portion of the hypopharynx. This is a site of webs and postcricoid carcinoma, which is, curiously for head and neck cancers, more common in women.

The walls of the hypopharynx are made up of the inferior constrictor. There is an anatomical dehiscence in the fibres of the inferior constrictor which is known as Killian's dehiscence. It is through this defect that pharyngeal pouches (Zenker's diverticula) appear. The inferior constrictor is therefore split into two separate aggregations. The upper is called the thyropharyngeus and the lower, which forms the upper oesophageal sphincter, is known as the cricopharyngeus.

Larynx

The larynx is made up of three single cartilaginous structures and three small paired cartilages (Fig. 3.54). The leaf-like epiglottis forms a lid to the laryngeal inlet, the shield-like thyroid cartilage makes up the main laryngeal

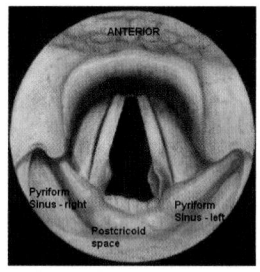

Fig. 3.53 The larynx and hypopharynx. The hypopharynx lies posterior and lateral to the larynx. It is divided into the postcricoid space posteriorly and the 'pear-shaped' pyriform sinuses laterally.

211

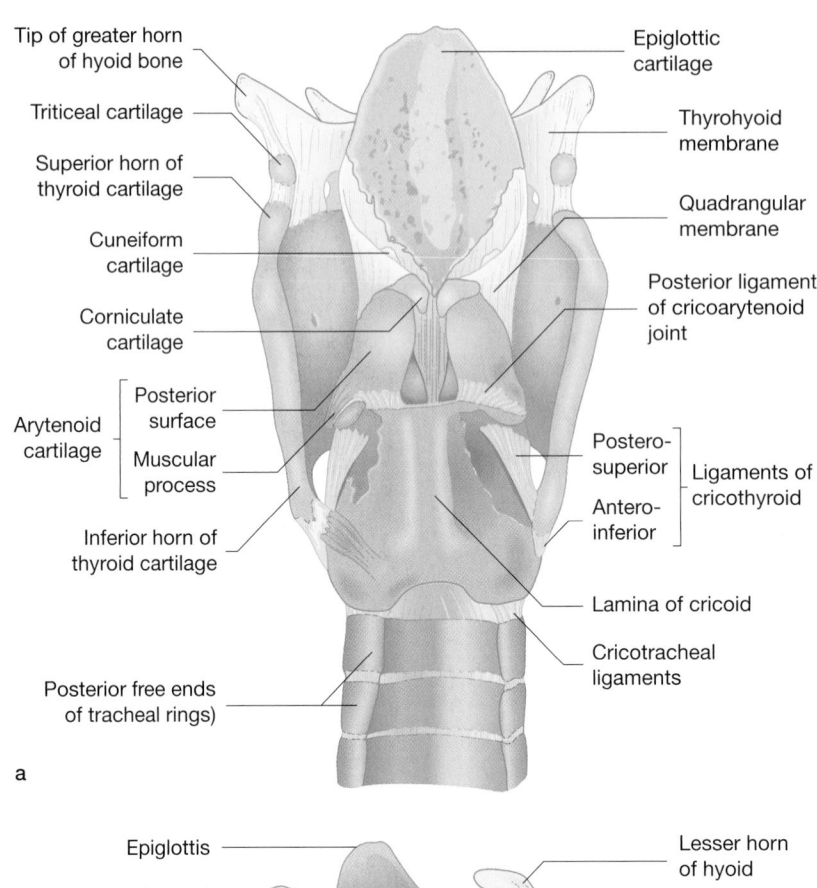

Tip of greater horn of hyoid bone

Triticeal cartilage

Superior horn of thyroid cartilage

Cuneiform cartilage

Corniculate cartilage

Arytenoid cartilage
- Posterior surface
- Muscular process

Inferior horn of thyroid cartilage

Posterior free ends of tracheal rings)

Epiglottic cartilage

Thyrohyoid membrane

Quadrangular membrane

Posterior ligament of cricoarytenoid joint

Ligaments of cricothyroid
- Postero-superior
- Antero-inferior

Lamina of cricoid

Cricotracheal ligaments

a

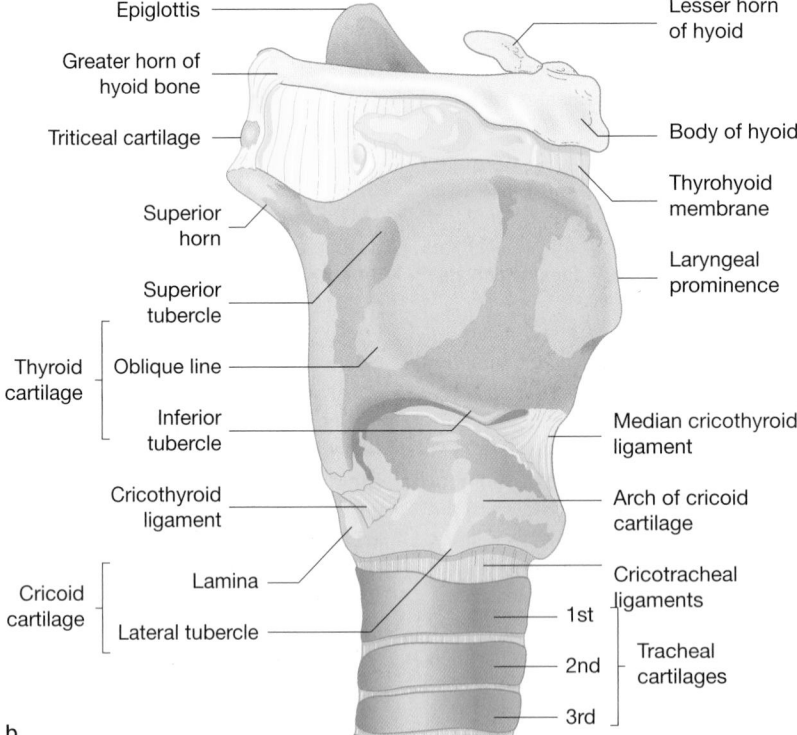

Epiglottis

Greater horn of hyoid bone

Triticeal cartilage

Superior horn

Superior tubercle

Thyroid cartilage
- Oblique line
- Inferior tubercle

Cricothyroid ligament

Cricoid cartilage
- Lamina
- Lateral tubercle

Lesser horn of hyoid

Body of hyoid

Thyrohyoid membrane

Laryngeal prominence

Median cricothyroid ligament

Arch of cricoid cartilage

Cricotracheal ligaments

1st

2nd   Tracheal cartilages

3rd

b

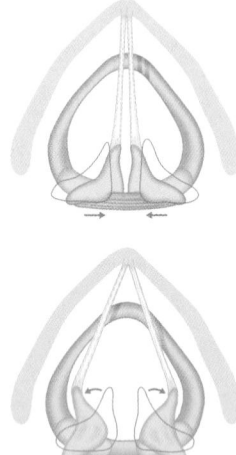

Fig. 3.55 Superior view of the larynx and vocal fold movements. Rotation and gliding of the arytenoid cartilages on the cricoid cause abduction and adduction of the vocal folds.

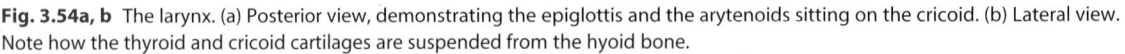

Fig. 3.54a, b The larynx. (a) Posterior view, demonstrating the epiglottis and the arytenoids sitting on the cricoid. (b) Lateral view. Note how the thyroid and cricoid cartilages are suspended from the hyoid bone.

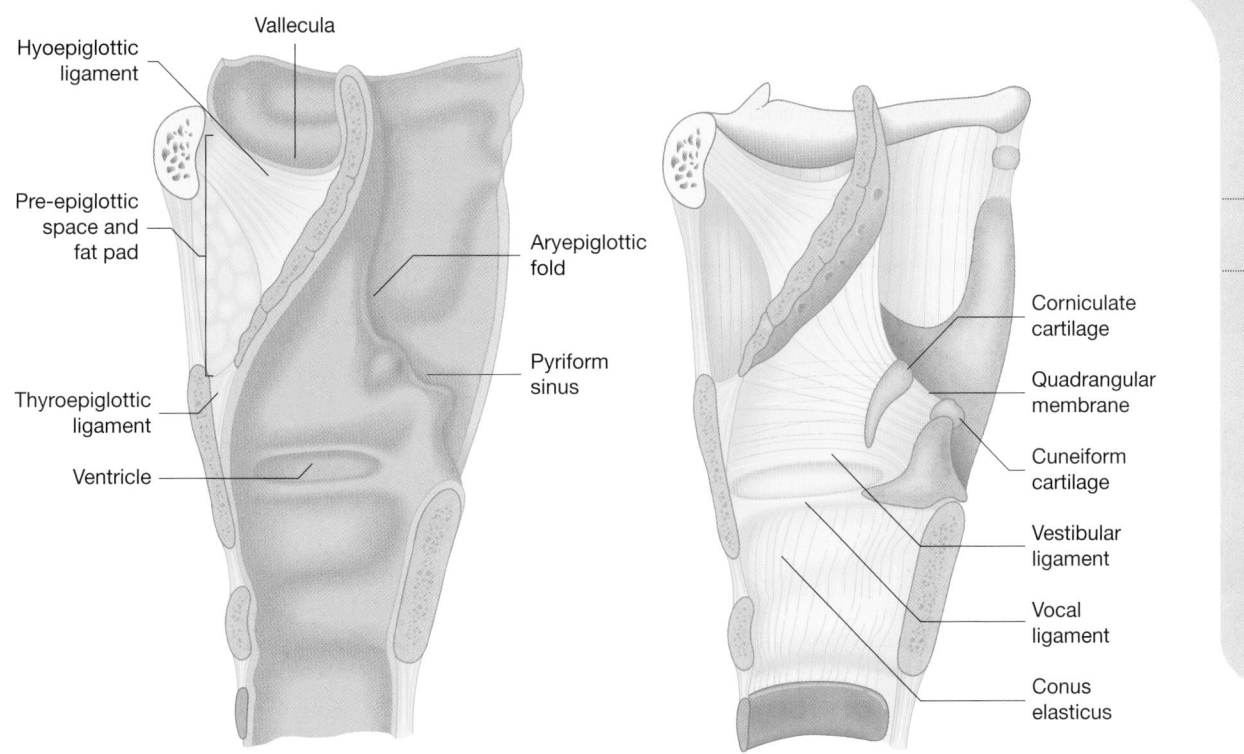

Applied basic sciences
of the throat

**Symptoms of throat
disease**

Examination of
the throat

Fig. 3.56 Sagittal section of the larynx. The larynx is divided into the supraglottis, glottis and subglottis for descriptive purposes.

Physiology

Swallowing

Swallowing or deglutition occurs in two phases. The first is voluntary and the second is entirely involuntary under reflex control. Following mastication, a soft food bolus which has been moistened by saliva is passed posteriorly from the oral cavity into the oropharynx. This is achieved by the tongue, which rises to push the bolus against the palate.

As the bolus passes into the oropharynx over the smooth dorsum of the posterior third of the tongue, the involuntary phase of swallowing commences. The hyoid bone and larynx are drawn up and this brings the epiglottis down passively to close off the laryngeal inlet. The soft palate rises simultaneously to seal off the nasopharynx and prevent nasal regurgitation of food and fluid. The bolus then passes into the valleculae and laterally into the pyriform fossae. Eventually the bolus enters the cervical oesophagus where further propulsion occurs by peristalsis.

Speech

Speech is produced in three phases. The first is the pulmonary phase in which the lungs produce a jet of air that passes out into the subglottis. The second phase is the laryngeal phase where passage of air across the glottis creates a mucosal wave that generates sound. This is called phonation. The sound produced is then turned into speech by the articulators (e.g. tongue, soft palate and mouth). This is known as the oral phase. The pharynx, nasal cavity and paranasal sinuses are important resonating chambers that give speech its individual distinctive quality.

Symptoms of throat disease

Pain arising from the larynx or pharynx is often non-specific in its location. Patients frequently relate the pain to the anterior neck. Lateralization of pain is often the case when lesions are above the cricoid cartilage. Pain with phonation is suggestive of laryngeal pathology, and pain on swallowing is usually indicative of pharyngeal or upper oesophageal pathology.

Sensation in the ear and upper aerodigestive tract (UADT) is supplied by both the glossopharyngeal and vagus nerves. This explains the phenomenon of referred otalgia, where pathology in the upper aerodigestive tract causes pain in the ear. When unilateral, this helps the clinician locate the primary pathology. A common cause of referred otalgia is tonsillitis or pain following a tonsillectomy.

Pharyngeal symptoms

Dysphagia

Dysphagia refers to difficulty in swallowing. This can be related to food or fluids, and the patient often has to 'double swallow', drink copious amounts of water, or soften food. When pain is associated with difficulty swallowing, the term odynophagia is used. Dysphagic patients often exhibit weight loss.

Globus

When the sensation of a lump in the throat is present at all times, the term globus is used. A globus sensation may not be associated with any true dysphagia, but may still indicate organic pathology.

Regurgitation

Regurgitation is the production of undigested food that has been swallowed. This contrasts with vomiting where partially digested gastric contents are produced. Regurgitation is the hallmark of a pharyngeal pouch and an obstruction in the oesophagus which prevents food passing into the stomach.

Laryngeal symptoms

Fortunately, most pathology in the larynx produces symptoms early on. This is because small lesions disrupt the mucosal wave or cause narrowing of the airway.

Hoarseness

Hoarseness or dysphonia is the subjective perception of abnormality in the quality of one's voice. There is often an element of strain. Objective voice analysis may show increased irregularity in voice pitch and intensity. Virtually everyone has suffered from hoarseness of voice at some point in their lives. When hoarseness persists for more than 6 weeks, particularly in a smoker, urgent referral to an ENT specialist is mandatory.

Stridor and stertor

Respiratory sounds are produced from the upper airway when it is narrowed or obstructed. Stertor is a polyphonic sound that is produced by supralaryngeal obstruction. This is often heard in patients with adenoidal hypertrophy. Stridor, by contrast, is monophonic and almost 'melodious' in nature. It arises from the larynx or trachea.

Stridor may be present on inspiration alone, on expiration alone, or during both phases of breathing (biphasic). When stridor is inspiratory, it is said to be caused by narrowing in the supraglottis or glottis. Subglottic and extrathoracic tracheal narrowing produces biphasic stridor, whilst narrowing of the intrathoracic tracheobronchial tree produces expiratory stridor.

Stridor is a more worrying symptom than stertor as it may suggest impending total airway obstruction.

Examination of the throat

Inspection of the oral cavity and oropharynx is simple, but examination of the hypopharynx and larynx requires considerable skill and experience.

Inspection

Examination of the oral cavity and oropharynx is performed with a good light source and a tongue depressor. ENT surgeons normally use a head-mounted mirror that reflects light from a lamp placed just above the patient's left shoulder. This allows the surgeon to use both hands to examine the oral cavity (Fig. 3.57). Two angled metal tongue depressors (Lacks speculae) are used to depress the tongue or retract the cheeks. Systematic examination of the oral cavity and oropharynx ensures that no lesion is missed. The posterior pharyngeal wall, tonsils, soft and hard palate, dentition, tongue, floor of mouth, bucco-alveolar sulcus (the area where the cheek mucosa meets the gums) and retromolar trigone (gum behind the last lower molars) are inspected in turn.

Glossopharyngeal and hypoglossal nerve palsies are missed if the patient is not asked to say 'ah' or protrude the tongue.

Palpation

Bimanual digital palpation is an important part of oral cavity examination. Masses in the floor of the mouth, areas of lingual thickening or nodularity, and tonsillar irregularities become more evident with a finger in the mouth.

Indirect laryngoscopy

Examination of the tongue base, valleculae, larynx and hypopharynx may be performed indirectly with a warmed, downward-facing laryngeal mirror placed up against the soft palate. The patient is asked to protrude the tongue and breathe through the mouth whilst the examiner gently holds the tip of the tongue in one hand (Fig. 3.58). In most patients, indirect laryngoscopy is well tolerated if performed gently with clear instructions. In some, gagging will make this procedure impossible.

The larynx and hypopharynx may be carefully inspected. The mirror gives a good view of these structures with great clarity.

Flexible laryngoscopy

A flexible fibreoptic laryngoscope may be used to examine the upper airway. This flexible scope is passed through the nose into the nasopharynx and then down to the larynx

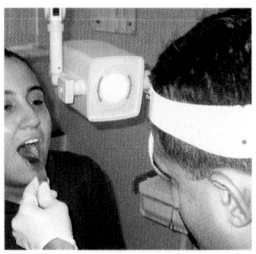

(a)

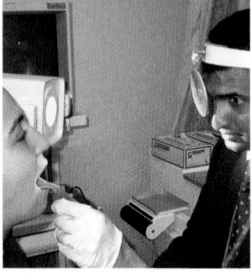

(b)

Fig. 3.57a, b Examination of the throat. The head-mounted bull's eye mirror reflects light from a lamp placed just above the patient's left shoulder, to free the examiner's hands. The hole in the head mirror sits over the surgeon's right eye, preserving binocular vision which is important for assessing depth.

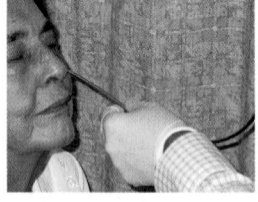

Fig. 3.59 Flexible nasoendoscopy can be performed in clinic and allows the surgeon to view the postnasal space, tongue base, hypopharynx and larynx with ease and clarity.

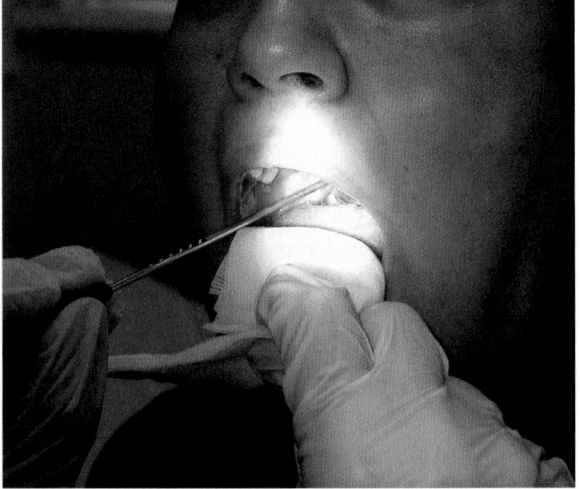

Fig. 3.58 Indirect laryngoscopy. The patient's oral cavity is examined with a laryngeal mirror placed against the soft palate and the tongue being held by the examiner.

and hypopharynx (Fig. 3.59). Topical anaesthetic and a decongestant are usually sprayed into the nose to make this examination better tolerated.

Flexible laryngoscopy allows the examiner to inspect the upper airway during quiet respiration, phonation, snoring and swallowing. These investigations provide abundant information about pathology affecting the upper airway and the options available for treatment.

Stroboscopy

Stroboscopy is a useful technique to assess the mucosal wave that forms on the vocal folds during phonation. A rigid 70 or 90 fibreoptic scope is placed just beside the uvula and allows visualization of the larynx below. The xenon light source attached to the scope then flashes at a rate of 2 Hz, 2 ms out of synchronization with phonation, whilst images of the vibrating vocal folds are captured on video. The images captured are out of phase with the mucosal wave and allows different phases of the wave to be studied (Fig. 3.60).

Stroboscopy is used in the voice clinic to analyze benign pathology of the larynx and to help ENT surgeons and speech therapists to plan treatment and assess response to therapy. Modern stroboscopes are coupled to laryngographs that measure the parameters of voice simultaneously.

SECTION 3.11 Investigations for throat disease

Diagnostic imaging

Lateral neck X-ray

A simple and useful way of imaging the larynx and pharynx is a soft tissue lateral radiograph of the neck. The penetration is reduced to give better detail of the upper airway. In particular, the hyoid bone, thyroid and cricoid cartilages, epiglottis and prevertebral soft tissue are easily identified. Foreign bodies in the upper airway which are radio-opaque may be seen with clarity. Swelling of the epiglottis secondary to epiglottitis, swelling of prevertebral soft tissues from a retropharyngeal abscess, or soft tissue swelling may be apparent.

Calcification of the laryngeal apparatus often causes confusion and is frequently mistaken for a foreign body. Calcification of the stylohyoid ligament may have the appearance of a long thin bone extending from the pharynx into the skull base.

Contrast studies

Various contrast studies may be employed to image the pharynx and oesophagus. The most common of these is the barium swallow. It gives good detailed images of the oesophagus but also provides some information about the hypopharynx (Fig. 3.61). When there is clinical suspicion of a pharyngeal or oesophageal perforation, or aspiration into an airway, a water-soluble contrast medium should be used instead of barium.

The process of swallowing may be imaged by videofluoroscopy in patients who have difficulties following surgery or a stroke. This involves taking a video of a radio-opaque bolus of food or fluid being swallowed. It gives useful information for clinicians and speech therapists to advise patients about the cause of their difficulties and to devise strategies to overcome these difficulties (e.g. chin-tucking during swallowing).

Physiological investigations

pH manometry

pH manometry involves passing a fine probe through the nose into the oesophagus and securing it in place for 24 hours. The probe measures luminal pressure and pH over this period and is an effective way of identifying episodes of gastro-oesophageal reflux. Reflux is a common cause of laryngeal complaints.

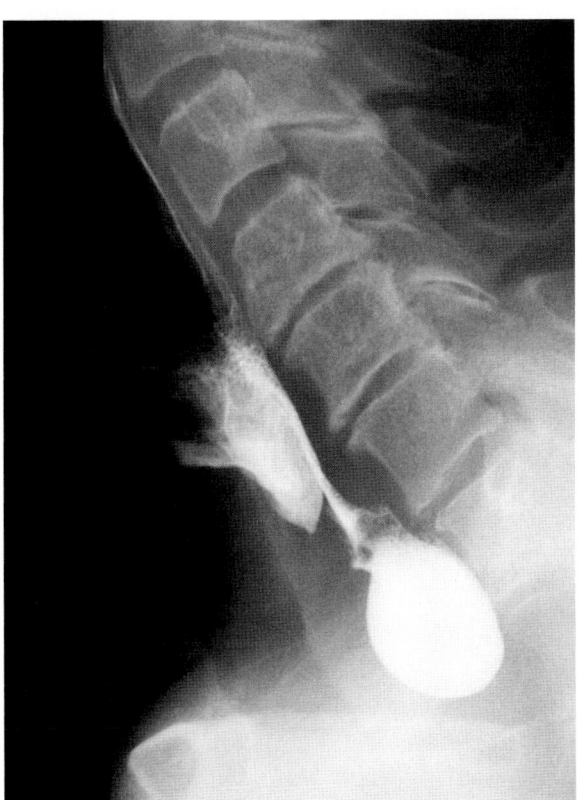

Fig. 3.61 Barium swallow. A radio-opaque bolus is swallowed and radiographic images are taken to trace its flow through the aerodigestive tract. This study demonstrates a pharyngeal pouch.

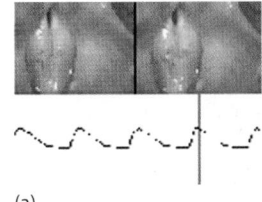

(a)

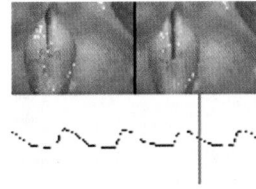

(b)

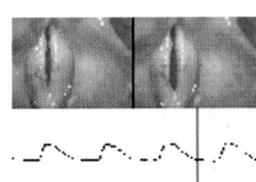

(c)

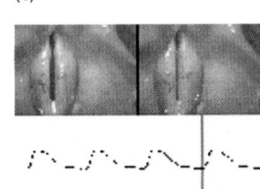

(d)

Fig. 3.60a–d Strobe images of the vocal folds in different phases of the mucosal wave.

Diseases of the throat

Foreign bodies in the throat

Foreign bodies in the upper aerodigestive tract vary in severity depending on the site of impaction. For the most part, foreign bodies in the throat that present to the emergency department are not life threatening in the immediate term.

Epidemiology

In the United States, acute airway obstruction by a foreign body causes 3000 deaths per year. This is often called the 'café coronary'; the Heimlich manoeuvre administered by a passer-by may be life saving.

Pathology

The majority of foreign bodies in patients who attend an emergency department are impacted in the oropharynx. Most commonly, fishbones are impaled in the tonsils. Once past the oropharynx, foreign bodies may lodge in the valleculae, pyriform fossae or cricopharyngeal sphincter. Within the oesophagus, impaction may occur at the natural point of narrowing 25 cm from the incisors. Benign or malignant strictures may also cause foreign body or food bolus impaction. Indeed, many strictures may present for the first time in this manner.

Foreign bodies that obstruct the glottis may be cleared by expectoration or the Heimlich manoeuvre. If neither occurs, respiratory arrest and death may ensue. Objects that are inhaled past the glottis often pass into the main bronchi. The right main bronchus lies more vertically and is therefore more commonly obstructed.

Scope of disease

Sharp foreign bodies such as fishbones may perforate the pharynx and oesophagus and cause a neck space infection or mediastinitis. Rarely, they may undergo extraluminal migration and form a fistula to major vessels in the neck or chest. Obstruction of a bronchus may cause an intractable lobar pneumonia that does not respond to antibiotics. This is often seen in the elderly.

Clinical features

Pharyngo-oesophageal foreign bodies usually present with symptoms from the onset. The most common culprit in most countries is a fishbone. Patients who have an impacted bone often have immediate symptoms. Patients usually reliably indicate the level and side of the obstruction when this is above the level of the cricoid cartilage. When a foreign body obstructs the oesophagus completely, patients present with total dysphagia and drooling.

In cases of laryngeal or tracheobronchial obstruction, the history may be vague. Children in particular may simply be noted to have a choking fit and then present with stridor or unilateral wheezing. If a foreign body is lodged in a bronchus, it may create a ball-valve effect and lead to hyperexpansion of the affected side. This can cause severe respiratory and then cardiac embarrassment when the mediastinum is shifted.

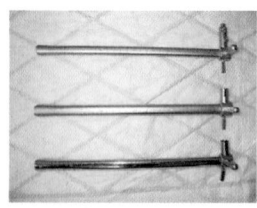

(a)

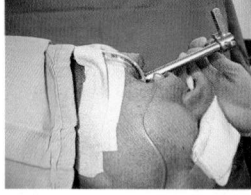

(b)

Fig. 3.63a, b
Oesophagoscopy. Rigid hollow scopes with illumination (a) allow the surgeon to inspect the lumen of the pharynx and oesophagus, and remove any objects with a grasping forceps (b).

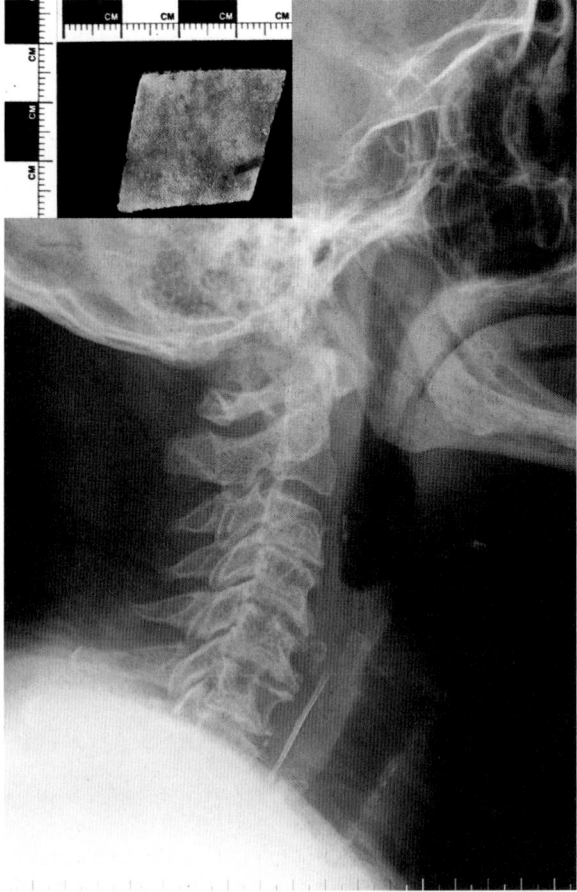

Fig. 3.62 Foreign body in the oesophagus. A soft tissue lateral neck X-ray demonstrates the piece of lamb bone lodged in this patient's cervical oesophagus visible between the trachea or cervical spine.

Initial investigations

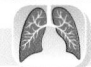

Fibreoptic laryngoscopy

Careful examination of the oropharynx, hypopharynx and larynx with flexible fibreoptic scopes will identify most foreign bodies. In oesophageal obstruction, pooling of saliva in the pyriform fossae and valleculae will be noted.

Lateral neck X-ray

A soft tissue lateral neck X-ray will reveal any radio-opaque foreign bodies (Fig. 3.62). Trapping of air in the upper oesophagus is a vital clue to a foreign body in the upper oesophagus. Foreign bodies that impale the retropharyngeal tissues will produce a wider prevertebral soft tissue shadow.

Chest and abdominal X-ray

Imaging is helpful if the foreign body is radio-opaque. If a coin has been ingested, a chest X-ray should be obtained to image the entire oesophagus.

Initial management

Endoscopic removal of foreign bodies

Removal of most oropharyngeal foreign bodies may be undertaken with topical anaesthesia in the clinic. Rigid oesophagoscopy and bronchoscopy allows the surgeon to visualize the lumen of the oesophagus and bronchus respectively. Grasping forceps permit the removal of any obstructing object. The 'ventilating' bronchoscope allows for ventilation of the anaesthetized patient whilst the tracheobronchial tree is examined.

Prognosis

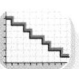

Most foreign bodies are successfully removed with endoscopic procedures; rarely, open surgery may be required when endoscopic procedures fail.

Tonsillitis

The palatine tonsils consist of lymphoid tissue and make up part of Waldeyer's ring. This ring guards the entrance to the aerodigestive tract and helps collect antigens for immune processing. The tonsils are found between the anterior and posterior faucial pillars on the lateral wall of the oropharynx (see Fig. 3.51). They are present at birth and are hypertrophic in early childhood.

Epidemiology

Inflammation of the palatine tonsils, or tonsillitis, is a common childhood disorder. It is unusual for a child not to suffer one or two episodes in early life. Recurrent tonsillitis is less common. The incidence in the population has not been accurately documented. In the United Kingdom, primary care physicians deal with 10 000 cases of sore throat per 100 000 of the population. Most of these cases represent generalized pharyngitis. Tonsillitis makes up a minority of cases and fewer still suffer recurrent episodes.

Pathology

Of the causative organisms of acute tonsillitis, rhinoviruses, adenoviruses and enteroviruses probably constitute 50%, although it is hypothesized that many cases of tonsillitis begin as viral infections before secondary bacterial infection supervenes. Of the bacteria responsible for acute tonsillitis, β-haemolytic streptococci, *Streptococcus pneumoniae* and *Haemophilus influenzae* are the most common. Many anaerobic bacteria are often isolated on throat swabs; their significance is doubtful.

Other important but less common causes of tonsillitis include infectious mononucleosis (glandular fever) as a result of infection by the Epstein–Barr (EB) virus; diphtheria, which is uncommon in the West due to vaccination but may be seen in the developing world, and tonsillar infiltration from acute lymphoblastic leukaemia.

Scope of disease

Infection in a tonsil may pass deep to its capsule and spread to the loose areolar tissue that surrounds it. This cellulitis, or peritonsillitis, may develop into a peritonsillar abscess (quinsy). Septicaemia, septic arthritis, endocarditis and meningitis are rare consequences of untreated cases. Rheumatic fever (p. 36) can occur with group A β-haemolytic streptococci infection.

Clinical features

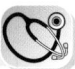

Whilst the most common symptom of tonsillitis is a sore throat, not all sore throats are due to tonsillitis. This distinction is pivotal in selecting patients for tonsillectomy. Tonsillitis is often accompanied by fever, malaise and anorexia. Referred otalgia is a common symptom and often misdiagnosed as acute otitis media. Severe pain, trismus, dysphagia and drooling with a spiking fever are symptoms suggestive of a peritonsillar abscess.

On examination, the cervical lymph nodes are often enlarged and tender to palpation. Inspection of the oropharynx will reveal swollen, inflamed tonsils and associated inflammation and oedema of the soft palate and uvula. The crypts of the tonsils often contain debris and pus. This gives the classical appearance of 'follicular tonsillitis' (Fig. 3.64). Examination of the pharynx in patients with peritonsillar abscesses may be difficult, but if successful reveals a bulging soft palate and a uvula that is displaced from the midline (Fig. 3.65).

A grey-white exudate over the tonsils is often seen in glandular fever (infectious mononucleosis; Fig. 3.66). There may be associated petechiae of the soft palate, or splenomegaly.

A thick white membrane over the oropharynx in a child of 2–3 years is a classical sign of diphtheria. Ecchymoses of the soft palate and uvula, accompanying tonsillitis, may be a feature of acute lymphoblastic leukaemia.

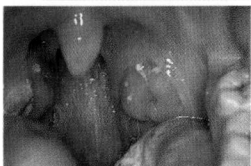

Fig. 3.64 Follicular tonsillitis. Bacterial tonsillitis with exudative pus coating inflamed tonsils.

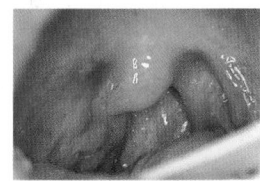

Fig. 3.65 A developing peritonsillar abscess or quinsy, requiring surgical drainage.

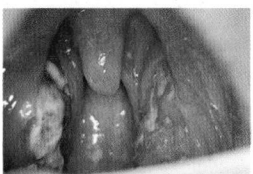

Fig. 3.66 Glandular fever. A grey-white coating of the tonsils is highly suggestive of Epstein–Barr viral infection causing glandular fever.

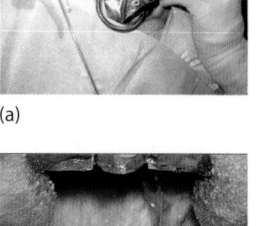

(a)

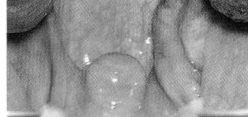

(b)

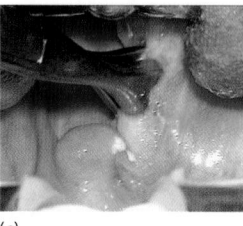

(c)

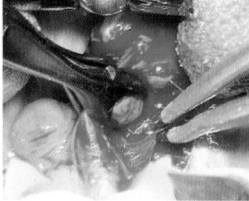

(d)

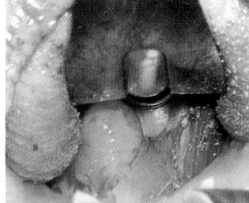

(e)

Fig. 3.67a–e Tonsillectomy. The mouth of the supine patient is held open by a Boyle–Davis gag. This is supported by Draffin rods in a tripod configuration. Bipolar diathermy is used to dissect the tonsils from the oropharynx.

Initial investigations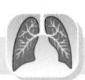

Investigations are generally not required in patients with mild symptoms.

Further investigations

Full blood count

The white count is often raised, and a blood film is indicated when leukaemia (p. 801) is suspected.

Monospot test

The monospot or Paul–Bunnell test for heterophile antibodies is useful in confirming glandular fever, but may only be positive in the second week of infection.

Initial management

Rehydration

Patients who come to urgent medical attention are often dehydrated due to poor oral intake and pyrexia. Patients with severe dehydration should be admitted for intravenous fluid resuscitation.

Analgesia

Effective analgesia is important in managing acute tonsillitis. Paracetamol is safe and effective. The use of anaesthetic gargles may provide good symptomatic relief and allow the patient to re-establish oral intake.

Medical management

Antibiotic therapy

Treatment of tonsillitis with antibiotics will reduce the severity of an episode but have no effect on the outcome, e.g. prevention of rheumatic sequelae or peritonsillar abscess. Phenoxymethylpenicillin is the best first-line antibiotic. Until glandular fever is excluded, it is best to avoid ampicillin-type antibiotics as these produce an idiosyncratic rash.

Diphtheria antitoxin

The airway is at risk in patients with diphtheria and urgent treatment with antitoxin is critical in patients with suspected disease.

Immunomodulation

In severe glandular fever, where there is difficulty breathing, intravenous dexamethasone will improve symptoms dramatically.

Surgical management

Tonsillectomy

Patients who suffer five or more episodes of tonsillitis in one year, or who have severe episodes which prevent normal functioning, are best served by tonsillectomy. Surgical removal of the tonsils is undertaken intra-orally, and a Boyle–Davis gag is inserted following intubation of the anaesthetized patient (Fig. 3.67a). The tonsils may be excised by a variety of methods. These include 'cold steel' dissection, diathermy, laser excision, cold ablation (coblation) or harmonic scalpel dissection.

The surgeon stands at the head of the patient, viewing the oropharynx from above. The gag is held in place by rods, leaving her hands free to operate. The tongue-blade of the gag at the top of the picture keeps the tongue and endotracheal tube out of view (Fig. 3.67b) and the tonsil is grasped and pulled medially (Fig. 3.67c). The blood vessels from the lateral wall to the tonsil are diathermized using bipolar forceps (Fig. 3.67d). After removal of the first tonsil, the muscle fibres of the superior constrictor are seen (Fig. 3.67e), and eventually both tonsils are removed. The day after surgery, the uvula is oedematous and a coating of yellow slough covers the bed of the tonsils. This is not an infection. Re-epithelialization takes 2 weeks (Fig. 3.68).

Up to 97% of patients derive benefit from this procedure. There is, however, a 2% morbidity rate, principally due to postoperative haemorrhage.

Prognosis

Full recovery is the general rule after an episode of tonsillitis; few patients go on to develop recurrent disease.

---

i FURTHER INFORMATION

Management of sore throat and indications for tonsillectomy. Scottish Intercollegiate Guidelines Network (SIGN) publication no. 34 (ISBN 1899893 66 0). See also www.sign.ac.uk

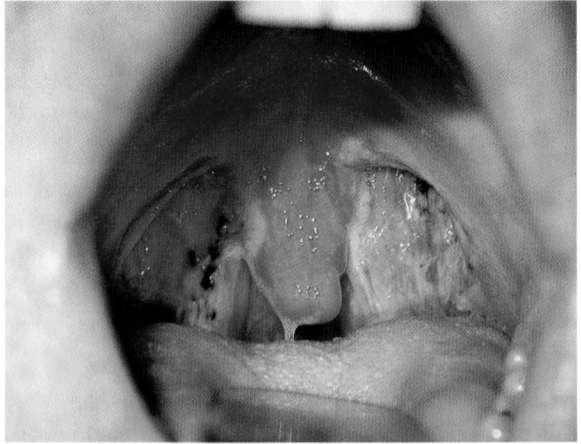

Fig. 3.68 A postoperative view of the tonsillar fossae following tonsillectomy. Slough forms soon after surgery and gradually clears after 5–7 days. This appearance is often mistaken for infection. It does not warrant antibiotics.

Laryngitis

Laryngitis is inflammation of the mucosa of the larynx. It may be acute, recurrent or chronic.

Epidemiology

Laryngitis is a common condition and is associated to some extent with all cases of upper respiratory tract infections. No accurate data are available on its incidence but it tends to affect young adults and is equally common in both sexes.

Pathology

Acute laryngitis is usually accompanied by hyperaemia and oedema of the vocal folds. This is most commonly due to a viral infection as part of an upper respiratory tract infection. Vocal fold abuse, e.g. shouting at a football match, may also cause these changes. Other predisposing factors are smoking, alcohol consumption, use of steroid inhalers and gastro-oesophageal reflux disease. Patients with gastro-oesophageal reflux develop a distinct disease entity known as laryngopharyngeal reflux (LPR), which is treated by antireflux medication (p. 253).

Recurrent or chronic laryngitis is more common in people who use their voice regularly. Teachers and singers are particularly susceptible as they are unable to rest their voice during an acute episode, often resulting in the development of recurrent or chronic laryngitis.

When vocal fold abuse continues or irritants such as tobacco smoke, industrial fumes, alcohol and gastric refluxate persist, chronic laryngitis supervenes and irreversible pathological changes occur. Most commonly, oedema of the intermediate layer of the vocal folds develops resulting in swollen, boggy vocal folds. This condition is known as Reinke's oedema and is commonly seen in smokers (Fig. 3.69).

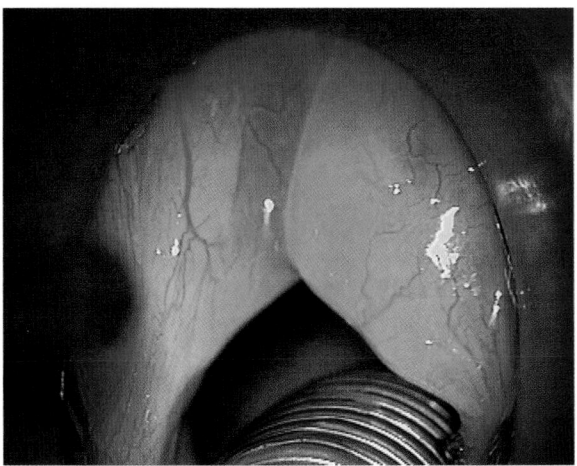

Fig. 3.69 Reinke's oedema is commonly seen in smokers and produces a 'rough' voice.

Scope of disease

Metaplasia of the squamous epithelium covering the vocal folds may occur producing keratinizing epithelium. The vocal folds become hypertrophic and thickened, with white plaques (leukoplakia). If left untreated, this progresses to dysplasia (mild, moderate or severe), intra-epithelial neoplasia or carcinoma in situ. Severe laryngitis can also lead to upper airway obstruction.

Clinical features

Laryngitis causes hoarseness or dysphonia. In severe forms, episodes of complete voice loss (aphonia) may occur. Pain is seldom severe but there is often some discomfort with swallowing. Haemoptysis is uncommon. Patients may have concurrent flu or report symptoms of heartburn. A monophonic inspiratory sound or stridor is not a sign of simple laryngitis but a hallmark of epiglottitis or supraglottitis and suggests impending airway obstruction.

Examination may reveal lymphadenopathy in the neck and pain on palpation of the thyroid cartilage. Inspection of the pharynx may reveal inflamed mucous membrane suggesting a coexisting pharyngitis. All patients with unresolving dysphonia for 6 weeks should be referred urgently to an ENT department for laryngoscopy. This examination will exclude neoplasia and identify Reinke's oedema or leukoplakia.

Initial management

Laryngitis is managed with adequate voice rest, adequate lubrication of the vocal folds and removal of any irritants to the larynx.

Voice rest

Patients are advised to rest the voice for a few days until the symptoms resolve.

Analgesia

Aspirin gargles and simple analgesics may be indicated. Steam inhalation may provide additional symptomatic relief.

Identify and correct any underlying cause

In chronic cases, it is vital to remove any persistent irritant such as tobacco smoke, steroid inhalants or gastric reflux. A simple method of helping asthmatics on inhalers is to encourage them to gargle with water after delivery of inhaled steroids.

A postnasal drip from chronic rhinosinusitis often perpetuates a throat-clearing habit that is damaging to the vocal folds. Speech therapy may help to identify and modify this and other abusive vocal habits.

Medical management

Antibiotics

Occasionally, a secondary bacterial infection may supervene and necessitate treatment with antibiotics.

Surgical management

Suspension microlaryngoscopy

Surgery is undertaken only when conservative measures have failed or malignancy is suspected. Suspension microlaryngoscopy is performed under general anaesthesia with the assistance of an operating microscope. A laryngoscope is inserted orally and suspended (Fig. 3.70); areas of keratosis that have developed on the vocal folds are excised. Similarly, Reinke's oedema may be aspirated or areas of polypoidal change excised with microlaryngoscopy. This surgery must be undertaken delicately as scarring and web formation between the vocal folds may leave a patient dysphonic for life.

Prognosis

In general, vocal folds are able to return to their normal vitality once irritants are removed or vocal abuse modified.

Vocal fold palsy

All the intrinsic muscles of the larynx, except the posterior cricoarytenoid, bring together (adduct) the vocal folds. The posterior cricoarytenoid muscles abduct the vocal folds. Paralysis of the vocal folds may selectively affect the adductors and cause the vocal fold to lie in a lateral position (adductor palsy). Alternatively, the posterior cricoarytenoid may be weaker than the adductors, leaving the vocal fold in the paramedian position (abductor palsy).

Epidemiology

The epidemiology of vocal fold palsy is variable, as it is related to the underlying cause.

Pathology

Vocal fold palsies are most commonly the result of damage to the nerve supply to the intrinsic muscles of the larynx. Specifically, this may be due to damage in the brainstem or anywhere along the length of the vagus nerve or the recurrent laryngeal nerve (Table 3.6). Rarely, myopathies of the intrinsic muscles of the larynx or arthritis affecting the synovial cricoarytenoid joints may produce 'vocal fold palsy'. When no cause is found, the palsy is described as idiopathic in nature. It is postulated that the majority of these cases are actually due to infection by a neuropathic virus.

Scope of disease

Vocal fold palsies can lead to dysphonia, and aspiration is likely to be problematic in patients with bilateral palsies. As the cough reflex is likely to be ineffective, chronic aspiration may lead to recurrent pneumonias. Acute airways obstruction can also occur as a complication of bilateral palsies.

Table 3.6	Causes of a vocal cord palsy
Peripheral lesions (>80%)	
Malignant neoplasms	
Lung	
Thyroid	
Larynx	
Oesophagus	
Trauma	
Neck trauma	
Surgery	
Thyroidectomy	
Lung surgery	
Surgery of the aorta	
Central lesions	
Neurological (rare)	
Poliomyelitis	
Pseudobulbar palsy	
Bulbar palsy	
Multiple sclerosis	
Infarction of the posterior inferior cerebellar artery (Wallenberg's syndrome)	
Idiopathic (10%)	

Clinical features

In adductor palsy, the vocal fold lies in an abducted, or lateral, position. In these cases, the voice is often weak and breathy. The cough in adductor palsies is sometimes likened to that of a cow ('bovine' cough).

In abductor palsy, the paralyzed vocal fold lies in the paramedian position. Voice production is often not a problem but voice frequently tires easily. In bilateral cases, where both vocal folds lie adducted, breathing is surprisingly not compromised until an upper airway infection causes oedema and narrows the airway further. Stridor may then herald acute airway obstruction.

Initial investigations

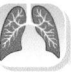

Indirect and flexible fibreoptic laryngoscopy

A thorough evaluation of the airway is critical in the management of patients with vocal fold palsy. Indirect laryngoscopy or flexible fibreoptic laryngoscopy offers a good view of the vocal folds at rest and in phonation. The paralyzed fold often appears atrophic and shorter than its normal fellow. The apparent shortening is due to the arytenoid cartilage prolapsing forwards. The paralyzed fold also appears to lie at a higher level (Fig. 3.71). Upon phonation, compensation by the normal fold may be seen.

Further investigations

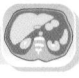

CT or MRI of the neck and upper mediastinum

A search for a cause is mandatory. This invariably involves imaging of the brainstem and the length of the recurrent laryngeal nerve by CT or MRI.

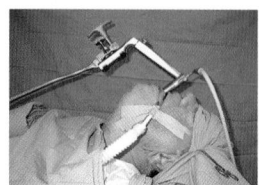

(a)

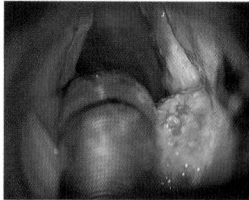

(b)

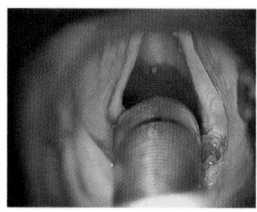

(c)

Fig. 3.70a–c Microlaryngoscopy and excision of a keratotic plaque. A laryngoscope is sited over the glottis and suspended, leaving the surgeon's hands free to manipulate fine surgical instruments. Here a keratotic plaque is excised; it proved to be squamous cell carcinoma.

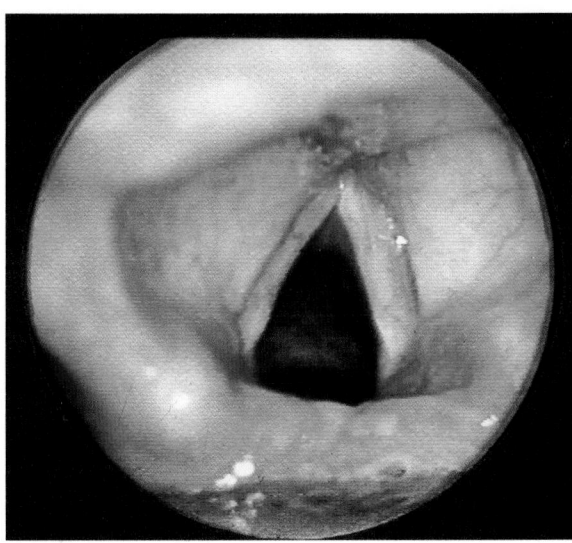

Fig. 3.71 Left vocal fold palsy showing the paralyzed atrophic fold lying at a lateral lower level.

Laryngeal electromyography

Where there is a need to exclude a possible myopathy, laryngeal electromyography is useful.

Examination under anaesthesia

Cricoarytenoid joint fixation may be excluded by direct laryngoscopy under general anaesthesia and joint palpation to assess mobility.

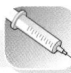

Initial management

Speech therapy

In cases where there are no voice problems, aspiration or breathing difficulties, conservative measures may be employed. Speech therapists often teach patients vocal fold adduction exercises to keep muscle tone from deteriorating and to facilitate compensation.

Surgical management

The indications for surgery include protection of the airway (tracheostomy), improvement of symptoms of upper airways obstruction (laser arytenoidectomy), management of chronic aspiration (laryngeal diversion) and improving phonation (vocal fold medialization procedures).

Tracheostomy

Surgical tracheostomy (more correctly termed a tracheotomy) is the only solution to providing a safe airway in patients with acute breathing difficulties. Tracheostomy may be performed surgically or percutaneously using the Seldinger technique. Mini-tracheostomy may be performed if the main indication is bronchial toilet.

General anaesthesia is required for a surgical tracheostomy (Figs 3.72 and 3.73). The patient is positioned supine with a roll under the shoulders and the neck extended. The cricoid cartilage is identified, and an incision line falling in a skin crease halfway between this and the suprasternal notch is marked (Fig. 3.72a). The incision is made through skin, subcutaneous tissue and platysma (Fig. 3.72b), and the strap muscles are separated in the midline to reveal the trachea (Fig. 3.72c). A fenestration is made below the first tracheal ring (Fig. 3.72d) and a cuffed tracheostomy tube is inserted as the endotracheal tube is withdrawn from the trachea (Fig. 3.72e).

Laser arytenoidectomy

In cases where breathing limits normal activity, a laser arytenoidectomy with partial resection of one arytenoid creates a large posterior glottic space to improve breathing. The anterior segments of both vocal folds, which are necessary for phonation, remain unaffected.

Laryngeal diversion

Chronic aspiration is difficult to manage. Changing the consistency of fluids ingested may minimize aspiration. In some cases, a laryngeal diversion procedure or a laryngectomy is the only solution. Tracheostomy is often a poor solution for aspiration; the presence of a tracheostomy may actually perpetuate aspiration.

Vocal fold medialization

When voice is a problem, a variety of vocal fold medialization procedures are available. The best established procedure is a 'medialization thyroplasty' in which a piece of Silastic is implanted through a window cut in the thyroid cartilage (Isshiki's type I thyroplasty). This effectively pushes a paralyzed vocal fold medially towards its normal fellow.

RECENT ADVANCES

Advances in endolaryngeal surgery have facilitated the injection of biologically inert materials into the paralyzed vocal fold to effect medialization.

Prognosis

Recovery of a vocal fold palsy, where no cause or a reversible cause is found, may occur up to one year following onset. Any irreversible treatment should therefore not be performed until this period of time has elapsed.

Pharyngeal pouch

Pharyngeal pouches (Zenker's diverticula) are diverticula that usually arise from the posterior wall of the lowest part of the pharynx or hypopharynx.

Epidemiology

Pharyngeal pouches are more common in northern than southern parts of Europe. Incidence is higher in North

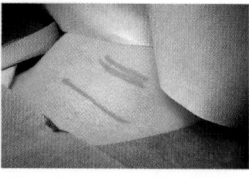
(a)

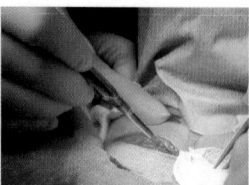
(b)

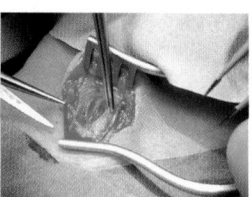
(c)

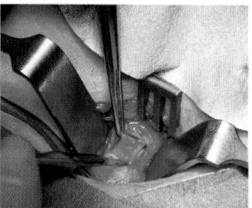
(d)

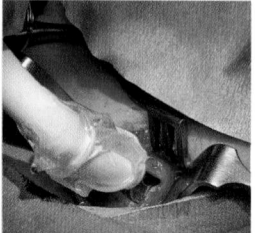
(e)

Fig. 3.72a–e Tracheostomy.

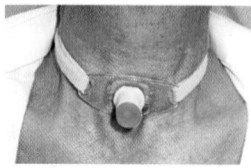

Fig. 3.73 Patient with a completed tracheostomy. The tracheostomy tube is also shown in situ.

America and Australia than in Japan and Indonesia. A community study in the United Kingdom suggested an incidence of 2 per 100 000 per year. The condition is uncommon below the age of 40, with most patients presenting in the seventh decade of life. There is a clear male preponderance.

Pathology

A pharyngeal pouch is a protrusion of hypopharyngeal mucosa through the posterior or posterolateral wall of the pharynx. The pathogenesis may be that of a pulsion diverticulum arising from high hypopharyngeal pressures secondary to increased cricopharyngeal tonicity.

The site of herniation between the thyropharyngeal and cricopharyngeal fibres of the inferior constrictor is known as Killian's dehiscence (Fig. 3.74). The pouch is lined by stratified squamous epithelium and varies in size. Small pouches may only be visible on contrast videofluoroscopic assessment of swallowing; large pouches may be palpable.

Scope of disease

There have been reports of carcinoma or carcinoma in situ arising in the fundus of a pharyngeal pouch. Chronic aspiration often leads to cough, halitosis and dysphonia. In addition, chronic aspiration in elderly patients predisposes to pneumonias.

Clinical features

Pouches consistently produce symptoms of dysphagia. Regurgitation of undigested food is pathognomonic but often not forthcoming in the history. Borborygmi of the neck, chronic cough, bronchospasm, chronic aspiration, halitosis and dysphonia are other common features. Large pouches may produce severe malnutrition and emaciation. Rapid deterioration of symptoms, pain and haemoptysis may suggest malignancy.

Clinical examination is often fruitless. Occasionally, a swelling in the neck that gurgles on palpation (Boyce's sign) is noted. The diagnosis is often reached with the use of contrast studies.

Initial investigations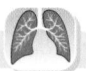

Barium swallow
A barium swallow is the gold standard (Fig. 3.75) for the diagnosis of a pharyngeal pouch.

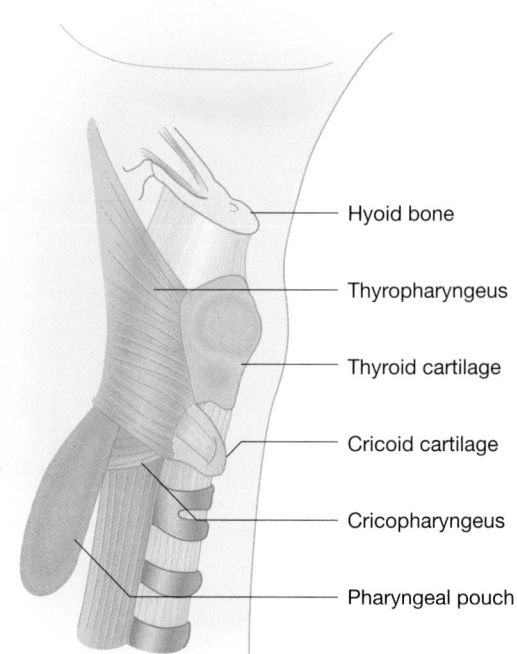

- Hyoid bone
- Thyropharyngeus
- Thyroid cartilage
- Cricoid cartilage
- Cricopharyngeus
- Pharyngeal pouch

Fig. 3.74 Lateral view of the pharynx. Killian's dehiscence is a site of natural weakening of the inferior constrictor, between the thyropharyngeal and cricopharyngeal fibres.

Upper gastrointestinal endoscopy
On rigid or flexible endoscopy, a double oesophageal lumen is noted. It is important to pass the endoscope into the anterior lumen to avoid entering the pouch and perforating it.

Surgical management

Endoscopic cricopharyngeal myotomy
Endoscopic treatment modalities offer a quicker and safer procedure, and rapid recovery. This method involves division of the 'muscular septum' between the oesophageal and pouch lumens. The pouch is not excised, but its wider neck prevents it filling with food and fluid. Division of the septum may be undertaken by laser or diathermy. Satisfaction rates with this procedure are high. More recently,

endoscopic stapling has been introduced as a safer and equally effective method. The muscular septum is stapled together before being cut (Fig. 3.76).

The obvious concern with all endoscopic techniques is the possibility of missing a malignancy in the fundus of the pouch.

Diverticulectomy

Surgical excision was the only method of treatment of pharyngeal pouches before the advent of endoscopic techniques. This involved an 'open' neck procedure in which the pouch was inverted or excised (diverticulectomy). This procedure has a high complication rate. It may result in severe mediastinitis in patients who are often frail and elderly, resulting in death.

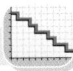

Prognosis

The symptoms produced by a pharyngeal pouch relate to its size. Most patients with small pouches have few or no symptoms. Pouches usually increase in size gradually. The results are often good in the small proportion that eventually require surgery.

ℹ FURTHER INFORMATION

Siddiq M A, Sood S, Strachan D. Pharyngeal pouch (Zenker's diverticulum). Postgraduate Medical Journal 2001; 77: 506–511.

Foreign bodies in the throat

Tonsillitis

Laryngitis

Vocal fold palsy

Pharyngeal pouch

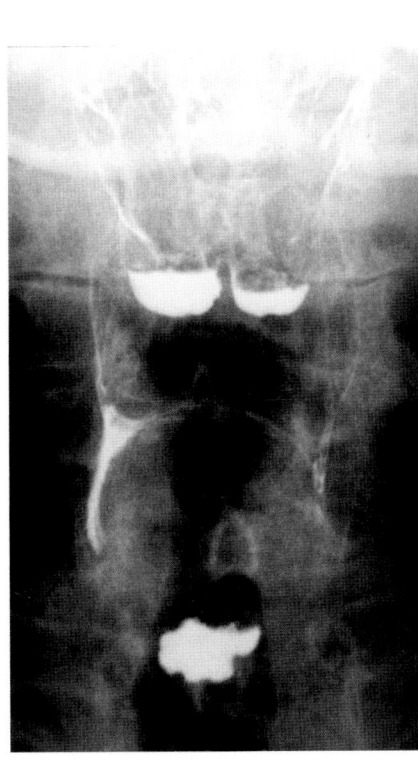

(a)

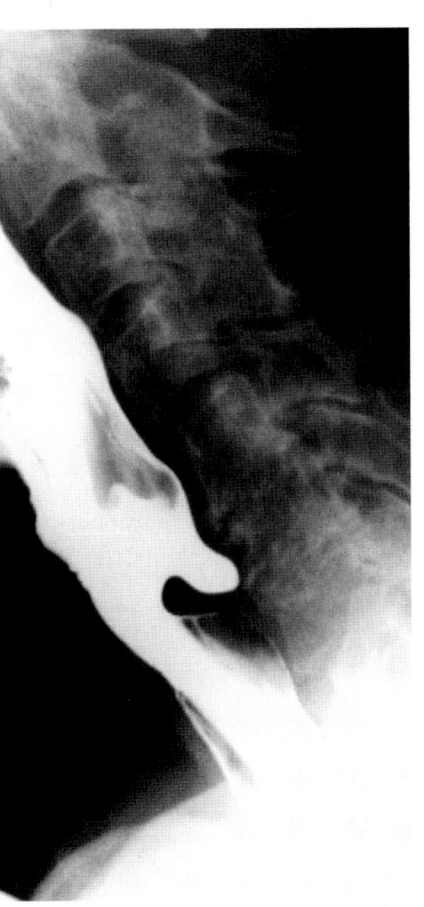

(b)

Fig. 3.75a, b Barium swallow of a pharyngeal pouch. (a) Frontal view; (b) lateral view.

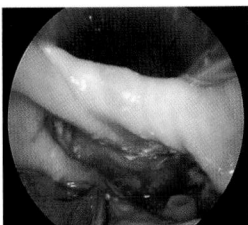

(a)

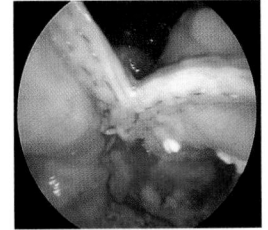

(b)

Fig. 3.76 Endoscopic stapling. The muscular septum or bar seen on rigid endoscopy in (a) with the lumen of the oesophagus above and the pouch below, and the appearance after stapling (b).

Head and neck

Head and neck cancers

A variety of histological malignancies can affect the skin of the head and neck, the upper aerodigestive tract (nose, oral cavity, larynx and pharynx), paranasal sinuses, thyroid and parathyroid glands and the salivary glands.

Head and neck squamous cell cancers arise from the mucosal surface of the upper aerodigestive tract. The larynx and the oral cavity are the two most common sites.

Epidemiology

There is a wide variation in geographical incidence. Countries such as France, Spain, Italy, the USA, Thailand and Poland have high rates of laryngeal and hypopharyngeal cancers, and the Indian subcontinent has a high rate of oral cavity cancers. In the United Kingdom, head and neck squamous cell cancers make up 3% of new cancers diagnosed each year.

The peak incidence of head and neck squamous cell cancers is the seventh decade of life. For nasopharyngeal cancers, the peak incidence in the 40s reflects the genetic, environmental and dietary factors that contribute to its development. Head and neck squamous cell cancers affect more men than women; however, the incidence in women is rising fast as more women take up smoking.

Pathology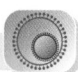

The main aetiological factors in the development of head and neck squamous cell cancers are summarized in Table 3.7. Cigarette smoking and alcohol consumption act independently and synergistically in a dose-dependent manner. It has been demonstrated that the relative risk of head and neck squamous cell cancers in smokers of <7 and >25 cigarettes/day over non-smokers is 2.4 and 16.4 respectively. Consuming 7–21 units of alcohol per week confers a 3.0 relative risk of head and neck squamous cell cancers over non-drinkers, but this risk drops to 0.5 when a third of the alcohol consumed is wine. Drinking more than 21 units a week increases both these figures.

Nasopharyngeal carcinoma has a high incidence amongst Southern Chinese. There is a clear genetic predisposition amongst these people as they carry their risk with them, albeit reduced, when they emigrate. Salted fish that are high in nitrosamines and EBV infection are the other key aetiological factors.

Nasopharyngeal carcinoma arises in the cleft between the eustachian tube cushion and the posterior nasopharyngeal wall (fossa of Rosenmüller) and may remain submucosal for some time, eluding endoscopic diagnosis. The tumour has three distinct histological types: keratinizing, non-keratinizing and undifferentiated. Spread to the draining lymph nodes tends to occur early, first to the retropharyngeal node of Rouviere before passing to the posterior triangle nodes (level V).

There are a variety of premalignant lesions of the oral cavity. Leukoplakia (meaning white plaque) shows mild to moderate dysplasia in 10% of lesions and severe dysplasia or carcinoma in situ in 5%. Erythroleukoplakia, which is

Table 3.7	Risk factors for head and neck squamous cancer

Principal carcinogens
Smoking
Alcohol

Site-specific carcinogens
Oral cavity
   Betel nut in Indian subcontinent, Taiwan and south-east Asia
Paranasal sinuses
   Hardwood dust causing adenocarcinoma
Nasopharynx
   Nitrosamines in salted fish diet
Nose, larynx, lung and sinuses
   Chromate and nickel dust

Viruses
HPV types 6, 18 and 33
EBV—nasopharyngeal carcinoma cells contain EBV genome.
   Serum levels of IgA against the EBV viral capsid antigen (VCA) are elevated before clinical symptoms are evident

Iron deficiency
Paterson–Brown–Kelly syndrome (iron deficiency, glossitis, koilonychia and an upper oesophageal web) is associated with a 4–16% risk of postcricoid carcinoma

Familial risks
First-degree relatives of patients with head and neck squamous cell carcinoma have a 3.5–3.8 relative risk of disease

an erythematous variant of leukoplakia, has a higher premalignant potential. Similarly, lichen planus, which is an immunologically mediated disorder, produces white reticulated striae in the buccal mucosa and has a 4% malignant transformation rate over a patient's lifetime. Growths on the lip, tongue, buccal mucosa and gingiva may represent head and neck squamous cancers of the oral cavity. These may be ulcerative and deeply infiltrating or exophytic in verrucous squamous cell carcinoma. Oropharyngeal tumours may arise from the tonsil, tongue base or posterior pharyngeal wall. The consumption of betel nut in some societies increases the incidence of oral cavity squamous cell cancer. The chewed mixture of betel nut, lime and tobacco is often 'kept' in the bucco-gingival sulcus for prolonged periods of time where it acts as a carcinogen.

Clinical features

Depending on the primary site, head and neck squamous cancers may remain silent for some time before causing any symptoms. Typically, cancers of the supraglottis, pyriform sinuses, tongue base and nasopharynx may cause no problems until fairly advanced. Commonly, the first presentation may be with an enlarged neck node as a result of metastatic spread (Fig. 3.77).

All primary care physicians should be well acquainted with the early signs of head and neck cancer and refer patients urgently to the appropriate specialists (Table 3.8).

Table 3.8	Referral guideline for suspected head and neck cancer*

Urgent referral

An unexplained neck lump, of recent onset, or a previously diagnosed lump that has changed over a period of 3–6 weeks

An unexplained persistent swelling in the parotid or submandibular gland

An unexplained persistent sore or painful throat

Unilateral unexplained pain in the head and neck area for more than 4 weeks, associated with otalgia (earache) but normal otoscopy

Unexplained ulceration of the oral mucosa or mass persisting for more than 3 weeks

Unexplained red and white patches (including suspected lichen planus) of the oral mucosa that are painful or swollen or bleeding

For patients with persistent symptoms or signs related to the oral cavity in whom a definitive diagnosis of a benign lesion cannot be made, refer or follow-up until the symptoms and signs disappear. If the symptoms and signs have not disappeared after 6 weeks, make an urgent referral

Urgent referral for chest X-ray

Patients with persisting hoarseness for more than 3 weeks, particularly smokers aged older than 50 years and heavy drinkers

If there is a positive finding, refer urgently to a team specializing in the management of lung cancer. If there is a negative finding, refer urgently to a team specializing in head and neck cancer

*National Institute for Health and Clinical Excellence, UK

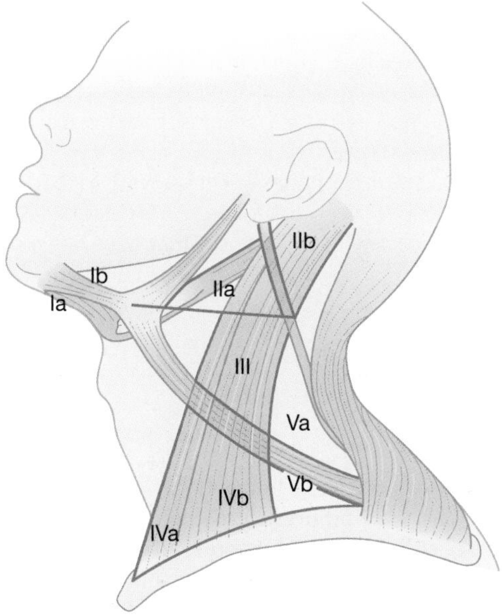

Fig. 3.77 The cervical lymph nodes that drain the head and neck are divided into seven groups or levels. Cancers from different sites have a predilection to spread to specific levels first. Level VI are the paratracheal nodes adjacent to the thyroid gland, and level VII nodes are in the upper mediastinum.

Laryngeal cancer

Squamous cell carcinoma of the larynx presents early and metastasizes late (Fig. 3.78). It causes persistent hoarseness in a smoker and may cause some discomfort. Referred pain to the ear (referred otalgia) is sometimes reported. In advanced cases, commonly seen in the self-neglected, stridor and airway obstruction may occur.

Nasopharyngeal cancer

The tumour's proximity to the eustachian tube orifice often causes dysfunction of middle ear ventilation and produces an effusion. Hence, unilateral conductive deafness and posterior cervical lymphadenopathy, particularly in Southern Chinese, is nasopharyngeal cancer until proven otherwise.

Tumours of the oral cavity and oropharynx

These tend to produce pain and referred otalgia. When oropharyngeal tumours cause trismus, they have usually infiltrated the medial pterygoid muscles and may be inoperable.

Tumours of the hypopharynx

Tumours of the postcricoid space and pyriform sinuses often grow to an advanced stage before producing any symptoms. Commonly, infiltration of the larynx produces hoarseness, which brings the patient to medical attention.

225

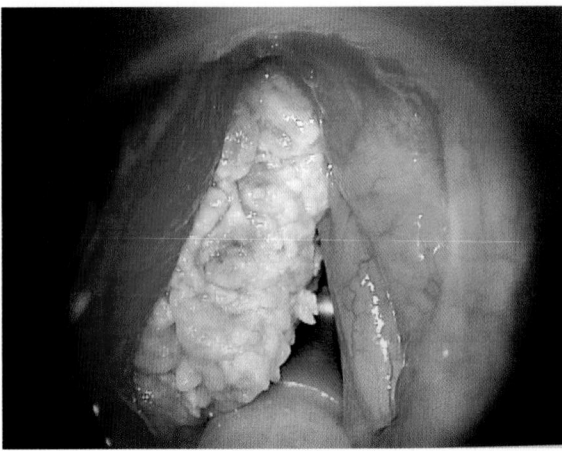

Fig. 3.78 T2 tumour of the larynx. A verrucous squamous cell carcinoma of the left vocal fold. The entire length of the fold is involved by this exophytic growth.

The association with Paterson–Brown–Kelly syndrome makes postcricoid carcinoma more common in women than in men.

Initial investigations

Aspiration of lymph nodes
All enlarged neck nodes should be subjected to fine-needle aspiration cytology before any attempt is made at excision (Fig. 3.79).

Fibreoptic ENT examination
A thorough ENT examination with flexible fibreoptic endoscopy is important. Often rigid endoscopy and biopsy under general anaesthesia is warranted. Imaging of the neck and chest is mandatory.

CT scan of the head and neck
A CT scan is usually sufficient and should be performed before any biopsies are taken. The incidence of second

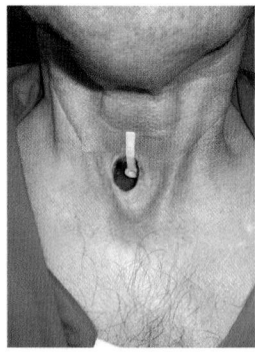

Fig. 3.80 An end stoma following laryngectomy. The one-way valve on the posterior tracheal wall allows for voicing.

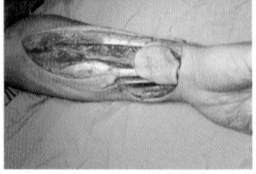

Fig. 3.81 A radial forearm free flap raised for use in reconstructing defects following surgical resection.

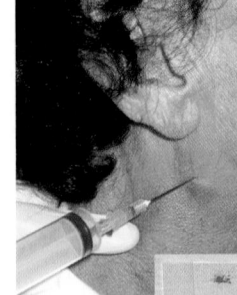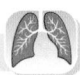

Fig. 3.79a, b Fine-needle aspiration (a) and smearing of slides (b) for cytological analysis of a neck lump.

primaries or synchronous tumours (i.e. tumours diagnosed within 6 months of each other) can be as high as 15%, particularly in cases where the index primary is in the larynx.

Further investigations

PET scan
In cases where the primary is unknown, positron emission tomography scanning is increasingly useful in finding occult lesions.

Surgical management

Treatment of head and neck squamous cancers is by surgery or radiotherapy, or a combination of both. The principle of treatment is to use the same modality for both the primary and cervical metastases where possible. Organ preservation is also a key consideration.

Laryngectomy
Surgical treatment aims to remove the primary tumour and draining lymph nodes as a single en bloc dissection. In laryngeal squamous cell cancers, this involves a laryngectomy in which the trachea is exteriorized as a stoma at the base of the neck (Fig. 3.80). The defect in the pharynx is closed primarily. Patients are unable to speak postoperatively, but this can be aided by oesophageal speech, artificial larynx speech (with a phonation device) or tracheo-oesophageal speech.

Resection of the tongue and pharynx
In larger resections of the tonsil, tongue or pharynx, it is necessary to reconstruct any defect with tissue transferred from elsewhere. Reconstruction may be performed using a pedicled myocutaneous flap such as the pectoralis major muscle or using free-tissue transfer such as a radial forearm free flap (Fig. 3.81).

Malignant lymph nodes are removed as part of an operation known as a neck dissection. This is occasionally done prophylactically for tumours that have not metastasized but are known to have high metastatic potential (e.g. tongue and supraglottis).

Medical management

Radiotherapy
When surgery is the primary treatment, radiotherapy may be used as adjuvant treatment if resection has not been complete or in aggressive tumours. In some cancers, primary radiotherapy offers a better survival and functional outcome. This is particularly so in early glottic cancers.

Ionizing radiation may also be used to treat tumours that cannot be resected safely without significant morbidity. The radiation dose is delivered as small fractions on a daily basis or twice daily (hyperfractionation). The total dose is delivered over 6–7 weeks and varies between 60 and 70 Gy. The patient has a mask moulded to help keep the head and neck immobile during the irradiation.

Radiotherapy causes mucositis, which may be very severe. Damage to the salivary glands may cause permanent oral dryness (xerostomia). Fibrosis of the larynx may cause glottic stenosis, laryngeal incompetence or aspiration, whilst fibrosis of the pterygoids may cause trismus.

Chemotherapy

The addition of chemotherapy (concomitant chemoradiotherapy) improves disease-free survival but increases the morbidity of treatment. Chemotherapy is often an adjunct to radiotherapy. Agents used are 5-fluorouracil or cisplatin. In recurrent disease, chemotherapeutic agents may be useful in palliation.

Prognosis

Approximately 50% of patients with head and neck squamous cell cancers die within 4 months of presentation if left untreated. The remainder may survive up to 4 years but have a very poor quality of life. In treated patients, survival and disease-free survival depend on the TNM stage and histological grade of the tumour, as well as the completeness of surgical resection and response to chemoradiotherapy.

There has been little improvement in mortality rates from head and neck squamous cancers in the past 20 years despite the innovations in surgery and chemoradiotherapy. The overall 5-year survival is 60%; for each year of survival following treatment, there is a 4–7% risk of a second (metachronous) primary.

227

Diseases of the gastrointestinal system

4

Roger Ackroyd, David S Sanders

SECTION 4.1 **Introduction**

Applied basic sciences of the gastrointestinal system

Anatomy and physiology

Oesophagus

The oesophagus is a muscular tube that connects the pharynx to the stomach. Anatomically, it is divided into cervical, thoracic and abdominal components. From the lumen outwards, the layers of the oesophagus consist of the mucosa (epithelium, lamina propria and inner longitudinal muscularis mucosa), submucosa (blood vessels, nerves and mucous glands) and muscularis externa (outer circular muscle layer). Appreciation of the tissue organization is important for T staging of oesophageal cancer (p. 258).

There are four sites of narrowing of the oesophagus at which foreign bodies may potentially lodge; the distances are measured from the incisors (as they have been derived from upper gastrointestinal endoscopic measurements): the commencement of the oesophagus (15 cm), the level of the aortic arch (22 cm), the level of the left main bronchus (28 cm) and the diaphragm (40 cm).

The lower oesophagus is smooth muscle that becomes continuous with the stomach. The epithelial lining is squamous until the oesophagogastric junction, where it becomes columnar. In long-standing reflux, premalignant change of the stratified squamous lining to metaplastic columnar degeneration above the gastro-oesophageal junction is known as Barrett's oesophagus.

On swallowing, waves of primary peristalsis are initiated at the pharynx and push food distally. Closure of the upper oesophageal sphincter is maintained by contraction of the cricopharyngeal muscle (Fig. 4.1a). The lower oesophageal sphincter has a high resting tone to prevent gastric contents refluxing into the oesophagus (Fig. 4.1b). The sphincter is controlled by vagal nerve and hormonal influences, and decreased tone pressure predisposes to oesophageal reflux.

A food bolus culminates in the relaxation of the lower oesophageal sphincter to allow passage of the food into the stomach. Secondary peristalsis is a locally induced phenomenon that allows food residue to be cleared from the oesophagus. The presence of abnormal tertiary waves can impair motility. This occurs typically in the elderly.

Stomach

The stomach is a muscular 'bag' comprised of mucosa (epithelium, gastric glands, lamina propria, inner circular and outer longitudinal layers of the muscularis mucosa), submucosa (blood vessels and nerves), muscularis externa (inner oblique, middle circular and outer longitudinal layers) and serosa (visceral peritoneum). Appreciation of the tissue organization is important for T staging of gastric cancer (p. 266).

Anatomically, the stomach is divided into the fundus (stomach that lies above the cardiac orifice), the body (the main part of the stomach) and the antrum (the distal portion that leads to the duodenum). Predominantly along the greater curve the mucosal surface displays thickened folds called rugae (Fig. 4.1c). The pyloric sphincter controls the passage of food into the duodenum.

The stomach acts as a food reservoir and is also involved in absorption by mixing food and initiating the

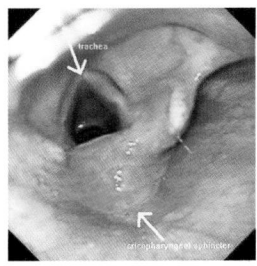

(a)

Fig. 4.1a Endoscopic view of the cricopharyngeal sphincter. Note the trachea lying anteriorly.

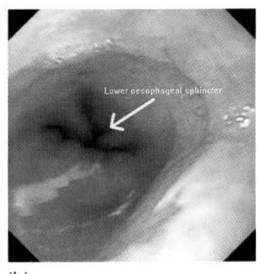

(b)

Fig. 4.1b Endoscopic view of the lower oesophageal sphincter (LOS). Note the change in mucosa from squamous to columnar.

emulsification of dietary fat. Acid is produced by parietal cells and pepsinogen by the chief cells; both these cell types are found within the mucosal surface of the upper two-thirds of the stomach. The G-cells within the antrum produce gastrin which stimulates parietal cells (to produce acid) and contraction of stomach muscles. The presence of acid within the stomach has a negative feedback effect on gastrin release. Parietal cells also produce intrinsic factor, which combines with vitamin B_{12} to facilitate absorption in the terminal ileum.

Small intestine

The small intestine is the major organ of absorption and is approximately 5–7 metres long. The mucosal surfaces have finger-like projections called villi that increase 20-fold the surface area for absorption (Fig. 4.1d). On the epithelial surface there is a brush border of microvilli to further enhance absorption.

Anatomically, the small intestine is divided into the duodenum, jejunum and ileum. The duodenojejunal flexure is supported by the ligament of Treitz, an arbitrary point used by clinicians to distinguish upper (proximal to the ligament of Treitz) from lower gastrointestinal bleeding. The jejunum is slightly thicker and has a greater number of mucosal folds compared to the ileum (Fig. 4.1e).

Peristalsis is initiated by a pacemaker situated in the lower part of the stomach and duodenum, and the absorption of nutrients, salt and water is promoted by passive diffusion (movement from areas of high concentration to low), facilitated diffusion (energy dependent) and active transport (which involves the sodium/potassium ATPase pump).

Water and electrolytes are usually absorbed from the upper jejunum in combination with monosaccharides and amino acids. However, the ileum and right side of the colon may also be involved in regulating this process. Carbohydrates are hydrolyzed to monosaccharides initially by pancreatic amylase and thereafter by brush border enzymes. They are then actively transported using the sodium/potassium ATPase transport system. Protein is initially digested to pepsin within the stomach and then by a number of pancreatic enzymes (trypsin, chymotrypsin and elastase) until it becomes oligopeptides. Thereafter, brush border enzymes (peptidases) convert oligopeptides to free amino acids which are finally absorbed using many of the available transport systems. Fat emulsification is initiated within the stomach and continued thereafter by bile salts (secreted by the contracting gall bladder). Pancreatic amylase hydrolyzes triglycerides until monoglycerides and fatty acids are produced. Bile salts allow the monoglycerides and fatty acids to cross the mucosal cell membrane by creating a water-soluble micelle. Bile salts are then reabsorbed at the terminal ileum to allow them to re-enter the entero-hepatic circulation.

Colon

The colon or large bowel extends from the distal ileum to the anus and is divided into the caecum, ascending colon, transverse colon, descending colon, sigmoid colon and rectum (Fig. 4.2). The appendix is located on the posterior medial wall of the caecum.

The layers of tissue in the colon consist of the mucosa (columnar epithelium, lamina propria, muscularis mucosa), submucosa, muscularis externa (outer longitudinal, inner circular layer) and serosa (visceral peritoneum). The incomplete outer longitudinal layer of the muscularis externa results in the taeniae coli, which can be seen radiologically as a haustral pattern. Unlike the small bowel, the mucosa of the colon does not have villi and is flat.

The absorption of fluids and electrolytes is predominantly regulated in the right side of the colon. When a stool enters the rectum this results in relaxation of the internal sphincter and puborectalis muscle. The urge to defecate is experienced when a quantity of stool (perhaps greater than 100 mL) is present within the rectum. The rectum is emptied by relaxation of the external anal sphincter, which is under voluntary control. Increased abdominal pressure (straining) may relieve this process.

The inguinal canal

The inguinal canal is an oblique passage situated superior to the inguinal ligament. It is approximately 4 cm long and runs from the deep (laterally) to the superficial (medially) inguinal ring.

The deep inguinal ring is bounded medially by the inferior epigastric artery, and the superficial ring lies above and lateral to the pubic tubercle. The inguinal canal is defined by the following boundaries: anterior (external oblique aponeurosis), lateral (conjoint tendon), posterior (transversalis fascia), medial (insertion of the conjoint tendon), inferior (inguinal ligament) and superior (conjoint tendon developed from the fusion of transversus abdominis and internal oblique muscles).

In the male the spermatic cord runs down through the inguinal canal, containing the testicular artery, veins and vas deferens. In the female, the cord is replaced by the round ligament. An inguinal hernia appears at the superficial ring of the inguinal canal, which in the male is formed by the passage of the testis through the muscle layers of abdominal wall.

The femoral canal

The femoral canal is defined by the following boundaries: anterior (inguinal ligament), posterior (pectineus muscle), medial (lacunar ligament) and lateral (femoral vein). A femoral hernia passes beneath the inguinal ligament into the thigh, via the femoral canal.

Symptoms of gastrointestinal disease

History taking and examination are essential components in the recognition of gastrointestinal disease. These may help to provide the clinician with a differential diagnosis and to direct subsequent investigations.

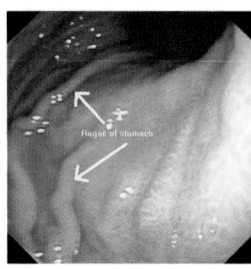

(c)

Fig. 4.1c Endoscopic view of the rugae of the stomach running along the greater curve.

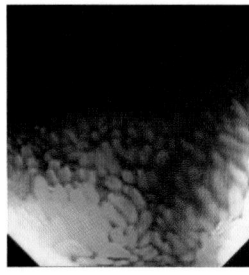

(d)

Fig. 4.1d Endoscopic view of small bowel using water immersion as a means of magnifying mucosal views. Also, the mucosa has been sprayed with indigo carmine dye spray to further enhance mucosal views. Note the magnified image of normal villi.

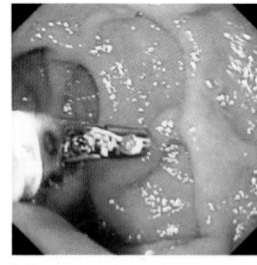

(e)

Fig. 4.1e Endoscopic view of normal folds of the small bowel. Note the open biopsy forceps just prior to taking a small bowel biopsy.

Abdominal pain

Pain is a common symptom. It should be categorized according to site, severity, radiation, character (for example, sharp or dull), duration and exacerbating or relieving factors. Pain may be caused by the stretching of smooth muscle or organ capsules. An important distinction is the difference between acute and chronic abdominal pain.

Pain from a peptic ulcer is usually experienced in the epigastrium and may radiate into the back. It may be gnawing or dull in character with mild to moderate severity, lasting for hours at a time with periods of no symptoms (remission) lasting for week or months before the next bout. Acute pancreatitis can also produce epigastric pain, which may radiate to the back.

Acute cholecystitis pain is experienced in the epigastrium or right hypochondrium and may radiate to the scapula or right shoulder tip (due to the inflamed gall bladder irritating the diaphragm whose innervation is derived from the phrenic nerve). The pain is constant and severe, lasting for several hours. The periodicity is unpredictable and may depend on the passage of a gallstone that may have impacted within the cystic duct.

Non-gastrointestinal causes can also produce abdominal pain. Ureteric colic may be experienced as flank pain radiating into the groin, and rarely diabetic ketoacidosis, acute intermittent porphyria, lead colic and tabes dorsalis may present with acute abdominal pain. Pain from conditions such as acute myocardial infarction, aortic aneurysm, vertebral collapse and herpes zoster may also falsely localize to the abdomen.

Upper gastrointestinal symptoms

Dysphagia

Dysphagia is difficulty in swallowing; it is usually caused by lesions in the oropharynx or oesophagus or a neurological cause (such as a stroke). Progressive dysphagia is a worrying symptom and may suggest oesophageal malignancy.

Odynophagia

Odynophagia is pain on swallowing (particularly with hot or cold liquids). This symptom may represent a structural lesion or severe oesophagitis.

Nausea, retching and vomiting

Nausea is the sensation of wanting to vomit, retching is an involuntary effort to vomit, and vomiting is the actual expulsion of gastric contents. Vomiting may be secondary to gastrointestinal disorders (e.g. gastroenteritis), central nervous system disease (e.g. raised intracranial pressure), metabolic causes (e.g. diabetic ketoacidosis) or drugs (e.g. opiates).

Heartburn, reflux and water brash

Heartburn is retrosternal burning or discomfort, often attributed to the passage of acid from the stomach into the oesophagus. Reflux is often described as the sensation of the passage of gastric fluid or contents into the oesophagus. Water brash is the excessive production of saliva prior to the symptoms of reflux, or a term sometimes used to describe the bitter or salty taste associated with the reflux of gastric contents.

Dyspepsia and indigestion

Dyspepsia (described by the clinician) and indigestion (described by the patient) are terms used to describe upper abdominal pain.

Lower gastrointestinal symptoms

Altered bowel habit

Altered bowel habit refers to any change in defecation frequency. Often patients may not be describing a true change in bowel habit but rather a change in the consistency or appearance of the stool, for example patients with hard stools may complain of constipation and patients with *true steatorrhoea* may describe this as diarrhoea. Constipation and diarrhoea are defined on pages 246 and 245.

Steatorrhoea

Steatorrhoea is pale, offensive-smelling bulky stools that are difficult to flush (because they float as a result of the high fat content). Steatorrhoea occurs because fat is inadequately absorbed or digested, a feature of malabsorption (p. 241) that suggests small bowel or pancreatic disease.

Abdominal distension

Abdominal distension refers to an increase in abdominal girth. This can occur with fat, fluid (ascites), intra-abdominal organomegaly, intestinal obstruction and chronic constipation.

Examination of the gastrointestinal system

When examining a patient for gastrointestinal system symptoms, the patient is positioned supine with the head resting on one pillow and the torso exposed from nipples to hernial orifices.

The abdomen is subdivided into nine areas (Fig. 4.3) delineated by lines following superficial anatomical landmarks. The upper horizontal plane (transpyloric) lies midway between the suprasternal notch and the pubis. The lower horizontal plane runs along the upper borders of the iliac crest. The sagittal or vertical planes run midway (on either side) between the anterior superior iliac spines and pubis.

Inspection

An overall inspection of the patient's abdomen can be very informative. Occasionally, distension (flatus, fat, faeces, fluid and fetus), intra-abdominal mass or organomegaly can be seen from the end of the bed as asymmetry. Operative scars may also be identified.

Applied basic sciences of the gastrointestinal system

Symptoms of gastrointestinal disease

Examination of the gastrointestinal system

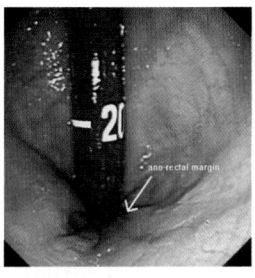

Fig. 4.2 Endoscopic view of the rectum. This particular view involves retroflexing the colonoscope (J-manoeuvre) to allow assessment of the ano-rectal margin.

231

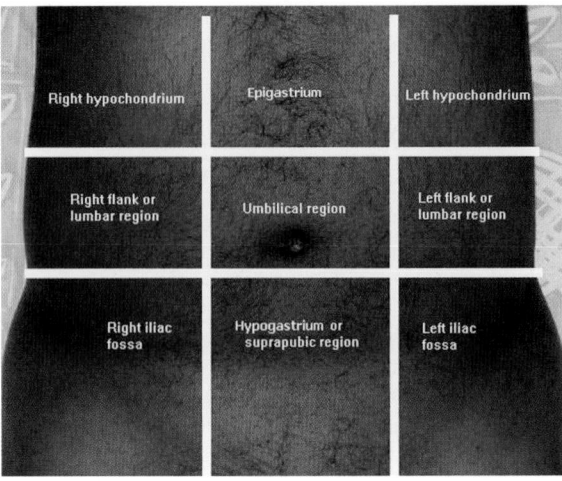

Fig. 4.3 Schematic diagram of the nine abdominal regions.

The fingers should be inspected for clubbing, and the palmar creases should be assessed for pallor (anaemia). Asterixis (liver disease) should be ascertained by asking the patient to hold the hands out, cock the wrists back and close the eyes. The conjunctiva can be inspected for pallor, and the mouth inspected for ulceration, stomatitis and angular cheilitis. The tongue should be visualized to ensure there is no glossitis.

Palpation and percussion

It is important to enquire about abdominal pain prior to palpation. Initially, light palpation should be performed in all nine areas to ensure that there are no signs of rebound tenderness (occurring on the rapid withdrawal of the hand) that may indicate peritonism. Light palpation may also delineate significant abnormal masses or organomegaly. Deep palpation allows recognition and further examination of any abnormality detected. The site, size, shape, consistency, degree of movement, mobility and tenderness of the mass can be assessed, and deep palpation for specific organs performed.

Palpation of the liver begins in the right iliac fossa (significant hepatomegaly can extend to this level). The patient is asked to take deep breaths (as the liver moves with respiration) and a sharp edge is palpable if there is hepatomegaly. The consistency of the liver (firm or soft), presence of irregularities (for example, a craggy surface can occur in malignancy), tenderness (which may occur in congestion secondary to right heart failure) and degree of enlargement (measured by centimetres or fingerbreadths from the costal margin at the midclavicular line) should be assessed. A pulsatile liver may be a feature in tricuspid regurgitation. Percussion of the liver allows the size to be confirmed and should be performed from the right iliac fossa upwards as well as downwards from the anterior chest wall. The upper border of the liver normally lies at the

level of the intercostal space below the fifth rib. This can be counted down to by using the suprasternal notch as a landmark. Chest disease such as emphysema may result in hyperexpansion of the lungs which displaces the liver downwards and can falsely give the impression of hepatomegaly.

Normally the spleen lies against the posterolateral wall of the abdominal cavity beneath the ninth to eleventh ribs. Its anterior border reaches the midaxillary line. Palpation commences in the right iliac fossa, moving diagonally across to the left hypochondrium. If no grossly enlarged spleen is palpable, the left hand should be placed in the left renal angle with the right hand lying over the left hypochondrium. A moderately enlarged spleen can be detected by lifting the left hand, which will push the spleen against the right hand. The spleen is distinguished by its position, movement with respiration and, occasionally, a palpable splenic notch. When inserting the fingers between the spleen's upper border and the left costal margin, the examiner should not be able to get above it. With the patient on his/her right-hand side, and inserting the fingers between the posterior margin of the spleen and the paraspinal muscles, the examiner should be able to get behind it. This allows the spleen to be distinguished from the left kidney. Percussion may be used to discriminate between kidney and spleen: the kidney is retroperitoneal so there should be a band of resonance whilst percussion of the spleen will be dull.

Bimanual palpation of the kidneys is required. This involves placing one hand posteriorly between the twelfth rib and iliac crest and the other hand in the iliac fossa on the same side. A palpable kidney will move with respiration and has a rounded lower margin. Percussion is performed to distinguish the kidney from the spleen.

Auscultation

Normal bowel sounds (borborygmi) are audible by placing the diaphragm of the stethoscope on the abdominal wall and listening for 1 minute. When peritonitis is present or perforation has occurred the bowel sounds may be absent. Tinkling bowel sounds (high pitched) may be heard in the presence of intestinal obstruction. In pyloric obstruction a succussion splash may be demonstrated without the use of the stethoscope; the patient's abdomen is moved gently from side to side to elicit this sign.

Additional examination

Occasionally, the bladder or uterus may be palpated in the suprapubic region. Palpation or percussion to demonstrate a fluid thrill or shifting dullness may be performed when ascites is suspected. For completion, examination of the groin for femoral pulses, lymph nodes, genitalia and hernial orifices is necessary. Digital examination of the anus and rectum is also performed for the presence of anal tags, haemorrhoids, fissures, fistula, prostatic abnormalities and rectal masses.

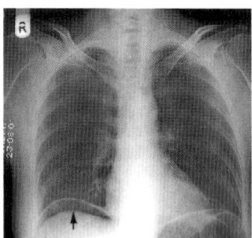

Fig. 4.4 Chest X-ray showing free air under the hemidiaphragm.

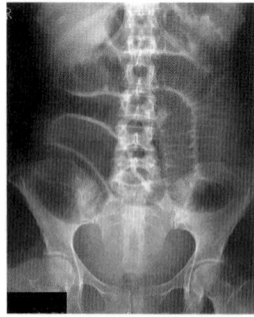

Fig. 4.5 Plain abdominal film revealing dilated small bowel loops consistent with small bowel obstruction.

Investigations for gastrointestinal disease

Diagnostic imaging

Plain abdominal film

The standard images for the plain abdominal film are the supine and erect antero-posterior views. The main advantage of the erect view is to detect air–fluid levels in the bowel (not visible on supine films). Air is normally visible in the stomach (classically it is absent in achalasia), colon and (less commonly) small bowel. Air outside the bowel lumen (pneumoperitoneum) in the absence of surgery usually indicates perforation of a viscus. It is not seen on a plain abdominal film, but as free air under the diaphragm on a chest X-ray (Fig. 4.4).

Bowel loops may be visible, and distinguishing small from large bowel in the presence of gross distension can be difficult. In general, small bowel loops are situated centrally in the abdomen and have haustra that run all the way across the lumen (Fig. 4.5).

Ultrasound scan

Abdominal ultrasound scanning is commonly used to investigate liver, biliary, pancreatic and renal disease. Occasionally it is used to ascertain the location and structure of intra-abdominal masses, to identify acute appendicitis (non-compressible thickened appendix, Fig. 4.6), and also to screen for pelvic pathology in women who present with lower abdominal pain.

Endoscopic ultrasound scan of the oesophagus is currently being investigated for staging oesophageal cancer.

Computed tomography

The main use of CT scanning is in the setting of the acute abdomen and for staging gastrointestinal malignancies (Fig. 4.7). A CT of the chest is performed to evaluate the oesophagus, and occasionally as a screening investigation for pulmonary metastasis in gastrointestinal malignancies.

Magnetic resonance imaging

MRI has a significant advantage over CT as there is no ionizing radiation. It is particularly useful for the assessment of the perineum in patients with inflammatory bowel disease.

Contrast studies

Endoscopy has superseded barium studies in the investigation of a number of gastrointestinal diseases as it allows a diagnostic as well as interventional approach; however, there are still many clinical scenarios in which a radiological approach is used.

Barium sulphate is a contrast medium that coats mucosal surfaces, allowing the identification of mucosal defects (ulceration), filling defects (space occupying lesions) and strictures. Continuous fluoroscopic imaging is used to allow real time visualization of the passage of barium in order to distinguish fixed stenoses from normal peristalsis. In a single contrast barium study, the bowel is only filled with barium. A double contrast study (more useful) enhances mucosal views by insufflating air into the bowel.

In situations such as perforation where there is a risk of barium leaking out of the bowel lumen, water-soluble contrast such as Gastrografin is preferred.

Barium swallow

The barium swallow is an investigation of the oesophagus. It is a useful initial screening investigation for dysphagia when a motility disorder is suspected, as real-time imaging of the passage of the contrast can be obtained and peristalsis evaluated. It is also useful in initial investigation of a pharyngeal pouch as endoscopy risks perforation. The anatomy distal to a stricture that cannot be passed by an endoscope can also be visualized.

Barium meal

A barium meal is the standard contrast study to examine the stomach and duodenum, but it is now rarely required due to advances in endoscopy. It is, however, still valuable in recognizing linitis plastica, a rare presentation of gastric cancer which may be missed at endoscopy as the stomach may not distend optimally and the limited peristalsis may obliterate the mucosal folds. These features are subtle but more easily recognized by performing a barium meal. Hiatus hernia or gastric outlet obstruction or gastroparesis (resulting in delayed gastric emptying) are also readily identified with a barium meal.

Barium small bowel follow-through

Given the limitations of endoscopic imaging of the small bowel, the barium small bowel follow-through remains an important investigation for small bowel disease. It takes approximately 2–3 hours for the swallowed barium to reach the small bowel. Abnormalities such as strictures, bowel dilatation, fistulae, ulceration and other mucosal abnormalities can be seen.

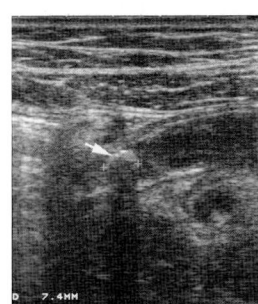

Fig. 4.6 Abdominal ultrasound. A dilated appendix with an impacted faecalith is visible.

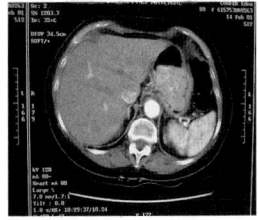

Fig. 4.7 CT scan of the abdomen. A gastric carcinoma is visible within the lumen of the stomach.

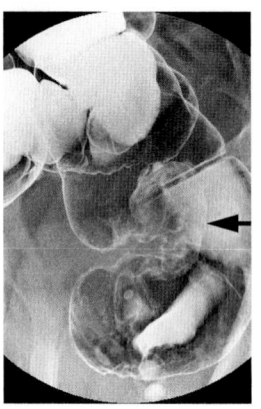

Fig. 4.8 A barium enema demonstrating a stricture from a mid-rectal tumour.

Barium enema

Currently, most clinicians prefer colonoscopy to barium enema for the investigation of diseases of the colon. The barium enema is usually performed after unsuccessful endoscopy (patient intolerance, stricture or tortuous bowel).

Barium is introduced into the rectum via gravity through a tube, and air is insufflated to produce a double contrast study to visualize strictures (Fig. 4.8), filling defects, colonic dilatation, mucosal ulceration, diverticula and fistulae.

SECTION 4.3 Diagnostic procedures

Gastrointestinal endoscopy

The development of fibre-optic endoscopy revolutionized the ability to investigate the gastrointestinal tract. Flexible endoscopes often have a diameter of less than 1 cm, with a control head (Fig. 4.9) and a flexible shaft with a manoeuvrable tip. The head is connected to a light source and can transmit images to a video image screen.

All endoscopes have multiple small lumens allowing transmission of air and water and for suction. The suction channel can also be used for the passage of interventional devices, for example biopsy forceps. The ability to transmit air (insufflation) allows the endoscopist to inflate the lumen to obtain optimal views. The water channel provides a means of washing mucosal surfaces, and suction may be used to remove pools of fluid within the gastrointestinal tract, thus ensuring that all mucosal surfaces are inspected.

RECENT ADVANCES

The combination of gastroscopy and colonoscopy does not provide views of the whole of the small bowel. The length of visualized bowel can be increased by using an enteroscope. An enteroscope is longer than a gastroscope and it may be passed into the upper gastrointestinal tract, allowing views of up to 1–1.5 m of small bowel.

Further visualization of small bowel is now possible due to the development of the gastrointestinal video endoscopy capsule. This mini-camera is swallowed by the patient and takes multiple pictures of the whole of the small bowel. Its only limitation is the inability to procure biopsies (Fig. 4.10).

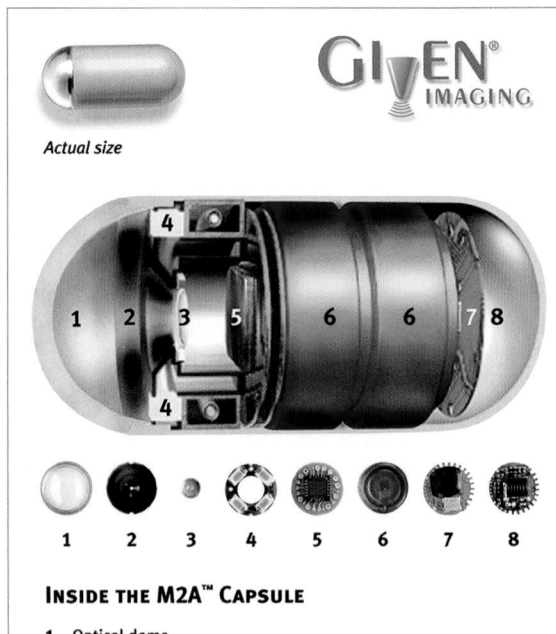

Actual size

INSIDE THE M2A™ CAPSULE

1. Optical dome
2. Lens holder
3. Lens
4. Illuminating LEDs (Light Emitting Diode)
5. CMOS (Complementary Metal Oxide Semiconductor) imager
6. Battery
7. ASIC (Application Specific Integrated Circuit) transmitter
8. Antenna

Fig. 4.10 Schematic representation of a gastrointestinal video endoscopy capsule (© Given Imaging, with permission).

Upper gastrointestinal endoscopy

Indications

Diagnostic indications include the investigation of dysphagia, upper gastrointestinal bleeding, anaemia (iron deficient, folate or vitamin B_{12}), upper abdominal pain, gastro-oesophageal reflux (diagnostic investigation or surveillance endoscopy of Barrett's oesophagus) and coeliac disease (biopsies).

Therapeutic procedures that can be undertaken include mucosal biopsy, polypectomy, therapy for gastrointestinal

---

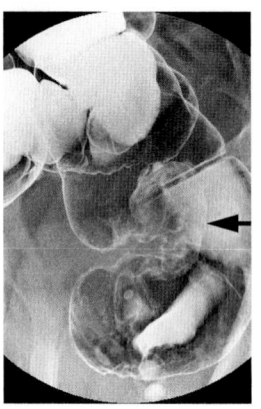

Fig. 4.9 The head of a colonoscope. This is the control panel which the endoscopist digitally manipulates whilst performing endoscopy.

ℹ️ FURTHER INFORMATION

Eisen GM, Baron TH, Dominitz JA, et al. American Society for Gastrointestinal Endoscopy. Complications of upper GI endoscopy. Gastrointestinal Endoscopy 2002; 55; 784–793.

Dominitz JA, Eisen GM, Baron TH, et al. American Society for Gastrointestinal Endoscopy. Complications of colonoscopy. Gastrointestinal Endoscopy 2003; 57; 441–445.

bleeding, laser therapy for neoplastic or bleeding lesions, percutaneous entero-gastrotomy or jejunostomy (PEG or PEJ) insertion, stent insertion for strictures, dilatation of strictures and banding for oesophageal varices.

Patient preparation

Informed consent is required, and patients are fasted for 4–6 hours prior to the procedure. Although most patients do not require sedation, the choice is offered and discussed. Sedation involves the use of a short-acting benzodiazepine which provides a sedative and amnesic effect. Monitoring is required (pulse oximetry) with sedation due to the risk of respiratory depression. Antibiotic prophylaxis is administered to patients with heart valve disease to prevent bacterial endocarditis.

Procedure

A mouthguard is used. The endoscope is introduced into the pharynx, then the oesophagus. Patients may retch during this procedure. The endoscope is progressively introduced to inspect the oesophagus, stomach and proximal small bowel (duodenum).

Complications

The overall complication rate is approximately 1 per 1000 with a mortality rate of approximately 1 per 25 000. Complications include bleeding, perforation and respiratory arrest (a complication of sedation).

Post procedure care

Patients are monitored in a recovery area until safe for discharge.

Lower gastrointestinal endoscopy

Indications

The indications for lower gastrointestinal endoscopy include the investigation of altered bowel habit, lower gastrointestinal bleeding, iron deficiency anaemia, lower abdominal pain and cancer surveillance.

Patient preparation

Informed consent is required, and patients are given bowel preparation with a laxative such as sodium picosulfate prior to the procedure. Antibiotic prophylaxis is administered to patients with heart valve disease to prevent bacterial endocarditis.

Procedure

The endoscope (Fig. 4.11) is introduced into the anus and progressively advanced into the rectum and sigmoid colon, through the entire colon to the caecum and up to 50 cm of the ileum.

Complications

The overall complication rate is approximately 1 in 300, with a mortality of approximately 1 per 16 000. Complications include bleeding and perforation of the bowel.

Post procedure care

Patients are usually discharged shortly after the procedure.

Rigid sigmoidoscopy

Indications

Rigid sigmoidoscopy can be easily performed as an outpatient procedure with similar indications to lower gastrointestinal endoscopy. However, the examination is limited to the rectum and sigmoid colon, and the views may be poor as bowel preparation is not usually performed.

Patient preparation

The procedure is explained to the patient, and the consenting patient is placed in a lateral position with the knees retracted up to the chest.

Procedure

The sigmoidoscope is lubricated and introduced in a posterior direction into the anus. Insufflation of air is performed and the scope gradually advanced further under direct vision.

Complications

Complications of rigid sigmoidoscopy include bleeding and perforation of the bowel.

Post procedure care

Patients are usually discharged as soon as they are comfortable after the procedure.

Proctoscopy

The proctoscope is a rigid tube which allows inspection of the anal canal and may be specifically valuable in the treatment and identification of haemorrhoids or anal fissures. It is lubricated and introduced gently into the anus to visualize the anus and rectum.

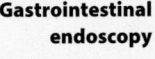

Gastrointestinal endoscopy

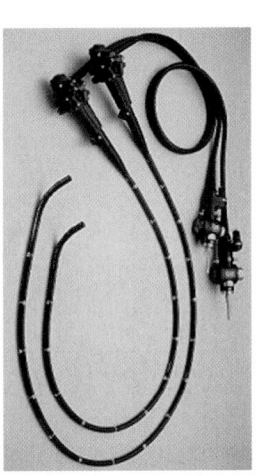

Fig. 4.11 Colonoscopes (lower gastrointestinal endoscopy).

Therapeutic procedures

Nasogastric tube insertion

Indications

The main indications for nasogastric tube insertion are feeding and drainage (decompression) of the stomach.

Patient preparation

The patient should sit upright and be asked to maintain his or her head in a neutral position (looking neither up nor down) by fixing the gaze at a point horizontally in front. A glass of water should be provided to the patient.

Procedure

A nasogastric tube should be lubricated. The tube is inserted through the nostril, pointing inferiorly to follow the anatomical direction of the nasal cavity. Once the nasogastric tube has reached the oropharynx, the patient should place his or her chin onto the chest wall to promote the passage of the tube into the oesophagus rather than the trachea. If the patient can sip water, it may help in traversing the oropharynx and thereafter passage into the stomach. The tube is then fixed to the side of the patient's face with adhesive tape.

The position of the nasogastric tube within the stomach is confirmed by aspiration of gastric contents or injecting 50 mL of air and auscultating for the sound of bubbling. The diaphragm of the stethoscope is placed slightly to the (patient's) left of the epigastrium.

Complications

Inadvertent passage of the tube into the trachea can occur.

Post procedure care

A chest X-ray is performed to confirm correct positioning in the stomach (this is mandatory if the nasogastric tube is to be used for feeding).

Percutaneous endoscopic gastrostomy (PEG) tube insertion

Indications

The main indication for PEG tube insertion is the requirement for prolonged feeding. This may occur in patients with degenerative neurological disease (advanced dementia, multiple sclerosis, motor neurone and Parkinson's disease) and brain damage due to head injury in which swallowing is impaired.

Relative contraindications include bleeding disorders, gastric or other metastatic cancer, extensive gastric ulceration, intestinal obstruction or ascites.

Patient preparation

Patients require assessment for fitness for endoscopy, light sedation and informed consent. Most patients are elderly with significant comorbidity, and many patients with neurological disease have impaired ventilatory function and are prone to aspiration. Abdominal examination may reveal evidence of prior surgery, organomegaly or subcutaneous fluid infusions that may make PEG placement more difficult or hazardous. A clotting screen should be performed and abnormal clotting corrected.

A broad-spectrum prophylactic antibiotic (either a cephalosporin or co-amoxiclav) is usually administered prior to the procedure.

Procedure

An endoscope is passed into the stomach, and then a needle is introduced from the abdominal wall into the stomach where the tube should be sited. Through the needle, a fine wire is passed into the stomach, grasped by the endoscope and pulled out through the mouth. The needle is removed and a wider incision made over the needle entry site. The PEG tube is attached to the wire and introduced through the mouth into the stomach. It is then pulled through the incision and secured onto the abdominal wall (Fig. 4.12).

Complications

Minor complications such as tube blockage, leakage or inadvertent removal, local sepsis and granulation tissue formation or damage to the fixation device or Y connector occur in about 10% of patients. Major complications include aspiration pneumonia; these occur in about 5%.

The PEG tube lasts for approximately 6 months, after which the tubing begins to wear and may pull away from the stomach causing a leak.

Post procedure care

Patients are monitored in the recovery area for potential complications. They should be educated about the care and use of the PEG tube. A formal dietician assessment is required to plan for the type and amount of feed that is to be introduced via the PEG tube. Nutritional assessment of PEG patients should continue following discharge, as many continue to have protein–energy malnutrition. The swallowing of some patients may recover sufficiently to allow PEG removal (up to a fifth of dysphagic stroke patients).

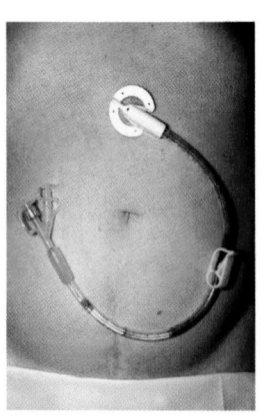

Fig. 4.12 A PEG tube in situ.

Manifestations of gastrointestinal disease

Upper gastrointestinal haemorrhage

Acute upper gastrointestinal haemorrhage is defined as bleeding that occurs proximal to the ligament of Treitz, the peritoneal fold that is attached to the third and fourth part of the duodenum. It can present with haematemesis, melaena, haematochezia (fresh blood per rectum) or incidental anaemia.

Epidemiology

Upper gastrointestinal haemorrhage is common with an overall incidence of 103 per 100 000 adults per year, increasing with age from 23 per 100 000 per year in patients less than 30 years to 485 per 100 000 per year in those aged over 75.[1] It is twice as common in males as compared to females.

Pathology

A cause for upper gastrointestinal haemorrhage can be identified in approximately 65%. Peptic ulceration is the most common cause; others include gastroduodenal erosions, oesophagitis, oesophageal varices and Mallory–Weiss tears (Table 4.1).

Scope of disease

Depending on the rate of blood loss, the manifestations can range from incidental anaemia to circulatory shock from severe bleeding.

Table 4.1	Causes of upper gastrointestinal bleeding
Peptic ulcer	
Gastroduodenal erosions	
Oesophagitis	
Varices	
Mallory–Weiss tears*	
Vascular malformations*	
Upper gastrointestinal malignancy*	

* Less common causes.

Clinical features

Patients may present with typical haematemesis (the vomiting of bright or dark red blood) or 'coffee ground vomiting', which is the term used to describe the granular and black-tinged appearance of blood that has been altered by gastric acid. Melaena is the passage of black tarry stool, due to blood from the upper gastrointestinal tract. Torrential upper gastrointestinal haemorrhage can occasionally present as bright red rectal bleeding (p. 240).

It is important to screen for the conditions listed in Table 4.1 in the past medical history. A drug history to screen for anticoagulants or non-steroidal anti-inflammatory drugs (NSAIDs) is important. Concurrent oral iron therapy can produce faeces that have a similar appearance to melaena.

On examination, high pulse rate and postural hypotension are reliable indicators of hypovolaemia. Clinical features of chronic liver disease may suggest oesophageal varices as the underlying cause, and upper abdominal pain may indicate peptic ulcer disease. A rectal examination may identify melaena.

Risk stratification

Re-bleeding from peptic ulcer disease is the single most important determinant of death. The Rockall risk score is used to identify patients at high risk for re-bleeding and death by adding the separate scores obtained for each individual variable as listed in Table 4.2.

Initial investigations

Full blood count

Anaemia may be present with chronic blood loss. It is important to note that anaemia will not be present with acute severe blood loss until haemodilution occurs.

Urea and electrolytes

An increased urea to creatine ratio can be caused by upper intestinal absorption of blood, a marker of gastrointestinal bleeding.

Liver profile

A liver profile should be performed to screen for hepatic failure as varices can result from portal hypertension.

Table 4.2 The Rockall risk score*

Variable	0	1	2	3
Age (years)	<60	60-79	>80	
Shock	Systolic BP >100 mmHg Heart rate <100 bpm	Systolic BP >100 mmHg Heart rate >100 bpm	Systolic BP <100 mmHg	
Comorbidity	No major comorbidity		Cardiac failure Ischaemic heart disease Any major comorbidity	Renal failure Liver disease Disseminated malignancy
Diagnosis	Mallory–Weiss tear No lesion identified No stigmata of recent haemorrhage	All other diagnoses	Malignancy of upper gastrointestinal tract	
Major stigmata of recent haemorrhage	None Dark spot sign		Blood in upper gastrointestinal tract Adherent clot Visible or spurting vessel	

The risk of re-bleeding if the Rockall score is 0 is 5%, and 40% when the Rockall score is >8.
* Rockall TA, Logan RF, Devlin HB, Northfield TC. Risk assessment after acute upper gastrointestinal haemorrhage. Gut 1996; 38: 316–321.

Coagulation screen

A coagulation screen should be performed as impaired coagulation can occur in patients with liver disease and those who are taking anticoagulants.

Group and crossmatch

Blood should be crossmatched for patients who are actively bleeding, or for those with significant blood loss. Otherwise a group and save should be performed.

Initial management

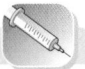

Optimal management involves a multidisciplinary approach and patients should be managed in a centralized bleed unit where available.

Intravenous access and fluid replacement

The initial priority is circulatory resuscitation. Patients are kept nil by mouth and large-bore intravenous cannulae are sited for fluid replacement. Blood transfusion may be required depending on the severity of blood loss and the presence of cardiorespiratory disease that would render a patient more susceptible to the effects of acute anaemia.

With blood losses of less than 20% of circulating volume, haemodynamic stability is usually achieved at initial resuscitation. With blood losses between 20% and 40% of the circulating volume, transient haemodynamic improvement to resuscitative measures occurs with subsequent deterioration. This scenario commonly represents ongoing bleeding or inadequate resuscitation. No response to initial fluid replacement occurs with severe volume depletion or rapid continuous bleeding.

Proton pump inhibitor therapy

As peptic ulceration is the most common cause for upper gastrointestinal haemorrhage, patients should be commenced on intravenous proton pump inhibitor therapy. This is associated with lower rates of re-bleeding and surgical intervention.[2]

Upper gastointestinal endoscopy

Endoscopy is useful for diagnosis, therapy and risk stratification, but should only be performed after adequate resuscitation. Usually the site and cause of bleeding is visible such as gastric (Fig. 4.13) or duodenal ulcerations or Dieulafoy lesions (Fig. 4.14) which are vascular malformations. Any clot or adherent mucus or debris is washed away to locate the bleeding vessel.

Endoscopic therapies include thermal coagulation with bipolar or thermal probes, or injection of vasoconstrictors such as epinephrine (1:10000) solution. Other forms of haemostasis include injection of fibrin glue (derived from individually prepared fibrinogen and thrombin), NdYAG (neodymium–yttrium–aluminium–garnet) non-contact laser ablation, and endoclip assisted haemostasis (Fig. 4.15). A check endoscopy is usually performed 24 hours later following successful haemostasis.

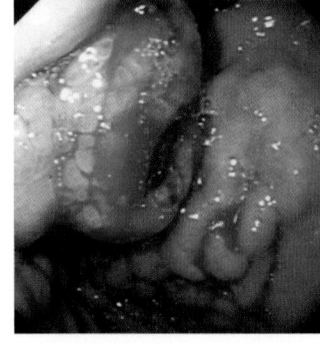

Fig. 4.13 Endoscopic view of a gastric ulcer. Fundic gastric ulcer with rolled margin and deep ulcer crater (see overlying clot and fibrin debris). Note an associated non-bleeding gastric fundic varix adjacent to the lateral ulcer margin.

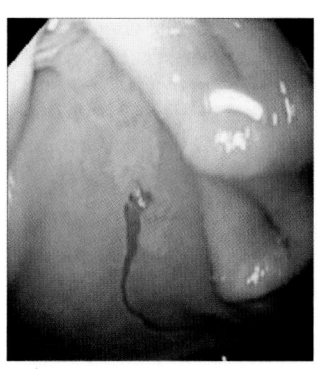

Fig. 4.14 Endoscopic view of a Dieulafoy lesion. Bleeding peri-ampullary Dieulafoy lesion (view obtained from a side viewing duodenoscope).

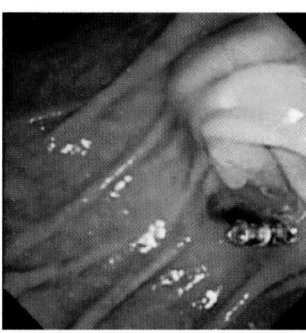

Fig. 4.15 Endoscopic haemostasis using endoclip closure method.

involving the left gastric artery, is more difficult to treat endoscopically and is hence more likely to present for surgical intervention. In this scenario, excision of the lesser curve (Pauchet's manoeuvre) is indicated. Formal total gastrectomy may be unnecessary. High lesser curve ulcers can be treated by direct ulcer excision (not a minor procedure).

Prognosis

Despite advances in medical and endoscopic intervention there has been no demonstrable improvement in mortality. The overall mortality is 14% (11% for emergency admissions and 33% for haemorrhage in inpatients).[1] The mortality for patients under 60 in the absence of malignancy or organ failure at presentation is 0.8%.[1]

Patients who test positive for *H. pylori* should receive eradication therapy, which lowers the re-bleeding rate in patients with peptic ulcers.[3]

Endoscopic haemostasis can be difficult if there are large amounts of intraluminal debris or free blood such as in posterior duodenal ulceration with brisk bleeding from the gastroduodenal artery. If no lesion is found in a patient with major bleeding, then selective mesenteric angiography, small-bowel capsular imaging or enteroscopy needs to be performed.

Surgical management

Early surgical referral is required for high-risk patients for joint management with the gastroenterologist. Surgery is indicated if re-bleeding occurs after initial successful endoscopic treatment, or if it is impossible to control the bleeding endoscopically, or if the bleeding arises from posterior duodenal ulceration. An upper midline laparotomy is performed; the exact surgical procedure depends on the location of the bleed (variceal haemorrhage is described on p. 237).

Duodenal source of bleeding

Most duodenal ulcers requiring surgery are chronic posterior wall ulcers involving the gastroduodenal artery. Initially a longitudinal duodenotomy is performed distal to the pyloric ring. If active arterial bleeding is noted, finger pressure is applied immediately to achieve haemostasis. Access can be improved by mobilizing the duodenum using Kocher's manoeuvre. The vessel is then under-run using Vicryl or Dexon sutures.

Gastric source of bleeding

Bleeding gastric ulcers are conventionally treated by a partial gastrectomy. The chronic high lesser curve ulcer,

FURTHER INFORMATION

British Society of Gastroenterology Endoscopy Committee. Non-variceal upper gastrointestinal haemorrhage: guidelines. Gut 2002; 51(suppl IV): iv1–iv6.

Barkun A, Bardou M, Marshall JK. Consensus recommendations for managing patients with nonvariceal upper gastrointestinal bleeding. Annals of Internal Medicine 2003; 139: 843–857.

REFERENCES

(1) *Rockall TA, Logan RF, Devlin HB, Northfield TC. Incidence of and mortality from acute upper gastrointestinal haemorrhage in the United Kingdom. Steering Committee and members of the National Audit of Acute Upper Gastrointestinal Haemorrhage. BMJ 1995; 311: 222–226.*
(2) *Leontiadis GI, McIntyre L, Sharma VK, Howden CW. Proton pump inhibitor treatment for acute peptic ulcer bleeding (Cochrane Review). The Cochrane Library. Issue 3. Chichester: John Wiley & Sons, 2004.*
(3) *Gisbert JP, Khorrami S, Carballo F, Calvet X, Gene E, Dominguez-Munoz JE. H. pylori eradication therapy vs. antisecretory non-eradication therapy (with or without long-term maintenance antisecretory therapy) for the prevention of recurrent bleeding from peptic ulcer. Cochrane Database of Systematic Reviews 2004: CD004062.*

Lower gastrointestinal bleeding

Lower gastrointestinal bleeding (haematochezia) is defined as bleeding that occurs distal to the ligament of Treitz, the peritoneal fold that is attached to the third and fourth part of the duodenum.

Epidemiology

The epidemiology of lower gastrointestinal bleeding varies according to the aetiology and the wide range of severity.

Pathology

The causes of lower gastrointestinal bleeding are detailed in Table 4.3. The colon is the most common site for lower gastrointestinal bleeding, and upper gastrointestinal bleeding is responsible for approximately 10% of patients presenting with 'lower gastrointestinal bleeding'.

Scope of disease

Complications relate to the severity of the bleeding and the presence of comorbid conditions. Severe bleeding can lead to circulatory shock.

Clinical features

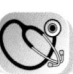

Anorectal bleeding results in fresh bright red blood passed either on the toilet paper or in the toilet pan. It tends to be separate from the stool or coats the surface. Bleeding that occurs more proximally in the bowel (for example the sigmoid colon) results in dark red blood often mixed in with the stool. The further proximal the bleeding point, the less likely the blood is to be detected by the patient. If the bleeding is from the stomach or small bowel, then it will present as melaena (black tarry stool) rather than as fresh red blood.

It is important to screen for coexistent diseases listed in Table 4.3 that predispose to lower gastrointestinal bleeding, and also to screen for any comorbid conditions. A

Table 4.3	Causes of lower gastrointestinal bleeding
Anorectal	
Haemorrhoids	
Fissure in ano	
Colon	
Diverticular disease	
Angiodysplasia	

Colitis
    Inflammatory bowel disease
    Ischaemic colitis	

Colorectal cancer	
Small bowel	
Crohn's ileitis	
Meckel's diverticulum	
Small bowel tumours	
Upper gastrointestinal*	
Gastric/duodenal ulcers	
Variceal bleeding	

* Upper gastrointestinal haemorrhage is responsible for approximately 10% of 'lower gastrointestinal bleeding'.

detailed drug history should be performed to enquire about anticoagulants and NSAIDs (gastric ulcers).

On examination, tachycardia, hypotension or postural hypotension may indicate significant blood loss. Abdominal tenderness may occur with Crohn's ileitis, diverticular disease and ischaemic colitis. Haemorrhoids and anal fissures are visible on anal examination.

Initial investigation

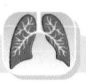

Full blood count
Anaemia may be present with chronic blood loss. It is important to note that anaemia will not be present with acute severe blood loss until haemodilution occurs.

Urea and electrolytes
Urea may be elevated in patients with active gastrointestinal bleeding.

Liver profile
A liver profile should be performed to screen for hepatic failure as varices can result from portal hypertension.

Coagulation screen
A coagulation screen should be performed as impaired coagulation can occur in patients with liver disease and those who are taking anticoagulants.

Group and crossmatch
Blood should be crossmatched for patients who are actively bleeding, or in those with significant blood loss. Otherwise a group and save should be performed.

Sigmoidoscopy and proctoscopy
The investigation of lower gastrointestinal bleeding begins with rigid sigmoidoscopy and proctoscopy. This will identify any anorectal cause and visualizes the large bowel up to the sigmoid.

Further investigations

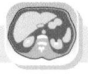

Selective mesenteric angiography
Mesenteric angiography is reserved for patients in whom colonoscopy is unable to identify the source of bleeding or where significant bleeding would obscure the view at colonoscopy. Mesenteric angiography cannot detect small amounts of bleeding; a rate of bleeding of at least 1 mL per minute is usually required. Therapeutic options include intra-arterial injection of vasoconstrictors and therapeutic embolization.

Initial management

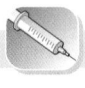

Intravenous access and fluid replacement
Patients are kept nil by mouth, and large-bore intravenous cannulae are sited for fluid replacement. Blood transfusion

may be required depending on the severity of blood loss and the presence of cardiorespiratory disease that would render a patient more susceptible to the effects of acute anaemia.

Colonoscopy

If the lesion cannot be identified on sigmoidoscopy, then colonoscopy will be able to visualize the large bowel up to the caecum. Endoscopic therapy includes thermal coagulation and injection of vasoconstrictors into the bleeding sites.

Surgical management

The management of lower gastrointestinal bleeding depends on the underlying cause. In the majority, colonoscopy can identify and treat the source of bleeding.

Colonic resection

In the emergency situation when severe uncontrollable haemorrhage occurs, a colonic resection may be the only means of arresting the bleeding.

Prognosis

The prognosis varies according to the amount and cause of bleeding.

---

i FURTHER INFORMATION

Zuccaro G, Jr. Management of the adult patient with acute lower gastrointestinal bleeding. American College of Gastroenterology. Practice Parameters Committee. American Journal of Gastroenterology 1998; 93: 1202–1208.

Malabsorption

Malabsorption is the inability to absorb nutrients adequately from the gastrointestinal tract.

Epidemiology

As diseases of the small intestine are frequently accompanied by a degree of impairment of absorptive function, the exact epidemiology of malabsorption is not well documented.

Pathology

Diseases such as coeliac disease (p. 267), tropical sprue (which has similar histological features to coeliac disease but is endemic in tropical areas) and giardiasis that cause small bowel mucosal lesions can result in malabsorption. Rare diseases that result in mucosal abnormalities (similar to villous atrophy) include Whipple's disease, Zollinger–Ellison syndrome (p. 262) and hypogammaglobulinaemia.

Small bowel lymphoma may present with malabsorptive symptoms and can also be seen in association with coeliac disease. Intestinal lymphangiectasia can be primary or secondary to constrictive pericarditis or malignancy (causing obstruction of the lymphatic system).

Eosinophilic gastroenteritis can also affect any part of the gastrointestinal tract but typically affects the gastric antrum and proximal small bowel. Associations with hypersensitivity conditions such as asthma, urticaria and eczema have been described.

Other causes of malabsorption include bacterial overgrowth, which can occur as a result of a structural lesion or as a complication after gastric surgery (particularly if there is a blind loop), diabetic gastroparesis, systemic sclerosis and radiation enteritis. Fistulae between the colon and small bowel (which may occur in Crohn's disease) will introduce faecal flora to the small bowel and may have the same effect.

Small bowel surgery with short bowel syndrome or resection of the terminal ileum (where vitamin B_{12} and bile salts are absorbed) may also result in malabsorptive symptoms.

Scope of disease

Complications related to malabsorption vary according to the underlying cause, site and extent of disease. Oral symptoms, particularly of pain, are related to nutritional deficiencies causing aphthous ulcers, stomatitis (inflammation of the whole lining of the mouth), angular stomatitis (inflammation at the corners of the mouth which may result in fissures), glossitis (inflammation of the tongue) and cheilitis (inflammation of the lips).

Anaemia can result from deficiency of iron, vitamin B_{12} or folate. Tetany is a rare complication of hypocalcaemia, and osteomalacia can result from vitamin D deficiency. Impaired clotting (spontaneous bruising) may occur as a result of vitamin K deficiency and peripheral neuropathy with vitamin B_{12} deficiency.

Clinical features

The patient with malabsorption typically complains of steatorrhoea and diarrhoea that may be accompanied by abdominal pain or discomfort, depending on the underlying cause (Table 4.4). A history of significant weight loss usually indicates organic disease, and tiredness or fatigue can result from anaemia.

On examination, peripheral oedema may be due to hypoalbuminaemia. Abdominal examination is usually unremarkable.

Initial investigations
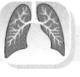

Full blood count
A full blood count may reveal anaemia due to nutritional deficiencies.

Table 4.4	Causes of malabsorption
Small bowel mucosal lesions	
Coeliac disease	
Tropical sprue	
Giardiasis	
Whipple's disease	
Zollinger–Ellison syndrome	
Hypogammaglobulinaemia	
Small bowel lymphoma	

Intestinal lymphangiectasia
    Constrictive pericarditis
    Malignancy	

Amyloidosis	
Eosinophilic gastroenteritis	
Structural lesions	
Crohn's disease	
Jejunal diverticulosis	
Other causes	
Bacterial overgrowth	
Intestinal fistulae	

Small bowel surgery
    Short bowel syndrome
    Resection of the terminal ileum	

Erythrocyte sedimentation rate and C-reactive protein

These non-specific markers of inflammation may be raised with active disease (e.g. Crohn's).

Liver profile

Low albumin may be noted with chronic malabsorption.

Haematinic studies

Screening for vitamin B_{12}, folate and iron deficiencies (p. 781) is particularly relevant in the presence of anaemia.

Calcium

Serum calcium may be low secondary to malabsorption.

Coeliac serology

Serology for coeliac disease (p. 261) should be performed in areas with a high prevalence of disease.

Further investigations

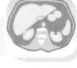

A diagnostic algorithm for further investigations is presented in Figure 4.16.

Carbon breath tests

Carbon breath tests assess the rate of excretion of radio-labelled carbon dioxide following the ingestion of a radio-labelled compound. ^{14}C-triolein absorption quantifies both absorption and lipolysis. A 20 g radio-labelled fat load is given to the patient (for this reason it is not recommended in patients with obesity, diabetes or liver disease), and reduced rate of $^{14}CO_2$ excretion occurs in patients with malabsorption.

Urinary D-xylose testing

Xylose is an inert sugar absorbed by passive diffusion. If the small bowel mucosa is damaged then there will be increased absorption (as an indicator of intestinal permeability). The excretion is measured in the urine.

Schilling test

The Schilling test assesses the absorptive pathway for vitamin B_{12}. Initially, vitamin B_{12} forms a complex with an 'R' binder and then intrinsic factor (which is produced in the stomach). Vitamin B_{12} is then liberated at the mucosal surface in the terminal ileum but intrinsic factor remains within the lumen.

In the Schilling test the patient is given an oral radio-active dose of vitamin B_{12} (1 µg of ^{58}Co-B_{12}). Then 1000 µg of non-radioactive vitamin B_{12} are injected intramuscularly to saturate binding proteins and displace the ^{58}Co-B_{12}. Normal individuals will excrete more than 10% of the radioactive dose, which is measured by a 24-hour urinary collection. If the level of excretion is abnormal then oral intrinsic factor is given to the patient. If excretion is still abnormal this suggests a terminal ileal lesion or the presence of bacterial overgrowth.

^{75}Se HCAT (selenium homo taurocholate)

This test for bile acid or bile salt malabsorption involves the ingestion of ^{75}Se HCAT, which is a synthetic analogue of the natural conjugated bile acid taurocholic acid. Normal individuals who reabsorb their bile acids will have a retained fraction of greater than 15% at 7 days. Lower values indicate bile acid malabsorption. Bile acid replacement therapy with cholestyramine can alleviate symptoms.

Direct pancreatic function tests

Computed tomography (CT), endoscopic retrograde cholangiopancreatography (ERCP) and magnetic resonance cholangiopancreatography (MRCP) have replaced the need for tests that stimulate pancreatic function. ERCP is currently considered the most valuable for diagnosing chronic pancreatitis but studies comparing the diagnostic yield of MRCP may in due course result in this non-invasive test superseding ERCP.

Serum lipase, trypsin and amylase

These pancreatic enzymes have all been assessed but their diagnostic accuracy is only valuable in the presence of significant pancreatic insufficiency.

Faecal pancreatic elastase

Faecal pancreatic elastase (FPE), a recently described marker of pancreatic insufficiency, is not degraded during intestinal transit and low levels may indicate pancreatic insufficiency (suggesting the production of pancreatic elastase is reduced).

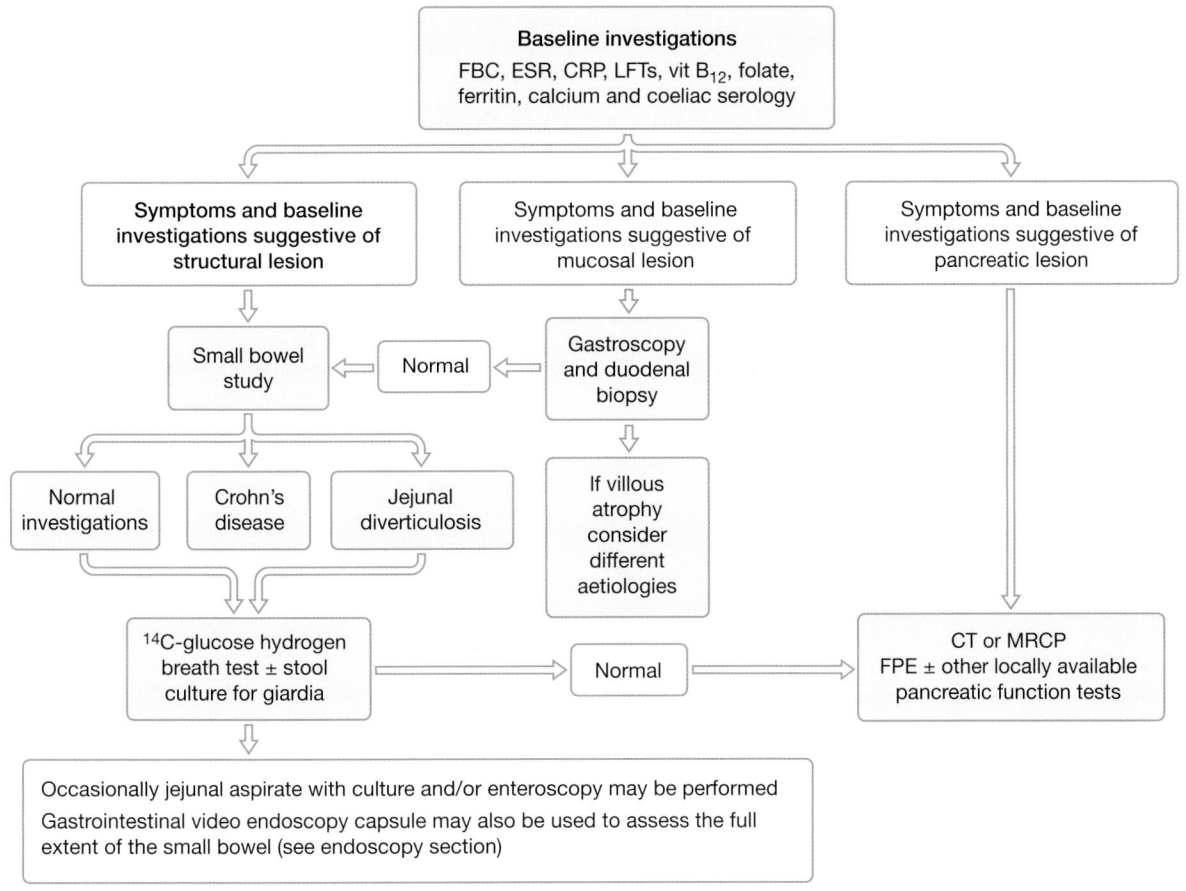

Fig. 4.16 Investigation for malabsorption. CRP, C-reactive protein; CT, computed tomography; ESR, erythrocyte sedimentation rate; FBC, full blood count; FPE, faecal pancreatic elastase; LFTs, liver function tests; MRCP, magnetic resonance cholangiopancreatography.

Management

The causes of malabsorption are diverse, and management is described under individual causes.

 FURTHER INFORMATION

Thomas PD, Forbes A, Green J, et al. Guidelines for the investigation of chronic diarrhoea, 2nd edn. Gut 2003; 52(suppl v): v1–v15.

Undernutrition

Undernutrition arises from failure to meet nutritional requirements. It is common in hospitalized patients and has an important impact on morbidity and mortality.

Epidemiology

Undernutrition has been estimated to occur in up to 40% of hospitalized patients,[1] however the estimates vary according to definition.

Pathology

Undernutrition can result from inadequate nutritional intake, failure of absorption or a catabolic response in which increased cell metabolism and turnover causes energy demands to exceed supply, or any combination of these factors (Table 4.5).

Clinical features

The wide-ranging effects of malnutrition are not always appreciated and may include apathy, loss of concentration, depression, impaired respiratory and cardiac function, impaired cell-mediated and humoral immunity, poor wound healing, increased incidence of sepsis, prolonged hospital stay and increased morbidity and mortality.

Investigation

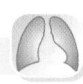

Anthropometric measurements

Anthropometric measurements of body mass index (BMI), triceps skinfold thickness, mid-arm circumference, mid-arm muscle circumference, and weight loss are common indicators of protein–energy malnutrition. The

243

Table 4.5	Causes of undernutrition in hospital

Increased requirement
  Malignancy
  Sepsis

Reduced absorption
  Inflammatory bowel disease
  Short bowel syndrome (after small bowel resection where
    less than 100 cm of small bowel remains)

Reduced intake
  Oesophageal cancer
  Anorexia/bulimia

criteria used by McWhirter and Pennington are listed in Table 4.6.

Management

Management requires a multidisciplinary approach with the help and advice of hospital dieticians. Specific nutrition support teams often manage the care of patients on total parenteral nutrition.

Treat the underlying cause

An important aspect of the management of undernutrition is the attempt to identify and treat any underlying cause such as sepsis and anorexia nervosa.

Improving oral calorie intake

This may be achieved by the use of high-energy meals and the addition of high-calorie and high-protein snacks based on the consumption of meat and fish, starch foods, milk and dairy products, fats and sugars and fluid. In addition, food can be fortified by adding milk powder or by using butter, cream and grated cheese in food preparation.

Commercial sip feeds are available as whole protein (polymeric), predigested or 'chemically defined' and disease-specific diets. Whole protein sip feeds are commonly used and contain an energy density of 1 kcal/mL (1.5 kcal/mL in high-energy feeds) and a nitrogen concentration of 5–7 g/L. The predigested or 'chemically defined' diets contain synthetic L-amino acids (elemental diet) or oligopeptides as the nitrogen source. They are mainly used in the treatment of active Crohn's disease, and occasionally in exocrine pancreatic insufficiency or short bowel syndrome. The benefits are largely theoretical as absorption studies have not shown a clear difference between polymeric and elemental diets.

Enteral tube feeding

Tube feeding (Fig. 4.17) may be used in any malnourished patient who cannot attain his or her requirements orally, for example due to anorexia or dysphagia due to oesophageal cancer. The most common indication for short-term outpatient nasoenteral tube feeding is the administration of elemental or semi-elemental feeds for the treatment of Crohn's disease in those who find the diet too unacceptable to take orally. The main contraindications are paralytic ileus, gastrointestinal obstruction and major intra-abdominal sepsis.

A nasogastric tube is usually inserted at the bedside (p. 286). In patients with impaired consciousness without a gag reflex (e.g. stroke) or impaired gastric emptying (e.g. diabetic gastroparesis), nasojejunal (post-pyloric) tube feeding is preferred to minimize the risk of aspiration.

Complications of enteral feeding relate to the tube (blockage), the feed (abdominal discomfort, nausea, vomiting, diarrhoea, regurgitation, pulmonary aspiration) and metabolic disorders (hyperglycaemia, hypokalaemia, hypomagnesaemia and hypophosphataemia). Complications may be minimized by checking the positioning of the tube (on chest film), continuous feeding (as opposed to bolus feeding) and adjustment of the feed contents based on regular assessment of serum electrolytes.

Percutaneous endoscopic gastrostomy feeding

A PEG tube is the preferred route of administration for long-term enteral feeding (more than a few weeks). The most common indications for PEG insertion (p. 236) and feeding are dysphagic stroke and oropharyngeal malignancies. PEG feed is infused directly into the tube; this can be performed by the patient.

As many as 40% of patients continue to have protein–energy malnutrition after discharge and regular monitoring is required to adjust the feed in the light of the patient's nutritional status and to assess the need for continuing PEG feed. The swallowing reflex recovers sufficiently in approximately 20% of dysphagic stroke patients to allow for PEG removal.

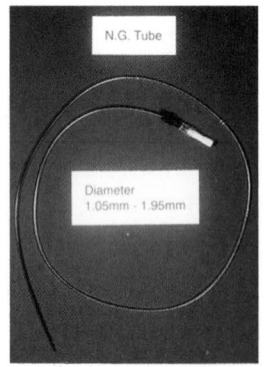

N.G. Tube

Diameter
1.05mm - 1.95mm

Fig. 4.17 A nasogastric tube.

Table 4.6	Classification of undernutrition

	Body mass index (BMI)	Triceps skinfold thickness	Mid-arm circumference
Mild undernutrition	<20	<15th centile	<15th centile
Moderate undernutrition	<18	<5th centile	<5th centile
Severe undernutrition	<16	<5th centile	<5th centile

Unintentional weight loss before illness of more than 10% in the 6 months before admission and values for grip strength below 85% of standard are considered additional evidence of undernutrition.

Total parenteral nutrition

Total parenteral nutrition refers to the administration of nutrition via a long-term intravenous catheter placed in a central vein. Common indications include Crohn's disease, ischaemic gut disorders, motility disorders, radiation enteritis, congenital bowel disorders, malignancy and acquired immune deficiency syndrome.

Complications include line blockages, catheter-related sepsis and central vein thrombosis. Line blockages may be treated by thrombolytic agents, but ultimately line replacement may be required. Catheter exit-site infection, tunnel infection or catheter-related septicaemia may occur. Antibiotic therapy and line removal may be required in severe infections.

Prognosis

Oral and enteral protein–energy nutritional supplementation is associated with improvements in weight gain, anthropometric measures and significant improvement in survival of hospitalized patients.[2]

REFERENCES

(1) *McWhirter JP, Pennington CR. Incidence and recognition of malnutrition in hospital. BMJ 1994; 308: 945–948.*
(2) *Potter J, Langhorne P, Roberts M. Routine protein energy supplementation in adults: systematic review. BMJ 1998; 317: 495–501.*

Diarrhoea

Diarrhoea may be described as an increase in the frequency, watery consistency, volume or weight of stool. It is (arbitrarily) classified as chronic if it persists for 4 weeks or more. The definition of chronic diarrhoea is the abnormal passage of three or more loose or liquid stools per day for more than 4 weeks and/or a stool weight of greater than 200 g per day (measurement of stool weight is normally reserved for difficult cases of chronic diarrhoea or when factitious diarrhoea is suspected).

Epidemiology

Diarrhoea can occur at any age and in either sex. The incidence of acute diarrhoea varies according to geography. It has a major impact on public health, especially in developing countries with poor sanitation and lack of clean drinking water. The prevalence of chronic diarrhoea has been estimated at 14 000 per 100 000 (14%) of the elderly population.[1]

Pathology

The causes of diarrhoea are listed in Table 4.7.

Clinical features

Whilst the definition of diarrhoea may be straightforward, patients may present with other symptoms that they attribute to diarrhoea. It is important to distinguish diarrhoea from steatorrhoea and faecal incontinence.

A detailed drug history is required to exclude diarrhoea as a side effect or result of medication, and assessment should include screening for clinical features of any associated diseases (Table 4.7).

Table 4.7	Causes of diarrhoea

Acute (less than 4 weeks)

Infective

Bacterial (*E. coli, Staphylococcus, Campylobacter, Salmonella, Cholera, Shigella*)

Viral (rotavirus, hepatitis virus)

Protozoa (giardiasis, *Entamoeba*)

Worms (threadworm—Fig. 4.18)

All other causes of chronic diarrhoea

Chronic (4 weeks or more)

Colonic

Colonic carcinoma

Diverticular disease

Inflammatory bowel disease

Small bowel

Malabsorption

Mesenteric ischaemia

Pancreatic

Exocrine pancreatic failure

Parasitic or bacterial

Traveller's diarrhoea

Pseudomembranous colitis (antibiotic-associated diarrhoea)

Protozoal

Giardiasis

Hookworm infection

Hereditary

Lactase deficiency

Endocrine

Hyperthyroidism

Hypoparathyroidism

Addison's disease

Hormone-secreting tumours (for example, VIPoma, carcinoid and gastrinoma)

Autonomic neuropathy

Diabetes

Drugs

Laxatives

Iatrogenic

Small bowel resection

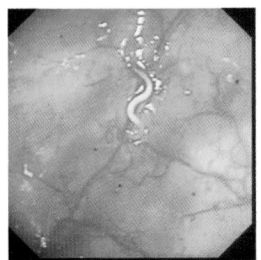

Fig. 4.18 Endoscopic image of a threadworm.

Investigations

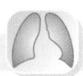

In view of the numerous causes of diarrhoea, investigations should be directed by the clinical features. In most cases of acute diarrhoea of mild to moderate severity, no investigations are required on the presumption of an infective cause.

Initial management

Rehydration

Maintenance of hydration is important and hospital admission for intravenous fluid replacement may be required when severe vomiting prevents adequate oral fluid intake. In developing countries, WHO oral rehydration solutions have reduced mortality associated with acute diarrhoea. Reduced osmolarity oral rehydration solution (224 mmol/L), however, is associated with fewer unscheduled intravenous fluid infusions, lower stool volume and less vomiting compared to standard WHO preparations (311 mmol/L).[2]

Medical management

The most important aspect of treatment is to diagnose and treat the specific cause of the diarrhoea.

Probiotic therapy

A probiotic is a live microbial supplement such as *S. thermophilus*, *L. casei* or *Lactobacillus GG*. Administration of a probiotic in infective diarrhoea reduces the risk of diarrhoea at 3 days (relative risk 0.66) and the mean duration of diarrhoea by 30 hours.[3]

Antibiotics

In general, antibiotics are not appropriate in the management of acute infectious diarrhoea. Antibiotics prolong the carriage of *Salmonella*, worsen the outcome of *E. coli* O157 infections, and lead to the emergence of drug-resistant organisms.

The use of antibiotics should be guided by positive microbiology in symptomatic *Campylobacter* infection and bacteraemia with salmonellosis. Empirical use of antibiotics (e.g. quinolones such as ciprofloxacin) in traveller's diarrhoea improves the cure rate at 3 days (odds ratio 5.9) and reduces severity of symptoms.[4] However, the incidence of adverse reactions such as rash and nausea was more than doubled (odds ratio 2.37). Giardiasis should be treated with metronidazole.

Antidiarrhoeal agents

An antimotility agent such as loperamide provides faster symptomatic benefit (complete relief of symptoms in 24 hours as opposed to 45 hours), but leads to an increased risk of constipation (absolute risk increase 18%).[5]

Prognosis

The mortality from diarrhoea in developed countries is low. However, diarrhoeal diseases are associated with increased mortality in the elderly and have an important impact on the global mortality in children under 5 years of age, accounting for 21% of deaths at a rate of 4.9 children per 1000 per year.[6]

REFERENCES

(1) Talley NJ, O'Keefe EA, Zinsmeister AR, Melton LJ III. *Prevalence of gastrointestinal symptoms in the elderly: a population-based study.* Gastroenterology 1992; 102: 895–901.

(2) Hahn S, Kim S, Garner P. *Reduced osmolarity oral rehydration solution for treating dehydration caused by acute diarrhoea in children.* Cochrane Database of Systematic Reviews 2002: CD002847.

(3) Allen SJ, Okoko B, Martinez E, Gregorio G, Dans LF. *Probiotics for treating infectious diarrhoea.* Cochrane Database of Systematic Reviews 2004: CD003048.

(4) De Bruyn G, Hahn S, Borwick A. *Antibiotic treatment for travellers' diarrhoea.* Cochrane Database of Systematic Reviews 2000: CD002242.

(5) Hughes IW. *First line treatment in acute non-dysenteric diarrhoea: clinical comparison of loperamide oxide, loperamide and placebo.* British Journal of Clinical Practice 1995; 49: 181–185.

(6) Kosek M, Bern C, Guerrant RL. *The global burden of diarrhoeal disease, as estimated from studies published between 1992 and 2000.* Bulletin Of The World Health Organization 2003; 81: 197–204.

Constipation

Constipation is an ill-defined term often used by the patient to describe infrequent defecation, straining during defecation, hard stool or the sensation of incomplete evacuation. The definition is arbitrary, and symptoms such as infrequency or hard stool consistency may be normal for some individuals.

In order to standardize the definition (to assist in diagnosis and treatment), the Rome II criteria are used (Table 4.8).

Epidemiology

The prevalence of constipation is approximately 20 000 per 100 000 (20%) and increases with age.[1]

Table 4.8	Rome II criteria for functional constipation*

Any symptoms of at least 12 weeks in the preceding year (need not be consecutive), or two or more symptoms that occur in more than a quarter of all defecations

1. Straining

2. Lumpy or hard stool

3. Sensation of incomplete evacuation

4. Sensation of anorectal obstruction or blockage

5. Manual manoeuvres to facilitate evacuation

6. Less than 3 defecations per week

* Thompson WG, Longstreth GF, Drossman DA, Heaton KW, Irvine EJ, Muller-Lissner SA. Functional bowel disorders and functional abdominal pain. Gut 1999; 45: 43ii–47.

Pathology

Constipation may be primary (idiopathic) or secondary to underlying disease. The causes are listed in Table 4.9.

Scope of disease

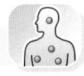

Complications of severe constipation can include large bowel obstruction from faecal impaction. Associated conditions related to or worsened by chronic straining on defecation include haemorrhoids and inguinal herniae.

Clinical features

Patients usually complain of an alteration in the normal bowel habit that may include a combination of symptoms such as infrequent defecation, straining during defecation, hard stool or the sensation of incomplete evacuation. In addition, patients may already be taking laxatives or performing manoeuvres for evacuation of stool.

A detailed drug history is required to identify any medication associated with constipation.

On examination, abdominal distension may be present with faeces palpable as left-sided abdominal masses that indent with pressure. A rectal examination is very important, as the presence of impacted faeces on digital examination will guide appropriate management.

Table 4.9	Causes of constipation
Primary	
Idiopathic constipation	
Secondary	
Drugs	
Opiates	
NSAIDs	
Diuretics	
Antihistamines	
Colonic	
Neuromuscular disorders (Hirschsprung's disease or megacolon)	
Strictures (tumour, diverticular, ischaemia)	
Endocrine	
Hypothyroidism	
Diabetes mellitus	
Metabolic	
Hypocalcaemia of any origin	
Neurological	
Stroke	
Spinal injury	
Autonomic neuropathy	
Psychological	
Anorexia nervosa	
Bulimia nervosa	
Affective disorders	

It is important to screen for features of any underlying secondary cause for constipation (Table 4.9).

Initial investigations

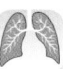

In the majority of patients without clinical features to suggest underlying disease, no investigations are required.

Further investigations

Further investigations are reserved for patients with chronic severe constipation or if an underlying cause is suspected.

Rigid sigmoidoscopy

Examination of the rectum and sigmoid may reveal the mucosal appearance of melanosis coli which occurs with constant use of laxatives, as demonstrated in Figure 4.19 where the mucosa is so deeply pigmented that the stool appears as light brown by comparison.

Colonoscopy or barium enema

Further imaging investigation of the colon is performed if a malignant or diverticular stricture is suspected, particularly in the elderly with a sudden change in bowel habit.

Colonic transit study

Radio-opaque markers are ingested (no laxative should be taken during the test) and a single plain abdominal film is performed at 120 hours post ingestion. The patient's degree of retention of the markers can then be compared against a normal range.

Anorectal manometry

A balloon inserted in the rectum and dilated to 50 mL allows assessment of the patient's ability to tolerate rectal distension. Patients with constipation can tolerate larger volumes than normal individuals. Anal sphincter pressure and waveform can also be observed. A normal individual should develop a relaxed sphincter with increasing rectal distension. Hirschsprung's disease is characterized by unchanged anal sphincter pressure with considerable balloon dilatation.

Defecating proctogram

A defecating proctogram assesses the dynamics of defecation. The patient defecates (or tries to) whilst videoradiography is performed. Abnormalities such as rectal mucosal prolapse or excessive pelvic floor descent may be identified.

Initial management

Lifestyle modification

Initial advice is often to increase dietary fibre, fluid intake and exercise, but evidence to support these recommendations is limited. Ideally, patients should stop any drugs that may cause constipation. If this is not practical, then substitution for another drug or concomitant laxatives may be required.

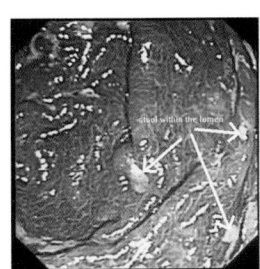

Fig. 4.19 Endoscopic view of severe melanosis coli.

Medical management

The majority of patients may already be self-administering laxatives that are widely available over the counter. The treatment of constipation is modified according to the presence of faecal impaction on rectal examination.

Oral laxatives

Although these agents are widely used, data from randomized trials are available only for bulking agents and osmotic laxatives. It would be reasonable to use these agents as first- and second-line treatment, and change to any of the others if treatment fails or the patient is troubled by adverse effects.

Bulking agents

Bulking agents increase dietary fibre and subsequent faecal mass. This results in stimulation of peristalsis but may take several days to have an effect. Bulking agents have been shown to improve bowel frequency (mean increase 1.4 bowel movements per week) and reduce abdominal pain.[2] However, flatulence and bloating are recognized adverse effects. Examples are ispaghula and wheat bran.

Osmotic laxatives

Osmotic laxatives act by retaining fluid within the colon by osmosis or increasing the volume of fluid in the faeces, leading to an improvement in bowel frequency and reduction in abdominal discomfort.[2] Examples are lactulose and magnesium sulphate.

Stimulant laxatives

Stimulant laxatives enhance colonic motility and may cause unwanted abdominal cramping. Prolonged use can result in an atonic, non-functioning colon. Examples are senna and bisacodyl.

Faecal softeners

Faecal softeners can be used orally or rectally. Examples include docusate sodium and liquid paraffin. Excessive use of liquid paraffin can result in anal seepage and irritation.

Suppositories and enemas

Glycerin suppositories and phosphate enemas are usually reserved for patients with evidence of faecal impaction. Both agents exert an osmotic effect by drawing water into the lower bowel; the resulting distension promotes bowel evacuation. In addition to its lubricant properties, glycerin also works by having a mild irritant effect.

Manual evacuation of faeces

In severe cases, manual evacuation of faeces may be the only means to dislodge faecal impaction.

Prognosis

In the majority, constipation is a self-limiting condition, or resolves with a course of laxatives.

REFERENCES

(1) *Thompson WG, Longstreth GF, Drossman DA, Heaton KW, Irvine EJ, Muller-Lissner SA. Functional bowel disorders and functional abdominal pain. Gut 1999; 45: 43ii–47.*
(2) *Petticrew M, Rodgers M, Booth A. Effectiveness of laxatives in adults. Quality in Health Care 2001; 10: 268–273.*

Intestinal obstruction

Intestinal obstruction is the partial or complete blockage of the bowel, obstructing the normal passage of the intestinal contents.

Epidemiology

The epidemiology of intestinal obstruction varies according to the underlying causes. Small bowel obstruction is a common surgical emergency.

Pathology

Mechanical obstruction

The causes of intestinal obstruction are classified as intraluminal, intramural and extramural, and are presented in Table 4.10. Common causes of small bowel obstruction are adhesions (60%), tumours and herniae, and for large bowel obstruction, colorectal cancer (60%), diverticulitis and volvulus.

With mechanical obstruction, the proximal bowel becomes hyperdynamic with increased peristaltic contractions in an attempt to overcome the blockage. This causes the proximal gut to distend whilst the distal bowel becomes collapsed.

Table 4.10	Causes of intestinal obstruction
Intraluminal	
Faecal impaction	
Foreign body	
Gallstones (gallstone ileus)	
Intramural	
Tumours (benign/malignant)	
Inflammatory strictures, e.g. Crohn's disease	
Extramural	
Adhesion bands	
Obstructed herniae	
Tumours (primary/secondary)	
Volvulus	
Intussusception	

Pseudo-obstruction (paralytic ileus)

With paralytic ileus, there is no blockage of the bowel. Normal peristaltic activity is absent leading to pseudo-obstruction. The most common cause is abdominal surgery, where handling of the intestines leads to a short-lived (5 days) paralytic ileus. Other causes include electrolyte abnormalities, drugs, sepsis, abdominal trauma, acute pancreatitis, haemoperitoneum and spinal injuries.

Scope of disease

The wall of the obstructed gut becomes congested and oedematous, and a large amount of fluid is lost (secreted) into the bowel lumen. This causes dehydration and electrolyte imbalance.

'Closed loop obstruction' can occur with obstructive lesions of the colon if the ileocaecal valve is competent (approximately 20%). Progressive distension can lead to ischaemia, perforation and sepsis. If the ileocaecal valve is incompetent, reflux into the ileum relieves the pressure on the colon. Other causes of bowel ischaemia that can lead to perforation are strangulation (bands, adhesions, obstructed herniae), volvulus, intussusception and mesenteric infarction.

Clinical features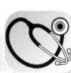

The four cardinal features of acute mechanical intestinal obstruction are colicky abdominal pain, vomiting, absolute constipation (neither faeces nor flatus) and distension.

The site of the colicky pain depends on the location of the obstruction (umbilical pain for midgut obstructions, hypochondrium pain for hindgut obstructions). Pain is usually more acute with small bowel obstruction, and may be minimal for large bowel obstruction. Severe, constant localized pain due to parietal peritoneal irritation suggests infarction or impending perforation (e.g. right lower quadrant pain with impending caecal perforation).

Early vomiting is a feature of small bowel obstruction, and is usually bile stained (proximal obstruction) or altered small bowel content (distal obstruction). With large bowel obstruction, vomiting occurs late and may be faeculent.

Once distal faeces have been evacuated, absolute constipation develops. This occurs late with proximal obstruction and is an early feature with distal obstruction.

On examination, the patient may be severely dehydrated (tachycardia, hypotension, loss of skin turgor). The abdomen is distended and tympanitic. Localized tenderness is indicative of infarction or impending perforation. In cases of mechanical obstruction, peristalsis may be visible and bowel sounds are increased ('tinkling' in nature), whilst in paralytic ileus they are both absent. Rectal examination usually reveals an empty rectum.

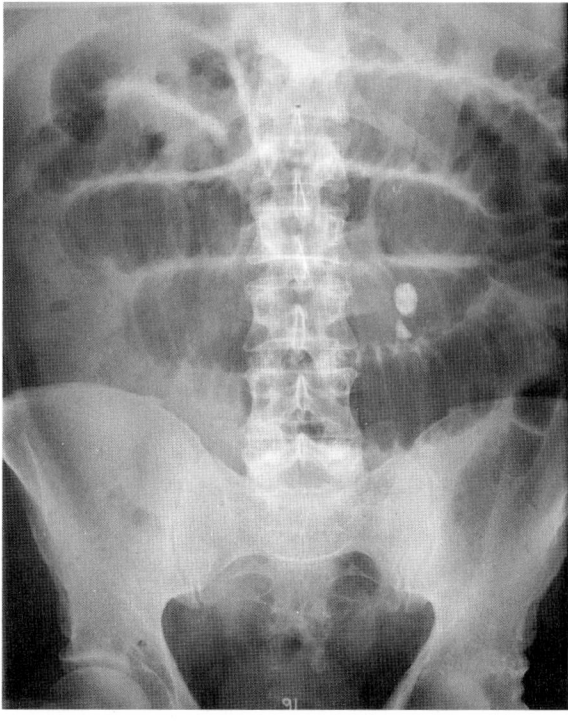

Fig. 4.20 Plain abdominal film of small bowel obstruction. In this image, small bowel is identified by the central position and valvulae conniventes that traverse the width of the bowel lumen.

Initial investigations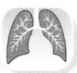

Full blood count

The haemoglobin and haematocrit may be raised due to haemoconcentration, a consequence of dehydration. The white cell count may be elevated.

Urea and electrolytes

There are usually marked electrolyte disturbances depending on the site and severity of the obstruction. Raised urea and creatinine indicate renal impairment, usually as a result of dehydration.

Plain abdominal film

The plain abdominal film will show grossly distended loops of bowel. Small bowel distension can be distinguished from large bowel distension by the valvulae conniventes traversing the whole width of the small bowel wall (Fig. 4.20), as opposed to the colonic haustrae, which pass only part way across the bowel wall (Fig. 4.21). With paralytic ileus, both large and small bowels are dilated. The risk of caecal perforation increases as the maximum diameter increases above 10 cm.

Some advocate the use of supine and erect abdominal films, the latter to demonstrate air–fluid levels, but a supine film is normally adequate.

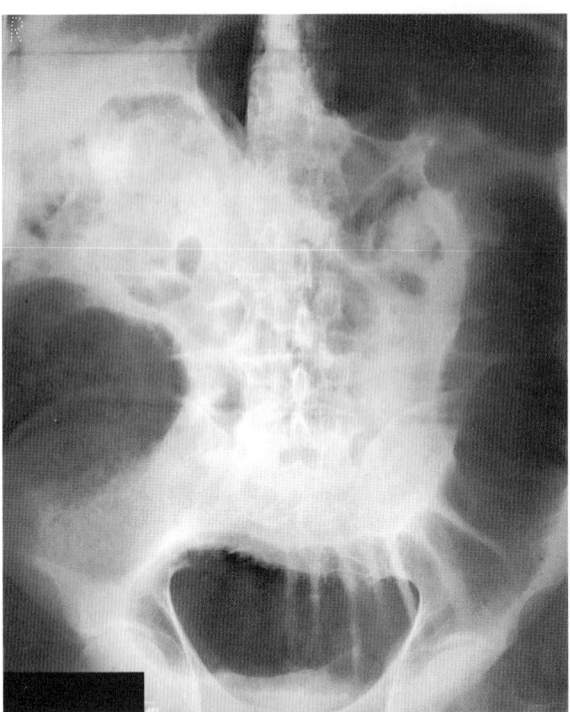

Fig. 4.21 Plain abdominal film of large bowel obstruction. In this image, large bowel is identified by the peripheral position and haustrae that pass only part way across the bowel lumen.

Erect chest X-ray

An erect chest film is necessary to exclude perforation, which will be apparent as free air beneath a raised hemi-diaphragm (p. 232).

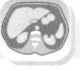

Further investigations

CT abdomen

A CT scan of the abdomen may be required to localize the site, extent and cause of the obstruction.

Initial management

Nasogastric tube

The patient is kept nil by mouth and a nasogastric tube is passed to decompress the proximal bowel and reduce nausea and vomiting.

Fluid and electrolyte replacement

Fluid replacement and the correction of any electrolyte abnormalities are an important aspect of the management.

Antibiotics

Intravenous antibiotics (cefuroxime and metronidazole) are usually administered if there are features to suggest bowel perforation.

Medical management

Initial conservative management is appropriate for patients with paralytic ileus, and patients with suspected small bowel obstruction due to adhesions.

Surgical management

The indications for surgery (Fig. 4.22) are clinical features of strangulation, impending perforation, peritonitis, progressive disease despite medical therapy and the presence of any surgically correctable lesions (incarcerated hernia, carcinoma). The definitive surgical procedure depends on the underlying cause.

Prognosis

The prognosis depends on the underlying cause. Obstruction due to malignancy has a very poor prognosis. Recurrent obstruction is unusual unless the cause is adhesions.

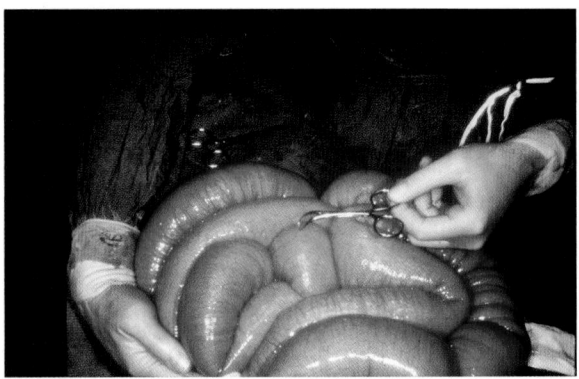

Fig. 4.22 Intraoperative image of small bowel obstruction.

Irritable bowel syndrome

Irritable bowel syndrome is a common functional bowel disorder, a condition defined by symptoms in the absence of known structural pathology.

Epidemiology

The community-based prevalence of irritable bowel syndrome has been estimated at 10.5% (10 500 per 100 000): 14% of women and 7% of men.[1] The estimates of prevalence vary according to definition, and no consistent associations have been reported with age or race.

Pathology

Although no known structural pathology has been identified, proposed aetiologies include gastrointestinal infection, stress, psychological morbidity, abnormal illness behaviour and food sensitivity.[2]

Scope of disease

Apart from gastrointestinal symptoms, irritable bowel syndrome can impact on the patient's quality of life due to psychological morbidity (anxiety, restriction of social activities) and sleep disturbance.

Clinical features

Typical symptoms are recurrent abdominal pain associated with a change in the frequency or appearance of the stool. The clinical presentation may be subdivided into diarrhoea predominant, constipation predominant or alternating symptoms in the absence of sinister symptoms such as weight loss, rectal bleeding, anaemia and nocturnal diarrhoea (Table 4.11). Associated symptoms include lethargy, poor sleep, dyspareunia, frequency and urgency of micturition. A careful dietary and drug history should be undertaken to identify any precipitating causes. Clinical examination should be normal.

As the clinical features overlap considerably with known organic disease, the diagnosis should be one of exclusion, particularly in those individuals over the age of 45 where the risk of significant disease is greater.

Table 4.11	Rome II diagnostic criteria for irritable bowel syndrome*

At least 12 weeks, which need not be consecutive, in the preceding 12 months of abdominal discomfort or pain that has two of three features:

1. Relieved with defecation; and/or

2. Onset associated with a change in frequency of stool; and/or

3. Onset associated with a change in form (appearance) of stool.

Supportive symptoms that cumulative suggest irritable bowel disease

1. Fewer than three bowel movements a week

2. More than three bowel movements a day

3. Hard or lumpy stools

4. Loose (mushy) or watery stools

5. Straining during a bowel movement

6. Urgency (having to rush to have a bowel movement)

7. Feeling of incomplete bowel movement

8. Passing mucus (white material) during a bowel movement

9. Abdominal fullness, bloating or swelling

Diarrhoea-predominant

1 or more of 2, 4, or 6 and none of 1, 3, or 5

Constipation-predominant

1 or more of 1, 3, or 5 and none of 2, 4, or 6

* Thompson WG, Longstreth GF, Drossman DA, Heaton KW, Irvine EJ, Muller-Lissner SA. Functional bowel disorders and functional abdominal pain. Gut 1999; 45: 43ii–47.

Initial investigations

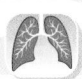

Investigations in general are not required for patients less than 45 years with a typical history of fluctuating disease without any features of organic disease.

Further investigations

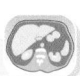

Lower gastrointestinal endoscopy

Rigid sigmoidoscopy can be performed at the bedside to examine the rectum for colitis in patients who present with diarrhoea. Patients over the age of 45 years or those presenting with blood in the stool should have a formal lower gastrointestinal endoscopy to screen for colon cancer.

Initial management

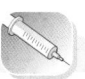

Patient education

Making a definitive diagnosis is important for the patient and the physician. Listening to the patient and accepting his or her symptoms are also important aspects of management. Patients should be encouraged to keep a symptom diary as well as document their food intake to identify any possible associations.

Medical management

Antispasmodics

This group of drugs consists of smooth muscle relaxants such as dicycloverine, mebeverine and alverine. Mean symptom improvement was 38% with placebo and 56% with a smooth muscle relaxant.[3]

Antidepressants

Antidepressants can have an action on the bowel as well as the central nervous system. Imipramine slows small bowel transit in patients with diarrhoea predominant irritable bowel syndrome, whilst paroxetine can accelerate small bowel transit.

Antidiarrhoeal agents

Loperamide or codeine may be prescribed for patients with troublesome diarrhoea.

Laxatives

Laxatives are useful for the management of patients with constipation as the predominant symptom.

> **RECENT ADVANCES**
>
> *The effects of the 5-hydroxytryptamine (5-HT) receptor antagonist alosetron and the 5-HT$_4$ receptor partial agonist tegaserod are superior to placebo in the treatment of irritable bowel syndrome.*[4,5]

Prognosis

Irritable bowel syndrome is a chronic relapsing condition; whilst initial treatment can be effective, the beneficial effects often wear off.

 FURTHER INFORMATION

Jones J, Boorman J, Cann P, et al. British Society of Gastroenterology guidelines for the management of the irritable bowel syndrome. Gut 2000; 47: 1ii–19.

REFERENCES

(1) Wilson S, Roberts L, Roalfe A, Bridge P, Singh S. Prevalence of irritable bowel syndrome: a community survey. British Journal of General Practice 2004; 54: 495–502.
(2) Jones J, Boorman J, Cann P, et al. British Society of Gastroenterology guidelines for the management of the irritable bowel syndrome. Gut 2000; 47: 1ii–19.
(3) Poynard T, Regimbeau C, Benhamou Y. Meta-analysis of smooth muscle relaxants in the treatment of irritable bowel syndrome. Alimentary Pharmacology and Therapeutics 2001; 15: 355–361.
(4) Cremonini F, Delgado-Aros S, Camilleri M. Efficacy of alosetron in irritable bowel syndrome: a meta-analysis of randomized controlled trials. Neurogastroenterology and Motility 2003; 15: 79–86.
(5) Evans BW, Clark WK, Moore DJ, Whorwell PJ. Tegaserod for the treatment of irritable bowel syndrome. Cochrane Database of Systematic Reviews 2004: CD003960.

SECTION 4.6 — Diseases of the oesophagus

Gastro-oesophageal reflux disease

Spontaneous gastro-oesophageal reflux occurs as a normal event, and gastro-oesophageal reflux disease (GORD) is defined as symptoms (dyspepsia) and/or tissue damage caused by retrograde flow of gastric contents into the oesophagus.

Epidemiology

Symptoms of GORD have been reported in approximately 44% of a surveyed population, but the precise prevalence varies according to the definition of the disease.[1] The incidence increases with age and peaks at the age of 55–64 years,[2] with an approximately equal sex distribution.

Pathology

The normal anti-reflux mechanism involves both anatomical and physiological factors: the lower oesophageal sphincter, angle of His, crura of the diaphragm, mucosal rosette, swallowed saliva (lubrication and neutralization of acid), antegrade oesophageal peristalsis and normal gastric motility/emptying.

A mild degree of reflux is experienced in most normal individuals, but a major cause of significant GORD is inappropriate transient lower oesophageal sphincter relaxations (not preceded by a primary propagated oesophageal contraction initiated by swallowing). Other causes include hiatus hernia and delayed gastric emptying.

Although a greater proportion of patients with symptoms of GORD smoke and consume alcohol, clinical studies confirm that traditional risk factors of increasing age, male sex, smoking and alcohol consumption are not strongly associated with symptoms of GORD.[3]

Scope of disease

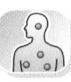

The majority have mild disease without oesophagitis (non-erosive reflux disease). Symptoms can arise with minimal gastric reflux due to increased sensitivity of the oesophagus to acid. Moderate disease is associated with oesophagitis, and severe chronic disease results in the development of Barrett's oesophagus (defined as metaplastic columnar degeneration above the gastro-oesophageal junction). This is a premalignant condition, with a 0.5% per patient-year risk of malignant change to adenocarcinoma.[4]

Severe or prolonged reflux can lead to ulceration, bleeding or perforation. Healing occurs by fibrosis and may lead to stricture formation. Severe reflux may also produce a hoarse voice from laryngitis. If the refluxate is aspirated, pneumonia may develop.

Clinical features

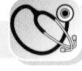

Most patients complain of heartburn, characterized by retrosternal burning pain, precipitated by meals. It may be aggravated by posture (lying flat, stooping, bending forwards) and conditions that raise intra-abdominal pressure (sneezing and coughing). It is often relieved by antacids and may be associated with water brash, the excessive secretion of saliva preceding reflux.

Atypical symptoms include back pain, cardiac-type chest pain, chronic wheeze, nocturnal 'asthma' or recurrent chest infections (due to aspiration), sore throat, hoarse voice, halitosis or dental decay. Dysphagia may occur with oesophageal strictures from chronic disease.

Initial investigations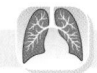

In general, the history can lead to a confident diagnosis of GORD and initial treatment can commence for uncomplicated cases. Older patients, or those who experience weight loss, dysphagia or haematemesis will require further investigations.

Further investigations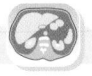

Upper gastrointestinal endoscopy

Oesophagoscopy is appropriate for patients with symptoms suggestive of complications (weight loss, dysphagia, haematemesis), when the diagnosis is unclear, when symptoms cannot be adequately controlled on medical therapy, or for screening for Barrett's epithelium (in patients over 50 with chronic symptoms).

Oesophageal abnormalities that can be diagnosed at endoscopy include hiatus hernia, oesophagitis, Barrett's oesophagus, strictures and tumours. The severity of reflux oesophagitis can also be assessed at endoscopy, and biopsies can be taken. GORD cannot be excluded by a normal endoscopy.

24-hour pH measurement

Intra-oesophageal pH measurement may be required to diagnose GORD if the initial endoscopy is normal or if symptoms do not respond to medical therapy. It is usually performed as an ambulatory test over a 24-hour period, facilitating the diagnosis of GORD by assessment of the duration, frequency and severity of reflux attacks in relation to the pH of the oesophagus. It does not provide any information as to the aetiology of GORD and may be normal (false negative) in patients with significant bile or volume reflux.

Oesophageal manometry

Oesophageal manometry is a useful investigation to assess oesophageal function when planning surgical intervention, especially if achalasia and other oesophageal motility disorders are suspected. It is possible to determine the length and position of the lower oesophageal sphincter and to measure the sphincter pressure. A short or weak lower oesophageal sphincter is often a major contributing cause of reflux oesophagitis.

Initial management

Lifestyle modification

Suggestions that may improve symptoms include weight loss for obese patients, stopping smoking, frequent small meals, avoiding foods that are known to precipitate symptoms, avoiding eating for several hours before bedtime, and raising the head of the bed. However, evidence for improvement associated with these measures is scarce.

Medical management

There are three pharmacological approaches to controlling symptoms of GORD: neutralization of acid (antacids and alginates), reduction in acid production (H_2-receptor blockers, proton pump inhibitors) and increasing gastrointestinal motility (metoclopramide).

Step-up therapy

Most agents for initial therapy are available without prescription, and pharmacists offer the first-line management of GORD in a step-up regimen (starting from the simplest, most cost-effective agent).

Antacids and alginates

Antacids, such as bicarbonate, act by reducing the acidity within the stomach and lower oesophagus. Alginate preparations (such as Gaviscon) act by coating the top of the gastric contents to reduce the effect of acid on the oesophageal mucosa. Both these agents are effective,[5] but the effects are often short-lived and suitable only for patients with mild symptoms.

H_2-receptor antagonists

H_2-receptor antagonists (e.g. cimetidine, ranitidine) block the H_2-receptors in gastric mucosa, leading to a marked reduction in gastric acid production. Initial symptomatic relief is experienced in approximately 60%.[6]

Step-down therapy

Patients who seek medical attention may already be on a combination of antacids, alginates and H_2-receptor antagonists. Current consensus favours step-down therapy (starting with the most effective agent), as it is associated with greater symptomatic relief and fewer treatment failures and physician consultations.[7]

Proton pump inhibitors

The proton pump inhibitors (e.g. omeprazole, lansoprazole) act by blocking the proton pump within the gastric mucosa, almost completely abolishing gastric acid production. Initial symptomatic relief is experienced in approximately 83%.[6] An initial 2–4-week course is recommended followed by maintenance therapy. Failure to respond to initial therapy is an indication for further investigations (endoscopy, pH studies) to confirm and assess the severity of the disease.

Prokinetic agents

Due to the superiority of proton pump inhibitors, the role of prokinetic agents (metoclopramide) is ill defined. Prokinetic agents are usually reserved for use in combination with proton pump inhibitor for step-up therapy, or in combination with an H_2-receptor blocker for long-term maintenance step-down therapy.

Maintenance therapy

After 6 months of initial therapy 75% of patients experience symptom relapse.[8] A trial of withdrawal of drug therapy may be initiated[7] but the majority will require maintenance therapy either by step-down treatment (long-term H_2-receptor blocker) or intermittent on-demand proton pump inhibitor therapy, a 2–4-week course each time symptoms recur.[9]

Surgical management

Before considering anti-reflux surgery, upper gastrointestinal endoscopy, 24-hour pH studies and oesophageal manometry are required for confirmatory diagnosis and documentation of the presence and severity of reflux.

Anti-reflux surgery provides effective long-term treatment of GORD with symptomatic control equivalent to medical therapy but lower rates of oesophagitis.[10] The indications for surgery are failure of medical treatment or development of complications (ulceration, strictures, Barrett's oesophagus or respiratory complications). Relative indications include volume reflux (i.e. excessive volume rather than acid content) and patient preference.

Anti-reflux surgery has a 90% initial success rate. Complications of surgery include dysphagia (usually short-lived) in about 10%, inability to belch, the so-called 'gas bloat syndrome' (20%) and excessive flatus.

Nissen fundoplication

The most common operation is the Nissen (360 degree) fundoplication, which can be performed via an abdominal incision (midline laparotomy) or laparoscopically. The hiatus of the diaphragm is repaired, the lower oesophagus is mobilized, then the greater curvature of the stomach via division of the short gastric arteries. The fundus of the stomach is wrapped completely around the lower oesophagus.

To reduce the risk of dysphagia, various partial fundoplications have been described, including the anterior partial (Watson), posterior partial (Toupet) and Lind (270 degree) subtotal fundoplications.

Collis–Nissen procedure

This uncommon procedure is reserved for situations where the gastro-oesophageal junction cannot be reduced below the diaphragm. An abdominal approach is used and a linear stapler is used to 'lengthen' the oesophagus by incorporating the cardia of the stomach prior to creating the wrap.

Management of benign strictures

A barium swallow is often performed to delineate the site and extent of the stricture, followed by endoscopy and biopsies to determine the aetiology. The treatment of benign strictures consists of bougie dilatation, and several sessions may be required for resistant strictures. Further treatment options include resection or bypass of the stricture and long-term intubation of the oesophagus.

Following oesophageal dilatation, the patient is kept nil by mouth if symptoms such as chest or back pain or surgical emphysema develop. A chest film is performed to exclude a pneumomediastinum, which will suggest oesophageal perforation.

Prognosis

GORD is a chronic relapsing condition. Long-term studies report 10-year recurrence rates (based on use of anti-reflux medications) in 62% of surgically treated and 92% of medically treated patients. If Barrett's oesophagus develops, regular endoscopic surveillance for dysplasia is required.

REFERENCES

(1) Fass R. Epidemiology and pathophysiology of symptomatic gastroesophageal reflux disease. American Journal of Gastroenterology 2003; 98: S2–7.

(2) El-Serag HB, Sonnenberg A. Associations between different forms of gastro-oesophageal reflux disease. Gut 1997; 41: 594–599.

(3) Lagergren J, Bergstrom R, Lindgren A, Nyren O. Symptomatic Gastroesophageal Reflux as a Risk Factor for Esophageal Adenocarcinoma. New England Journal of Medicine 1999; 340: 825–831.

(4) Shaheen N, Ransohoff DF. Gastroesophageal Reflux, Barrett Esophagus, and Esophageal Cancer: Scientific Review. JAMA 2002; 287: 1972–1981.

(5) Farup PG, Weberg R, Berstad A, et al. Low-dose antacids versus 400 mg cimetidine twice daily for reflux oesophagitis. A comparative, placebo-controlled, multicentre study. Scandinavian Journal of Gastroenterology 1990; 25: 315–320.

(6) DeVault KR, Castell DO. Updated guidelines for the diagnosis and treatment of gastroesophageal reflux disease. The Practice Parameters Committee of the American College of Gastroenterology. American Journal of Gastroenterology 1999; 94: 1434–1442.

(7) Dent J, Brun J, Fendrick AM, et al. An evidence-based appraisal of reflux disease management—the Genval Workshop Report. Gut 1999; 44: 1S–16.

(8) Carlsson R, Dent J, Watts R, et al. Gastro-oesophageal reflux disease in primary care: an international study of different treatment strategies with omeprazole. International GORD Study Group. European Journal of Gastroenterology and Hepatology 1998; 10: 119–124.

(9) Bardhan KD. Intermittent and on-demand use of proton pump inhibitors in the management of symptomatic gastroesophageal reflux disease. American Journal of Gastroenterology 2003; 98: S40–48.

(10) Allgood PC, Bachmann M. Medical or surgical treatment for chronic gastroesophageal reflux? A systematic review of published evidence of effectiveness. European Journal of Surgery 2000; 166: 713–721.

Oesophageal motility disorders

Oesophageal motility disorders are disorders of oesophageal function, which result in chest pain or disturbed swallowing.

Epidemiology

These disorders are relatively uncommon, with an incidence that increases with age. Males and females are equally affected and there is no particular geographical variation. Achalasia is the most common oesophageal motility disorder with a prevalence of 1 per 100 000.

Pathology

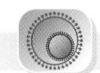

The three most common primary oesophageal motility disorders are achalasia, diffuse oesophageal spasm and nutcracker oesophagus (symptomatic peristalsis). These disorders are caused by paralysis, spasm or uncoordinated oesophageal muscular activity, and they may be related to degeneration of the myenteric nerve plexus or interruption to the extrinsic nerve supply.

In achalasia, peristalsis is absent from the lower two-thirds of the oesophagus and there is incomplete relaxation of the lower oesophageal sphincter. This leads to gross dilatation of the proximal oesophagus, producing the so-called 'baggy' oesophagus. Diffuse oesophageal spasm is characterized by repetitive simultaneous contractions of the oesophageal body, which can be of high amplitude and are often prolonged. In nutcracker oesophagus, also known as symptomatic peristalsis, oesophageal manometry shows normal peristalsis but the amplitude of the peristaltic contractions is very high (often in excess of 150 mmHg).

Motility disorders can also be secondary to underlying disease such as scleroderma, diabetes, Chagas' disease (*Trypanosoma cruzi* infection) and neuromuscular disorders such as myasthenia gravis.

Scope of disease

Complications are uncommon and include weight loss or malnutrition (due to dysphagia) and aspiration pneumonia (due to regurgitation and overspill of oesophageal contents into the respiratory tract). The most important complication is the long-term increased risk of squamous cell carcinoma of the oesophagus, which occurs in around 5% of patients with achalasia.

Clinical features

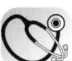

Oesophageal motility disorders usually present with dysphagia or retrosternal pain. The dysphagia is often intermittent and (usually) slowly progressive. It is equally severe or worse for liquids than solids, which may differentiate it from other causes of dysphagia. The chest pain can be quite severe and is often triggered by eating or anxiety. It may occur spontaneously. Marked regurgitation can occur, especially at night, which may present with food soiling of the pillow.

Initial investigations

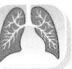

Upper gastrointestinal endoscopy

Upper gastrointestinal endoscopy allows visualization of the oesophageal lining and gastro-oesophageal junction and is a useful investigation to exclude any secondary causes of dysphagia, in particular oesophageal carcinoma. The endoscope should pass into the stomach without resistance and the mucosa should appear normal. In advanced achalasia, the oesophagus may appear 'baggy'.

Barium swallow

A barium swallow is particularly useful when assessing oesophageal motility disorders, as oesophageal function as well as anatomy can be evaluated. With well-developed achalasia, the barium swallow appearance is often diagnostic (Fig. 4.23). Diffuse oesophageal spasm is classically seen as a 'corkscrew oesophagus' (Fig. 4.24). When more subtle changes are present, the addition of marshmallow or bread soaked in barium may help.

Oesophageal manometry

This is the most important investigation in the assessment of oesophageal motility disorders. In achalasia, the lower oesophageal sphincter pressure is high and it does not fully relax on swallowing. Diffuse oesophageal spasm is seen as simultaneous, often high-amplitude contractions in the oesophageal body, which may be prolonged or repetitive. In the nutcracker oesophagus, manometry displays prolonged high-amplitude oesophageal body contractions.

Medical management

Medical therapy is often ineffective, although long-acting nitrates, calcium channel blockers or local injection of botulinum toxin (to disrupt neuromuscular function) may help to some extent.

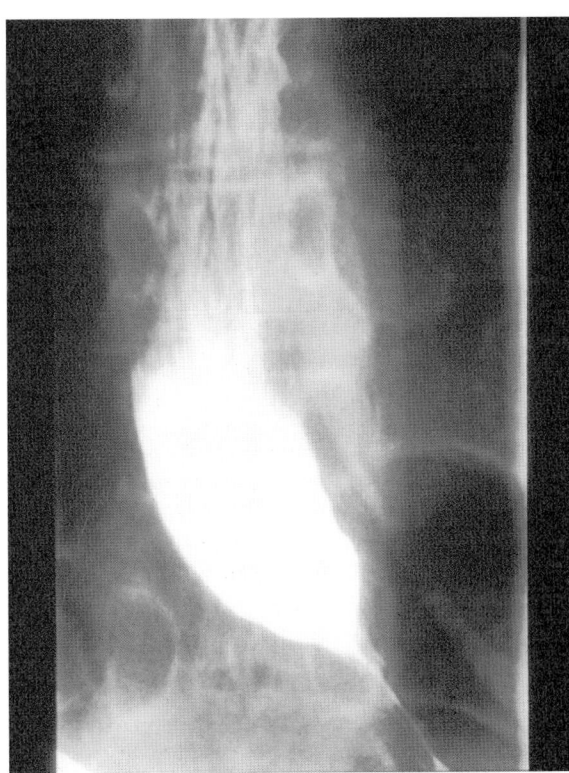

Fig. 4.23 A barium swallow of achalasia. The barium swallow reveals a dilated oesophagus with a 'rat tail' appearance.

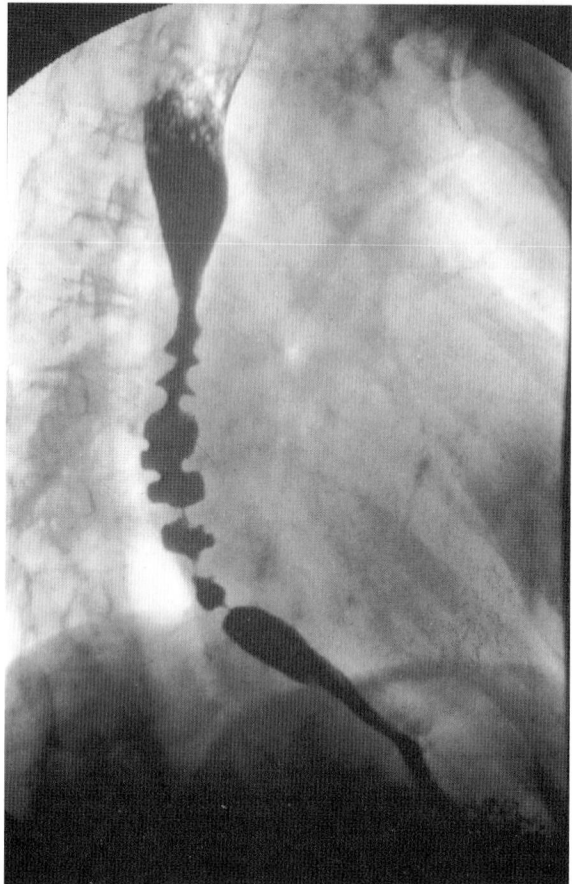

Fig. 4.24 A barium swallow of diffuse oesophageal spasm. The barium swallow reveals a 'corkscrew' appearance.

Oesophagoscopy and dilatation

Achalasia can be effectively treated with forceful balloon dilatation to disrupt the integrity of the lower oesophageal sphincter and carries a success rate for symptom control of 51%.[1]

Surgical management

Heller's cardiomyotomy

The most effective treatment for achalasia is a Heller's cardiomyotomy, in which the fibres of the lower oesophageal sphincter are divided down to the oesophageal mucosa. This can be performed through either chest or abdomen, although the latter is by far the most common approach. The success for symptom control is reported to be 95%.[1]

RECENT ADVANCES

Laparoscopic surgery allows a Heller's myotomy to be performed via a minimally invasive approach. The outcome appears more effective and long-lasting than other methods of treatment.

Oesophagectomy

Oesophagectomy is reserved for patients with severe symptoms and a markedly dilated oesophagus (when Heller's cardiomyotomy is ineffective) and for patients with squamous cancer as a complication of chronic disease.

Prognosis

The prognosis of these disorders depends on the underlying cause. Primary oesophageal motility disorders are rarely life threatening unless a carcinoma develops in long-standing achalasia. They can, however, be notoriously difficult to treat and can have a long and protracted course.

REFERENCE

(1) *Spiess AE, Kahrilas PJ. Treating achalasia: from whalebone to laparoscope. JAMA 1998; 280: 638–642.*

Oesophageal tumours

Benign oesophageal tumours

Epidemiology

Benign tumours of the oesophagus are rare, and account for less than 1% of oesophageal tumours.

Pathology

The most common of the benign oesophageal tumours is the leiomyoma. It is a slow-growing tumour that may be asymptomatic for years. Complications can include dysphagia, ulceration and bleeding.

Clinical features

The slow-growing benign oesophageal tumour may be asymptomatic and detected as an incidental finding. Patients can present with slowly progressive dysphagia.

Investigations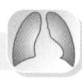

Clinical features cannot reliably distinguish benign from malignant oesophageal tumours, therefore investigations should be performed as for oesophageal carcinoma on page 257.

Management

Expectant management

Expectant management is suitable for asymptomatic patients. Prophylactic surgery is not required.

Surgical resection

Once confirmatory histological diagnosis has been obtained, surgery (enucleation or local resection) may be offered to patients with dysphagia.

Prognosis
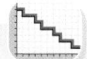

Benign oesophageal tumours are usually slow growing. It is extremely rare for leiomyomas to develop into leiomyosarcomas.

Oesophageal carcinoma

Epidemiology

There is a wide geographical variation in the incidence of oesophageal cancer, with the highest incidence ranging from 7.1 to 11.9 per 100 000 per year in South Africa, China and Asia.[1]

It is a disease of middle and old age with a 3:1 male preponderance. Worldwide, squamous cell carcinoma is most common, particularly in China, Russia, Iran and South Africa. In the West, adenocarcinoma (secondary to Barrett's oesophagus) is now the most common histopathological subtype.

Pathology

Squamous carcinoma

Smoking and high alcohol intake are established risk factors for squamous carcinoma. Some epidemiological studies support the association of a high carbohydrate and low protein and vegetable intake with squamous oesophageal cancer. Environmental carcinogens are thought to be the cause of the striking differences in worldwide incidence. Nitrosamines and their precursors (nitrite and nitrates) have been implicated in the high incidence in China and Iran.

Less common predisposing conditions include achalasia, tylosis (a familial syndrome that includes hyperkeratosis of the palms and feet) and Plummer–Vinson or Paterson–Brown-Kelly syndrome (post-cricoid web associated with iron-deficiency anaemia).

Adenocarcinoma

Adenocarcinoma is strongly associated with long-standing gastro-oesophageal reflux and usually arises in the metaplastic columnar epithelium of Barrett's oesophagus.

Scope of disease

Local

Progressive intraluminal obstruction causes dysphagia. Bleeding and ulceration can result in haematemesis. Infiltration of the trachea can cause a tracheo-oesophageal fistula resulting in chronic cough and chest infection. Recurrent laryngeal nerve involvement can lead to hoarseness.

Metastatic

Common sites of metastatic spread are the liver, lungs, bones and kidney.

Paraneoplastic

Dysphagia in association with anorexia and cachexia of malignancy can lead to rapid severe weight loss and malnutrition.

Clinical features
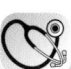

The most common features are dysphagia and weight loss. Dysphagia is progressive, initially for solids then both liquids and solids. Less common features include cough, retrosternal chest pain, odynophagia (painful swallowing), haematemesis and hoarse voice.

Initial investigations
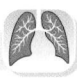

Full blood count

Abnormalities on full blood count are usually non-specific. Occasionally a microcytic anaemia can result from chronic blood loss or from chronic disease.

Liver profile

Raised transaminases may indicate liver metastasis, and raised alkaline phosphatase from either liver or bony metastasis.

Chest X-ray

With advanced disease, a wide mediastinum or tracheal compression may be seen. Pulmonary consolidation may be suggestive of aspiration pneumonia, or infiltration of the trachea. Rarely, pulmonary metastasis may be visible.

Upper gastrointestinal endoscopy

Oesophago-gastro-duodenoscopy is the investigation of choice. It directly visualizes the oesophagus and stomach and allows biopsies for histological examination.

Barium swallow

Alternatively, a barium swallow may be performed when upper gastrointestinal endoscopy is not readily available, or the history is suggestive of a neuromuscular disorder. The classic appearance of oesophageal carcinoma is of a narrowed lumen with 'shouldering' (Fig. 4.25). A barium swallow that suggests oesophageal carcinoma requires follow-up with an upper gastrointestinal endoscopy and biopsies for confirmatory diagnosis.

Further investigations
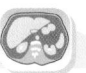

Having obtained histological diagnosis of oesophageal carcinoma, the next step is to evaluate the stage of disease.

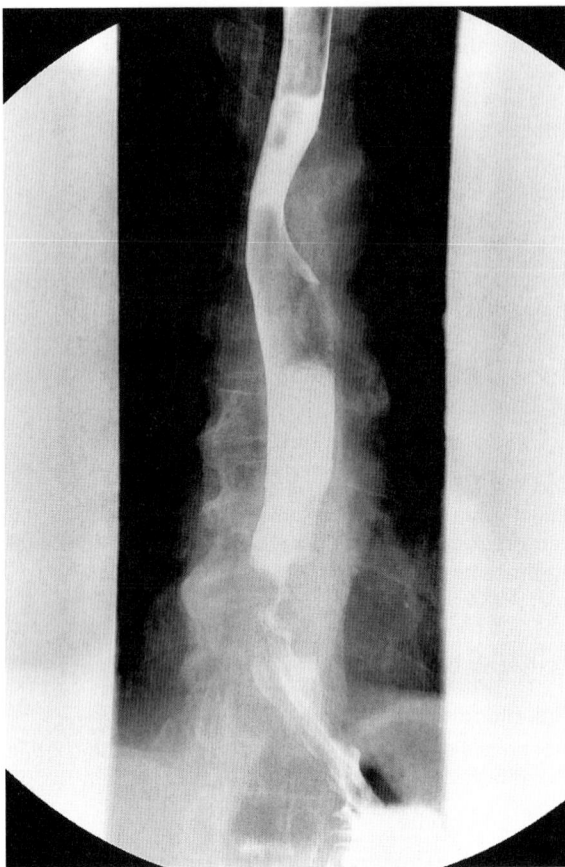

Fig. 4.25 Barium swallow of oesophageal carcinoma. The barium swallow reveals an irregular narrow stricture at the distal oesophagus, with 'shouldering' where the contrast tapers into the stricture.

TNM staging for oesophageal carcinoma

Primary tumour

T1	Tumour invades lamina propria or submucosa
T2	Tumour invades muscularis propria
T3	Tumour invades adventitia
T4	Tumour invades adjacent structures

Regional lymph nodes

N0	No regional lymph node metastases
N1	Regional lymph node metastases

Distant metastases

M0	No distant metastases
M1	Distant metastases

Stage grouping

Stage I	T1, N0, M0
Stage IIA	T2, N0, M0
	T3, N0, M0
Stage IIB	T1, N1, M0
	T2, N1, M0
Stage III	T3, N1, M0
	T4, any N, M0
Stage IV	Any T, any N, M1

CT chest and abdomen

A CT scan is required to assess the anatomical extent of the disease, providing information on local and intrathoracic or abdominal spread (Fig. 4.26).

Endoluminal ultrasound

Endoluminal ultrasound allows better assessment of local spread and fixation to surrounding structures (indicators of inoperable disease). It also gives a better view of lymphadenopathy, suggestive of lymphatic spread.

Bronchoscopy

Bronchoscopy is required to screen for tracheal or main bronchus invasion (inoperable disease) if there is a history of chronic cough or recurrent chest infections.

Initial management

If initial staging investigations suggest that the patient has operable disease, it is important to screen for comorbid disease as part of preoperative assessment of overall operative risk. Patients can be dehydrated and malnourished and may require admission for intravenous fluid and enteral or parenteral (TPN) feeding prior to surgery.

Surgical management

The mainstay of treatment for oesophageal carcinoma is surgical resection, which should be offered to patients with T1 disease. Combination therapy (neoadjuvant therapy followed by curative surgery) should be offered to patients with T2 disease. The best management for patients with T3 N1 disease is not yet determined and this subset should be offered the opportunity to participate in clinical trials.[2] Patients with advanced disease (T4) should be offered palliative therapy (approximately 60%).

There is no consensus on the best operation, and the type of procedure performed depends on the individual surgeon's experience.

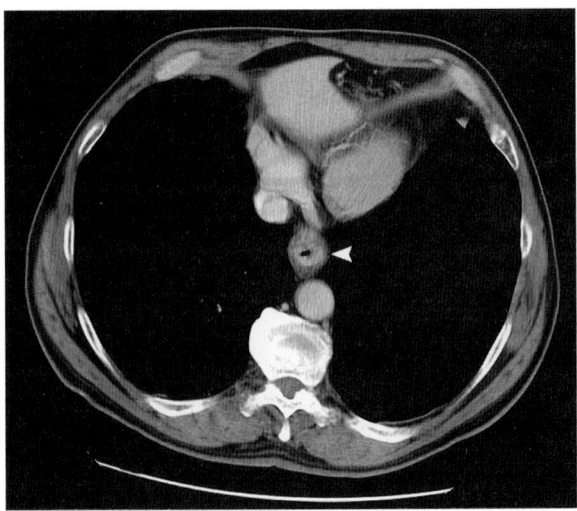

Fig. 4.26 This CT thorax shows thickening of the oesophagus.

Ivor Lewis oesophago-gastrectomy

This is a commonly performed two-stage operation. The first stage is a laparotomy to mobilize the abdominal oesophagus and stomach, and the second stage is a right thoracotomy to mobilize and resect the oesophagus. The resected oesophagus is replaced with stomach (fashioned into a tube), or occasionally either jejunum or colon.

Transhiatal oesophagectomy

An alternative approach is the transhiatal oesophagectomy. An abdominal laparotomy is performed and an incision is made in the left side of the neck. The oesophagus is dissected from below upwards through the hiatus of the diaphragm and from above downwards via the neck incision. The diseased segment is resected and a handsewn anastomosis is fashioned in the neck. Similarly, the resected oesophagus is replaced with stomach, or occasionally either jejunum or colon.

The overall operative mortality is 12%, with 20% developing respiratory (infection, failure) complications and 11% developing cardiac complications (failure, arrhythmia, ischaemia). Approximately 10% will require a second operation due to anastomotic or other enteric (e.g. chyle) leak.[3]

Medical management

After complete surgical resection, neither chemotherapy nor radiotherapy confers additional improvement to survival.

Chemotherapy

The indications for chemotherapy are either as neoadjuvant (preoperative) or as palliative therapy. Preoperative chemotherapy (in conjunction with radiotherapy) has been shown to improve 3-year survival rates after surgery; however, this was at the cost of increased operative mortality.[4]

In the setting of advanced disease, despite less than 20% tumour response rates, improvement in pain control, weight loss, dysphagia and oesophageal reflux was observed in over 64% on fluorouracil-based regimens.[5]

Palliative therapy

In patients unfit for surgery or with unresectable disease, options for the palliation of dysphagia include the insertion of oesophageal stents, ablation therapy using thermal laser, argon plasma coagulation or photodynamic therapy (PDT). Palliative radiotherapy is also used to improve dysphagia.

Prognosis

Oesophageal carcinoma has a dismal prognosis, with an overall 5-year survival rate of less than 5%. Even after potentially curative surgery, the survival rate is around 30%.

FURTHER INFORMATION

Allum WH, Griffin SM, Watson A, Colin-Jones D. Guidelines for the management of oesophageal and gastric cancer. Gut 2002; 50 Suppl 5: v1–23.

REFERENCES

(1) Parkin DM, Pisani P, Ferlay J. Global cancer statistics. CA: A Cancer Journal for Clinicians 1999; 49: 33–64.

(2) Allum WH, Griffin SM, Watson A, Colin-Jones D. Guidelines for the management of oesophageal and gastric cancer. Gut 2002; 50 Suppl 5: v1–23.

(3) McCulloch P, Ward J, Tekkis PP. Mortality and morbidity in gastro-oesophageal cancer surgery: initial results of ASCOT multicentre prospective cohort study. BMJ 2003; 327: 1192–1197.

(4) Fiorica F, Di Bona D, Schepis F, et al. Preoperative chemoradiotherapy for oesophageal cancer: a systematic review and meta-analysis. Gut 2004; 53: 925–930.

(5) Tebbutt NC, Norman A, Cunningham D, et al. A multicentre, randomised phase III trial comparing protracted venous infusion (PVI) 5-fluorouracil (5-FU) with PVI 5-FU plus mitomycin C in patients with inoperable oesophago-gastric cancer. Annals of Oncology 2002; 13: 1568–1575.

SECTION 4.7 Diseases of the stomach and duodenum

Helicobacter pylori

Helicobacter pylori colonizes approximately 60% of the global population. Recognition and understanding of *H. pylori* as a major pathogen is one of the most important advances in diseases of the upper gastrointestinal tract.

Epidemiology

There is marked disparity in the prevalence of *H. pylori* colonization between Western and developing countries (Fig. 4.27). Colonization is usually acquired in childhood and persists for decades, although the route of transmission has not yet been established. In the West, the prevalence is falling with a childhood acquisition rate of 0.3–1% per year.

Pathology

H. pylori is a Gram-negative microaerophilic, spiral flagellate bacterium (Fig. 4.28). It has a variety of virulence factors such as urease, which converts urea to ammonia, creating a local alkaline environment that allows the bacterium to survive in the stomach. Flagellae, which help the bacterium to migrate to the mucus layer of the stomach, and vacuolating cytotoxins and their products (Cag-A and Vac-A) may be related to its pathogenicity in humans. *H. pylori* adheres to the gastric epithelium, sitting in grooves between the epithelial cells within the mucus layer (Fig. 4.29).

Scope of disease

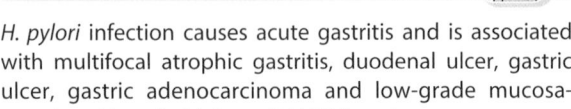

H. pylori infection causes acute gastritis and is associated with multifocal atrophic gastritis, duodenal ulcer, gastric ulcer, gastric adenocarcinoma and low-grade mucosa-associated lymphoid tissue (MALT) lymphoma.

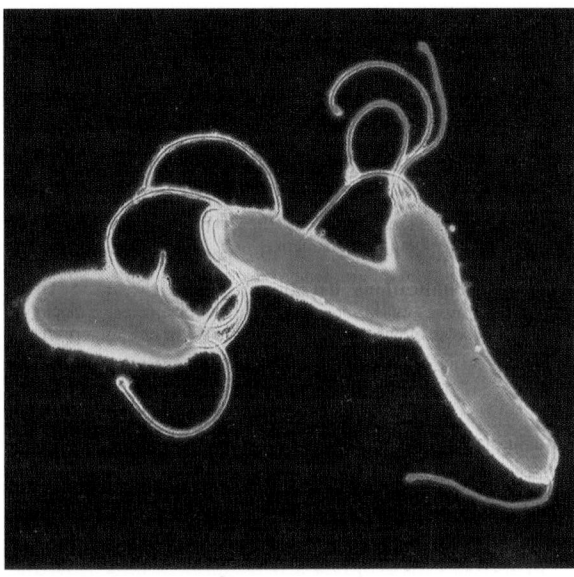

Fig. 4.28 Coloured transmission electron micrograph of *H. pylori*, showing the flagellae which make it highly motile.

Developing countries — Developed countries

Fig. 4.27 Prevalence of *H. pylori*. Serological prevalence by age and economic status.

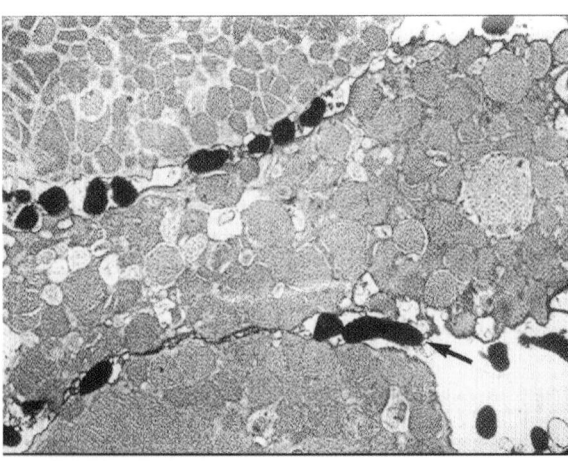

Fig. 4.29 Electron microscopy of *H. pylori* on gastric epithelium surface denoted by the arrow.

Clinical features

Most people colonized with *H. pylori* will not develop symptomatic disease, but have histological antral gastritis. Clinical features of gastritis (p. 263), peptic ulcer disease (p. 262), and gastric cancer (p. 264) are detailed in the respective sections.

Initial investigations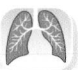

Investigations for *H. pylori* are usually indicated in patients with symptomatic disease.

H. pylori serology

Serology (a blood test) is frequently used as first-line primary care assessment of patients with dyspepsia who are aged less than 45 years with no sinister symptoms. Most commercially available tests are enzyme immunoassay (EIA) based and detect IgG to a mixture of purified antigens from several strains. *H. pylori* antigen can also be detected in stool; this has the advantage of confirming current infection.

Further investigations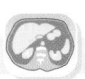

Upper gastrointestinal endoscopy

The key investigation for patients with dyspeptic symptoms is upper gastrointestinal endoscopy. At the time of gastroscopy, antral biopsies for histology, CLO test and culture should be undertaken to identify *H. pylori* (Fig. 4.30). Multiple biopsies should be taken to minimize sampling error, especially in the presence of gastric atrophy and intestinal metaplasia, and to increase sensitivity histology specimens should be stained with modified Giemsa or Warthin–Starry silver stain.

Rapid urease tests (CLO test) have a specificity of 97% and sensitivity of 90%. The test can be performed in the endoscopy room using a biopsy specimen placed into a urea-based gel (Fig. 4.30). A pH indicator will give a positive reaction within 3–4 hours.

Samples sent for culture allow the assessment of antibiotic sensitivities to guide eradication therapy (if indicated). Ideally the specimen should reach the microbiology laboratory in saline or distilled water and be plated within 4–6 hours of biopsy being taken to prevent false negative results. The organism is slow growing and antibiotic sensitivity results will not be available to the clinician for several days.

Carbon-labelled urea breath test

To evaluate the success of eradication or as a diagnostic test in itself, the carbon-labelled urea breath test has excellent sensitivity (98%) and specificity (97%). The test relies on the ability of *H. pylori* to break down ^{13}C- or ^{14}C-labelled urea to carbon dioxide. It is the best non-invasive method for checking eradication. Assessment by reduction in antibody levels or re-endoscopy and biopsy post treatment are less acceptable methods.

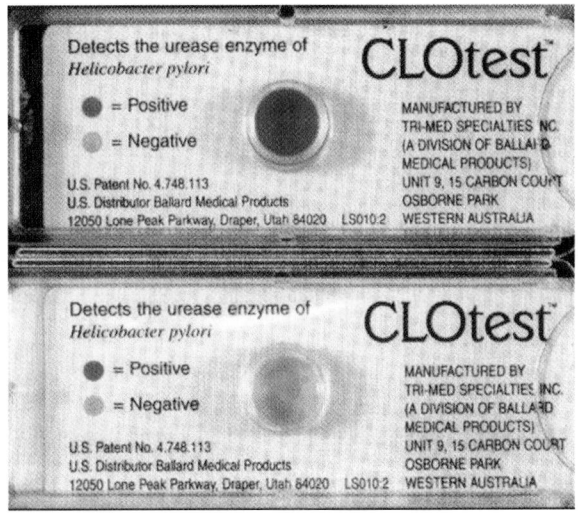

Fig. 4.30 Detection of *H. pylori* using a rapid urease test (CLOtest™). The gastric mucosal sample is placed within the 'well'. A colour change from yellow to red indicates the presence of *H. pylori* (CLOtest™ manufactured by Tri-med Specialties Inc.).

RECENT ADVANCES

A more recent development in diagnostic tools is the H. pylori faecal antigen enzyme immunoassay (HpSA). This test has greater than 90% sensitivity and specificity and may be useful to verify the result of eradication therapy.

Medical management

Initial triple therapy

First-line triple therapy for *H. pylori* eradication consists of a proton pump inhibitor with either clarithromycin and amoxicillin or clarithromycin and metronidazole. Although many combinations and treatment durations have been proposed, the most effective are the twice-daily dosing, 1-week duration regimens such as omeprazole 20 mg bd, amoxicillin 1 g bd and clarithromycin 500 mg bd.[1]

Initial eradication regimens progressively change due to failure rates associated with the development of antibiotic-resistant strains of *H. pylori*. Currently metronidazole-resistant strains are common and clarithromycin resistance is increasing. Dual therapy often fails to eradicate *H. pylori* and promotes emergence of resistant organisms.

Rescue therapy

Rescue therapy for failed initial eradication should consist of a different combination of antibiotics to that used for initial treatment, administered for 10–14 days. Selection of further antibiotic treatment should be based on anti-microbial susceptibilities from primary or secondary endoscopy biopsy culture results.

RECENT ADVANCES

Trials of vaccination against H. pylori are underway.

261

Prognosis

The therapeutic results of eradication therapy are considered separately under each disease heading below.

REFERENCE

(1) Ford A, Moayyedi P. *How can the current strategies for Helicobacter pylori eradication therapy be improved? Canadian Journal of Gastroenterology* 2003; 17 Suppl B: 36B–40B.

Peptic ulcer disease

Although a peptic ulcer is a lesion in the mucosa of the stomach or duodenum in which acid and pepsin play a major role, the term is often used to encompass any gastric or duodenal ulceration. This includes ulceration that may occur from drugs (NSAIDs) or excessive gastrin production (Zollinger–Ellison syndrome).

Epidemiology

Peptic ulcer disease is common: the prevalence of self-reported cases in an unselected cohort of 30-year-olds was 2290 per 100 000.[1] In patients with symptoms of dyspepsia, peptic ulceration is found in 5% on endoscopy.[2] It usually presents after the age of 15 and is equally common in both sexes.

Pathology

Although the term peptic ulceration suggests that the main aetiological factor is increased acid secretion, patients with peptic ulcer disease usually have normal acid secretion rates.

The currently most widely accepted aetiological agent is *H. pylori*. Approximately 95% of duodenal ulcers and 70% of gastric ulcers are associated with *H. pylori* (but only 15% of *H. pylori* colonized individuals will develop peptic ulcer disease). The odds of developing peptic ulceration are increased 2-fold in *H. pylori* positive patients. Peptic ulceration is also more common in patients on NSAIDs (36%) as compared to patients who are not on NSAIDs (8%) in clinical studies.[3] Weaker associations of peptic ulcer disease include smoking, alcohol, family history and blood group O.

Rare causes of peptic ulceration include hyperparathyroidism and Zollinger–Ellison syndrome, which results from a gastrinoma that usually arises from the G-cells in the pancreas, resulting in excess gastrin production and increased gastric acid secretion.

Scope of disease

Complications of peptic ulcer disease include dyspepsia, upper gastrointestinal haemorrhage (p. 237) and gastric or duodenal perforation. Chronic or recurrent ulceration may result in peptic strictures of the oesophagus or gastric outflow obstruction (pyloric stenosis).

Clinical features

Dyspepsia (recurrent upper abdominal pain) is the most common symptom. The pain may be related to meals and may occur at night. Associated symptoms include nausea and vomiting. Although attempts have been made to differentiate gastric from duodenal ulceration from the history, this has proved to be inaccurate and does not influence subsequent management.

Warning symptoms of significant disease or potential complications are dysphagia, weight loss and haematemesis. Patients with these symptoms or those who are over 35 years at initial presentation require urgent upper gastrointestinal endoscopy to screen for complications or malignancy (oesophageal, gastric).

Initial investigations
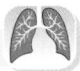

Screening for *H. pylori*
No investigations apart from screening for *H. pylori* colonization are required for young patients without any warning symptoms, as empirical treatment can commence on clinical diagnosis. Screening tests are detailed on page 261.

Further investigations
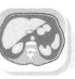

Upper gastrointestinal endoscopy
Upper gastrointestinal endoscopy (Fig. 4.31) is required for patients with warning symptoms and those over 35 years to screen for complications or oesophageal or gastric cancer.

Initial management

Risk factor modification
Ideally patients should stop taking NSAIDs, but often this may not be possible; alternatives include the concomitant long-term use of a proton pump inhibitor. General advice involves stopping smoking and reducing alcohol intake, but there is little evidence to support the efficacy of these recommendations.

H. pylori eradication
Triple therapy (p. 261) is recommended for all patients who are *H. pylori* positive. In patients with duodenal ulcers, eradication therapy was associated with a lower relative risk of persistent ulcer (0.66) compared to acid suppression alone, but no differences were found for patients with gastric ulcers (1.32), nor does eradication therapy prevent recurrences in patients with duodenal ulcers (compared to acid suppression alone).[4]

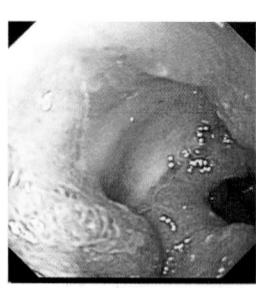

Fig. 4.31 Endoscopic view of an acute duodenal ulcer in the first part of the duodenum

Medical management

Proton pump inhibitors

A proton pump inhibitor is currently the standard treatment, and part of triple therapy. Thereafter, symptomatic patients, those with complicated peptic ulcer disease (presenting with bleeding, stricture or perforation) and those patients who require NSAIDs may still require long-term proton pump inhibitor therapy. Intermittent on-demand therapy is suitable for patients without complications for the control of symptoms.

Surgical management

Peptic ulcer surgery

Peptic ulcer surgery is now extremely rare for failed medical therapy due to the powerful acid suppression by proton pump inhibitors. Currently surgery is usually reserved for the development of complications such as perforation, severe bleeding and rarely stricture formation.

In patients with gastric or duodenal perforation, a primary oversew repair is usually performed on laparotomy. A pyloroplasty to increase the diameter of the gastric outlet may be performed for patients with pyloric stenosis due to peptic stricture. A longitudinal incision is performed through the pylorus and closed as a transverse defect. Alternatively, a gastroenterostomy may be performed to bypass the narrowed pylorus. Gastrectomy is rarely performed unless there is evidence of malignancy (p. 265).

Prognosis

Peptic ulcer disease is a chronic relapsing condition. Symptom control with proton pump inhibitor therapy is usually achieved in the vast majority. Up to 15% may suffer with upper gastrointestinal haemorrhage requiring hospital admission, and less than 5% will require surgical intervention.

REFERENCES

(1) *Ehlin AGC, Montgomery SM, Ekbom A, Pounder RE, Wakefield AJ. Prevalence of gastrointestinal diseases in two British national birth cohorts. Gut 2003; 52: 1117–1121.*

(2) *Thomson AB, Barkun AN, Armstrong D, et al. The prevalence of clinically significant endoscopic findings in primary care patients with uninvestigated dyspepsia: the Canadian Adult Dyspepsia Empiric Treatment - Prompt Endoscopy (CADET-PE) study. Alimentary Pharmacology and Therapeutics 2003; 17: 1481–1491.*

(3) *Huang J-Q, Sridhar S, Hunt RH. Role of Helicobacter pylori infection and non-steroidal anti-inflammatory drugs in peptic-ulcer disease: a meta-analysis. Lancet 2002; 359: 14–22.*

(4) *Ford AC, Delaney BC, Forman D, Moayyedi P. Eradication therapy in Helicobacter pylori positive peptic ulcer disease: systematic review and economic analysis. American Journal of Gastroenterology 2004; 99: 1833–1855.*

Gastritis

Gastritis is inflammation of the stomach. It is relatively common but is usually an endoscopic or histological diagnosis. The most common cause of antral gastritis is *H. pylori*; other injurious agents leading to gastritis include drugs (NSAIDs) and bile reflux. Gastritis and stress ulcerations can also result from any acute severe illness or occur after trauma/surgery. The usual clinical features are dyspepsia (recurrent upper abdominal pain) or upper gastrointestinal bleeding. Treatment should be directed to the underlying cause, and proton pump inhibitor therapy to suppress acid production is usually recommended.

Benign gastric tumours

Benign tumours of the stomach are rare and include gastric adenomas, leiomyomas and gastric polyps. The most common polyps are regenerative hyperplastic ones; these are seen with gastritis and increasingly with proton pump inhibitor therapy. Once the histological diagnosis is confirmed, these tumours do not require treatment unless symptoms develop, in which case surgical excision can be considered.

Malignant gastric tumours

The most important malignant tumour of the stomach is gastric carcinoma; others include lymphoma and rare smooth muscle tumours.

Gastric carcinoma

Epidemiology

Gastric carcinoma is the second most common cancer in the world. The incidence is highest in Japan, China, Eastern Asia and Eastern Europe, ranging between 36.3 and 77.8 per 100 000 in men and 16.8 and 33.3 per 100 000 in women, an approximate 2:1 male preponderance.[1] It is primarily a disease of the elderly, with a peak incidence at age 70–80.

Pathology

Approximately 90% of stomach cancers are adenocarcinomas (the remaining 10% are non-Hodgkin's lymphomas and leiomyosarcomas). Adenocarcinomas are subdivided histologically into intestinal and diffuse histological types (Lauren classification).[2] The intestinal variety arises from a background of chronic gastritis and is generally well circumscribed. The diffuse type usually arises within apparently normal gastric mucosa and tends to be poorly localized, infiltrating beneath the mucosa through the muscle of the stomach wall. In the advanced stage, this leads to a thickened and shrivelled stomach known as linitis plastica (leather bottle stomach). Unfortunately it is this type of disease that is often seen in the younger patient.

263

Risk factors for intestinal-type gastric carcinoma (those for the diffuse type are largely undefined) include smoking[3] and diet (in particular high consumption of preserved food and high salt intake);[4] there is a weak association with excess alcohol intake.[5] Other diseases associated with gastric carcinoma are pernicious anaemia, atrophic gastritis, gastric adenomatous polyps and *H. pylori* infection, an increasingly important risk factor associated with a 2-fold increase in risk of gastric cancer.[6]

Scope of disease

Local
In the early stages, when the disease is confined to the mucosa or submucosa, it may be either a prominent nodule or a depressed ulcer. Excavated cancers may cause upper gastrointestinal bleeding and anaemia, whilst large exophytic growths near the cardia can (rarely) produce dysphagia.

Metastatic
The majority of tumours present with local or with lymph node metastases. Spread may be lymphatic, haematogenous (to the liver, lungs and brain) or transcoelomic to the peritoneum, omentum or ovaries (Krukenberg tumour).

Paraneoplastic
Specific paraneoplastic manifestations of gastric carcinomas are uncommon.

Clinical features

A common presentation is that of new-onset dyspepsia in a middle-aged patient (over 45 years). Symptoms are often non-specific such as epigastric discomfort, post-prandial fullness, loss of appetite or vague indigestion. Other symptoms include dysphagia, nausea or vomiting (especially after eating), weight loss and those of iron deficiency anaemia.

Clinical examination is often unremarkable in early stage disease. In advanced disease, clinical findings may include an epigastric mass, hepatomegaly, lymphadenopathy, classically in the left supraclavicular fossa (Virchow's node, Troisier's sign), ascites and jaundice.

> ### ⚡ CLINICAL ALERT
> *Non-specific symptoms of gastric carcinoma often 'respond' to antacid therapy. It is important not to ignore initial complaints in the older patient.*

Initial investigations

Full blood count
Abnormalities on full blood count are usually non-specific. Occasionally anaemia can result from chronic blood loss or from chronic disease.

Liver profile
Raised liver enzymes may indicate liver metastasis, and raised alkaline phosphatase may result from bony metastasis.

Upper gastrointestinal endoscopy
A high index of suspicion is required in the older patient with new-onset dyspepsia, and the investigation of choice is an upper gastrointestinal endoscopy, which allows direct visualization of the stomach lining and facilitates biopsies for histological examination.

Barium swallow
Where facilities are not available for gastrointestinal endoscopy, a barium swallow (Fig. 4.32) may suggest gastric carcinoma if an ulcerated area or a narrowed distorted region is identified.

Further investigations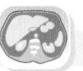

Having established the diagnosis, further investigation is needed to stage the disease and plan further management.

Staging CT abdomen
A CT scan of the abdomen is the main staging investigation, giving an indication of local extent and any intra-abdominal spread (Fig. 4.33).

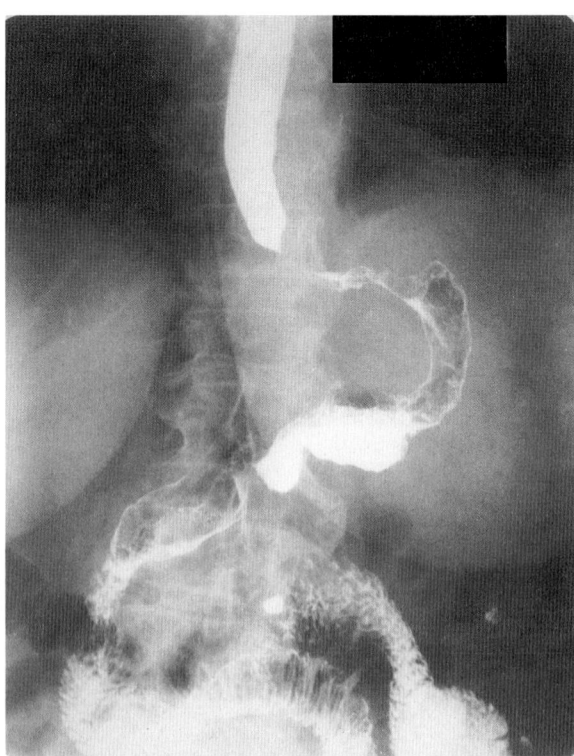

Fig. 4.32 Barium swallow of stomach cancer. Diffuse stomach cancer (linitis plastica) gives rise to the fixed contracted appearance.

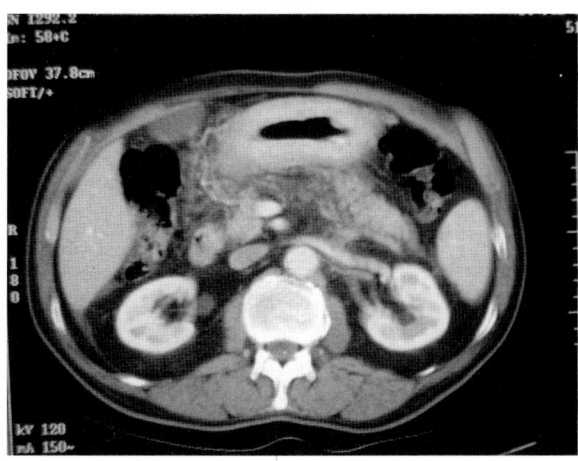

Fig. 4.33 CT of the abdomen showing the thickened wall of the stomach due to infiltrating tumour.

Staging laparoscopy

Prior to major surgery, most surgeons tend to perform a staging laparoscopy to screen for peritoneal metastasis or local fixity of the tumour, as these would preclude gastric resection.

RECENT ADVANCES

Endoluminal ultrasound is able to assess accurately the depth of tumour invasion and is gaining in popularity.

Initial management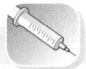

Surgery is the only curative management option for patients with gastric carcinoma. Prior to surgery, it is necessary to evaluate pulmonary function and any concomitant disease that may increase the risk of operative mortality.

The options for patients not suitable for curative surgery include palliative gastrectomy, gastric bypass procedures and chemotherapy.

RECENT ADVANCES

Japanese surgeons have defined an early gastric carcinoma as a lesion confined to the mucosa or submucosa, usually detected on screening upper gastrointestinal endoscopy, and are currently evaluating the results of endoscopic mucosal resection.[7]

Surgical management

Gastrectomy

The aims of curative surgery are to excise the lesion with adequate resection margins and to remove local and regional lymph nodes. In the majority of cases it is possible to perform the necessary resection through a midline laparotomy incision. Occasionally a left thoraco-abdominal incision may be required.

A *subtotal gastrectomy* is appropriate for well-circumscribed T2 tumours located away from the cardia. A *total gastrectomy* is required for tumours located in close proximity to the cardia and for infiltrative lesions (5 cm resection margins are required). In general, the first tier of draining lymph nodes is also excised (D1 resection) for curative resection.

The stomach is mobilized en bloc with the greater omentum and local lymph nodes. Proximally, the upper stomach is closed (usually with a linear stapler), or in a total gastrectomy the lower oesophagus is transected. The first part of the duodenum is stapled closed and usually over-sewn. Reconstruction is usually by a Roux loop or a Polya (Billroth II) gastroenterostomy.

Although widely advocated by Japanese surgeons, no survival benefit has been demonstrated with excision of the second tier of lymph nodes (D2 resection),[8] or prophylactic excision of the spleen and pancreas.[9]

Palliative surgery

For unresectable lesions of the antrum, gastric bypass surgery in the form of a gastro-enterostomy (i.e. stomach to intestine) may be more appropriate. Non-curative gastrectomy often provides the best form of palliation and is usually necessary in patients with bleeding or obstructive lesions.

Medical management

Chemotherapy

Adjuvant chemotherapy (after curative resection) is not established treatment. The impact of current regimens on survival is small (9% improvement at 3 years).[10] The adverse effects of chemotherapy, however, may be justified in patients with higher stage (T2 or N1) disease. The effects of neoadjuvant therapy (before surgery) are still under investigation.

Radiotherapy

Radiotherapy has a limited role in the treatment of gastric cancer. It is occasionally used to treat residual disease from unsuccessful surgery. Combination chemo-radiotherapy has been shown to improve median survival by 9 months, and may be considered in patients at high risk of recurrence.[11]

Palliative endoscopic therapy

For patients unfit for surgery, or those with unresectable disease, various endoscopic therapies are available. Local tissue coagulation with laser or argon plasma coagulation may be helpful to control symptoms of upper gastrointestinal bleeding. Expandable metal stents or intubation with a rigid prosthesis may be employed to relieve gastric outflow obstruction.

Prognosis

Gastric carcinoma has a poor prognosis, with an overall 5-year survival rate of around 5%. Results after surgery by stage are presented below.

TNM staging for gastric carcinoma

Primary tumour

T1   Tumour invades lamina propria or submucosa

T2   Tumour invades muscularis propria or subserosa

T3   Tumour invades serosa without adjacent structures

T4   Tumour invades adjacent structures

Regional lymph nodes

N0   No lymph node metastases

N1   Metastases in 1–6 regional lymph nodes

N2   Metastases in 7–15 regional lymph nodes

N3   Metastases in more than 15 regional lymph nodes

Distant metastases

M0   No distant metastases

M1   Distant metastases

Stage grouping		5-year survival*
Stage IA	T1, N0, M0	78%
Stage IB	T1, N1, M0	58%
	T2, N0, M0	
Stage II	T1, N2, M0	34%
	T2, N1, M0	
	T3, N0, M0	
Stage IIIA	T2, N2, M0	20%
	T3, N1, M0	
	T4, N0, M0	
Stage IIIB	T3, N2, M0	8%
Stage IV	T4, N1–3, M0	7%
	T1–3, N3, M0	
	Any T, any N, M1	

Post-surgery survival by stage, from Hundahl SA, Phillips JL, Menck HR. The National Cancer Data Base Report on poor survival of U.S. gastric carcinoma patients treated with gastrectomy, 5th edn. American Joint Committee on Cancer staging, proximal disease, and the "different disease" hypothesis. Cancer 2000; 88: 921–932.

FURTHER INFORMATION

Allum WH, Griffin SM, Watson A, Colin-Jones D. Guidelines for the management of oesophageal and gastric cancer. Gut 2002; 50 Suppl 5: v1–23.

REFERENCES

(1) *Parkin DM, Pisani P, Ferlay J. Global cancer statistics. CA: A Cancer Journal for Clinicians 1999; 49: 33–64.*
(2) *Lauren P. The two histological main types of gastric carcinoma: diffuse and so-called intestinal type carcinoma. Acta Pathologica et Microbiologica Scandinavica 1965; 64: 31–49.*

REFERENCES—cont'd

(3) *Gonzalez CA, Pera G, Agudo A, et al. Smoking and the risk of gastric cancer in the European Prospective Investigation Into Cancer and Nutrition (EPIC). International Journal of Cancer 2003; 107: 629–634.*
(4) *Tsugane S, Sasazuki S, Kobayashi M, Sasaki S. Salt and salted food intake and subsequent risk of gastric cancer among middle-aged Japanese men and women. British Journal of Cancer 2004;90:128–134.*
(5) *Sasazuki S, Sasaki S, Tsugane S. Cigarette smoking, alcohol consumption and subsequent gastric cancer risk by subsite and histologic type. International Journal of Cancer 2002; 101: 560–566.*
(6) *Eslick GD, Lim LL, Byles JE, Xia HH, Talley NJ. Association of Helicobacter pylori infection with gastric carcinoma: a meta-analysis. American Journal of Gastroenterology 1999; 94: 2373–2379.*
(7) *Ono H, Kondo H, Gotoda T, et al. Endoscopic mucosal resection for treatment of early gastric cancer. Gut 2001; 48: 225–229.*
(8) *Bonenkamp JJ, Hermans J, Sasako M, van de Velde CJ. Extended lymph-node dissection for gastric cancer. Dutch Gastric Cancer Group. New England Journal of Medicine 1999; 340: 908–914.*
(9) *Cuschieri A, Weeden S, Fielding J, et al. Patient survival after D1 and D2 resections for gastric cancer: long-term results of the MRC randomized surgical trial. Surgical Co-operative Group. British Journal of Cancer 1999; 79: 1522–1530.*
(10) *Earle CC, Maroun J, Zuraw L. Neoadjuvant or adjuvant therapy for resectable gastric cancer? A practice guideline. Canadian Journal of Surgery 2002; 45: 438–446.*
(11) *Macdonald JS, Smalley SR, Benedetti J, et al. Chemoradiotherapy after surgery compared with surgery alone for adenocarcinoma of the stomach or gastroesophageal junction. New England Journal of Medicine 2001; 345: 725–730.*

Gastric lymphoma

Although gastric lymphoma is much less common than gastric carcinoma, the stomach is the most common site of extranodal lymphoma. Primary gastric lymphoma arises from the mucosa-associated lymphoid tissue (MALT), and *H. pylori* has been implicated in the pathogenesis. The clinical presentation is similar to that of gastric cancer, the predominant symptoms including dyspepsia, nausea and vomiting, anorexia, weight loss and occasionally diarrhoea. Some tumours present acutely with bleeding or perforation. Treatment usually involves surgery (a major determinant of improved prognosis) followed by chemotherapy or radiotherapy. Unresectable disease is treated with chemoradiotherapy. The prognosis is much better than for gastric cancer.

Gastro intestinal stromal tumours

Gastro intestinal stromal tumours (GIST) are most common in the stomach and until recently could only be treated by surgical resection. They usually present with haemorrhage due to ulceration, and are treated by partial or total gastrectomy. A targeted drug to the c-kit oncogene activated in GIST now allows treatment of advanced or recurrent disease and has improved prognosis.

Diseases of the small intestine and appendix

Coeliac disease

Coeliac disease or gluten-sensitive enteropathy is a state of heightened immunological responsiveness to ingested gluten in genetically susceptible individuals.

Epidemiology

Coeliac disease is a disease of Europe and occurs in populations of European migration (America, Australia). The prevalence varies by location and stage of diagnosis (symptomatic disease, asymptomatic seropositive disease and genetic predisposition), a concept known as the coeliac iceberg (Fig. 4.34). In the UK, the prevalence of endomysial antibody positive patients is 1200 per 100 000 (1.2%).[1] Coeliac disease is twice as common in females, and presentation in adulthood (typically the fourth to sixth decade) is now more common than in childhood.[2]

Pathology

There is a strong genetic component to coeliac disease: almost all patients are either HLA DQ2 or DQ8 positive (Fig. 4.34), and 15% of first-degree relatives may be affected (Table 4.12).

Gluten is a high molecular weight heterogeneous compound found in the endosperm (white flour portion) of wheat, rye and barley. In patients with coeliac disease, the ingestion of gluten results in an immunological response and causes small bowel inflammation. Raised antibody titres in untreated coeliac disease include gliadin, reticulin, endomysium and tissue transglutaminase.

The histological features of coeliac disease are classified in concordance with the revised Marsh criteria (Table 4.13) and tend to be more severe in the duodenum and jejunum, possibly due to greater proximal gluten load.

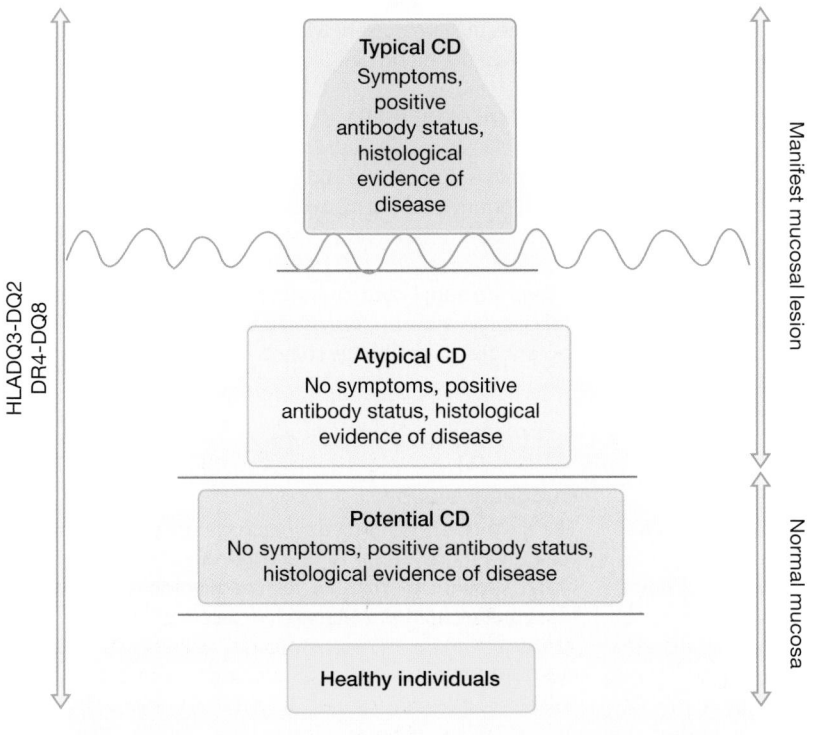

Fig. 4.34 The coeliac iceberg. Patients with typical or atypical coeliac disease have histological evidence of villous atrophy. Individuals with *potential* coeliac disease have positive antibody status but normal histology.

Table 4.12	Conditions associated with coeliac disease*

Associated diseases	Prevalence of coeliac disease
Family history (first-degree relative)	5–15%
Type 1 diabetes	3–5%
Autoimmune thyroid disease	3–8%
Selective IgA deficiency	2–5%
Irritable bowel syndrome	3–5%
Primary biliary cirrhosis	3%
Cryptogenic hypertransaminasaemia (deranged liver function, particularly AST and ALT)	9%
Idiopathic peripheral neuropathy or ataxia	6–9%
Female infertility	3%
Osteoporosis	3%

*Other diseases have also been reported, for example epilepsy (with cerebral calcification), rheumatoid disease and Sjögren's syndrome, but these associations are less well described.

Table 4.13	Revised Marsh criteria*

Marsh I

A Marsh I lesion comprises of normal mucosal architecture in which the villous epithelium is markedly infiltrated by lymphocytes. The lymphocytosis score is greater than 30 lymphocytes per 100 enterocytes

Marsh II

Marsh II is a hyperplastic lesion (with crypt hyperplasia)

Marsh III

Marsh III is subdivided into grades:

a. partial villous atrophy (PVA)

b. subtotal villous atrophy (SVA)

c. total villous atrophy (TVA)

* The revised Marsh criteria describe the progressive histopathological features due to coeliac disease.

Scope of disease

Patients with unrecognized coeliac disease can have nutritional deficiencies of iron (iron deficiency anaemia), vitamin B_{12} or folate. Up to 60% may have reduced bone mineral density (osteoporosis or osteopenia) due to inadequate calcium absorption. Most complications are avoidable or reversible on a gluten-free diet.

Patients with coeliac disease have a higher risk of gastrointestinal malignancy (small bowel lymphoma). There is also an association with splenic aplasia and other autoimmune diseases (Table 4.12).

Clinical features

Patients with coeliac disease may be asymptomatic (silent) or present with atypical symptoms (atypical form). The median delay from the onset of symptoms to diagnosis is approximately 5 years.[2]

The classic symptoms of coeliac disease occur soon after the introduction of wheat cereals into infant feed. Children present with soft, clay-coloured, bulky and offensive stool, resulting from steatorrhoea. Malabsorption results in failure to thrive, anorexia and muscle wasting. Diarrhoea and abdominal pain occasionally occur.

In adults, the mode of presentation is varied with non-specific symptoms of diarrhoea, abdominal pain, bloating, nausea and vomiting. Alternative presentations relate to the complications of glossitis, anaemia, osteoporosis, bleeding diathesis (vitamin K deficiency), weight loss and dermatitis herpetiformis.

On examination, patients may be of short stature from chronic malnutrition. Anaemia may be evident, as may koilonychia from iron deficiency. There may be stomatitis and a blistering pruritic symmetrical skin rash on the elbows, knees, scalp, face, neck and sacral areas (dermatitis herpetiformis). Abdominal examination may reveal ascites from hypoproteinaemia.

Initial investigations

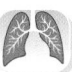

The most important investigational aspect of coeliac disease is a high index of suspicion.

Full blood count and blood film

Anaemia may be present with target cells and Howell–Jolly bodies on the blood film.

Serological markers

The profile of antibodies requested consists of endomysial, tissue transglutaminase and antigliadin antibodies (IgG and IgA). Endomysial and tissue transglutaminase are specific investigations, however IgA and IgG antigliadin antibodies are more sensitive in less severe disease (partial or subtotal villous atrophy) and in patients with concurrent IgA deficiency (where endomysial, tissue transglutaminase and IgG antigliadin antibodies may be negative).

Further investigations

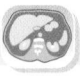

Duodenal biopsy

The diagnosis is confirmed by performing gastroscopy and duodenal biopsy. Prior to undertaking a duodenal biopsy, blood should be screened for coagulation abnormalities that could result from vitamin K deficiency.

Haematinic studies

Further studies for iron, B_{12} and red cell folate levels will be required in patients with anaemia to characterize the aetiology. Bone marrow aspiration may be required in selected patients with megaloblastic anaemia.

DEXA scan

A bone mineral density scan is required to screen for osteopenia in patients with confirmed disease.

Screening for gastrointestinal lymphoma

Patients with persistent symptoms despite compliance with a gluten-free diet should be screened for small bowel lymphoma using enteroscopy (deeper endoscopic viewing of the small bowel), and gastrointestinal video capsule endoscopy.

Initial management

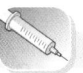

Education

Patients should be educated about their disease and encouraged to join national support groups for information and advice such as Coeliac UK (www.coeliac.co.uk) and Celiac.com (www.celiac.com). They should also be counselled about the possible complications and the risk of coeliac disease in their first-degree relatives

Diet

The cornerstone of management for coeliac disease is a gluten-free diet, and referral to a dietician is mandatory. The removal of gluten from the diet may result in complete resolution of symptoms, improvement of nutritional deficiencies and avoidance of complications. Duodenal biopsies may be repeated 3–6 months after commencement on a gluten-free diet to assess for evidence of histological improvement.

Nutritional supplementation

Dietary supplementation is required for iron and folate deficient patients. Regular B_{12} injections may be required for B_{12} deficiency, although serum levels often improve with a gluten-free diet. Calcium supplementation is required for patients with osteopenia, especially postmenopausal women.

Pneumococcal vaccination

Pneumococcal vaccination is recommended due to the association of coeliac disease with splenic atrophy, although the benefit remains to be proven.

> **RECENT ADVANCES**
>
> *A new concept of gluten sensitivity is emerging. Patients who do not have histological changes of coeliac disease but have a positive antibody result may be classified as potential coeliac disease. Long-term follow-up (with repeat antibody testing and duodenal biopsy) will determine whether they develop typical coeliac disease.*

Medical management

Immunosuppression

In general, long-term steroids are not indicated unless there is persistent severe hypoalbuminaemia to regain control of a protein-losing enteropathic state. Corticosteroids are usually reserved for the treatment of coeliac crisis, characterized by severe malabsorption (diarrhoea, weight loss, ascites and hypoproteinaemia). This condition is now rarely seen as antibody testing means that patients are often recognized at an earlier stage in the disease process. The management of refractory coeliac disease (without lymphoma) may require both corticosteroids and other immunosuppressants (azathioprine and anti-TNF antibody).

Surgical management

The role of surgery is limited and confined to refractory coeliac disease with lymphomatous change or when overt lymphoma develops, when surgical resection may be required.

Prognosis

The mortality of patients with coeliac disease is modestly increased compared to controls, with an overall hazard ratio for death of 1.17.[3] The risk of gastrointestinal and haematological malignancies is also increased (gastrointestinal lymphoma occurs in approximately 6% and manifests in the sixth decade).

Symptom control is generally good as long as patients are compliant and adhere to a gluten-free diet. The less compliance with a gluten-free diet, the greater is the likelihood of the development of complications.

Screening

There is no accepted screening programme for coeliac disease. There is currently controversy on whether population screening should be provided, given that the prevalence may be as high as 1%.

ℹ FURTHER INFORMATION

Ciclitira PJ, King AL, Fraser JS. AGA technical review on celiac sprue. American Gastroenterological Association. Gastroenterology 2001; 120: 1526–1540.

Scott EM, Gaywood I, Scott BB. (British Society of Gastroenterology) Guidelines for osteoporosis in coeliac disease and inflammatory bowel disease. Gut 2000; 46(suppl I): i1–i8.

REFERENCES

(1) *West J, Logan RFA, Hill PG, et al. Seroprevalence, correlates, and characteristics of undetected coeliac disease in England. Gut 2003; 52: 960–965.*
(2) *Sanders DS, Hurlstone DP, Stokes RO, Rashid F, Milford-Ward A, Hadjivassiliou M, Lobo AJ. Changing face of adult coeliac disease: experience of a single university hospital in South Yorkshire. Postgraduate Medical Journal 2002; 78: 31–33.*
(3) *West J, Logan RFA, Smith CJ, Hubbard RB, Card TR. Malignancy and mortality in people with coeliac disease: population based cohort study. BMJ 2004; 329: 716–719.*

Acute appendicitis

Acute appendicitis is inflammation of the vermiform appendix, an important surgical condition that should be easily recognized and treated in the majority of cases.

Epidemiology

Appendicitis is the most common surgical emergency in the developed world. The incidence has been estimated at 86 per 100 000 per year, with a peak in the age group 13–40 years; it is equally common in both sexes.[1] It is rare in the elderly and in children under 2 years.

Pathology

Acute appendicitis is thought to arise as a result of a faecolith obstructing the appendicular lumen, causing secondary infection in the appendix. However, this is not always the case and luminal obstruction is not invariably present. In some cases, it may be due to viral infection, causing lymphoid hyperplasia, mucosal ulceration and consequent bacterial invasion.

Infection is almost invariably of mixed origin, with both anaerobes (*Bacteroides, Clostridia*) and Gram-negative aerobes (*E. coli, E. faecalis*).

Scope of disease

Complications of acute appendicitis include perforation leading to peritonitis, intra-abdominal, pelvic or liver abscess formation, peritoneal adhesions and portal pyaemia (pylephlebitis). Intra-abdominal adhesions may lead to small bowel obstruction in later life and sterility due to blocked fallopian tubes in women.

Clinical features

The classical history is initial central colicky abdominal pain (visceral pain from the foregut), followed by nausea and vomiting then localized pain in the right iliac fossa several hours later (irritation of the parietal peritoneum). Anorexia and general malaise are usually present.

It is the position of the appendix that dictates the subsequent localization of pain. The most common caecal position gives rise to right iliac fossa pain; a retrocaecal appendix may not present with pain localizing to the right iliac fossa, but pain on extension of the hip due to irritation of the iliopsoas muscle; and a pelvic appendix may present with dysuria or diarrhoea due to irritation of the bladder and rectum respectively.

On examination, the patient may appear flushed and mildly pyrexial (classically around 37.5°C) with a tachycardia. The tongue is often furred and the patient may have a distinctive breath odour. Abdominal examination reveals tenderness with guarding and rebound tenderness, maximal over McBurney's point (one third the way along a line from the anterior superior iliac spine to the umbilicus) when the appendix is in the caecal position.

If the appendix has perforated, more generalized peritonitis may be present. If the patient presents late, then an appendix mass (abscess) may be palpable. Digital rectal examination often reveals right-sided tenderness, particularly if the inflamed appendix lies in the pelvis.

The differential diagnosis of acute appendicitis is provided in Table 4.14.

Initial investigation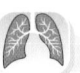

Screening investigations are usually performed as part of the diagnostic workup for an acute abdomen (p. 230–231).

Full blood count
A full blood count almost invariably reveals a raised white cell count, usually a neutrophil leukocytosis.

Urea and electrolytes
Urea and electrolytes are performed routinely to screen for evidence of severe dehydration (raised urea, occasionally raised creatinine) and to assess renal function prior to proposed surgery.

Further investigations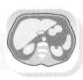

Further investigation is often unnecessary, as the diagnosis is usually straightforward.

Abdominal ultrasound
When the clinical picture is obscured by the possibility of concomitant pelvic pathology, an abdominal ultrasound scan is the investigation of choice. It is usually sufficient to rule out any other pelvic pathology and may occasionally be able to visualize a thickened appendix (suggestive of inflammation).

Initial management

Fluid resuscitation
Patients are normally kept nil by mouth until a decision for theatre is undertaken. Meanwhile, appropriate fluids should

Table 4.14	Differential diagnosis of acute appendicitis
Mesenteric lymphadenitis (especially in children)	
Urinary tract infection	
Pelvic inflammatory disease	
Ruptured ovarian cyst	
Ectopic pregnancy	
Crohn's disease	
Meckel's diverticulitis	
Acute cholecystitis	
Perforated duodenal ulcer	
Diverticulitis (right-sided)	
Acute non-specific abdominal pain	

be administered to replace losses in dehydrated patients, and for maintenance therapy.

Antibiotics

Antibiotic therapy reduces postoperative infection, the development of intra-abdominal abscesses and length of hospital stay.[2] Intravenous antibiotics (cefuroxime and metronidazole are a popular choice) should be administered routinely.

Surgical management

Once the diagnosis has been made, the patient should be taken to theatre as soon as possible. Intravenous antibiotics are usually given at induction of anaesthesia and may be continued postoperatively in cases of perforation.

Appendicectomy

The operation is usually performed through a Lanz incision in the right iliac fossa using a muscle-splitting ('grid-iron') approach. The caecum is found and the inflamed appendix is delivered into the wound and excised. Laparoscopy should be performed in women of child bearing age to confirm the diagnosis.

RECENT ADVANCES

Laparoscopic appendicectomy is a technique that is gaining in popularity. Although wound infection is decreased by half, intra-abdominal abscesses increase by a factor of 2.7. Return to normal activities was 6 days faster than with conventional surgery. Overall this procedure adds substantially to cost.[3]

Medical management

Antibiotic therapy

Conservative management is reserved for patients who present late with an appendix mass. Intravenous fluids, antibiotic therapy and regular clinical observations are undertaken. However, if the patient's condition deteriorates, urgent surgery will be required. Radiological drainage of an abscess is an option for patients with poor operative risk, and an interval appendicectomy may be performed a few months later.

Prognosis

Providing the diagnosis is made early and the patient is treated appropriately, the outcome following acute appendicitis is complete recovery. It is usually only where an incorrect or late diagnosis has been made or when the appendix has perforated that any long-term sequelae such as adhesions and infertility occur.

REFERENCES

(1) *Korner H, Sondenaa K, Soreide JA, Andersen E, Nysted A, Lende TH, Kjellevold KH. Incidence of acute nonperforated and perforated appendicitis: age-specific and sex-specific analysis. World Journal of Surgery 1997; 21: 313–317.*
(2) *Andersen BR, Kallehave FL, Andersen HK. Antibiotics versus placebo for prevention of postoperative infection after appendicectomy. Cochrane Database of Systematic Reviews 2003: CD001439.*
(3) *Sauerland S, Lefering R, Neugebauer EA. Laparoscopic versus open surgery for suspected appendicitis. Cochrane Database of Systematic Reviews 2002: CD001546.*

Benign intestinal tumours

Epidemiology

Small intestinal tumours are uncommon, accounting for less than 5% of all gastrointestinal tumours.

Pathology

Benign adenomas are seen as part of various familial polyposis syndromes, such as Familial Polyposis Coli (FAP), Peutz Jeugher's syndrome and Turcot's syndrome (familial polyposis and brain tumours).

Clinical features

The majority are symptomatic; occasionally tumours may present with bleeding (anaemia) or intussusception.

Investigations

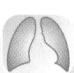

As these tumours are rare, the diagnosis is rarely suspected from the history and examination.

Small bowel contrast study

The small bowel is difficult to visualize endoscopically and so a barium meal or small bowel enema is usually the investigation of choice.

CT abdomen

If a mass lesion is present, CT of the abdomen is useful to diagnose and stage the extent of disease.

RECENT ADVANCES

Visualization of the small bowel has recently been made much easier with the development of an endoscopic capsule, which is swallowed by the patient and then passes through the whole gastrointestinal tract, allowing direct visualization of the small bowel mucosa (p. 234).

Management

Small bowel resection

The mainstay of treatment is surgery for patients with symptomatic disease.

Prognosis

Patients with benign small bowel tumours have a good prognosis and may remain asymptomatic for long periods.

Malignant intestinal tumours

Epidemiology

Malignant small intestinal tumours are uncommon and tend to occur in patients over 40 years.

Pathology

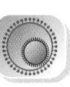

Lymphoma is the most common primary malignancy of the small bowel. It originates from mucosa-associated lymphoid tissue (MALT). Carcinoid tumours are of intermediate malignancy, originating from enterochromaffin cells. These neuroendocrine tumours may secrete serotonin (5-HT) and other hormones. Adenocarcinoma of the small bowel is rare.

Clinical features

Malignant tumours tend to present late, often with obstruction (p. 248). Patients with hormone-producing carcinoid tumours that have metastasized to the liver may experience a combination of symptoms of carcinoid syndrome: flushing, colicky abdominal pain, diarrhoea, bronchospasm, skin rashes and right-sided heart valve lesions.

Investigations

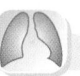

Investigations are similar to those for benign small intestinal tumours (p. 249).

24-Hour urinary 5-hydroxyindoleacetic acid

Elevated levels of urinary 5-HIAA are suggestive of carcinoid syndrome.

Management

Small bowel resection

Small bowel resection is the mainstay of treatment. Adjuvant chemotherapy or radiotherapy is required for lymphoma after surgical resection, and may also be administered as primary treatment for inoperable disease.

Octreotide

Patients with symptoms of carcinoid symptoms are best treated with this long-acting somatostatin analogue.

> **RECENT ADVANCES**
>
> *Recent trials have suggested that the addition of interferon-alpha to octreotide may retard tumour growth in patients with inoperable midgut carcinoid tumours.[1]*

Prognosis

In general, the prognosis of patients with malignant tumours is poor. Midgut carcinoid tumours, however, are slow-growing tumours with a 5-year survival of 77%.[2]

REFERENCES

(1) *Kolby L, Persson G, Franzen S, Ahren B. Randomized clinical trial of the effect of interferon alpha on survival in patients with disseminated midgut carcinoid tumours. British Journal of Surgery 2003; 90: 687–693.*
(2) *Sjoblom SM. Clinical presentation and prognosis of gastrointestinal carcinoid tumours. Scandinavian Journal of Gastroenterology 1988; 23: 779–787.*

SECTION 4.9 Inflammatory bowel disease

Ulcerative colitis and Crohn's disease are the two major forms of chronic idiopathic inflammatory bowel disease. Approximately 5% of patients with colonic disease have features of both conditions and remain unclassifiable (indeterminate colitis).

The precise aetiology of inflammatory bowel disease is unknown. Currently it is thought that normal bowel functions with a degree of 'physiological inflammation', and that inflammatory bowel disease results from uncontrolled persistent activation of the mucosal immune system by normal gut flora.

The contribution of genetic factors is suggested by the different prevalence among different populations (higher in Ashkenazi Jews) and the increased risk in first-degree relatives. A number of candidate genes have been proposed, but none has been sufficiently specific for clinical application.

Table 4.15   Comparison of ulcerative colitis and Crohn's disease

	Ulcerative colitis	Crohn's diseas
Clinical features		
Pyrexia	Common	Common
Abdominal pain	Common	Common
Diarrhoea	Common	Common
Rectal bleeding	Common	Common
Gastrointestinal disease		
Perianal disease	None	Common
Colon	Common	Common
Ileum	Rare (backwash ileitis)	Common
Jejunum	None	Uncommon
Duodenum	None	Uncommon
Stomach	None	Uncommon
Oesophagus	None	Uncommon
Aphthous mouth ulcerations	Occurs	Common
Extraintestinal disease		
Erythema nodosum	Occurs	Occurs
Pyoderma gangrenosum	Occurs	Occurs
Clubbing	Occurs	Occurs
Seronegative arthritis	Occurs	Occurs
Sacroiliitis	Occurs	Occurs
Uveitis	Occurs	Occurs
Episcleritis	Occurs	Occurs
Obstructive uropathy	None	Uncommon
Renal calculi	Uncommon	Uncommon
Pulmonary fibrosis	Rare	Rare
Bronchiectasis	Rare	Rare
Amyloidosis	Rare	Uncommon
Cirrhosis	Rare	Rare
Sclerosing cholangitis	Occurs	Occurs
Endoscopic features		
Friable mucosa	Occurs	Common
Cobblestone appearance	None	Common
Linear ulceration	Occurs	Common
Pseudopolyps	Common	Rare
Radiological features		
Distribution	Continuous	Segmented
Ulceration	Fine, superficial	Deep
Fissures	None	Common
Fistula	None	Common
Pathological features		
Inflammation	Superficial and continuous	Transmural with skip lesions
Granuloma	Rare	Common
Goblet cell mucus depletion	Common	Absent
Crypt abscesses	Common	Uncommon

Crohn's disease

Ulcerative colitis

273

The concordance in identical twins has been reported to be only 45%, suggesting a significant environmental contribution. It is possible that the genetically determined variations in mucosal function reflect different susceptibility to the disease, caused by mucosal activation from gut bacteria and persistent amplified inflammation resulting from cytokine-mediated self-reinforcing activation of select T-helper subtypes, macrophages and other antigen-presenting cells.[1]

The diagnosis and differentiation of ulcerative colitis from Crohn's disease depend on clinical, radiological, endoscopic and pathological criteria (Table 4.15).

REFERENCE

(1) *Podolsky DK. Inflammatory bowel disease. New England Journal of Medicine 2002; 347: 417–429.*

Crohn's disease

Crohn's disease is a systemic disorder with predominant gastrointestinal involvement characterized by patchy, transmural inflammation, which may affect any part of the gastrointestinal tract from 'mouth to anus'.

Epidemiology

The incidence of Crohn's disease varies with geographical location. It is common in Europe and North America with an incidence of approximately 5–10 per 100 000 per year and a prevalence of 50–100 per 100 000.[1] It is uncommon in Asia, Africa and South America. The disease can arise at any age but tends to present in the second to fourth decades and equally in both sexes. In contrast to the stable incidence of ulcerative colitis, the incidence of Crohn's disease is rising.

Pathology

The characteristic feature of Crohn's disease is sharply delimited transmural inflammation of the bowel. Although any part of the gastrointestinal tract may be involved, in the majority the disease is located in the terminal ileum and colon.

The disease process may be described by location (terminal ileal, colonic, ileocolic, upper gastrointestinal), or by pattern of disease (inflammatory, fistulating, or stricturing).

Scope of disease

Intestinal

Complications of Crohn's disease include the formation of strictures (bowel obstruction), fistulae (from bowel to perineal skin, bladder, vagina or another segment of bowel) and intra-abdominal abscesses (abdominal mass, peritonitis). There is an increased risk of colorectal cancer.

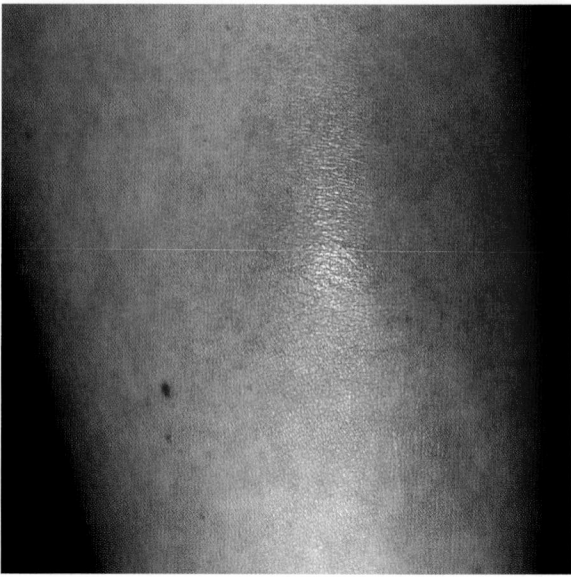

Fig. 4.35 Erythema nodosum.

Extraintestinal

Extraintestinal manifestations include non-erosive arthritis of large joints, ankylosing spondylitis, erythema nodosum (Fig. 4.35), pyoderma gangrenosum (Fig. 4.36), iritis, primary sclerosing cholangitis and chronic active hepatitis.

Clinical features

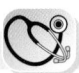

Symptoms of Crohn's disease are varied but typically include abdominal pain, diarrhoea and weight loss. Other systemic symptoms are malaise, anorexia and fever. Patients may also present with perianal abscess due to fistula formation and intestinal obstruction (p. 292) due to stricture formation.

On examination there may be tachycardia, pyrexia, anaemia, evidence of dehydration due to fluid depletion, abdominal tenderness or palpable masses. Examination of the mouth may reveal aphthous ulceration (Fig. 4.37) and perineal examination may reveal an abscess due to fistula formation.

Initial investigations

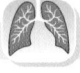

Full blood count

Anaemia may be present, and a raised white count or platelet count may indicate active disease.

Markers of inflammation

Erythrocyte sedimentation rate (ESR) and C-reactive protein (CRP) are usually elevated in active disease and may be used to monitor clinical progression in the acute phase.

Urea and electrolytes

Urea may be elevated with dehydration, and if sufficiently severe may lead to renal impairment.

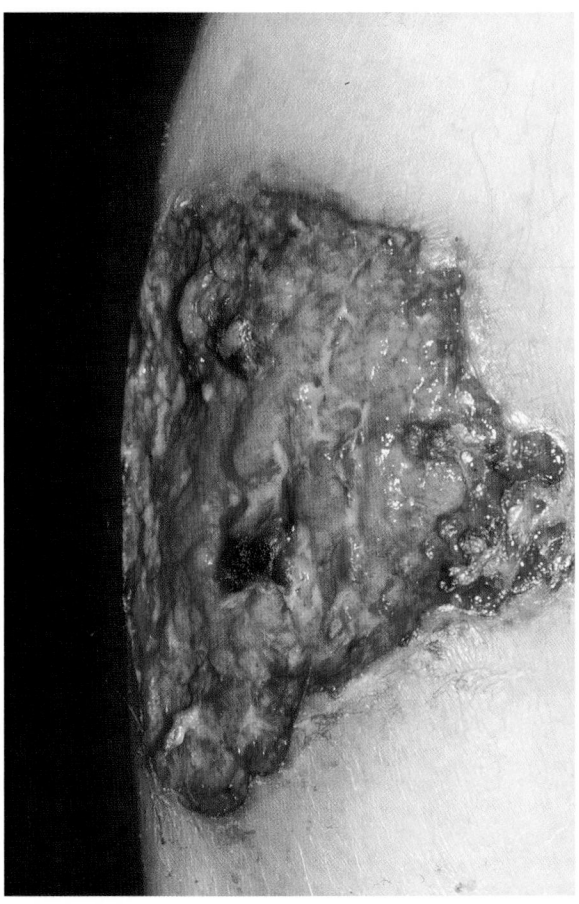

Fig. 4.36 Pyoderma gangrenosum.

Liver profile
Low serum albumin is a marker of poor nutritional status and suggests active disease.

Stool culture
Stool cultures are required to exclude infectious diarrhoea such as *Clostridium difficile*.

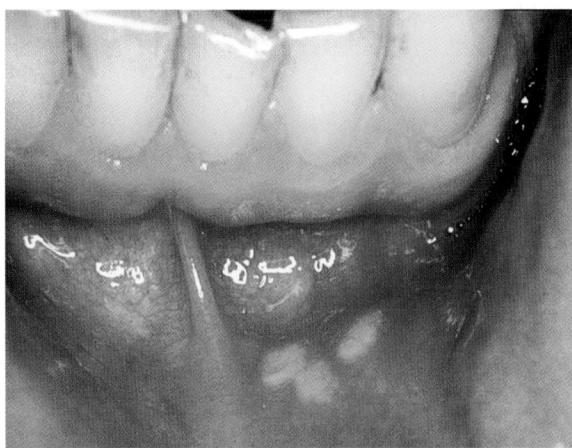

Fig. 4.37 Aphthous ulceration with Crohn's disease

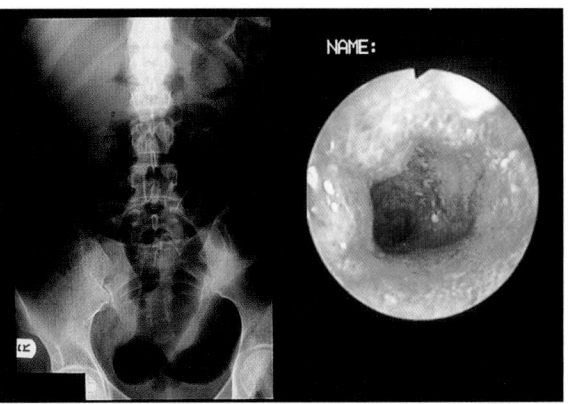

Fig. 4.38 Plain abdominal film and endoscopic view of Crohn's disease.

Abdominal film
A plain abdominal film may reveal a right-sided abdominal mass or visible small bowel loops.

Rigid sigmoidoscopy
Macroscopic features of inflammatory bowel disease may include inflamed, ulcerated and friable mucosa (Fig. 4.38). It is not possible to differentiate between ulcerative colitis and Crohn's disease on inspection and a rectal biopsy from the lower aspect of posterior wall of rectum may reveal microscopic changes even in the absence of macroscopic disease.

Further investigations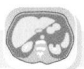

In Crohn's disease, assessment of disease severity is more difficult as gastrointestinal disease can occur from mouth to anus.

Colonoscopy
In general, a colonoscopy with visualization of the terminal ileum is performed with biopsies of the terminal ileum.

Small bowel follow-through
Small bowel barium studies are performed to screen for ulcerations (cobblestone appearance), strictures (string sign), inflammatory masses and fistulae.

Initial management

Fluid and electrolyte replacement
Intravenous fluid and electrolyte replacement is required to correct or prevent dehydration and electrolyte imbalance.

Blood transfusion
Blood transfusion is required to maintain a haemoglobin concentration of at least 10 g/dL.

Nutritional support
An elemental or polymeric diet may result in remission of disease, although this is less effective than corticosteroids.

Crohn's disease

Ulcerative colitis

275

Parenteral feeding is required for patients with fistulating disease or malabsorption and malnutrition from extensive disease.

Thromboprophylaxis

Subcutaneous heparin is required to reduce the risk of thromboembolism for patients admitted to hospital.

Smoking cessation

Patients who are smokers should be advised to stop.

Medical management

Therapeutic decisions depend on disease activity, site and extent. Disease activity should be evaluated objectively using the Crohn's disease activity index (CDAI; Table 4.16). Patients with severe disease will require hospital admission, whilst those with mild to moderate disease may be managed as outpatients.

Aminosalicylates

High-dose oral aminosalicylates (e.g. mesalazine) may be sufficient to induce remission in patients with mild ileo-colonic involvement. However, the evidence for long-term use of aminosalicylates in Crohn's is much less convincing than for ulcerative colitis, and the aminosalicylates do not have an important role in maintenance of remission.

Table 4.16	Crohn's disease activity index*						
				Day			
	1	2	3	4	5	6	7
Soft/liquid stools							
Abdominal pain							
(0 = none, 1 = mild, 2 = moderate, 3 = severe)							
Well being							
(0 = well, 1 = unwell, 2 = poor, 3 = very poor, 4 = terrible)							
Arthritis/arthralgia (Y/N)							
Iritis/uveitis (Y/N)							
EN/PG/aphthous stomatitis (Y/N)							
Anal fissure/fistula/abscess (Y/N)							
Other fistula (Y/N)							
Fever >37.8 C in last week (Y/N)							
Loperamide for diarrhoea (Y/N)							
Abdominal mass (Yes/Possible/No)							
Haematocrit							
Weight (kg)							

* Best WR, Bectel JM, Singleton JW, Kern F. Development of the Crohn's disease activity index. Gastroenterology 1976; 70: 439–444.

Corticosteroids

Prednisolone 40 mg should be added to mesalazine in patients with moderate to severe disease and weaned according to severity and patient response over 8 weeks. If oral intake is not possible, intravenous corticosteroids can be administered. Topical steroids may be given to patients with oral Crohn's disease. Long-term corticosteroids do not appear to be effective in the maintenance of remission.

Other immunosuppressants

Azathioprine or mercaptopurine can be used as adjunctive therapy or as alternative immunosuppressants to maintain remission in patients whose disease flares up on the reduction or withdrawal of steroids (chronic active steroid-dependent disease). Low-dose weekly methotrexate is an alternative for those who cannot tolerate or fail to respond to azathioprine or mercaptopurine.

Antibiotics

Metronidazole or ciprofloxacin is reserved for patients with simple perianal fistulae.

RECENT ADVANCES

Infliximab, an anti-tumour necrosis factor (TNF) monoclonal antibody, has potent anti-inflammatory effects. By 12 weeks, 41% of patients treated with infliximab compared with 12% of untreated patients have been reported to achieve disease remission.[2]

Surgical management

The indications for surgery in patients with Crohn's disease are failure of medical therapy or the onset of complications (small bowel obstruction, fistulae, abscess formation, fulminating colitis, severe haemorrhage, carcinoma of the colon).

Bowel resection

Prior to making an incision, a site for a potential stoma is selected and marked. A midline incision is usually performed and localized resection of the affected bowel is undertaken. In severe cases of Crohn's colitis, a total colectomy may be required with the construction of an ileostomy. In elective cases of Crohn's colitis an ileo-anal anastomosis can be considered if there is minimal rectal and perianal disease.

Stricturoplasty

For patients with multiple strictures and inactive disease, multiple stricturoplasties can be performed to widen the lumen of the bowel without having to resort to bowel resection.

Incision and drainage of peri-anal abscesses

The management of peri-anal abscesses and fistulae is detailed on pages 292 and 291 respectively. In very severe cases, a colonic resection may be required with the construction of an ileostomy to divert the faecal flow.

Prognosis

The overall mortality of Crohn's disease is slightly higher than the normal population and is greatest in the 2 years after diagnosis or in those with upper gastrointestinal disease. The clinical course of Crohn's disease is characterized by exacerbations and remission. Approximately 75% of patients are capable of work in the year after diagnosis, and 15% of patients are unable to work after 5–10 years.

Surgery is not curative and management is directed to minimizing the impact of disease. At least 50% of patients require surgical treatment in the first 10 years of disease and approximately 70–80% will ultimately require surgery.

---

i **FURTHER INFORMATION**

Carter MJ, Lobo AJ, Travis SPL. Guidelines for the management of inflammatory bowel disease in adults. Gut 2004; 53: v1–16.

REFERENCES

(1) *Carter MJ, Lobo AJ, Travis SPL. Guidelines for the management of inflammatory bowel disease in adults. Gut 2004; 53: v1–16.*
(2) *Targan SR, Hanauer SB, van Deventer SJH, et al, The Crohn's Disease cA2 Study Group. A short-term study of chimeric monoclonal antibody cA2 to tumor necrosis factor α for Crohn's disease. New England Journal of Medicine 1997; 337: 1029–1036.*

Ulcerative colitis

Ulcerative colitis is a diffuse disease of the colon characterized by inflammation and ulceration that is usually confined to the mucosa and submucosa.

Epidemiology

The incidence of ulcerative colitis varies with geographical location. It is common in Europe and North America with an incidence of approximately 10–20 per 100 000 per year and a prevalence of 100–200 per 100 000.[1] It is uncommon in Asia, Africa and South America. The disease can arise at any age but tends to present in the second to fourth decades, equally in both sexes.

Pathology

The disease process tends to start distally in the rectum or rectosigmoid colon and extends in a continuous manner proximally; in severe cases it can involve the entire colon. Unlike Crohn's, the disease tends to be limited to the colon, but occasionally ulcerative colitis can also involve the terminal ileum (backwash ileitis).

'Distal disease' is the most common anatomical distribution (80%), involving the rectum (proctitis) or rectosigmoid colon (proctosigmoiditis). With more severe disease, 'left-sided colitis' (up to the splenic flexure), 'extensive colitis' (up to the hepatic flexure) and pancolitis (entire colon) can occur.

Scope of disease

Intestinal
Complications of ulcerative colitis include diarrhoea leading to dehydration, haemorrhage, perforation, toxic megacolon and increased risk of colorectal cancer.

Extraintestinal
Extraintestinal manifestations are less common compared to Crohn's disease and include non-erosive arthritis of large joints, ankylosing spondylitis, erythema nodosum, pyoderma gangrenosum, iritis, primary sclerosing cholangitis and chronic active hepatitis.

Clinical features

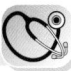

The cardinal symptom is bloody diarrhoea and this may be accompanied by urgency of defecation, tenesmus and colicky lower abdominal pain. Assessment of severity should include stool frequency, consistency, rectal bleeding, mucus, the presence of abdominal pain, malaise, fever and weight loss. Symptoms of extra-intestinal manifestations should be enquired about.

On examination there may be tachycardia, pyrexia, anaemia, evidence of dehydration due to fluid depletion, abdominal tenderness or palpable masses. Perineal examination is usually unremarkable.

Initial investigations

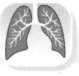

Full blood count
Anaemia may be present, and a raised white count or platelet count may indicate active disease.

Markers of inflammation
ESR and CRP are usually elevated in active disease and may be used to monitor clinical progression in the acute phase.

Urea and electrolytes
Urea may be elevated with dehydration, and if sufficiently severe may lead to renal impairment.

Liver profile
Low serum albumin is a marker of poor nutritional status and suggests active disease.

Stool culture
Stool cultures are required to exclude infectious diarrhoea such as *Clostridium difficile*.

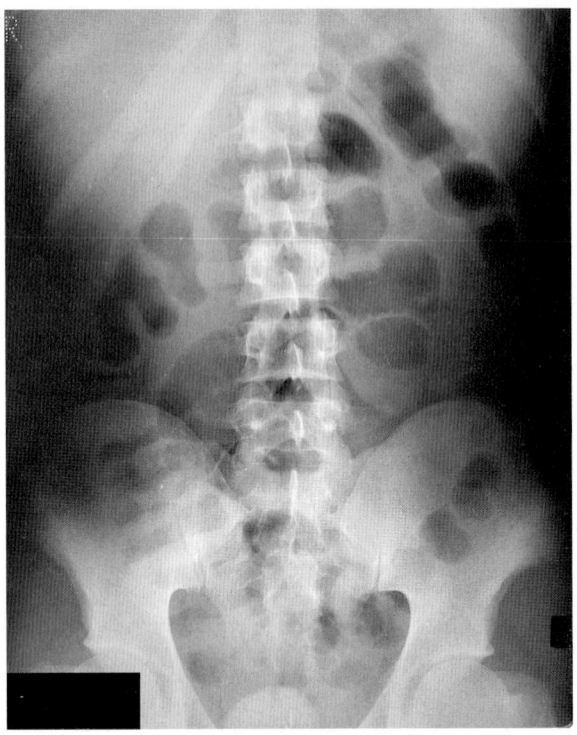

Fig. 4.39 Plain abdominal film of a patient with severe colitis.

Abdominal film

A plain abdominal film (Fig. 4.39) is performed to screen for toxic dilatation and may identify proximal constipation.

Rigid sigmoidoscopy

Macroscopic features of ulcerative colitis include inflamed, ulcerated and friable mucosa. A rectal biopsy should be taken for histological analysis.

Further investigations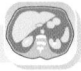

Once the diagnosis of inflammatory bowel has been established on initial investigation, an assessment of disease severity is required.

Colonoscopy

Colonoscopy is able to assess the full extent of disease, but in moderate to severe cases there is a higher risk of bowel perforation. Under these circumstances flexible sigmoidoscopy is safer, or investigation may be deferred until the clinical condition improves.

Initial management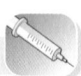

Fluid and electrolyte replacement

Intravenous fluid and electrolyte replacement is required to correct or prevent dehydration and electrolyte imbalance.

Blood transfusion

Blood transfusion is required to maintain a haemoglobin concentration of at least 10 g/dL.

Nutritional support

Enteral or parenteral feeding is required if the patient is malnourished.

Thromboprophylaxis

Subcutaneous heparin is required to reduce the risk of thromboembolism for patients admitted to hospital.

Prevention of toxic megacolon

Anticholinergic and antidiarrhoeal agents, NSAIDs and opiates should be stopped in severe illness to reduce the risk of toxic dilatation.

Medical management

Aminosalicylates

All the aminosalicylate drugs (e.g. sulfasalazine, mesalazine) aim to deliver the active component 5-aminosalicylic acid (5-ASA) to the lower bowel. High-dose oral aminosalicylates are used in active disease to induce remission. Following that, life-long maintenance therapy is generally recommended for all patients, especially those with left-sided or extensive disease, and those with distal disease who relapse more than once a year. Discontinuation of medication may be reasonable for those with distal disease who have been in remission for 2 years and are averse to such medication.

Corticosteroids

Oral corticosteroids (e.g. prednisolone 40 mg) are used in patients with active disease when a prompt response is required or when initial mesalazine treatment is unsuccessful. In order to limit systemic adverse effects, corticosteroids can be administered locally for patients with distal disease. Enema preparations can deliver the drug as far as the splenic flexure (for patients with rectosigmoid involvement), while suppositories are useful in those with proctitis.

Prednisolone should be weaned (according to severity and patient response) over 6–12 weeks; it is not an effective agent for maintenance of remission.

Other immunosuppressants

Azathioprine, mercaptopurine and methotrexate are alternative immunosuppressants that can be administered to maintain remission in patients who develop active disease on the reduction or withdrawal of steroids (chronic active steroid-dependent disease).

Surgical management

Colonic resection

Surgery may be indicated as an emergency or an elective procedure. In the acute phase, perforation, severe haemorrhage, toxic megacolon (more than 5.5 cm in diameter or 9 cm at the caecum) or failure to respond to medical therapy (tachycardia, pyrexia, frequent stool, increasing abdominal girth) after 3 days of treatment are indications for surgery. Elective surgery is indicated for patients with persistent disease that does not respond to medical therapy (poor control or frequent exacerbations) or the presence of dysplasia or early carcinoma.

The extent of resection depends on the distribution and severity of disease and patient preference.

A panproctocolectomy with a permanent ileostomy is a definitive procedure that involves excision of the rectum and colon leaving the ileum as a stoma. The operation removes all bowel that could be affected by ulcerative colitis and eliminates the risk of bowel cancer, but it leaves the patient with a permanent stoma.

Less extensive procedures can be performed such as a colectomy with an ileo-anal anastomosis in patients who do not have severe rectal disease. The operation leaves the rectum in situ and preserves anal continence but leaves the patient susceptible to distal disease and the risk of colorectal cancer. Alternatively, a panproctocolectomy can be performed and an ileo-anal pouch constructed. This operation removes all the bowel that could be affected by ulcerative colitis and preserves anal continence by creating a W or J shaped loop of ileum. A period of 'pouch training' may be required to preserve anal continence; diarrhoea is a common complication. Unfortunately, patients may develop inflammatory disease at the pouch (pouchitis); if this is sufficiently severe, complete resection and ileostomy can be performed at a later stage.

The mortality associated with surgery increases with the urgency of the operation and severity of disease. With elective surgery, the mortality rate is 0.5%, and approximately 10% of patients will progress to permanent ileostomy due to pouch failure by 7 years,[2] due to pelvic sepsis, pouchitis or poor function.

Prognosis

The clinical course is marked by exacerbation and remission. The yearly relapse rate is approximately 50%, with an appreciable minority having more frequently relapsing or chronic, continuous disease. Approximately 30% will require surgery.

Currently, the disease carries only a slight excess of mortality in the first year after diagnosis compared to the normal population. An attack of severe ulcerative colitis is still a serious and potentially life-threatening illness.

The value of surveillance colonoscopy for dysplasia and early colorectal cancer is unclear and still under debate.

FURTHER INFORMATION

Carter MJ, Lobo AJ, Travis SPL. Guidelines for the management of inflammatory bowel disease in adults. Gut 2004; 53: v1–16.

REFERENCES

(1) *Carter MJ, Lobo AJ, Travis SPL. Guidelines for the management of inflammatory bowel disease in adults. Gut 2004; 53: v1–16.*
(2) *Tulchinsky H, Hawley PR, Nicholls J. Long-term failure after restorative proctocolectomy for ulcerative colitis. Annals of Surgery 2003; 238: 229–234.*

Diseases of the colon and rectum

Diverticular disease

Diverticular disease (or diverticulosis) develops as a result of mucosal and submucosal herniations through the circular muscle fibres of the colon.

Epidemiology

Diverticular disease is very common in the Western world and the prevalence increases with age from less than 10% in people younger than 40 years to 50–66% in those older than 80 years.[1] It is equally common in both sexes and is rare in developing countries.

Pathology

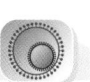

The high prevalence of diverticular disease in the developed world is thought to be due to low dietary fibre intake leading to constipation and increased colonic intraluminal pressure, resulting in herniation of the mucosa through the muscle of the colonic wall. This usually occurs at the weak points where the branches of the marginal artery penetrate the colon. The diverticula thus emerge between the taenia coli, usually in the sigmoid colon, which is often shortened and thickened.

Scope of disease

The most common complications are acute inflammation (diverticulitis), haemorrhage, perforation, stricture, large bowel obstruction and fistula formation. Colonic perforation may lead to peritonitis or intra-abdominal abscess formation. Fistula formation is due to the inflamed colon lying next to adjacent organs, with consequent erosion into structures such as small bowel, bladder and vagina.

Clinical features

Diverticular disease is usually asymptomatic. Chronic left lower quadrant pain, bloating, constipation, diarrhoea or mucus in the stools are often attributed to diverticular disease. However these symptoms overlap considerably with irritable bowel syndrome (p. 250) and the presence of diverticula on investigations should not lead automatically to attribution of these symptoms to diverticular disease as diverticula are very common in the elderly.[2]

Symptoms usually occur when there is a complication such as acute diverticulitis. Colonic strictures may present with symptoms of large bowel obstruction (p. 248). A fistula into the small bowel presents as diarrhoea, one into the bladder may cause a urinary tract infection or occasionally air in the urine (pneumaturia), and a colo-vaginal fistula can cause vaginal discharge of faecal material.

Initial investigations
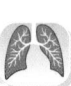

Colonoscopy
Colonoscopy is a useful investigation for patients with chronic left lower quadrant pain and non-specific symptoms. Apart from identifying diverticula, it is a useful screening investigation for colorectal cancer, as the symptoms often overlap. It is also required in patients who present with rectal bleeding. The presence of diverticula should not lead automatically to attribution of the symptoms to diverticular disease as diverticula are very common in the general population.

Colonoscopy is generally avoided in patients who present with acute diverticulitis due to the risk of colonic perforation from insufflation of air.

Barium enema
A barium enema (Fig. 4.40) can identify the presence and location of diverticula but does not give information on their clinical significance. This used to be the investigation of choice, but currently colonoscopy is preferred due to the diagnostic error rate of the barium enema.[2]

Initial management
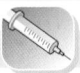

High dietary fibre intake
Patient should be advised to take a diet high in dietary fibre, particularly fruit, vegetables and bran. However, evidence of the efficacy of this measure is lacking.

Surgical management

Surgery is rarely necessary for uncomplicated diverticular disease. Fistulae are usually treated by colonic resection and excision of the fistula tract with or without a covering stoma.

Prognosis

In the majority, diverticular disease is benign and self-limiting.

i FURTHER INFORMATION

Stollman NH, Raskin JB. Diagnosis and management of diverticular disease of the colon in adults. Ad Hoc Practice Parameters Committee of the American College of Gastroenterology. American Journal of Gastroenterology 1999; 94: 3110–3121.

REFERENCES

(1) Stollman N, Raskin PJB. Diverticular disease of the colon. Lancet 2004; 363: 631–639.
(2) Stollman NH, Raskin JB. Diagnosis and management of diverticular disease of the colon in adults. Ad Hoc Practice Parameters Committee of the American College of Gastroenterology. American Journal of Gastroenterology 1999; 94: 3110–3121.

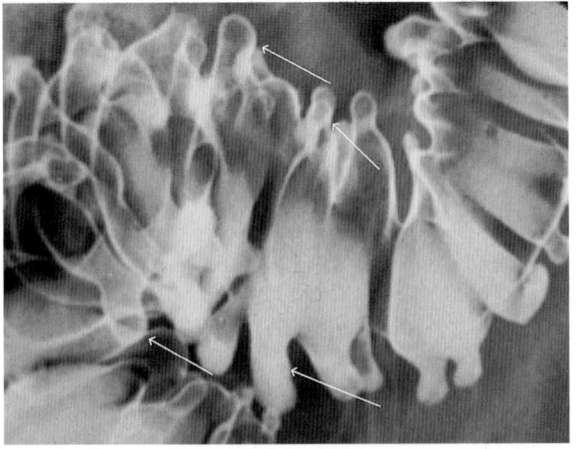

Fig. 4.40 Barium enema of diverticular disease.

Acute diverticulitis

Clinical features

Acute diverticulitis presents with left iliac fossa pain, anorexia, fever and general malaise. There may also be associated urinary frequency or haematuria due to adjacent bladder involvement. Abdominal examination usually reveals local tenderness, distension and possibly a left iliac fossa mass.

Haemorrhage will present as rectal bleeding (p. 240). Localized colonic perforation may present with signs and symptoms of an intra-abdominal collection (pyrexia, malaise, abdominal mass), but many cases of perforation produce generalized peritonitis with severe acute abdominal pain and a rigid abdomen.

Initial investigations

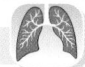

Full blood count

A high white cell count is usually present, and an estimation of haemoglobin is required in patients with rectal bleeding.

Plain abdominal film

Large or small bowel dilatation may be visible with colonic obstruction. Areas of increased density may suggest intra-abdominal collections.

Chest X-ray

A chest film is performed to screen for bowel perforation, which is seen as free air under the diaphragm (Fig. 4.41).

Further investigations

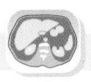

CT abdomen

The CT scan of the abdomen is a useful investigation to image disease within the bowel wall, intra-abdominal disease and adjacent structures.

Abdominal ultrasound

An ultrasound scan is useful to identify bowel wall thickening, diverticula or intra-abdominal abscess.

Contrast enema

A barium enema is not usually performed in acute disease due to the risk of barium leaking into the abdomen in the presence of colonic perforation. In cases of suspected left colonic obstruction, as seen on a plain abdominal film, a water-soluble contrast enema may be helpful.

Once the acute inflammation has settled, a barium enema (or colonoscopy) is usually performed to assess the severity of diverticular disease.

Colonoscopy

Colonoscopy may identify the site of colonic bleeding in patients with rectal bleeding. Epinephrine may be injected into the bleeding area to stop the haemorrhage.

Selective mesenteric angiography

In cases of severe bleeding where colonoscopy has failed to identify the site, selective mesenteric angiography and therapeutic embolization of the culprit artery may be attempted.

Initial management

Intravenous fluids

Patients are kept nil by mouth and intravenous fluids are administered.

Intravenous antibiotics

Antibiotics (usually cefuroxime and metronidazole) are administered.

Surgical management

Percutaneous drainage of abscess

An intra-abdominal collection may be treated by radiologically guided percutaneous drainage.

Left colonic resection

Resection of the affected segment of the left colon is usually necessary for perforation or obstruction and occasionally in cases of severe haemorrhage (p. 278–279). If there is no faecal soiling of the peritoneal cavity, resection followed by primary anastomosis is the procedure of choice. If there is gross faecal contamination, then resection with proximal colostomy and distal colonic closure (Hartmann's procedure) is usually a safer option. Bowel continuity may then be restored at a later date.

Prognosis

Approximately 38% of patients admitted with acute diverticulitis will require surgery, with an overall surgical mortality rate of 2%.[1]

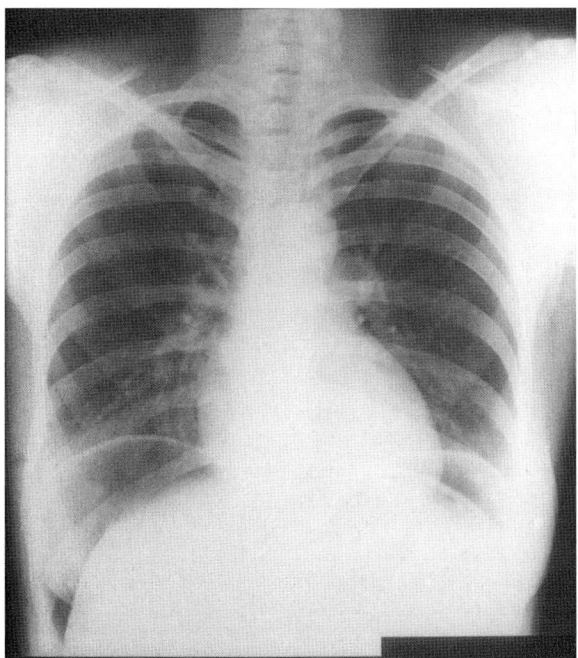

Fig. 4.41 Abdominal film of perforated diverticula. Free air can be seen under both hemidiaphragms from perforated diverticula.

REFERENCE

(1) Bahadursingh AM, Virgo KS, Kaminski DL, Longo WE. *Spectrum of disease and outcome of complicated diverticular disease. American Journal of Surgery* 2003; 186: 696–701.

Colorectal carcinoma

Colorectal cancer is an adenocarcinoma of the colon or rectum.

Epidemiology

Colorectal carcinoma is common. The incidence is highest in Australia, North America, Japan and Western Europe, ranging from 39 to 45 per 100 000 per year.[1] The frequency increases with age and whilst the overall incidence is similar for both sexes, rectal tumours are more common in men.

Pathology

The most important aetiological factor is believed to be the low-fibre, high-fat diet of Western civilization. Predisposing diseases include ulcerative colitis and Crohn's disease, and strongly associated hereditary conditions include familial adenomatous polyposis (FAP), hereditary non-polyposis colorectal cancer syndromes (HNPCC or Lynch I and II syndromes), Peutz–Jeghers syndrome and juvenile polyposis.

Two thirds of carcinomas occur in the rectum and sigmoid colon, with about half of the rest being found in the caecum.

Scope of disease

Local

Colorectal cancer may develop as an ulcerating lesion, an exophytic growth, a diffuse infiltrating tumour or a stenosing annular constriction within the bowel lumen. Constrictive lesions in the left colon where faeces are more solid may result in altered bowel habit (constipation). Ulcerative lesions may bleed and lead to anaemia. Rectal lesions can produce mucus and give rise to the sensation of tenesmus. Tumour infiltration into adjacent structures can result in fistula formation.

Metastatic

Metastases can be local (direct extension, transcoelomic within the abdominal cavity) or distant (lymphatic or haematogenous spread to the liver or lungs). Each can produce site-specific symptoms.

Paraneoplastic

Hypercalcaemia of malignancy can occur.

Clinical features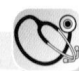

Clinical presentation depends on the site. Tumours of the ascending colon rarely produce alteration of bowel habit, but rather iron deficiency anaemia due to chronic blood loss. Tumours of the transverse or upper descending colon often give rise to colicky abdominal pain or even dyspeptic symptoms. On the other hand, left-sided colonic tumours tend to give rise to more obvious changes in bowel habit, often alternating constipation and diarrhoea, and sometimes dark red rectal bleeding mixed in with the motions.

Rectal lesions tend to bleed or secrete mucus, which is passed per rectum, and patients may also present with tenesmus (a feeling of incomplete evacuation) in addition to bloody diarrhoea. Other features of advanced disease include weight loss, anorexia and malaise. Clinical examination is often normal, except in advanced disease, when an abdominal mass, hepatomegaly or ascites may be found. Digital rectal examination may reveal the presence of low rectal lesions.

Initial investigations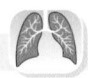

Full blood count

Anaemia can result from chronic lower gastrointestinal bleeding.

Liver profile

Raised transaminases may indicate liver metastasis. Raised alkaline phosphatase may result from either liver or bony metastasis.

Serum calcium

Serum calcium levels may be raised from bony metastasis or (rarely) ectopic parathyroid hormone production.

Rigid sigmoidoscopy

Direct visualization of the rectum and sigmoid by rigid sigmoidoscopy may detect neoplasms in this area.

Colonoscopy

Colonoscopy allows direct visualization of the mucosa and facilitates the taking of biopsies for tissue analysis. However, in a patient with a long and tortuous sigmoid colon, often with associated diverticular disease, it may prove difficult to get all the way around the colon at colonoscopy, in which case a barium enema may be the only option.

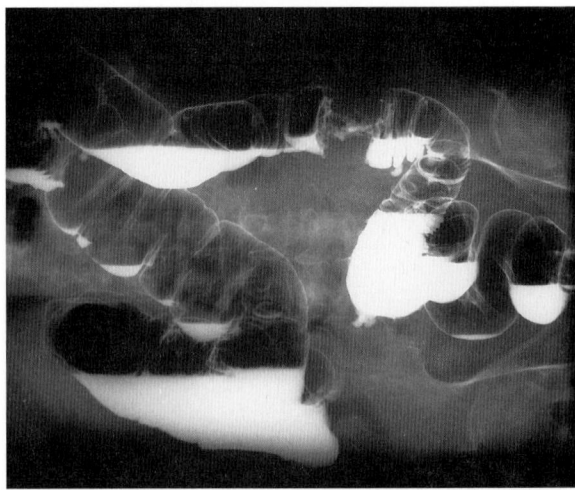

Fig. 4.42 Barium enema of colorectal cancer. The tumour can be seen in the descending colon giving rise to the classic apple core appearance.

Barium enema

Barium enema should be arranged if complete visualization of the colon cannot be achieved by colonoscopy. The classic barium enema appearance of an annular carcinoma of the colon is that of an 'apple core' lesion (Fig. 4.42).

RECENT ADVANCES

If both colonoscopy and barium enema are difficult, a new alternative, CT pneumocolography, may prove useful.

Further investigations

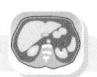

Once a histopathological diagnosis confirming colon cancer has been acquired, the next step is to stage the tumour to decide the best treatment option.

▶▶▶ TNM Staging of colorectal carcinoma

Primary tumour (T)

T1	Tumour invades submucosa
T2	Tumour invades muscularis propria
T3	Tumour invades through the muscularis propria into the subserosa, or into non-peritonealized pericolic or perirectal tissues
T4	Tumour directly invades other organs or structures, and/or perforates visceral peritoneum

Regional lymph nodes (N)

N0	No regional lymph node metastasis
N1	Metastasis in 1–3 regional lymph nodes
N2	Metastasis in 4 or more regional lymph nodes

Distant metastasis (M)

M0	No distant metastasis
M1	Distant metastasis

Stage grouping

UICC/AJCC				Dukes
Stage 0	Tis	N0	M0	—
Stage I	T1	N0	M0	A
	T2	N0	M0	A
Stage IIA	T3	N0	M0	B
Stage IIB	T4	N0	M0	B
Stage IIIA	T1–2	N1	M0	C
Stage IIIB	T3–4	N1	M0	C
Stage IIIC	Any T	N2	M0	C
Stage IV	Any T	Any N	M1	D*

UICC, Union Internationale Contre le Cancer (International Union Against Cancer); AJCC, American Joint Committee on Cancer.
* The term Dukes' D is not part of the original classification, but an often used term referring to the presence of distant metastases.

Staging chest radiograph

A plain chest film is a useful initial screening investigation for pulmonary metastases.

Staging abdominal ultrasound

Abdominal ultrasound may be used to screen for liver or lymph node metastases, although the sensitivity is lower than that of a CT scan.

Staging CT chest and abdomen

If there is any suspicion of metastatic disease on initial screening investigations, a CT scan of chest and abdomen would be required to confirm or exclude evidence of metastatic disease.

MRI of the liver

In selected patients with limited liver metastases, concomitant liver resection may be considered. In these patients, preoperative MRI provides detailed soft tissue imaging to assess the extent of liver involvement.

Carcinoembryonic antigen (CEA)

CEA levels are documented as a baseline. The poor sensitivity and specificity of this test limit its use in the diagnosis of colorectal cancer. However, it can be a useful marker of recurrent disease.

Surgical management

Surgery is the definitive management option for approximately 80%.[2] The operation performed is dependent on the site and extent of the tumour. The general principle of colorectal cancer surgery is resection with adequate margins and regional lymph node clearance. Good bowel preparation is essential so that the surgeon has a clean operating field and the empty bowel facilitates the anastomosis.

A midline laparotomy or transverse incision is usually performed and the site and extent of resection is governed by the location of the tumour.

Right hemicolectomy

Tumours of the caecum and ascending colon are treated by right hemicolectomy. The right hemicolon is mobilized from the peritoneal reflection and supplying arterial and venous branches of the superior mesenteric artery and vein are ligated. The segment of colon is transected and an anastomosis formed between the ileum and transverse colon (ileo-transverse anastomosis).

Transverse colectomy

The transverse colon is usually mobile and the supplying arterial and venous branches are ligated. The segment of colon is transected with incorporation of both the hepatic and splenic flexures in the resection specimen, and an anastomosis may be formed between the right and left hemicolon. More usually tumours of the transverse colon or splenic flexure are often best treated by an extended right hemicolectomy, with an ileo-descending colonic anastomosis.

Left hemicolectomy

Tumours of the left colon and upper sigmoid are treated by left hemicolectomy. The left hemicolon is mobilized from the peritoneal reflection, and the supplying arterial and venous branches of the inferior mesenteric artery and vein are ligated. The diseased segment is resected and an anastomosis is formed between the descending colon and the rectum.

Anterior resection of the rectum

Rectal and rectosigmoid junction lesions should undergo anterior resection of the rectum. The extent of the resection depends on the location of the tumour. Rectosigmoid junction tumours are excised as a high anterior resection, whilst those in the mid rectum usually need a low anterior resection for adequate clearance.

If the tumour is low, a covering stoma (loop ileostomy or colostomy) is often fashioned to defunction the anastomosis. The bowel proximal to the anastomosis is led out onto the anterior abdominal wall to allow the bowel content to discharge such that no faeces are present at the site of the anastomosis. The stoma is closed only after satisfactory healing has been proven.

> **RECENT ADVANCES**
>
> *It was previously thought that 5 cm of tumour clearance was necessary to effect cure; currently a 2 cm margin is thought to be sufficient. This realization, together with the advent of circular stapling instruments, has meant that most rectal tumours can now be excised and the bowel re-anastomosed at the same procedure.*

Abdomino-perineal resection of the rectum

Very low rectal tumours may require abdomino-perineal resection in order to achieve good clearance. In this procedure the rectum and anus are excised. Restoration of bowel continuity cannot be achieved and a permanent end colostomy is required.

> **RECENT ADVANCES**
>
> *In all rectal cancer operations, the current standard is total mesorectal excision. This procedure involves excision of the rectum and mesorectum (containing the lymphatic supply, the most common site of local recurrence) down to at least 5 cm below the tumour. Using this technique, the rate of local tumour recurrence has been reported as 8.2% at 5 years; with the addition of preoperative radiotherapy the recurrence reduces to 2.4%.[3]*

Management of colonic obstruction/perforation

Occasionally patients may present as an emergency with left colonic obstruction, with or without perforation, with the bowel unprepared. In this situation primary anastomosis may carry an unacceptably high anastomotic leakage rate. Therefore, following resection of the diseased segment, an end colostomy is favoured with the distal bowel being closed off and dropped back into the pelvis (Hartmann's procedure).

Currently, more surgeons are moving towards resection, on-table colonic lavage and primary re-anastomosis to avoid a stoma and obviate the need for a second operation. However, this should not be performed in the presence of gross faecal contamination, or on a very ill patient, or if the surgeon lacks the necessary expertise. In these situations, Hartmann's operation is the preferred option.

Management of liver metastases

Increasingly, colorectal liver metastases are being surgically resected. This is one of the secondary liver cancers where surgical resection offers any hope of cure. With careful patient selection, a 5-year survival of 30% can be achieved. Equally, colorectal lung metastases may be amenable to resection (p. 153).

Medical management

Chemotherapy

Chemotherapy is being used increasingly in both the adjuvant and palliative settings, with some, if small, survival benefit being seen. Most chemotherapy regimens are 5-fluorouracil based, often in combination with other agents, such as leucovorin. Pooled meta-analyses now suggest survival benefit for all patients with stage II and III disease.[4] Combination treatments include irinotecan (which works by its interaction with topoisomerase I) and oxaliplatin (a third-generation platinum derivative) with a 5-fluorouracil based derivative; however, the best combination and sequence of treatment is still unknown.

Radiotherapy

Radiotherapy, with or without chemotherapy, has been used both in the adjuvant and neoadjuvant (preoperative) setting. It has been shown to reduce the incidence of local recurrence of rectal cancer[3] (with a minimal role in colon cancer), but effects on long-term survival are not clear. Combination treatment carries a relatively high incidence of morbidity such as anastomotic breakdown and non-healing perineum.

Palliative therapy

Endoscopic therapies are available for patients unfit for surgery or with unresectable disease. These include intubation with expandable metal stents, ablation therapy with thermal laser, argon plasma coagulation or photodynamic therapy (PDT).

> **RECENT ADVANCES**
>
> *Currently, researchers are investigating the use of monoclonal antibodies against vascular endothelial growth factor (bevacizumab) and epidermal growth factor receptor (cetuximab). Monoclonal antibodies have minimal toxicity and can be used for chemoresistant colorectal cancers. Early results indicate improvements to disease-free survival.[5]*

Prognosis

The overall 30-day mortality for surgery for colorectal carcinoma is 7.5%, although this varies according to age, urgency of operation and extent of disease.[6] The overall 3-year survival by Dukes' stage in Europe is 73% (A and B), 45% (C), and 11% (D), where 82% of patients underwent surgical resection (Table 4.17).[2]

Postoperative surveillance and treatment of recurrent disease (colonoscopy, CT scans or CEA levels) improves survival of patients with a risk ratio for death of 0.81 compared to control.[7]

Table 4.17	Modified Dukes' staging of colorectal carcinoma and associated 5-year survival rate	
Dukes' stage	Disease extent	5-year survival
A	Tumour confined to muscularis propria	90%
B1	Tumour breaches muscularis propria but no nodal involvement	70%
B2	Tumour involves serosa but no nodal involvement	60%
C1	Tumour involves regional lymph nodes, but apical node negative	35%
C2	Tumour involves regional lymph nodes and apical node positive	25%
D	Metastatic disease	11%

REFERENCES

(1) Parkin DM, Pisani P, Ferlay J. Global cancer statistics. CA: A Cancer Journal for Clinicians 1999; 49: 33–64.
(2) Gatta G, Capocaccia R, Sant M, et al. Understanding variations in survival for colorectal cancer in Europe: a EUROCARE high resolution study. Gut 2000; 47: 533–538.
(3) Kapiteijn E, Marijnen CAM, Nagtegaal ID, et al, the Dutch Colorectal Cancer Group. Preoperative radiotherapy combined with total mesorectal excision for resectable rectal cancer. New England Journal of Medicine 2001; 345: 638–646.
(4) Gill S, Loprinzi CL, Sargent DJ, et al. Pooled analysis of fluorouracil-based adjuvant therapy for stage II and III colon cancer: who benefits and by how much? Journal of Clinical Oncology 2004; 22: 1797–1806.
(5) Slevin M, Payne S. New treatments for colon cancer. BMJ 2004; 329: 124–126.
(6) Tekkis PP, Poloniecki JD, Thompson MR, Stamatakis JD. Operative mortality in colorectal cancer: prospective national study. BMJ 2003; 327: 1196–1201.
(7) Renehan AG, Egger M, Saunders MP, O'Dwyer ST. Impact on survival of intensive follow up after curative resection for colorectal cancer: systematic review and meta-analysis of randomised trials. BMJ 2002; 324: 813.

Colonic volvulus

A volvulus occurs when part of the bowel becomes twisted on its mesentery. It can affect any part of the bowel that has a mesentery (e.g. gastric volvulus) but the most common site is the colon.

Epidemiology

Colonic volvulus is relatively common, affecting the elderly and often confused patient.

Pathology

The caecum and the sigmoid colon are the two most commonly affected locations. A caecal volvulus results from poor fixation of the caecum in the right iliac fossa, whilst a sigmoid volvulus usually occurs where a long redundant sigmoid loop is found on a relatively narrow mesentery (allowing it to twist on the mesenteric axis).

Scope of disease

A closed loop obstruction can occur with the risk of ischaemic necrosis and perforation. This can lead to faecal peritonitis.

Clinical features

The clinical features are those of intestinal obstruction with abdominal pain, vomiting, absolute constipation and abdominal distension.

On examination the abdomen is usually tender and distended. If perforation has occurred, the patient presents with signs and symptoms of acute peritonitis (p. 318).

Initial investigations

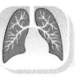

Investigations should be performed as for intestinal obstruction (p. 249–250).

Plain abdominal film
A grossly distended loop of colon arising from the left or right iliac fossa may be seen (Fig. 4.43). In the case of caecal volvulus, the classic appearance is that of a 'coffee bean' (Fig. 4.44).

Further investigations

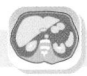

Further investigations are rarely necessary, as the diagnosis is usually apparent from the plain abdominal film.

CT abdomen
If there is any doubt, a CT scan will confirm the diagnosis and is the further investigation of choice.

Contrast enema
An instant (unprepared) contrast enema may help.

Initial management

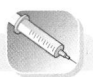

Fluid and electrolyte replacement
Fluid replacement and the correction of any electrolyte abnormalities are an important aspect of the management.

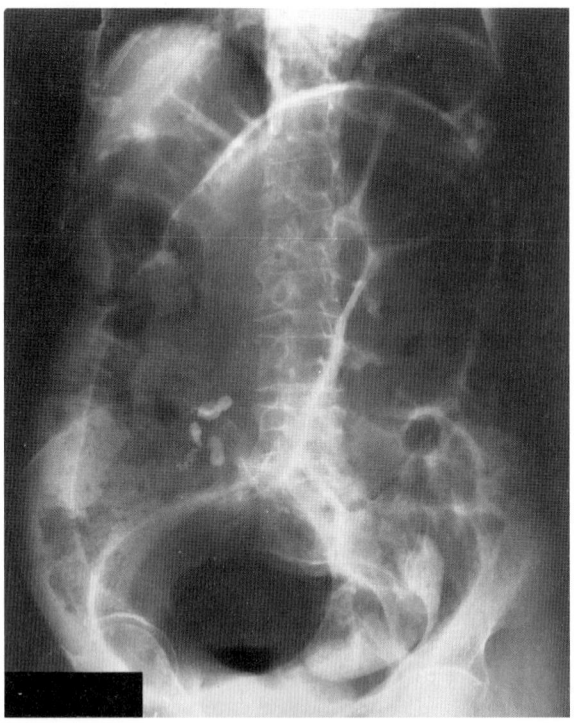

Fig. 4.43 Barium enema of a sigmoid volvulus.

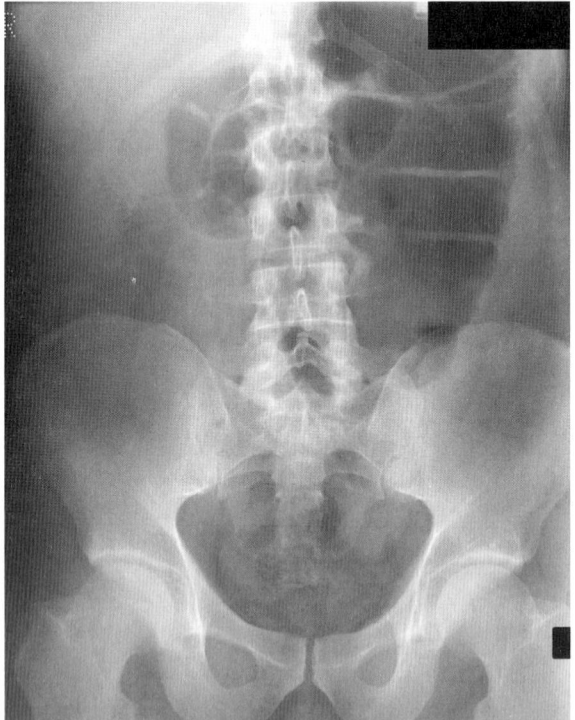

Fig. 4.44 Caecal volvulus

Colonic decompression

Colonic decompression can be achieved using a rigid sigmoidoscope and flatus tube or a flexible sigmoidoscope.

A flatus tube is usually left in place for 1–2 days to allow resolution.

Surgical management

Laparotomy and fixation

Laparotomy is required to untwist the bowel in patients who fail to respond to initial therapy or if there are signs of impending rupture. If the bowel is viable, simple fixation to the abdominal wall (caecopexy, sigmoidopexy) usually suffices; if not, colonic resection may be necessary. In patients with recurrent volvulus, elective colonic resection may be required to prevent recurrence.

> **RECENT ADVANCES**
>
> *Recently colonic deflation and fixation to the anterior abdominal wall using a percutaneous technique has been successfully employed as a means of treating and preventing recurrence of volvulus.*[1]

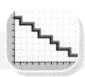
Prognosis

Volvulus is a benign condition and has a low recurrence rate once surgical fixation has been undertaken. Emergency colonic surgery in the elderly patient carries risk of morbidity and mortality.

REFERENCE

(1) *Pinedo G, Kirberg A. Percutaneous endoscopic sigmoidopexy in sigmoid volvulus with T-fasteners: report of two cases. Diseases of the Colon and Rectum 2001; 44: 1867–1869; discussion 1869–1870.*

Angiodysplasia of the colon

Epidemiology

Angiodysplasia of the colon is uncommon; the prevalence is 830 per 100 000.[1] Although it can present at any age, it tends to be more common in the elderly. There is no particular sex or geographical variation.

Pathology

Angiodysplastic lesions are vascular abnormalities that occasionally bleed into the colonic lumen. They are most commonly seen in the caecum and right colon. Chronic blood loss can lead to anaemia, and acute severe blood loss can present with rectal bleeding.

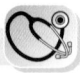
Clinical features

In the majority these lesions are asymptomatic and are evident only on investigation for anaemia or rectal bleeding.

Investigations

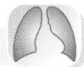

Full blood count
A full blood count may reveal anaemia.

Colonoscopy
Colonoscopy will reveal small vascular lesions on direct inspection of the bowel lumen.

Selective mesenteric angiography
Selective mesenteric angiogram is indicated if colonoscopy cannot adequately visualize the right hemicolon, or in cases of acute severe bleeding. The site of bleeding may be identified and therapeutic embolization can be undertaken.

Management

In the majority, angiodysplasia is a benign condition. Treatment is usually only indicated in acute bleeding.

Intra-arterial vasopressin/embolization
Acute bleeding from angiodysplasia may be treated by selective intra-arterial infusion of vasopressin or embolization of the mesenteric 'feeding' vessels during mesenteric angiography.

Colonic resection
Emergency colonic resection may be necessary when intra-arterial infusion of vasopressin or embolization fails to control the bleeding, or when the bleeding is severe.

Prognosis

The natural history of angiodysplasia is benign, and the risk of bleeding in incidentally diagnosed lesions is very low.[1]

REFERENCE

(1) Foutch PG, Rex DK, Lieberman DA. Prevalence and natural history of colonic angiodysplasia among healthy asymptomatic people. American Journal of Gastroenterology 1995; 90: 564–567.

Ischaemic colitis

Epidemiology

Precise figures of the epidemiology are not available. In general, ischaemic colitis tends to be more common in the elderly, patients with risk factors for atherosclerosis and patients with chronic renal failure.[1] There is no particular sex or geographical variation.

Pathology

Colonic ischaemia can result from atherosclerosis of the mesenteric vessels or an embolus causing sudden vascular occlusion. Occasionally, colonic ischaemia results from prolonged hypotension (shock), increased plasma viscosity or iatrogenic damage of a mesenteric vessel during surgery. Acute ischaemic colitis may lead to gangrene and perforation (with consequent peritonitis). Chronic ischaemia may produce mesenteric angina or colonic stricture.

Clinical features

Acute ischaemic colitis usually presents with abdominal pain and bloody diarrhoea. Symptoms and signs of perforation are discussed on page 280. Chronic ischaemia usually causes malabsorption or mesenteric angina (abdominal pain after eating). Post-ischaemia colonic stricture can cause change in bowel habit (constipation) or present with intestinal obstruction (p. 250).

Investigations

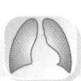

The diagnosis may be suspected from the history and examination. Investigations are usually directed by the presenting complaint.

Full blood count
The white cell count is usually elevated.

Arterial blood gas
An arterial blood gas may reveal acidosis due to necrotic bowel.

Plain abdominal film
A plain abdominal film may demonstrate distended bowel loops and 'thumb printing' (indentations) of the colonic wall, due to mucosal oedema in acute ischaemia of the colon (Fig. 4.45).

Barium enema
A barium enema is the investigation of choice when a colonic stricture is suspected.

Selective mesenteric angiography
A selective mesenteric arteriogram is often diagnostic.

Management

Less severe forms of colonic ischaemia may be treated conservatively with intravenous fluids and antibiotics in the acute phase, on the presumption of reversible ischaemia.

Colonic resection
Approximately half of the patients presenting with acute ischaemic colitis will require emergency laparotomy and colonic resection, usually when gangrene or perforation is suspected. Of those that are treated initially with conservative management, approximately 24% will require surgery.[1] Ischaemic strictures are also usually treated by surgical resection.

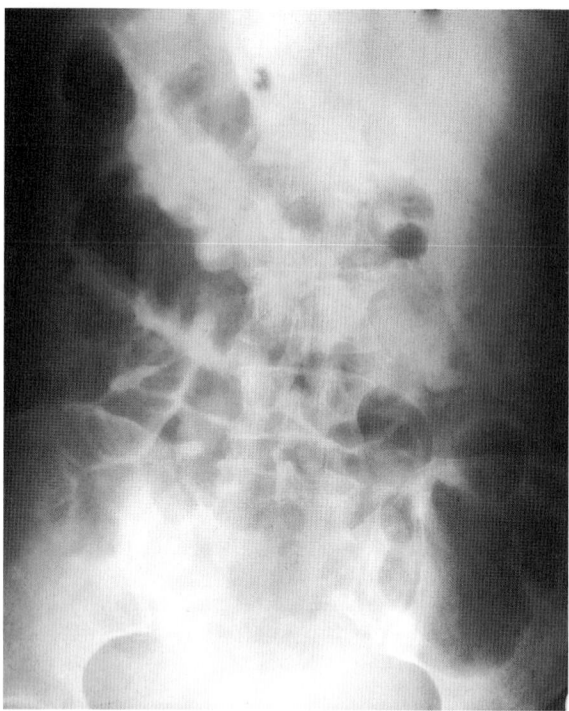

Fig. 4.45 Plain abdominal film of ischaemic bowel showing classic thumbprinting.

Prognosis

The mortality rate in patients with disease that does not require emergency surgery is 9%, and the mortality rate of patients who require emergency surgery is 48%.[1]

REFERENCE

(1) *Scharff JR, Longo WE, Vartanian SM, Jacobs DL, Bahadursingh AN, Kaminski DL. Ischemic colitis: Spectrum of disease and outcome. Surgery 2003; 134: 624–629.*

Rectal prolapse

Full thickness rectal prolapse is the complete eversion of the rectum through the anal canal.

Epidemiology

Little is known of the incidence of rectal prolapse. Although it can occur at any age, it is more common in elderly women.

Pathology

Predisposing factors to rectal prolapse include rectal intussusception (perhaps due to a change in calibre from the sigmoid into the rectum), poor sphincter tone and a lax pelvic floor following childbirth.

Scope of disease

A major complication of prolapse is irreducibility, leading to strangulation and necrosis. Faecal incontinence can occur if the anal sphincter is lax.

Clinical features

Patients usually present with a swelling that prolapses on defecation. It either reduces spontaneously or requires manual reduction. The prolapse is often accompanied by rectal bleeding, mucus discharge and occasionally faecal incontinence.

Digital rectal examination is essential and the patient should be asked to bear down (as though straining at stool) to induce rectal prolapse.

Initial investigations

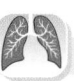

Investigation is rarely necessary, as the diagnosis is clinical.

Surgical management

Surgery should be offered to all patients with acceptable operative risk. There are two approaches, transabdominal and perineal. Recurrence rates are low (5%) with the various rectopexy procedures; there is a risk of postoperative faecal incontinence or constipation.

Posterior rectopexy

The most frequently employed abdominal operation is the posterior rectopexy. A midline incision is performed and the rectum mobilized, followed by fixation to the sacrum. This is performed directly with sutures or using synthetic material (Marlex mesh or Ivalon sponge).

Resection rectopexy

In patients with severe constipation, the rectopexy is usually best combined with a sigmoid resection.

Delorme's rectopexy

The Delorme's rectopexy is achieved via a perineal approach. The mucosa of the prolapsed rectum is excised, and the muscle is plicated and reduced.

RECENT ADVANCES

Laparoscopy has revolutionized abdominal rectopexy, speeding up recovery and reducing postoperative pain, but producing equally good results to open surgery.[1]

Prognosis

Rectal prolapse is a benign but distressing condition. Recurrence rates are low after surgery.

REFERENCE

(1) *Solomon MJ, Young CJ, Eyers AA, Roberts RA. Randomized clinical trial of laparoscopic versus open abdominal rectopexy for rectal prolapse. British Journal of Surgery 2002; 89: 35–39.*

Haemorrhoids

Haemorrhoids (or piles) result from the fragmentation, descent and engorgement of the fibrovascular cushions that line the anal canal.

Epidemiology

Haemorrhoids are common. The estimated prevalence is 4.4% (4400 per 100 000), occurring at a peak age of 45–65 years.[1] They are thought to be more common in men although the prevalence in females increases after childbirth.

Pathology

The three fibrovascular cushions that line the normal anal canal are located at the 3, 7 and 11 o'clock positions (when the anus is viewed in the lithotomy position). They are thought to play a role in the maintenance of anal continence.

The most commonly held theory implicated in the pathogenesis of haemorrhoids is low dietary fibre intake. This leads to constipation and repeated straining during defecation causing descent and engorgement of the fibrovascular cushions.

Haemorrhoids are classified as internal if the origin is above the dentate line and external if the origin is below the dentate line.

Scope of disease

Inflammation or erosion of the surface epithelium of haemorrhoids can lead to bleeding, and thrombosis leads to acute painful haemorrhoids. Occasional rectal varices from portal hypertension may be mistaken for haemorrhoids.

Clinical features

The majority of haemorrhoids are asymptomatic. Those that come to medical attention present with intermittent bright red rectal bleeding (on the toilet paper or in the toilet pan), perianal irritation, pruritus ani (itchy anus) or prolapse. When thrombosed and incarcerated (irreducible), haemorrhoids are acutely painful.

On examination, a swelling may be seen just inside or outside the anal verge, as in the case of prolapsing piles (Fig. 4.46). There may be surrounding excoriation of the skin due to scratching by the patient. It is important to classify the severity of the haemorrhoids (Table 4.18) as it is used as a guide to treatment.

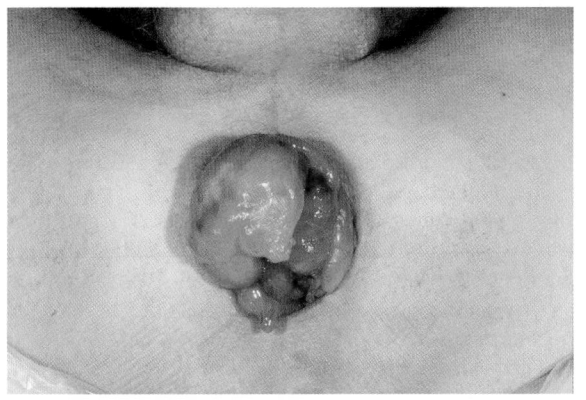
Fig. 4.46 Prolapsing haemorrhoids.

Initial investigations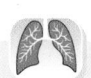

Sigmoidoscopy and proctoscopy

Rigid sigmoidoscopy should be performed to exclude other anorectal causes for the irritation such as an anal fissure or fistula. Then proctoscopy should be performed to visualize the piles.

Initial management

Dietary modification

A high-fibre diet should be recommended to reduce the frequency of constipation.

Medical management

Laxatives

For patients with first-degree haemorrhoids, administration of a bulk laxative may be effective in the treatment and prevent further haemorrhoids. There is little evidence to support the efficacy of topical creams often prescribed for anal irritation or soreness.

Surgical management

Various outpatient procedures are available for patients with symptomatic second- or third-degree haemorrhoids.

Table 4.18	Classification of the severity of haemorrhoids
First degree	Haemorrhoids that do not prolapse
Second degree	Haemorrhoids that prolapse but reduce spontaneously
Third degree	Haemorrhoids that remain prolapsed unless manually reduced
Fourth degree	Acutely thrombosed incarcerated internal haemorrhoids or thrombosed haemorrhoids that involve the circumference of the rectum

The procedure with the lowest recurrence rate is rubber band ligation.[2,3]

Rubber band ligation

Rubber band ligation may be used for second- or third-degree haemorrhoids. It involves the application of a tight rubber band (Barron's band) to the base of the pile, above the dentate line, which cuts off the blood supply and causes sloughing of the pile about 10 days later. Rubber bands placed below the dentate cause severe pain; they are therefore unsuitable for external haemorrhoids.

The recurrence rate is 12% at 2 years. Complications are experienced in 18%, the most common being pain and bleeding.[4] Other complications include abscess formation, slipping of the rubber bands, and thrombosis of adjacent haemorrhoids.

Injection sclerotherapy

The most commonly employed agent is 5% phenol in oil injected submucosally into the base of the pile haemorrhoid, leading to sclerosis of connective tissue and shrinkage of the haemorrhoid. The recurrence rate is 43% at 6 months and may not be any different from laxatives alone.[5]

Coagulation therapy

Other outpatient coagulation procedures include diathermy, electrocautery, infrared photocoagulation and laser photocoagulation, all of which cause mucosal injury (heat, electricity or laser) leading to shrivelling and sloughing of the haemorrhoid. Pain and bleeding are common complications and the results are not as effective as rubber band ligation. Multiple procedures may be required.

Milligan–Morgan haemorrhoidectomy

Haemorrhoidectomy is reserved for third-degree haemorrhoids or failure of non-operative treatment. Patients are placed in a lithotomy position, and three primary haemorrhoids are excised by careful dissection off the internal anal sphincter to leave three raw areas, which are usually left to heal rather than being sutured (for the Ferguson haemorrhoidectomy, each component is sutured). In general, it is important to leave a skin 'bridge' between each of the excised piles in order to prevent anal stenosis and to avoid damage to the anal sphincter.

Complications include delayed bleeding ('reactionary' haemorrhage usually occurs after 10 days), infection, anal stenosis and postoperative faecal incontinence.

RECENT ADVANCES

Surgical treatment of haemorrhoids has been simplified with the introduction of the stapled haemorrhoidectomy technique. This simple operation, in which the haemorrhoids are excised using a circular stapling device inserted into the anus, results in faster recovery and shorter hospital stay.[6]

Prognosis

Haemorrhoids are a benign disease but are characterized by frequent recurrences, depending on the treatment modality. The lowest recurrence rates occur with haemorrhoidectomy.[3]

REFERENCES

(1) Johanson JF, Sonnenberg A. *The prevalence of hemorrhoids and chronic constipation. An epidemiologic study.* Gastroenterology 1990; 98: 380–386.
(2) Johanson JF, Rimm A. *Optimal nonsurgical treatment of hemorrhoids: a comparative analysis of infrared coagulation, rubber band ligation, and injection sclerotherapy.* American Journal of Gastroenterology 1992; 87: 1600–1606.
(3) MacRae HM, McLeod RS, Johanson JF, Rimm A. *Comparison of hemorrhoidal treatment modalities. A meta-analysis.* Diseases of the Colon and Rectum 1995; 38: 687–694.
(4) Komborozos VA, Skrekas GJ, Pissiotis CA. *Rubber band ligation of symptomatic internal hemorrhoids: results of 500 cases.* Digestive Surgery 2000; 17: 71–76.
(5) Senapati A, Nicholls RJ. *A randomised trial to compare the results of injection sclerotherapy with a bulk laxative alone in the treatment of bleeding haemorrhoids.* International Journal of Colorectal Disease 1988; 3: 124–126.
(6) Sutherland LM, Burchard AK, Matsuda K, et al. *A systematic review of stapled hemorrhoidectomy.* Archives of Surgery 2002; 137: 1395–1406; discussion 1407.

Anal fissure

An anal fissure is a linear tear in the mucosa of the anal canal below the dentate line.

Epidemiology

Anal fissure is an exceedingly common complaint. It can occur at any age, but the highest incidence is in the third and fourth decades, with a slight male preponderance.

Pathology

The exact cause of anal fissure is unknown. It may be due to local anal trauma during evacuation of a constipated stool. Spasm of the internal anal sphincter is a consistent finding and is occasionally so severe that the resulting pain and the midline location are thought to originate from sphincter ischaemia.

Scope of disease

Anal fissure itself may lead to constipation due to fear of pain on defecation.

Clinical features

The most common symptom is severe 'tearing' pain on defecation that may persist for a few hours afterwards and change in character to a 'burning' pain. Defecation is often associated with bright red rectal bleeding, usually a streak on the toilet paper. This may be accompanied by pruritus and a mucous discharge.

On examination, most anal fissures occur in the midline posteriorly. At the distal end, a skin tag known as a sentinel pile is often seen. Digital rectal examination is painful, due to stretching of the split mucosa.

Initial investigation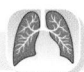

Sigmoidoscopy or proctoscopy

Although external inspection of the anus is usually sufficient to make the diagnosis, visualization of the distal sigmoid and rectum is essential to exclude any other pathology.

Initial management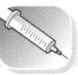

Laxatives

Stool-softening agents such as lactulose or a bulk laxative (e.g. senna) are useful to reduce the pain associated with defecation.

Topical anaesthetic

Local anaesthetic gel can be applied for symptomatic relief.

Medical management

Topical glyceryl trinitrate

The use of 0.2% glyceryl trinitrate ointment applied topically twice daily reduces anal sphincter tone and may be associated with fissure healing. Although a number of randomized trials reported improvements, when a systematic review was restricted to high-quality trials, the odds ratio for improvement of 0.73 compared to placebo was not statistically significant.[1] Headache is the main side effect of glyceryl trinitrate treatment.

Surgical management

Lateral anal sphincterotomy

Lateral anal sphincterotomy is recommended when medical management fails; this is particularly common in chronic fissures. Lateral sphincterotomy allows a much more controlled sphincter injury and is preferred by most surgeons. It is performed by making a small incision adjacent to the anal margin followed by a controlled division of the lower third of the internal sphincter (below the level of the dentate line). The results are superior to glyceryl trinitrate therapy with a comparative odds ratio for recurrence of 0.11. Faecal incontinence occurs in approximately 6%.[2]

Anal dilatation has been largely abandoned as a surgical procedure due to uncontrolled damage to the internal sphincter, with a consequent risk of incontinence.

Excision of anal fissure and flap reconstruction

More resistant fissures may require excision and flap reconstruction using either VY advancement flaps or rhomboid island flaps.

Prognosis

Although they cause distressing symptoms, anal fissures are largely successfully treated with a low recurrence rate of 5%.[2]

REFERENCES

(1) Nelson R. Non surgical therapy for anal fissure. Cochrane Database of Systematic Reviews 2003: CD003431.
(2) Hoffmann DC, Goligher JC. Lateral subcutaneous internal sphincterotomy in treatment of anal fissure. British Medical Journal 1970; 3: 673–675.

Anal fistulae

An anal fistula is an abnormal communication between the anorectum and the external perianal skin. Pus often discharges on to the skin or into the bowel.

Epidemiology

Anal fistulae are common, particularly in the third to fifth decades (occurring at an earlier age in Afro-Caribbeans). Anal fistula is approximately 2–4 times more common in men, and on the Asian subcontinent.

Pathology

Most fistulae occur as a consequence of anorectal sepsis. An inadequately treated perianal abscess may fistulate simultaneously into the bowel lumen and on to the skin, producing a tract of granulation tissue.

Fistulae may also occur secondary to ulcerative colitis or Crohn's disease. The latter is more common and often gives rise to multiple external openings ('watering can' perineum). Tuberculosis is a rare cause.

Anal fistulae are classified into low (internal opening below the dentate line) or high (internal opening above the dentate line) to aid subsequent management.

Clinical features

Symptoms of anal fistulae are intermittent pain and chronic purulent perianal discharge. Occasionally flatus or even stool may be passed via the external opening. On examination, an external orifice is usually seen adjacent to the anus.

Initial investigation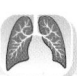

The diagnosis is clinical, but investigations are often necessary to assess the nature and extent of the fistula.

Sigmoidoscopy and proctoscopy

Direct visualization may reveal a low internal opening of the fistula.

Further investigations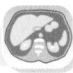

MRI pelvis

MRI of the pelvis is a useful investigation for patients with complex or high fistulae or recurrent fistulae to delineate the anatomy of the fistulae prior to surgery.

Endoanal ultrasound

Where feasible, endoanal ultrasound is also a useful investigation to delineate the anatomy of complex or recurrent fistulae.

Surgical management

The first step in the management of fistulae is an examination under anaesthetic (EUA), at which time the fistula tract is usually probed to assess the anatomy. The following procedures may be required.

Fistulotomy and marsupialization

A low fistula (internal opening below the dentate line) can be either laid open or excised and then allowed to heal from deep to superficial.

Seton placement

If the internal opening is high, it is not safe to lay open the fistula due to the risk of injury to the anal sphincter and consequent faecal incontinence. In such cases, a seton suture may be placed through the fistula tract and tied. A seton may be either tight, slowly cutting the tissues and allowing healing behind as it goes, or loose, acting as a drain for any residual sepsis.

Defunctioning colostomy

In the case of very high or complex fistulae, a defunctioning colostomy may be necessary to divert the faecal stream and promote healing; this is in addition to seton placement or local surgery.

Prognosis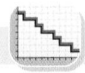

The overall recurrence rate after surgical treatment is 8%. Recurrence usually occurs in complex or recurrent fistulae.[1]

REFERENCE

(1) *Garcia-Aguilar J, Belmonte C, Wong WD, Goldberg SM, Madoff RD. Anal fistula surgery. Factors associated with recurrence and incontinence. Diseases of the Colon and Rectum 1996; 39: 723–729.*

Perianal abscess

A perianal abscess is a collection of pus adjacent to the anal canal.

Epidemiology

Perianal abscesses are very common. They can present at any age in either sex but are more common in young men.

Pathology

Perianal abscesses originate from a focus of bacterial infection in the anal glands between the internal and external anal sphincters. Infection spreads to the perianal tissues, where an abscess develops. Should the infection track laterally, an ischiorectal abscess may develop.

Clinical features

The patient presents with acute pain and swelling adjacent to the anus; this may be accompanied by a fever. If an ischiorectal abscess develops, the patient is often more unwell with systemic signs of infection. Clinical examination reveals a tender, red and hot swelling beside the anal canal.

Investigations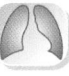

The diagnosis is clinical and investigations are only required if there is a suspected underlying fistula (p. 291).

Surgical management

Incision and drainage

Treatment is by urgent incision and drainage of the abscess. This can be achieved by a simple incision into the abscess or a cruciate incision with deroofing (removal of an ellipse of skin over the abscess). A swab should be taken for microscopy, culture and sensitivity, and the wound should be washed out and if necessary curetted to remove any focus of sepsis or necrotic tissue. The cavity is then packed and regular dressing changes are required to allow the abscess to heal from deep to superficial, minimizing the risk of a residual cavity and recurrent abscess formation.

If an underlying fistula is present, this will require definitive surgery at a later date to prevent recurrence of the abscess.

Prognosis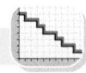

Simple drainage is usually an effective cure, although recurrent abscess formation occasionally occurs.

Diseases of the abdominal wall and herniae

Divarication of recti

Divarication of recti is the midline separation of the two rectus abdominis muscles in the epigastrium.

Epidemiology

Divarication is a relatively common complaint occurring equally in both sexes. It can occur at any age.

Pathology

Divarication is not a true hernia but may result from congenital weakness in the anterior abdominal wall or acquired weakness in the linea alba (e.g. multiple pregnancies).

Scope of disease

Complications are rare.

Clinical features

The patient may present with an intermittent sausage-shaped swelling in the epigastrium. It can be unsightly but rarely causes discomfort. When the anterior abdominal muscles are tensed by raising the legs or head off the bed, the defect becomes more prominent.

Initial investigations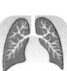

This is a clinical diagnosis and investigations are not required.

Initial management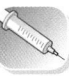

Reassurance
The patient should simply be reassured about the nature of the problem.

Surgical management

Surgical repair
Surgery is reserved for symptomatic or large defects. Usually a Keel suture repair is used, similar to the approach for an incisional hernia.

Prognosis

Divarication is benign and complications are rare.

Umbilical hernia

A true umbilical hernia occurs when a sac of peritoneum protrudes through a defect in the umbilicus, whilst a paraumbilical hernia is one that protrudes through the abdominal wall adjacent to the umbilicus.

Epidemiology

True umbilical herniae are more common in infants, especially on the African subcontinent. In adults, true umbilical herniae are rare, and the paraumbilical hernia is the more common subtype. Both types of hernia are equally common in both sexes.

Pathology

An infant (true) umbilical hernia is due to persistence of the umbilical defect in utero. In adults, chronically raised intra-abdominal pressure (multiple pregnancies, ascites, obesity) may cause reopening of the umbilical defect leading to a true umbilical hernia. A paraumbilical hernia is due to a weakness in the abdominal wall adjacent to the umbilicus.

Scope of disease

Umbilical herniae may be associated with pain on coughing. The neck of the defect is usually small, therefore intestinal obstruction and strangulation (of omentum or bowel) are important complications.

Clinical features

The patient may present with a swelling in or immediately adjacent to the umbilicus. This may be transient and associated with a dragging sensation or pain on coughing.

Feature of intestinal obstruction are presented on page 250, and severe pain or erythema over the swelling is suggestive of strangulation.

Initial investigations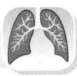

Umbilical hernia is a clinical diagnosis; investigations are not required.

Surgical management

Open hernia repair
In general, all adults with umbilical herniae require hernia repair for symptoms or as a prophylactic measure for

complications. Repair is usually performed through a short transverse incision just above or below the umbilicus. The hernia is reduced and any excess tissue may need excising before repair is performed. If necrotic tissue is found, it will require excision; if non-viable bowel is identified, then bowel resection will be necessary. Best results are currently obtained by tension-free open mesh repair with a 5-year recurrence rate of 1%.[1] Postoperative complications include seroma, haematoma and wound infection.

Prognosis

In general, the prognosis is excellent and recurrence rates after surgery are low.

REFERENCE

(1) Arroyo A, Garcia P, Perez F, Andreu J, Candela F, Calpena R. Randomized clinical trial comparing suture and mesh repair of umbilical hernia in adults. British Journal of Surgery 2001; 88: 1321–1323.

Inguinal hernia

An inguinal hernia is a protrusion of a sac of peritoneum (with or without abdominal content) through a weakness in the abdominal wall of the groin.

Epidemiology

Inguinal herniae are common: the incidence is 130 per 100 000 per year, with a lifetime prevalence of 27% in men and 3% in women.[1] Although herniae can occur at any age, there are two peaks, in infants (congenital herniae) and in the elderly. There is little racial or geographical variation.

Pathology

There are two types of inguinal hernia, direct and indirect. The indirect hernia is the most common type in either sex and at any age.

An indirect hernia protrudes *indirectly* through the abdominal wall as the sac passes through the deep ring, down the inguinal canal before emerging at the superficial inguinal ring. The sac may continue down into the scrotum (Fig. 4.47).

A direct inguinal hernia occurs due to a weakness of the posterior wall of the inguinal canal (i.e. in the transversalis fascia). This type of hernia protrudes *directly* through the abdominal wall and does not descend into the scrotum. It tends to be seen in elderly patients.

Scope of disease

The complications of inguinal hernia are pain, incarceration (when a hernia does not reduce back into the

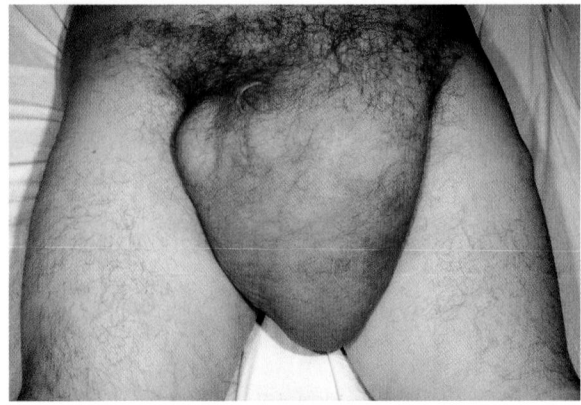

Fig. 4.47 A large left indirect hernia extending into the scrotum.

abdominal cavity, usually due to a small neck or the formation of adhesions), obstruction (when a loop of bowel becomes obstructed within the sac) and strangulation (when a loop of bowel or omentum becomes trapped in the sac in a manner that compresses the blood supply rendering the bowel ischaemic and necrotic).

Variants on the content and complications give rise to a plethora of terms such as a Richter's hernia (where only a knuckle of bowel is trapped and ischaemic without intestinal obstruction) and sliding hernia (or hernia en glissade, when a retroperitoneal structure such as the bladder becomes trapped in the sac).

Clinical features

Symptoms of an uncomplicated inguinal hernia include discomfort (dragging sensation) in the groin associated with a groin swelling. Associated symptoms of complications such as intestinal obstruction are presented on page 250. There may be a history of a precipitating event such as heavy lifting that coincided with the onset of the hernia. Symptoms of exacerbating factors such as chronic cough, constipation and prostatism should be sought.

On examination, an inguinal hernia presents with a groin swelling above and medial to the pubic tubercle. Unless it is incarcerated, a cough impulse is palpable. Severe pain, redness or tenderness over the site of a hernia suggests strangulation.

Once reduced, an indirect hernia can be controlled by pressure over the deep inguinal ring, whereas a direct hernia cannot be controlled in this way. Distinction can only be confirmed during surgery, when an indirect hernia emerges lateral to the inferior epigastric vessels, and a direct hernia medial to these vessels.

Initial investigations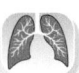

Inguinal hernia is a clinical diagnosis and investigation is rarely needed.

Further investigations

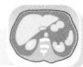

Herniogram

A herniogram may be helpful if there is doubt about the diagnosis. Radio-opaque contrast medium is injected through the anterior abdominal wall and the patient is asked to stand to allow the contrast to flow down into any hernial sac. A plain X-ray is taken and will delineate the outline of a hernia (Fig. 4.48).

Initial management

Addressing exacerbating factors

The underlying cause of any exacerbating factors such as chronic cough, constipation or prostatism should be addressed.

Surgical management

As herniae are progressive, surgery is recommended for patients with symptoms. Elderly patients with poor operative risk and asymptomatic herniae can be safely managed with a truss (hernia support).

Open hernia repair

The operation can be performed as a day case under local anaesthesia, under regional (e.g. spinal) or general anaesthesia (overnight stay). A short skin crease incision is made just above the inguinal ligament and dissection is taken down through subcutaneous fat and Scarpa's fascia to the external oblique aponeurosis. This is then opened along the line of the fibres to expose the inguinal canal and spermatic cord. The ilioinguinal nerve should be identified and preserved, prior to mobilizing the cord.

At this stage, it is necessary to differentiate an indirect from a direct hernia. An indirect sac is dissected free from the cord, opened (Fig. 4.49), emptied, twisted and transfixed at the base. Occasionally the contents of the sac are stuck to the wall of the sac, a so-called 'sliding hernia', in which case the sac is simply reduced as it is. The contents of a hernia sac can include omentum and bowel (Fig. 4.50). A direct hernia sac does not need opening and is simply pushed back through the abdominal wall defect. Plication of the transversalis muscle may help keep back the reduced hernia to facilitate repair.

Although the actual hernia repair (herniorrhaphy) can be performed in many different ways, the Bassini and Shouldice repair are now largely confined to historical interest. In view of the extremely low recurrence rates, the Liechtenstein repair, in which a flat synthetic mesh is sutured over the defect (allowing for a tension-free repair), is the current standard.

The overall recurrence rate is 3%. Other complications include persisting pain (19%), haematoma (11%), superficial wound infection, deep mesh infection (rare) and numbness.[2]

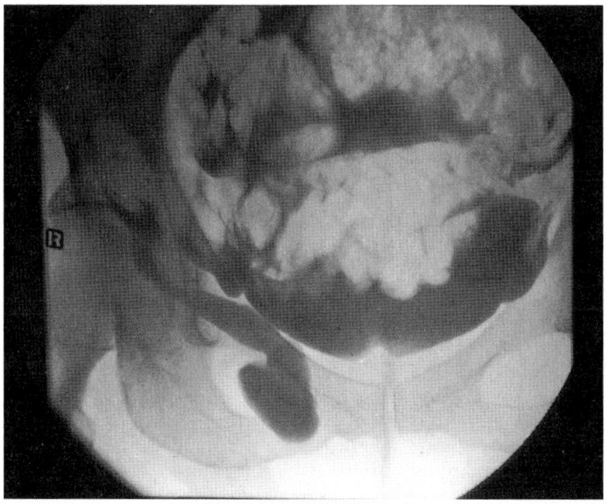

Laparoscopic hernia repair

The main indications for laparoscopic hernia repair are simultaneous bilateral herniae and recurrent herniae. Laparoscopic repair can be performed using either a trans-abdominal preperitoneal approach (TAPP) in which the hernia is accessed via the abdominal cavity and a mesh inserted through the peritoneum to cover potential hernia sites, or a totally extraperitoneal (TEP) approach in which the hernia is accessed through the preperitoneal plane without entering the abdominal cavity.

Recurrence rates with laparoscopic hernia repair are similar to those with open repair, and the recovery time is shorter with less persisting pain and numbness. However, this technique is more expensive, takes longer, and carries higher serious complication rates in respect of visceral (especially bladder) and vascular injuries compared to open repair.[2]

Prognosis

The prognosis in general is excellent and recurrence rates should be less than 3%.

REFERENCES

(1) *Primatesta P, Goldacre MJ. Inguinal hernia repair: incidence of elective and emergency surgery, readmission and mortality. International Journal of Epidemiology 1996; 25: 835–839.*
(2) *McCormack K, Scott NW, Go PM, Ross S, Grant AM. Laparoscopic techniques versus open techniques for inguinal hernia repair. Cochrane Database of Systematic Reviews 2003: CD001785.*

Femoral hernia

A femoral hernia is the protrusion of the extraperitoneal fat and peritoneum, with or without abdominal contents, through the femoral canal.

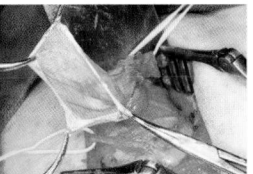

Fig. 4.49 A hernia sac.

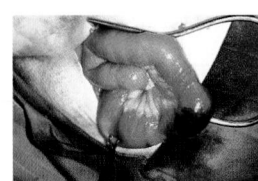

Fig. 4.50 A hernia containing gangrenous small bowel.

Fig. 4.48 A herniogram showing a right indirect hernia sac.

Epidemiology

Femoral hernia tends to occur after middle age (50 years) and is much more common in women than men, especially in the elderly (it should be noted that in women it is still less common than inguinal hernia).

Pathology

Little is known of the aetiology of femoral herniae. The hernial sac passes down through the femoral canal and appears in the groin below and lateral to the pubic tubercle; it may contain omentum or bowel.

Scope of disease

The complications are similar to those of inguinal hernia (p. 294) but strangulation is more common.

Clinical features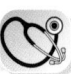

The patient may present with pain and a swelling in the groin. Associated symptoms of complications such as intestinal obstruction are described on page 250.

On examination, the neck of the hernia is below and lateral to the pubic tubercle. Unlike an inguinal hernia, it is often not completely reducible. Severe pain, redness or tenderness over the site of a hernia suggests strangulation. The differential diagnosis includes saphena varix, femoral artery aneurysm, lymphadenopathy and psoas abscess.

Initial investigation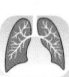

This is a clinical diagnosis and investigation is rarely needed, although ultrasound may be helpful.

Further investigations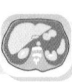

Herniogram
If there is any doubt about the diagnosis, a herniogram (Fig. 4.51) may be helpful.

Ultrasound scan
An ultrasound scan may be required to distinguish between nodes, a saphena varix or femoral artery aneurysm.

Surgical management

Unless there is prohibitive operative risk, all femoral herniae should be repaired to prevent potential complications.

Open hernia repair
Open repair is usually performed through a short groin crease incision. The hernia is reduced and any excess tissue may need excising before repair is performed using several interrupted non-absorbable sutures, usually using a J-shaped needle. Alternatively, the defect may be closed with a mesh plug.

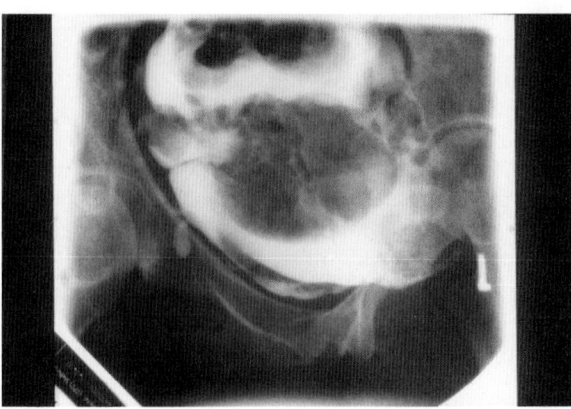

Fig. 4.51 A herniogram revealing a small right femoral hernia.

Resection is necessary for necrotic tissue or infarcted bowel. If bowel entrapment is suspected, a high approach through the back of the inguinal canal gives better surgical access.

Prognosis

The recurrence rate is very low, and the prognosis is usually excellent.

Incisional hernia

An incisional hernia is a hernia through an acquired scar.

Epidemiology

Incisional herniae are common, although the frequency of this complication varies according to the site and type of operation. There is no sex predilection, and such herniae are slightly more common in the elderly.

Pathology

Predisposing factors to incisional hernia include wound infection, suture failure, poor tissue (in the elderly and patients with malignant disease) and poor surgical technique.

Scope of disease

Abdominal incisional herniae may contain omentum or bowel, which often adheres to the sac. The risk of intestinal obstruction or strangulation is related to the size of the neck of the hernia sac: the smaller the neck, the greater the risk.

Clinical features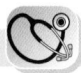

The patient presents with a swelling (intermittent or irreducible) over or adjacent to the scar of a previous wound (Fig. 4.52). It often causes discomfort and may be painful.

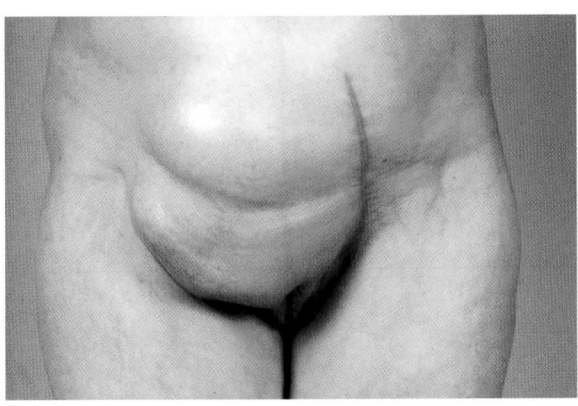

Fig. 4.52 An incisional hernia. The hernia can be seen to the patient's right of the laparotomy scar.

Symptoms of intestinal obstruction or strangulation are presented on page 250.

Initial investigation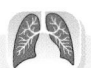

Incisional hernia is a clinical diagnosis and investigation is rarely needed.

Surgical management

Open hernia repair

The indications for surgical repair are the onset of symptoms or risk of intestinal obstruction. The wound is reopened and the sac is dissected off the surrounding tissues. It may be necessary to divide any adhesions within the sac so that clean edges of the defect can be produced.

The edges may be simply apposed or overlapped (Mayo repair). Other repairs are the Keel repair, in which the edges are apposed and a second layer of sutures tightens and strengthens the repair, or an interrupted 'near and far' suture. The important factors are adequate freshening up of the edges of the defect and the use of interrupted sutures.

Alternatively, a mesh repair may be used, especially for large defects where the edges of the defect cannot be directly apposed. Even where the edges have been pulled together, a mesh over the sutures to further strengthen the repair is associated with lower recurrence. It is usually wise to insert a suction drain to prevent haematoma formation.

> **RECENT ADVANCES**
>
> *Incisional herniae may now be repaired using laparoscopic techniques. A mesh is placed inside the peritoneal cavity to cover the defect. It is held in place either with sutures or tacks. Patient recovery may be more rapid with less pain, but randomized trials are awaited.*

Prognosis

Recurrence rates following surgical repair are low and the prognosis in general is excellent.

Rare abdominal herniae

Other abdominal herniae are relatively uncommon and are classified according to anatomical site.

An *epigastric hernia* is a midline hernia in the epigastric region that occurs through a defect in the linea alba between the rectus muscles. A *Spigelian hernia* is seen at the lateral edge of the rectus abdominis, emerging through a defect in the transversus and internal oblique fascia midway between the umbilicus and symphysis pubis. It is uncommon and can be difficult to diagnose as it is covered by the external oblique muscle. An *obturator hernia* emerges through the obturator foramen and is found in the perineal area. A *gluteal hernia* protrudes between the muscles in the gluteal region and presents in the buttock area, and a *lumbar hernia* comes out between the muscles of the lumbar region, presenting in the flank.

Apart from the epigastric hernia, diagnosis of these herniae can be difficult and may require imaging with ultrasound, CT or MRI. Surgical repair is usually required upon the diagnosis of these rare herniae.

Diseases of the liver, biliary system and pancreas

5

Christopher Callaghan, Wing-Kin Syn, Monz Ahmed, Paul Gibbs

Diseases of the liver

SECTION 5.1 Introduction

Applied basic sciences of the hepatobiliary system

Anatomy

The liver lies in the upper right part of the abdominal cavity, extending up to the left lateral line. It is usually divided into a left and a right lobe based on the falciform ligament and fissure of the ligamentum teres. On the inferior surface there are two prominences, the caudate and the quadrate lobes, which are separated by the porta hepatis. The gallbladder lies in a shallow fossa of the quadrate lobe. Although the liver has four lobes (right, left, caudate and quadrate), in terms of vascular supply and physiological function it is divided into eight physiological segments, numbered I to IV in the left liver and V to VIII in the right liver (Fig. 5.1). Anatomical knowledge of liver segmentation is applied to liver resections.

The liver receives 20% of the cardiac output via the hepatic artery and portal vein. The hepatic artery delivers about 33% of the blood flow while the portal vein delivers the rest. The portal vein and hepatic artery divide into left and right branches, with further subdivisions beyond the porta hepatis. Hepatic arterioles and portal venules then drain into sinusoids. Blood flows from the portal triad along sinusoids towards the hepatic venules. These hepatic venules form three major hepatic veins, right, middle and left, which drain into the inferior vena cava.

Hepatocytes near the portal triad are called periportal hepatocytes. This area is also known as zone 1 in Rappaport's concept. Hepatocytes near the hepatic veins are called perivenular hepatocytes and are located in zone 3. Zone 2 refers to hepatocytes located in between. The location of hepatocytes is important because those in zone 3 are more susceptible to drug and toxic effects and vascular-related conditions.

Physiology

The liver takes part in a wide variety of metabolic processes that include carbohydrate, fat and protein metabolism. All plasma proteins (including clotting factors) except part of gamma globulin are produced in the liver; thus, assessment of the synthetic function of the liver includes the measurement of serum albumin and assessment of the coagulation profile. In addition to metabolism, the liver also acts as the storage organ for vitamins, especially A, B_{12} and D. Iron is usually stored in the liver as ferritin. The excretory functions of the liver include removal of bile (Fig. 5.2), hormones and drugs.

299

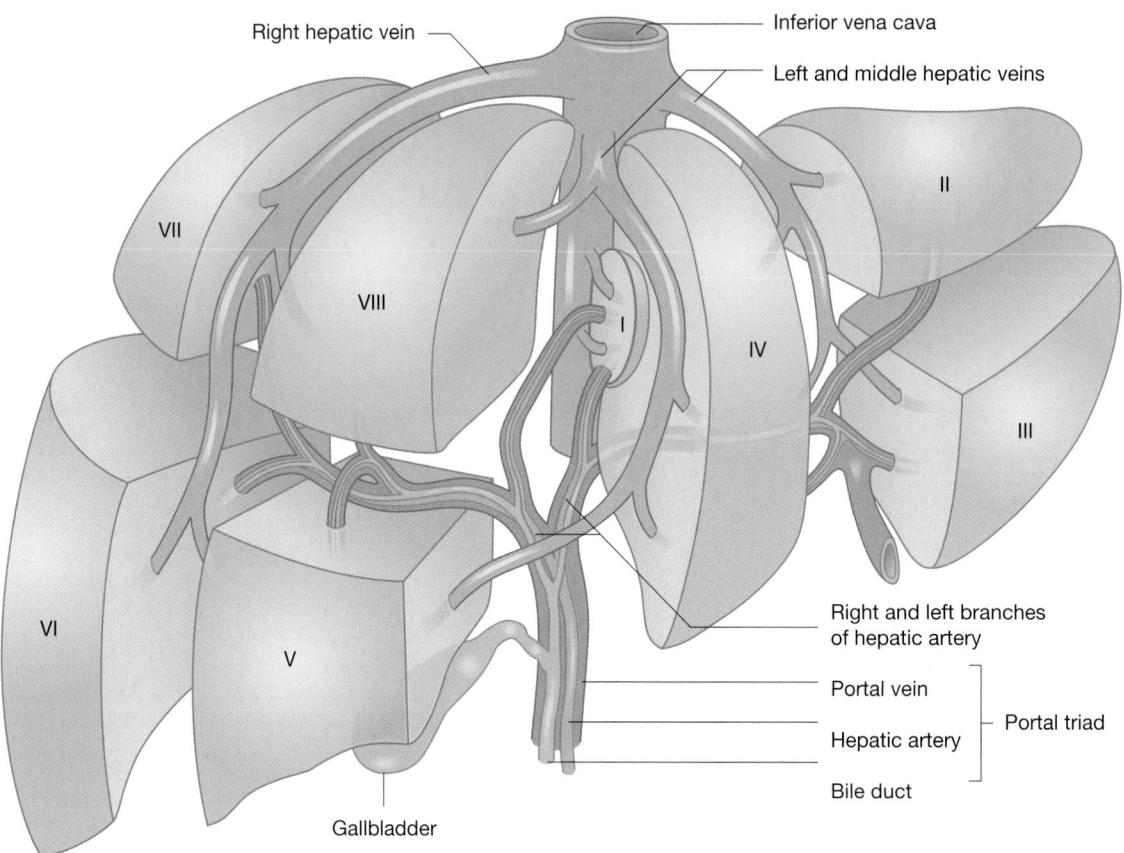

Fig. 5.1 Liver segmentation. There are eight hepatic segments divided on the basis of their separate arterial and portal venous supply and biliary drainage. Segment I is also known as the caudate lobe. The right, middle, and left hepatic veins drain multiple segments. The falciform ligament marks the boundary between the left lateral segment (segments II and III) and the rest of the liver.

Symptoms of hepatobiliary disease

Abdominal pain

Abdominal pain can be a symptom of liver or biliary disease. Right upper quadrant pain can occur with biliary colic, a common misnomer as the pain is usually constant. Right upper quadrant pain can also occur with cholecystitis and cholangitis. Tender hepatomegaly can occur with hepatitis and rarer manifestations of hepatic vascular disease. Dragging abdominal pain can be a feature of hepatomegaly.

Abdominal distension

Abdominal distension can occur with moderate to severe ascites.

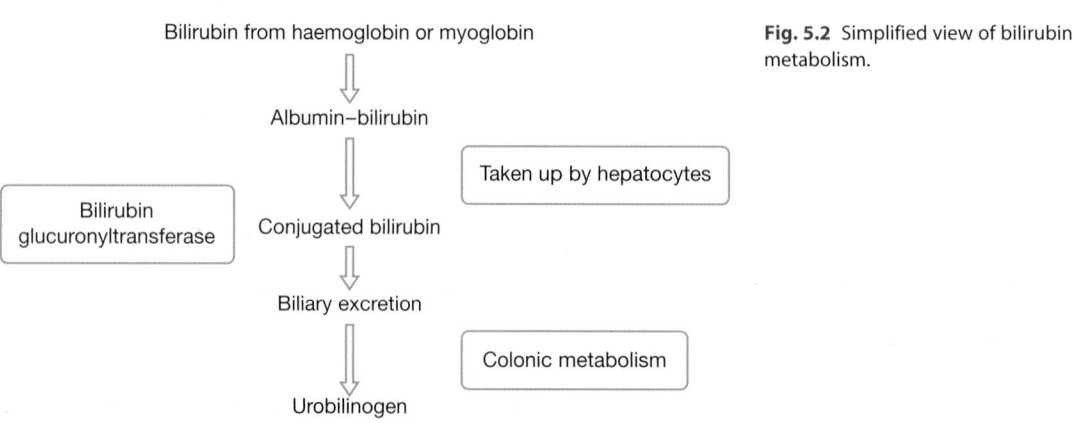

Fig. 5.2 Simplified view of bilirubin metabolism.

Appetite or weight change

Nausea and anorexia can be a non-specific symptom of liver disease. An unpleasant taste in the mouth classically occurs with hepatitis, and patients may even stop smoking. Cachexia can be associated with advanced malignancy.

Jaundice

Jaundice is a common symptom with biliary and severe liver disease and is presented in detail on page 310.

Bruising

Bruising of skin can occur with prolonged coagulation from impaired synthesis of coagulation factors by the liver.

Confusion

Severe liver failure can result in encephalopathy (Table 5.1) and coma.

Occupation and travel history

During history taking, it is very important to enquire about occupation, travel and recreational history: diseases such as leptospirosis are more common in sewage workers, and travel to hepatitis endemic areas would increase the clinical suspicion for hepatitis. In addition, risk factors for hepatitis include a job in health care, intravenous drug abuse and sexual contacts.

Examination of the hepatobiliary system

Inspection

The examination begins with the assessment of the patient's mental state and ability to communicate. Deficiencies in communication or orientation may suggest encephalopathy or other neurological deficits. The nutritional state can be assessed generally by inspection. Cachexia is common with liver disease (tumours, alcohol). The abdomen should be inspected for any distension, mass or scars.

Clubbing is non-specific. It can be secondary to chronic liver disease (alcoholic liver disease, primary biliary cirrhosis), coeliac disease, lymphoma, inflammatory bowel

disease and malignancy. Nail changes should be carefully noted. Koilonychia (spoon-shaped nails) suggests iron deficiency, and leukonychia (pale nails) is indicative of hypoalbuminaemia. Palmar erythema occurs in alcoholic liver disease, sepsis, pregnancy, hyperthyroidism and with the use of the oral contraceptive pill. Dupuytren's contractures (p. 539) may be associated with alcohol excess.

The arms are inspected for tattoos and intravenous puncture sites (risk factors for hepatitis C and human immunodeficiency virus—HIV). Spontaneous bruising may occur with significant liver impairment due to impaired synthetic function.

Excess alcohol consumption may cause a Cushingoid appearance (p. 422) and parotid enlargement. Cholesterol deposits occur around the eyelids with cholestatic diseases. Jaundice (yellow pigmentation of the sclerae) may be detectable when bilirubin levels are above 50 µmol/L (Fig. 5.3). Pallor of the conjunctiva suggests anaemia.

Spider naevi (dilated arterioles with small radiating vessels in the distribution of the superior vena cava) may be seen and usually indicate liver disease (possibly due to excess oestrogen). Hereditary haemorrhagic telangiectasia is associated with arterio-venous malformations in the liver, biliary obstruction and portal hypertension. Gynaecomastia (enlargement of breast tissue) occurs in cirrhosis, due to excess oestrogen levels. Body hair is often lost in end-stage liver disease. Peripheral oedema occurs with hypoalbuminaemia.

In the abdomen, scars from previous surgery may aid the clinical diagnosis; for example, previous major surgery with features of portal hypertension could be related to portal venous thrombosis. Dilated collaterals on the anterior abdominal wall are present in inferior vena cava obstruction and portal venous hypertension. Direction of venous flow, however, differs. In inferior vena cava obstruction, blood flows superiorly towards the heart, whilst in portal hypertension blood flows inferiorly (away from the umbilicus). Distension of the abdomen may represent ascites formation or organomegaly.

Palpation

During examination it is important to ensure that the patient is not in any discomfort and that privacy is maintained at all times. Light palpation is essential to determine areas of peritonism. Deep palpation is then performed to determine the presence of masses. Each quadrant of the abdomen is systematically examined so as not to miss any lesion, paying attention to the spleen, liver, kidneys and organs originating from the pelvis.

Starting from the right iliac fossa, the liver edge is palpated using the lateral border of the index finger. The liver will move inferiorly during chest inspiration, therefore the liver edge is best palpated during inspiration. The causes of hepatomegaly are listed in Table 5.2.

The spleen moves inferiorly with inspiration towards the right iliac fossa. Palpation should start from the right upper quadrant and proceed towards the left upper quadrant.

Table 5.1	Grading of hepatic encephalopathy
Grade 0	Normal mental state
Grade 1	Mental changes such as lack of awareness, anxiety, eutrophia, inability to add and subtract
Grade 2	Lethargy, disorientation, personality changes, inappropriate behaviour
Grade 3	Stupor, gross disorientation, confusion
Grade 4	Coma

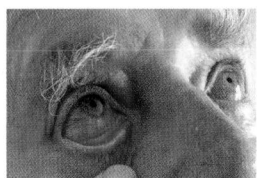

Fig. 5.3 Jaundice.

301

Table 5.2	Causes of hepatomegaly
Hepatitis (inflammation/infective)	
Malignancy (primary and secondary)	
Vascular congestion (heart failure)	
Early cirrhosis (liver disease)	
Fatty liver	
Haematological disease	
Storage diseases	

Table 5.3	Causes of splenomegaly
Portal hypertension	
Infection (malaria, kala-azar)	
Haematological disease (lymphoma or myelofibrosis or leukaemia or haemolysis)	
Splenic vein thrombosis	
Storage disease	

Once palpable, the spleen is already enlarged to twice its normal size. It is essential to differentiate masses in the left iliac fossa, particularly between the left kidney and spleen. The spleen moves inferiorly and towards the right iliac fossa with inspiration; it also has a notch on the medial border. One cannot get above the spleen during palpation. Unlike the kidney, the spleen is dull to percussion, and the kidney is ballotable while the spleen is not. The causes of splenomegaly are listed in Table 5.3.

Percussion

Dullness to percussion of the flanks suggests the presence of ascites. When the patient is rolled, the fluid will shift with gravity and the dullness in the flank that is superior will disappear (shifting dullness). Usually at least 2 L of ascites is present when shifting dullness is elicited.

Another method of confirming fluid in the abdominal cavity is the fluid thrill. The patient is asked to place his hand (medial border) in the middle of the anterior abdom-inal wall. Then with one hand on the flank of the abdomen, the opposite flank is 'flicked' with a finger. The vibration is transmitted by the ascites to the opposite flank and hand. The purpose of the patient's hand is to reduce any transmission of vibration along the cutaneous tissues. Generally, this can only be elicited when a large amount of ascites is present.

Auscultation

Absence of bowel sounds suggests paralytic ileus or large-volume ascites. Liver bruits can occur with vascular tumours, including hepatocellular carcinoma.

Additional procedures

Inspection of the urine and stool is useful. Pale stools and dark urine occur with obstructive jaundice. Dark sticky stool (melaena) suggests upper gastrointestinal bleeding (e.g. from oesophageal varices), while fresh blood suggests lower gastrointestinal bleeding (rectal varices). Scrotal examination should be performed as testicular atrophy occurs in the setting of chronic liver disease.

SECTION 5.2	**Investigations for hepatobiliary disease**

Blood tests

The liver profile

The standard liver biochemical profile (Table 5.4) is often termed 'liver function tests', but many of the measures do not assess liver function. The pattern of abnormalities in the liver profile can suggest an underlying disease process or be used to monitor the course of disease or response to therapy.

It is important that the results of the liver profile should be interpreted in a clinical context: the results may be abnormal without liver involvement (e.g. renal failure), and the biochemical abnormalities may not relate to the clinical state of the patient.

Table 5.4	The standard liver biochemistry panel
Bilirubin	
Alkaline phosphatase (ALP)	
Gamma (γ)-glutamyltransferase (GGT)	
Aspartate aminotransferase (AST)	
Alanine aminotransferase (ALT)	
Albumin/total protein	

Table 5.5	Types of liver injury	
	Hepatocyte predominant	Cholestatic predominant
AST and ALT	↑↑↑	↑
ALP and GGT	↑ or ↑↑	↑↑↑
Bilirubin	↑ or ↑↑	↑↑ or ↑↑↑
Examples	Autoimmune	Extrahepatic biliary obstruction
	Drugs	Intrahepatic cholestasis
	Viral hepatitis	Alcoholic hepatitis
	Ischaemic hepatitis	
	Metabolic diseases	

Injuries to the liver are never isolated to hepatocytes or biliary epithelium. In the majority of cases, most liver enzymes are elevated. In general the degree of AST and ALT elevation can help differentiate between the two processes, but the clinical context is usually a better means.

Blood tests

Investigations of encephalopathy

Diagnostic imaging

Tests of liver synthetic function

The only tests in the standard liver profile that may reflect the true function or reserve of the liver are the serum albumin and prothrombin time.

Serum albumin

Low levels of serum albumin may indicate a poor liver synthetic function and correlate with the severity of chronic liver disease (p. 299). However, serum albumin levels are also affected by nutrition, renal disease and catabolic states.

Prothrombin time

The liver synthesizes most clotting factors, including the vitamin K-dependent factors. Liver impairment can lead to deficiency of clotting factors and a prolonged prothrombin time (assuming that vitamin K levels are normal). Vitamin K clotting factors have a shorter half-life than albumin, therefore the prolonged prothrombin time arises before the drop in serum albumin.

Tests for hepatocellular damage

Aspartate and alanine aminotransferases

Aspartate (AST) and alanine (ALT) aminotransferases are intracellular enzymes that are released during hepatic necrosis. They are useful markers of hepatocellular injury that are elevated in inflammatory, focal and diffuse diseases of the liver. In addition, mild elevations also occur with obstructive biliary tract disease. Marked elevations of the aminotransferases (>1000 i.u.) are usually due to drug-induced, viral, or ischaemic hepatitis.

AST is less specific than ALT as it can also be released from the heart and skeletal muscle. In general, point estimates of both aminotransferases do not correlate well with prognosis or severity of liver disease; the monitoring of the trends is more useful (Table 5.5).

Tests of biliary stasis/cholestatic injury

Alkaline phosphatase

Alkaline phosphatase (ALP) is a group of enzymes involved in the transfer of phosphate. Alkaline phosphatase is a membrane-derived enzyme, therefore hepatic parenchymal damage will result in mild elevations. Alkaline phosphatase production is also stimulated by bile acids, and alkaline phosphatase can be markedly elevated when there is obstruction to bile acid flow.

Alkaline phosphatase is also produced in the bones, intestine and placenta. Although the specific isoenzymes can help determine the source, in practice clinicians rely on the clinical context and other supporting investigations.

Gamma-glutamyltransferase

Gamma (γ)-glutamyltransferase (GGT) is found in hepatocytes and the biliary epithelium. It is the most sensitive (but not specific) indicator of hepatobiliary disease. It is elevated in other diseases of the kidney, pancreas and the heart. Elevated levels of γ-glutamyltransferase can be induced by alcohol and certain drugs. The source of an elevated alkaline phosphatase level is more likely to be hepatic when there is an accompanying rise in glutamyltransferase.

Other investigations in the liver profile

Bilirubin

Bilirubin is not a liver enzyme, it is a pigment produced by the breakdown of red cells. Bilirubin is normally bound to albumin, conjugated by liver and excreted as bile. Levels of bilirubin can be elevated (causing jaundice) in a number of conditions (p. 320). Laboratories normally measure total bilirubin, and fractionation of bilirubin (unconjugated and conjugated fractions) can be helpful in determining the source of the defect in the metabolism or excretion.

Lactate dehydrogenase

Lactate dehydrogenase may be part of the liver profile, but by itself it is not a specific marker of liver disease (it is elevated in many conditions). It is a useful marker in ischaemic and haematological diseases of the liver.

Glucose

Hypoglycaemia is a useful indicator of the severity of liver injury when the gluconeogenesis and glycogenolysis functions of the liver become impaired.

Lactic acid/pH

The liver normally metabolizes lactate, producing carbon dioxide. In acute liver failure the metabolic function becomes impaired, resulting in lactic acidosis. Unfortunately, high levels of lactic acid are not a specific marker of liver impairment, as lactic acid is also produced by anaerobic respiration. Therefore any impairment of circulation and perfusion (including dehydration) can give rise to lactate production.

Total protein

Apart from albumin, other proteins such as fibrinogen, transferrin, globulins and albumin are also produced by the liver. Low total protein levels can occur with liver impairment, but this is not specific to liver disease. Low protein levels can also occur with poor nutrition and renal impairment. In catabolic states (sepsis), there may be a shift in production from albumin to globulin.

Bile acids

Bile acids are useful in the assessment of pregnancy-related liver disease.

Full blood count

The full blood count is a useful investigation in liver disease. Portal hypertension and hypersplenism can lead to pancytopenia. Alcohol excess is associated with folate deficiency (pancytopenia and high mean corpuscular volume—MCV), and Wilson's disease is associated with haemolysis.

Immunoglobulins

IgA is elevated in alcohol-related liver disease and non-alcoholic steatohepatitis. IgM is elevated in primary biliary cirrhosis, and IgG is elevated in autoimmune hepatitis.

Autoantibodies

Specific autoantibodies associated with liver disease are anti-smooth muscle antibody (autoimmune hepatitis), antimitochondrial antibody (primary biliary cirrhosis) and antinuclear antibody (autoimmune hepatitis). It is important to note that antibodies are present in many overlapping conditions and a full panel is required to exclude associated conditions.

Iron studies

Iron studies are usually performed for the investigation of haemochromatosis (p. 331) and consist of the estimation of serum iron, ferritin and transferrin saturations (iron-binding capacity).

Copper studies

Copper studies are performed for the investigation of Wilson's disease and consist of serum caeruloplasmin and serum copper. In addition, 24-hour copper excretion and 24-hour copper excretion after penicillamine challenge is also performed.

Tumour markers

Tumour markers such as alpha (α)-fetoprotein are elevated in some patients with hepatocellular carcinoma and liver inflammation (hepatitis). CA19-9 is elevated in pancreatic malignancies, cholangiocarcinoma, cholangitis and hepatocellular carcinoma and can be falsely elevated in the presence of ascites or pleural effusions.

Investigations of encephalopathy

Serum ammonia

Serum ammonia is elevated in liver dysfunction due to failure of the breakdown of ammonia (shunting of blood in portal hypertension) and is believed to have a role in the pathogenesis of hepatic encephalopathy (despite poor correlation of ammonia levels and neuropsychiatric state).

Number connection test

The number connection test documents the minimum time taken for a subject to join a series of numbers in ascending order. Repeated tests can be done to assess for any changes in higher cortical function from encephalopathy.

Copying 5-pointed star test

Constructional apraxia results in the inability to copy a 5-pointed star.

Electroencephalogram (EEG)

The EEG can be used to diagnose hepatic encephalopathy.

Diagnostic imaging

Abdominal ultrasound

Abdominal ultrasound is usually the first-line imaging modality for the liver, as it is radiation free and relatively inexpensive. Ultrasound can readily image the size and texture of the liver and detect any focal lesion of more than 1 cm.

Doppler examination is able to detect flow abnormalities (thrombus) in the portal and hepatic vessels. Assessment of blood flow is particularly important after liver transplantation and for the detection of collateral vessels in portal hypertension. Microbubbles can be used to assist the evaluation of hepatic artery flow.

In addition, ultrasound imaging can assist in aspiration of ascites, placement of pigtail drains and targeting difficult liver biopsies or specific abnormalities of the liver.

CT of the liver

CT scanning provides more detailed imaging of the liver and adjacent structures, although it involves exposure to radiation. Injection of lipoidal contrast can be performed to identify hepatocellular carcinomas. CT is also used for the drainage of abdominal collections, placement of hepatic drains and guiding liver biopsies.

MRI of the liver

Magnetic resonance imaging is increasingly used to image the hepatobiliary tree and vessels. It allows for focused imaging and three-dimensional reconstructions. It is free from radiation. New contrast agents such as manganese are taken up by hepatocytes and can be used to facilitate the detection of hepatocellular carcinoma.

Liver biopsy

Endoscopic retrograde cholangio-pancreatography

Percutaneous transhepatic cholangiography

Diagnostic procedures

Liver biopsy

Indications

Liver biopsy is an important part of the assessment of liver disease. It can be a diagnostic procedure or be utilized for the assessment of disease severity or viability of allograft liver transplants. The indications and contraindications are presented in Tables 5.6 and 5.7, respectively.

Patient preparation

Patients are admitted to hospital. A full blood count, coagulation screen and a group and save are performed. A single dose of oral ciprofloxacin (500 mg) is administered as antibiotic prophylaxis (for patients with previous biliary reconstruction).

In patients with an elevated prothrombin time (impaired hepatic synthetic function) fresh frozen plasma is administered prior to the procedure. Platelet transfusion is performed if the platelet count is between 40 and 60×10^9/L. In patients with a platelet count of less than 40×10^9/L, a transvenous approach to liver biopsy should be undertaken.

Table 5.6	Indications for liver biopsy
Diagnosis	
Investigation of hepatomegaly	
Investigation of abnormal liver function tests	
Suspected cirrhosis	
Biopsy of focal liver lesions (except suspected hepatocellular carcinoma, due to risk of tumour seeding)	
Assessment of disease severity	
Pretreatment for viral hepatitis	
Chronic hepatitis	
Drug-related hepatitis	
Storage diseases	
Assessment of the viability of liver transplant	

Table 5.7	Contraindications to blind percutaneous liver biopsy
Absolute	
Uncooperative patient (untoward movements can result in capsular tears and bleeding)	
Uncorrected prolonged coagulation times (PT/INR)	
Uncorrected thrombocytopenia	
Dilated biliary system (risk of biliary peritonitis; the transvenous route should be used)	
Bacterial cholangitis (increased risk of peritonitis and shock)	
Cystic lesions (increased risk of biliary peritonitis)	
Relative	
Amyloidosis (increased bleeding risk)	
Ascites (increased bleeding risk and technical failure; paracentesis or laparoscopic procedures should be used)	

PT, prothrombin time; INR, international normalized ratio.

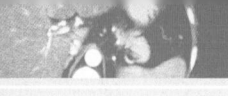
The patient should also have a liver ultrasound prior to the procedure to rule out anatomical variations, or in conjunction with the procedure to identify focal lesions and to guide the liver biopsy

Procedure

Percutaneous liver biopsy

The transthoracic approach is most commonly used. The patient lies supine and the liver borders are identified by percussion or ultrasound. The target should be at the centre of dullness (between both borders) and along the midaxillary line. The area is prepared and 10 mL of 1% lidocaine is injected into the liver capsule. The patient is asked to hold his breath on expiration and 1–3 biopsies are undertaken using either a Menghini or Tru-Cut needle. This process is also performed with ultrasound guidance when available.

Complications include mortality (0.3%), intraperitoneal bleeding (leading to laparotomy), pneumothorax, intra-abdominal organ injury (gallbladder, bowel, kidneys) leading to haemobilia (0.5%) and peritonitis. Fracture of the biopsy needle can occur, as can failure to obtain an adequate sample.

Transvenous liver biopsy

A transvenous approach is recommended in patients with a significant risk of bleeding (coagulopathy, thrombocytopenia). If bleeding should occur, the blood extravasates into the intravascular space. Access is obtained using a catheter inserted into the internal jugular or femoral vein.

Under fluoroscopy, the catheter is advanced into the hepatic veins. A biopsy needle is passed through the catheter and advanced into the liver parenchyma to acquire biopsy specimens.

Complications include transient and usually self-terminating arrhythmias (as the right atrium is traversed) and perforation of the liver capsule.

Laparoscopic and open liver biopsy

This is rarely undertaken and involves surgical exploration for the acquisition of a biopsy specimen. Either laparoscopy or a laparotomy (in patients with previous abdominal surgery) is performed, and the liver capsule is identified. A section of the liver is then obtained under direct vision. Any bleeding is arrested during this procedure, and routine closures of the wounds are performed. Intraperitoneal bleeding is an unusual complication from surgical liver biopsies.

Post procedure care

Pain is a common complaint and regular analgesics are required. The majority of complications occur in the first 3 hours after biopsy. Patients are advised to stay for 6 hours after the procedure, during which time regular monitoring of the blood pressure and pulse is undertaken.

Endoscopic retrograde cholangio-pancreatography

Endoscopic retrograde cholangio-pancreatography (ERCP) is an endoscopic procedure to examine the biliary tree and pancreatic ducts. Through the use of specialized instruments and techniques, ERCP can also be used for crushing and extracting stones, dilating strictures and placing stents.

Indications

The indications for ERCP are numerous (Table 5.8). Contraindications include anaphylaxis to contrast agents and severe cardiorespiratory disease. Previous gastric surgery, abnormal anatomy of the duodenal papilla, and pathology of the ampulla (e.g. tumour, stricture) can prevent papillary cannulation and result in ERCP failure in 5–10%.

Patient preparation

Patients are admitted to hospital. A full blood count, urea and electrolytes, liver function tests, serum amylase, coagulation screen and a group and save are performed. Fresh frozen plasma may be required for patients with prolonged prothrombin time and platelets are required for patients with a platelet count less than 60×10^9/L. Intravenous fluids are given and patients are fasted for 6 hours before the procedure.

A prophylactic antibiotic such as cefuroxime, ciprofloxacin or Tazocin may be given an hour before the procedure, especially in patients who are at high risk of infection (e.g. previous cholangitis or an obstructed biliary system).

Table 5.8	Indications for endoscopic retrograde cholangio-pancreatography (ERCP)

Diagnostic

Common bile duct and hepatic duct stones

Strictures in the biliary tree

Ampullary lesions

Head of pancreas lesion

Investigation of haemobilia

Investigation of an obstructed biliary tree

Confirm primary or secondary sclerosing cholangitis

Anatomical variants (e.g. pancreas divisum)

Brushings and aspirates for cytology (false negative rates of 40–50%)

Therapeutic

Sphincterotomy to allow passage of stones

Balloon trawl or baskets to remove stones

Mechanical lithotripsy to crush stones

Dilatation of strictures

Placement of pancreatic or biliary stents

Management of post-cholecystectomy bile leaks

Management of severe acute pancreatitis (with biliary dilatation)

Procedure

The patient lies in the left lateral position. The left arm is placed behind the patient's back. The right arm/hand is free, hence the cannula is placed here.

Sedation and analgesia are given to keep the patient comfortable. A simple regimen includes midazolam 5 mg i.v., pethidine 50 mg i.v. and hyoscine butylbromide 20 mg i.v. (to reduce bowel contractions). A side-viewing duodenoscope is passed into the oesophagus, stomach and duodenum. Biopsy and cytology samples can be taken from these regions if required. The major duodenal papilla is identified and cannulated. The common bile duct or pancreatic duct can be selectively catheterized by altering the angle of entry into the papilla. Contrast is injected and filling of the intra- and extrahepatic biliary tree and pancreatic duct can be achieved by tilting the table and altering the patient's position (Fig. 5.4).

Instrumentation or stenting of the pancreatic or biliary ducts usually requires ablation of the sphincter of Oddi with electrocautery to allow access (sphincterotomy). Biliary stents are often placed for tumours of the ampulla or pancreatic head (Fig. 5.5). Temporary dilatation of the sphincter can be achieved with balloon inflation (endoscopic balloon sphincteroplasty). Pancreatic or biliary stones can be removed using a wire (Dormia) basket or balloon catheter. Stone crushing can also be performed.

Complications

ERCP is associated with a complication rate of 5–10% (Table 5.9) and mortality of 0.1% (from severe acute pancreatitis or acute cholangitis). Complication and mortality rates are twice as high when sphincterotomy is performed.[1] The most common complication is acute pancreatitis, but most cases are mild and resolve in a few days. Transient

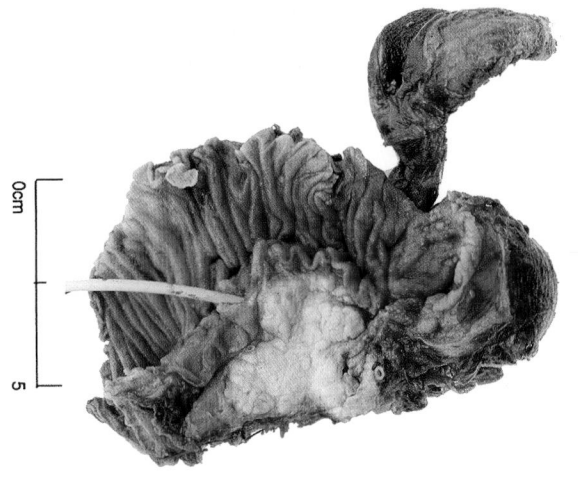

Fig. 5.5 Biliary stent. Pathology specimen of a pancreatic head adenocarcinoma with a green stent protruding out of the major papilla. The gallbladder is also seen. Courtesy Dr S. Davies, Addenbrooke's Hospital, Cambridge, UK.

asymptomatic hyperamylasaemia occurs in 50%, but has no clinical importance. Reactions to sedative drugs and/or contrast agents can also occur.

RECENT ADVANCES

Newer, less invasive techniques (magnetic resonance cholangio-pancreatography—MRCP, spiral CT, endoscopic ultrasound) have begun to replace ERCP for diagnosis alone (Table 5.10). Gabexate, somatostatin, glyceryl trinitrate and diclofenac have been shown to reduce the rate of ERCP-induced pancreatitis, though none is presently in routine use. Insertion of temporary pancreatic stents and the use of alternative investigations (e.g. MRCP, endoscopic ultrasound) may also help to avoid post-ERCP pancreatitis.[2]

REFERENCES

(1) *Freeman ML, Nelson DB, Sherman S, et al. Complications of endoscopic biliary sphincterotomy. New England Journal of Medicine 1996; 335: 909–918.*
(2) *Freeman ML. Prevention of post-ERCP pancreatitis: pharmacologic solution or patient selection and pancreatic stents? Gastroenterology 2003; 124: 1977–1980.*

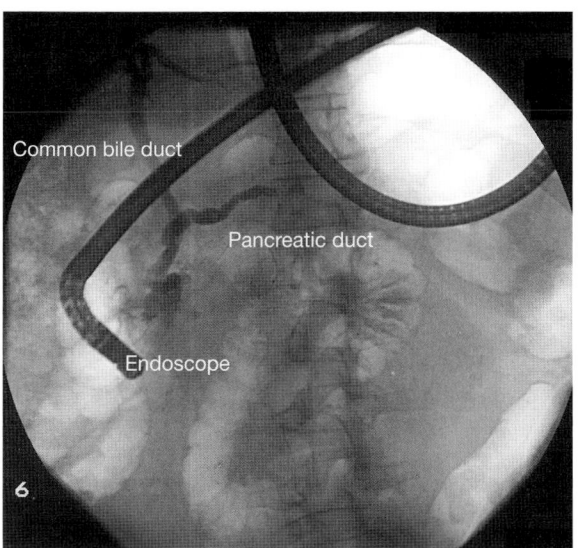

Fig. 5.4 Endoscopic retrograde cholangio-pancreatography (ERCP). A normal ERCP showing contrast in the biliary and pancreatic ducts.
Copyright Addenbrooke's Hospital, Cambridge, UK.

Table 5.9	Complications of ERCP and their approximate frequency
Type of complication	**Frequency (%)**
Pancreatitis	2–5
Cholangitis	1–2
Haemorrhage	1–2
Cholecystitis	0.5
Bowel perforation	0.5
Death	0.1

Liver biopsy

Endoscopic retrograde cholangio-pancreatography

Percutaneous transhepatic cholangiography

307

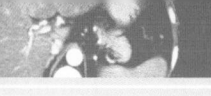

Table 5.10	Magnetic resonance cholangio-pancreatography (MRCP) versus endoscopic retrograde cholangio-pancreatography (ERCP)

Advantages of MRCP over ERCP

Non-invasive, therefore no increased risk of acute pancreatitis, cholangitis, pseudocyst infection, haemorrhage, etc.

No anaesthesia or premedication required

No contrast agent or ionizing radiation required

Can be performed on patients with abnormal pancreaticobiliary anatomy, e.g. after pancreatic, gastric or biliary surgery

Simultaneous examination of the liver, retroperitoneum, and lymph nodes for staging of malignancies

Advantages of ERCP over MRCP

Inspection of the oesophagus, stomach and duodenum

Superior demonstration of main pancreatic duct and side branches

Direct inspection of papilla for diagnosis of ampullary tumours

Allows cytology, biopsy and culture of biliary and pancreatic fluid

Permits performance of therapeutic manoeuvres, e.g. stone removal, sphincterotomy, stent insertion

Percutaneous transhepatic cholangiography

Percutaneous transhepatic cholangiography (PTC) is a radiological technique to image the biliary tract. It is less commonly used since the advent of ERCP.

Indications
The main indications are diagnostic (for the investigation of obstructive jaundice when ERCP fails or is unsuitable due to occluded common ducts or post-surgical recon-struction of the biliary tract), as part of a combined procedure with ERCP to aid the passage of a guidewire, or therapeutic (percutaneous drain insertion for drainage of the biliary system, and stent placement for malignant or benign strictures).

Patient preparation
Patients are admitted to hospital. A full blood count, coagulation screen and a group and save are performed. A single dose of oral ciprofloxacin (500 mg) is administered as antibiotic prophylaxis. In patients with elevated prothrombin time (impaired hepatic synthetic function) fresh frozen plasma is administered prior to the procedure. Platelet transfusion is performed if the platelet count is between 40 and 60×10^9/L.

Procedure
Percutaneous transhepatic cholangiography is performed under fluoroscopic guidance by an experienced radiologist. A needle is inserted through the intercostal space into the liver with the aim of cannulating an intrahepatic duct. Contrast is used to delineate the ducts and biliary tree to confirm the position of the needle. Once access to the biliary system is confirmed, a cholangiogram can be performed and a drain or stent can be introduced.

Complications
Pain is a common complication. Other less common complications are bleeding, bile leak and sepsis (cholangitis), pneumothorax and death (from sepsis or bleeding). In the longer term, percutaneous drains can become blocked and stents can occlude or fracture.

Post procedure care
Bed rest is advised for 6 hours with monitoring of blood pressure, pulse and temperature. Post procedure antibiotics are administered due to the risk of infection, especially with percutaneous drains.

Therapeutic procedures

Insertion of a Sengstaken–Blakemore tube

Indications

Balloon tamponade is used to control oesophageal variceal bleeding when initial measures (octreotide, vasopressin, sclerotherapy or banding) have failed. Such control is only temporary as a bridge to definitive treatment (endoscopy, transjugular intrahepatic portosystemic shunt (TIPSS) or surgery). Various balloons are available, the most common of which is the Sengstaken–Blakemore tube.

Patient preparation

Bleeding is often torrential and it is essential that the patient be adequately resuscitated via wide-bore intravenous cannulas. Insertion of the Sengstaken–Blakemore tube or other similar tubes should be undertaken when the patient is under sedation or general anaesthetic. Preferably, the patient should be intubated to protect the airway, as there are risks of aspiration. A mouth-guard is placed to prevent biting of the tube.

It is recommended that the Sengstaken tube should be cooled (they are usually kept in the fridge) prior to insertion to increase stiffness and aid insertion. The balloon is checked to ensure patency and absence of leak, and then lubricated with jelly.

Procedure

If awake, the patient is asked to swallow the tube; alternatively, the tube is pushed gently through the mouth into the oesophagus. At least 45 cm of tube should be inserted before inflating the gastric balloon with 300 mL of water. Some Gastrografin can be added to aid identification on a chest X-ray. The gastric port should then be clamped and the Sengstaken tube pulled back till resistance is felt; this indicates that the gastric balloon is abutting the gastro-oesophageal junction. The oesophageal balloon should not be used as most variceal bleeding occurs at the gastro-oesophageal junction and is controlled by the gastric balloon. If bleeding continues despite appropriate gastric balloon position, the oesophageal balloon can be inflated with air to 30 mmHg.

The position of the tube should be marked and the tube taped to the side of the face. Weights for traction are not recommended due to the risk of lip necrosis.

Balloon tamponade is highly effective, controlling variceal haemorrhage in nearly 90% of cases. It is important that a more definitive strategy is in place as 50% re-bleed on deflation of the balloon.

Complications

There is a risk of trachea intubation and aspiration, which may be reduced by pre-procedure endotracheal intubation. If the oesophageal balloon is inflated, there is a risk of oesophageal perforation from ischaemia, especially in patients with ulcerated oesophagus from previous endoscopic therapy.

Post procedure care

A chest X-ray must always be obtained to confirm the position of the tube. The oesophageal balloon should be deflated regularly to prevent oesophageal ulceration and perforation. Gastric balloons should be deflated after 12–24 hours to allow repeat endoscopy.

Paracentesis

Patients with chronic liver disease have a potent salt-retaining state. This is the result of secondary hyperaldosteronism. Portal hypertension and hypoalbuminaemia contribute to the formation of ascites.

Indications

The indications for paracentesis can be diagnostic (investigation of ascites of unknown aetiology) or therapeutic to drain ascites. The initial treatment of ascites is with a low salt intake, diuretics and fluid restriction. However, when these fail (ascites uncontrolled by diuretics, recurrent ascites) or there are complications associated with diuretic use (in the form of renal impairment or electrolyte imbalance) therapeutic paracentesis is an option.

Patient preparation

Patients are advised to stop diuretics 48 hours prior to hospital admission. On arrival, baseline urea and electrolytes, liver function tests and a coagulation screen are performed. Coagulation and electrolyte abnormalities should be corrected prior to paracentesis to minimize the post-procedure risks of bleeding and encephalopathy respectively. It helps to ensure that the bladder has been emptied prior to the procedure.

Procedure

The patient should be in a supine position. The abdomen is percussed to determine the level of ascites. The best sites of drainage are in the flanks, below the level of the umbilicus and lateral to the inferior epigastric artery. Alternatively, drainage can be performed in the midline.

309

Local anaesthetic is infiltrated at the site of catheter placement. A stab incision is then made to ease insertion of a pigtail (Bonanno) catheter. The trocar is withdrawn once the catheter has penetrated the peritoneal cavity. There should be free drainage of ascites. Sutures are not required. The catheter is firmly attached to the patient with tape and then connected to an intravenous giving set that drains into a urine collection bag (this facilitates accurate fluid measurement).

The ascitic fluid is sent for protein analysis, cell count, microbiological culture and cytology.

Complications

Rapid shifts of fluid and electrolytes can precipitate encephalopathy. Haemodynamic instability and renal dysfunction can be addressed by aggressive intravascular fluid replacement with 20% albumin. Infection can occur with long-term catheterization; removing the catheter after 6–8 hours may lower infection rates.

Post procedure care

Ascites should be allowed to drain freely and the catheter removed after 6–8 hours, irrespective of the volume of drainage. Slow or interrupted drainage increases the risk of infection. Intravascular volume repletion should be undertaken with 20% salt-poor albumin (100 mL of 20% albumin for every 3 litres of ascites drained). This can be increased if the urine output falls or there is incipient renal impairment. Blood pressure, urine output and ascitic drainage should be monitored hourly.

| SECTION 5.5 | **Manifestations of liver disease** |

Jaundice

Jaundice refers to the yellow discolouration of the sclera or skin resulting from elevated bilirubin levels. Clinically, jaundice is usually detectable when bilirubin levels are more than 50 μmol/l. Discolouration of the sclera occurs because bilirubin has a strong affinity for elastin.

The causes of jaundice are divided into pre-hepatic, hepatic and post-hepatic (cholestatic) in origin (Tables 5.11 and 5.12). In theory, pre-hepatic causes result in unconjugated hyperbilirubinaemia, post-hepatic causes result in conjugated hyperbilirubinaemia, and hepatic causes result in a mixed picture. In practice, determining the origin based on the presence of unconjugated or conjugated bilirubin is not straightforward as the proportions are often variable and multiple pathways resulting in jaundice can occur with single disease processes.

History

A good history is essential, and should enquire into the speed of onset and duration of jaundice. Pale stools and dark urine suggest a post-hepatic origin for the jaundice. Abdominal pain can occur with gallbladder stones or any cause of acute hepatitis. Rigors and night sweats may indicate cholangitis.

A drug history may reveal offending drugs associated with hyperbilirubinaemia, and the amount of alcohol intake should be documented to assess the risk of development of alcoholic liver disease. The ingestion of herbal medications or broad (fava) beans may be associated with haemolysis and jaundice. Intravenous drug abuse or tattoos from endemic areas are risk factors for viral hepatitis. A family history of haematological disorders may help direct investigations, or patients may be completely well, as in Gilbert's disease.

A travel history may reveal visits to endemic areas of hepatitis, and a sexual history needs to be obtained due to the risk of sexual transmission. A transfusion history is relevant, along with any past medical history that may warrant repeated blood transfusions to screen for haemolytic anaemia and risk of acquired hepatitis.

Examination

Patients with cirrhosis may have features of chronic liver disease such as spider naevi, hepatosplenomegaly, caput medusae (collateral veins) and ascites. Abdominal scars from previous biliary surgery may suggest an obstructive cause. A rectal examination is performed; pale stools suggest a cholestatic cause.

Investigations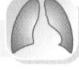

Full blood count

Anaemia occurs with haemolysis.

Liver profile

Elevated alanine and aspartate transaminases suggest a hepatic origin of the jaundice. The alkaline phosphatase levels are elevated in post-hepatic cholestasis. Gamma-glutamyltransferase is elevated in post-hepatic causes as well as alcoholic liver disease. Disproportionately elevated levels of unconjugated bilirubin would suggest a pre-hepatic cause. Serum albumin is low in patients with impaired synthetic function of the liver.

Urine analysis

Dark urine suggests a cholestatic cause; dipstick testing of the urine may reveal urobilinogen.

Ultrasound of the abdomen

Ultrasonography is usually the initial investigation to detect extra-hepatic causes such as stones and masses.

Table 5.11	Causes of jaundice
Pre-hepatic causes of jaundice	
Increased bilirubin production	
Haemolytic anaemia (haemolysis)	
Resorption of blood from haematoma	
Reduced hepatic uptake	
Reduced hepatic conjugation of bilirubin	
Gilbert's syndrome	
Crigler–Najjar syndrome (I and II)	
Hepatic causes of jaundice	
Liver cirrhosis	
Hepatitis	
Viruses	
Alcohol	
Autoimmune	
Drugs	
Infiltrative malignancy	
Liver congestion	
Cardiac failure	
Hepatic vascular disease	
Hepatic ischaemia	
Dubin–Johnson syndrome	
Post-hepatic causes of jaundice	
Biliary obstruction	
Stones	
Biliary malignancy	
Biliary strictures	
External compression	
Primary sclerosing cholangitis	

Table 5.12	Causes of postoperative jaundice
Pre-hepatic causes of jaundice	
Haemolysis (incompatible blood transfusion)	
Resorption of haematoma	
Hepatic causes of jaundice	
Drug (halothane anaesthesia)	
Systemic infection	
Hepatic ischaemia or infarction	
Post-hepatic causes of jaundice	
Residual stones after cholecystectomy	
Ischaemic strictures after biliary procedures	
Anastomotic strictures after liver transplantation	

A dilated biliary tree strongly suggests an extra-hepatic cause. Ultrasound may detect intrahepatic causes such as tumours.

CT of the abdomen

CT may be helpful to assess the biliary tree or provide better imaging if initial ultrasonography is unhelpful.

Endoscopic retrograde cholangio-pancreatography

Endoscopic retrograde cholangio-pancreatography or magnetic resonance cholangio-pancreatography (MRCP) may be needed to confirm an extra-hepatic cause in the presence of a dilated biliary tree.

Further investigations

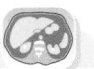

Depending on the clinical presentation the following tests may be needed: haemolytic screen, paracetamol levels, viral serology, autoimmune screen, copper studies and iron studies. A liver biopsy may be required in chronic liver disease of unknown aetiology.

Acute liver failure

Acute liver failure is a multisystem disorder that results in encephalopathy and coagulopathy following a massive insult to the liver.

History

The most common causes of acute liver failure are paracetamol overdose (40% in the UK), drug reactions and infection with hepatitis A or B. Less common causes include Wilson's disease and Budd–Chiari syndrome.

Patients may present with a clear history of the underlying cause for acute liver failure, or with severe encephalopathy and coma.

Examination

The severity of the encephalopathy can be graded (p. 316); in addition, there may be severe jaundice, ascites and bruising from coagulopathy.

Investigations

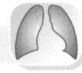

Liver profile

Transaminases are usually elevated with low serum albumin. The liver profile is of limited use in the classification of the severity of liver failure.

Coagulation screen

The prothrombin time is prolonged in acute liver failure.

Urea and electrolytes

Renal failure with elevated serum creatinine can accompany hepatic failure.

311

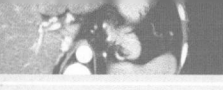
Serum blood sugar

Hypoglycaemia can develop with severe hepatic impairment.

Paracetamol levels

If a history is unavailable, screening for paracetamol levels is required to diagnose paracetamol overdose.

Hepatitis serology

A serological screen should be sent for viral hepatitis.

Further investigations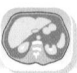

Further investigations should be performed according to the suspected underlying cause. Ultrasound would be helpful to diagnose Budd–Chiari syndrome. Copper studies may be performed to screen for Wilson's disease. Autoantibodies can be tested to screen for autoimmune hepatitis.

Management

Management of patients with severe liver failure is best undertaken by a multidisciplinary team in centres where liver transplantation facilities are available.

Address any underlying cause

The most important aspect in the management is to identify and address any underlying cause. Paracetamol overdose should be managed with N-acetyl cysteine. Penicillamine may be of use in patients with Wilson's disease, and immunomodulation should be commenced for patients with autoimmune hepatitis.

Supportive treatment

Hypoglycaemia should be corrected with glucose infusion. Hypovolaemia can be corrected with appropriate fluid resuscitation or may require inotropic support. Bleeding associated with coagulopathy can be corrected with clotting products. Patients with grade 3 or more severe encephalopathy may require intubation and ventilation. Renal replacement therapy may be required for patients in renal failure.

Liver support systems

The role of artificial liver support systems including albumin dialysis (molecular adsorbents recirculating system—MARS) and plasmapheresis is still under evaluation with some reports of success.

Liver transplantation

Approximately 50% of patients with acute liver failure will require liver transplantation (p. 347).

 FURTHER INFORMATION

O'Grady JG. Acute liver failure. Postgraduate Medical Journal 2005; 81: 148–154.

Hepatitis

Hepatitis is inflammation of the liver parenchyma. Causes are listed in Table 5.13. Hepatitis may be subclinical, acute or chronic. Rarely, it can lead to hepatic failure and death.

Acute hepatitis refers to liver inflammation of less than 6 months. There may be clinical, biochemical and histological evidence of hepatic parenchymal inflammation. Mild cases can be managed conservatively in the outpatient department. Symptomatic patients with profound abnormalities in synthetic function should be admitted. No treatment is necessary in most cases (unless fulminant hepatic failure ensues), and all hepatotoxic drugs or toxins such as alcohol should be withdrawn. Acute hepatitis usually resolves spontaneously. Acute hepatitis may lead to chronic

Table 5.13	Causes of hepatitis
Acute	
Viruses	
Hepatitis A, B, C, D	
Epstein–Barr virus (EBV)	
Coxsackie virus	
Herpes simplex	
Mycoplasma	
Leptospirosis	
Drugs	
Paracetamol	
Halothane	
Carbamazepine	
Rifampicin	
Toxins (mushrooms)	
Alcohol	
Autoimmune	
Ischaemia	
Wilson's disease	
Chronic	
Alcohol	
Viruses	
Hepatitis B, C, D	
Autoimmune	
Metabolic	
Haemochromatosis	
Wilson's disease	
α_1-Antitrypsin deficiency	
Primary biliary cirrhosis	
Primary sclerosing cholangitis	
Drugs	
Non-alcoholic steatohepatitis	
Cryptogenic	

hepatitis, hence long-term follow-up is required. It can also (rarely) lead to fulminant hepatic failure.

Chronic hepatitis refers to continued inflammation and necrosis of the liver parenchyma. This may be non-progressive or progressive, leading to further damage such as scarring and cirrhosis. The diagnosis is histological, characterized by parenchymal, portal and periportal inflammation. Treatment is determined by the underlying cause. Most cases can be managed in the outpatient department. Patients with chronic hepatitis should be kept under review as progression to cirrhosis can occur.

History

A good history is essential. Recent exotic travel, food intake or social habits may indicate a viral cause. The ingestion of herbal medications or even seemingly benign medication may cause acute hepatitis. Continued excessive alcohol consumption may suggest alcoholic hepatitis, although this usually occurs in the setting of chronic liver disease.

Patients may be asymptomatic, as in many cases of hepatitis A and C infections. Other hepatotropic viruses such as cytomegalovirus and Coxsackie viruses can also cause asymptomatic infections. In other causes, patients may complain of non-specific constitutional symptoms such as lethargy, arthralgia, headaches and fevers. These are often followed by jaundice, which is frequently first noticed by a friend or relative. Patients may notice discolouration of the urine and stools.

Chronic hepatitis is often asymptomatic and detected on routine biochemistry. Some patients may complain of right upper abdominal discomfort, anorexia, weight loss or pruritus. Others may be diagnosed by liver function tests as part of the investigative workup for epilepsy, chorea (Wilson's disease), blistering skin disease (porphyria cutanea tarda in haemochromatosis), alcoholic liver disease, hepatitis C, HIV and arthritis (haemochromatosis).

Examination

Examination may be normal. In acute hepatitis, some patients may have hepatosplenomegaly or even features of chronic liver disease (in alcoholics). There may be a mild pyrexia. Severe cases of acute hepatitis may lead to hepatic failure with encephalopathy, coagulopathy and renal failure. Features of chronic liver disease (cirrhosis and its complications) include spider naevi, splenomegaly, ascites and bruising.

Investigations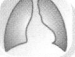

Liver function tests
Liver enzymes such as ALP, GGT, AST, ALT and bilirubin may be elevated. Serum albumin is a test of liver synthetic function, and may be low.

Coagulation screen
The prothrombin time is also a test of liver synthetic function (production of coagulation factors).

Full blood count
A full blood count should be performed to screen for anaemia.

Urea and electrolytes
Renal function is assessed to screen for hepatorenal syndrome (p. 317).

Random blood glucose
Blood sugar levels may be low in severe liver disease.

Viral serology
Viral serology is performed to identify any potential source of infection that may lead to hepatitis.

Immunology
Serology (p. 329) may identify antibodies associated with an autoimmune aetiology.

Toxicology (acute hepatitis)
Serum paracetamol levels must be assessed when an overdose is suspected.

Ultrasound of the abdomen
Ultrasonography may demonstrate hepatomegaly in acute hepatitis, splenomegaly in EBV infection or chronic liver damage.

Liver biopsy
Liver biopsy is required for the investigation of chronic hepatitis when there is doubt about the aetiology or for the assessment of disease severity.

Cirrhosis

Oesophageal varices

Portal hypertension results in the development of venous collaterals between the portal and systemic venous circulation. Blood flow bypasses the liver parenchyma and essentially serves to decompress the portal system (and portal pressure). However, as flow in the venous collaterals increases, they develop into dilated, tortuous, thin-walled vessels known as varices. The gastro-oesophageal junction is an important site for varices as patients can present with torrential upper gastrointestinal bleeding. Other sites of venous collaterals are the rectum, the retroperitoneal space, and the falciform ligament of the liver with the umbilical or abdominal veins. The mortality associated with bleeding oesophageal varices is approximately 50%.

History

Approximately 50% of patients with varices will experience an episode of upper gastrointestinal bleeding (the risk of bleeding is increased if the pressure gradient between the portal and hepatic veins is greater than 10 mmHg). Most patients present with haematemesis due to the volume of

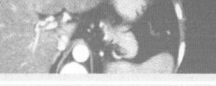

blood loss. Anaemia with chronic bleeding is unusual. Patients with oesophageal varices usually have an existing history of liver impairment and cirrhosis. In addition, symptoms of hepatic encephalopathy may coexist with the diversion from blood (and toxins) from the liver with portosystemic shunting.

Examination

Patients may have signs of chronic liver disease (p. 312). In addition, they may be cold, clammy and sweating due to shock from blood loss. Tachycardia and hypotension may be evident.

Investigations

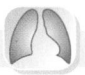

Full blood count
In the acute setting, the haemoglobin concentration cannot be used as a reliable indicator of the severity of blood loss. It is usually within the normal range as there is insufficient time for haemodilution to occur.

Urea and electrolytes
Blood loss into the gut can lead to a raised urea level. In addition, volume depletion can result in renal impairment with elevated serum creatinine.

Liver profile
The liver profile is usually deranged in the pattern reflective of the underlying cause of liver cirrhosis.

Coagulation screen
A coagulation screen is essential as the prothrombin time may be prolonged with failure of the synthetic function of the liver.

Crossmatch
Urgent crossmatch of 6 units of blood is usually requested due to the severity of the volume of blood loss.

Management

> **CLINICAL ALERT**
>
> *Bleeding can be torrential. Large-bore intravenous access should be obtained and immediate fluid resuscitation should commence (Gelofusine or blood). If crossmatched blood is not available, O-negative blood can be obtained as an emergency. The airway should be protected by intubation if the patient has a Glasgow Coma Score (GCS) of 8 or less.*

Somatostatin analogues
Terlipressin (Glypressin), a somatostatin analogue, acts as a potent splanchnic vasoconstrictor and may reduce blood loss. The usual dose is 2 mg i.v. four times daily for 72 hours.

The use of octreotide is less common due to the side effects of diarrhoea. Somatostatin carries the risk of angina and myocardial infarction.

Balloon tamponade
Balloon tamponade with either a Sengstaken–Blakemore tube (p. 309) or a Minnesota tube may be undertaken if endoscopy services are unavailable or if endoscopic methods fail to achieve haemostasis.

Upper gastrointestinal endoscopy
Early endoscopy should be arranged to confirm the source of bleeding. The varices can also be treated with endoscopic therapies. The risk of re-bleeding is highest within the first 7 days, and a repeat endoscopy should be performed to ensure that all significant varices have been attended to and to check if any previous bands have slipped.

Endoscopic banding
Endoscopic banding can be performed in the setting of acute bleeding or as prophylactic therapy. It is performed with a ligator-cap device fitted over the tip of the endoscope which releases a rubber band. The varix is sucked into the adaptor and the trip wire is triggered, releasing a rubber band over the varix that cuts off its blood supply causing necrosis and sloughing of the varix. Complications include the development of oesophageal stricture, perforation and aspiration during the procedure.

Endoscopic sclerotherapy
Sclerotherapy can be performed in the setting of acute bleeding or as prophylactic therapy. Approximately 2 mL aliquots of sclerosants are injected into the varix using a standard endoscope and a retractable needle. The most common sclerosing agents are sodium tetradecyl sulphate (STD) and ethanolamine oleate; these cause local fibrosis and eradication of the varix. Meta-analysis suggests a higher rate of complications and lower efficacy than banding. Complications include the development of oesophageal strictures, ulceration at the injection sites, perforation of the oesophagus and further bleeding following injection.

Endoscopic glue injection
Histoacryl is a substance that polymerizes with water to form a hardened complex. Direct injection of Histoacryl glue has been used in the management of gastric and oesophageal varices. Results with gastric varices have been promising, but with oesophageal varices there appears to be a higher rate of stricture and ulceration.

Endoscopic argon-plasma coagulation
Endoscopic coagulation of the varices (and other vascular lesions such as vascular ectasia and tumours) can be performed using an argon-plasma coagulation probe. A high-frequency electrical current is conducted through argon, an inert, ionized gas. The thermal effects are devitalization, coagulation, desiccation and shrinking of varices.

The maximum effect is between 3 and 4 mm, thereby reducing the risks of unwanted organ damage. Complications include oesophageal perforation and mediastinal emphysema.

Transjugular intrahepatic portosystemic shunt

A transjugular intrahepatic portosystemic shunt (TIPSS) reduces portal pressure by creating an artificial bypass between the portal and systemic blood flow. It is very effective in controlling variceal bleeds. Complications include hepatic encephalopathy and shunt occlusion; 6-monthly ultrasound or venography is required to confirm patency.

Surgical shunt

Surgical shunts (splenorenal) are often used as a last resort to reduce the portal pressure; morbidity and mortality are high. Complications include hepatic encephalopathy, mediastinitis, perforation and death. Scar formation after surgery may preclude liver transplantation. Other surgical methods include devascularization and oesophageal transection.

Secondary prevention

Recurrent bleeding occurs in approximately 50%. Propranolol, a non-selective beta-blocker, can be used successfully to reduce portal pressures to reduce the risk of further bleeding. If beta-blockers are contraindicated, isosorbide mononitrate or an ACE inhibitor may be prescribed. Regular endoscopy should be performed to screen for and treat any further varices.

Ascites

Ascites is the accumulation of fluid in the peritoneal cavity. Liver disease is the most common cause (Table 5.14).

Table 5.14	Causes of ascites
Serum–ascites albumin gradient more than 11 g/L	
Chronic liver disease	
Cardiac failure	
Nephrotic syndrome	
Malabsorption	
Hepatic vascular obstruction	
Hypothyroidism	
Serum–ascites albumin gradient less than 11 g/L	
Inflammatory conditions	
Infections	
Pancreatitis	
Hepatic ischaemia	
Malignancy	
Peritoneal malignancy	
Intra-abdominal tumour	

History

Abdominal swelling and peripheral oedema have usually developed. Any history of malignancy in the abdomen or pelvis is relevant. Cirrhosis of the liver may result from excess alcohol consumption, previous hepatitis, Wilson's disease, primary and secondary biliary cirrhosis and haemochromatosis.

Examination

Classical features are shifting dullness and a fluid thrill. Evidence of liver disease would be suggested by the presence of jaundice, spider naevi, loss of body hair, gynaecomastia, palmar erythema or caput medusae. The jugular venous pressure (JVP) is elevated in the presence of cardiac failure. Hepatomegaly and splenomegaly can occur with portal hypertension and hepatic tumours. Peripheral oedema can occur with cirrhosis, cardiac failure, malabsorption or obstruction of lymphatic flow due to intra-abdominal malignancy.

Investigations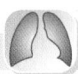

Ultrasound scan of the abdomen

Usually, clinical examination is sufficient to detect ascites, but smaller volumes of ascites can be revealed on ultrasound, as can other features of portal hypertension or portal vein thrombosis.

Paracentesis

A diagnostic tap (p. 309) should be taken in all cases of ascites. A bloody tap suggests malignancy or bleeding. Milky ascites may be chylous in nature (lymphatic source). Samples must be assessed for protein (albumin) counts, amylase, cell counts (microbiology) and cytology. Amylase will be significantly elevated in pancreatitis. A serum–ascites albumin gradient (serum albumin to ascitic albumin level) of more than 11 g/L suggests portal hypertension.

Cytology is useful to confirm peritoneal disease but abnormal cells are seen in less than 10% of patients with malignant ascites, thus a negative result does not exclude malignancy.

A significant proportion of patients with ascites from liver disease have spontaneous bacterial peritonitis. These patients may be asymptomatic. A white cell count >250/mm^3 indicates spontaneous bacterial peritonitis.

Management

The most important aspect in the management of ascites is to identify and treat any underlying cause. Often, when the underlying cause is addressed, ascites resolves. The remainder of this section specifically discusses the *management of ascites due to liver disease*.

Low-sodium diet

In patients with ascites due to liver disease, the general aim is to reduce the overall sodium load by reducing intake and increasing excretion. Corresponding reductions of

315

ascitic fluid occur, and the aim is to reduce the patient's weight by 500 g per day. A low-sodium diet is recommended with restriction of salt intake to less than 80 mmol/day.

Fluid management

Water restriction may be needed to maintain blood sodium levels. The rapid correction of hyponatraemia may cause fits and central pontine myelinosis. When intravascular volume is low, 5% dextrose or colloids (20% albumin, Gelofusine, 10% HAES-steril) are used in preference to normal saline or dextrose saline to reduce sodium load.

Diuretics

Spironolactone and furosemide increase sodium and free water excretion. Spironolactone antagonizes the renin–angiotensin–aldosterone system and is the drug of choice. It is started at 100 mg per day, increasing to a maximum of 400 mg per day. Furosemide is usually added for its synergistic effects, and 90% of patients with ascites respond to such measures. Side effects of diuretic therapy include electrolyte abnormalities, renal failure and precipitation of hepatic encephalopathy.

Paracentesis

When ascites is refractory to diuretic therapy, paracentesis is the next treatment option (p. 309). Adequate intravascular replacement with albumin solution is essential to reduce the risks of renal impairment and cardiovascular compromise.

Transjugular intrahepatic portosystemic shunt

A transjugular intrahepatic portosystemic shunt (p. 315) is a highly effective treatment option for patients who require regular paracentesis. The use of surgical shunts is less common as no survival benefit is conferred by the more invasive surgical procedure.

Liver transplantation

If end-stage liver disease is the cause of refractory ascites, liver transplantation should be considered (p. 347).

Prognosis

Ascites associated with liver disease carries a poor prognosis, the 5-year survival is usually less than 30%.

i FURTHER INFORMATION

Arroyo V, Gines P, Gerbes AL, et al. Definition and diagnostic criteria of refractory ascites and hepatorenal syndrome in cirrhosis. Hepatology 1996; 23: 164–176.

Lebrec D, Giuily N, Hadengue A, et al. Transjugular intrahepatic portosystemic shunts: comparison with paracentesis in patients with cirrhosis and refractory ascites: a randomized trial. Journal of Hepatology 1996; 25: 135–144.

i FURTHER INFORMATION—cont'd

D'Amico G, Morabito A, Pagliaro L, Marubini E. Survival and prognostic indicators in compensated and decompensated cirrhosis. Digestive Diseases and Sciences 1986; 31: 468–475.

Runyon BA, Montano AA, Akriviadis EA, et al. The serum-ascites albumin gradient is superior to exudates-transudate concept in the differential diagnosis of ascites. Annals of Internal Medicine 1992; 117: 215–220.

Schrier RW, Arroyo V, Bernardi M, et al. Peripheral vasodilation hypothesis: a proposal for the initiation of renal sodium and water retention in cirrhosis. Hepatology 1988; 8: 1151–1157.

Cattau EL Jr, Benjamin SB, Knuff TE, Castell DO. The accuracy of the physical examination in the diagnosis of suspected ascites. JAMA 1982; 247: 1164–1166.

Hepatic encephalopathy

Hepatic encephalopathy is a spectrum of neuropsychiatric disturbances associated with liver dysfunction. Loss of the detoxification function of the liver due to acute liver failure or from the shunting of blood in chronic liver failure (microcirculatory changes secondary to fibrosis and cirrhosis) can lead to the accumulation of toxins that interfere with normal cerebral function. Some of these toxins include ammonia, gamma (γ)-aminobutyric acid (GABA) and endogenous opiates.

History

Hepatic encephalopathy is divided into a subclinical, acute or chronic (>4 weeks in duration) presentation. The neurological changes are non-specific and vary from sleep disturbance to personality changes and deterioration in day-to-day function.

It is important to be able to establish liver disease as the underlying cause and to exclude other diseases that may give rise to confusion such as hypoglycaemia, hypomagnesaemia, hyponatraemia, sepsis, epilepsy, Wernicke's encephalopathy and intracranial haematoma.

Once liver disease is established as the underlying cause, it is important to determine any precipitating cause such as non-compliance with existing medication, drugs, electrolyte abnormalities, bleeding, infection (particularly bacterial peritonitis), constipation, development of malignancy (particularly hepatocellular carcinoma), portal vein thrombosis or the insertion of a portosystemic shunt.

Examination

Physical changes in encephalopathy include asterixis (flapping tremor when arms are outstretched and wrists hyperextended), hyper-reflexia and a positive Babinski sign (extension of the big toe when the sole of the foot is scratched along its lateral border). There may even be Parkinsonian features.

Investigations
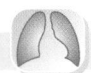

Investigations are performed to exclude other causes of encephalopathy and identify precipitating factors for hepatic encephalopathy.

Full blood count

Anaemia may be caused by blood loss (a precipitant for encephalopathy).

Urea and electrolytes

Sodium or potassium levels should be assessed. Other electrolytes that should be estimated include magnesium, calcium, glucose and zinc.

Liver profile

Severe deterioration in liver function may be the underlying cause of encephalopathy.

Blood cultures

Blood cultures should be performed to screen for bacteraemia.

Chest X-ray

A chest film should be performed if pneumonia is suspected.

Ultrasound scan of the abdomen

Ultrasound with Doppler examination should be performed to exclude venous occlusion (hepatic vein, portal vein thrombosis).

CT of the head

CT of the head is performed to exclude stroke, intracranial bleed or any other space-occupying lesion that might account for the symptoms.

Upper gastrointestinal endoscopy

Upper gastrointestinal endoscopy is performed to screen for bleeding varices, as this is a known precipitant of encephalopathy.

Electroencephalogram (EEG)

An EEG is usually performed to identify subclinical cases of encephalopathy.

Management

Airway

Airway management is essential in patients with grade 3 and 4 encephalopathy, as there is a significant risk of aspiration. If necessary, patients may require intubation and ventilation if they are unable to protect their own airway.

Identify and correct any underlying cause

This may include correction of any electrolyte abnormalities, treatment of upper gastrointestinal bleeding, and administration of naloxone if there is a suggestion of opiate use. Correction of the underlying cause may itself correct the encephalopathy.

Antibiotics

Prophylactic antibiotics, including antifungals, should be administered to patients with ascites or a history of bacterial peritonitis.

Gut cleansing

Enemas and lactulose are administered to decrease bowel transit time (to three good bowel movements per day) to reduce the amount of ammonia produced from gut fermentation available for reabsorption.

Thiamine/parenteral vitamin B and C

Patients should receive thiamine and parenteral vitamin B and C as Wernicke's encephalopathy may occasionally account for the symptoms of 'hepatic encephalopathy'.

Flumazenil

Flumazenil may be administered. It is associated with short-term improvements in neuropsychiatric function.[1] Neomycin is less commonly used due to the risks of drug toxicity.

Liver transplantation

Transplantation should be actively considered in a patient with end-stage liver disease and recurrent or chronic encephalopathy.

REFERENCE

(1) *Goulenok C, Bernard B, Cadranel JF, Thabut D, Di Martino V, Opolon P, Poynard T. Flumazenil vs placebo in hepatic encephalopathy in patients with cirrhosis: a meta-analysis. Alimentary Pharmacology and Therapeutics 2002; 16(3): 361–372.*

Hepatorenal syndrome

Hepatorenal syndrome is renal failure in association with advanced liver disease and portal hypertension without any evidence of intrinsic renal disease. The pathogenesis is multifactorial; it is thought to be due to failure of the hepatic metabolism of vasodilatory toxins resulting in splanchnic vasodilatation and reduced renal perfusion pressure. The reflex activation of the vasoconstrictive systems (sympathetic nervous system and vasoactive mediators) results in impaired renal perfusion and renal dysfunction in the absence of intrinsic renal disease.

History

Hepatorenal syndrome is divided into two subtypes. Type 1 is characterized by a rapid, progressive deterioration of renal function in less than 2 weeks; type 2 is characterized by a gradual fluctuation in renal function with general deterioration. The diagnosis is essentially biochemical and patients may be asymptomatic.

It is important to exclude other causes of renal impairment such as hypovolaemia (acute tubular necrosis), drugs, infections and intrinsic renal disease (glomerulonephritis) (Table 5.15).

317

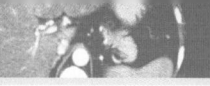

Table 5.15	Diagnostic criteria for hepatorenal syndrome*
Presence of advanced liver disease and portal hypertension	
Abnormal renal function defined by creatinine >200 μmol/L or reduced glomerular filtration rate (creatinine clearance <40 mL/min)	
No improvement despite fluid resuscitation with at least 1.5 L of saline	
Exclusion of possible causes of hypovolaemia, sepsis or drug-related cause	
Exclusion of significant proteinuria (<500 mg/dL) and normal renal ultrasound	

* From Arroyo V, Gines P, Gerbes AL, et al. Definition and diagnostic criteria of refractory ascites and hepatorenal syndrome in cirrhosis. Hepatology 1996; 23: 164–176.

Examination

Patients may have evidence of chronic liver disease. The coexistence of renal impairment does not normally carry any additional physical signs.

Investigations

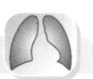

Urea and electrolytes, 24-hour urinary collection
Type 1 hepatorenal syndrome is diagnosed with a serum creatinine more than 200 μmol/L or 50% reduction in creatinine clearance to less than 20 mL/min. The urine sodium concentration is low and the urine osmolality is high.

Urine analysis
Microscopy is performed to exclude red cell casts, which suggest glomerulonephritis.

Septic screen
Blood, urine and sputum cultures are done to screen for any evidence of infection or sepsis that can result in renal impairment.

Initial management

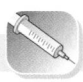

Identify and address any precipitating factor
Diuretics should be stopped, and circulating volume status and blood pressure should be corrected.

Monitoring
Strict fluid balance charts are kept. A central venous line may be required to assess filling pressures. Urinary catheterization is required to monitor hourly urine output.

Paracentesis
If there is tense ascites, paracentesis may improve renal perfusion by reducing tamponade on the renal veins. Volume replacement in the form of albumin/colloid is essential to prevent further cardiovascular and renal compromise.

Medical management

Vasopressors
Antidiuretic hormone (ADH) analogues such as terlipressin act by increasing renal perfusion through splanchnic circulation vasoconstriction and have been shown to improve the course of hepatorenal syndrome.[1] Noradrenaline can also be used (in the ICU setting) but takes up to a week to achieve a response. It is important to ensure that patients are well hydrated as there is a risk of organ ischaemia. Albumin is often used in conjunction to increase intravascular volume.[2]

Renal replacement therapy
In acute liver failure or hepatitis, haemofiltration may be required during the period of liver regeneration.

Liver support
A new liver support system, the molecular adsorbents recirculating system (MARS), has been shown to improve outcome in patients with hepatorenal syndrome[3].

Surgical management

Liver transplantation
As the underlying cause for renal failure is hepatic failure, liver transplantation is the most effective treatment.

Prognosis

Almost all patients with type 1 hepatorenal syndrome die without liver transplantation. Medical therapy in the form of albumin and vasopressors may reverse the deterioration in some, allow time for liver regeneration in others, or act as a bridge to transplantation.

REFERENCES

(1) Guevera M, Gines P, Fernandez-Esparrach G, et al. Reversibility of hepatorenal syndrome by prolonged administration of ornipressin and plasma volume expansion. Hepatology 1988; 27: 35–41
(2) Gines P, Ortega R, Uriz J, et al. Effect of terlipressin administration with and without albumin in hepatorenal syndrome (HRS). A phase-II study. Hepatology 2001; 34: 186A (abstract)
(3) Mittzer SR, Stange J, Klammt S, et al. Improvement of hepatorenal syndrome with extracorporeal albumin dialysis MARS. Result of a prospective, randomized, controlled clinical trial. Liver Transplantation 2000; 6: 277–286

Spontaneous bacterial peritonitis

Spontaneous bacterial peritonitis results from bacterial infection of ascitic fluid in patients with cirrhosis. It is a common condition, affecting up to 33% of patients with ascites due to bacterial translocation from the gut to the blood stream (bacteraemia) and into the ascitic fluid (bacterascites). The organisms responsible are usually Gram-negative, aerobic, enteric bacteria such as *E. coli*, *Klebsiella* and *Enterococcus* species. The long-term prognosis of patients who develop spontaneous bacterial peritonitis is poor, with less than 50% survival at 1 year.

History

Some patients have asymptomatic infection while others may complain of abdominal discomfort, fever, malaise and night sweats (sepsis) or confusion (encephalopathy). A high index of suspicion is necessary to diagnose bacterial peritonitis. Risk factors include a history of gastrointestinal bleeding, previous spontaneous bacterial peritonitis, fulminant hepatic failure, low ascitic total protein (<10 g/L) and low serum complement levels (C3).

Examination

There may be evidence of chronic liver disease and ascites may be detectable. Patients may be pyrexial. Palpation of the abdomen may reveal diffuse non-specific tenderness.

Investigations

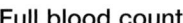

Full blood count
The white cell count may be elevated.

Urea and electrolytes
Renal failure is an important complication and carries a poor prognosis.

Liver profile
The liver profile is usually deranged in a pattern specific to the underlying cause of cirrhosis (p. 302).

Septic screen
Blood, urine and sputum cultures should be taken.

Paracentesis
An ascitic neutrophil count of more than 250 cells/mm^3 is a sensitive indicator for bacterial peritonitis. Immediate treatment is warranted. Low ascitic protein levels are a risk factor for spontaneous bacterial peritonitis.

Gram staining does not usually identify the presence of bacteria despite the presence of infection. Culture results typically demonstrate infection by a single organism. Polymicrobial infection usually suggests secondary peritonitis (e.g. perforated viscus).

Management

Antibiotics
Empirical treatment is usually started with a cephalosporin and fluoroquinolone (cefotaxime and ciprofloxacin) for a week. Antibiotics may be tailored according to the culture results. Antibiotics lead to resolution of infection in 90%. Those who are unresponsive to treatment have a high mortality rate.

Albumin replacement
Intravenous 20% albumin is administered at a volume of 1.5 g/kg, reducing to 1 g/kg by day 3 to reduce the risk of renal impairment and death.[1]

REFERENCE

(1) Sort P, Navasa M, Arroyo V, et al. *Effect of intravenous albumin on renal impairment and mortality in patients with cirrhosis and spontaneous bacterial peritonitis. New England Journal of Medicine* 1999; 341: 403–409.

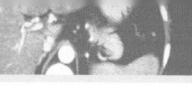

SECTION 5.6 # Disorders of bilirubin metabolism and excretion

Gilbert's syndrome

Up to 10% of the population is affected by Gilbert's syndrome. It is a common cause of hyperbilirubinaemia, due to partial deficiency of the enzyme bilirubin glucuronosyltransferase. Most of the bilirubin is unconjugated, due to the failure of conjugation, and a small amount of haemolysis may exist.

Diagnosis of this condition is made usually by exclusion as there are no systemic features apart from mild jaundice. Liver function tests are usually normal apart from the elevated bilirubin. The level of bilirubin may rise on fasting, infection and with alcohol consumption. No treatment is required for Gilbert's syndrome and reassurance is important.

Crigler–Najjar syndrome

Crigler–Najjar syndrome exists in two forms. Type I is a rare, autosomal recessive condition characterized by the absence of the enzyme glucuronosyltransferase. It leads to kernicterus and most affected patients die in the first year of life. Type II is an autosomal dominant condition with partial deficiency of the enzyme glucuronosyltransferase. The levels of bilirubin are higher than in Gilbert's syndrome, but kernicterus rarely occurs.

Dubin–Johnson syndrome

Dubin–Johnson syndrome is a rare, benign condition characterized by a defect in hepatic excretion of bilirubin, resulting in predominantly conjugated hyperbilirubinaemia.

Patients with Dubin–Johnson syndrome are usually asymptomatic; in particular, pruritus and steatorrhoea are absent. Some patients may suffer with constitutional symptoms of being unwell. Cholangiography is often abnormal and pigmented hepatocytes may be seen on a liver biopsy. In general the disease is benign and the prognosis is good.

SECTION 5.7 # Alcoholic liver disease

Chronic excessive consumption of alcohol results in liver damage that exists as a continuous spectrum from simple steatosis to hepatitis to cirrhosis.

Epidemiology

Alcohol-related liver disease is very common. Approximately 20% of heavy alcohol drinkers develop histological features of chronic liver disease. Alcoholic cirrhosis (Laënnec's cirrhosis) is the most common cause of cirrhosis in North America and Europe. It is the final stage of alcohol-induced liver damage and accounts for nearly 75% of deaths from alcoholism.

Pathology

The volume and duration of alcohol consumption leading to pathological changes vary considerably among gender and population. Women are generally more susceptible to alcohol injury, and twin studies suggest a strong genetic component. Polymorphisms of the anti-oxidative systems and immune-mediated injury are believed to be important factors in the development of alcoholic liver disease. Acetaldehyde from alcohol metabolism results in cell membrane damage through T-lymphocyte activation.

Alcoholic fatty disease (steatosis) is the most common manifestation of alcoholic liver disease, characterized by fatty infiltration of the liver from altered fatty acid metabolism. Macroscopically, the liver is yellow, greasy and filled with fat. Microscopically, hepatocytes are swollen with fat vacuoles displacing the nucleus. This must be distinguished from non-alcoholic steatohepatitis.

Alcoholic hepatitis is suggested by features of liver cell necrosis and inflammation on liver biopsy with polymorphs, fatty change and the presence of Mallory's hyaline in liver cells.

Alcoholic cirrhosis is characterized by micronodular cirrhosis on liver biopsy. Deposition of collagen in the periportal and pericentral areas is due to alcohol-mediated injury and the associated inflammatory response. The septations eventually merge, and ongoing regeneration causes the liver to develop a nodular and shrunken appearance.

Scope of disease

Alcoholic liver disease is only a single manifestation of the systemic effects of alcohol abuse. Other organ systems that are also affected include the kidney (renal failure), brain (alcohol dependency, psychiatric manifestations), heart (cardiomyopathy), blood (macrocytosis) and an impaired immune system.

Clinical features

High alcohol intake (>80 g of alcohol per day for men and >60 g of alcohol per day for women) is common to the three manifestations of alcoholic liver disease, although some patients may deny a history of excessive alcohol consumption. The history may be suggestive of symptoms of alcohol withdrawal and social disruptions.

Patients with alcoholic fatty disease are asymptomatic. On examination, tender hepatomegaly may be detectable due to capsular distension of the liver.

Patients with alcoholic hepatitis may complain of abdominal discomfort, abdominal swelling or upper gastrointestinal symptoms including nausea. They may notice the yellow discolouration of their sclera or discolouration of the urine. On examination, spider naevi, palmar erythema, parotid and abdominal swelling (ascites) may be present. There may be bruising from coagulopathy. Hepatic flap (asterixis) suggests hepatic encephalopathy. Poor urine output may result from hepatorenal syndrome or tubular necrosis from concomitant sepsis and intravascular volume depletion. The increased susceptibility to infection is usually due to malnourishment.

Patients with alcoholic cirrhosis usually have silent disease for many years. Early symptoms include fatigue and a poor appetite. In the later stages, features of liver failure and portal hypertension develop. Examination findings in the late stage of disease are similar to those of alcohol hepatitis.

Initial investigations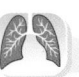

Full blood count
The full blood count is usually normal with fatty change, and there may be evidence of macrocytosis. With hepatitis, there is usually a polymorph leukocytosis. Haemolysis may develop from spur-cell anaemia. With cirrhosis, pancytopenia can result from a combination of marrow suppression, hypersplenism and B_{12} deficiency. The blood film may reveal acanthocytes with hyperlipidaemia.

Urea and electrolytes
Renal function may be impaired in alcoholic hepatitis and cirrhosis.

Liver profile
Gamma-glutamyltransferase is elevated from alcohol consumption. The aspartate (AST) and alanine (ALT) aminotransferases are elevated, usually in a ratio of 2:1 in fatty change. Levels are usually below 300 i.u./L even in patients with hepatitis. Serum bilirubin is usually greatly elevated.

Coagulation screen
The prothrombin time is normal with fatty change but can be prolonged in hepatitis and cirrhosis due to impairment of the synthetic function of the liver.

Blood alcohol levels
Blood alcohol levels are performed to screen for continued alcohol intake.

Viral serology
It is essential to exclude other causes of liver disease, including infection with viral hepatitis.

Ultrasound of the abdomen
With fatty change, ultrasound of the liver shows increased echogenicity. With cirrhosis, a small, shrunken liver may be evident. Ultrasound is also able to assess the size of the spleen, pressure in the portal veins and the presence of subclinical ascites. Biliary disease can be excluded as a differential diagnosis.

Further investigations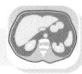

Liver biopsy
A liver biopsy is not essential in all patients. It is performed if other causes of liver impairment are suspected, or if the underlying aetiology of alcoholic hepatitis is uncertain. Features suggestive of alcoholic hepatitis are hepatocyte necrosis and inflammation with polymorph infiltration, fatty changes and Mallory's hyalin. Performance of a percutaneous liver biopsy should be undertaken with respect to the risks of bleeding. A transjugular liver biopsy may be considered in patients with coagulopathy.

Initial management

There is no cure for alcoholic liver disease. The mainstay of management is abstinence from alcohol, supportive treatment and management of complications.

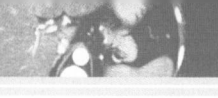
Patient education

The importance of abstinence from alcohol must be stressed. It is usually sufficient to reverse the changes of a fatty liver.

Alcohol withdrawal

Patients who require admission to hospital may suffer severe alcohol withdrawal. Prophylactic treatment with chlordiazepoxide is usually administered over 5 days. Benzodiazepines may also be required. Management of withdrawal symptoms may require specialist psychiatric services and, in the longer term, independent alcoholic support groups (Alcoholics Anonymous).

Nutrition

Review by a dietician is appropriate to address vitamin deficiencies and malnutrition. The recommended protein intake is between 1 and 1.5 g/kg. Supplementation with vitamin B complex helps reduce Wernicke–Korsakoff syndrome. In addition, hypomagnaesemia, hypokalaemia and hypophosphataemia should be corrected. Patients with severe nutritional deficiency may require nasogastric (enteral) feeding.

Prophylactic antibiotics

There is an increased risk of sepsis in patients with hepatitis and cirrhosis, and prophylactic antibiotics in the form of ciprofloxacin and fluconazole should be given.

Medical management

Immunomodulation

The use of steroids in active hepatitis is controversial. Currently no statistically significant benefit has been demonstrated.[1]

Pentoxifylline

Tumour necrosis factor is elevated in acute alcoholic hepatitis. Pentoxifylline is a tumour necrosis factor (TNF) synthesis inhibitor that improves short-term survival in patients with alcoholic hepatitis.[2]

RECENT ADVANCES

The molecular adsorbents recirculating system is a form of extracorporeal liver support that attempts to remove toxins from the circulation, allowing the liver to regenerate and recover from acute alcoholic hepatitis. A pilot study has demonstrated encouraging results.[3]

Surgical management

Portosystemic shunt

Transjugular or formal surgical portosystemic shunts may be required to decrease the portal pressure in patients with portal hypertension. The main indications are for patients with refractory ascites or recurrent variceal bleeds.

Liver transplantation

Liver transplantation (p. 347) should be considered in patients who have been abstinent and are highly motivated with appropriate social support

Prognosis

A fatty liver resolves completely with 4 weeks of continued abstinence from alcohol. A fatty liver can also occur in the setting of alcoholic hepatitis or cirrhosis, in which case outcome depends on the degree of steatohepatitis or severity of chronic liver disease.

The prognosis in alcoholic hepatitis relates to the severity of disease. It ranges from potentially reversible disease (mild alcoholic hepatitis) to death (severe hepatitis). Short-term mortality ranges from 10% to 60% for mild and severe cases respectively. Variables associated with poor outcome are increasing age, urea, bilirubin, prothrombin time, low serum albumin and high leukocyte count.

The prognosis of patients with alcoholic cirrhosis varies significantly. Abstinence may arrest the disease process and allow some functional improvement. Patients with compensated cirrhosis have a relatively good prognosis compared to patients with decompensated disease.

REFERENCES

(1) *Christensen E, Gluud C. Glucocorticoids are ineffective in alcoholic hepatitis: a meta-analysis adjusting for confounding variables. Gut 1995; 37: 113–118.*
(2) *Akriviadis E, Botla R, Briggs W, Han S, Reynolds T, Shakil O. Pentoxifylline improves short-term survival in severe acute alcoholic hepatitis: a double-blind, placebo-controlled trial. Gastroenterology 2000; 119: 1637–1648.*
(3) *Jalan R, Sen S, Steiner C, Kapoor D, Alisa A, Williams R. Extracorporeal liver support with molecular adsorbents recirculating system in patients with severe acute alcoholic hepatitis. Journal of Hepatology 2003; 38: 24–31.*

Non-alcoholic fatty liver disease

Non-alcoholic fatty liver disease is a spectrum of liver disease ranging from fatty infiltration of the liver (steatosis) to inflammation (non-alcoholic steatohepatitis) to fibrosis and cirrhosis.

Epidemiology

Hepatic steatosis is a very common benign condition. Autopsy studies suggest that the prevalence of non-alcoholic steatohepatitis is 15 000 per 100 000 obese individuals and up to 5000 per 100 000 of individuals with normal body weight.[1] It is more common in middle-aged obese women.

Pathology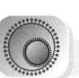

The diseases associated with hepatic steatosis and non-alcoholic steatohepatitis are listed in Table 5.16. The pathogenesis is unclear but is believed to be due to abnormal fatty acid metabolism with reduced oxidation but increased delivery and synthesis of free fatty acids in the liver. It is characterized by macrovesicular steatosis with polymorph, monocyte and lymphocyte infiltration of the portal tracts and hepatocytes. There may be hyaline deposits and fibrosis leading to cirrhosis. Iron can be found on staining, but the hepatic iron index is low (excluding haemochromatosis).

Table 5.16	Diseases associated with hepatic steatosis and non-alcoholic steatohepatitis
Obesity	
Diabetes	
Hypothyroidism	
Hyperlipidaemia	
Pregnancy	
Jejuno-ileal bypass	
Short bowel syndrome	
Total parenteral nutrition	

Drugs
  Steroids
  Amiodarone
  Methotrexate
  Tamoxifen
  Sodium valproate
  Non-steroidal anti-inflammatory drugs	

Clinical features

Patients with hepatic steatosis are asymptomatic and often diagnosed because of abnormal transaminases. Occasional symptoms include right upper quadrant discomfort from liver capsule distension. More commonly, patients are identified through abnormal liver biochemistry.

On examination, mild hepatomegaly may be felt in the minority, and features of portal hypertension are rare.

Investigations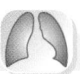

Liver profile
There is a mild elevation of AST and ALT. The AST/ALT ratio is typically <1 (unlike alcoholic hepatitis). ALP is raised and the bilirubin is normal.

Serum lipid profile
Hyperlipidaemia may be present.

Screening for other causes of hepatitis
Serum autoantibodies, viral antibodies, copper, caeruloplasmin (Wilson's disease) and iron studies are normal.

Ultrasound of the liver
Ultrasound imaging can detect fatty infiltration.

Liver biopsy
The liver biopsy is the gold standard for diagnosing steatohepatitis. Biopsy will confirm fatty infiltration but is not always needed in very mild cases with an obvious cause. The presence of microvesicular steatosis or steatohepatitis may predict progressive disease.

Management

Patient education
Obese patients are advised to lose weight, and diabetics are encouraged to have a tight glucose control.

Identify and treat any underlying disease
An important aspect is to identify and stop any offending drug, or to treat any associated disease. Hyperlipidaemia should be treated.

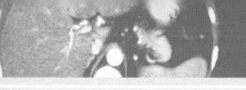

Liver transplantation

Liver transplantation may be required for patients with end-stage cirrhosis.

Prognosis

Hepatic steatosis and steatohepatitis are less benign than previously thought. Those with significant inflammation and fibrosis are more likely to progress to cirrhosis (10%).

There have been reports of recurrences of non-alcoholic steatohepatitis after liver transplantation.

REFERENCE

(1) *Wanless IR, Lentz JS. Fatty liver hepatitis and obesity: an autopsy study with analysis of risk factors. Hepatology 1990; 12: 1106–1110.*

SECTION 5.9 Viral hepatitis

Hepatitis A

Epidemiology

Hepatitis A is endemic throughout the world, especially in areas of poor sanitation.

Pathology

Hepatitis A is a non-enveloped RNA virus. It is transmitted by the faecal–oral route, and the incubation period is 2–6 weeks. During the incubation period, the patient is infectious due to faecal shedding of the virus. There is no carrier state and hepatitis A does not progress to chronic liver disease.

Clinical features

Many patients are asymptomatic. Some may develop a self-limiting acute hepatitis with non-specific symptoms such as anorexia, arthralgia and myalgia. On examination, patients may be pyrexial and jaundiced with hepatosplenomegaly.

Investigations

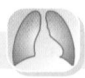

Liver profile

Liver transaminases (ALT and AST) are markedly elevated. Serum bilirubin may be elevated.

Hepatitis serology

The presence of specific hepatitis A IgM confirms the diagnosis. The level rises at around the same time as the serum bilirubin. The presence of hepatitis A IgG antibodies marks life-long immunity.

Management

Patient education

There is no specific treatment for HAV infection. Patients are advised to have bed rest and fluids, and to avoid alcohol. Hygiene in the form of hand washing and proper sanitation should be strongly encouraged.

Monitoring

In patients with deteriorating clinical state, monitoring of liver function tests, full blood count and coagulation screen are required to screen for the development of incipient hepatic failure.

Prevention

Prevention is difficult as virus shedding occurs in the incubation period. Good personal hygiene, careful food handling and a clean water supply are essential. Hepatitis A vaccine is available and should be offered for travellers to endemic areas. Vaccination lasts at least 10 years.

Prognosis

Most patients recover spontaneously. Hepatitis A rarely results in fulminant hepatic failure.

Hepatitis E

Epidemiology

Hepatitis E is endemic to Asia, the Middle East and Africa.

Pathology

Hepatitis E virus is a single-stranded RNA virus that is transmitted by the faecal–oral route (similar to hepatitis A).

Clinical features

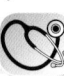

As in hepatitis A, many patients are asymptomatic. Some may develop a self-limiting acute hepatitis with non-specific symptoms such as anorexia, arthralgia and myalgia. On examination, patients may be pyrexial and jaundiced with hepatosplenomegaly. Fulminant hepatitis may occur in pregnant patients, especially in the third trimester.

Investigations

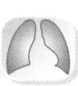

Hepatitis serology
Detection of antibodies to hepatitis E virus or RNA confirms hepatitis E infection.

Management

Patient education
Generally, only supportive treatment is required. Patients are advised to have bed rest and fluids, and to avoid alcohol. Hygiene in the form of hand washing and proper sanitation should be strongly encouraged.

Monitoring
In the rare cases of hepatic failure, patients should be managed in a specialist liver unit.

Prevention
Recombinant vaccines are currently undergoing phase III clinical trials.

Prognosis

Hepatitis E infection is self-limiting in the majority. In the third trimester of pregnancy, there is a high mortality.

Hepatitis B

Epidemiology

Hepatitis B is a common infection worldwide. Over 400 million have been affected by this virus, mainly in Asia, Africa and the Indian subcontinent.

Pathology

In low endemic areas, the main route of transmission is via blood (intravenous drug use, blood transfusions, occupational exposure), semen (sexual contacts) and saliva. In high endemic areas, transmission is predominantly from mother to fetus (vertical transmission).

After acquisition of infection with hepatitis B, the incubation period can be as long as 6 months. Usually, the first virological marker detectable in the serum is HBsAg (hepatitis B surface antigen, an envelope protein expressed on the outer surface of the virion). There are two other important antigens for the hepatitis B virus, the core antigen (HBcAg) and the 'e' antigen (HBeAg). The core antigen (HBcAg) is not directly detectable but its corresponding antibody is useful as an early marker of infection (anti-HBc) as antibodies to HBs take several months to develop. HBeAg corresponds to high levels of viral replication and is used as a marker of infectivity.

Scope of disease

Infection with hepatitis B is self-limiting in the majority. However, patients may progress to fulminant liver failure, chronic infection and cirrhosis, and are at an increased risk of developing hepatocellular carcinoma.

Clinical features

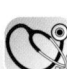

The majority of patients are asymptomatic (especially in childhood). Symptoms of acute hepatitis include headache, malaise, nausea, vomiting, right upper quadrant discomfort, jaundice, and occasionally a rash (viral exanthem) or joint pains. On examination, patients may be pyrexial and jaundiced with tender hepatomegaly. The stool may be clay coloured and the urine may be dark.

Chronicity is indicated by the failure of resolution of symptoms, biochemical features (liver transaminases), immunological markers of infectivity (HBsAg, HBeAg) or the histological appearance of bridging necrosis 6 months or more after the initial infection.

Initial investigations

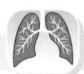

Full blood count
Low neutrophil and lymphocyte count occurs transiently with the acute illness. A haemolytic anaemia may be present.

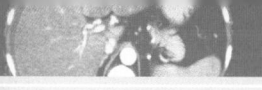

Liver profile

Liver transaminases and bilirubin are elevated. Serum albumin, a marker of the synthetic function of the liver, may be low.

Coagulation screen

The prothrombin time may be prolonged with severe liver disease due to impairment of the production of clotting factors.

Hepatitis serology

Circulating HBsAg precedes the clinical and biochemical features (raised serum transaminases) of hepatitis B infection and resolves 2 months after the onset of jaundice. Only at this stage do IgM antibodies to HBsAg (anti-HBs) become detectable, and they remain detectable indefinitely, being useful as a marker of immunity. IgM anti-HBs antibodies are not useful as a marker of infection within the first 2 months.

Anti-HBc antibodies are detectable within the first 2 weeks and are used to diagnose hepatitis B infection early in the course of the disease. HBsAg and HBeAg are markers of active infection (viral replication); they disappear when the acute infection clears (Fig. 5.6). Chronicity is suggested when HBsAg is detected 6 months after the initial infection, and the presence of HBeAg at this time indicates ongoing replication.

Rare variants of the hepatitis B virus do not produce HBeAg. These escape immune surveillance and are therefore free to cause liver damage. Patients with such mutations are negative for HBeAg and HBe antibodies. They may have ongoing liver inflammation as manifested by abnormal liver function tests and abnormal liver biopsies. The presence of a pre-core mutant is suspected in patients who are HBeAg negative but have high levels of serum hepatitis B DNA.

Initial management

Patient education

Patients with acute hepatitis B infection do not require antiviral treatment. Patient education, avoidance of alcohol and reduction of high-risk activities are important. Intra-

venous drug abusers should be educated about the risk of sharing of needles. Patients should be informed about the use of barrier contraception.

Medical management

Overall management aims to suppress inflammation of the liver and reduce long-term liver damage and complications.

Lamivudine

Lamivudine acts by inhibiting viral reverse transcription. It is administered to patients with a persistently high viral load (hepatitis B viral DNA >105), elevated ALT (twice normal), infection with pre-core mutant strains and those with decompensated liver disease or cirrhosis. It is prescribed as oral therapy for at least 1 year. There is a 30% response rate (assessed by the absence of HBeAg). Approximately 30% develop lamivudine resistance after 12 months; adefovir, another antiviral agent, can then be used instead.

Interferon treatment

Interferon-alfa or pegylated interferon can be administered to patients with a persistently high viral load or elevated ALT (twice normal). It is administered as subcutaneous injections and requires a shorter duration of treatment. It is not useful for patients with decompensated liver disease. The response rate is approximately 10% at 1 year.

RECENT ADVANCES

Thymosin α-1 is a new agent that stimulates stem cell differentiation, increases T lymphocytes, reduces apoptosis of T lymphocytes, increases IL-2 and interferon-γ and reduces IL-4 and IL-10.

Surgical management

Liver transplantation

Patients who subsequently develop fulminant liver failure may require liver transplantation (p. 347).

Prognosis

In approximately 90%, acute hepatitis B resolves spontaneously. Approximately 1% develop acute liver failure, and 15% develop chronic disease (hepatitis for >6 months). The development of chronic disease is more common in men, Asians and those who are infected when young. In those with chronic disease, HBeAg clearance occurs spontaneously at a rate of 20% per year.

Prevention

Active vaccination is indicated for those in high-risk categories such as health-care workers. Passive vaccination may be given to babies in high-risk births.

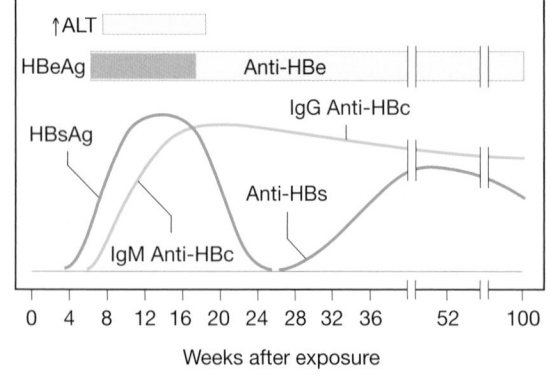

Fig. 5.6 Timing of clinical features and hepatitis serology.

Hepatitis D

Hepatitis D (or delta agent) is a single-stranded circular RNA virus that occurs only in the presence of hepatitis B infection. Approximately 5% of chronic hepatitis B carriers are infected with hepatitis D. The acquisition of hepatitis D infection (superinfection) results in a more severe hepatitis and higher risk of cirrhosis and hepatocellular carcinoma in patients with chronic hepatitis B. Acute liver failure develops in 20%, and the majority develop chronic hepatitis D infection. Co-infection refers to the acquisition of both hepatitis B and D at the same time. There is more severe acute hepatitis and a higher incidence of acute liver failure. Unlike superinfection, the majority of patients with co-infection clear both viruses at a rate that is similar to that for hepatitis B infection alone.

Hepatitis C

Epidemiology

Over 150 million people are infected with hepatitis C worldwide. Different genotypes correlate closely to the geographical area of origin. In Asia, genotypes 2 and 3 predominate, whilst in Europe and North America genotype 1 predominates.

Pathology

The hepatitis C virus (HCV) is an enveloped, single-stranded RNA virus. The most important route of transmission is parenteral; this includes the sharing of needles by intravenous drug abusers, acquisition from tattoos and blood transfusion (prior to screening). Sexual transmission is unusual, and no obvious risk factor is identified in 25%. The majority of patients (80%) who are infected with hepatitis C develop chronic liver disease. Chronic infection is a slow, progressive disease of variable duration (mean 20–30 years). The disease process may be accelerated in those who are co-infected with HIV or hepatitis B, those who consume excess alcohol and those who acquire hepatitis C later in life.

Clinical features

The majority of patients with acute and chronic hepatitis C infection are asymptomatic. Patients with chronic infection may present with features of chronic liver disease (splenomegaly, ascites and varices). The diagnosis is mainly serological.

Investigations

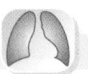

Hepatitis serology

Anti-hepatitis C antibodies develop within 6 months of acute infection and are detected by enzyme-linked immunosorbent assay (ELISA) or recombinant immunoblot assay (RIBA). The gold standard for detecting the presence of active infection is by polymerase chain reaction (PCR) for hepatitis C RNA.

Liver biopsy

Liver biopsy should be performed to assess the degree of inflammation and fibrosis.

Management

The aim of treatment is to eradicate HCV and therefore reduce the complications of liver disease.

Interferon 2 and ribavirin

In acute hepatitis, combination therapy with interferon-2α or β and ribavirin may reduce the risk of chronicity. Combination therapy is also recommended for patients with chronic disease with persistent levels of hepatitis C RNA and moderate to severe hepatitis or compensated cirrhosis. Those with mild disease assessed by biochemical and histological features may not require treatment (approximately 20% spontaneously recover).

The duration of treatment is 1 year in patients with genotype 1 hepatitis C, and 6 months in patients with genotype 2. Combination therapy (using conventional interferon) increases sustained virological response to approximately 40%.

Pegylated interferon

Pegylated interferon (attachment of the polyethylene glycol chain to the interferon molecule) improves pharmacokinetics and is superior to standard interferon. Single-agent therapy with pegylated interferon is administered to patients intolerant of ribavirin or when ribavirin is contraindicated (the patient is expected to conceive). The use of pegylated interferon improves overall success rates, especially in the treatment of genotype 1 disease.

> **RECENT ADVANCES**
>
> *Preliminary studies on thymosin α-1 have shown promising results, with improved viral clearance and histological scores and sustained response in combination with interferon.*

Prognosis

The majority of patients infected with hepatitis C progress to chronic liver disease. Approximately 20% resolve spontaneously, with medical therapy increasing the resolution rate to approximately 40%. The prognosis is also influenced by the genotype.

Autoimmune hepatitis

Autoimmune hepatitis is a chronic, progressive liver disease characterized histologically by interface hepatitis associated with autoantibodies and hypergammaglobulinaemia.

Epidemiology

There is marked geographical variation in autoimmune hepatitis. It is more common in the Caucasian population, and accounts for 20% of chronic hepatitis in Europe. In the United Kingdom, the incidence is 1 per 100 000 per year. Similar to other autoimmune conditions, it is more common in women (four fold).

Pathology

The precise aetiology is unclear. Autoimmune hepatitis is thought to result from an initiated inflammatory response in predisposed individuals with loss of immune self-tolerance leading to the production of autoantibodies (Table 5.17). The association with HLA-D3 suggests a genetic component of this disease. Autoantibodies associated with autoimmune hepatitis have not been shown to have a pathogenic role and neither is there a correlation between the levels of the autoantibodies and disease severity. The disease can, however, be subtyped according to the type of autoantibodies identified (1, 2 and 3; Table 5.18).

Autoimmune hepatitis behaves as a chronic hepatitis usually lasting more than 6 months and progressing to cirrhosis. Histological features include interface hepatitis (piecemeal necrosis) with disruption of the portal tract limiting plate, lobular hepatitis, plasma cell infiltration of

Table 5.17	Conditions associated with autoimmune hepatitis
Thyroiditis	
Ulcerative colitis	
Renal tubular acidosis	
Synovitis	
Coeliac disease	
Insulin-dependent diabetes mellitus	
Coombs' haemolytic anaemia	
Pernicious anaemia	
Rheumatoid arthritis	
Sjögren's syndrome	
Myasthenia gravis	

Table 5.18	Classification of autoimmune hepatitis
Type 1 (positive SMA)	
Represents majority of autoimmune hepatitis in Europe and US	
Majority are below 30 years of age	
Anti-nuclear antibodies (ANA) may also be positive	
Type 2 (positive anti-LKM-1)	
Represents 4% of autoimmune hepatitis in the US	
Usually occurs in the young, less than 15 years	
May be other antibodies such as anti-thyroid, anti-parietal cells	
Strong autoimmune presence	
Serum IgA may be low	
May develop a fulminant course	
Type 3 (positive anti-SLA/LP)	
Possibly a variant of type 1 autoimmune hepatitis	

SMA, anti-smooth muscle antibodies; anti-LKM-1, anti-liver/kidney microsome type 1 antibodies; anti-SLA/LP, anti-soluble liver antigen/liver-pancreas.

portal tracts and centrilobular (zone 3) necrosis. The presence of bridging necrosis indicates a poorer prognosis as there is a greater risk of cirrhosis.

Scope of disease

Autoimmune hepatitis can progress to liver cirrhosis with the development of portal hypertension and end-stage liver disease. Acute liver failure can (rarely) occur. Patients who develop autoimmune hepatitis are also predisposed to hepatocellular carcinoma. Autoimmune hepatitis often coexists with other conditions (overlap syndromes) such as primary biliary cirrhosis, primary sclerosing cholangitis and autoimmune cholangitis.

Clinical features

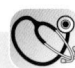

The presenting symptoms are often vague with lethargy, malaise, anorexia and right upper quadrant discomfort. Jaundice is uncommon in the early stages of the disease. A proportion of patients present with an acute illness (rarely with fulminant hepatic failure) before settling to a more indolent stage. Cirrhosis is present in about 25%, and occasionally patients may present late in the course of disease with the complications of cirrhosis. There are usually features of other autoimmune diseases. A social and drug history is necessary to exclude other causes of liver impairment such as alcohol- or drug-related hepatitis.

On examination there may not be any obvious features of liver disease. In those with examination findings, spider naevi and palmar erythema are most common. Jaundice or features of portal hypertension (ascites, splenomegaly, encephalopathy) occur late in the disease. Occasionally, tender hepatomegaly may be noted. Encephalopathy and bruising indicate the development of fulminant hepatitis.

Initial investigations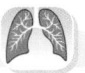

The diagnosis of autoimmune hepatitis requires the exclusion of other causes of hepatitis as their clinical presentations are very similar. Some may be straightforward while others are difficult, especially when antibody titres fluctuate and may even disappear.

Full blood count
Anaemia may be secondary to autoimmune haemolysis.

Liver profile
Liver transaminases are markedly elevated. Serum albumin and the prothrombin time are usually normal, except in the acute setting and with end-stage disease.

Serum autoantibodies
The antibodies associated with autoimmune hepatitis include anti-nuclear antibodies, anti-smooth muscle antibodies (SMA), anti-liver/kidney microsome (LKM) type 1 antibodies, anti-soluble liver antigen/liver-pancreas (SLA/LP) and anti-double-stranded DNA (dsDNA).

Hepatitis viral serology
Viral serology is often performed to exclude hepatitis A, B, C, cytomegalovirus (CMV) and Epstein–Barr virus (EBV) hepatitis as a differential diagnosis.

Serum caeruloplasmin
Serum copper and caeruloplasmin are assessed to exclude Wilson's disease as a differential diagnosis.

Iron studies
Iron studies (ferritin, iron, transferrin) are performed to exclude haemochromatosis as a differential diagnosis.

Serum α_1-antitrypsin
Serum levels of α_1-antitrypsin are estimated to exclude deficiency as a cause of hepatitis.

Ultrasound of the abdomen
The presence of a small liver suggests the development of cirrhosis. Hyperechogenicity suggests fatty infiltration.

Further investigations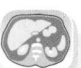

Liver biopsy
A liver biopsy may show features typical of autoimmune hepatitis or may be useful to diagnose overlap syndromes. In addition, a liver biopsy may help to exclude other causes of chronic hepatitis. As the histological improvement lags biochemical improvement (by up to 6 months), a liver biopsy is useful to grade the treatment response before it is reflected in the blood tests, to confirm remission and to determine the risk of relapse.

Initial management

Supportive treatment
Not all patients require treatment; patients without significant disease as assessed on liver biochemistry and biopsy do not require medical therapy.

Medical management

Immunomodulation
Immunomodulation therapy is reserved for patients with significant inflammation as assessed by liver biochemistry or histology.

Steroids (prednisolone) and azathioprine are the mainstay of treatment. They can be administered as monotherapy or combination therapy. Both regimens are equally effective but the combination therapy allows a lower dose of steroid to be prescribed and therefore reduces the potential side effects of steroid therapy (especially in postmenopausal women).

High-dose prednisolone is started for monotherapy, at 40–60 mg/day. This is reduced weekly and kept at the lowest dose to maintain remission (usually 10–20 mg/day).

For combination therapy, azathioprine is started at 1 mg/kg with prednisolone at 30 mg per day. Prednisolone is gradually reduced as in monotherapy, weekly, and maintained at about 10 mg per day. Azathioprine can cause bone marrow suppression. It should be avoided in those with thiopurine methyltransferase deficiency.

Single or combination therapy is continued for about 1–2 years because of a high relapse rate. Prior to considering withdrawal of treatment, a liver biopsy should be performed to confirm the absence of ongoing inflammation.

Surgical management

Liver transplantation
Liver transplantation (p. 347) should be considered in patients who do not respond to therapy and those with fulminant hepatic failure, decompensated cirrhosis and a high Child–Pugh score. Patients should remain on steroids post transplantation to reduce the recurrence of autoimmune hepatitis in the transplanted liver.

Prognosis

In the majority of cases, autoimmune hepatitis is a progressive disease with periods of remission. Cirrhosis ensues in the majority of patients who are not treated.

Features on the liver biopsy help to predict prognosis. The presence of periportal hepatitis and bridging necrosis is associated with the development of cirrhosis in 20% and 80% respectively by 5 years. The development of cirrhosis is associated with a high mortality rate.

Failure of improvement of hyperbilirubinaemia within 2 weeks in a background of multilobular necrosis is predictive of high short-term mortality, and failure of remission within 2 years of treatment carries a 50% chance of the development of decompensation.

Liver transplantation for autoimmune hepatitis has an excellent 5-year survival but carries a higher risk of rejection.

> **FURTHER INFORMATION**
>
> Alvarez F, Berg PA, Bianchi FB, et al. International Autoimmune Hepatitis Group Report: review of criteria for diagnosis of autoimmune hepatitis. Journal of Hepatology 1999; 31: 929–938.

SECTION 5.11 Haemochromatosis

The iron overload syndromes may be classified as primary (genetic) or secondary haemochromatosis (Table 5.19). Currently the term 'haemochromatosis' refers to genetic haemochromatosis.

Epidemiology

Genetic haemochromatosis is the most common inherited metabolic defect in Northern Europeans. It is inherited in an autosomal recessive manner with a gene frequency of 10%. It is more common in men, and the age at presentation is usually between 40 and 60 years.

Pathology

The gene responsible for genetic haemochromatosis is located on chromosome 6 and codes for a major histocompatibility complex type 1 protein. Numerous mutations exist, the most common of which is a cysteine tyrosine substitution in position 282. Homozygosity of this mutation is the principal defect in 90% of patients with genetic haemochromatosis.

The body contains about 4 g of total iron, the majority contained within haemoglobin. Approximately 10% of ingested iron is absorbed from the villi of the small intestine (1.5 mg of iron per day). In haemochromatosis, mucosal absorption amounts to 4 mg per day or more and leads to elevated plasma iron, saturation of transferrin and elevation of plasma ferritin.

Excess iron in the body is deposited in the parenchyma of the liver, pancreas and heart, leading to oxidative stress and organelle damage. In the liver, activation of Kupffer cells leads to the production of pro-inflammatory cytokines. These inflammatory mediators stimulate stellate cells to produce fibrogenic material causing organ damage. Early in the disease, iron deposition occurs in a periportal and hepatocellular distribution. With progressive accumulation, the hepatocellular distribution of iron is predominant, with iron also present in the Kupffer and biliary cells. Eventually, repeated liver injury leads to micronodular cirrhosis.

Scope of disease

Iron deposition in the liver leads to hepatitis, fibrosis and cirrhosis. Patients with cirrhosis are also at an increased risk of hepatocellular carcinoma. Systemic iron deposition leads to organ-specific manifestations such as diabetes mellitus (pancreas), cardiomyopathy (heart), hypogonadism (testes), hypopituitarism (pituitary), arthritis and arthralgia (joints).

Clinical features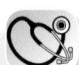

Most patients are asymptomatic and identified through routine biochemistry or family screening for haemochromatosis. Symptoms of haemochromatosis are non-specific and include malaise, lethargy, weight loss and anaemia. Jaundice, ascites and hepatomegaly can occur with iron deposition in the liver. Symptoms associated with iron

Table 5.19	Causes of iron overload
Primary	
Genetic haemochromatosis	
Secondary	
Iron-loading anaemias (repeated blood transfusions)	
Thalassaemia	
Chronic haemolytic anaemia	
Sideroblastic anaemia	
Chronic liver disease	
End-stage liver disease	
Alcoholic liver disease	
Hepatitis C	
Dietary iron overload	

deposition in other organs include dyspnoea (cardiac failure), joint swellings, typically of the second and third metacarpophalangeal joints, and a skin rash (porphyria cutanea tarda).

It is important to exclude secondary causes of iron overload such as repeated transfusions for haemolytic anaemias, excess alcohol intake and herbal medications that might contain iron.

Initial investigations

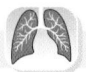

Full blood count
Polycythaemia may be present.

Liver profile
The liver function tests are generally normal in the early stages of the disease. Cirrhosis usually leads to elevated transaminase and bilirubin levels.

Fasting blood sugar
A fasting blood sugar level is performed to screen for diabetes. If this is equivocal, a formal glucose tolerance test should be performed.

Iron studies
In genetic haemochromatosis, serum ferritin is elevated and transferrin saturation and the iron-binding capacity is usually more than 50%. Transferrin saturation is more specific for genetic haemochromatosis. Other causes of elevated iron or ferritin include alcoholic liver disease, viral hepatitis and inflammatory conditions. Occasionally, these disorders may coexist. Iron studies are also performed for screening.

Hepatitis serology
Elevated iron studies can also occur with viral hepatitis, therefore it is important to perform these screening investigations.

Further investigations

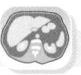

Genetic analysis
Genetic analysis for specific mutations should be performed. Patients who are homozygous for the *C282Y* mutation or are compound heterozygous with *C282Y/H63D* and *C282Y/S65C* mutations are likely to have iron overload due to genetic haemochromatosis. By themselves, *H63D* and *S65C* gene mutations do not cause iron overload.

Liver biopsy
A liver biopsy should be undertaken to exclude coexisting conditions and to assess the degree of fibrosis or cirrhosis. This is important in patients over 40 years and those with abnormal liver function tests. Perls' stain is used to aid identification of iron deposition, and the iron concentration can be determined on histology. A hepatic iron index (hepatic iron concentration in μmol/g divided by age in

years) of more than 2 suggests the diagnosis of genetic haemochromatosis. Values below 2, however, do not exclude the disease. The presence of cirrhosis should identify those at risk of developing hepatocellular carcinomas.

Serum α-fetoprotein
Elevated levels of α-fetoprotein may occur in patients with the secondary complication of hepatocellular carcinoma.

Ultrasound of the liver
A liver ultrasound is a useful investigation for patients with suspected hepatocellular carcinoma.

Initial management

Patient education
Patients should be advised to avoid iron supplements, excessive consumption of vitamin C (promotes iron absorption) and excessive alcohol intake as the degree of liver injury increases in the presence of alcohol and iron excess.

Screening
All first-degree relatives should be offered screening through the combination of iron studies and genetic testing. Gene mutations are present in more than 90% of patients with genetic haemochromatosis, therefore it is possible to identify those at risk. Early treatment prevents the development of complications from iron overload.

Medical management

Venesection
Weekly venesection of 1 unit of blood (approximately 250 mg of iron) may be required for up to 2 years before tissue iron stores are reduced. Patients with serum ferritin >100 and haemoglobin >10 g/dL require continued weekly venesection. If the serum ferritin is >100 and haemoglobin <10 g/dL or if there is a more than 2 g/dL fall in haemoglobin, the frequency or volume of venesection is reduced. When serum ferritin falls below 100, patients can be moved to maintenance venesection therapy (1 unit of blood every 2–3 months) using the same criteria as above.

Improved physical well-being and energy levels are often experienced after venesection therapy, even in previously asymptomatic patients. Serum transaminase levels may improve (reduce), and glucose intolerance may be more easily managed.

Chelation therapy
Intravenous desferrioxamine may be administered to reduce weekly iron stores by 10–20 mg. As venesection is the more cost-effective and safer option, desferrioxamine is reserved for patients with anaemia severe enough to preclude venesection.

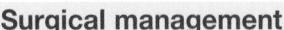

Surgical management

Liver transplantation

Liver transplantation should be considered in patients with end-stage liver disease. Those who develop hepatocellular carcinoma should be assessed early (p. 339).

Prognosis

In general, the prognosis is good if there is no organ damage. Some patients have continued deterioration of liver function despite treatment. Once end-organ damage

(cirrhosis, diabetes mellitus, arthritis) has occurred, it is irreversible. The development of cirrhosis or hepatocellular carcinoma is associated with a poor prognosis.

---

i FURTHER INFORMATION

Dooley J, Worwood M. Genetic haemochromatosis guidelines. British Committee for Standards in Haematology. Abingdon, Oxford: Darwin Medical Communications, 2000.

SECTION 5.12 Wilson's disease

Wilson's disease is an autosomal recessive neurodegenerative disorder of copper metabolism, also known as hepatolenticular degeneration. The abnormal gene (*ATP7B*) is found on chromosome 13 and codes a membrane-spanning copper-transport protein.

Epidemiology

Wilson's disease is a rare disorder, with a prevalence reported to be around 1 in 30 000. It affects both sexes equally, and peaks in the age range of 8–20 years.

Pathology

Wilson's disease results in intrahepatic copper accumulation due to impaired excretion. Possible mechanisms include the failure of intracellular copper transport due to abnormal proteins or enzymes. As the accumulated copper is released, other organs such as the brain, eyes and kidneys can be affected.

Scope of disease

Liver disease results from excess copper accumulation and can lead to cirrhosis and fulminant hepatitis. Other manifestations of copper accumulation include hypothyroidism, arthropathy (pseudo-gout), nephrolithiasis, renal tubular acidosis, haemolytic anaemia, neuropsychiatric disturbances and movement disorders.

Clinical features

In young patients, liver impairment is the principal feature and is usually asymptomatic. Diagnosis from incidental abnormal liver function tests accounts for 50% of the mode of presentation. Clinical examination is often normal until later in the disease when features of chronic liver disease (p. 299) develop. Copper deposition in the nails may cause azure lunulae.

Older patients tend to present with neuropsychiatric symptoms, liver impairment and movement disorders such as tremor, chorea, incoordination and Parkinsonian symptoms. Depression and schizophrenia are known psychiatric manifestations. On examination, Kayser–Fleischer rings, copper-coloured rings at the periphery of the cornea, are common, although their identification usually requires slit-lamp examination. It is important to note that cholestasis from any cause can also result in hepatic copper accumulation and pigmented corneal rings.

Initial investigations

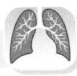

Full blood count
A haemolytic anaemia may be present.

Liver profile
Liver transaminases and bilirubin may be elevated with the development of hepatitis or cirrhosis.

Serum caeruloplasmin
Serum caeruloplasmin is low (<200 mg/L) in 90% of patients with Wilson's disease. When initial samples are non-diagnostic, repeat samples should be taken.

Serum copper
Serum copper is usually low, but this is not diagnostic.

Ophthalmic assessment
Slit-lamp examination may reveal Kayser–Fleischer rings in the majority.

Further investigations

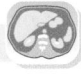

24-Hour urinary copper level
This is requested if the initial tests are abnormal or non-diagnostic but high clinical suspicion remains. A level over

100 µg in 24 hours is suggestive of Wilson's disease and this can be confirmed with a penicillamine challenge.

Liver biopsy

If urinary and serum levels are not diagnostic, a liver biopsy is performed to measure the amount of copper deposition. A concentration more than 250 µg/g is confirmatory. Liver biopsy also allows histopathological assessment of disease severity.

Screening

Screening for Wilson's disease by means of serum caeruloplasmin levels should be offered to all first-degree relatives.

RECENT ADVANCES

Genetic techniques for diagnosis are currently under development. Their clinical use is still limited as numerous polymorphisms exist.

Initial management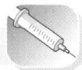

Patient education

Patients are advised to avoid foods that are high in copper, such as liver, shellfish and nuts.

Medical management

Penicillamine

D-Penicillamine is the initial copper chelating agent of choice. It is prescribed at a starting dose of 20 mg/kg/day in conjunction with pyridoxine 20 mg/day. It is essential that the patient be warned of the possibility of deterioration in his or her neurological state. Treatment is usually life-long and regular monitoring of liver function should be undertaken.

Trientine

An alternative chelating agent is trientine. This is prescribed to patients who develop intolerance to penicillamine or worsening neurological function whilst receiving penicillamine.

Zinc sulphate

Zinc sulphate can be prescribed to patients whose copper stores are not reduced by penicillamine or trientine, or for women of child-bearing potential. It should not be prescribed in conjunction with either penicillamine or trientine, as their effects are neutralized.

Immunomodulation

In rare cases of autoimmune-like hepatitis, a trial of prednisolone should be started at 30–40 mg/day until clinical improvement occurs.

Surgical management

Liver transplantation

Liver transplantation should be considered for patients with fulminant hepatic failure or in patients with end-stage disease with no response to medical therapy.

Prognosis

With medical therapy, an asymptomatic state can be achieved indefinitely. Neurological and psychiatric symptoms usually respond with the treatment of the underlying disease. Some residual neurological deficits, however, may persist.

SECTION 5.13 Alpha-1-antitrypsin deficiency

Alpha-1-antitrypsin is a serine protease inhibitor that inactivates elastase, collagenase and trypsin. It is also an acute phase protein synthesized in the liver and by macrophages (lesser extent). The main clinical manifestations of α_1-antitrypsin deficiency are pulmonary emphysema and liver cirrhosis.

Epidemiology

Alpha-1-antitrypsin deficiency is a genetic disorder occurring mainly in Caucasian populations with a gene frequency of 1 in 2000. The heterozygous state has a prevalence of approximately 10 000 per 100 000 of the population. It is more difficult to estimate the prevalence of the clinical manifestations in carriers of the gene mutation.

Pathology

The gene for α_1-antitrypsin is located on chromosome 14; there are more than 70 allelic variants. Only some, such as the S and Z protease inhibitor types, are associated with liver and lung disease. The phenotype MM is normal whilst the ZZ phenotype results in the lowest levels of α_1-antitrypsin; 25% of these patients subsequently develop liver disease.

Liver injury is caused by the hepatotoxic effects of mutant α_1-antitrypsin polymer sheets that accumulate within cells leading to cell death and cirrhosis. Pulmonary emphysema is caused by uninhibited proteolytic damage to elastic tissue in the lung parenchyma.

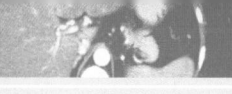
Scope of disease

Continuing liver damage results in cirrhosis, portal hypertension and an increased risk of hepatocellular carcinoma. Other organs that may be affected are the lungs (bronchiectasis, emphysema) and the kidney (glomerulonephritis).

Clinical features

Clinical features are dependent on the severity of α_1-antitrypsin deficiency. Infants can be asymptomatic or present with neonatal jaundice and elevated transaminases.

Most adults are asymptomatic; some are diagnosed from incidental abnormal liver function tests. Later in the disease, patients may present with features or complications of chronic liver disease such as variceal haemorrhage. On examination, hepatosplenomegaly may be evident.

Initial investigations

Serum α_1-antitrypsin

A level lower than 2.5 g/L suggests α_1-antitrypsin deficiency and further tests for phenotyping should be performed.

Alpha-1-antitrypsin phenotyping

Currently, α_1-antitrypsin phenotyping is the gold standard for diagnosis and identifies the specific abnormal mutation.

Further investigations

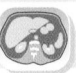

Liver biopsy

Liver biopsy can also help in establishing the diagnosis. Characteristic globules can be identified in hepatocytes with periodic acid–Schiff (PAS) diastase staining.

Initial management

Patient education

Treatment is supportive for those without chronic liver disease. Patients are advised against excess alcohol intake and smoking. Risk factors for viral hepatitis should be discussed and discouraged. Nutritional advice and high calorie intake are recommended, especially in those with liver impairment.

Screening

Screening by serum α_1-antitrypsin levels should be offered to first-degree relatives.

Surgical therapy

Liver transplantation

Orthotopic liver transplantation should be considered for those with advanced disease (hepatic decompensation) and impaired quality of life. The α_1-antitrypsin phenotype switches to that of the transplanted liver.

Prognosis

The prognosis depends on the severity of lung or liver disease. For patients with liver disease, there is no effective treatment apart from transplantation. Post transplantation, α_1-antitrypsin levels usually return to normal.

REFERENCE

(1) *Lomas DA, Mahadeva R. Alpha1-antitrypsin polymerization and the serpinopathies: pathobiology and prospects for therapy. Journal of Clinical Investigation 2002; 110: 1585–1590.*

Liver cysts

Simple liver cysts

Non-parasitic simple cysts of the liver have a prevalence of about 1% and are more common in women. The cysts are lined by columnar epithelial cells that resemble biliary epithelium, although there is no connection with the intrahepatic biliary tree. Simple liver cysts are often multiple and unilocular (contain no septa). Most patients with simple cysts are asymptomatic, although huge cysts can compress biliary or vascular structures leading to obstructive jaundice or portal hypertension respectively. Intracystic haemorrhage or infection can also occur. Thin walls, lack of septa and daughter cysts differentiate simple cysts from hydatid cysts on ultrasonography. Asymptomatic cysts require no treatment. Symptomatic or complicated cysts should undergo treatment with either percutaneous drainage and sclerotherapy or surgical fenestration (Fig. 5.7).[1]

> **REFERENCE**
>
> **(1)** Cowles RA, Mulholland MW. Solitary hepatic cysts. *Journal of the American College of Surgeons* 2000; 191: 311–321.

Hydatid liver cysts

Hydatid disease is a zoonosis caused by larval stages of the tapeworm Echinococcus. Although four species of Echinococcus cause disease in humans, the majority are due to infection with *E. granulosus*.

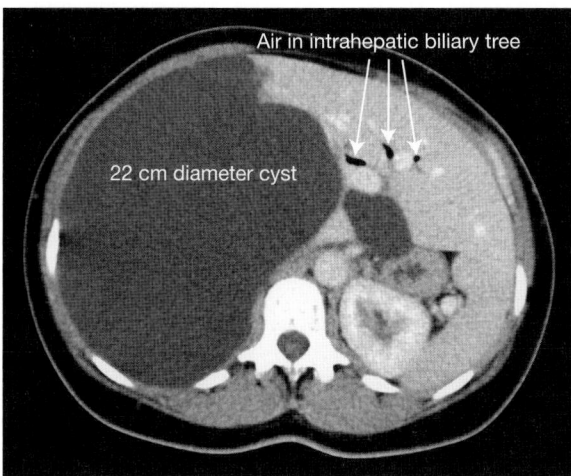

Fig. 5.7 CT scan showing multiple simple liver cysts and air in the intrahepatic biliary tree (pneumobilia).
Copyright Addenbrooke's Hospital, Cambridge, UK.

Epidemiology

The annual incidence of liver hydatid cysts is highly variable, ranging from <1 to 220 cases per 100 000. The disease occurs worldwide, but principally in sheep-grazing areas.

Pathology

Dogs are the definitive hosts of *E. granulosus* and are infected by ingesting infected offal from intermediate hosts (usually sheep). Eggs are passed in canine faeces, and humans become infected via the oral route after ingesting faecally contaminated water or coming into contact with contaminated objects. Activation and maturation of the eggs in the human duodenum leads to penetration of the intestinal mucosa and carriage via the portal vein to the liver. Hydatid cysts most commonly affect the liver (66%), but they can occur in the lungs (20%) or elsewhere in the body (14%).

Scope of disease

Complications include secondary bacterial infection, pressure effects on nearby structures, or rupture causing disease spread. Rupture can lead to minor allergic symptoms such as pruritus and urticaria, or rarely to anaphylaxis and death.

Clinical features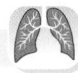

The symptoms of liver hydatid cysts depend on the size and location of the cysts. In general, cysts are slow growing (1–2 cm annually) and are asymptomatic in the early stages of the disease. Patients with large cysts may present with right upper quadrant pain and jaundice. Hepatomegaly and jaundice are the most common features on examination.

Initial investigations

Ultrasound of the liver
Ultrasound reveals the cystic nature of the lesion. Septa are present and the demonstration of multiple 'daughter' cysts inside or outside the main cyst cavity is diagnostic.

Echinococcus serology
Echinococcus serology can confirm the diagnosis in patients with suspicious cysts.

CT of the liver
CT will also be able to delineate the location of the liver cysts in preparation for surgery or percutaneous drainage.

Initial management

Antibiotics
Medical therapy with albendazole or mebendazole is curative in only 30%, and is therefore indicated for disseminated disease, or before surgery or percutaneous drainage to reduce disease spread.

Medical management

Conservative management
Patients with a small central cyst can be treated conservatively and monitored with regular ultrasound scans.

Percutaneous drainage
Percutaneous drainage in general is contraindicated due to the risk of transmission of infection. However, in patients who are unfit for surgery, percutaneous drainage with injection and instillation of hypertonic saline may be performed.[1]

Surgical management

Hepatectomy/cystectomy
Surgery is curative and is the recommended treatment for symptomatic, large or peripheral liver cysts prone to rupture. Surgery can be radical (partial hepatectomy) or conventional with aspiration of the cyst contents, instillation of a parasiticidal agent (e.g. hypertonic saline) and cystectomy.[2] Spillage of cyst contents must be avoided.

Prognosis

With appropriate treatment, mortality is 2–4%.

i FURTHER INFORMATION

Guidelines for treatment of cystic and alveolar echinococcosis in humans. WHO Informal Working Group on Echinococcosis. Bulletin of the World Health Organization 1996; 74(3): 231–242.

REFERENCES

(1) *Khuroo MS, Wani NA, Javid G, et al. Percutaneous drainage compared with surgery for hepatic hydatid cysts. New England Journal of Medicine 1997; 337: 881–887.*
(2) *Yorganci K, Sayek I. Surgical treatment of hydatid cysts of the liver in the era of percutaneous treatment. American Journal of Surgery 2002; 184: 63–69*

SECTION 5.15 **Liver abscesses**

Liver abscesses are focal collections of pus in the liver parenchyma due to bacterial, fungal or amoebic infection. Worldwide, the most common form is amoebic liver abscess, but in developed countries pyogenic liver abscesses are predominant.

Pyogenic liver abscess

Pyogenic liver abscesses result from bacterial or, rarely, fungal infection. Causes are listed in Table 5.20.

Epidemiology

The incidence is 20 per 100 000 hospital admissions with an equal gender distribution.

Pathology

Multiple abscesses are present in 50% of patients.[1] Abscesses are commonly caused by mixed infection from gut commensals such as *Escherichia coli, Klebsiella pneu-moniae* and *Enterococcus* species that enter the liver by different routes. Anaerobic organisms are also commonly involved but are less frequently identified on routine culture. Iatrogenic immunosuppression or AIDS predisposes to fungal or mycobacterial abscesses.

Scope of disease

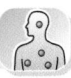

Complications occur in 10–20%, with metastatic septic emboli, haemobilia, subphrenic abscess formation, or rupture into the pleural, peritoneal or pericardial cavities.

Clinical features

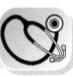

The clinical features of a patient with a solitary pyogenic liver abscess are non-specific and may include fever, malaise and vague abdominal pain. Patients with multiple abscesses are often septicaemic with fever, sweats and rigors. Only 33% have the classic signs of right upper quadrant tenderness and pyrexia.[2] Patients may also have clinical features from the site of primary infection.

Pyogenic liver abscess

Table 5.20	Frequency and underlying causes of pyogenic liver abscesses

Biliary tract obstruction and ascending infection (60%)
  Gallstones
  Pancreatic head adenocarcinoma
  Cholangiocarcinoma

Cryptogenic (10%)

Haematogenous spread via the hepatic artery from systemic infection (10%)
  Pneumonia
  Urinary sepsis
  Bacterial endocarditis

Haematogenous spread via the portal vein from gastrointestinal tract disease (7%)
  Appendicitis
  Diverticulitis
  Crohn's disease

Trauma and subsequent bacterial seeding (5%)

Direct extension from adjacent structures (3%)
  Subphrenic abscess
  Gallbladder empyema

Miscellaneous (5%)
  Iatrogenic (liver biopsy, biliary stents)
  Secondary infection of liver cysts
  Secondary infection of liver tumours (primaries or metastases)

Initial investigations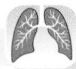

Full blood count
Neutrophilia and mild anaemia are present on full blood count.

Markers of inflammation
Erythrocyte sedimentation rate (ESR) and C-reactive protein (CRP) are markedly raised.

Urea and electrolytes
Raised urea and creatinine can occur with renal impairment.

Liver function tests
Raised liver enzymes with mild bilirubinaemia are common.

Coagulation screen
The prothrombin time may be elevated due to hepatic impairment.

Blood cultures
Blood cultures are performed before commencing antibiotics.

Viral and amoebic serology
Amoebic serology and viral hepatitis serology should be taken to exclude amoebiasis and hepatitis.

Chest X-ray
Right pleural effusion, right lower lobe atelectasis or raised right hemidiaphragm is present on half of chest radiographs.

Liver imaging
Imaging with either ultrasound or CT is diagnostic for liver abscess (Fig. 5.8). Radiologically guided aspiration of pus confirms the diagnosis of pyogenic liver abscess and enables microbiological culture. CT is marginally more sensitive than ultrasound (99% versus 94%)[3] and can also detect causative abdominal lesions.

Further investigations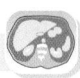

Endoscopic retrograde cholangio-pancreatography (ERCP)
If biliary obstruction is present on imaging (dilated bile ducts), ERCP can localize the site of obstruction and drain any biliary sepsis.

Initial management

Intravenous fluids, analgesia and nutritional care are important aspects of initial management.

Antibiotics
Once pyogenic liver abscess is suspected, empirical broad-spectrum intravenous antibiotics should be started. Anaerobic, Gram-negative, and Gram-positive aerobic bacterial infection should be covered, e.g. with metronidazole, gentamicin, and ampicillin. Treatment should be tailored to the specific organism if cultures are positive.

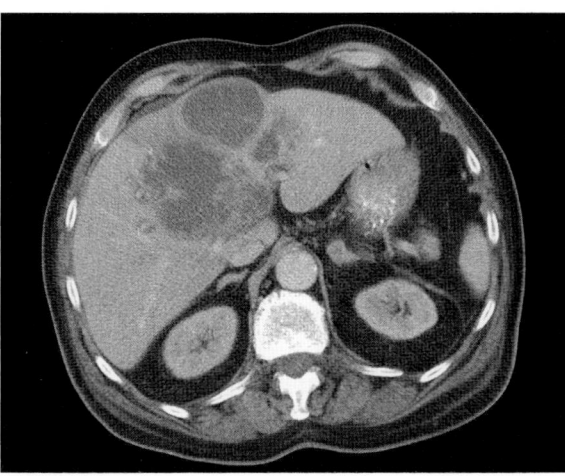

Fig. 5.8 CT of pyogenic liver abscess. Contrast-enhanced CT shows multiple ill-defined liver lesions which suggested liver abscesses. The patient's history is important as liver metastases can often look similar to abscesses on CT.
Courtesy of Dr M. Bennie, Norfolk and Norwich University Hospital, UK.

Antibiotic penetration into abscess cavities is poor, so intravenous antibiotics should be continued for at least 2 weeks. A further 2–4 weeks of oral treatment may be needed depending on the clinical course.

Surgical management

Abscess cavities should be drained, either percutaneously under radiological guidance or surgically.

Percutaneous drainage
Percutaneous techniques are the first-line treatment as they are less invasive and have equivalent efficacy to surgery. Pus should be sent for urgent microbiological examination.

Laparotomy and surgical drainage
Laparotomy is indicated if percutaneous treatment cannot completely drain the abscess cavities or if surgery is already required for an underlying abdominal source for the sepsis. Severe hepatic destruction may require partial hepatectomy.

Prognosis

Prognosis is dependent on the underlying diagnosis. The overall mortality is up to 30%

REFERENCES

(1) *Huang CJ, Pitt HA, Lipsett PA, et al. Pyogenic hepatic abscess. Changing trends over 42 years. Annals of Surgery 1996; 223: 600–607.*
(2) *Seeto RK, Rockey DC. Pyogenic liver abscess. Changes in etiology, management, and outcome. Medicine (Baltimore) 1996; 75: 99–113.*
(3) *Alvarez Perez JA, Gonzalez JJ, et al. Clinical course, treatment, and multivariate analysis of risk factors for pyogenic liver abscess. American Journal of Surgery 2001; 181: 177–186.*

SECTION 5.16 Liver tumours

Tumours in the liver can be benign or malignant. Malignant tumours can be primary or, more commonly, secondary (metastatic).

Benign liver tumours

The three most common benign hepatic tumours are cavernous haemangiomas, liver cell adenomas, and focal nodular hyperplasia. All three are usually asymptomatic and are often found incidentally during radiological examinations. Symptoms may arise from mass effects, necrosis, thrombosis, haemorrhage or rupture. Liver function tests and serum α-fetoprotein are characteristically normal. Diagnosis can usually be made radiologically with ultrasound, CT or MRI. Biopsies are often inconclusive, so lesions that cannot be diagnosed radiologically should undergo resection.

Liver cell adenomas

Liver cell adenomas occur predominantly in young women taking the combined oral contraceptive pill (COCP). The estimated annual incidence in COCP users is 3–4 per 100 000 if taken for more than 2 years. The tumours are usually solitary. Microscopically, the tumours are highly vascular with neoplastic cells closely resembling normal hepatocytes. Spontaneous rupture and bleeding into the peritoneum occasionally occur. Large liver cell adenomas have a potential for malignant transformation into hepatocellular carcinomas. Some surgeons recommend that small, asymptomatic lesions may be observed once exogenous oestrogen has been withdrawn. Others favour consideration of resection for all adenomas. Symptomatic or large (>5 cm diameter) adenomas should be resected (Fig. 5.9). If α-fetoprotein is raised, or if the adenoma occurs in the presence of a cirrhotic liver, the lesion should be treated as a hepatocellular carcinoma.

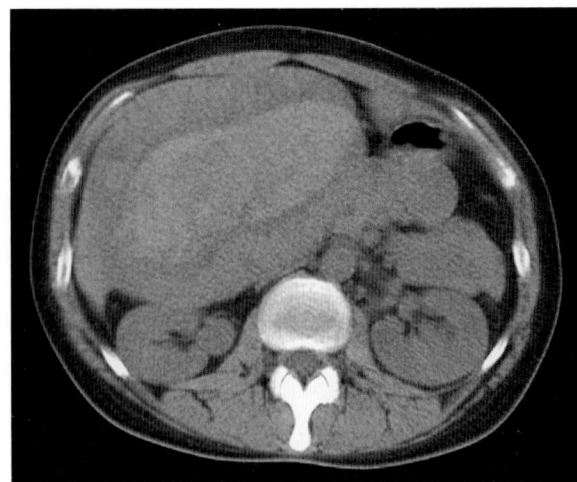

Fig. 5.9 Unenhanced CT showing spontaneous haemorrhage into a liver adenoma.
Courtesy of Dr M. Bennie, Norfolk and Norwich University Hospital, UK.

Focal nodular hyperplasia

Focal nodular hyperplasia (FNH) is found in 3% of livers at autopsy and is more common in females. FNH is commonly a single tumour and consists of a central scar surrounded by normal hepatocytes and Kupffer cells (Fig. 5.10). Differentiation from liver cell adenomas may be difficult radiologically, although the central scar can sometimes be seen on MRI scanning. Asymptomatic tumours do not require treatment if a confident diagnosis can be made radiologically.

Cavernous haemangiomas

Cavernous haemangiomas are benign tumours of vascular endothelium found in 10–15% of livers. They occur in all age groups and are more common in women. Although the aetiology and pathogenesis are unknown, female sex hormones are thought to have some influence. The majority of patients with liver haemangiomas do not require treatment. Surgical excision should be considered for those with complications, rapid growth or large haemangiomas on the liver surface with a potential for rupture. Malignant transformation has not been reported.

Malignant liver tumours

Malignant tumours can be primary or, more commonly, secondary (metastatic, Fig. 5.11). Primary liver malignancies usually arise from hepatocytes (hepatocellular carcinoma) or biliary epithelium (intrahepatic cholangiocarcinoma, see p. 370). Primary malignant liver tumours from other tissue types are rare.

Hepatocellular carcinoma

Hepatocellular carcinomas (hepatic adenocarcinomas, hepatomas) are the most common primary liver malignancy.

Epidemiology

Hepatocellular carcinoma is the fifth most common malignancy worldwide. The incidence is highest in Asia and Africa, reflecting high rates of hepatitis B infection. In developed countries, the incidence is 2.4 per 100 000 per year and rising due to the increase in hepatitis C infection.[1] Men are affected at least twice as often as women.

Pathology

The strongest risk factor for hepatocellular carcinoma is chronic hepatitis infection (B and C). Cirrhosis is also an important risk factor, as the increased cell turnover predisposes to the production of abnormal hepatocytes. Cirrhosis

is present in more than 80% of patients with hepatocellular carcinoma (Fig. 5.12), although the risk of hepatocellular carcinoma varies considerably with the underlying cause of cirrhosis. Ingestion of aflatoxin, a naturally occurring fungal metabolite found on corn and nuts, is also an established risk factor for hepatocellular carcinoma.

Like colorectal cancer, hepatocellular carcinoma develops in a stepwise manner, from liver cell hyperplasia to dysplasia and then carcinoma.

Scope of disease

Local

Enlargement of the liver from hepatocellular carcinoma can compress vascular structures leading to hepatic vein thrombosis (Budd–Chiari syndrome) or portal vein thrombosis.

Metastatic

The lung is the most common site of metastatic disease.

Paraneoplastic

Rarely, hepatocellular carcinoma can cause hypoglycaemia, polycythaemia or hypercalcaemia.

Clinical features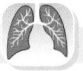

Hepatocellular carcinoma is usually detected in patients with one of three distinct presentations: a right upper quadrant mass, worsening liver function in established cirrhosis, or as a result of screening or other incidental radiological investigations in stable cirrhotic patients.

Patients with a right upper quadrant mass usually complain of malaise, right upper quadrant pain and anorexia. Patients with cirrhosis and new onset hepatocellular carcinoma may present with worsening jaundice, ascites or complications of portal hypertension such as variceal bleeding.

Initial investigations

Liver profile

Serum transaminases and bilirubin may be markedly elevated in patients with existing cirrhosis or hepatitis.

Alpha-fetoprotein

The serum α-fetoprotein level is elevated in the majority of patients with hepatocellular carcinoma. However, it is also elevated in patients with cirrhosis and hepatitis without hepatocellular carcinoma.

Ultrasound of the liver

Combining α-fetoprotein measurement with abdominal ultrasound improves diagnostic accuracy. Ultrasound is highly specific (85–95%) in detecting lesions more than 5 cm in diameter. Smaller lesions are difficult to detect.

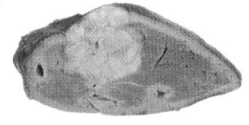

Fig. 5.10 Pathology specimen of focal nodular hyperplasia. The central scar of the liver with focal nodular hyperplasia is clearly seen. Courtesy of Dr S. Davies, Addenbrooke's Hospital, Cambridge, UK.

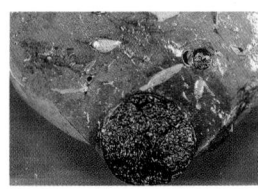

Fig. 5.11 Post mortem specimen showing malignant melanoma metastases in the liver. Courtesy of Dr S. Davies, Addenbrooke's Hospital, Cambridge, UK.

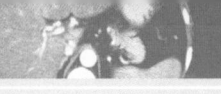

A significantly raised serum α-fetoprotein level in conjunction with a liver mass on ultrasound has a sensitivity of 60% and specificity of 90% for the diagnosis of hepatocellular carcinoma.[2]

Chest X-ray

Chest radiography should be performed to exclude lung metastases.

Further investigations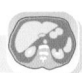

CT of the liver

CT is indicated for patients with suspected hepatocellular carcinoma after α-fetoprotein and ultrasound investigations. Hepatocellular carcinomas produce characteristic appearances on CT angiography due to their arterial supply (Fig. 5.13). MRI can also be used as an alternative investigation with similar diagnostic ability.

Liver biopsy

Liver biopsy can be performed if the diagnosis remains in doubt, but it carries a risk of bleeding and tumour seeding of the needle track.

Hepatic angiography

Angiography is performed to assess the anatomical blood supply for liver resection.

Initial management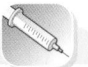

Patients presenting acutely with decompensated liver failure require specialist hepatological management. Management principles include attention to nutrition, careful fluid balance and treatment of portal hypertension.

Surgical management

Liver resection and transplantation are the only potentially curative therapies for hepatocellular carcinoma but are suitable for only 10–20% of patients. Contraindications to both include significant comorbid medical conditions and extrahepatic metastases.

Liver resection

Liver resection is undertaken in non-cirrhotic patients or those with Child–Pugh grade A cirrhosis when the tumour is technically resectable (1 cm resection margin). Also, the remaining liver must be able to support life. For a normal liver, a maximum of 70% can be removed due to rapid liver regeneration. This value is much less in cirrhotic patients but is difficult to determine preoperatively. The resection can be a hemi-hepatectomy (right or left), segmentectomy or non-anatomical resection, depending on the patient's suitability for major surgery and the tumour size and distribution.

Postoperative mortality from liver resection is 5–10%, mainly due to liver failure.[3]

Liver transplantation

Transplantation should be considered in patients with Child–Pugh grade B or C cirrhosis with single lesions of ≤5 cm diameter or up to three lesions ≤3 cm diameter in the absence of vascular invasion on imaging studies (Milan criteria).[4]

Medical management

Non-surgical treatment options

There are a variety of medical and interventional treatments (Table 5.21). Preference varies between centres. At present, they are all considered to be palliative; however, the outcomes after percutaneous ethanol injection and percutaneous radiofrequency ablation may be comparable to surgery.[5,6] Randomized trials comparing percutaneous therapy with liver resection and transplantation are needed.

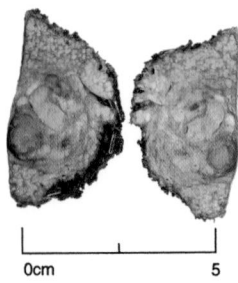

Fig. 5.12 Pathology specimen of hepatocellular carcinoma in a cirrhotic liver. Courtesy of Dr S. Davies, Addenbrooke's Hospital, Cambridge, UK.

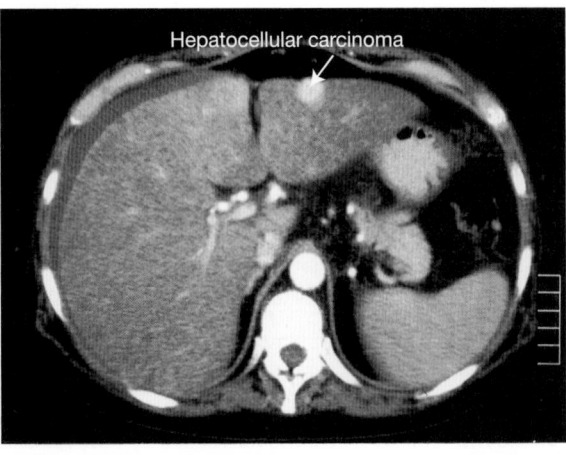

Hepatocellular carcinoma

Fig. 5.13 Hepatocellular carcinoma shown during the arterial phase of a contrast-enhanced CT scan.
Copyright Addenbrooke's Hospital, Cambridge, UK.

Table 5.21	Non-surgical treatments for hepatocellular carcinoma

Percutaneous ablation
  Ethanol injection
  Radiofrequency ablation
  Microwave coagulation	

Chemoembolization	
Systemic chemotherapy	
Cryosurgery	
Hepatic artery chemotherapy infusion	
Immunotherapy with interferon-alpha or -beta	

Prognosis

Clinical staging systems (Table 5.22) have greater prognostic value than the TNM classification, as TNM system does not take account of the underlying liver disease. Five-year survival after liver resection ranges from 30% to 40%, with 75% 4-year survival after transplantation.[4] Worldwide, overall 5-year survival is less than 5%.

TNM Staging of hepatocellular carcinoma

Primary tumour(s)

T1   Solitary tumour without vascular invasion

T2   Solitary tumour with vascular invasion or multiple tumours, none greater than 5 cm diameter

T3   Multiple tumours more than 5 cm diameter or tumour involving a major branch of the portal or hepatic vein(s)

T4   Tumour(s) invades adjacent organs (other than the gallbladder) or perforation of the visceral peritoneum

Regional lymph nodes

N0   No regional lymph node metastasis

N1   Regional lymph node metastasis

Distant metastases

M0   No distant metastasis

M1   Distant metastasis

Stage grouping

Stage I	T1	N0	M0
Stage II	T2	N0	M0
Stage IIIA	T3	N0	M0
Stage IIIB	T4	N0	M0
Stage IIIC	Any T	N1	M0
Stage IV	Any T	Any N	M1

Table 5.22	Okuda hepatocellular carcinoma staging system and prognosis without treatment*

	Points	
Parameter	1	0
Tumour size	>50% of liver	<50%
Ascites	Yes	No
Albumin	<30 g/L	>30 g/L
Bilirubin	>30 mg/L	<30 mg/L
Stage	**Points**	**Median survival (months)**
I	0	8.3
II	1 or 2	2.0
III	3 or 4	0.7

* Okuda K, Ohtsuki T, Obata H, et al. Natural history of hepatocellular carcinoma and prognosis in relation to treatment. Study of 850 patients. Cancer 1985; 56(4): 918–928.

Screening and prevention

The best prospects for reducing the incidence of hepatocellular carcinoma lie in prevention such as vaccination against hepatitis B. Surveillance of high-risk patient groups with 6-monthly abdominal ultrasound examination and serum α-fetoprotein measurement aims to detect tumours at an early stage (Table 5.23).

i FURTHER INFORMATION

Ryder SD. Guidelines for the diagnosis and treatment of hepatocellular carcinoma (HCC) in adults. Gut 2003; 52 Suppl 3: iii1–8.

REFERENCES

(1) *El-Serag HB, Mason AC. Rising incidence of hepatocellular carcinoma in the United States. New England Journal of Medicine 1999; 340: 745–750.*
(2) *Daniele B, Bencivenga A, Megna AS, Tinessa V. Alpha-fetoprotein and ultrasonography screening for hepatocellular carcinoma. Gastroenterology 2004; 127: S108–112.*
(3) *Fong Y, Sun RL, Jarnagin W, Blumgart LH. An analysis of 412 cases of hepatocellular carcinoma at a Western center. Annals of Surgery 1999; 229: 790–799; discussion 799–800.*
(4) *Mazzaferro V, Regalia E, Doci R, et al. Liver transplantation for the treatment of small hepatocellular carcinomas in patients with cirrhosis. New England Journal of Medicine 1996; 334: 693–699.*
(5) *Livraghi T, Giorgio A, Marin G, et al. Hepatocellular carcinoma and cirrhosis in 746 patients: long-term results of percutaneous ethanol injection. Radiology 1995; 197: 101–108.*
(6) *Lau WY, Leung TW, Yu SC, Ho SK. Percutaneous local ablative therapy for hepatocellular carcinoma: a review and look into the future. Annals of Surgery 2003; 237: 171–179.*

Table 5.23	Indications for surveillance for hepatocellular carcinoma*
Those with established cirrhosis due to HBV, HCV, genetic haemochromatosis	
Those with alcohol-related cirrhosis who are abstinent or likely to comply with treatment	
Males with cirrhosis due to primary biliary cirrhosis	

* Adapted from: Ryder SD. Guidelines for the diagnosis and treatment of hepatocellular carcinoma (HCC) in adults. Gut 2003; 52 Suppl 3: iii1–8.

Liver metastases from colorectal cancer

The liver is a common site of metastasis for a wide variety of tumours. Unlike most other types of cancer, liver metastases from colorectal adenocarcinoma (Fig. 5.14) may be amenable to curative treatment.

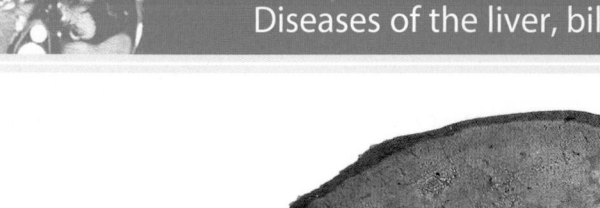

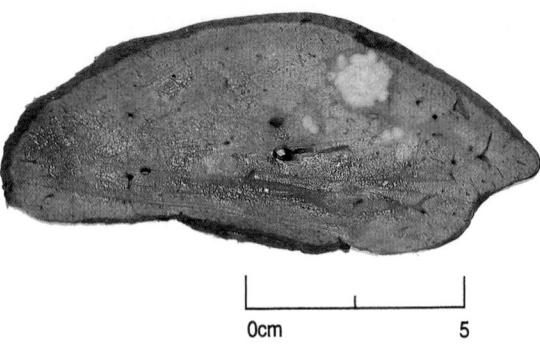

Fig. 5.14 Multiple colorectal cancer metastases are seen in a resected liver specimen.
Courtesy of Dr S. Davies, Addenbrooke's Hospital, Cambridge, UK.

Epidemiology

Colorectal cancer is the third most common cancer in the developed world. Liver metastases are the main cause of death in patients with colorectal cancer and are present in 15–25% of patients at detection of the primary tumour.

Pathology

Liver metastases seed from colorectal primary tumours via the portal vein. As the metastases grow they derive their blood supply from the hepatic artery (the normal liver is primarily supplied by the portal vein), aiding their identification on contrast-enhanced CT scans.

Scope of disease

Complications of colorectal cancer liver metastases include direct spread into adjacent organs (e.g. diaphragm, stomach), compression of hollow structures (e.g. common bile duct) and further metastatic spread.

Clinical features

Asymptomatic liver metastases may be discovered during staging investigations of the primary colorectal tumour or on follow-up surveillance investigations after colorectal surgery.

Symptoms from colorectal cancer liver metastases include weight loss, right upper quadrant discomfort, and symptoms of obstructive jaundice (pruritus, pale urine, dark stools, jaundice).

On examination, a liver mass may be palpable and jaundice may be present. The presence of ascites, lymphadenopathy or haemoptysis suggests extrahepatic metastases.

Initial investigations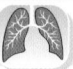

Ultrasound of the liver

Liver metastases can be confirmed by ultrasound. Liver biopsies may lead to metastatic seeding and should be avoided.

Further investigations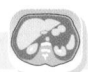

Further investigations are required for patients who are potential candidates for surgical resection. The aims are to assess general fitness for surgery, confirm local control of the primary colorectal tumour, and screen for the presence of extrahepatic disease (i.e. staging investigations).

Colonoscopy

A colonoscopy is performed to exclude primary recurrence or development of a metachronous tumour within the colon or rectum.

CT scan

A contrast-enhanced CT scan of the chest, abdomen and pelvis is performed to ensure that the metastatic deposits are confined to the liver.

Laparoscopy

Some centres use laparoscopy with laparoscopic ultrasound to confirm resectability before proceeding to liver resection.

> **RECENT ADVANCES**
>
> *Positron emission tomography (PET) with 18-fluoro-2-deoxyglucose (^{18}F-FDG) images tumours based on increased glucose uptake by tumour cells (Fig. 5.15). ^{18}F-FDG PET is more sensitive and specific than CT at detecting colorectal metastases (95% and 100% versus 74% and 85%, respectively).[1] Although not widely available, this is expected to become the gold standard investigation for detecting extrahepatic metastases.*

Surgical management

Liver resection

Surgical resection is the only potentially curative treatment for patients with colorectal cancer liver metastases. However, only 15% fulfil the criteria for surgery (Table 5.24). The anatomy of liver resection is based on Couinaud's findings of eight hepatic segments (Fig. 5.1). Liver resections are named according to the segments removed (Table 5.25). The caudate lobe (segment I) is rarely removed.

An inverted T incision is made in the upper abdomen, and the abdominal cavity is explored for signs of extrahepatic malignancy. The liver is mobilized by division of the falciform ligament, and the right and left triangular ligaments. Blood loss is minimized with the use of argon beam coagulation, transient occlusion of the hepatic blood

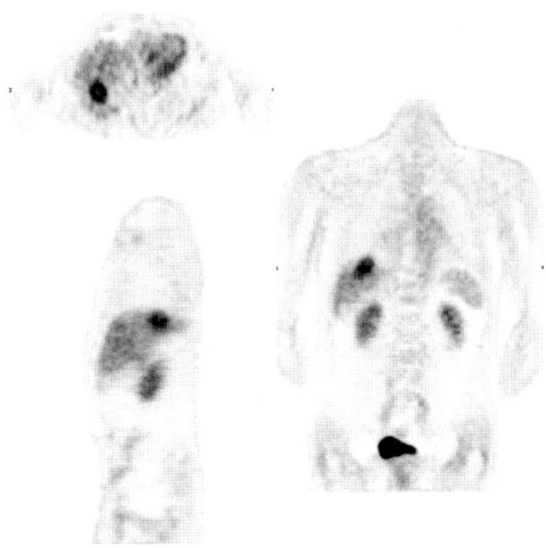

Fig. 5.15 18F-FDG PET scan. A solitary colorectal cancer metastasis is seen in the liver in transverse, coronal and sagittal planes. Excreted 18F-FDG is seen in the kidneys and bladder. Courtesy of Dr K. Balan, Addenbrooke's Hospital, Cambridge, UK.

Table 5.24	Resection criteria for colorectal cancer liver metastases

Primary colorectal cancer removed with negative resection margins

No extrahepatic disease present (resectable lung metastases may be an exception)

1 cm tumour-free margin around all liver metastases

Adequate liver parenchyma after resection (minimum of 25–30% of normal liver)

Patient fit enough to undergo major surgical procedure

Table 5.25	The nomenclature of segmental liver resections

Name	Segments removed
Right hemi-hepatectomy	V, VI, VII, VIII
Left hemi-hepatectomy	II, III, IV
Extended right hepatectomy	Right hemi-hepatectomy + IV
Extended left hepatectomy	Left hemi-hepatectomy + affected (V or VIII)
Left lateral segmentectomy	II, III
Segmentectomy	One segment only

supply, and anaesthetic techniques to reduce hepatic venous pressure. For right or left hemi-hepatectomy, the portal vein and hepatic artery branch supplying the side of the liver to be resected can be tied off. Hepatic parenchyma can be divided using clamp fracture and ultrasonic dissection. Small metastases in the liver periphery can be removed with a wedge of tissue (non-anatomical resection).

In some patients the left lobe (segments II, III, IV) is too small to provide enough liver function after right hemi-hepatectomy. Pre-operative interventional radiological embolization of the right portal vein leads to compensatory enlargement of the left lobe and allows subsequent right hemi-hepatectomy.

Operative mortality is 2–7% and is commonly due to haemorrhage, sepsis and hepatic failure. The role of adjuvant chemotherapy after surgery is controversial.

Medical management

As with hepatocellular carcinoma, a number of techniques exist for palliation of non-resectable colorectal cancer liver metastases (Table 5.26). Currently, there is little to choose between them, although percutaneous radiofrequency ablation may be shown to be a promising non-surgical therapy in the future.

Radiofrequency ablation

Percutaneous insertion of a radiofrequency electrode into the metastases under radiological guidance allows generation of heat causing tissue necrosis. Randomized controlled trials comparing these techniques with surgical resection are needed.

Systemic chemotherapy

Patients with extensive liver metastases or extrahepatic disease can be treated with palliative chemotherapy (e.g. 5-fluorouracil plus folinic acid, irinotecan, oxaliplatin) to improve the duration and quality of remaining life. Delivery of chemotherapy directly into the hepatic artery via a cannula does not appear to result in prolonged survival.[2]

Prognosis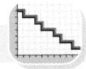

The median survival of patients with untreated colorectal liver metastases is 9 months, and the 5-year survival is less than 2%. Chemotherapy extends the median survival to 15 months but is non-curative.[2] Patients who are suitable for hepatic resection have 5-year survival rates of 30–40%.

Table 5.26	Non-surgical treatments for colorectal cancer liver metastases

Percutaneous ablation
  Radiofrequency ablation
  Microwave coagulation

Systemic chemotherapy

Cryosurgery

Hepatic artery chemotherapy infusion

Liver cell adenomas

Focal nodular hyperplasia

Cavernous haemangiomas

Hepatocellular carcinoma

Liver metastases from colorectal cancer

343

FURTHER INFORMATION

Yoon SS, Tanabe KK. Surgical treatment and other regional treatments for colorectal cancer liver metastases. Oncologist 1999; 4: 197–208.

Ruers T, Bleichrodt RP. Treatment of liver metastases, an update on the possibilities and results. European Journal of Cancer 2002; 38: 1023–1033.

REFERENCES

(1) *Ogunbiyi OA, Flanagan FL, Dehdashti F, et al. Detection of recurrent and metastatic colorectal cancer: comparison of positron emission tomography and computed tomography. Annals of Surgical Oncology 1997; 4: 613–620.*

(2) *Kerr DJ, McArdle CS, Ledermann J, et al. Intrahepatic arterial versus intravenous fluorouracil and folinic acid for colorectal cancer liver metastases: a multicentre randomised trial. Lancet 2003; 361: 368–373.*

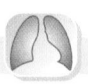

SECTION 5.17   Hepatic vascular disease

The delivery of blood to the liver is via the hepatic artery (33%) and portal vein (67%), and blood leaves via the inferior vena cava. Diseases of the liver vasculature may result from the obstruction of the normal flow of blood from the liver to the inferior vena cava (Budd–Chiari syndrome, veno-occlusive disease) or from the impairment of blood delivery (portal vein thrombosis, ischaemic hepatitis, hepatic artery thrombosis).

Hepatic vein thrombosis

Hepatic vein thrombosis is also known as Budd–Chiari syndrome.

Epidemiology

Hepatic vein thrombosis is rare.

Pathology

Thrombosis of the hepatic veins leads to obstruction, venous congestion and sinusoidal dilatation. Necrosis can occur in severe cases. Acute thrombosis can lead to fulminant hepatic failure, whilst more chronic complications include hepatic fibrosis and cirrhosis.

As the caudate lobe has a separate venous outflow (dorsal hepatic veins) that drain directly into the inferior vena cava, it hypertrophies to increase the amount of functioning liver. The risk factors for hepatic vein thrombosis are listed in Table 5.27.

Clinical features

With acute thrombosis, patients may present with right upper quadrant pain and ascites. On examination, tender hepatomegaly may be evident. Rarely patients may present with fulminant hepatic failure.

Patients with chronic thrombosis may present with gradual ascites or portal hypertension (p. 365).

Investigations

Ultrasound of the liver

Ultrasonography with Doppler assessment of hepatic venous flow may reveal a thrombus in the hepatic vein or a reduction in or absence of hepatic venous outflow.

Hepatic vein angiography

Hepatic vein angiography is the gold standard investigation and allows thrombolysis or direct interventions such as dilatation of the hepatic vein.

Transthoracic echocardiography

An echocardiogram is important to assess right ventricular function as patients with right ventricular failure or pericardial effusion can present with a similar picture.

Screening for thrombophilia

After the initial event has resolved, it is important to screen for diseases associated with thrombophilia (p. 829).

Table 5.27	Risk factors for hepatic vein thrombosis

Thrombophilia
    Factor V Leiden deficiency
    Protein C and S deficiency
    Antithrombin III deficiency
    Anti-cardiolipin antibodies
    Myeloproliferative disease	

Malignancy	
Trauma	
Drugs Oral contraceptive pill	
Pregnancy	

Management

Identification and treatment of underlying cause

It is important to correct any underlying cause that predisposes the patient to thrombosis.

Anticoagulation

Initially, heparin is commenced, followed by warfarin to maintain the international normalized ratio (INR) between 3 and 4.5.

Thrombolysis

Thrombolytic therapy should be considered in the acute setting.

Hepatic vein dilatation/stenting

Angioplasty dilatation or stenting of the hepatic veins can be considered (depending on local availability) to decompress the vascular system. There is a high risk of re-occlusion if the underlying condition is not corrected.

Portosystemic shunt

The creation of a portosystemic shunt is a useful procedure to reduce portal hypertension. This can be performed via a transjugular route (TIPSS) or by formal surgical portosystemic shunt.

Liver transplantation

Liver transplantation is an option for patients with acute hepatic vein thrombosis and fulminant hepatic failure and chronic hepatic vein thrombosis with cirrhosis.

Prognosis

The prognosis in general is poor. Survival after liver transplantation is improving, although recurrence may occur.

Veno-occlusive disease

Veno-occlusive disease refers to occlusion of small hepatic veins, usually by connective tissue. The larger-calibre vessels are unaffected.

Epidemiology

Veno-occlusive disease is rare.

Pathology

The cause is unknown. In early disease, there is extravasation of red cells into the space of Disse. Hepatic congestion develops with hepatocellular damage. Disease progression leads to perivenular fibrosis, scarring, bridging and eventually cirrhosis. The risk factors for veno-occlusive disease are listed in Table 5.28.

Table 5.28	Risk factors for veno-occlusive disease
Bone marrow transplantation	
Liver irradiation (dose-dependent)	
Hepatitis C infection	
Systemic infections	

Drugs
    Azathioprine
    Ciclosporin
    Busulfan
    Cyclophosphamide	

Ingestion of 'bush tea' (pyrrolizidine alkaloids)	
Oral contraceptives (rare)	

Clinical features

The acute presentation is with rapid abdominal swelling, tender hepatomegaly and, in some, progression to acute liver failure. A more chronic presentation (long-term bush tea ingestion, drug usage, bone marrow transplantation) is with progressive jaundice, abdominal pain and swelling.

It is important to screen for clinical features of right heart failure as the presentation can be similar. A detailed drug and medical history is crucial to ascertain risk factors for the development of veno-occlusive disease.

Investigations

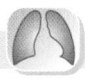

Ultrasound of the liver

An ultrasound scan of the liver is initially performed to exclude large (main) hepatic vein thrombosis. If this is negative, then a liver biopsy is performed.

Liver biopsy

A liver biopsy is required to confirm the diagnosis of veno-occlusive disease.

Management

Identify and treat underlying cause

The underlying cause or associated risk factors should be identified and corrected if possible.

Acute disease

Patients presenting with acute liver failure may need to be admitted to the intensive care unit. Defibrotide has been shown to be effective in patients with severe veno-occlusive disease.

Chronic disease

For patients with chronic disease, management should be directed to the complications of chronic liver disease. Transjugular intrahepatic portosystemic shunts have been used, but results are poor, especially in the severe group.

Liver transplantation is an option in early disease. In patients with multi-organ failure, the outcome of liver transplantation is poor.

Prognosis

In general, the prognosis is poor, especially in patients with severe disease, encephalopathy and multi-organ failure.

Portal vein thrombosis

Epidemiology

Portal vein thrombosis is rare.

Pathology

In the majority, no cause is identified. The risk factors associated with portal vein thrombosis are listed in Table 5.29. The main complication of portal vein thrombosis is the development of portal hypertension and the associated complications.

Clinical features

Patients may be asymptomatic or present with features of portal hypertension such as variceal bleeding, encephalopathy and sudden onset of ascites. On examination, the patient may be pyrexial with right upper quadrant tenderness.

Investigations

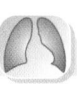

Liver profile
A liver profile is performed to assess the degree of hepatic impairment in patients with cirrhosis.

Ultrasound of the liver
Ultrasonography (Doppler) is able to quantify the absence of blood flow within the portal vein.

CT abdomen
A CT (or MR) venogram can confirm a thrombus within the portal vein.

Angiography
Formal angiography is able to measure hepatic and portal pressures, and assess regional venous outflows such as splenic and mesenteric veins.

Upper gastrointestinal endoscopy
An upper gastrointestinal endoscopy is performed to screen for oesophageal varices.

Management

Identify and treat underlying condition
Any underlying cause or risk factor should be identified and corrected if possible.

Management of chronic disease
The management of chronic disease is focused on the complications of portal hypertension such as varices (p. 309) and encephalopathy (p. 317). TIPSS is not usually technically possible, and a formal surgical portosystemic shunt may be required.

Prognosis

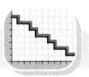

The prognosis in general is poor. In patients with established cirrhosis, shunt surgery may cause worsening of hepatic function, and liver transplantation may be difficult or impossible.

Hepatic artery thrombosis

Thrombosis of the hepatic artery is rare. The causes are listed in Table 5.30. Acute onset is associated with hepatic infarction, but chronic onset leads to less infarction as there may be time for collateral arteries to form. The complications associated with hepatic artery thrombosis are hepatic failure, sepsis and biliary strictures. Patients may present acutely with right upper quadrant pain, fever and liver failure, whereas patients with chronic disease may be asymptomatic or present with symptoms from biliary strictures or hepatic abscesses. The liver transaminases are usually elevated, and hepatic artery thrombosis can be identified on ultrasound. Patients with acute liver failure should be managed on the intensive care unit and may require transplantation. Infection should be treated aggressively with broad-spectrum antibiotics. The prognosis in general is poor.

Table 5.29	Risk factors for portal vein thrombosis
Thrombophilia states	
Malignancy	
Intra-abdominal infection	
Pancreatitis	
Trauma	
Cirrhosis	

Table 5.30	Causes of hepatic artery thrombosis
Vasculitides	
Abdominal aneurysm	
Sepsis	
Trauma	
Post liver transplant (split grafts, abnormal donor artery)	
Drugs (sirolimus)	

Liver transplantation

Liver transplantation is the treatment of choice for both end-stage chronic and acute liver failure. In adults, the most common causes of liver failure that result in transplantation are chronic cirrhosis and acute liver failure from hepatitis or paracetamol overdose. In children, biliary atresia, acute hepatitis and metabolic diseases are the common aetiologies of liver failure that require transplantation.

Indications

Patients with acute liver failure are selected on the King's College Hospital criteria (Table 5.31). Patients with chronic liver disease can be considered for transplantation when the severity is Child–Pugh grade C. Patients with Child–Pugh grade B or C cirrhosis with hepatocellular carcinomas that meet the Milan criteria (see p. 329) are also considered for transplantation.

Patient preparation

Recipient selection is a multidisciplinary procedure involving surgeons, hepatologists, anaesthetists and psychiatrists, with criteria based on the disease severity and subsequent prognosis.[1]

Procedure

Donor procedure

Abdominal organ retrieval is via a midline laparotomy incision. The liver is mobilized and flushed with cooled University of Wisconsin (UW) preservation solution via the aorta and portal vein. The liver is removed, packed in a sterile bag with further cooled UW solution, and transported in an icebox. The removed liver is able to withstand a maximum of 20 hours of cold ischaemia, although most centres try to limit this to 14 hours.

Recipient procedure

For the recipient procedure (Fig. 5.16) the patient is positioned supine and an inverted T incision is made supra-umbilically to the xiphisternum. The recipient hepatectomy begins with mobilization of the liver and dissection of the porta hepatis and inferior vena cava (IVC). Removal of the liver requires cross-clamping of the suprahepatic IVC, and if the patient's haemodynamic status deteriorates, veno-venous bypass (infra-hepatic IVC and portal vein to internal jugular vein) can be used. The recipient liver is removed and the donor liver is implanted by anastomosing the suprahepatic IVC, infra-hepatic IVC, portal vein, hepatic artery and common bile duct (Fig. 5.17).

Table 5.31	Criteria for transplantation in acute liver failure*

Paracetamol-induced acute liver failure

Arterial pH <7.3 *or*

The presence of the following:
  Prothrombin time >100 s *and*
  Grade III/IV encephalopathy *and*
  Serum creatinine >300 μmol/L

Non-paracetamol-induced acute liver failure

Prothrombin time >100 s *or*

The presence of any three of the following:
  Age <10, or >40 years
  Non-A, non-B hepatitis or drug/halothane-induced liver
    failure
  Bilirubin >300 μmol/L
  Duration of jaundice before onset of encephalopathy
    >7 days
  Prothrombin time >50 s

* O'Grady J, Alexander G, Hayllar K, Williams R. Early indicators of prognosis in fulminant hepatic failure. Gastroenterology 1989; 97: 439–445.

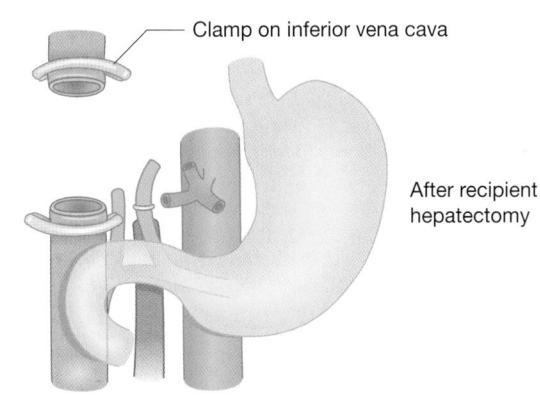

Clamp on inferior vena cava

After recipient hepatectomy

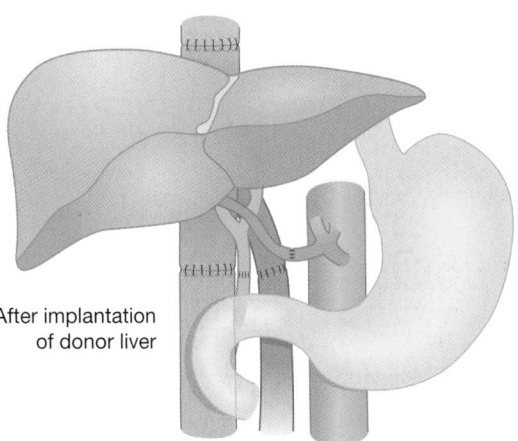

After implantation of donor liver

Fig. 5.17 Liver transplant anastomoses.

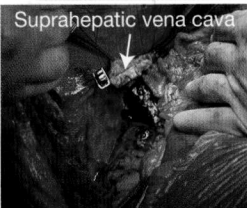

Suprahepatic vena cava

(a)

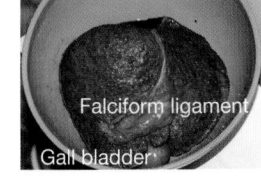

Falciform ligament

Gall bladder

(b)

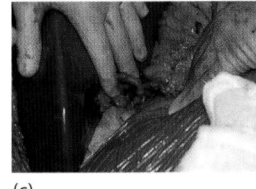

(c)

Fig. 5.16 a–c Liver transplantation. The recipient's liver (a) has been excised and the clamp across the suprahepatic inferior vena cava is seen. The excised cirrhotic liver is explanted (b) and the new liver (c) implanted, with the hepatic artery anastomosis demonstrated. Copyright Addenbrooke's Hospital, Cambridge, UK.

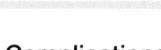

Complications

Infection and rejection are the two most common complications after liver transplantation. Other acute complications and their management are listed in Table 5.32. Late complications include side effects of immunosuppression and disease recurrence.

Post procedure care

Patients require intensive care postoperatively for 24–48 hours for ventilation and monitoring. A calcineurin inhibitor (ciclosporin or tacrolimus), azathioprine and prednisolone are prescribed for immunosuppression to prevent organ rejection. However, unlike other organ transplants, immunosuppression can occasionally be withdrawn without adverse effects.[2]

Prognosis

The UK 1-year patient survival rate is 90%, with 5- and 10-year patient survival rates of 75% and 60%, respectively. Quality of life is improved and 55% regain employment at one year post transplant. Long-term survival is lower for those transplanted for cancer than either cirrhosis or acute liver failure.

RECENT ADVANCES

The shortage of donor organs has stimulated innovative approaches in an attempt to satisfy increasing demand. The liver can be surgically split along anatomical planes to provide smaller grafts with individual blood supplies as well as venous and biliary drainage, enabling multiple recipients for a single liver. Alternatively, family members can donate a segment of their liver to paediatric or adult recipients. These techniques accounted for 15% of liver transplants in the UK in 2001.

Hepatocyte infusion via the portal vein has successfully treated a small number of patients with inherited metabolic disorders, though the risk of rejection remains and this treatment remains experimental at present.

 FURTHER INFORMATION

Devlin J, O'Grady J. Indications for referral and assessment in adult liver transplantation: a clinical guideline. Gut 1999; 45(Suppl VI): VI1–VI22.

REFERENCES

(1) *Neuberger J, James O. Guidelines for selection of patients for liver transplantation in the era of donor-organ shortage. Lancet 1999; 354: 1636–1639.*
(2) *Goddard S, Adams DH. New approaches to immunosuppression in liver transplantation. Journal of Gastroenterology and Hepatology 2002;17:116–126.*

Table 5.32 — **Early complications of liver transplantation and their management**

Complication	Management
Postoperative infection (60%)	Antimicrobials, drainage of sepsis
Acute rejection (30%)	Corticosteroids, antibody therapy
Biliary leak or stenosis (10–15%)	Operative correction or stent via ERCP
Haemorrhage (10–15%)	Coagulopathy correction, re-operation
Primary non-function of liver (<5%)	Urgent re-transplantation
Hepatic artery thrombosis (5%)	Thrombectomy, re-transplantation

Diseases of the biliary system

SECTION 5.19 Introduction

Applied basic sciences of the biliary system

Anatomy

The biliary tract

The biliary tract develops from the foregut. The cystic duct and gallbladder arise from a diverticulum of the bile duct. The biliary tract consists of intrahepatic and extrahepatic biliary systems (Fig. 5.18). Together these are known as the biliary tree.

The intrahepatic system begins at the level of the biliary canaliculi that lie between adjacent hepatocytes (p. 299). The canaliculi drain to bile ductules, eventually combining to form right and left hepatic ducts.

The extrahepatic system starts as the right and left hepatic ducts exit the liver and unite to form the common hepatic duct. The common hepatic duct (CHD) is joined by the cystic duct from the gallbladder to form the common bile duct (CBD).

The CBD continues posterior to the first part of the duodenum and runs in a groove behind the pancreas to meet with the main pancreatic duct at the ampulla of Vater. The ampulla is surrounded by the sphincter of Oddi, controlling bile and pancreatic fluid flow. The ampulla empties into the second part of the duodenum. The blood supply of the CBD is from small branches of the cystic, hepatic and gastroduodenal arteries.

Parasympathetic fibres from the vagus (cranial nerve X) stimulate contraction of the gallbladder and relaxation of the sphincter of Oddi. Pain fibres from the CBD and gallbladder run with sympathetic nerves and enter the spinal cord at T7–9. Some pain fibres from the gallbladder may be carried by the right phrenic nerve (C3–5). Pain from the biliary tract and gallbladder is felt in the right upper quadrant and epigastrium, and may radiate posteriorly in the distribution of dermatomes T7–9. Because of the phrenic nerve supply, pain may also be referred to the right shoulder.

The gallbladder

The gallbladder is a pear-shaped organ with a capacity of 30–40 mL. It is adherent to the undersurface of the liver. The fundus of the gallbladder is in contact with the parietal peritoneum of the anterior abdominal wall and is the site of maximal abdominal tenderness during gallbladder disease. The fundus is adjacent to the transverse colon, while the body of the gallbladder touches the first part of the duodenum. Gallstones may erode the wall of the gallbladder to enter the duodenum (cholecysto-duodenal fistula) and cause gallstone ileus (p. 355). The neck of the gallbladder continues into the cystic duct, and in pathological gallbladders, a small pouch may form between the neck and the cystic duct (Hartmann's pouch). A gallstone may become impacted here, causing biliary colic or acute cholecystitis.

The blood supply of the gallbladder is from the cystic artery, a branch of the right hepatic artery, and from small vessels from the hepatic bed. The cystic artery runs in the triangle formed by the liver edge, CHD and cystic duct (Calot's triangle, Fig. 5.19). This triangle is an important anatomical landmark during laparoscopic cholecystectomy (p. 358).

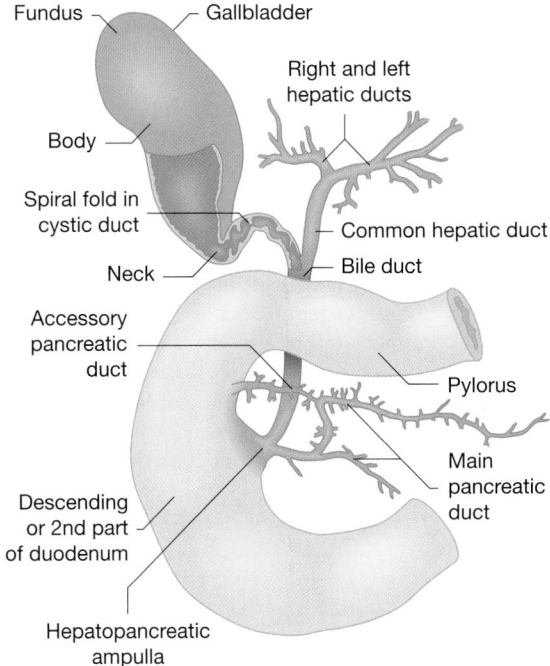

Fundus — Gallbladder
Right and left hepatic ducts
Body
Spiral fold in cystic duct
Common hepatic duct
Neck — Bile duct
Accessory pancreatic duct
Pylorus
Main pancreatic duct
Descending or 2nd part of duodenum
Hepatopancreatic ampulla

Fig. 5.18 Anatomy of the biliary tract.

349

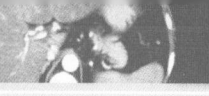

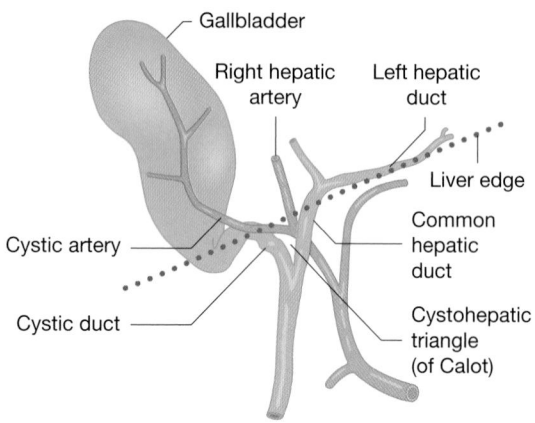

Fig. 5.19 Calot's triangle. The cystic artery usually arises from the right hepatic artery, although variations occur in 25%.

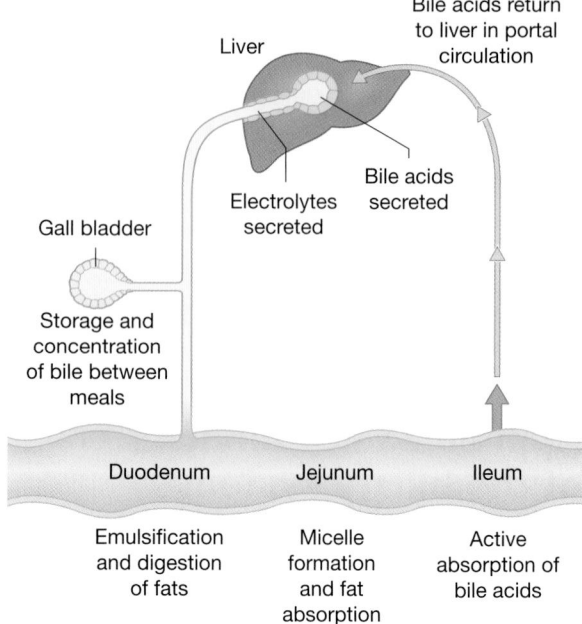

Fig. 5.20 The enterohepatic circulation.

Physiology

Bile is made up of water, bicarbonate (HCO_3^-), bile salts, cholesterol, lecithin, bile pigments and metabolized hormones and drugs (Table 5.33). Bicarbonate-rich fluid is secreted by the epithelial cells lining the duct system; the other components of bile are produced by the hepatocytes.

Bile acids are synthesized from cholesterol and are conjugated with taurine or glycine to form bile salts. Bile salts act as detergents, emulsifying fats and increasing the surface area available for pancreatic lipase to convert triglycerides to free fatty acids and 2-monoglycerides. Lecithin aids this emulsification process. Bile salts, lecithin, cholesterol, fat-soluble vitamins (A, D, E, K) and lipid degradation products form mixed micelles. These are absorbed by microvilli of the duodenal and jejunal epithelium. Bile salts are absorbed in the terminal ileum by simple diffusion and active transport mechanisms. They are trans-

ported back to the liver via the portal circulation, where they are avidly taken up by hepatocytes. Up to 90% of the bile salts secreted into the small intestine are returned to the liver via this enterohepatic circulation (Fig. 5.20). The most potent stimulators of bile salt secretion are bile salts themselves. Parasympathetic fibres from the vagus play a minor role. Secretin, released as a result of acid chyme in the duodenum, increases the production of the HCO_3^- – rich secretion from the duct cells.

The function of the gallbladder is to store and concentrate bile. Between meals, the high resting tone of the sphincter of Oddi diverts bile to the gallbladder. Gallbladder epithelium actively transports Na^+, Cl^-, and HCO_3^-. Water follows down the osmotic gradient. In this way bile acids are concentrated 5–20-fold, converting the 5000 mL of bile produced by the liver per day to the 500 mL of bile released into the duodenum.

Like other gastrointestinal organs, gallbladder motility is controlled by combined hormonal and neural mechanisms. During the cephalic and gastric phases of digestion, relaxation of the sphincter of Oddi and contraction of the gallbladder are mediated by the vagus nerve and gastrin released by the stomach. Cholecystokinin (CCK) is the strongest stimulus for gallbladder contraction. CCK is released into the blood stream by duodenal epithelial cells after coming into contact with products of digestion during the intestinal phase.

Table 5.33	Components of bile and their function
Component	**Function**
Bicarbonate	Neutralization of acid chyme from the stomach
Bile salts	Emulsification of fats Excretion of cholesterol Lowering the optimum pH of pancreatic lipase from 9.0 to 6.7
Lecithin	Assists bile salts in fat emulsification
Cholesterol	Excretion aids cholesterol homeostasis
Bile pigments	Excretion of haem breakdown products

Investigations of the biliary system

Blood tests

Liver profile

The standard liver profile is also used for the diagnosis and monitoring of diseases of the biliary system.

Tumour markers

A highly sensitive and specific serum tumour marker for cholangiocarcinoma has not yet been identified. Carbohydrate antigen (CA) 19-9 and carcinoembryonic antigen (CEA), either alone, or in combination, are the most widely used markers, but both have significant false negative and false positive rates and are better used for monitoring treatment rather than diagnosis.

Endoscopy

Endoscopic ultrasound

Endoscopic ultrasound (EUS) is a relatively non-invasive technique in which an endoscope fitted with an ultrasound probe is passed into the oesophagus, stomach and duodenum. The close proximity of the pancreas, extrahepatic biliary tree, portal vein, superior mesenteric vein and artery allows accurate imaging of these structures. The hepatic parenchyma and intrahepatic biliary tree are less well seen. EUS is >95% sensitive and specific for the detection of bile duct stones and is useful in the assessment of resectability of distal biliary masses (e.g. cholangiocarcinoma). EUS-guided fine-needle aspiration can be performed but is associated with a significant false positive rate.

Endoscopic retrograde cholangio-pancreatography

Endoscopic retrograde cholangiography (ERC) of the biliary tree is commonly performed simultaneously with ERCP of the pancreas. The basic procedure, contraindications and complications are listed on page 307.

If ERCP fails, or is not possible because of anatomical abnormalities, MRCP (Table 5.10) percutaneous transhepatic cholangiography (PTC) can be performed (see below).

Diagnostic imaging

Plain abdominal film

Plain radiography is usually unhelpful in the investigation of biliary tract pathology. Gallstones with a high calcium content are radio-opaque, but these are found in just 10–15% of patients with gallstones (Fig. 5.21). Severe acute cholecystitis may result in air in the gallbladder wall (gangrenous or emphysematous cholecystitis) but this is difficult to see on plain films. Air within the biliary tree (pneumobilia) may also be seen on plain radiography. A calcified gallbladder silhouette indicates a porcelain gallbladder (rare). A full triad of radiographic signs may occasionally be seen in gallstone ileus (distended loops of small bowel, air in the biliary tree, and a radio-opaque gallstone), but more commonly only signs of bowel obstruction are present.

Abdominal ultrasound

Transabdominal ultrasonography is the method of choice for the initial radiological investigation of the biliary tree, and is particularly accurate at diagnosing gallbladder stones (>95% sensitivity and specificity), polyps and gallbladder adenocarcinoma. Gallbladder stones appear as mobile, echogenic lesions with acoustic shadows (Fig. 5.22). Acute calculous cholecystitis appears as a thickened gallbladder containing gallstones with pericholecystic fluid

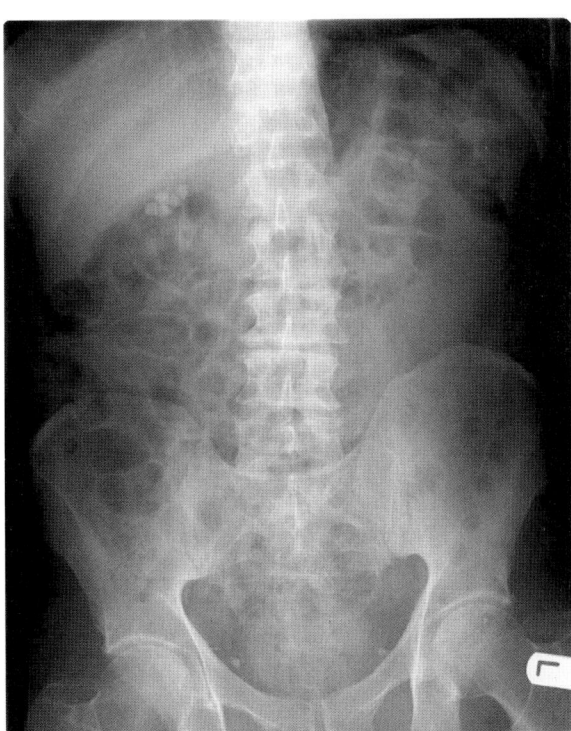

Fig. 5.21 Radio-opaque gallstones are seen in the right upper quadrant on plain abdominal radiography.
Courtesy of Dr M. Bennie, Norfolk and Norwich University Hospital, UK.

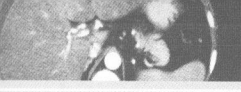
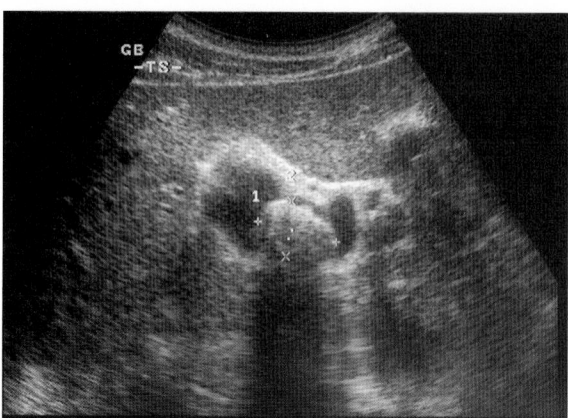

Fig. 5.22 Ultrasound scan of gallbladder with gallstone. The gallbladder is seen in a transverse section with the gallstone reflecting the ultrasound waves and casting an acoustic shadow over deeper structures.
Copyright Addenbrooke's Hospital, Cambridge, UK.

and localized tenderness over the gallbladder (sonographic Murphy's sign). Sensitivity is relatively low at 70–80%, and hepatobiliary iminodiacetic acid (HIDA) scanning or CT scanning can be performed if acute calculous cholecystitis is suspected clinically despite a negative ultrasound scan. Ultrasonography is relatively poor (sensitivity 60–70%) at detecting stones within the common bile duct (choledo-cholithiasis), especially stones <1 cm diameter and those in the distal CBD. This is due to air in the overlying duodenum. Obesity and/or ascites may also make ultrasound exami-nation difficult. Obstruction of the CBD (e.g. by stones or tumour) causes CBD dilatation (>8 mm diameter) that is easily detected on ultrasound. Despite these limitations, abdominal ultrasound remains the method of choice for the diagnosis of CBD stones due to its widespread avail-ability and non-invasive nature.

Oral cholecystogram

Oral or intravenous administration of contrast material that is excreted in the bile has historically been used to diagnose gallbladder stones or cystic duct obstruction. With the widespread use of ultrasound, which avoids ionizing radia-tion, both oral and intravenous cholecystography have become almost obsolete. Oral cholecystography has a minor role in assessing which gallstones are suitable for treatment with oral bile acids, as only floating radiolucent stones are likely to represent cholesterol stones amenable to bile acid therapy.

CT abdomen

Computed tomography is less sensitive than ultrasound for visualizing gallbladder wall abnormalities and can miss cholesterol gallstones which have a similar radiographic density to bile. CT has a similar sensitivity to ultrasound for the detection of choledocholithiasis, and other investiga-tions are therefore preferred if choledocholithiasis is suspected (i.e. ERCP, magnetic resonance cholangio-pancreatography). CT is used for staging biliary tumours as

it enables the assessment of the retroperitoneum, liver, pelvis and chest in a single examination. CT is also less operator-dependent than ultrasound and the images generated are more readily understood by non-radiologists.

Magnetic resonance cholangio-pancreatography

Magnetic resonance cholangio-pancreatography (MRCP) uses T2-weighting during a single breath-hold to visualize the static columns of fluid within the biliary and pancreatic ducts without using contrast material. These stagnant fluids appear bright compared to solid tissue and fast-flowing blood (Fig. 5.23). Ductal stones appear as filling defects (black). MRCP is beginning to replace ERCP for diagnosis alone, although controversy still exists as to its exact role. MRCP is highly sensitive (>95%) and specific (>95%) for the detection of biliary obstruction and defining the site of obstruction, but it is slightly less sensitive at detecting stones within the biliary tree (sensitivity 92%) and differentiating benign from malignant obstruction (sensitivity 88%).[1] Surgical clips around the biliary tree may produce artefacts. Like ERCP, stones may be difficult to distinguish from intraductal tumours, blood clots or gas bubbles on MRCP. Complications from MRCP are very rare due to its non-invasiveness and avoidance of contrast medium and sedatives. Other advantages of MRCP over ERCP include its speed (20–30 minutes) and reduced operator dependence. In addition, because MRCP does not depend on the flow of contrast within the ducts, as do ERCP and PTC, it can show ducts both proximal and distal to an obstruction. Standard contraindications to magnetic resonance imaging (MRI) apply.

Abdominal MRI using T1-weighting can also be performed during the same examination to provide staging informa-tion for suspected malignancy, although CT remains the

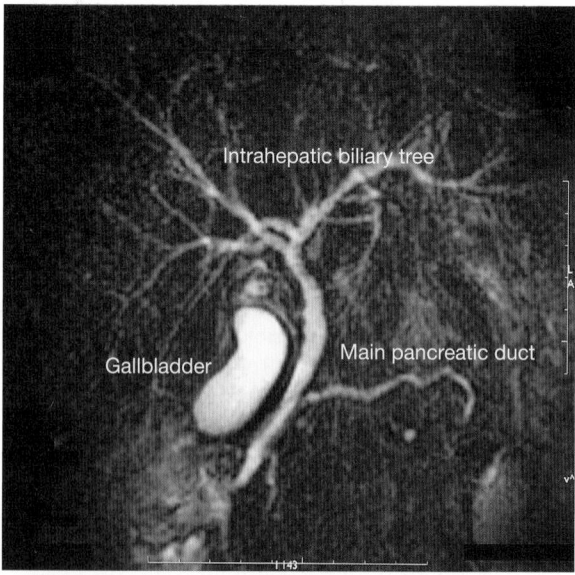

Intrahepatic biliary tree

Gallbladder

Main pancreatic duct

Fig. 5.23 Magnetic resonance cholangio-pancreatography (MRCP) of normal biliary tree and pancreatic duct.
Copyright Addenbrooke's Hospital, Cambridge, UK.

preferred abdominal cross-sectional imaging modality at present. The administration of intravenous contrast medium (usually chelates of gadolinium) allows magnetic resonance angiography (MRA) to be performed to assess tumour invasion and define vascular anatomy.

Percutaneous transhepatic cholangiogram

Percutaneous transhepatic cholangiography (PTC) is performed under local anaesthetic and involves passing a fine, flexible needle through the abdominal wall into the liver (see p. 308). Intrahepatic duct dilatation on transabdominal ultrasonography must be demonstrated first to ensure that PTC is feasible.

Hepatobiliary iminodiacetic acid (HIDA) scan

Hepatobiliary scintigraphy can be performed with radioactive technetium-99m labelled acid that is injected intravenously, taken up by the liver and excreted in the bile over 1–4 hours. Decay of the radiopharmaceutical leads to emission of gamma rays, allowing biliary imaging with a gamma camera. The most common indication for HIDA scanning is for the diagnosis of acute calculous cholecystitis when abdominal ultrasound is non-diagnostic. Acute calculous cholecystitis is visualized as lack of filling of the gallbladder due to obstruction of the cystic duct by the gallstone.

HIDA scanning is more accurate than ultrasound for the diagnosis of acute calculous cholecystitis (sensitivity of >95% and specificity 90% versus sensitivity of 90% and specificity of 80%)[2] but is a second- or third-line investigation due to its greater inconvenience, patient exposure to radiation, and inability to diagnose alternative abdominal pathologies. HIDA scanning can also be used to visualize biliary leaks or fistulae after trauma or surgery.

Positron emission tomography

Positron emission tomography (PET) scanning for cholangiocarcinoma appears promising but has not yet been shown to have a definite role.

> ### *i* FURTHER INFORMATION
>
> Baillie J, Paulson EK, Vitellas KM. Biliary imaging: a review. Gastroenterology 2003; 124: 1686–1699.

> ### REFERENCES
>
> **(1)** *Romagnuolo J, Bardou M, Rahme E, Joseph L, Reinhold C, Barkun AN. Magnetic resonance cholangiopancreatography: a meta-analysis of test performance in suspected biliary disease. Annals of Internal Medicine 2003; 139: 547–557.*
> **(2)** *Chatziioannou SN, Moore WH, Ford PV, Dhekne RD. Hepatobiliary scintigraphy is superior to abdominal ultrasonography in suspected acute cholecystitis. Surgery 2000; 127: 609–613.*

Acute acalculous cholecystitis

Mirizzi's syndrome

Gallstone ileus

Acute cholangitis

Common bile duct stones (choledocholithiasis)

Porcelain gallbladder

Biliary colic and chronic cholecystitis

SECTION 5.21   Gallstones and associated conditions

Gallstones are very common but with wide geographical variation in their occurrence. The overall prevalence is 12 000 per 100 000 in the West, 4000 per 100 000 in Asian populations. In African populations they are rare.[1] These differences are probably due to dietary and genetic factors.

The prevalence of gallstones increases with age: in the West, gallstones are present in 20–30% of those over the age of 75. They are approximately twice as common in women as men. Whilst numerous risk factors apply (Table 5.34), the typical patient with gallstones has been described as 'fat, female, fecund, and forty'.

Whilst gallstones are common, complications occur in only 30% (Table 5.35). The most common complication by far is biliary colic (90%). Because the risk of serious complications is low, asymptomatic gallstones discovered incidentally do not require treatment.

Gallstones can be divided into cholesterol and pigment stones. Cholesterol stones can be made up of cholesterol alone ('pure' cholesterol stones), or, more commonly, contain small amounts of bile salts and calcium. These are known as 'mixed' cholesterol stones (Fig. 5.24).

Bile salts and lecithin increase the solubility of cholesterol in aqueous solution. Increased cholesterol secretion, or a reduction in the excretion of bile salts or lecithin, leads to bile being supersaturated with cholesterol. This by itself may not be enough to cause cholesterol stone formation. Biliary mucus, protein and calcium act as 'nucleating agents'. This allows cholesterol to precipitate from solution as crystals. Gallbladder stasis encourages contact between nucleating agents and cholesterol crystals and promotes cholesterol stone growth.

Pigment gallstones are classified as 'black' or 'brown'. Both types contain calcium salts of unconjugated bilirubin. Insoluble, unconjugated bilirubin normally makes up less than 1% of the total bilirubin found in bile.

Black pigment stones are formed when ionized calcium combines with excess unconjugated bilirubin. This occurs when the conjugating capacity of the liver is exceeded, e.g. in liver failure or chronic haemolysis. These stones are usually found in the gallbladder. Brown stones are found in the ducts of infected biliary systems, when the bacterial enzyme β-glucuronidase hydrolyzes conjugated bilirubin to the unconjugated form. Combination with ionized calcium occurs, and stone formation can go on to cause further stasis and infection.

Most gallstones form in the gallbladder (cholecystolithiasis). Gallstones found in the bile ducts (choledocholithiasis) commonly originate from the gallbladder but

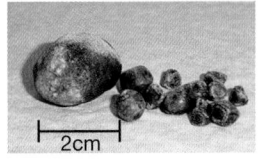

Fig. 5.24 Mixed cholesterol gallstones. Copyright Addenbrooke's Hospital, Cambridge, UK.

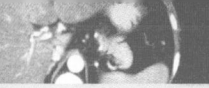

Table 5.34	Factors associated with increased gallstone formation
Risk factor	**Mechanism**
Age	Increased biliary cholesterol excretion Biliary stasis due to decreased sensitivity to CCK
Ethnicity, e.g. Pima Indians, USA	Exact mechanism unknown
Female gender Pregnancy Women of child-bearing age	Oestrogen increases hepatic synthesis of cholesterol Progesterone relaxes smooth muscle, leading to decreased gallbladder motility and biliary stasis
High cholesterol diet Obesity Hyperlipidaemia	Increased cholesterol excretion in bile
Starvation Total parenteral nutrition	Lack of CCK leads to decreased gallbladder motility and biliary stasis
Vagotomy for gastric ulceration Diabetic vagal neuropathy	Lack of vagal tone leads to decreased gallbladder motility and biliary stasis
Ileal disease 　Crohn's disease 　Surgical resection	Decreased absorption of bile salts leading to reduced production by the liver
Chronic haemolytic disease 　Sickle cell disease 　Thalassaemia 　Hereditary spherocytosis	Excessive release of bilirubin
Biliary tract infections 　E. coli 　B. fragilis	Production of β-glucuronidase by bacteria deconjugates bilirubin

Table 5.35	Scope of gallstone disease
Complication	**Pathology**
Biliary colic	Transient obstruction of the gallbladder
Chronic cholecystitis	Recurrent transient obstruction of the gallbladder (pathological diagnosis)
Acute calculous cholecystitis	Obstruction of the gallbladder with chemical or bacterial inflammation
Mucocele	Obstruction of the gallbladder without chemical or bacterial inflammation
Gallbladder empyema	Obstruction of the gallbladder with severe bacterial inflammation
Acute cholangitis	Stone from the gallbladder becoming lodged in the CBD, leading to obstruction and acute infection
Obstructive jaundice	Stone from the gallbladder becoming lodged in the CBD, leading to obstruction without infection
Acute pancreatitis	Stone from the gallbladder becoming lodged in the distal CBD, obstructing the pancreatic duct
Gallstone ileus	Large gallbladder stone eroding through the gallbladder into the duodenum, obstructing the small intestine
Mirizzi's syndrome	Acute cholecystitis with obstruction of the common hepatic duct due to inflammation or direct pressure
Porcelain gallbladder	Calcification of the gallbladder wall (associated with gallstones, but mechanism unknown)
Gallbladder carcinoma	Possibly due to chronic gallstones in the gallbladder
Cholangiocarcinoma	Possibly due to chronic gallstones in bile ducts

CBD, common bile duct.

may develop within the ducts if biliary stasis is present. Some small gallstones (<5 mm diameter) probably pass unnoticed into the duodenum but larger stones may impact in the duct or ampulla of Vater, causing pain, obstructive jaundice, acute pancreatitis or acute cholangitis. Stones may also impact in Hartmann's pouch, and the secondary inflammation can obstruct the normal flow of bile into the common bile duct (Mirizzi's syndrome). The development of a fistula between the gallbladder and the duodenum can allow the passage of large gallstones leading to intestinal obstruction (gallstone ileus). Chronic complications of gallstones include the development of a porcelain gallbladder and, rarely, gallbladder cancer.

Removal of the gallbladder (cholecystectomy) alters biliary physiology. Loss of the concentrating function of the gallbladder leads to an increased flow of bile into the duodenum that may result in biliary reflux into the stomach and biliary gastritis. After cholecystectomy, mild dilatation of the common bile duct occurs. The loss of storage function may decrease fat absorption, leading to diarrhoea.

> **REFERENCE**
>
> (1) *Kratzer W, Mason RA, Kachele V. Prevalence of gallstones in sonographic surveys worldwide. Journal of Clinical Ultrasound 1999; 27: 1–7.*

Acute acalculous cholecystitis

Epidemiology

Approximately 10% of patients with acute cholecystitis do not have detectable gallstones (acute acalculous cholecystitis). This usually occurs in critically ill patients. Spontaneous cases can occur, especially in patients with diabetes.

Pathology

In critically ill patients (usually with sepsis or shock), acute acalculous cholecystitis may result from microvascular occlusion within the gallbladder resulting in ischaemia and infection.

Clinical features

A high index of suspicion is required, as clinical diagnosis is difficult due to coexistent pathology and comorbidity of the patient.

Investigations
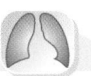

Abdominal ultrasound
Ultrasonography shows a thickened, distended gallbladder with pericholecystic fluid but without gallstones.

HIDA scan
A HIDA scan (p. 353) may be more accurate, with 95–98% sensitivity, but is difficult to perform in critically ill patients.

CT of the abdomen
CT scanning is useful to exclude other intra-abdominal causes of abdominal pain or sepsis.

Management

Emergency cholecystectomy
Treatment is with broad-spectrum intravenous antibiotics and emergency cholecystectomy if the patient is fit enough for a general anaesthetic.

Percutaneous cholecystostomy
In patients who are not fit for surgery the gallbladder can be decompressed via percutaneous cholecystostomy.

Prognosis

Mortality is high, up to 50%, usually due to the poor condition of the patient.

Mirizzi's syndrome

Mirizzi's syndrome describes impaction of a gallstone in the neck of the gallbladder or cystic duct resulting in common hepatic duct obstruction due to direct mechanical compression or inflammation. It is found in approximately 1% of patients undergoing biliary surgery. Patients with Mirizzi's syndrome may present with recurrent biliary colic, painful obstructive jaundice, acute cholangitis or acute cholecystitis. Preoperative diagnosis is difficult, even with ERCP or MRCP. Surgery is the treatment of choice, but failure to recognize the presence of Mirizzi's syndrome during cholecystectomy carries a high risk of common bile duct or common hepatic duct injury.

> ℹ **FURTHER INFORMATION**
>
> Abou-Saif A, Al-Kawas FH. Complications of gallstone disease: Mirizzi syndrome, cholecystocholedochal fistula, and gallstone ileus. American Journal of Gastroenterology 2002; 97: 249–254.

Gallstone ileus

Gallstone ileus occurs when a large gallstone from the gallbladder (or, rarely, the common bile duct) enters the gastrointestinal tract and causes small bowel obstruction.

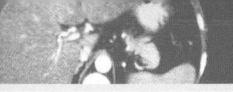

Epidemiology

Gallstone ileus typically occurs in those over 65 years of age, and accounts for approximately 4% of all cases of intestinal obstruction.

Pathology

Gallstones enter the gut via a fistula between the gallbladder and duodenum (cholecysto-duodenal fistula) in 75% of cases, and usually cause obstruction in the terminal ileum where the small bowel is narrowest.

Clinical features

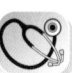

Patients present with symptoms and signs of small bowel obstruction (p. 248). There may be a history of previous episodes of right upper quadrant pain consistent with biliary colic.

Investigations

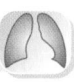

Plain abdominal film

Abdominal radiography shows dilated small bowel loops. A radio-opaque gallstone may be seen in the bowel (Fig. 5.25). Occasionally, air can be seen in the biliary tree (pneumobilia).

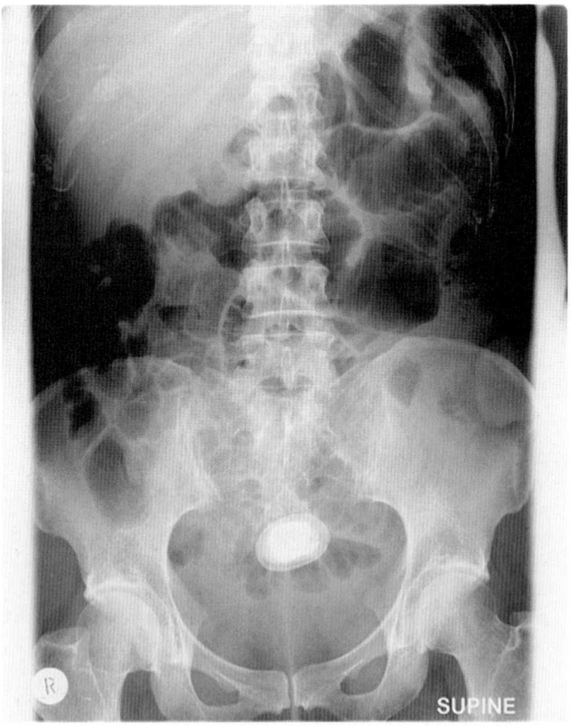

Fig. 5.25 Abdominal film of gallstone ileus. A laminated, calcified gallstone is seen in the pelvis with evidence of small bowel obstruction. Air in the biliary tree is not seen.
Courtesy of Dr M. Bennie, Norfolk and Norwich University Hospital, UK.

Management

Laparotomy and entero-lithotomy

Laparotomy with removal of the gallstone from the intestine (entero-lithotomy) is required. In high-risk patients, simple entero-lithotomy is the appropriate management. In patients who are generally fit, cholecystectomy and fistula closure may be considered.

Prognosis

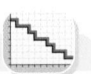

Mortality is high (15–18%) due to the advanced age and comorbidities of most patients.

---

i **FURTHER INFORMATION**

Rodriguez-Sanjuan JC, Casado F, Fernandez MJ, Morales DJ, Naranjo A. Cholecystectomy and fistula closure versus enterolithotomy alone in gallstone ileus. British Journal of Surgery 1997; 84: 634–637.

Reisner RM, Cohen JR. Gallstone ileus: a review of 1001 reported cases. American Surgeon 1994; 60: 441–446.

Acute cholangitis

Although normal bile is sterile, stasis or poor biliary flow renders bile susceptible to bacterial infection (bactibilia) resulting in acute cholangitis. This is also known as ascending cholangitis.

Epidemiology

Of all hospital admissions due to gallstone-related disease, acute cholangitis is responsible for 10%. The usual age at presentation is 60–70 years, and both sexes are equally affected.

Pathology

Acute cholangitis results from biliary obstruction. This is most commonly caused by common bile duct stones (50%) or malignant strictures (30%). Other causes of biliary obstruction are listed in Table 5.36. The combination of bacterial colonization and complete obstruction results in acute cholangitis. With partial obstruction, however, chronic low-grade infection occurs. Increased pressure within the biliary tree leads to reflux of bacteria through hepatic veins and lymphatics into the systemic circulation. Gram-negative aerobes (*E. coli*, *Klebsiella* species), *Enterococcus* species, and the Gram-negative anaerobe *Bacteroides fragilis* are common causative organisms. Blood and bile cultures are positive in 30% and 70% of cases, respectively.

Table 5.36	Causes of biliary obstruction leading to cholangitis

Gallstone(s)

Blocked biliary stent

Tumour
  Pancreatic
  Ampullary
  Duodenal
  Bile duct
  Gallbladder
  Liver

Benign stricture
  Idiopathic inflammatory
  Post cholecystectomy
  Stenosed biliary–enteric anastomosis
  Traumatic
  Post radiotherapy

Pancreatic pseudocyst

Chronic pancreatitis

Mirizzi's syndrome

Congenital
  Biliary atresia
  Choledochal cyst

Primary sclerosing cholangitis

Haemobilia

Parasitic infestation of the bile ducts (common in the Far East)
  Ascaris lumbricoides
  Clonorchis sinensis

Scope of disease

Direct spread of infection can lead to intrahepatic abscess formation or infection of the portal vein (pyelophlebitis) and subsequent portal vein thrombosis. In severe cholangitis, systemic release of bacterial toxins and inflammatory mediators can lead to disseminated intravascular coagulation, septic shock and multi-organ dysfunction. Long-standing bacterial colonization promotes formation of intraductal stones by enzymatic deconjugation of bilirubin. A vicious cycle of obstruction and infection ensues. Chronic infection also leads to irreversible fibrosis of the biliary system and secondary biliary cirrhosis.

Clinical features

Patients present with variable degrees of illness. Fever is present in more than 90% of cases, but abdominal pain can be quite mild and is not always localized to the right upper quadrant. A history of rigors is present in about half and symptoms of obstructive jaundice may occur. Specific questions about a history of gallstones, previous biliary surgery or biliary stenting should be asked.

Examination findings are also variable. The patient is febrile, often dehydrated and jaundiced (66%). Tenderness is present in the right upper quadrant, but is less marked than in acute cholecystitis. Septic shock, con-fusion or obtundation can occur with severe cholangitis. Fever, jaundice and right upper quadrant pain (Charcot's triad) are present in only 25% of patients with confirmed cholangitis.

Severe acute cholangitis occurs in 20–30%, and is diagnosed on the presence of septic shock or persisting/intermittent fever despite appropriate antibiotic therapy.[1]

Initial investigations

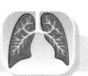

Full blood count
Full blood count almost invariably shows an elevated white cell count. The platelet count is reduced with disseminated intravascular coagulation.

C-reactive protein
C-reactive protein is elevated.

Urea and electrolytes
Urea may be elevated with dehydration, and renal impairment with elevated creatinine can occur with severe dehydration.

Liver profile
Liver enzymes are raised with an obstructive pattern (raised alkaline phosphatase, γ-glutamyltransferase, and bilirubin).

Coagulation screen
Prolonged prothrombin time and activated partial thromboplastin time occur with disseminated intravascular coagulation.

Serum amylase
Amylase may be mildly raised.

Blood, sputum and urine cultures
A bacteraemia is present in 30%. Other cultures are sent to exclude concomitant infection or other potential sources of infection that may present like cholangitis.

Abdominal ultrasound
Transabdominal ultrasonography is a non-invasive and sensitive investigation for biliary tree dilatation, although it is less sensitive at detecting the cause of the obstruction (e.g. choledocholithiasis or malignant stricture). In a septic patient with right upper quadrant pain, the presence of a dilated biliary tree strongly suggests biliary obstruction with acute cholangitis. The diagnosis is a clinical one until bactibilia is confirmed.

Further investigations

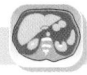

Hepatitis serology
Viral hepatitis should be excluded with serological tests if the transaminases are also elevated.

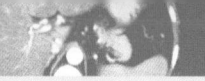

Chest X-ray

A chest film is performed if right lower lobe pneumonia remains a differential diagnosis.

Plain abdominal film

Plain abdominal radiography is rarely helpful, but occasionally pneumobilia due to gas-forming organisms or a biliary–enteric fistula may be seen.

Endoscopic retrograde cholangio-pancreatography

Bile culture and definitive diagnosis of the cause of the obstruction is usually provided by endoscopic retrograde cholangio-pancreatography (ERCP) (Fig. 5.26).

Initial management

This is summarized in Figure 5.27.

Rehydration

Prompt recognition of dehydration and rehydration with intravenous fluids is vital.

Antibiotics

Empiric intravenous antibiotics (e.g. ciprofloxacin 200 mg 12-hourly and metronidazole 500 mg 8-hourly) should be prescribed.

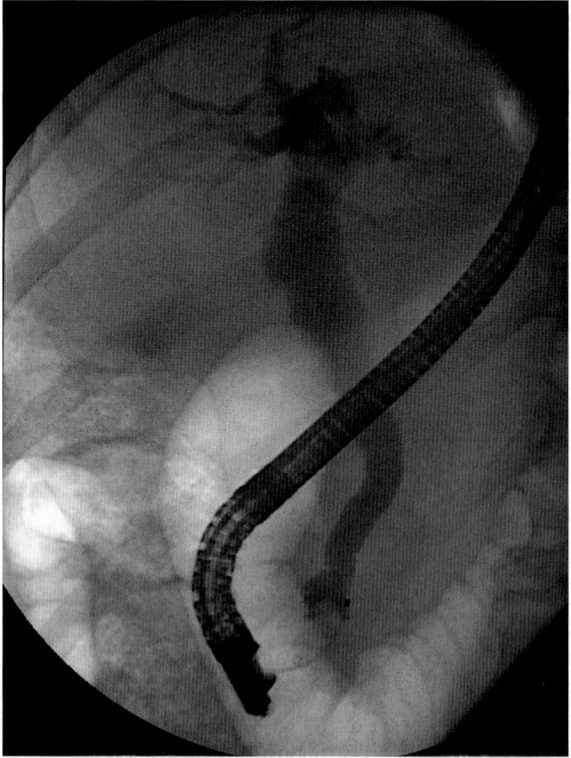

Fig. 5.26 Dilated, obstructed biliary tree on ERCP. Copyright Addenbrooke's Hospital, Cambridge, UK.

ICU admission

Severe sepsis or septic shock may require admission to intensive care, invasive monitoring and administration of inotropic agents. Early discussion and involvement of the ICU team is important.

Medical management

Conservative management

Antibiotics alone control cholangitis in 80% of patients. Cholangiography, relief of obstruction, and definitive treatment can be performed on an elective basis once the fever has resolved.

Cholangiography and biliary decompression

Patients with severe acute cholangitis require emergency biliary decompression of the infected biliary tree. The priority is to drain sepsis, as gallstone extraction and gallbladder removal can be performed at a later date when the patient's clinical state improves. Cholangiography and biliary decompression can be achieved percutaneously (PTC), endoscopically (ERCP) or surgically.

Percutaneous transhepatic cholangiography (PTC)
PTC is preferred to ERCP if the obstructing lesion is near the liver hilum, or if a previous biliary–enteric anastomosis has been performed. A needle is passed percutaneously into the liver and advanced into a bile ductule. The position is confirmed with cholangiography and a catheter is introduced into the bile ductule allowing direct drainage of bile.

Endoscopic retrograde cholangio-pancreatography
In patients with severe acute cholangitis due to bile duct stones, ERCP with nasobiliary drainage is superior to surgery.[1] Nasobiliary drainage allows irrigation, cholangiographic imaging and collection of bile. The nasobiliary drain is removed once the fever settles. Biliary stents can be inserted instead of nasobiliary drainage or for the management of malignant obstructions.

Extraction of common bile duct stones can also be achieved via ERCP. The gallbladder should be removed, e.g. with laparoscopic cholecystectomy, at a later date to prevent recurrence.[2]

Surgical management

Surgical decompression and cholecystectomy

Emergency surgical decompression of the bile ducts is required for patients with severe acute cholangitis when percutaneous or endoscopic techniques are unavailable or unsuccessful.

If the patient is haemodynamically unstable during surgery, biliary drainage alone is performed. Drainage can be achieved with incision of the common bile duct (choledochotomy) and placement of a T-tube percutaneously. The T-tube allows drainage of the bile and injection of contrast to perform cholangiography. Once the drain tract matures, the T-tube

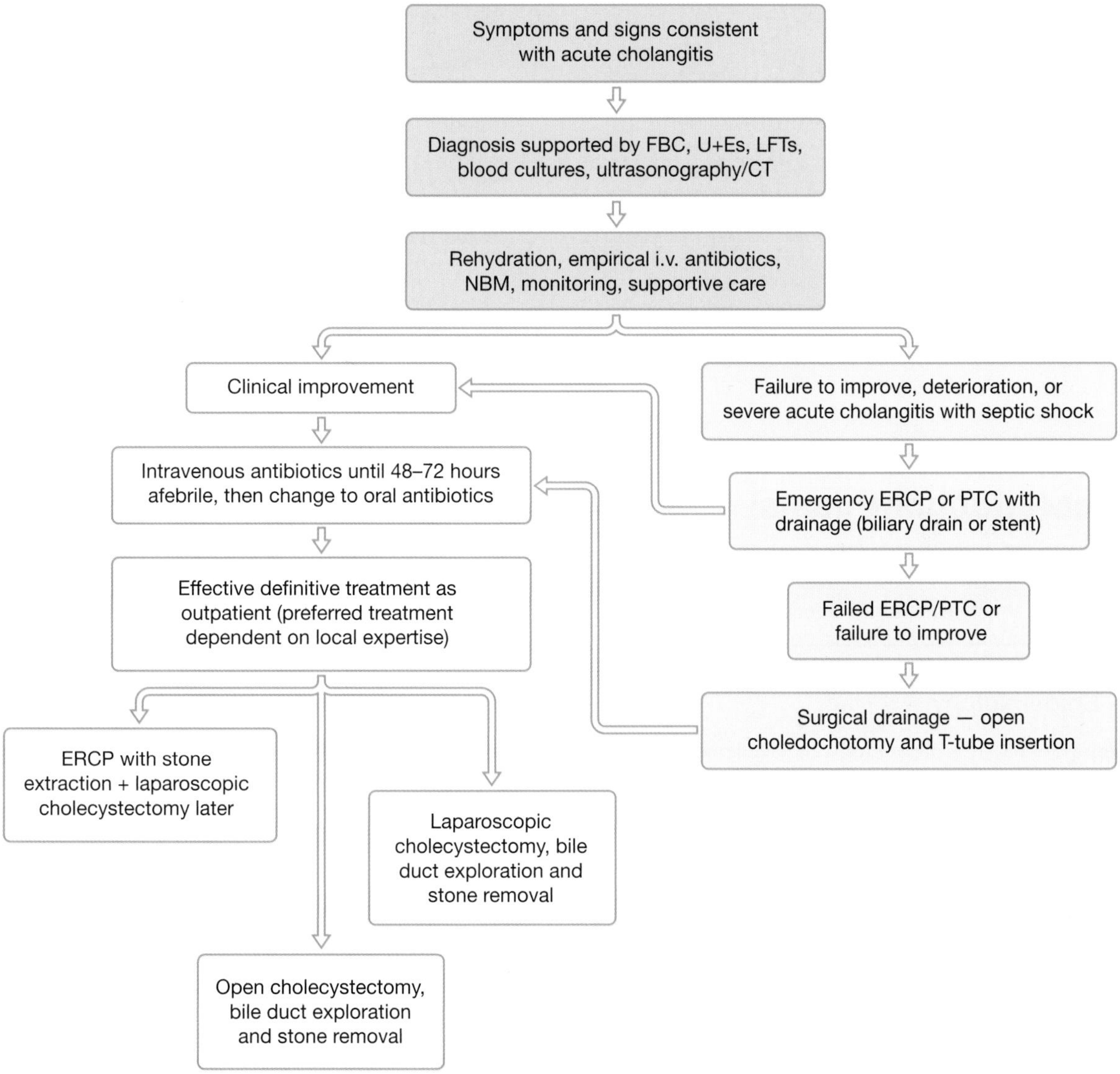

Symptoms and signs consistent
with acute cholangitis

⇩

Diagnosis supported by FBC, U+Es, LFTs,
blood cultures, ultrasonography/CT

⇩

Rehydration, empirical i.v. antibiotics,
NBM, monitoring, supportive care

Clinical improvement

Failure to improve, deterioration, or
severe acute cholangitis with septic shock

Intravenous antibiotics until 48–72 hours
afebrile, then change to oral antibiotics

Emergency ERCP or PTC with
drainage (biliary drain or stent)

Effective definitive treatment as
outpatient (preferred treatment
dependent on local expertise)

Failed ERCP/PTC or
failure to improve

ERCP with stone
extraction + laparoscopic
cholecystectomy later

Laparoscopic
cholecystectomy, bile
duct exploration and
stone removal

Surgical drainage — open
choledochotomy and T-tube insertion

Open cholecystectomy,
bile duct exploration
and stone removal

Fig. 5.27 Management of acute cholangitis due to choledocholithiasis. FBC, full blood count; U+Es, urea and electrolytes; LFTs, liver function tests; NBM, nil by mouth; ERCP, endoscopic retrograde cholangio-pancreatography; PTC, percutaneous transhepatic cholangiography.

can be removed, and the resulting biliary–cutaneous fistula will close spontaneously if no distal biliary obstruction is present.

In patients with milder forms of the disease, decompression with open or laparoscopic cholecystectomy and intraoperative gallstone removal is the definitive treatment. Surgery may be superior to endoscopic management in the initial treatment of mild acute cholangitis as additional procedures can be avoided.[3]

Prognosis

The overall mortality in acute cholangitis is 5%.[4] Severe acute cholangitis due to gallstones carries a mortality rate of 20%.[1] Short-term outcome is worse in malignant obstruction and the elderly. Long-term prognosis is dependent on the cause of the obstruction (i.e. benign versus malignant).

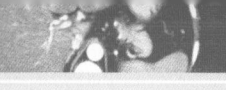

REFERENCES

(1) Lai EC, Mok FP, Tan ES, et al. Endoscopic biliary drainage for severe acute cholangitis. New England Journal of Medicine 1992; 326: 1582–1586.
(2) Poon RT, Liu CL, Lo CM, et al. Management of gallstone cholangitis in the era of laparoscopic cholecystectomy. Archives of Surgery 2001; 136: 11–16.
(3) Suc B, Escat J, Cherqui D, et al. Surgery vs endoscopy as primary treatment in symptomatic patients with suspected common bile duct stones: a multicenter randomized trial. French Associations for Surgical Research. Archives of Surgery 1998; 133: 702–708.
(4) Sugiyama M, Atomi Y. Treatment of acute cholangitis due to choledocholithiasis in elderly and younger patients. Archives of Surgery 1997; 132: 1129–1133.

Table 5.37	Features suggestive of common bile duct stones
Clinical features	
History of jaundice, acute pancreatitis or acute cholangitis	
Blood tests	
History of elevated alkaline phosphatase, bilirubin or amylase	
Ultrasound findings	
Dilated common bile duct (>8 mm)	

Common bile duct stones (choledocholithiasis)

Stones in the common bile duct can lead to a number of conditions such as obstructive jaundice, ascending cholangitis and pancreatitis. This section focuses mainly on the management of asymptomatic bile duct stones.

Epidemiology

Approximately 10% of patients with gallbladder stones will also have stones in the common bile duct.

Pathology

The majority of common bile duct stones originate from the gallbladder (secondary stones), although stones can also form within the bile ducts (primary stones), usually in the presence of infection or obstruction.

Clinical features

Gallstones in the common bile duct are commonly asymptomatic and, if less than 5 mm in diameter, may pass spontaneously through the sphincter of Oddi into the duodenum. The complications of common bile duct stones include right upper quadrant pain, obstructive jaundice, acute cholangitis and pancreatitis.

Investigations

Asymptomatic common bile duct (CBD) stones are difficult to detect as liver function tests are usually normal. Trans-abdominal ultrasonography is poor at detecting distal CBD stones but can detect a dilated CBD due to obstruction. In patients diagnosed with biliary colic, if ultrasonography shows gallbladder stones with a normal CBD diameter, then MRCP can be performed to screen for ductal stones. However, many surgeons would perform a cholecystectomy and exclude ductal stones with an intraoperative cholangiogram. Patients require further preoperative investigations if there is a raised suspicion of ductal stones (Table 5.37).[1,2]

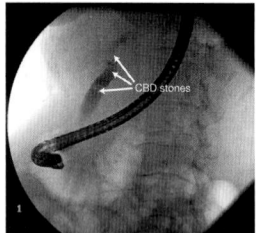

Fig. 5.28 Multiple common bile duct (CBD) stones are seen on ERCP. Copyright Addenbrooke's Hospital, Cambridge, UK.

Magnetic resonance cholangio-pancreatography

Magnetic resonance cholangio-pancreatography (MRCP) is non-invasive and has similar sensitivity and specificity to ERCP. MRCP is purely diagnostic, however, while ERCP can also be therapeutic.

Endoscopic retrograde cholangiopancreatography

Endoscopic retrograde cholangiopancreatography (ERCP) has a sensitivity of >90% for the detection of CBD stones (Fig. 5.28), but has an appreciable morbidity (p. 306). It is appropriate where there is a high probability of a therapeutic manoeuvre being required.

Intraoperative cholangiography

Intraoperative cholangiography can be performed during laparoscopic or open cholecystectomy, and is highly sensitive for the detection of choledocholithiasis.

Management

There are many options available for the management of CBD stones: endoscopic (ERCP), surgical (open or laparoscopic) or expectant (Table 5.38). With appropriate case selection, success rates are similar and there is no strong evidence supporting one technique over the others.

Endoscopic retrograde cholangio-pancreatography

ERCP and stone extraction is less invasive than surgery, but has the disadvantage that if the gallbladder has residual stones, recurrent biliary events can occur.[3]

Open cholecystectomy and common bile duct stone removal

Common bile duct stones can be removed laparoscopically but the techniques are difficult and are not widely available. Therefore, open cholecystectomy and common bile duct stone removal is a preferred option, but is now only performed when ERCP has failed.

Laparoscopic cholecystectomy and common bile duct stone removal

Laparoscopic cholecystectomy with routine intraoperative cholangiogram and laparoscopic common bile duct exploration is as effective as laparoscopic cholecystectomy alone with postoperative ERCP stone removal, and carries a

Technique	Advantages	Disadvantages
ERCP	Minimally invasive Good availability	Risk of ERCP-induced pancreatitis Long-term effects of sphincterotomy unknown Requires subsequent cholecystectomy May require repeated procedures
Laparoscopic bile duct exploration surgery	Preserves sphincter of Oddi Can remove gallbladder and CBD stones in one operation Minimally invasive	Technically difficult Not widely available
Open surgery	Wide availability Can remove gallbladder and CBD stone in one operation Preserves sphincter of Oddi	Invasive Longer recovery time
Expectant management ('wait-and-see')	Non-invasive	Risk of complications Only suitable for small stones

Table 5.38   Management options for common bile duct stones

ERCP, endoscopic retrograde cholangiopancreatography; CBD, common bile duct.

shorter hospital stay.[4] With improved surgical training, these laparoscopic techniques may become the definitive treatment of gallbladder stones with choledocholithiasis.

Expectant management

Small, asymptomatic common bile duct stones (<5 mm diameter) commonly pass into the duodenum spontaneously and in this situation a 'wait-and-see' policy may be appropriate.[5]

Screening for common bile duct stones

Before the introduction of laparoscopic cholecystectomy, common bile duct stones were removed during open cholecystectomy after routine intraoperative cholangiography. Currently, the main options for screening for common bile duct stones are MRCP, ERCP in selected cases with stone removal, or intraoperative cholangiography with postoperative ERCP for stone removal.

Prognosis

Small stones may pass spontaneously into the duodenum. Large stones (>5 mm diameter) causing complications usually require intervention for removal. The risk of recurrence is low after cholecystectomy.

FURTHER INFORMATION

Kristiansen VB, Rosenberg J. Laparoscopic treatment of uncomplicated common bile duct stones: what is the evidence? Scandinavian Journal of Gastroenterology 2002; 37: 993–998.

Eisen GM, Dominitz JA, Faigel DO, et al. An annotated algorithm for the evaluation of choledocholithiasis. Gastrointestinal Endoscopy 2001; 53: 864–866.

REFERENCES

(1) Abboud PA, Malet PF, Berlin JA, et al. Predictors of common bile duct stones prior to cholecystectomy: a meta-analysis. Gastrointestinal Endoscopy 1996; 44: 450–455.
(2) Prat F, Meduri B, Ducot B, et al. Prediction of common bile duct stones by noninvasive tests. Annals of Surgery 1999; 229: 362–368.
(3) Boerma D, Rauws EA, Keulemans YC, et al. Wait-and-see policy or laparoscopic cholecystectomy after endoscopic sphincterotomy for bile-duct stones: a randomised trial. Lancet 2002; 360: 761–765.
(4) Rhodes M, Sussman L, Cohen L, et al. Randomised trial of laparoscopic exploration of common bile duct versus postoperative endoscopic retrograde cholangiography for common bile duct stones. Lancet 1998; 351: 159–161.
(5) Ammori BJ, Birbas K, Davides D, et al. Routine vs "on demand" postoperative ERCP for small bile duct calculi detected at intraoperative cholangiography. Clinical evaluation and cost analysis. Surgical Endoscopy 2000; 14:1123–1126.

Porcelain gallbladder

Porcelain gallbladder (calcification of the gallbladder wall) is associated with recurrent attacks of right upper quadrant pain. A porcelain gallbladder may be discovered incidentally during radiography, when a calcified mass is seen in the right upper quadrant. Porcelain gallbladder is thought to be associated with gallbladder carcinoma and prophylactic cholecystectomy is recommended.

Biliary colic and chronic cholecystitis

Biliary colic is the most common symptom of patients with gallstones. Repeated low-grade inflammation can lead to chronic cholecystitis (a histological diagnosis), characterized by a thickened, shrunken and fibrosed gallbladder.

Epidemiology

Biliary colic is common. The incidence is 2000 per 100 000 per year in patients with gallstones.[1] The incidence decreases with time, to approximately half after 5 years as 30% of patients only ever experience one episode. The exact prevalence of biliary colic is difficult to determine as both gallstones and upper abdominal pain are common and often go undiagnosed.

Pathology

The symptoms of biliary colic arise from distension and spasm of the gallbladder from an impacted gallstone in the gallbladder neck obstructing the cystic duct and normal flow of bile. Once the impacted stone falls back from the gallbladder neck, the gallbladder empties and the pain ceases.

Scope of disease

Continued impaction of the stone results in chemical inflammation and can lead to acute cholecystitis. Recurrent episodes of biliary colic result in low-grade inflammation leading to chronic cholecystitis. Gallstone impaction in Hartmann's pouch when the gallbladder is empty may result in mucus secretion from the gallbladder leading to a mucocele.

Clinical features

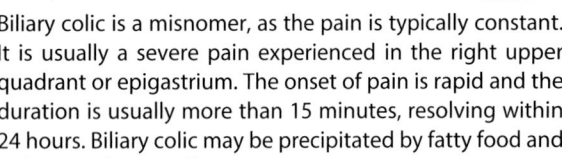

Biliary colic is a misnomer, as the pain is typically constant. It is usually a severe pain experienced in the right upper quadrant or epigastrium. The onset of pain is rapid and the duration is usually more than 15 minutes, resolving within 24 hours. Biliary colic may be precipitated by fatty food and radiate to the scapula.

Examination reveals right upper quadrant tenderness in an afebrile patient. Fever, jaundice, Murphy's sign, systemic upset or signs of peritoneal irritation indicate the development of other complications (Table 5.39). A palpable gallbladder suggests a mucocele.

Initial investigations

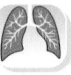

Full blood count, liver profile and amylase
Full blood count, liver profile and serum amylase are normal in biliary colic.

Ultrasound of the abdomen
Ultrasound scanning confirms the presence of gallstones in the gallbladder.

Further investigations

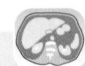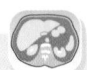

Upper gastrointestinal endoscopy
If ultrasonography is normal, upper gastrointestinal endoscopy should be performed to exclude peptic ulcer disease, gastritis and gastro-oesophageal reflux disease.

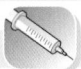

Initial management

Analgesia
Biliary colic is usually managed in the community with oral analgesics, but intramuscular diclofenac may prevent progression to acute cholecystitis.[2] If analgesia is inadequate, hospital admission for intravenous opiates is required until the pain settles.

Surgical management

Cholecystectomy
Elective cholecystectomy has become the standard therapy for gallstones causing biliary colic (other indications are listed in Table 5.39). The advantages over medical therapy are: no restrictions on the number, size or type of gallstone, rapid stone removal, prevention of recurrence and elimination of any risk of gallbladder cancer.

Cholecystectomy may be undertaken with a laparoscopic or open approach (Table 5.40). Over the last decade, laparoscopic cholecystectomy has become the operation of choice by surgeons and the general public, such that the open approach is now seldom performed as the first choice. This is despite randomized trials showing similar outcomes when a small incision open approach is compared to the laparoscopic approach.[3]

Laparoscopic cholecystectomy
There are no absolute indications to favour laparoscopic cholecystectomy over an open approach, although some surgeons would favour open cholecystectomy for patients with obesity, previous upper abdominal surgery and bleeding disorders, as they carry a higher risk of conversion to open surgery.

Laparoscopic cholecystectomy is performed under general anaesthesia with the patient supine. The first step is to create a pneumoperitoneum to improve vision and

Table 5.39	Indications for cholecystectomy
Symptomatic gallbladder stones	
Biliary colic	
Acute cholecystitis	
Complications of gallstone disease	
Acute pancreatitis	
Choledocholithiasis	
Cholangitis	
Early gallbladder cancer	
Other indications	
Symptomatic gallbladder polyps or >1 cm in length	
Chronic pancreatitis due to gallstones	
Chronic typhoid carrier	
Non-functioning gallbladder	

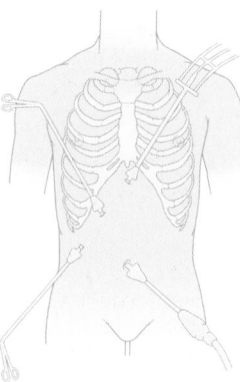

Fig. 5.29 Port placement for laparoscopic cholecystectomy.

Table 5.40	Comparison between laparoscopic and open cholecystectomy

Advantages of laparoscopic surgery compared with open cholecystectomy	Disadvantages of laparoscopic surgery compared with open cholecystectomy
Smaller incisions	Difficult to control haemorrhage
Less post-operative pain	Lack of depth perception
Better cosmesis	Slightly higher rate of CBD injury
Reduced hospital stay	Intraoperative cholangiography is technically demanding
Earlier return to work	Associated complications of laparoscopic surgery (e.g. unrecognized bowel injury, complications due to trocar introduction and insufflation)
Reduced respiratory complications	Complex technology
Overall decreased cost	Longer operating time

mobility within the abdomen. An open insertion of the first port is performed through an infra-umbilical incision (Hassan technique). Carbon dioxide is insufflated to a maximum pressure of 15 mmHg. Higher pressures result in decreased venous return, low blood pressure and low urine output.

The laparoscope (camera) is inserted and the abdominal and pelvic cavities are inspected, then three further ports are introduced (Fig. 5.29). Using laparoscopic dissectors, graspers and coagulators, adhesions are removed from the gallbladder and dissection is started at the neck of the gallbladder, proceeding along the cystic duct. The gallbladder is retracted superiorly and laterally to aid dissection (Fig. 5.30a). Once the cystic duct and cystic artery have been identified in Calot's triangle (p. 349) (Fig. 5.30b), a titanium clip is placed across the cystic duct. Intraoperative cholangiography is performed through a partial transection of the distal cystic duct by inserting a cholangio-catheter and injecting contrast (Fig. 5.31). Cholangiography

is important to identify any abnormal biliary anatomy, injuries to the biliary tree, and gallstones elsewhere in the biliary system.

Once the management of any common bile duct stones has been determined, the cystic duct is clipped distally and divided. The cystic artery is clipped and divided, and the gallbladder is dissected off the gallbladder fossa of the liver. Bleeding is controlled with diathermy. The gallbladder is removed via the epigastric port. The cannulae are removed and the incisions closed with sutures.

In young, fit patients with uncomplicated gallstone disease, laparoscopic cholecystectomy may be performed as day surgery. Most patients, however, require 2–3 days of hospitalization.

Laparoscopic cholecystectomy for biliary colic carries a mortality risk of 0.5% and a complication rate of 1–5% (Table 5.41).[4] The risks of complications are higher in the

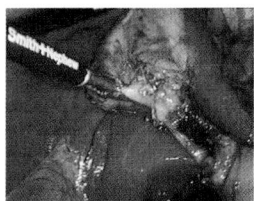

(a)

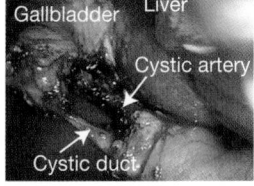

(b)

Fig. 5.30 a,b Intraoperative images of laparoscopic cholecystectomy. Courtesy of Mr A. Jah, Addenbrooke's Hospital, Cambridge. Copyright Addenbrooke's Hospital, Cambridge, UK.

Table 5.41	Complications of laparoscopic cholecystectomy

More common complications

Wound infection 1%
Pneumonia 1%
Haemorrhage 1%
Biliary tree injuries 0.5%

Uncommon complications

Bile spillage
Stone spillage
Incisional herniae
Acute pancreatitis
Pneumoperitoneum related CO$_2$ embolism Vasovagal reflex Hypercarbic acidosis
Trocar related Intestinal or vascular injuries Abdominal wall haematoma

Fig. 5.31 Intraoperative cholangiogram. Contrast is shown in the intra- and extra-hepatic biliary tree. No ductal stones are seen and the contrast has flowed into the duodenum.
Copyright Addenbrooke's Hospital, Cambridge, UK.

363

elderly, those with multiple comorbidities and in acute cholecystitis. Conversion to open surgery occurs in 5% due to bleeding, complications (e.g. bile duct injury), discovery of unexpected pathology or difficult dissection. The conversion rate rises to 30% in the setting of acute cholecystitis, due to the presence of inflammation.

RECENT ADVANCES

Laparoscopic cholecystectomy has been performed with robotic assistance, but remains an experimental technique at present.[5]

Open cholecystectomy

Although the indications for surgery are the same as for the laparoscopic approach, open cholecystectomy is most commonly performed as a conversion procedure from laparoscopic cholecystectomy.

Open cholecystectomy can be performed through a right subcostal (Kocher's) incision 3 cm below the costal margin, or through a smaller mini-laparotomy incision. The gallbladder can be removed using the retrograde or antegrade techniques. In the retrograde technique, dissection of Calot's triangle with ligation of the cystic duct and artery are performed before excision of the gallbladder. In the antegrade technique, the gallbladder is dissected off the liver followed by dissection of Calot's triangle with ligation of the cystic duct and artery.

The mortality rates for elective open cholecystectomy are similar to laparoscopic surgery. The operating time and complication rates in general are lower.

Medical management

Medical therapies for symptomatic gallbladder stones include oral bile acids, extracorporeal shock wave lithotripsy (ESWL) and dissolution therapy with methyl tert-butyl ether (MTBE) (Table 5.42). Medical therapies are not widely used due to their restrictive indications and the relative safety of laparoscopic cholecystectomy. These treatment options are usually reserved for patients in whom surgery cannot be safely performed or in patients who express a strong preference for non-surgical management.

Oral bile acids

Suitability for treatment with oral bile acids is assessed using oral cholecystography and abdominal radiography as only floating radiolucent stones are likely to represent cholesterol stones. Oral bile acids (e.g. ursodeoxycholic acid) decrease cholesterol secretion into bile and increase the solubility of cholesterol in bile. Bile acids may need to be taken for up to 2 years. Dissolution rates after 2 years range from 30% to 70% depending on the stone size and composition.

Extracorporeal shock wave lithotripsy

Lithotripsy uses acoustic shock waves to break up gallbladder stones into small pieces that can pass through the bile duct into the duodenum. Oral bile acids are given simultaneously to encourage fragment dissolution. Patients with solitary radiolucent stones less than 2 cm in diameter are the best candidates for extracorporeal shock wave lithotripsy as gallstones are successfully cleared in 90% within a year of treatment.

Methyl tert-butyl ether installation

MTBE is a contact solvent that dissolves cholesterol gallstones during instillation into the gallbladder. Instillation is via a catheter under ultrasound guidance.

Prognosis

Recurrence of biliary colic occurs in 50% of untreated patients after 1 year. Other biliary complications develop at a rate of 2% per year. In patients receiving only medical therapy, gallstones recur at a rate of 10% per year in the first 5 years. Biliary colic does not recur after cholecystectomy as the gallbladder has been excised. Rarely, stones may still form within the biliary tree.

Table 5.42	Non-operative management of symptomatic gallstone disease		
Therapy	**Indication**	**Advantage**	**Disadvantage**
Oral bile acids	Cholesterol gallstones less than 1.5 cm in diameter Mild biliary colic Good gallbladder function	Non-invasive Few side effects	Significant exclusion criteria Long duration of therapy Limited efficacy
Extracorporeal shock wave lithotripsy	Radiolucent stones with combined diameter of less than 3 cm Good gallbladder function	Non-invasive	Long duration of therapy Limited efficacy Oral bile acids required
Methyl tert-butyl ether (MTBE) instillation	Cholesterol stones	Rapid dissolution Number and size of stones not important Can be used in those with moderate–severe symptoms	Limited availability Invasive Complications if MTBE enters the peritoneal cavity or small intestine

FURTHER INFORMATION

Guidelines for the treatment of gallstones. American College of Physicians. Annals of Internal Medicine 1993; 119(7 Pt 1): 620–622.

REFERENCES

(1) *Ransohoff DF, Gracie WA. Treatment of gallstones. Annals of Internal Medicine 1993; 119: 606–619.*
(2) *Akriviadis EA, Hatzigavriel M, Kapnias D, Kirimlidis J, Markantas A, Garyfallos A. Treatment of biliary colic with diclofenac: a randomized, double-blind, placebo-controlled study. Gastroenterology 1997; 113: 225–231.*
(3) *Svanvik J. Results of laparoscopic compared with open cholecystectomy. European Journal of Surgery 2000; Suppl 585: 12–15.*
(4) *Hjelmqvist B. Complications of laparoscopic cholecystectomy as recorded in the Swedish laparoscopy registry. European Journal of Surgery 2000; Suppl 585: 18–21.*
(5) *Marescaux J, Leroy J, Gagner M, et al. Transatlantic robot-assisted telesurgery. Nature 2001; 413: 379–380.*

SECTION 5.22   Biliary cirrhosis

Primary biliary cirrhosis

Epidemiology

The prevalence of primary biliary cirrhosis varies with geography. It is more common in the Northern European countries. It mainly affects women in the fifth decade of life (it has not been described in children).

Pathology

Primary biliary cirrhosis is a chronic, progressive, cholestatic liver disease with an autoimmune aetiology and familial predisposition.

Primary biliary cirrhosis results in granulomatous bile duct destruction affecting mainly the middle-sized bile ducts. Characteristically, there is biliary epithelial damage, with infiltration of chronic inflammatory cells including granulomas within the portal tracts (stage 1), progressing to piecemeal necrosis, ductular proliferation and inflammation that extends beyond the portal tracts (stage 2) to fibrosis and bridging between portal tracts (stage 3) and micronodular liver cirrhosis (stage 4).

Scope of disease

The complications relate to liver cirrhosis, portal hypertension and cholestasis. Liver cirrhosis can lead to the development of ascites, encephalopathy and hepatocellular carcinoma. The complications of portal hypertension include oesophageal or gastric varices and splenomegaly. Cholestasis can lead to jaundice, malabsorption of fat-soluble vitamins (A, D, E and K), and osteoporosis (vitamin D deficiency).

Clinical features

Patients with early disease are asymptomatic and detected incidentally on biochemical screening. As the disease progresses, patients present with symptoms of lethargy and pruritus, and some may complain of right upper quadrant discomfort. Late in the disease, patients may develop jaundice (less than 20%) or features of decompensated liver disease (less than 5%) and portal hypertension (variceal bleeding and ascites). Patients may also have features of associated diseases (Table 5.43).

Examination may be normal in early disease. Pigmentation and excoriations may result with pruritus. Xanthomas and xanthelasma may be present, and examination of the cornea may reveal Kayser–Fleischer rings (normally associated with Wilson's disease). Clubbing may be present, and a significant proportion will have hepatosplenomegaly.

Table 5.43	Diseases associated with primary biliary cirrhosis
Endocrine disorders	
Hypothyroidism	
Addison's disease	
Myasthenia gravis	
Rheumatologic disorders	
Systemic sclerosis	
Dermatomyositis	
Sicca syndrome	
Respiratory disorders	
Pulmonary fibrosis	
Gastrointestinal disorders	
Coeliac disease	
Ulcerative colitis	

Jaundice, ascites and encephalopathy are complications of progressive disease.

Initial investigations

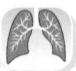

Liver profile

In early disease, the liver profile may be normal. Later, a cholestatic pattern emerges, characterized by elevated alkaline phosphatase, gamma glutamyltransferase and mildly elevated transaminases. Bilirubin rises late in the disease, and there are abnormalities of the markers of synthetic function (prothrombin time and albumin).

Immunoglobulins and autoantibodies

Immunoglobulins and autoantibodies are the mainstay of diagnosis of primary biliary cirrhosis. Serum IgM and possibly IgG levels are elevated. Anti-mitochondrial antibodies are elevated in 95%, and the M2 subset is highly specific for primary biliary cirrhosis. A small proportion of patients with primary biliary cirrhosis are anti-mitochondrial antibody negative (autoimmune cholangitis); they have a higher level of IgG and anti-nuclear antibodies (ANA).

Ultrasound of the abdomen

Ultrasound of the liver and biliary tree is performed to exclude extrahepatic biliary obstruction.

Further investigations

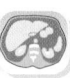

Liver biopsy

A liver biopsy is indicated if the diagnosis is in doubt, or to exclude other coexistent liver disease. It is not useful in the diagnosis of patients with a classical presentation, and the histological features have little prognostic value.

Magnetic resonance cholangio-pancreatography

In atypical cases, magnetic resonance cholangiography may be necessary to exclude primary sclerosing cholangitis (p. 369).

Initial management

Nutrition

Supplementation of the fat-soluble vitamins is important as malabsorption occurs with biliary obstruction. Calcium supplementation, bisphosphonates and hormone replacement therapy may be required in patients with osteoporosis.

Management of pruritus

Colestyramine is the most effective drug (taken at meal times), but a month may be required before any effect is observed. Mild gastrointestinal side effects may occur. Other drugs for pruritus include rifampicin, ursodeoxycholic acid, naloxone and naltrexone. Antihistamines are rarely effective.

Medical management

Ursodeoxycholic acid

Ursodeoxycholic acid administration leads to improvements in the liver profile and increases patient survival. The mechanism of action is unclear.

Immunomodulation

Prednisolone may lead to clinical improvement and is a useful drug for patients with coexistent autoimmune disease or cholangitis.

Management of portal hypertension

Prophylactic beta-blockers may be administered to patients with oesophageal varices.

Surgical management

Liver transplantation

Liver transplantation is indicated for patients with end-stage liver disease, impaired quality of life or with the development of early hepatocellular carcinoma. Liver transplantation has excellent survival rates, but recurrent disease may occur.

Prognosis

There is no specific feature that reliably predicts the rate of progression of disease. The majority of asymptomatic patients develop symptoms about 5 years after diagnosis, and patients who were symptomatic on presentation develop liver failure in about 10 years.

The most important prognostic factor is elevated serum bilirubin. Other poor prognostic variables (Mayo Clinic model) include increasing age, low serum albumin, prolonged prothrombin time and peripheral oedema.

ℹ️ FURTHER INFORMATION

Neuberger J. Primary biliary cirrhosis. Lancet 1997; 350: 876–879.

REFERENCE

(1) *Selmi C, Invernizzi P, Keeffe EB, et al. Epidemiology and pathogenesis of primary biliary cirrhosis. Journal of Clinical Gastroenterology 2004; 38: 264–271.*

Secondary biliary cirrhosis

Secondary biliary cirrhosis refers to biliary damage, subsequent hepatocyte damage, fibrosis and liver cirrhosis due to long-standing obstruction of the extrahepatic biliary tree.

Epidemiology

The epidemiology of secondary biliary cirrhosis is variable and reflects the prevalence of the underlying disease process (Table 5.44).

Pathology

Bile stasis from extrahepatic biliary obstruction leads to the dilatation of the interlobular bile ducts. When the interlobular bile ducts rupture, 'lakes' of bile are formed. Extravasation of bile into the periportal hepatocytes leads to reactive proliferation of ductules, infiltration of inflammatory cells (neutrophils) and periportal fibrosis. Progression of hepatic fibrosis gradually leads to micronodular cirrhosis and the associated complications (e.g. portal hypertension). Progression from biliary obstruction to liver cirrhosis may take up to a year. Patients with secondary biliary cirrhosis are also predisposed to recurrent ascending cholangitis.

Clinical features

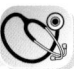

Pruritus is a prominent presenting feature, and unlike primary biliary cirrhosis, jaundice is common in early cases. There may be a history of previous biliary surgery or biliary colic. Fever, right upper quadrant discomfort, jaundice and night sweats or rigors could indicate the development of ascending cholangitis as a complication.

Investigations

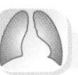

Liver profile
The liver profile usually reveals a cholestatic picture with markedly elevated alkaline phosphatase and bilirubin, and mildly elevated transaminases. In the setting of ascending cholangitis, the transaminases are markedly elevated.

Immunoglobulins and serum autoantibodies
As primary biliary cirrhosis is an important differential diagnosis, serum immunoglobulins and autoantibodies should be profiled; they are negative in secondary biliary cirrhosis.

Ultrasound of the abdomen
Ultrasound of the biliary system confirms dilated hepatic or biliary ducts (distal obstruction) and may identify the underlying cause (stones, tumour mass).

Further imaging
The biliary system should be further imaged with ERCP, MRCP or PTC to elucidate the cause of the obstruction. ERCP and MRCP are ideal for identification of choledochal cysts and extrahepatic primary sclerosing cholangitis.

   ERCP has the extra benefit of being a therapeutic procedure to remove stones or place biliary stents for the drainage of bile.

   PTC is useful for elucidating disease processes higher in the biliary tree. It can facilitate the placement of an external or internal drain to decompress the biliary system and also allows the placement of stents.

Management

Identify and treat the underlying cause
Relief of bile obstruction is the essential step in the prevention of secondary biliary cirrhosis. Strictures (benign and malignant) may be dilated or stented, and stones should be retrieved.

Surgery
Laparotomy and decompression of the bile ducts may be undertaken for distal obstruction (p. 370). Postoperative strictures may be repaired.

Liver transplantation
Patients with end-stage liver disease may require transplantation if there is deteriorating biochemistry or quality of life or complications of portal hypertension.

Antibiotics
Long-term ciprofloxacin or trimethoprim may be prescribed as prophylaxis for patients with recurrent attacks.

Table 5.44	Causes of secondary biliary cirrhosis
Postoperative strictures of the biliary system	
Gallstones	
Primary sclerosing cholangitis (extrahepatic disease)	
Chronic pancreatitis	
Cholangiocarcinoma	
Choledochal cysts	
Congenital biliary atresia	
Cystic fibrosis	

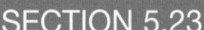

Primary sclerosing cholangitis

Primary sclerosing cholangitis is a chronic cholestatic condition characterized by progressive, inflammatory, sclerosing and obliterative processes of the extrahepatic and intrahepatic biliary system and pancreatic ducts.

Epidemiology

The prevalence of primary sclerosing cholangitis in North America and Europe is up to 10 per 100 000. Unlike primary biliary cirrhosis, it is twice as common in men and has a peak presentation between the ages of 20–40 years.

Pathology

The aetiology is unknown, but the pathogenesis involves an immune-mediated process in genetically predisposed individuals. There is an association with HLA-B8 and -DR4, and the disease process involves the activation of complement in the presence of perinuclear anti-nuclear cytoplasmic antibody (pANCA).

Approximately 75% of patients with primary sclerosing cholangitis suffer with inflammatory bowel disease (especially ulcerative colitis). Conversely, only about 5% of those with ulcerative colitis develop primary sclerosing cholangitis.

Early in the disease, there is enlargement of portal tracts, oedema, and an inflammatory cell infiltrate. Proliferation of the bile ducts occurs and subsequent fibrosis leads to loss of interlobular and septal bile ducts. Histologically, a typical 'onion skin' appearance occurs with fibrous obliterative cholangitis. Later in the disease process, progressive fibrosis and hepatocyte injury leads to loss of bile ducts and liver cirrhosis.

Primary sclerosing cholangitis is usually a diffuse disease, but it can be focal (causing strictures). Therefore, a normal liver biopsy would not exclude this diagnosis.

Scope of disease

The complications associated with primary sclerosing cholangitis relate to the development of biliary strictures, liver cirrhosis and malabsorption of fat-soluble vitamins (Table 5.45).

Clinical features

Primary sclerosing cholangitis presents very similarly to primary biliary cirrhosis. Patients may be asymptomatic early in the disease process and detected on incidental liver profiles. As the disease progresses, pruritus, lethargy, right upper quadrant discomfort and anorexia may occur.

Table 5.45	Complications and diseases associated with primary sclerosing cholangitis
Biliary strictures	
Malabsorption of fat-soluble vitamins (A, D, E, K)	
Recurrent cholangitis	
Biliary calculi formation	
Secondary biliary cirrhosis (SBC)	
Pancreatitis	
Cholangiocarcinoma	
Cirrhosis	
End-stage liver disease	
Portal hypertension	
Associated diseases	
Inflammatory bowel disease	
Colorectal cancer	
Retroperitoneal fibrosis (multifocal sclerosis syndromes)	

Rigors, sweats and jaundice suggest the development of ascending cholangitis. Jaundice is a late presentation. Steatorrhoea can occur from malabsorption, and weight loss may indicate the onset of malignancy (Table 5.45). In addition, there may be features of associated diseases such as ulcerative colitis.

On examination, 50% will have signs of chronic liver disease such as excoriation (pruritus), xanthomas and xanthelasma. Later in the disease process there may be features of decompensated liver disease.

Initial investigations

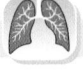

Liver profile
Typically a cholestatic picture develops with elevated alkaline phosphatase and γ-glutamyltransferase. Elevation of bilirubin occurs late in the disease. Albumin decreases late in the disease when cirrhosis develops.

Coagulation screen
The prothrombin time becomes prolonged late in the disease when the synthetic function of the liver is impaired.

Serum immunoglobulins
Serum immunoglobulins are negative (unless there is coexistent autoimmune hepatitis), but it is important to exclude primary biliary cirrhosis as a differential diagnosis.

Serum autoantibodies

The autoantibody profile is non-specific. There may be low but detectable levels of anti-nuclear and anti-smooth muscle antibodies. Serum pANCA is positive in 67%, but the diagnostic value is limited as there is considerable overlap with other conditions, and pANCA may be positive in the absence of primary sclerosing cholangitis.

Tumour markers

The levels of carcinoembryonic antigen (CEA) and α-fetoprotein are screened for colorectal cancer and hepato-cellular carcinoma respectively.

Endoscopic retrograde cholangio-pancreatography/magnetic resonance cholangio-pancreatography

Characteristics of primary sclerosing cholangitis are multiple strictures, beading and irregular sac-like dilatation of the biliary tree, or a localized dominant stricture. Brushings may also be obtained for cytology.

Further investigations
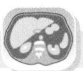

Ultrasound of the liver and biliary system

Regular ultrasound scanning is a useful screening tool for hepatocellular carcinoma. The progressive dilatation of the biliary tree with elevation of serum bilirubin may herald the onset of cholangiocarcinoma.

Liver biopsy

In the absence of dilated ducts, a liver biopsy may show classical features of primary sclerosing cholangitis (or reveal an alternative diagnosis such as cirrhosis).

Colonoscopy

Screening colonoscopy for inflammatory bowel disease is usually performed in patients with primary sclerosing cholangitis as there is a higher risk of colorectal cancers when both diseases coexist. Colon cancers in patients with both diseases tend to be proximal, hence the need for colonoscopy rather than sigmoidoscopy.

Initial management
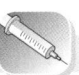

Colestyramine

Colestyramine is a useful agent for pruritus.

Vitamin supplementation

Supplementation of the fat-soluble vitamins is prescribed in patients with cholestasis.

Medical management

Ursodeoxycholic acid

There is no effective treatment for primary sclerosing cholangitis. Ursodeoxycholic acid may lead to improve-ments in the liver profile but has no effect on disease progression or survival. Immunosuppressive drugs have been ineffective.

Endoscopic retrograde cholangio-pancreatography

Although ERCP in patients with primary sclerosing cholangitis carries a higher risk of infective cholangitis, dilatation or stenting can be performed as part of the same procedure for localized/dominant extrahepatic strictures.

Surgical management
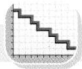

Resection of extrahepatic bile ducts

If endoscopic or percutaneous treatments fail, resection of the extrahepatic bile ducts may be appropriate for non-cirrhotic patients with primary sclerosing cholangitis and dominant extrahepatic biliary strictures.[1] However, surgery has 6% mortality and hilar scarring may complicate future liver transplantation.

Liver transplantation

Liver transplantation is the only effective treatment for primary sclerosing cholangitis.[2,3] The indications are end-stage liver disease and symptomatic portal hypertension, liver failure and recurrent or intractable bacterial cholangitis. Five-year survival rates of 85% have been reported, but recurrence of disease can occur in up to 20% after liver transplantation. Patients with primary sclerosing cholangitis with known cholangiocarcinoma before liver transplantation have a very poor outcome: most die by 5 years. However, the incidental discovery of a microscopic cholangiocarcinoma in the explanted liver does not alter long-term survival.

Prognosis

The median time from diagnosis to transplantation is about 10 years. Asymptomatic patients appear to have a better prognosis. The unpredictability of cholangiocarcinoma makes it difficult to predict the outcome of an individual patient.

REFERENCES

(1) *Ahrendt SA, Pitt HA, Kalloo AN, et al. Primary sclerosing cholangitis: resect, dilate, or transplant? Annals of Surgery 1998; 227: 412–423.*
(2) *Lee YM, Kaplan MM. Management of primary sclerosing cholangitis. American Journal of Gastroenterology 2002; 97: 528–534.*
(3) *Gow PJ, Chapman RW. Liver transplantation for primary sclerosing cholangitis. Liver 2000; 20: 97–103.*

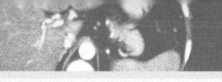

SECTION 5.24 Tumours of the biliary system

Cholangiocarcinoma

Cholangiocarcinomas are carcinomas of the intra- or extrahepatic bile ducts.

Epidemiology

Cholangiocarcinomas are rare with an incidence of 1.2 per 100 000 per year. Both sexes are equally affected.

Pathology

The risk factors for the development of cholangiocarcinomas are listed in Table 5.46, but molecular mechanisms of aetiology and pathogenesis are unknown. Approximately 50% of tumours occur at the confluence of the right and left hepatic ducts (Klatskin tumours, Fig 5.32), 25% are intrahepatic and 25% are distal extrahepatic. Adenocarcinoma is the predominant histological subtype (95%).

Clinical features

Klatskin and extrahepatic tumours commonly present with obstructive jaundice, but by this stage the disease is advanced. Intrahepatic cholangiocarcinomas and cancers obstructing an intrahepatic duct present late with malaise and weight loss. Biliary obstruction may also lead to cholangitis.

Investigations

Liver profile

There is usually an obstructive pattern. The prothrombin time may be increased if obstruction has been prolonged.

Table 5.46	Risk factors for cholangiocarcinoma
Primary sclerosing cholangitis (lifetime risk 5–15%)	
Increasing age	
Chronic ductal gallstones	
Liver fluke infection (*Opisthorchis viverrini, Clonorchis sinensis*)	
Bile duct adenomas and biliary papillomatosis	
Caroli's disease (congenital dilatation of intrahepatic bile ducts)	
Chronic typhoid carriers	
Choledochal cysts	
Chemical carcinogens	

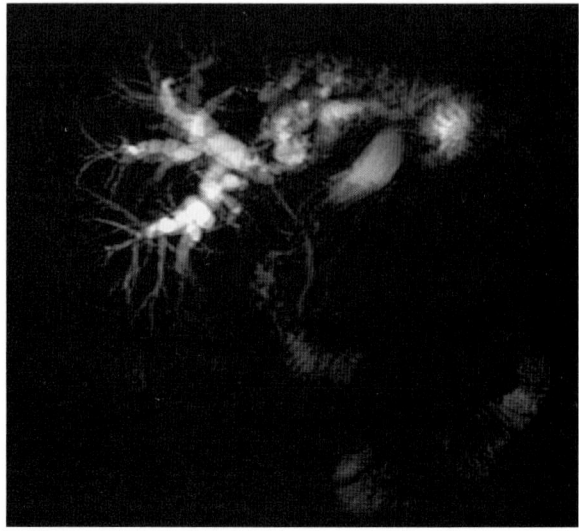

Fig. 5.32 MRCP of cholangiocarcinoma. Right and left hepatic ducts and intrahepatic ducts are dilated due to a cholangiocarcinoma at the confluence (Klatskin tumour). Courtesy of Dr M. Bennie, Norfolk and Norwich University Hospital, UK.

Tumour markers

Tumour markers such as CA19-9, CEA and CA-125 are elevated but are non-specific for cholangiocarcinoma.

Staging investigations

Ultrasound is the radiological first-line investigation of choice, with combined MRI/MRCP being the gold standard investigation for assessment of resectability. ERCP allows biopsy/cytology and stent insertion if there is evidence of acute cholangitis. In distal tumours, endoscopic ultrasound (EUS) may sometimes be useful. Clinical examination, CT/MRI and laparoscopy are performed for staging (Table 5.47).

Management

Surgical resection

Surgical resection is the only curative treatment but is rarely appropriate as patients usually present with metastases.

Relief of biliary obstruction and prevention of cholangitis is paramount. Intrahepatic disease requires liver resection (see p. 342). Klatskin tumours are treated with resection of the extrahepatic bile ducts and gallbladder with regional lymphadenectomy and hepaticojejunostomy to allow bile

Table 5.47	Simplified UICC/AJCC staging system for intra- and extrahepatic cholangiocarcinoma
Stage	**Description**
Stage 0	Carcinoma in situ
Stage I	Tumour invasion limited to the mucosa, muscle layer or ampulla
Stage II	Local invasion
Stage III	Stage I or II + metastases to regional lymph nodes
Stage IV	Extensive invasion of the liver, or invasion of adjacent organs, or distant metastases

NB: different staging systems exist for intra- and extrahepatic cholangiocarcinomas, therefore a simplified version is presented.

drainage. Hemi-hepatectomy may also be required. Distal cholangiocarcinoma can be removed with Whipple's operation (see p. 390).

Palliative management
Biliary stenting via ERCP or PTC to relieve jaundice should be considered for patients with inoperable disease and may be combined with photodynamic therapy. Palliative care teams should be involved at an early stage. Chemotherapy and radiotherapy may improve quality of life but have little survival benefit.

Prognosis

The 3-year survival for patients having curative surgery is 40%, and more than 95% of patients with inoperable disease are dead by 5 years.

 FURTHER INFORMATION

Khan SA, Davidson BR, Goldin R, et al. Guidelines for the diagnosis and treatment of cholangiocarcinoma: consensus document. Gut 2002; 51 Suppl 6: VI1–9.

Gallbladder carcinoma

Epidemiology

Carcinoma of the gallbladder is the most common malignancy of the biliary tract. The incidence is highly dependent on geography, varying from 2.5 per 100 000 in the USA to 10.1 per 100 000 in females in northern India. It afflicts women twice as often as men and its incidence increases with age.

Pathology

The precise aetiology and pathogenesis are unknown, although a number of factors associated with gallbladder carcinoma have been identified (Table 5.48). Up to 70% of patients with gallbladder cancer have gallstones, although only 1% of patients with gallbladder stones develop gallbladder cancer. Adenocarcinoma is the histological subtype in 95%. Direct invasion into the liver, duodenum or colon is the most common mode of spread.

Clinical features

Symptoms of early gallbladder carcinoma such as right upper quadrant pain and vomiting are easily mistaken for benign biliary tract disease. Gallbladder carcinoma is discovered incidentally during cholecystectomy or postoperatively by the pathologist in 20% of cases. Most patients present late with jaundice, weight loss and complications such as fistula or invasion of nearby organs. Late signs include a palpable gallbladder mass, hard nodular liver and malignant ascites.

Investigations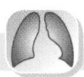

Liver profile
Serum bilirubin and alkaline phosphatase may be elevated if the biliary tract is obstructed.

Tumour markers
CEA and CA19-9 tumour markers may also be elevated.

Ultrasound of the abdomen
On ultrasound, gallbladder carcinoma appears as a thickened gallbladder with a fixed polypoidal mass. It may be difficult to distinguish between carcinoma and acute cholecystitis.

Staging CT
CT is used for staging the disease and to define the best treatment option.

Table 5.48	Risk factors for gallbladder carcinoma
Increasing age
Gallbladder stones
Calcification of the gallbladder ('porcelain gallbladder')
Large (>10 mm) gallbladder polyps
Abnormal junction of the pancreatic and biliary ducts
Chemical carcinogens
Chronic typhoid carrier

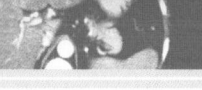

Simplified UICC/AJCC 2002 TNM classification and staging of gallbladder carcinoma

Primary tumour

Tis   Carcinoma in situ

T1   Invasion of lamina propria or muscle layer

T2   Invasion of perimuscular connective tissue, no extension beyond serosa or into liver

T3   Tumour perforates serosa or invades liver and/or one adjacent organ

T4   Invasion of portal vein or hepatic artery, or two or more extrahepatic organs

Regional lymph nodes

N0   No regional lymph node metastasis

N1   Regional lymph node metastasis

Distant metastasis

M0   No distant metastasis

M1   Distant metastasis

Stage grouping

Stage 0	Tis N0 M0
Stage IA	T1 N0 M0
Stage IB	T2 N0 M0
Stage IIA	T3 N0 M0
Stage IIB	T1, 2, or 3 N1 M0
Stage III	T4 Any N M0
Stage IV	Any T Any N M1

Management

Cholecystectomy

Surgery is the only potentially curative treatment, as radiotherapy and chemotherapy are not beneficial. Unfortunately, 75% of patients have inoperable disease. Cholecystectomy alone is sufficient for stages 0 and IA carcinoma. Radical cholecystectomy (removal of the gallbladder, gallbladder bed and draining lymphatics) should be considered in patients with stages IB and II disease. Other stages are considered inoperable.

Stenting and surgical bypass

Unresectable cancers that are obstructing the biliary system may require biliary stenting via ERCP or surgical bypass.

Prognosis

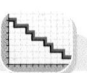

Overall 5-year survival is approximately 10%.

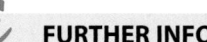

ℹ FURTHER INFORMATION

Misra S, Chaturvedi A, Misra NC, Sharma ID. Carcinoma of the gallbladder. Lancet Oncology 2003; 4: 167–176.

Diseases of the pancreas

SECTION 5.25   Introduction

Applied basic sciences of the exocrine pancreas

Anatomy

The pancreas is a retroperitoneal organ that lies at the level of the first and second lumbar vertebrae. It is subdivided into the head, neck and body on the basis of its relations to the superior mesenteric and portal veins (Fig. 5.33). The head lies lateral to the veins and lies in the C-shaped concavity of the second part of the duodenum, with the inferior vena cava behind it. The lowest part of the head continues medially and comes to lie posterior to the superior mesenteric vein and artery. This is the uncinate process of the head. The neck is defined as that portion of the pancreas directly anterior to the superior mesenteric and portal veins. To the left of the neck is the body, continuing laterally and slightly superiorly, and finishing adjacent to the spleen as the pancreatic tail.

The pancreas develops from ventral and dorsal buds lying opposite each other at the junction of the foregut and midgut. After rotation of the duodenum, the openings of the two buds lie beside each other and the two parts fuse to become a single organ (Fig. 5.34). The duct systems of

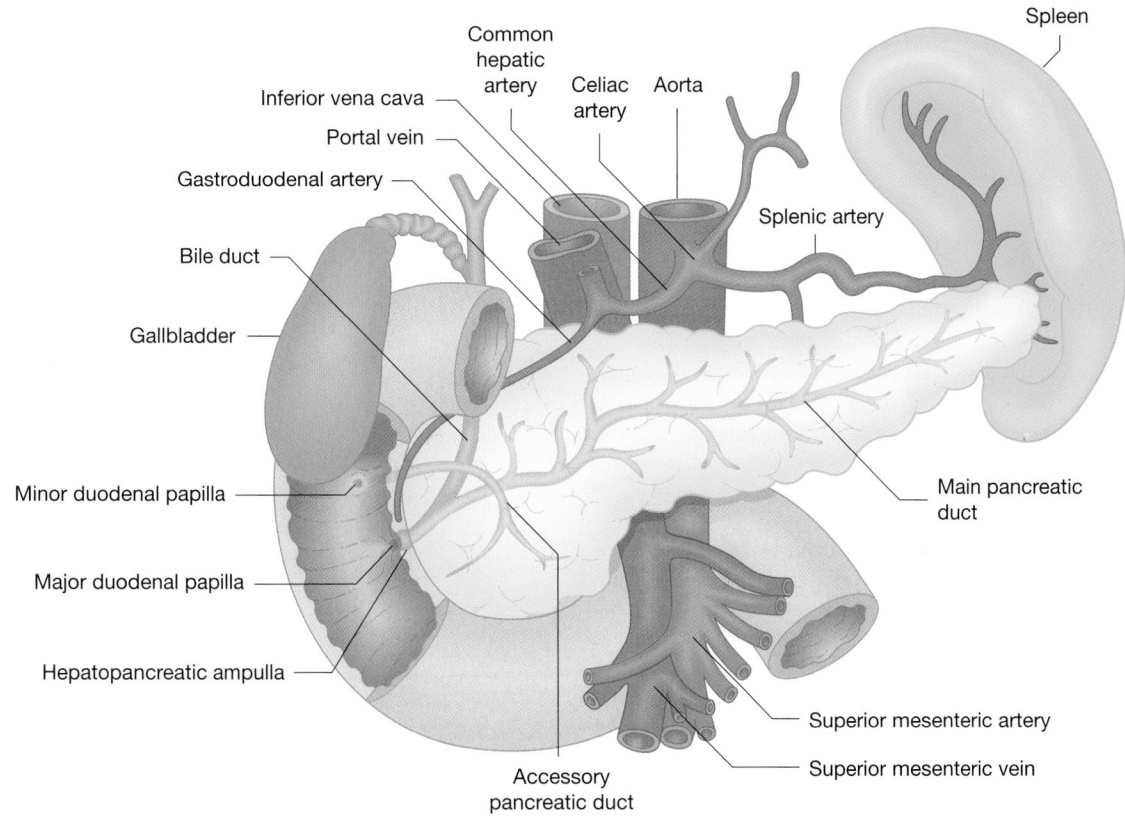

Fig. 5.33 Anatomy of the pancreas.

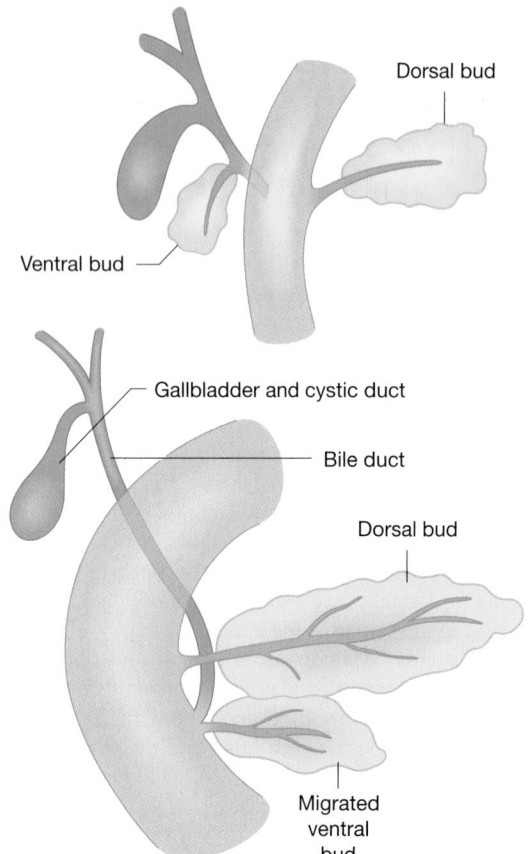

Fig. 5.34 Development of the pancreas. The ventral bud migrates dorsally and comes to lie inferior to the dorsal bud. The two systems fuse, and the main pancreatic duct is formed by the ventral bud and the distal part of the dorsal bud. The proximal part of the dorsal bud becomes the accessory pancreatic duct.

As expected from its development, the pancreas is supplied by branches of the arteries of the foregut (coeliac trunk) and midgut (superior mesenteric artery). From the coeliac trunk, the splenic artery supplies the neck, body and tail. The head is supplied by branches of the gastroduodenal artery (the superior pancreaticoduodenal artery) and superior mesenteric artery (the inferior pancreaticoduodenal artery). Venous return is via the splenic vein, superior pancreaticoduodenal vein and inferior pancreaticoduodenal vein. All drain eventually into the portal vein.

Pancreatic lymphatics follow the supplying arteries to terminate in the coeliac group and superior mesenteric group of aortic lymph nodes. The pancreatic nerve supply is from the autonomic nervous system. Parasympathetic nerves originate from the vagus (cranial nerve X) and stimulate exocrine secretion. Sympathetic vasoconstrictor nerves derive from splanchnic nerves from spinal cord segments T6–10. Afferent pain fibres accompany the efferent sympathetic supply, so that pancreatic pain may be referred to T6–10 dermatomes.

Physiology

The pancreas is a combined exocrine and endocrine organ; only the exocrine pancreas will be considered here. Pancreatic fluid is composed of enzymes and an alkaline aqueous component (Table 5.49).

Histologically, the exocrine pancreas is made up of clusters of microscopic spherical acini draining into ducts lined by columnar cells (Fig. 5.36). Systems of ducts eventually join to form the main pancreatic duct. Water and electrolytes are secreted by the ductal columnar cells, while enzymes come from the acinar cells.

The enzymes secreted by the acinar cells are important for digestion of all the major food classes (Table 5.50). To

the two buds join to form the main pancreatic duct of Wirsung, although the dorsal bud duct can persist as the accessory pancreatic duct of Santorini. The main pancreatic duct joins the common bile duct to become the hepatopancreatic ampulla (ampulla of Vater). The ampulla opens into the second part of the duodenum at the major duodenal papilla; the accessory pancreatic duct ends at the minor duodenal papilla. Surrounding the ampulla and the ends of the common bile duct and main pancreatic duct are sphincters, together known as the ampullary sphincter of Oddi (Fig. 5.35).

Pancreas divisum and annular pancreas are examples of abnormal pancreatic development that can cause acute pancreatitis. Pancreas divisum describes the abnormal fusion of the dorsal and ventral pancreatic ducts, so that the dorsal pancreas drains entirely via the duct of Santorini. It is seen in 5% of ERCP examinations. Stenosis of the accessory papilla may lead to acute pancreatitis. Annular pancreas is much rarer (1 in 7000) and occurs when the second part of the duodenum is encircled by pancreatic tissue. It is associated with acute pancreatitis and neonatal duodenal obstruction.

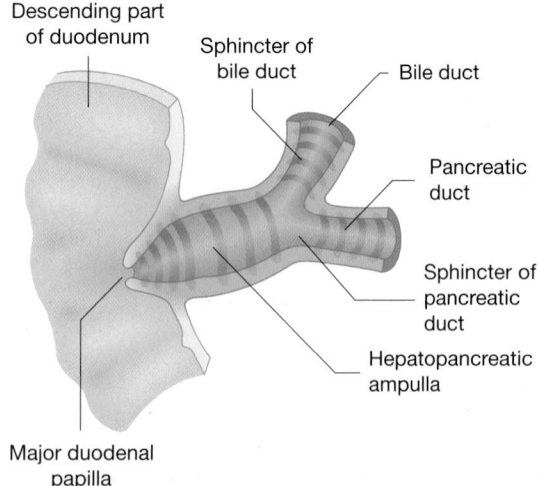

Fig. 5.35 Anatomy of the hepatopancreatic ampulla. The sphincters surrounding the hepatopancreatic ampulla, distal common bile duct and distal main pancreatic duct are collectively known as the sphincter of Oddi.

Table 5.49	Components of pancreatic fluid compared to plasma						
	Volume	Osmolality (mosmol/kg H_2O)	pH	Na^+ (mmol/L)	K^+ (mmol/L)	Cl^- (mmol/L)	HCO_3^- (mmol/L)
Plasma	3000 mL total	285	7.4	140	5	110	24
Pancreatic juice	1500 mL/day	285	7.8*	140	8	85*	60*

* Values vary significantly depending on flow rate.

Applied basic sciences of the exocrine pancreas

Table 5.50	Pancreatic enzymes		
Inactive proenzyme secreted by the pancreas	Enzyme	Activator	Enzyme function/substrate
Trypsinogen	Trypsin	Enterokinase, trypsin	Activation of other pancreatic proenzymes/ protein and polypeptides
Chymotrypsinogen	Chymotrypsin	Trypsin	Protein and polypeptides
Procarboxypeptidase	Carboxypeptidase	Trypsin	Protein and polypeptides
Proelastase	Elastase	Trypsin	Elastin
Not applicable	Amylase	Chloride	Starch, glycogen
Not applicable	Lipase	Emulsifying agents	Triglycerides
Prophospholipase A	Phospholipase A	Bile salts, trypsin	Lecithin

prevent pancreatic autodigestion, most enzymes are secreted as inactive proenzymes. These are stored in zymogen granules within the acinar cell. Proenzymes are activated upon reaching the duodenum when trypsin is generated from the action of enterokinase on trypsinogen. Enterokinase is found on intestinal epithelial cells.

The ionic concentration of the aqueous component of pancreatic juice varies with the rate of secretion. At high rates, bicarbonate concentration increases and chloride concentration decreases. This alkaline fluid neutralizes the acid chyme from the stomach and produces a favourable pH for pancreatic enzyme function.

Pancreatic secretions are under hormonal and neural control, and occur in three phases. Hormonal control is dominant. The sight and smell of food (the cephalic phase) is enough to stimulate pancreatic secretion via vagal stimulation. When food enters the stomach (the gastric phase) the hormone gastrin, released from the gastric antrum in response to distension, enhances secretion. During the intestinal phase, acid-rich chyme enters the duodenum and jejunum from the stomach. The presence of acid causes secretin to be released from the duodenal and jejunal mucosa, leading to stimulation of the pancreatic ductal epithelium and secretion of the fluid component of pancreatic juice. Peptides, amino acids and fatty acids in the upper small intestine elicit secretion of cholecystokinin (CCK) from intestinal cells. CCK stimulates the release of proenzymes from the pancreatic acinar cells. Exocrine secretion is inhibited by the sympathetic nervous system, glucagon and somatostatin.

Pancreatic trauma or surgery may lead to development of a fistula between the pancreatic duct and the skin. Daily losses of 1–2 litres of alkaline isotonic fluid can lead to metabolic acidosis and dehydration. Uncomplicated pancreatic fistulas will not cause skin digestion as the proenzymes remain inactivated. If infection occurs, trypsinogen can be activated and skin digestion results. Somatostatin analogues such as octreotide have been used to treat pancreatic fistulas in an attempt to reduce pancreatic secretion and allow the fistulae to heal.

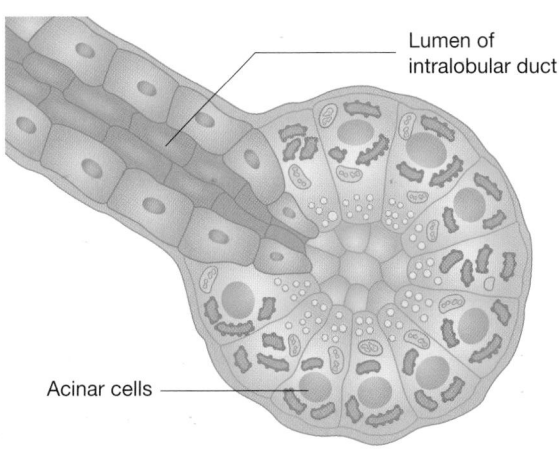

Lumen of intralobular duct

Acinar cells

Fig. 5.36 Histology of the exocrine pancreas.

SECTION 5.26 — Investigations for pancreatic disease

Blood tests

Serum amylase

Serum amylase is the most frequently used test for the diagnosis of acute pancreatitis. The normal range varies between laboratories but is usually 110–300 i.u./L. Amylase is a digestive enzyme that cleaves starch into smaller carbohydrates and is found predominantly in the pancreas and salivary glands. However, serum amylase can be elevated in a number of other conditions, reducing its specificity for the diagnosis of acute pancreatitis (Table 5.51).

Because amylase is a small molecule, it passes through the glomerulus and is detectable in the urine. Immuno-globulins may bind to amylase, preventing renal filtration and causing elevated serum amylase levels (macroamy-lasaemia). Low levels of urinary amylase differentiate this from true hyperamylasaemia.

Table 5.51	Sources and causes of elevated serum amylase
Source of amylase	**Condition associated with elevated amylase**
Pancreas	Acute and chronic pancreatitis Complications of acute pancreatitis (e.g. pseudocyst) Trauma (including surgery and ERCP) Pancreatic carcinoma
Salivary glands	Infection (e.g. mumps) Trauma (including surgery) Ductal obstruction
Gastrointestinal tract	Perforated peptic ulcer Bowel obstruction/perforation Acute bowel ischaemia Appendicitis Peritonitis
Liver	Hepatitis Cirrhosis
Gynaecological organs	Ruptured ectopic pregnancy Pelvic inflammatory disease
Miscellaneous	Ruptured abdominal aortic aneurysm Renal failure Macroamylasaemia Idiopathic, familial and non-familial Drug induced (e.g. azathioprine, furosemide) Cerebral trauma Anorexia nervosa

ERCP, endoscopic retrograde cholangio-pancreatography.

Serum lipase

Serum lipase is another useful test for acute pancreatitis. Lipases are mainly found in the pancreas but are also in the stomach and intestine. Although the lipase assay measures pancreatic lipase, false positives can still occur from non-pancreatic disease (Table 5.52). Lipase is reabsorbed in the proximal tubules and has a longer half-life than amylase.

Agreement is lacking on diagnostic thresholds for serum amylase and lipase, resulting in wide variability in quoted sensitivities and specificities for the diagnosis of acute pancreatitis. Lipase is equally sensitive but more specific than amylase (Table 5.53). As the test for lipase becomes increasingly available it may replace serum amylase as the preferred diagnostic blood test for acute pancreatitis. Neither serum amylase nor lipase has any prognostic value or correlation with the severity of pancreatitis.

Tumour markers

Carbohydrate antigen (CA) 19-9 is the most widely utilized tumour marker for pancreatic adenocarcinoma, with sensitivity and specificity of approximately 80% and 90%, respectively. Serum CA19-9 may also be raised in patients with cholangiocarcinoma, and occasionally in those with benign obstructive jaundice. Like tumour markers for other cancers, CA19-9 is not sensitive or specific enough to be used as a screening test, and is therefore used along with radiological and endoscopic investigations in a patient suspected of obstructive jaundice due to malignancy.

Diagnostic imaging

Plain abdominal film

Plain abdominal radiography is unremarkable in the majority of cases of acute pancreatitis. When radiographic abnor-

Table 5.52	Sources and causes of elevated serum lipase
Source of lipase	**Condition associated with elevated lipase**
Pancreas	Acute and chronic pancreatitis Trauma (including surgery and ERCP) Pancreatic carcinoma
Gastrointestinal tract	Perforated peptic ulcer Bowel obstruction or infarction Acute cholecystitis
Miscellaneous	Diabetic ketoacidosis Idiopathic

ERCP, endoscopic retrograde cholangio-pancreatography.

Table 5.53	Comparison of serum amylase with lipase in acute pancreatitis (AP)	
	Amylase	**Lipase**
Advantages	Widely available Easy to measure	Higher specificity Levels high in all causes of AP Long half-life (7–12 h), can be used in delayed presentation
Disadvantages	Lower specificity Levels lower in alcoholic AP and AP due to hyperlipidaemia Levels rapidly decrease due to short half-life (2 h)	Less widely available More difficult to measure
Time-course of rise	Rise within 6–24 h Peak at 48 h Normalize over 5–7 days	Rise within 4–8 h Peak at 24 h Normalize over 8–14 days

malities are present, they are relatively non-specific and may be subtle. These include a 'sentinel loop' (localized ileus of the duodenum), generalized gastrointestinal ileus, or isolated ileus of the transverse colon. In contrast, the presence of pancreatic calcification on plain radiography is highly suggestive of chronic pancreatitis. Plain radiography is of little use in the detection of pancreatic carcinoma.

Abdominal ultrasound

Transabdominal ultrasonography is a useful initial modality to investigate pancreatic disorders due to its relatively low cost, portability, non-invasiveness and lack of harmful ionizing radiation. Excellent definition of the pancreas, bile duct and surrounding blood vessels can be achieved by a skilful operator with an advanced machine. Unfortunately, patient obesity and the presence of overlying intestinal gas (common in acute pancreatitis due to ileus) can make visualizing the pancreas difficult.

Ultrasonography should be performed in all patients with suspected acute pancreatitis to detect biliary dilatation, gallstones and/or diagnostic pancreatic changes (pancreatic oedema and inflammation). It is the initial investigation of choice for the diagnosis and monitoring of pancreatic pseudocysts, which appear as echo-free smooth, round lesions. Ultrasonography in patients suspected of chronic pancreatitis may detect pancreatic calcification not visualized on plain radiography and may identify pancreatic duct dilatation. Pancreatic adenocarcinomas less than 1.0 cm in diameter are difficult to detect with ultrasound. Combining ultrasound with colour Doppler (colour duplex) allows visualization of vascular complications of acute pancreatitis (e.g. splenic artery pseudoaneurysm) and can be used to assess vascular infiltration in pancreatic malignancy.

Computed tomography (CT) of the abdomen

Spiral CT is presently the dominant radiological modality for visualizing the pancreatic parenchyma (Fig. 5.37). Spiral CT allows rapid image acquisition during a single patient breath-hold and thus substantially removes movement artefact. Intravenous contrast injection allows visualization of the pancreas in both arterial and portal venous phases (dual-phase). Acute pancreatitis appears as an enlarged, oedematous pancreas with peripancreatic fat stranding indicating inflammation. Peripancreatic effusions or free intraperitoneal fluid are commonly seen. Lack of enhancement of pancreatic tissue by contrast indicates pancreatic necrosis. Contrast-enhanced CT should be performed in patients with severe acute pancreatitis to confirm the diagnosis, detect pancreatic necrosis and other complications, and provide prognostic information.[1] CT scanning is more sensitive than plain radiography for the detection of pancreatic calcification and can identify pancreatic duct dilatation, parenchymal atrophy and pseudocysts. Dual-phase spiral CT is presently the preferred test for staging pancreatic tumours and determining resectability. Despite advances in technology, distinguishing between an inflammatory mass associated with chronic pancreatitis and pancreatic adenocarcinoma may still be difficult.

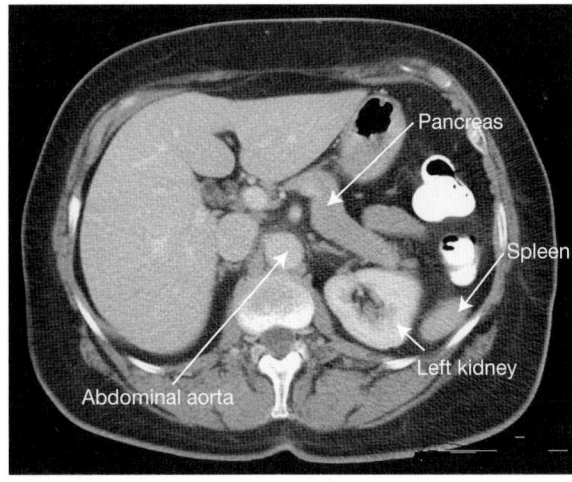

Fig. 5.37 CT of normal pancreas.
Courtesy of Dr M. Bennie, Norfolk and Norwich University Hospital, UK.

377

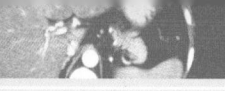

Magnetic resonance imaging (MRI) of the abdomen

MRI of pancreatic parenchyma appears to be as sensitive and specific as CT for the detection of pancreatic cancer. Gadolinium can be used as an intravenous contrast medium to allow detection of vascular invasion (magnetic resonance angiography—MRA).

Magnetic resonance cholangio-pancreatography

Stationary fluids such as bile and pancreatic juice have high signal intensity on T2-weighted MRI (magnetic resonance cholangio-pancreatography—MRCP). This enables non-invasive visualization of biliary and pancreatic ducts without the use of ionizing radiation. MRCP is therefore safer than ERCP. In the future, it is expected that MRCP combined with abdominal MRI and MRA, in a single examination, will replace other means of diagnosing and staging pancreatic carcinoma. MRCP alone does not allow cancer staging as only the ducts are imaged. MRCP has similar sensitivity and specificity to ERCP for the diagnosis of pancreatic carcinoma (84% sensitivity, 97% specificity for MRCP versus 70% and 94% for ERCP).[2] The role of MRCP/ MRI in acute and chronic pancreatitis is not yet determined.

Angiography

Conventional angiography is slowly being replaced by duplex ultrasound and dual-phase spiral CT for the diagnosis of major vascular involvement by pancreatic carcinoma. Angiography remains useful for allowing catheter embolization of bleeding pseudocysts and is probably the most sensitive technique for detecting insulinomas, which have a characteristic vascular blush (Fig. 5.38). Some units use it routinely prior to resection of a pancreatic carcinoma to enable detection of vascular anomalies (e.g. replaced or accessory right hepatic artery).

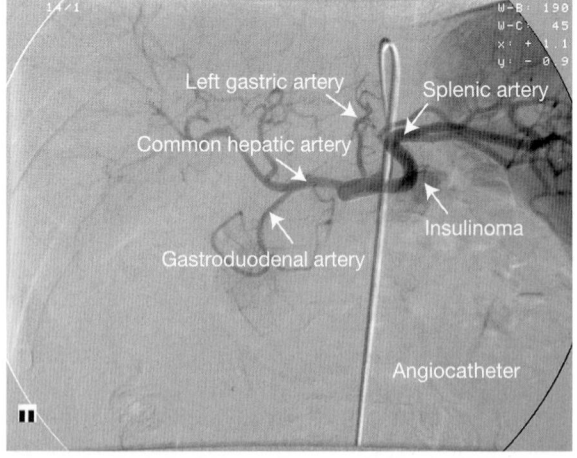

Fig. 5.38 A digital subtraction angiogram (DSA) of the coeliac trunk. The three branches of the coeliac trunk are seen (common hepatic artery, left gastric artery and splenic artery), as is the vascular blush of an insulinoma.
Copyright Addenbrooke's Hospital, Cambridge, UK.

Positron emission tomography (PET) scan

Increased uptake of fluorine-18-labelled fluorodeoxy-glucose (^{18}FDG) occurs in malignancies due to increased metabolism of glucose. This is the basis of the use of ^{18}FDG positron emission tomography (^{18}FDG-PET) in the diagnosis of pancreatic adenocarcinoma. Although the technique is highly sensitive (>90%) for the diagnosis of pancreatic malignancy,[3] generation of ^{18}FDG requires a cyclotron nearby. This technique is therefore limited by the very expensive and highly sophisticated technology required.

Percutaneous pancreatic biopsy

Percutaneous biopsy of the pancreas is reserved for patients with unresectable tumour masses in order to confirm the diagnosis and allow aggressive chemotherapy or radiotherapy if appropriate. Tissue diagnosis before surgery is not required in those with resectable masses as the best form of biopsy is surgical resection. Also, the probability of cancer is high if imaging suggests malignancy in the appropriate clinical setting. Percutaneous biopsy can be performed under CT or ultrasound guidance. Biopsy during endoscopic ultrasound is increasingly performed. Cytology brushings may be obtained from ERCP, but this results in low numbers of cells with a high false negative rate. Patients unexpectedly found to have unresectable pancreatic lesions at laparotomy should have frozen sections taken from the tumour mass, involved lymph node or secondary deposit. Confirmatory results should be awaited before proceeding to a palliative bypass or closing the abdomen.

Endoscopy

Endoscopic ultrasound (EUS)

Attachment of a small ultrasound probe to an endoscope enables close ultrasonographic examination of the pancreas through the duodenum and stomach. EUS is able to detect adenocarcinomas that are too small to be seen on CT or transabdominal ultrasound (<1 cm). Also, it can facilitate guided fine-needle aspiration cytology of suspected cancers or aspiration of cysts (e.g. pancreatic pseudocysts). Some disadvantages of EUS are that it cannot reliably detect liver metastases, it is difficult to perform and interpret, and requires expensive equipment.

The role of EUS in the investigation of the pancreas has not yet been clearly defined, but its high resolution, coupled with the ability to perform interventional procedures, means that its use is likely to expand.

Endoscopic retrograde cholangio-pancreatography (ERCP)

The use of ERCP as a diagnostic procedure for pancreatic disease is detailed on page 306.

Pancreatic function tests

Pancreatic function tests are reserved for those patients suspected of chronic pancreatitis where radiological investigations fail to make a diagnosis. Tests of exocrine function can be invasive or non-invasive (Table 5.54). The secretin–CCK stimulation test is considered to be the gold standard due to its ability to detect early disease. Intubation of the duodenum is required, making it uncomfortable for the patient and complex to perform. Its availability is therefore limited.

Non-invasive pancreatic function tests are relatively insensitive at diagnosing early or mild chronic pancreatitis due to the large functional reserve of the pancreas. Tests of the endocrine pancreas to assist in the diagnosis of chronic pancreatitis include fasting blood glucose and the oral glucose tolerance test.

FURTHER INFORMATION

Yadav D, Agarwal N, Pitchumoni CS. A critical evaluation of laboratory tests in acute pancreatitis. American Journal of Gastroenterology 2002; 97: 1309–1318.

Chowdhury RS, Forsmark CE. Review article: Pancreatic function testing. Alimentary Pharmacology and Therapeutics 2003; 17: 733–750.

REFERENCES

(1) *Balthazar EJ, Ranson JH, Naidich DP, Megibow AJ, Caccavale R, Cooper MM. Acute pancreatitis: prognostic value of CT. Radiology 1985; 156: 767–772.*
(2) *Adamek HE, Albert J, Breer H, Weitz M, Schilling D, Riemann JF. Pancreatic cancer detection with magnetic resonance cholangiopancreatography and endoscopic retrograde cholangiopancreatography: a prospective controlled study. Lancet 2000; 356: 190–193.*
(3) *Rose DM, Delbeke D, Beauchamp RD, et al. 18Fluorodeoxyglucose-positron emission tomography in the management of patients with suspected pancreatic cancer. Annals of Surgery 1999; 229: 729–737; discussion 737–738.*

Table 5.54   **Pancreatic exocrine function tests**

Test	Principle and comments
Invasive	
Secretin–cholecystokinin (CCK) test	Intravenous administration of secretin with or without CCK leads to the stimulation of pancreatic secretion. Aspiration of duodenal juice from a duodenal tube allows measurement of the bicarbonate and/or enzymes produced, depending on the hormone infused. Gold standard, but complex and invasive
Non-invasive	
PABA (bentiromide) test	Orally administered synthetic peptide* cleaved by chymotrypsin to Bz-Ty and PABA. PABA is absorbed into the blood stream and excreted in the urine. Blood and urinary PABA can be measured. Simple, but poor sensitivity in early disease
Faecal fat	A diet of 100 g of fat per day is administered for 2 days before and for 3 days during stool collection. More than 7 g/day of faecal fat is considered to be abnormal. Unpleasant for patient and laboratory staff. Insensitive in early disease
Faecal chymotrypsin or elastase	Proteolytic enzymes excreted by the pancreas measured in stool. Reduced levels found in late chronic pancreatitis. Simple. Faecal elastase more sensitive than faecal chymotrypsin, but neither is useful in early disease
$^{13}C/^{14}C$ breath tests	Various ^{13}C- or ^{14}C-labelled substrates have been developed that can be taken orally. Digestion by pancreatic enzymes leads to absorption of ^{13} or ^{14}C and excretion as ^{13} or $^{14}CO_2$
Pancreolauryl test	Orally taken fluorescein dilaurate is hydrolyzed by pancreatic elastase and absorbed. Fluorescein is measured in the urine or serum

*N-benzoyl-L-tyrosyl-p-aminobenzoic acid (Bz-Ty-PABA).

SECTION 5.27   # Pancreatitis

Acute pancreatitis

Acute pancreatitis is an inflammatory process of the pancreas secondary to enzymatic autodigestion. There is variable involvement of other regional tissues or remote organ systems. The Atlanta definition and other terms that relate to pancreatitis are listed in Table 5.55.

Epidemiology

The incidence of acute pancreatitis is 30 cases per 100 000 per year but depends on the local prevalence of gallstones and alcohol abuse.[1] It is equally common in both sexes.

Table 5.55	Atlanta definitions of selected terms relating to acute pancreatitis*
Term	**Definition**
Acute pancreatitis	An acute inflammatory process of the pancreas, with variable involvement of other regional tissues or remote organ systems
Mild acute pancreatitis	Associated with minimal organ dysfunction and an uneventful recovery. The predominant pathological feature is interstitial oedema of the gland
Severe acute pancreatitis	Associated with organ failure and/or local complications such as necrosis (with infection), pseudocyst or abscess. Most often this is an expression of the development of pancreatic necrosis, although patients with oedematous pancreatitis may manifest clinical features of a severe attack
Acute fluid collections	These occur early in the course of acute pancreatitis, are located in or near the pancreas, and always lack a wall of granulation or fibrous tissue. May develop into a pseudocyst
Pseudocyst ('pseudo' because it lacks the epithelial wall of a true cyst)	A collection of pancreatic juice enclosed in a wall of fibrous or granulation tissue that arises following an attack of acute pancreatitis. Formation requires 4 or more weeks from the onset of acute pancreatitis
Pancreatic necrosis and infected necrosis	A diffuse or focal area(s) of non-viable pancreatic parenchyma, which is typically associated with peripancreatic fat necrosis

* Adapted from Bradley EL III. A clinically based classification system for acute pancreatitis. Summary of the International Symposium on Acute Pancreatitis, Atlanta, Ga, September 11 through 13, 1992. Archives of Surgery 1993; 128: 586–590.

Pathology

Premature activation of trypsin within zymogen granules in pancreatic acinar cells is thought to be the essential event in the pathogenesis of acute pancreatitis. Release of proteolytic and lipolytic enzymes causes pancreatic auto-digestion and results in a systemic inflammatory cascade. Although the risk factors are well documented (Table 5.56), the mechanisms that stimulate the initial enzyme activation are unknown.

Scope of disease

Approximately 80% of patients with acute pancreatitis have mild disease, and 20% have severe disease. In severe attacks, shock and multi-organ failure can occur (Table 5.57). Local and systemic inflammation leads to significant fluid losses. Severe pancreatic inflammation leads to pancreatic necrosis and secondary infection from gut bacteria can lead to infected necrosis, trebling the risk of death.

Persistent pancreatic juice secretion and inflammation in the lesser sac can lead to pseudocyst formation (Fig. 5.39). Symptomatic pseudocysts can be drained endoscopically, percutaneously or surgically.

Clinical features

Patients commonly complain of continuous, poorly local-ized, upper abdominal pain that develops over hours and radiates to the back. It is often associated with vomiting. Bending forward may ease the pain. A history of risk factors such as gallstones, drug ingestion and recent heavy alcohol intake is important.

On examination, patients can have marked upper abdominal tenderness, but signs of peritonitis are absent in mild disease. Bruising of the flanks (Grey Turner's sign) or umbilicus (Cullen's sign) is rare.

Initial investigations

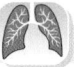

Initial investigations assist in the diagnosis, quantify the severity of disease and predict the risk of mortality. Full blood count, urea and electrolytes, serum calcium, serum glucose, liver function tests, serum lactate dehydrogenase (LDH) and an arterial blood gas sample should all be taken to allow risk scoring (Table 5.58). Other scoring systems include the Ranson score and APACHE II score.

Full blood count
A leukocytosis is usually present.

Urea and electrolytes
Electrolyte abnormalities arise from dehydration and systemic inflammation.

Serum calcium
Calcium combines with fatty acids released by the action of lipases on fat, leading to hypocalcaemia in patients with severe disease.

Liver profile
The liver profile is usually normal but elevated serum bilirubin is associated with gallstone pancreatitis.

Arterial blood gases
Hypoxaemia can result from atelectasis, or acute respira-tory distress syndrome with severe pancreatitis.

Table 5.56	Causes of acute pancreatitis and their frequency[a]

Obstruction of the pancreatic duct or papilla

Gallstones (45%)[b]

Pancreatic or ampullary tumours

Foreign bodies

Worms (*Ascaris lumbricoides*)

Pancreas divisum with obstruction of the duct of Santorini

Sphincter of Oddi hypertension (basal sphincter pressure >40 mmHg)

Toxins

Ethanol (35%)[b]

Methanol

Scorpion venom

Drugs

Azathioprine

Angiotensin-converting enzyme inhibitors

Sodium valproate

Oestrogens

Thiazide diuretics

Furosemide

Corticosteroids

Ranitidine

Paracetamol (acetaminophen)

Trauma

Blunt abdominal trauma (e.g. seatbelt injury in road traffic accident)

Iatrogenic trauma
    ERCP (5%)[b]
    Surgery

Metabolic abnormalities

Hypertriglyceridaemia

Hypercalcaemia

Infection

Viral (e.g. mumps, rubella, Coxsackie virus, cytomegalovirus, HIV, Epstein–Barr virus)

Parasitic (e.g. ascariasis, clonorchiasis)

Bacterial (e.g. *Mycoplasma, Campylobacter jejuni*)

Ischaemia

Hypotension (e.g. cardiopulmonary bypass during cardiac surgery)

Vasculitis (e.g. polyarteritis nodosa)

Miscellaneous

Hypothermia

Pregnancy

Penetrating peptic ulcer

Hereditary (familial) pancreatitis

Idiopathic[c] (10%)[b]

[a] Adapted from Steinberg W, Tenner S. Acute pancreatitis. New England Journal of Medicine 1994; 330: 1198–1210.
[b] The frequency of common causes is described. Remaining causes make up the final 5%.
[c] Investigations, including ERCP, have excluded the above causes.

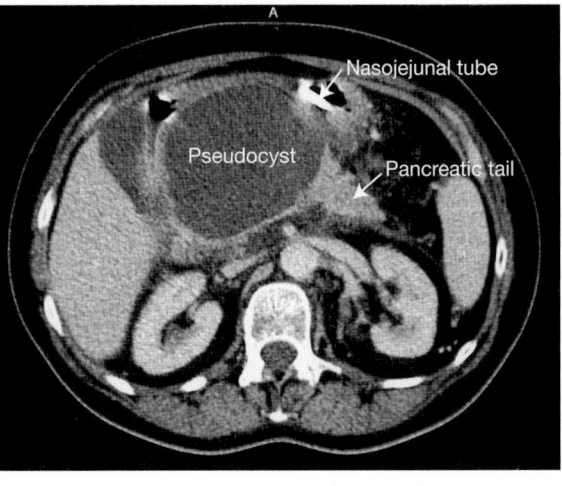

Fig. 5.39 CT of pancreatic pseudocyst. A large pseudocyst is seen in the head of the pancreas. A nasojejunal feeding tube is seen anterolaterally.
Copyright Addenbrooke's Hospital, Cambridge, UK.

Serum amylase

With the appropriate symptoms and signs, serum amylase greater than three times the upper limit of normal is diagnostic of acute pancreatitis.

Electrocardiogram

An ECG is necessary to exclude acute myocardial infarction as a differential diagnosis.

Erect chest and abdominal film

Chest and abdominal X-rays exclude a perforated viscus and intestinal obstruction, respectively. Chest X-ray may show atelectasis, pleural effusion or pneumonia. Acute respiratory distress syndrome (ARDS) can develop later. Abdominal X-ray may show a localized duodenal ileus (sentinel loop).

Ultrasound of the abdomen

Urgent abdominal ultrasonography should be performed to detect gallstones or common bile duct obstruction. Imaging of the pancreas is often poor due to overlying loops of bowel.

Further investigations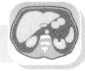

CT of the abdomen

Patients with severe acute pancreatitis should have contrast-enhanced CT scanning (Fig. 5.40) within 3–10 days of admission to screen for pancreatic necrosis or acute fluid collections.

RECENT ADVANCES

Activation of trypsinogen to trypsin during acute pancreatitis releases trypsinogen activation peptide (TAP). Urinary trypsinogen activation peptide is superior to C-reactive protein (CRP) as a marker of severity 24 hours after symptom onset,[2] and may become an important prognostic indicator.

Acute pancreatitis

Chronic pancreatitis

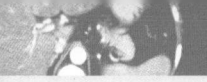

Table 5.57	Organ-specific and systemic complications of acute pancreatitis
Organ-specific	
Pancreas and retroperitoneum	Pancreatic fluid collections
	Pancreatic necrosis (sterile or infected)
	Pseudocysts
	Abscesses
	Digestion of peripancreatic blood vessels (haemorrhagic pancreatitis)
	Diabetes
	Pancreatic exocrine failure
Lungs	Atelectasis
	Pleural effusion
	Pneumonia
	Acute respiratory distress syndrome (ARDS)
Adjacent bowel/colon	Generalized ileus
	Inflammatory obstruction
	Fistulization into bowel
Gastrointestinal haemorrhage	Peptic stress ulcers
	Arterio-enteric fistula
Skin	Subcutaneous nodules of metastatic fat necrosis
Kidneys	Acute tubular necrosis
	Hydronephrosis due to retroperitoneal inflammation and fibrosis
Eyes	Purtscher's retinopathy (embolic retinopathy due to clumps of leukocytes, platelets and fibrin)
Heart	Dysrhythmias due to hypocalcaemia
Systemic	
Shock	Haemorrhage
	Sequestration of retroperitoneal fluid
	Sepsis
Disseminated intravascular coagulation (DIC)	SIRS/MODS
	Infective complications
Hypocalcaemia	Saponification of fat
	Hypoalbuminaemia

SIRS, systemic inflammatory response syndrome; MODS, multi-organ dysfunction syndrome.

Table 5.58	Modified Glasgow (Imrie) criteria for the classification of severity in acute pancreatitis*
Within 48 hours of admission	
Age >55 years	
White blood cell count >15 × 10⁹/L	

Within 48 hours of admission
Age >55 years
White blood cell count $>15 \times 10^9$/L
Glucose >10 mmol/L (no diabetic history)
Urea >16 mmol/L
$P_a O_2$ <8.0 kPa (60 mmHg)
Calcium <2 mmol/L
Albumin <32 g/L
Lactate dehydrogenase (LDH) >600 U/L
The presence of more than two risk factors predicts severe acute pancreatitis.

* Blamey SL, Imrie CW, O'Neill J, Gilmour WH, Carter DC. Prognostic factors in acute pancreatitis. Gut 1984; 25: 1340–1346.

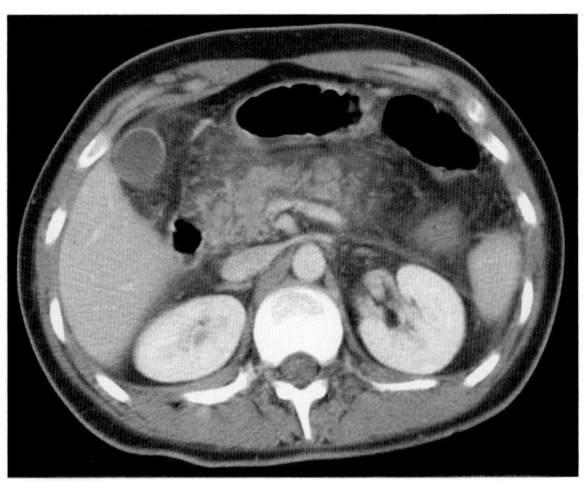

Fig. 5.40 CT of acute pancreatitis. The pancreas is oedematous and indistinct with inflammatory stranding of peripancreatic fat. The pancreas is enhanced on contrast with no evidence of necrosis. Courtesy of Dr M. Bennie, Norfolk and Norwich University Hospital, UK.

Initial management

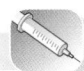

In general, the management of acute pancreatitis is supportive, with treatment directed at specific complications. No drug has been shown to prevent the development of severe acute pancreatitis. The initial management is guided by severity (Fig. 5.41).

Acute non-severe pancreatitis

Patients predicted to have mild disease (fewer than three markers of severity on the Glasgow criteria) can be managed on a general ward. Urinary catheterization is not usually necessary and a nasogastric tube is not required unless the patient suffers from severe vomiting or ileus. Prophylactic antibiotics are not beneficial.

Intravenous fluids

Patients are kept nil by mouth and hydration vigorously maintained with peripheral intravenous fluids. Once abdominal pain settles, oral fluids and food may slowly be reintroduced.

Analgesia

Parenteral opiates should be given for analgesia.

Acute severe pancreatitis

Patients with severe acute pancreatitis (more than two markers of severity on the Glasgow criteria) should be managed on a high-dependency or intensive care unit. Oxygenation a urinary catheter, nasogastric tube and a peripheral and central venous line are required. Some centres use somatostatin analogues such as octreotide to reduce pancreatic juice secretion.

Intravenous fluids

Patients are kept nil by mouth, and fluid resuscitation to maintain a urine output of 0.5 mL/kg/h is a priority.

Nutrition

Attention to nutrition is important. Enteral nutrition via a nasojejunal tube is cheaper and safer than total parenteral nutrition (TPN).[3]

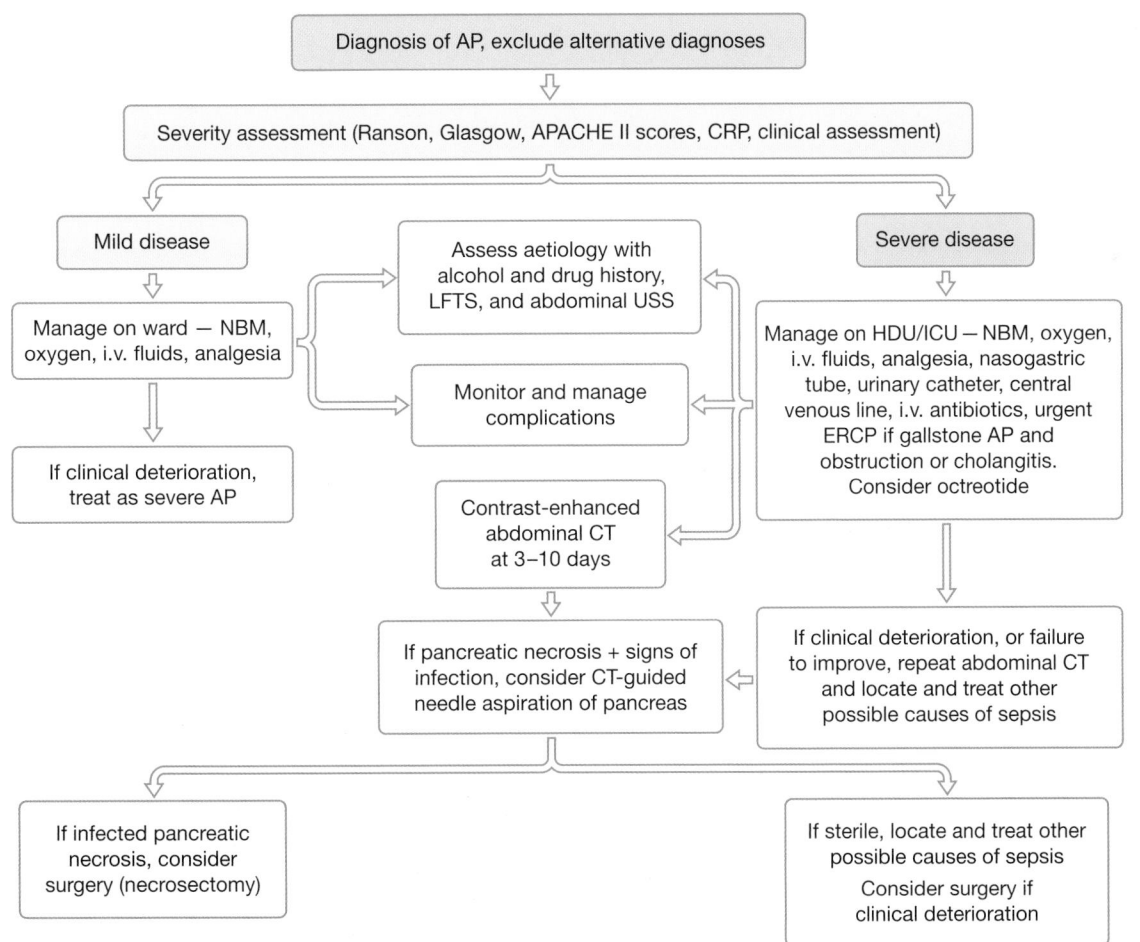

Fig. 5.41 Management of acute pancreatitis (AP). CRP, C-reactive protein; LFTs, liver function tests, USS, ultrasound; NBM, nil by mouth; ERCP, endoscopic retrograde cholangio-pancreatography.

Antibiotics

Prophylactic intravenous antibiotics should be given, e.g. cefuroxime or imipenem for 2–4 weeks, depending on the clinical course.[4]

Endoscopic retrograde cholangio-pancreatography

Urgent ERCP with sphincterotomy and stone extraction is beneficial for patients with severe gallstone pancreatitis with worsening liver profile or cholangitis.[5]

Prevention of further attacks

Patients with idiopathic mild pancreatitis should have their serum lipids and calcium corrected, and a CT scan to exclude a pancreatic tumour.

Endoscopic retrograde cholangio-pancreatography

Patients with severe or recurrent mild attacks with no obvious cause require ERCP to exclude occult common bile duct stones, pancreas divisum or a pancreatic carcinoma. MRCP or endoscopic ultrasound may also be used.

Cholecystectomy

Patients with gallstone pancreatitis should undergo cholecystectomy to prevent recurrent disease.

Surgical management

Necrosectomy

Sterile pancreatic necrosis is treated conservatively with intravenous antibiotics and supportive therapy. Surgical removal of necrotic pancreatic tissue (necrosectomy) is indicated for infected necrosis of the pancreas. Clinical deterioration despite medical treatment is also an indication for surgery.

Necrosectomy may be followed by repeated laparotomies for debridement or the abdominal wound left exposed to allow abdominal packs to be changed.

Prognosis

The mortality is related to the severity of the acute attack. The overall mortality is 15%, usually from multi-organ dysfunction syndrome. The majority (95%) of deaths occur in patients with severe acute pancreatitis.

i FURTHER INFORMATION

United Kingdom guidelines for the management of acute pancreatitis. British Society of Gastroenterology. Gut 2005; 54 Suppl 3: iii1–9.

REFERENCES

(1) Floyd A, Pedersen L, Nielsen GL, Thorladcius-Ussing O, Sorensen HT. Secular trends in incidence and 30-day case fatality of acute pancreatitis in North Jutland County, Denmark: a register-based study from 1981-2000. Scandinavian Journal of Gastroenterology 2002; 37: 1461–1465.
(2) Neoptolemos JP, Kemppainen EA, Mayer JM, et al. Early prediction of severity in acute pancreatitis by urinary trypsinogen activation peptide: a multicentre study. Lancet 2000; 355: 1955–1960.
(3) Imrie CW, Carter CR, McKay CJ. Enteral and parenteral nutrition in acute pancreatitis. Best Practice and Research Clinical Gastroenterology 2002; 16: 391–397.
(4) Schmid SW, Uhl W, Friess H, Malfertheiner P, Buchler MW. The role of infection in acute pancreatitis. Gut 1999; 45: 311–316.
(5) Folsch UR, Nitsche R, Ludtke R, Hilgers RA, Creutzfeldt W. Early ERCP and papillotomy compared with conservative treatment for acute biliary pancreatitis. The German Study Group on Acute Biliary Pancreatitis. New England Journal of Medicine 1997; 336: 237–242.

Chronic pancreatitis

Chronic pancreatitis is a progressive inflammatory disease resulting in permanent structural and/or functional pancreatic damage.[1]

Epidemiology

The prevalence of chronic pancreatitis in the West is approximately 15 per 100 000. It usually affects men aged 40–50 years.

Pathology

In the West, 70% of cases are due to alcohol and 20% are idiopathic (Table 5.59). The pathogenesis of chronic pancreatitis is poorly understood. Long-term alcohol abuse causes pancreatic epithelial damage and chronic obstruction due to intraductal protein plugs. Subsequent calcium carbonate precipitation causes pancreatic calcification. Ductal stones may also form. Pancreatic tumours or strictures of the main duct can lead to chronic obstruction and subsequent inflammation and fibrosis. Disease is often most severe in the head of the pancreas.

Scope of disease

Complications occur from loss of pancreatic exocrine and endocrine function and local inflammatory effects (Table 5.60). The exocrine pancreas has tremendous reserve capacity and requires 80–90% destruction before clinical effects occur. Pancreatic insufficiency leads to inadequate protein, fat and carbohydrate digestion. This impairs absorption, causing malnutrition and diarrhoea. Fat malabsorption causes steatorrhoea (pale, offensive, bulky stools) and deficiencies of fat-soluble vitamins (A, D, E and K).

Ductal hypertension and inflammation leads to pseudocyst formation in 20%. Patients with chronic pancreatitis have a 20–30 times higher risk of developing pancreatic

Table 5.59	Causes of chronic pancreatitis
Alcohol abuse	
Idiopathic	

Pancreatic duct stenosis/obstruction
    Periampullary tumour
    Post-traumatic
    Duodenal diverticulum
    Pseudocysts
    Pancreas divisum	

Tropical (nutritional) pancreatitis	
Hypertriglyceridaemia	
Hypercalcaemia	
Autoimmune disease Sjögren's syndrome	
Hereditary pancreatitis	

Table 5.60	Complications of chronic pancreatitis

Loss of pancreatic function
    Exocrine (malabsorption and steatorrhoea)
    Endocrine (diabetes mellitus)	

Local inflammatory effects
    Common bile duct strictures and obstruction
    Duodenal stenosis/occlusion
    Pancreatic duct strictures
    Portal vein thrombosis and portal hypertension
    Splenic vein thrombosis and gastric varices
    Erosion of peripancreatic vessels (pseudoaneurysm)
    Pancreato-colic fistula	

Pancreatic pseudocyst
    Haemorrhage
    Rupture (pancreatic ascites, pancreatico-pleural fistula)
    Infection
    Gastric outlet obstruction
    Duodenal obstruction
    Common bile duct obstruction	

Pancreatic adenocarcinoma	
Pancreatic abscess	

adenocarcinoma.[2] The two complications can coexist and distinguishing between them can be difficult.

Clinical features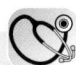

Intermittent upper abdominal pain is the dominant clinical feature. The pain usually occurs after food and radiates through to the back. It may be relieved by leaning forwards. As the disease progresses, the pain often becomes persistent and symptoms from exocrine (malabsorption) and endocrine (diabetes mellitus) pancreatic insufficiency such as weight loss, steatorrhoea, thirst and polyuria can occur. A long history of heavy alcohol consumption is common.

The examination is usually unremarkable apart from upper abdominal tenderness. A palpable epigastric mass

may be due to a pseudocyst, and jaundice can occur with bile duct obstruction due to strictures or pancreatic carcinoma. An acute exacerbation of chronic pancreatitis can be clinically indistinguishable from acute pancreatitis.

Initial investigations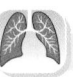

Histological diagnosis of chronic pancreatitis is not feasible due to the complications associated with pancreatic biopsy. Diagnosis therefore depends on radiological imaging and pancreatic function tests.

Serum amylase

Despite pancreatic inflammation, serum amylase and lipase are usually normal or slightly elevated, reflecting the loss of functioning pancreas.

Liver profile

The liver profile may reveal a cholestatic pattern (p. 370) due to common bile duct obstruction.

Random blood glucose

The blood sugar levels may be elevated with the onset of diabetes in late disease.

Plain abdominal film

Diffuse pancreatic calcifications on plain abdominal radiography are pathognomonic of chronic pancreatitis but are present in only 30% (Fig. 5.42).

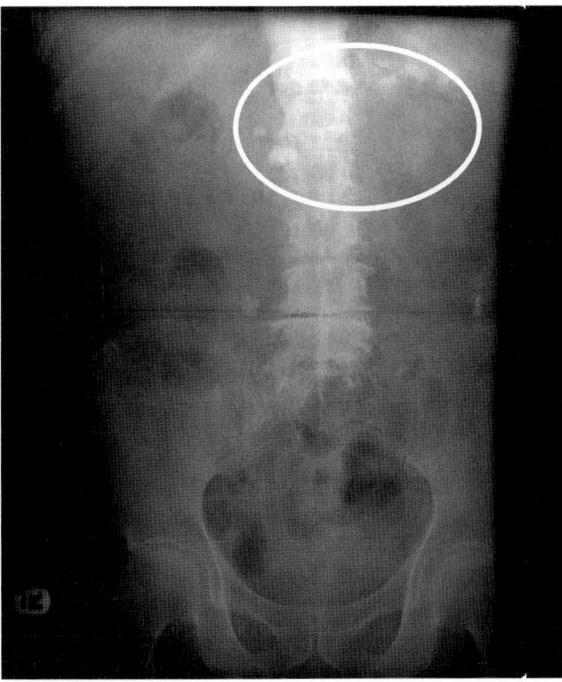

Fig. 5.42 Plain film of chronic pancreatitis. Calcification in the upper abdomen (circled) due to chronic pancreatitis.
Courtesy of Dr M. Bennie, Norfolk and Norwich University Hospital, UK.

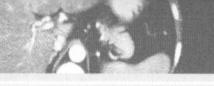

Endoscopic retrograde cholangio-pancreatography

ERCP is the gold standard test for the diagnosis of chronic pancreatitis, with a sensitivity of 80–95% and specificity >90%. ERCP reveals a combination of ectatic and strictured branch ducts with filling defects or calcified stones in the main pancreatic duct.

Further investigations

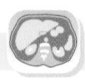

Abdominal ultrasound

Transabdominal ultrasound is not a useful investigation for chronic pancreatitis but is used to assess the size of the common bile duct and the presence of gallstone disease or pseudocysts.

Upper gastrointestinal endoscopy

Upper gastrointestinal endoscopy should be considered to rule out gastric carcinoma and peptic ulcer disease in patients with recurrent epigastric abdominal pain.

CT of the abdomen

CT can detect pancreatic calcification and screen for complications of chronic pancreatitis (Fig. 5.43).

Pancreatic function tests

Pancreatic function tests (p. 242) may reveal exocrine pancreatic insufficiency in patients with chronic pancreatitis, but it is an insensitive investigation in early disease.

Screening for pancreatic carcinoma

Clinically and radiologically it can be very difficult to exclude pancreatic carcinoma. ERCP with brush cytology, fine-needle aspiration biopsy and CA19-9 measurement

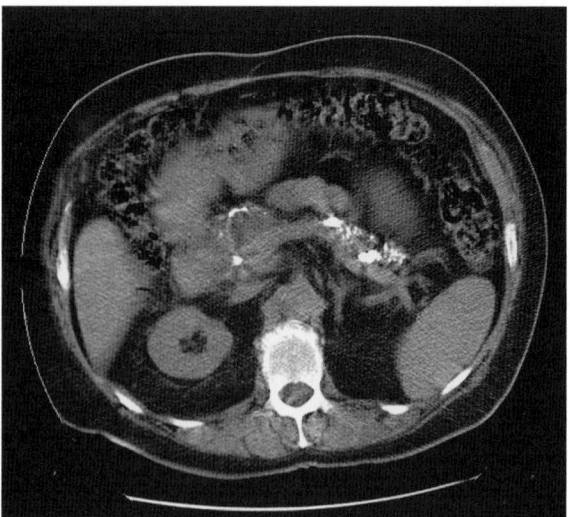

Fig. 5.43 CT of chronic pancreatitis. Atrophic pancreas with focal calcification.
Courtesy of Dr M. Bennie, Norfolk and Norwich University Hospital, UK.

may help. Endoscopic ultrasound is increasingly being used to rule out pancreatic carcinoma.

Initial management

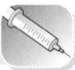

The outpatient management of patients with chronic pancreatitis focuses on pain relief and the detection and management of complications. Acute exacerbations require admission for gastrointestinal rest, analgesia and parenteral nutrition.

Patient education

Patients are advised to avoid fatty foods and smoking and to abstain from alcohol. Alcohol and narcotic addiction is common and patients may require counselling or psychiatric assessment and management.

Analgesia

Chronic pain is the most difficult symptom to manage. Regular simple oral analgesics (e.g. paracetamol, NSAIDs) are useful initially, with oral opioids during exacerbations. Some patients with intractable pain may require a coeliac plexus block or thoracoscopic sympathectomy. Progressive worsening of pain may herald the onset of complications (e.g. pancreatic carcinoma) and detailed investigations should be performed.

Pancreatic supplementation

Patients with malabsorption from exocrine failure are treated with enteric-coated pancreatic enzyme supplements. Oral pancreatic enzyme supplements may decrease pancreatic stimulation and also reduce pain, though their use for the purposes of pain relief alone is controversial.

Insulin

Diabetes mellitus eventually occurs in 30% and usually requires the administration of insulin.

Management of pancreatic duct stones

Endoscopic stone extraction, pancreatic duct stenting and extracorporeal shock wave lithotripsy may relieve intractable pain in those with pancreatic stones on ERCP.

Surgical management

Pancreaticojejunostomy

A longitudinal pancreaticojejunostomy can achieve pain relief in 70% of patients with dilated pancreatic ducts (suggestive of recurrent obstruction) and failed endoscopic therapy. The indications for surgery are listed in Table 5.61.

Whipple's procedure

Patients with severe disease in the pancreatic head without dilated ducts should be considered for the Whipple procedure or partial resection of the pancreatic head. Total pancreatectomy is rarely performed as it results in brittle diabetes and complete exocrine failure.

Prognosis

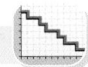

Chronic pancreatitis has a 20-year survival of 50%, mainly because of alcohol abuse and tobacco-related death.

Table 5.61	Indications for surgery in chronic pancreatitis

Severe, intractable pain

Local complications not amenable to medical or endoscopic management
    Distal common bile duct or duodenal stenosis
    Pseudocysts
    Pancreatic fistulae
    Pancreatic ascites
    Gastrointestinal haemorrhage due to splenic vein thrombosis
        and gastric varices

Suspicion of pancreatic malignancy

Progressive pancreatic destruction with conservative management

_i_   FURTHER INFORMATION

Steer ML, Waxman I, Freedman S. Chronic pancreatitis. New England Journal of Medicine 1995; 332: 1482–1490.

REFERENCES

(1) *Ammann RW. A clinically based classification system for alcoholic chronic pancreatitis: summary of an international workshop on chronic pancreatitis. Pancreas 1997; 14: 215–221.*
(2) *Malka D, Hammel P, Maire F, et al. Risk of pancreatic adenocarcinoma in chronic pancreatitis. Gut 2002; 51: 849–852.*

SECTION 5.28   Pancreatic tumours

Primary pancreatic tumours may be benign or malignant, exocrine or endocrine (Table 5.62). Secondary pancreatic tumours are uncommon. Ninety per cent of pancreatic tumours are pancreatic ductal adenocarcinomas.

Benign exocrine pancreatic tumours

Benign exocrine pancreatic tumours are rare but important, due to their variable potential for malignant transformation. Symptoms are often vague and these tumours are often incidental radiological findings. Mucinous cystadenomas and intraductal papillary mucinous tumours have high rates of malignant transformation and should be resected if suspected on imaging. Serous cystadenomas characteristically resemble a bunch of small grapes on ultrasound or CT. These can safely be observed, as serous cystadeno-carcinomas are extremely rare.

FURTHER INFORMATION

Brugge WR, Lauwers GY, Sahani D, Fernandez-del Castillo C, Warshaw AL. Cystic neoplasms of the pancreas. New England Journal of Medicine 2004; 351: 1218–1226.

Pancreatic ductal adenocarcinoma

Epidemiology

Pancreatic ductal adenocarcinoma (PDAC) is the sixth most common cause of cancer death in the UK with an age-adjusted incidence of 10 per 100 000 person-years. It is 1.5 times more common in men, and 80% occur in those aged over 60 years.

Table 5.62	Pancreatic tumours

Primary
Benign exocrine

Mucinous cystadenoma

Serous cystadenoma (microcystic adenoma)

Intraductal papillary mucinous tumours (benign variant)

Malignant exocrine

Ductal adenocarcinoma

Acinar cell adenocarcinoma

Mucinous cystadenocarcinoma

Intraductal papillary mucinous tumours (malignant variant)

Endocrine (variable risk of malignancy)

Insulinoma

Gastrinoma (Zollinger–Ellison syndrome)

Glucagonoma

Other

Lymphoma

Sarcoma

Secondary

Melanoma

Breast carcinoma

Lung carcinoma

Table 5.63	Risk factors for pancreatic ductal adenocarcinoma

Demographic factors

Increasing age

Males

Race, e.g. African Americans, New Zealand Maori

Lifestyle

Cigarette smoking

Meat and fish consumption

Occupational exposure to aromatic amines (e.g. hairdressing, rubber work)

Associated medical conditions

Chronic pancreatitis

Cystic diseases of the pancreas or pancreatic masses

Peutz–Jeghers syndrome

Familial adenomatous polyposis syndrome

Hereditary pancreatitis

Hereditary non-polyposis colorectal cancer syndrome (Lynch syndrome)

Familial atypical multiple mole melanoma syndrome

Pathology

Pancreatic ductal adenocarcinoma, PDAC, is thought to originate from areas of epithelial dysplasia that progress to infiltrating carcinoma. These foci of pancreatic intraepithelial neoplasia are similar to the precursor lesions found in cancer of the cervix or breast. Accumulation of multiple genetic alterations (*K-ras*, *p53* and *BRCA2* genes) is the proposed underlying mechanism.[1] The associated risk factors are listed in Table 5.63. Although the onset of diabetes after the age of 50 is associated with an increased risk of PDAC, it is probably PDAC that causes diabetes due to the destruction of islet cells by tumour infiltration.

Scope of disease

A summary is also listed in Table 5.64.

Local

Local tumour growth may obstruct and invade important vascular, neural and ductal structures. Obstruction of the common bile duct can lead to obstructive jaundice.

Metastatic

Distant metastases are present in more than 75% of patients at presentation (e.g. liver, lung, umbilicus and supraclavicular lymph nodes).

Table 5.64	Scope of disease of pancreatic adenocarcinoma

Complication	Manifestation
Common bile duct obstruction	Jaundice (usually painless)
Pancreatic duct obstruction	Acute pancreatitis Chronic pancreatitis Steatorrhoea
Duodenal obstruction	Post-prandial vomiting
Neural invasion	Intractable abdominal or back pain
Portal vein obstruction	Gastrointestinal haemorrhage, ascites
Coagulopathy	Recurrent or atypical venous thrombosis (Trousseau's syndrome)

Metastatic disease
  Liver
  Peritoneum
  Lungs
	Weight loss, malaise
	    Right upper quadrant
	    pain, jaundice
	  Ascites
	  Haemoptysis, dyspnoea

Pancreatic destruction	Steatorrhoea Symptoms of diabetes mellitus
Local vascular invasion	Upper gastrointestinal bleeding

Paraneoplastic

Trousseau's syndrome (migratory superficial thrombophlebitis) is classically due to pancreatic ductal adenocarcinoma.

Clinical features

Tumours in the head present earlier than tumours elsewhere in the pancreas as jaundice occurs due to the proximity of the common bile duct. Painless jaundice is present in half of patients with a potentially resectable lesion, whereas upper abdominal or back pain is present in 80% of those with advanced disease. Other symptoms include anorexia, early satiety, weight loss or other symptoms of obstructive jaundice. Steatorrhoea may occur in pancreatic head carcinoma.

In early disease, jaundice alone may be present on examination, possibly with a palpable distended gallbladder (Courvoisier's law). This 'law' states that a distended gallbladder is more likely to be from malignant common bile duct obstruction rather than obstruction due to common bile duct stones, as the stones originate in the gallbladder and cause fibrosis, preventing gallbladder distension.

In advanced disease, cachexia, supraclavicular lymph node enlargement (Virchow's node), umbilical metastases (Sister Mary Joseph's nodule), ascites, hepatic metastases or an epigastric mass may be found.

Initial investigations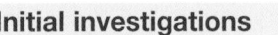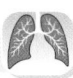

Full blood count

Mild anaemia is often present on full blood count.

Liver profile

Liver profile reveals an obstructive pattern and prothrombin time may be raised.

Serum amylase and lipase

Serum amylase and lipase may be non-specifically elevated.

CA19-9

The tumour marker CA19-9 lacks diagnostic sensitivity and specificity but may be used to monitor disease progression.

Chest X-ray

A chest X-ray should be performed to identify lung metastases.

Ultrasound of the abdomen

In pancreatic head carcinoma, ultrasonography will show a dilated common bile duct and may identify a pancreatic mass. Gallstones and hilar cholangiocarcinoma should be excluded.

Further investigations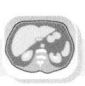

CT of the abdomen

In patients with symptoms suggestive of advanced pancreatic cancer a dual-phase spiral CT is an appropriate

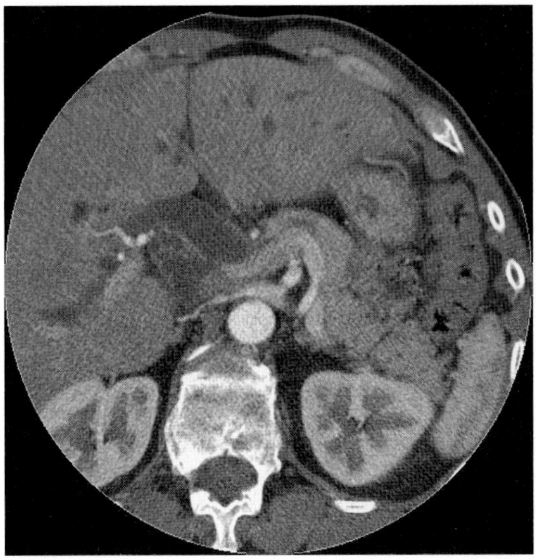

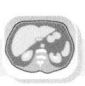

Fig. 5.44 CT of pancreatic adenocarcinoma. Close-up of contrast-enhanced CT showing a poorly enhancing mass in the head of the pancreas.
Courtesy Dr M. Bennie, Norfolk and Norwich University Hospital, UK.

> ### TNM staging system of pancreatic exocrine carcinomas[2]

T Primary tumour

Tis	Carcinoma in situ
T1	Tumour limited to pancreas, ≤2 cm diameter
T2	Tumour limited to pancreas, >2 cm diameter
T3	Tumour extends beyond pancreas, no coeliac axis or superior mesenteric artery involvement
T4	Tumour involves coeliac axis or superior mesenteric artery

N Regional lymph nodes

N0	No regional lymph node metastasis
N1	Regional lymph node metastasis

M Distant metastasis

M0	No distant metastasis
M1	Distant metastasis

Stage grouping

Stage 0	Tis	N0	M0
Stage IA	T1	N0	M0
Stage IB	T2	N0	M0
Stage IIA	T3	N0	M0
Stage IIB	T1, T2, or T3	N1	M0
Stage III	T4	Any N	M0
Stage IV	Any T	Any N	M1

initial imaging test. Spiral CT (Fig. 5.44) is currently thought to be the best imaging study to diagnose and stage PDAC with a sensitivity of 92%.

Endoscopic ultrasound

Endoscopic ultrasound (EUS) is better at detecting pancreatic masses than CT (sensitivity >95%) and allows accurate assessment of invasion into the superior mesenteric vessels and portal vein. However, EUS is operator dependent and is unable to stage the disease. The role of EUS is evolving but it is probably best used in patients with symptoms suggestive of PDAC with a normal CT. Some centres use it routinely to exclude vascular invasion in patients who are thought to have resectable disease on CT.

Laparoscopy and biopsies

CT or EUS may miss small peritoneal or hepatic metastases in 10–15% of patients thought to have resectable disease. Laparoscopy and biopsy of possible metastases may be used to stage the patient more accurately and therefore determine resectability.

Initial management

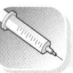

Nutrition

Adequate nutrition is an important aspect of management. Patients with exocrine pancreatic failure require enteric-coated pancreatic enzyme supplements.

Surgical management

Pancreatectomy

Surgical resection is the only potentially curative treatment. Unfortunately, 85% of patients present with unresectable advanced disease (Table 5.65). Patients with resectable masses should not have a biopsy as the best form of tissue diagnosis is surgical resection.

The Whipple partial pancreatoduodenectomy is the standard operation for operable pancreatic head tumours (Fig. 5.45). In specialist pancreatic centres mortality is 5%, with 30–50% morbidity (Table 5.66). Surgery should be followed by adjuvant chemotherapy with 5-fluorouracil.[3]

Distal pancreatectomy with splenectomy is used for carcinomas of the pancreatic body and tail, but only 5% are resectable due to late presentation.

Table 5.65	Contraindications to resection of pancreatic adenocarcinoma*
Severe comorbid illness	
Liver, peritoneal or distant metastases	
Metastases to lymph nodes not usually removed during surgery	
Encasement of superior mesenteric, coeliac, or hepatic arteries	
Encasement of superior mesenteric or portal veins	
Cirrhosis with portal hypertension	

* Adapted from Magee CJ, Ghaneh P, Neoptolemos JP. Surgical and medical therapy for pancreatic carcinoma. Best Practice and Research Clinical Gastroenterology 2002; 16: 435–455.

a

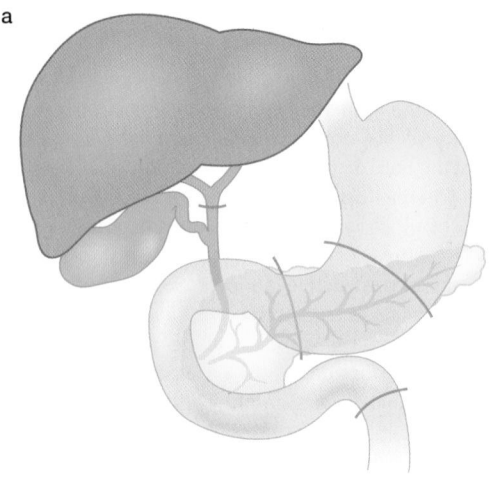

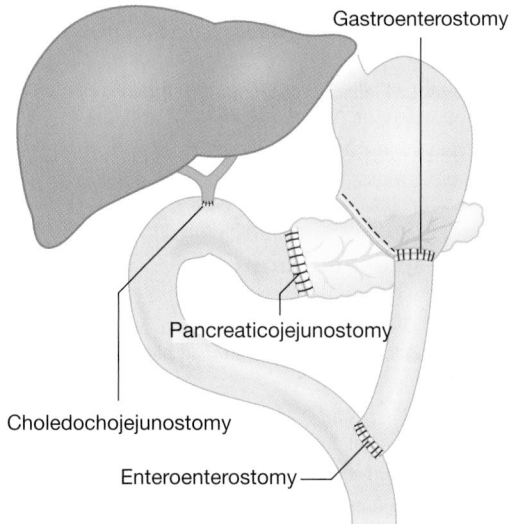

Gastroenterostomy

Pancreaticojejunostomy

Choledochojejunostomy

Enteroenterostomy

b

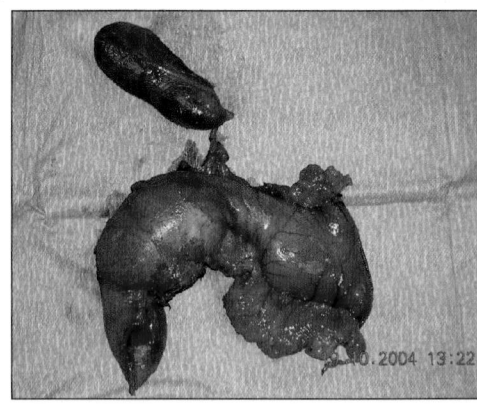

Fig. 5.45 a,b Whipple procedure for resection of pancreatic head adenocarcinoma. The duodenum, common bile duct and gallbladder, pancreatic head and distal stomach are removed (a). There are many different methods of re-attaching the remaining organs. A Roux-en-Y technique is shown. (b) The pancreatic carcinoma can be seen bulging into the second part of the duodenum.
Photograph courtesy of Mr R. Praseedom, Addenbrooke's Hospital, Cambridge, UK. Copyright Addenbrooke's Hospital, Cambridge, UK.

Table 5.66	Complications of a Whipple procedure
Complication	**Incidence**
Local	
Anastomotic leakage	10–20%
Delayed gastric emptying	10%
Sterile intra-abdominal fluid collection	10%
Wound infection	5%
Bleeding	5%
Re-operation	5%
Pancreatico-cutaneous fistula	5%
Cholangitis	3%
Postoperative pancreatitis	3%
Intra-abdominal abscess	3%
Systemic	
Sepsis	5%
Respiratory failure	4%
Shock	3%
Renal failure	3%

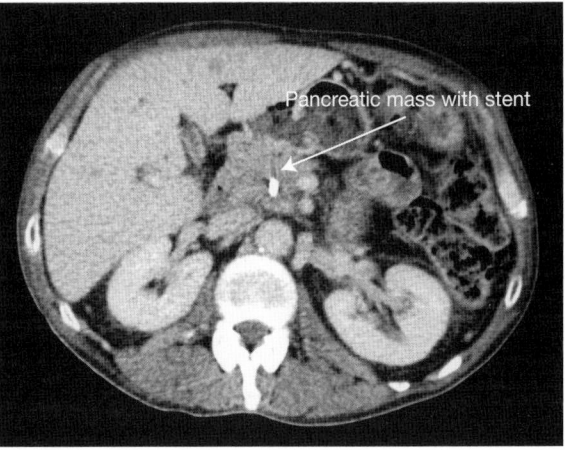

Fig. 5.46 Biliary stent. CT of the pancreas showing a pancreatic head mass surrounding a stent that had been inserted during ERCP to relieve obstructive jaundice.
Copyright Addenbrooke's Hospital, Cambridge, UK.

Prognosis

Patients undergoing resection have a 5-year survival rate of 20%. Those with inoperable disease have a median survival of 4–6 months. The overall 5-year survival is 1–3%.

i FURTHER INFORMATION

DiMagno EP, Reber HA, Tempero MA. AGA technical review on the epidemiology, diagnosis, and treatment of pancreatic ductal adenocarcinoma. American Gastroenterological Association. Gastroenterology 1999; 117: 1464–1484.

REFERENCES

(1) Hall P de L, Wilentz RE, de Klerk W, Bornman PP. Premalignant conditions of the pancreas. Pathology 2002; 34: 504–517.
(2) Sobin L, Wittekind C. TNM classification of malignant tumours, 6th edn. New York: Wiley, 2002.
(3) Neoptolemos JP, Stocken DD, Friess H, et al. A randomized trial of chemoradiotherapy and chemotherapy after resection of pancreatic cancer. New England Journal of Medicine 2004; 350: 1200–1210.

Total pancreatectomy is reserved for those with diffuse pancreatic involvement or insulin-dependent diabetics with pancreatic cancer.

Bypass procedures

Despite advances in imaging, some patients only have resectability confirmed at laparotomy. Patients found to have inoperable cancer intraoperatively should have a palliative surgical bypass procedure to prevent symptomatic common bile duct and duodenal obstruction.

Medical management

Patients not suitable for curative surgical resection require palliation of pain, obstructive jaundice and gastric outlet/duodenal obstruction, as well as treatment of exocrine pancreatic failure.

Chemotherapy and radiotherapy

Palliative radiotherapy and chemotherapy with 5-fluorouracil or gemcitabine alone can prolong median survival.

Pain control

Pain control can be difficult to achieve, even with regular oral or transcutaneous opioids. Coeliac plexus block or thoracoscopic splanchnicectomy provides relief in up to 75% of patients.

Relief of obstructive jaundice

Obstructive jaundice can be relieved endoscopically (ERCP) with stent insertion (Fig. 5.46).

Endocrine tumours of the pancreas

Endocrine tumours of the pancreas are rare and have variable malignant potential. Tumours arising from pancreatic islets may secrete substances normally produced by the islets (e.g. insulin, glucagon) or non-pancreatic hormones (e.g. gastrin). They occur sporadically or in association with multiple endocrine neoplasia 1 (MEN-1). Some may be found in extrapancreatic tissues (Table 5.67). Treatment is

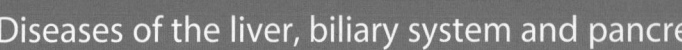
Table 5.67	Pancreatic endocrine tumours*			
Tumour and hormone produced	Pancreatic location	Malignant	Signs and symptoms	Diagnosis
Insulinoma (insulin)	>99%	<10%	Hypoglycaemic episodes	Hypoglycaemia, raised insulin/glucose ratio, elevated fasting C-peptide
Gastrinoma (gastrin)	25%	75%	Peptic ulceration, diarrhoea	Raised fasting serum gastrin, secretin provocation test
Glucagonoma (glucagon)	100%	70%	Diabetes, dermatitis	Elevated plasma glucagon

*Adapted from Mullan MH, Gauger PG, Thompson NW. Endocrine tumours of the pancreas: review and recent advances. ANZ Journal of Surgery 2001; 71: 475–482.

surgical excision, and even in patients with malignancies the prognosis is generally good. Non-functioning tumours present late, often with a palpable mass.

The insulinoma is the most common pancreatic endocrine tumour. Autonomous insulin secretion leads to hypoglycaemia-induced symptoms (e.g. hunger, tremor, altered behaviour, weakness, coma) and the classic diagnostic (Whipple's) triad of hypoglycaemic symptoms while fasting, a blood glucose less than 2.8 mmol/L, and symptomatic relief with glucose. Initial misdiagnosis is common. Gastrinomas cause peptic ulcers, severe diarrhoea and weight loss due to hypersecretion of gastrin (Zollinger–Ellison syndrome). Glucagonomas commonly metastasize and resection is possible in only 30%.

 FURTHER INFORMATION

Azimuddin K, Chamberlain RS. The surgical management of pancreatic neuroendocrine tumors. Surgical Clinics of North America 2001; 81: 511–525.

Diseases of the endocrine system

6

Marcus Simmgen, Yoon Kong Loke, Kevin Shotliff

Introduction

Applied basic sciences of the endocrine system

Hypothalamus and pituitary gland

Anatomy

The hypothalamus is located at the base of the brain surrounding the third ventricle. Specific populations of neural cells in the supraoptic and paraventricular regions of the hypothalamus produce hormones with releasing or inhibitory effects on the pituitary gland's endocrine function. Portal vessels within the stalk of the pituitary carry these hypothalamic hormones to the pituitary gland.

The pituitary gland consists of two distinct parts: the anterior and the posterior lobes. The anterior adenohypophysis/lobe develops from oropharyngeal ectoderm (Rathke's pouch) and ascends towards the skull base. The posterior neurohypophysis/lobe develops as an extension of the hypothalamus, descending towards the anterior part. Both lobes remain anatomically distinct whilst forming a single gland situated within the pituitary fossa.

The anterior lobe consists of cells producing growth hormone (GH), prolactin (PRL), adrenocorticotropic hormone (ACTH), luteinizing and follicle-stimulating hormone (LH/FSH), and thyroid-stimulating hormone (TSH), in descending order of abundance. Any such population of cells is referred to as '-troph', e.g. corticotroph for ACTH-producing cells. The posterior lobe consists of neuronal cells where the hypothalamic hormones vasopressin (antidiuretic hormone, ADH) and oxytocin are stored following their transport along the neural axons from the hypothalamus.

Physiology

Feedback regulation

The hypothalamus and pituitary gland represent the central unit regulating plasma levels of hormones secreted peripherally by the thyroid, adrenal and gonads.

'Long-loop' negative feedback mechanisms regulate most endocrine axes, with peripheral hormones suppressing their own stimulation at both hypothalamic and pituitary level. A 'short-loop' feedback refers to the direct effect of a pituitary hormone on its secretory cells and the hypothalamus.

An endocrine disturbance is considered 'primary' if it originates within the peripheral gland, 'secondary' with pituitary aetiology, and 'tertiary' if there is underlying hypothalamic pathology.

Simultaneous measurement of the corresponding peripheral and pituitary hormones (e.g. thyroxine and TSH) will distinguish between a primary and secondary disorder. Tertiary pathology can be evaluated by assessing the related hypothalamic releasing hormone (e.g. thyrotropin-releasing hormone, TRH), with TSH physiologically exerting a negative feedback on TRH secretion. Typical biochemical results of disorders of the thyroid axis are summarized in Table 6.1. In the same way the gonadal and the hypothalamic–pituitary–adrenal (HPA) axes can be evaluated.

Table 6.1	Biochemical results of disorders of the thyroid axis		
	Hormone	Deficiency	Excess
Primary disturbance (thyroid gland)	T_4	Low	High
	TSH	High	Low
	TRH	N/A	N/A
Secondary disturbance (pituitary gland)	T_4	Low	High
	TSH	Low	High
	TRH	High	Low
Tertiary disturbance (hypothalamus)	T_4	Low	High
	TSH	Low	High
	TRH	Low	High

T, thyroxine; TSH, thyroid-stimulating hormone; TRH, thyrotropin-releasing hormone; N/A, not applicable.

Anterior pituitary hormones

Single chain proteohormones

GH (somatotropin) consists of 191 amino acids (AA). GH stimulates the synthesis of insulin-like growth factor-1 (IGF-1) in the liver and other tissues, through which many GH effects are mediated. GH-releasing hormone (GHRH) and the inhibitory hormone somatostatin regulate GH secretion. Negative feedback on the hypothalamus and the pituitary is provided by both GH (short-loop) and by IGF-1 (long-loop).

PRL is structurally similar to GH and consists of 198 AA. It induces lactogenesis in breast tissue. Suckling, stress and sleep stimulate PRL secretion, as do a specific PRL-releasing peptide (PRP), TRH and oestrogen. PRL release is under tonic inhibition by dopaminergic neurones in the pituitary stalk, enhanced by a short-loop feedback by PRL on these neurones.

Heterodimeric proteohormones

LH, FSH, and TSH share a common α-subunit of 89 AA whilst the β-chain of around 115 AA is specific to each hormone. All molecules are glycosylated.

The gonadotropins LH and FSH are central to male and female fertility. Their secretion occurs under the influence of gonadotrophin-releasing hormone (GnRH). In men, testosterone provides inhibitory feedback, while in women, sex steroids can exert both positive and negative feedback on gonadotrophin secretion, depending on dose, time course and relation to the menstrual cycle. This mechanism is important for ovulation.

TSH regulates thyroid hormone secretion. TSH release is stimulated by TRH. The thyroid hormones provide negative feedback at pituitary and hypothalamic level.

Pro-opiomelanocortin (POMC) derived hormones

ACTH is a peptide of 39 AA cleaved from the large precursor protein pro-opiomelanocortin (POMC). Other hormones derived from POMC are α-melanocyte stimulating hormone (α-MSH), identical with the first 13 AA of ACTH, as well as lipotropin and endorphin. Their clinical relevance is limited.

ACTH controls adrenal glucocorticoid and androgen synthesis. It is released during stress and under the influence of corticotropin-releasing hormone (CRH). Glucocorticoids exert a negative feedback on ACTH secretion at both pituitary and hypothalamic level.

Posterior pituitary hormones

Vasopressin and oxytocin

Both vasopressin (ADH) and oxytocin are cyclical nonapeptides cleaved from their respective precursor molecule.

ADH increases the renal reabsorption of water in the ascending loop of Henle and the collecting ducts. It is released in response to a rise in plasma osmolality, a fall in blood pressure, and a range of environmental factors and drugs. Central osmoreceptors and cardiac baroreceptors mediate the main feedback mechanism.

Oxytocin causes smooth muscle contraction in the breast ducts and the uterus but has no defined role in men. It is released in response to suckling and during childbirth/parturition, thus increasing milk flow and reducing postpartum uterine blood loss. No specific feedback mechanism has been established for oxytocin.

The thyroid gland

Anatomy

The thyroid originates from pharyngeal epithelium, and progressive descent of the thyroid anlage gives rise to the thyroglossal duct from which thyroglossal cysts, ducts and accessory thyroid tissue (pyramidal lobe) can develop. The thyroid descends to the lower anterior neck between C5 and T1. The thyroid is encapsulated within the pretracheal layer of the deep cervical fascia; capsular invasion is an important determinant of staging in thyroid cancer (p. 415). The thyroid is a bilobed structure that weighs approximately 25 g. The lobes are conical and measure $5 \times 3 \times 2$ cm.

Microscopically, the thyroid is organized into follicles with a central colloid core (containing glucoprotein, iodothyroglobulin, triiodothyronine and thyroxine) surrounded by simple epithelium. A second parafollicular cell type, 'clear' or 'C' cells, secrete thyro-calcitonin and are the cell type from which medullary thyroid carcinoma arises.

The thyroid is supplied by the superior and inferior thyroid arteries, and occasionally a thyroid ima artery from the brachiocephalic trunk. The veins form a plexus on the surface and in front of the trachea and drain into the superior, middle and inferior thyroid veins. On the right, the recurrent laryngeal nerve ascends near the lower pole of the thyroid near the inferior thyroid artery and on the left it ascends between the thyroid and trachea. Injury to the recurrent nerve occasionally occurs during thyroid surgery leading to vocal fold palsy (p. 220).

Physiology

TSH controls thyroid function. It acts by binding to TSH receptors on thyroid follicular cells. Synthesis of thyroid hormone requires adequate quantities of iodine that is actively transported into the thyroid cell as iodide. Within the cell, iodide is converted into iodine. Thyroglobulin is iodinated to form mono-iodotyrosine and di-iodotyrosine (this step is inhibited by carbimazole and propylthiouracil). The iodotyrosines are coupled to form triiodothyronine (T_3) and thyroxine (T_4).

In the blood the majority of T_3 and T_4 are almost completely bound to thyroxine-binding globulin (TBG, transthyretin) and to a much lesser extent to albumin. Only the free hormone is metabolically active and available to the tissues. Thyroid hormone influences growth and maturation of tissues, cell respiration, turnover of substrates and total energy expenditure. The regulation of thyroid function is detailed on page 393.

The parathyroid glands

Anatomy
The parathyroid glands are intimately related to the thyroid gland and are typically found on the posterolateral aspect of the upper thyroid poles (superior parathyroid glands) and immediately adjacent to the inferior thyroid pole (inferior parathyroid glands). Each gland measures approximately $5 \times 2 \times 1$ mm and weighs between 30 and 75 mg. The glands develop from the third and fourth pharyngeal pouches and during development can descend with the thymus into the chest. The parathyroid contains chief cells responsible for the synthesis of parathyroid hormone. The blood supply is from the inferior thyroid arteries.

Physiology
The function of the parathyroid gland is the regulation of serum calcium concentrations via parathyroid hormone (PTH) production. PTH is secreted by all four glands; its effects are summarized in Table 6.2.

The adrenal glands

Anatomy
The adrenal glands are two small, flat, yellowish bodies situated superior to each renal pole. The right gland is an irregular tetrahedron whereas the left gland is semilunar;

Table 6.2	Actions of parathyroid hormone
System	**Action**
Kidney	Promotes calcium reabsorption in the loop of Henle and the proximal tubule
Gastrointestinal tract	Promotes production of 1,25-dihydroxyvitamin D Promotes absorption of calcium by the increased production of 1,25-dihydroxyvitamin D
Bone	Mobilization of calcium from the exchangeable bone pool Increased bone turnover and remodelling (this can weaken cortical bone such as long bones but preserves cancellous bone density such as the vertebrae)

both glands measure approximately $5 \times 3 \times 1$ cm. The adrenal gland has an outer cortex and an inner medulla. From externally to internally, the cortex has three zones, the zona glomerulosa (produces aldosterone), zona fasciculata and zona reticularis (both of which produce cortisol and androgens).

Physiology
In the plasma, cortisol can exist in a free state or bound to protein. Only free cortisol (less than 5%) is physiologically active. The daily cortisol secretion ranges from 40 to 80 µmol with a pronounced circadian cycle. The daily aldosterone production ranges between 0.1 and 0.7 µmol and varies according to salt intake. The main effects are to regulate extracellular fluid volume and potassium metabolism. The main androgen secreted by the adrenal gland is dehydroepiandrosterone (DHEA); there are smaller amounts of 11β-hydroxyandrostenedione. The adrenal medulla contains chromaffin cells that secrete catecholamines (epinephrine, norepinephrine and dopamine).

Symptoms of endocrine disease

As the endocrine system controls many functions of the body, symptoms of endocrine disease can be multiple and varied.

Appetite and weight change
An increase in appetite and weight occurs with Cushing's syndrome and hypothalamic disease. An increase in appetite with decreasing weight is characteristic of hyperthyroidism, and decrease in appetite but increasing weight can occur with hypothyroidism.

Temperature tolerance and sweating
Patients with hyperthyroidism tend to feel warm and sweaty, and patients with hypothyroidism tend to feel cold. Increased sweating despite no difference in temperature can occur with phaeochromocytoma and with any cause of hypoglycaemia.

Body hair distribution
Loss of body hair can occur with adrenal insufficiency or hypogonadism. A generalized increase in body hair (hypertrichosis) can occur with many causes (p. 927). Those associated with excess hair growth in a male pattern distribution (hirsutism) tend to be associated with excess androgen production (p. 426).

Energy
Patients with hyperthyroidism tend to be very energetic, whereas patients with hypothyroidism and Addison's disease tend to be lethargic.

Skin changes
The skin becomes dry and coarse with hypothyroidism. Soft tissue overgrowth occurs with acromegaly (p. 409). Skin pigmentation can occur with primary adrenal insufficiency,

Cushing's syndrome and acromegaly. Depigmentation can occur as part of an autoimmune process with associated disease such as Hashimoto's thyroiditis and Addison's disease.

Polyuria

Excess urine losses can occur with diabetes mellitus and diabetes insipidus.

Examination of the endocrine system

Due to the many different functions of the endocrine glands, a full examination of the entire endocrine system is rarely performed. Clinical examination is usually restricted to disease process, gland or axes of interest (e.g. thyroid gland or multiple axes in pituitary disease).

The thyroid axis

Inspection

Examination of the thyroid gland starts with inspection. Patients with hyperthyroidism may appear thin and restless, lid lag is present, and proptosis and exophthalmos may be evident as a feature of hyperthyroidism due to Graves' disease. Conversely, patients with hypothyroidism may appear obese and lethargic with loss of eyebrows in the outer thirds.

Inspection of the neck may reveal an enlarged thyroid gland, which moves with swallowing (Fig. 6.1). There may be an associated horizontal scar (Kocher's incision) from previous surgery.

It is usual to ask the patient to stretch his or her hands straight out, and to spread the fingers apart to assess for any tremor (associated with hyperthyroidism). The fingers are also inspected for clubbing, which is a rare manifestation of Graves' disease (thyroid acropachy). The palms may be warm and sweaty with thyrotoxicosis. Tachycardia or an irregular pulse (atrial fibrillation) is associated with hyperthyroidism, whereas bradycardia is associated with hypothyroidism. Proximal myopathy is assessed by asking the patient to rise from a chair without the aid of the arms. Pretibial, non-pitting oedema is associated with Graves' disease. The ankle reflex is very brisk in thyrotoxicosis, whereas it is delayed in hypothyroidism.

Palpation

Palpation of the thyroid gland is performed with the examiner standing behind the patient. The size, consistency and mobility with swallowing are noted. Thyroid gland enlargement may occur in an inferior direction (retrosternal extension) in which case the lower border of the thyroid gland may not be palpable. Diffuse enlargement can occur with Graves' disease and with iodine deficiency goitre. A single nodule may feel soft (adenoma, single nodule in multinodular goitre), or firm (cyst) or stony hard (carcinoma, calcified cyst) or fibrotic. Tenderness is usually a feature of thyroiditis.

It is also important to examine the trachea to determine if it is in a central position.

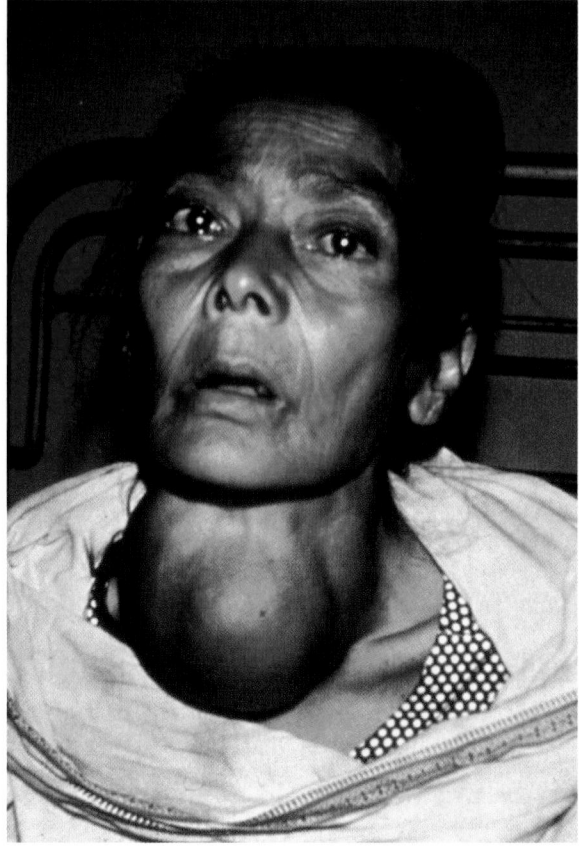

Fig. 6.1 Patient with a large goitre.

Auscultation

A bruit may be evident with Graves' disease.

The growth axis

Excessive secretion of growth hormone results in acromegaly.

Inspection

On first impression, the patient's facial features may appear coarsened with a prominent jaw, a prominent supraorbital ridge and thick lips. The tongue is large and the teeth are separated with malocclusion. The hands are enlarged and spade-like. Increased sweating may be noted due to increased metabolic rate. Skin tags may be evident, as may acanthosis nigricans which is indicative of insulin resistance (p. 435).

The eyes should be examined for a visual field defect that can occur with a pituitary adenoma (p. 399). The blood pressure should be taken to screen for hypertension, and a fasted blood glucose should be measured to screen for associated diabetes.

Palpation

The abdomen is examined for any evidence of organomegaly. The neck is examined for an enlarged thyroid gland (all organs are enlarged).

Auscultation

The lung fields are auscultated: coarse crepitations may be due to cardiac failure (p. 104).

The glucocorticoid axis

Patients with adrenocortical hypofunction (Addison's disease) tend to look cachectic, with pigmentation (p. 424) in the palmar creases, elbows and buccal mucosa. Vitiligo can occur as an associated autoimmune disease. Postural hypotension can occur due to mineralocorticoid deficiency.

The remaining section deals with the examination of patients with glucocorticoid excess (Cushing's syndrome).

Inspection

On inspection, patients may have facial fullness with central obesity and thin peripheries ('lemon on stick' appearance).

This is the characteristic appearance of steroid-induced fat redistribution. Thin skin, bruising and pink striae may be present, as may be acne and hirsutism. The patient may have difficulties rising from a squatting position due to a proximal myopathy. In the interscapular region there may be fat deposition leading to a 'hump'.

The visual fields should be inspected for defects, characteristically bitemporal hemianopia, associated with a pituitary adenoma. The blood pressure should be taken to screen for hypertension, and fasting blood glucose should be measured to screen for associated diabetes.

Palpation

The abdomen should be examined for any masses suggestive of an adrenal tumour, although enlargement sufficient to be detectable on clinical examination is rare.

SECTION 6.2 Investigations for endocrine disease

Tests of pituitary function

Basal anterior pituitary hormone profile

Evaluation of anterior pituitary endocrine function includes measurement of TSH, ACTH and FSH/LH levels that are assessed simultaneously with thyroxine, cortisol and oestrogen/testosterone, respectively. The test provides information on the endocrine feedback loops. PRL and insulin-like growth factor-1 (IGF-1, a marker for GH activity) are measured on their own.

Dynamic pituitary function tests

To determine the pituitary response to administered substances, stimulation tests are mostly used in suspected hormone deficiency and suppression tests in hormone excess. Dynamic function tests are used diagnostically and to assess response to therapy, especially postoperatively in pituitary surgery. Whilst hypothalamic releasing hormones (TRH, CRH, GnRH) provoke the pituitary secretion of TSH, ACTH and FSH/LH directly, an insulin tolerance test (ITT) acts indirectly by inducing hypoglycaemia, thereby triggering the counter-regulatory release of GH and ACTH. As an ITT is contraindicated in patients with established ischaemic heart disease or epilepsy, GH and ACTH reserve can alternatively be assessed by the glucagon test. GH release may also be assessed following the infusion of the amino acid arginine.

The glucocorticoid axis

24-hour urinary free cortisol

24-hour urinary free cortisol measurements serve as a screening test for hypercortisolaemia. Elevated levels correspond with cortisol excess. Normally the rate of urinary excretion is higher at night than in the day.

Low-dose dexamethasone suppression test

Dexamethasone suppression tests involve the measurement of cortisol after suppression of ACTH (trophic hormone).

The overnight dexamethasone suppression test is useful in the outpatient setting, in which 1 mg of dexamethasone administered at midnight normally suppresses the 9 a.m. cortisol level to less than 50 nmol/L. The false positive rate is <2% in normal individuals but can be as high as 20% in the obese or hospitalized patient.

The low-dose dexamethasone suppression test (0.5 mg 6-hourly for 48 h, with cortisol measurement at baseline and after 48 h) is preferred in obese or hospitalized patients. A normal result is a cortisol of <50 nmol/L at 48 hours. The loss of circadian rhythm in cortisol secretion can be demonstrated in the hospital by a detectable midnight cortisol (>50 nmol/L) taken while the patient is asleep.

Failure of cortisol suppression with low-dose dexamethasone implies autonomous cortisol secretion.

Basal plasma ACTH levels

Plasma levels of ACTH only reflect the instantaneous ACTH level. Low ACTH levels imply a pituitary defect or adrenal cortisol excess. High ACTH levels can arise from pituitary adenoma or ectopic sources.

High-dose dexamethasone suppression test

The high-dose dexamethasone suppression test is performed using 2 mg of dexamethasone administered 6-hourly for 48 h. Suppression (cortisol level <50% of the baseline value) implies a pituitary adenoma. Failure of suppression usually occurs with ectopic ACTH-secreting tumours that produce a large amount of ACTH. The high-dose dexamethasone suppression test has a false negative and false positive rate of 1%.

The mineralocorticoid axis

Mineralocorticoid suppression test

The aim of this test is to screen for autonomous aldosterone secretion. Intravenous normal saline is infused (500 mL over 4 hours) and normally suppresses plasma aldosterone to less than 220 pmol/L.

The thyroid axis

Free thyroxine

As the total thyroxine is not reflective of the metabolically active component, serum free thyroxine is the main clinical measurement. In hyperthyroidism, total and free thyroxine are increased, and the thyroid-binding globulin is decreased. The opposite happens with hypothyroidism.

Free triiodothyronine

Free T_3 is not routinely measured in thyroid function tests, as adequate information is obtained from TSH and free T_4. In the rare case where T_3 toxicosis is suspected, serum free T_3 can be assayed.

Thyroid-stimulating hormone

Measurement of basal TSH is the single most useful screening test for hyper- and hypothyroidism. TSH is low with hyperthyroidism and high with hypothyroidism.

Hypothalamic and pituitary disease

Hypothalamic disease

Diseases of the hypothalamus are rare. The functions of the hypothalamus include regulation of thirst, food intake, behaviour, the sleep–wake cycle and memory. Tumours affecting the hypothalamus include gliomas, craniopharyngiomas and germ cell tumours. Impairment of hypothalamic function only occurs when the disease process is bilateral, and symptoms of mass effects such as third ventricle obstruction or compression of the optic nerve, chiasm or optic tract can also occur.

Pituitary adenomas

Epidemiology

Pituitary adenomas are detected in 5–20% of autopsies. Clinically recognized adenomas are far less common, with an annual incidence estimated to be around 25 per million. Peak incidence is between 30 and 50 years of age with a possible female preponderance.

Pathology

The vast majority of pituitary tumours are benign: less than 0.5% of pituitary tumours are carcinomas. Pituitary adenomas are classified according to the predominant cell type and their immunohistochemical and electron microscopic properties into lactotrophs (PRL), somatotrophs (GH), corticotrophs (ACTH), gonadotrophs (LH, FSH), and thyrotrophs (TSH). Non-functioning adenomas (NFA) often contain secretory granules but do not cause endocrine excess, whilst other tumours may secrete more than one hormone. Anatomically, adenomas are arbitrarily defined by the size of greatest diameter as microadenomas (less than 10 mm) and macroadenomas (more than 10 mm).

NFA constitute the majority of macroadenomas and represent 25% of all pituitary adenomas. Lactotroph adenomas are predominantly microadenomas and are the most common functional cell type (40–50%), followed by somatotroph adenomas (30%), and corticotroph adenomas (20%). Gonadotroph and thyrotroph adenomas are rare, and up to 10% of adenomas may secrete more than one hormone.

Scope of disease

Mass effects

The optic chiasm lies above the pituitary fossa, and hence compression by a centrally enlarging gland can cause bitemporal hemianopia. Declining visual acuity and field defects confined to a single eye (due to asymmetrical tumour growth) may also occur. Overall, visual disturbances are present in up to 60% of patients. Headaches are usually due to the stretching of the dura mater overlying the pituitary fossa or, rarely, to hydrocephalus resulting from the obstruction of flow of cerebrospinal fluid (CSF). Lateral extension beyond the cavernous sinus can cause cranial nerve palsies and temporal lobe epilepsy (p. 605). Invasion into the hypothalamus may cause unusual symptoms such as increased appetite, thirst or coma. Ischaemic or haemorrhagic pituitary infarction (called apoplexy) occurs mostly in pre-existing adenomas. It frequently leads to hypopituitarism and uncommonly to acute compression of the optic chiasm by haemorrhagic enlargement of the gland.

Endocrine manifestations

Hypopituitarism is the most common endocrine disturbance associated with pituitary adenomas, followed by prolactin excess (p. 402). Growth hormone hypersecretion gives rise to acromegaly (p. 409), ACTH excess results in Cushing's disease (p. 423), and in very rare cases FSH or TSH secretion can lead to macro-orchidism or thyrotoxicosis, respectively.

Clinical features

The clinical presentation of patients with pituitary adenomas varies according to the symptoms related to mass effects and/or endocrine abnormalities. Frequently patients experience non-specific headaches and visual problems. Endocrine symptoms generally resemble the disorders of the target glands involved. Over- and underactivity of different axes often coexist and it is therefore essential to obtain a systematic endocrine history.

Physical examination also requires the screening of all endocrine axes for their potential involvement. Acromegaly and Cushing's syndrome may be evident due to their characteristic appearance, but the thyroid status requires formal assessment and signs of cortisol deficiency must be actively excluded.

Initial investigations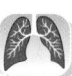

Basal anterior pituitary hormone profile

A complete evaluation of anterior pituitary endocrine function is necessary (p. 394) for the characterization of an adenoma and serves as a baseline for future monitoring of disease.

Dynamic function tests

Dynamic function tests (p. 397) are used diagnostically and to assess response to therapy, especially perioperatively to pituitary surgery. Whilst hypothalamic releasing hormones (TRH, CRH, GnRH) provoke the pituitary secretion of TSH, ACTH, FSH/LH directly, an insulin tolerance test (ITT) acts indirectly by inducing hypoglycaemia, thereby triggering the counter-regulatory release of GH and ACTH.

Perimetry

Although confrontational visual field testing at the bedside with a red pin is useful, formal Goldmann perimetry is required to detect subtle field defects and to allow their accurate comparison over time.

Magnetic resonance imaging (MRI) of the head

MRI is the modality of choice to visualize the soft tissues of the pituitary gland, the optic nerves and the peri-pituitary region. Non-malignant lesions in the pituitary fossa may also be detected on MRI. Pituitary adenomas may be of higher or lower signal intensity than the normally homogenous appearances of the normal pituitary gland (Fig. 6.2). Computed tomography (CT) may better delineate bone changes caused by tumour enlargement and calcifications within a suspected craniopharyngioma.

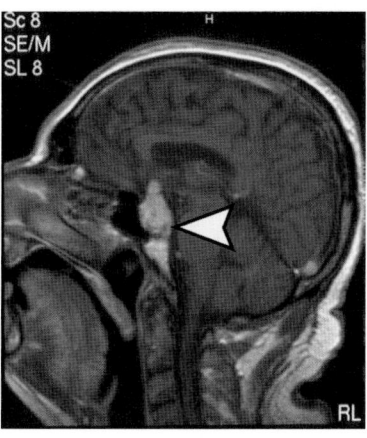

Fig. 6.2 MRI of the head illustrating a pituitary adenoma (arrow).

Medical management

For pituitary adenomas with normal endocrine function the relief of symptoms and avoidance of local complications due to mass effect is the primary therapeutic goal. Most tumours, however, require initial medical therapy to correct endocrine disturbances, followed by surgical resection and/or radiotherapy. Prolactinomas are usually managed by medical treatment alone.

Hormone replacement

In hypopituitarism (p. 400) the replacement of cortisol and thyroxine is of particular importance. The perioperative stress must be considered when deciding on the cortisol dose. Sex steroids and growth hormone can be replaced postoperatively if indicated.

Hormone antagonism

For hormone-producing adenomas specific drugs are available. Bromocriptine is effective in prolactinoma but the longer-acting cabergoline is more commonly used. Bromocriptine is also used in acromegaly as it inhibits GH release, but somatostatin analogues (octreotide and lanreotide) are more effective. Somatostatin analogues are the treatment of choice in TSH-producing adenomas. Whilst excess ACTH secretion in Cushing's disease cannot be suppressed at pituitary level, the adrenal glucocorticoid synthesis can be inhibited by metyrapone.

Surgical management

Transsphenoidal surgery

Transsphenoidal surgery refers to the surgical approach to the pituitary (transnasally through the sphenoid bone). It is indicated for virtually every type of pituitary tumour, including dopamine agonist-resistant prolactinomas and rapidly enlarging adenomas due to haemorrhagic infarction. Whilst microadenomas can often be completely removed, larger tumours with suprasellar extension may require a frontal craniotomy. This approach allows tumour debulking but is usually less successful in controlling

399

hormone excess. The mortality rate for transsphenoidal surgery is under 1%. Complications occur in 2%, consisting of persistent CSF rhinorrhoea with the risk of ascending infection, transient or permanent diabetes insipidus, oculomotor palsy and visual loss. Postoperative hypopituitarism develops in 3% of patients with a microadenoma. Therapeutic success and the need for postoperative hormone replacement are assessed by repeating the preoperative imaging and endocrine investigations. Follow-up of endocrine therapy and monitoring for tumour recurrence with visual field assessment is usually required for life.

Radiotherapy

External irradiation of the pituitary gland is an option if surgery is contraindicated or incomplete due to the size or anatomy of the tumour. It is usually performed through multiple fields. Radiotherapy takes effect over months and is most marked in the first two years, the regression slowing thereafter. Up to 50% of patients will have developed a degree of hypopituitarism 20 years following irradiation. As with pituitary surgery, life-long follow-up is indicated.

Prognosis

Non-functioning microadenomas can be cured by surgery alone in 80% or more. Large NFA treated with radiotherapy following surgery are cured in 95% or more.

Normalization of hormone excess following surgery alone has been reported for up to 90% of microadenomas but only for 65% of macroadenomas.

FURTHER INFORMATION

Pituitary tumours: recommendations for service provision and guidelines for management of patients. Consensus statement of a working party. London: Royal College of Physicians of London, 1997.

Hypopituitarism

Hypopituitarism is the deficiency of one or more of the pituitary hormones.

Epidemiology

The prevalence of hypopituitarism has been estimated at 29 per 100 000 with equal distribution in both sexes.[1] The average age at diagnosis is 45–46 years.[2]

Pathology

Hypopituitarism is often due to intrinsic pituitary disease, pituitary resection, radiotherapy or as a consequence of hypothalamic pathology. Non-functioning pituitary adenoma, craniopharyngiomas and prolactinomas account for the majority; other causes are listed in Table 6.3.

Table 6.3	Causes of hypopituitarism
Primary pituitary tumours	

Tumours adjacent to the pituitary
    Craniopharyngioma
    Meningioma
    Glioma
    Metastasis	

Iatrogenic
    Radiotherapy
    Neurosurgery	

Vascular
    Pituitary apoplexy
    Post-partum Sheehan's syndrome	

Infiltrative processes
    Sarcoid
    Haemochromatosis
    Langerhans' cell histiocytosis
    T-cell lymphocytic hypophysitis	

Infection
    Tuberculosis
    Abscess	

Traumatic	

Developmental
    Empty sella syndrome
    Posterior pituitary maldescent	

With pituitary tumours, hormone deficiencies often develop in a characteristic sequence over time. First affected is growth hormone, then the gonadotropins, followed by TSH and eventually ACTH. Prolactin may be elevated with stalk compression. Deficiency of posterior pituitary hormones is usually due to hypothalamic disease, as ADH and oxytocin can be secreted directly following synthesis.

CLINICAL ALERT

Chronic hypopituitarism has an insidious onset, but acute hypopituitarism is a medical emergency.

Clinical features

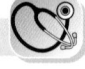

Presenting features of hypopituitarism depend on the endocrine axes affected (Table 6.4), as well as the severity and rate of onset of hormone deficiency. Clinical features may include secondary hypogonadism, reduced growth in children, secondary hypothyroidism, secondary adrenocortical deficiency and lactation failure.

Initial investigations

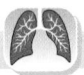

The aims of investigations are to confirm the presence of a hormone deficiency, exclude disease of the target organ and to test the pituitary hormone levels on maximum stimulation.

Table 6.4	Symptoms of hypopituitarism	
Hormone deficiency	**Symptoms**	**Hormone replacement**
ACTH	Symptoms of hypoadrenalism Fatigue Weight loss Nausea and vomiting Postural dizziness Circulatory compromise Pallor (simultaneous lack of α-melanocyte stimulating hormone) Hyperkalaemia does not occur as the mineralocorticoid production remains unaffected	Hydrocortisone
TSH	Symptoms of hypothyroidism Physical and mental lethargy Weight gain Constipation Susceptibility to the cold	L-thyroxine
LH/FSH	Oligo/amenorrhoea and vaginal dryness in women Erectile dysfunction and reduced secondary sexual hair (less frequent shaving) in men Reduced libido in both sexes	Oestrogen and progesterone for women, testosterone for men
Growth hormone	Fatigability Reduced sense of well-being Withdrawal from social contacts Difficulties coping with full-time employment	Growth hormone

ACTH, adrenocorticotropic hormone; TSH, thyroid-stimulating hormone; LH/FSH, luteinizing hormone/follicle-stimulating hormone.

Basal hormone levels

The screening profile includes cortisol (taken at 9 am), TSH and free T_4, LH, FSH and oestradiol (women) or testosterone (men), as well as prolactin and IGF-1.

Further investigations

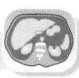

Combined pituitary stimulation test

This potentially dangerous investigation is indicated in patients with low target and trophic hormones on initial screening tests. After an overnight fast, insulin is injected to produce symptomatic hypoglycaemia. TRH and GnRH are injected and blood samples are taken. Normally, cortisol and growth hormone rise in response to hypoglycaemia, TSH and prolactin in response to TRH, and LH/FSH following GnRH administration.

Medical management

Management is generally directed to replacing the deficient hormones.

Hormone replacement

Hydrocortisone is used for glucocorticoid replacement, in two or three divided doses, to mimic the physiological plasma peaks and troughs, with the largest dose given on rising. Due to its longer half-life, prednisolone is less frequently used for this indication. Therapy is monitored clinically and by timed cortisol levels. Patients on glucocorticoid replace-ment must be educated never to stop treatment abruptly, to increase the dose during illness, to carry a steroid card and wear a MedicAlert bracelet. Replacement therapy with L-thyroxine is monitored according to clinical response and thyroxine levels as TSH is no longer a useful indicator. In women, sex steroid replacement therapy consists of oestrogen/progesterone preparations, whereas in men testosterone is given. Treatment should be monitored clinically and biochemically. If fertility is desired, pulsatile LH and FSH can be given in specialist centres. Adult growth hormone replacement therapy is available but costly. IGF-1 levels are used to monitor treatment. Symptoms of prolactin deficiency only occur in women during the post-partum period, when lactation fails. No replacement therapy is available.

Prognosis

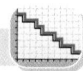

Patients with hypopituitarism have excess mortality, predominantly from vascular and respiratory disease. The median time of survival after diagnosis is 11 years for men and 10 years for women.[2]

REFERENCES

(1) *Regal M, Paramo C, Sierra SM, Garcia-Mayor RV. Prevalence and incidence of hypopituitarism in an adult Caucasian population in northwestern Spain. Clinical Endocrinology (Oxf) 2001; 55: 735–740.*
(2) *Tomlinson JW, Holden N, Hills RK, et al. Association between premature mortality and hypopituitarism. West Midlands Prospective Hypopituitary Study Group. Lancet 2001; 357: 425–431.*

Hyperprolactinaemia and prolactinoma

Epidemiology

Hyperprolactinaemia is the most common disorder of the anterior pituitary. Prolactinomas are the most common functional tumour of the pituitary, accounting for 30%. On post-mortem examination, up to 10% of the population have evidence of pituitary microadenomas staining for prolactin, the vast majority with no documented endocrine disturbance.

Pathology

Prolactin (PRL) secretion is under tonic inhibition by dopamine. Prolactin prepares the breast tissue for milk production. Hyperprolactinaemia interferes with GnRH and gonadotrophin release leading to disturbed sexual function and fertility. Consequent oestrogen deficiency may contribute to osteoporosis.

Hyperprolactinaemia can be caused by a wide range of conditions (Table 6.5), the most common of which are dopamine antagonistic drugs and untreated hypothyroidism (TRH stimulates prolactin release). Prolactinomas (and 30% of somatotroph adenomas) secrete prolactin autonomously whereas other pituitary or hypothalamic tumours can disrupt the inhibitory dopaminergic pathways by compression of the pituitary stalk leading to uninhibited prolactin secretion. Pre-menopausal women are more frequently found to have a microadenoma, probably because menstrual disturbances prompt earlier investigations. Post-menopausal women and men tend to present with larger tumours. Prolactinomas are the most common pituitary adenomas associated with multiple endocrine neoplasia type 1.

Table 6.5	Causes of hyperprolactinaemia

Dopamine antagonist drugs
  Antiemetics
  Neuroleptics
  Opiates
  Antihypertensives	

Raised thyrotropin-releasing hormone in primary hypothyroidism	

Physiological
  Stress
  Pregnancy
  Suckling
  Intercourse	

Prolactinoma	
Pituitary stalk compression	
Advanced renal failure (reduced clearance)	
Macroprolactinaemia	

Hyperprolactinaemia can also be due to the presence of macroprolactin, which is a high molecular weight IgG–prolactin complex with reduced bioactivity. Patients with macroprolactinaemia are asymptomatic and do not require treatment as prolactin levels measured after precipitation are often normal.

Clinical features

Spontaneous or expressible galactorrhoea is present in up to 80% of women and 20% of men. Oligo/amenorrhoea and symptoms of oestrogen deficiency are common in women of childbearing age. Men less frequently seek attention with loss of libido, erectile dysfunction or gynaecomastia. Reduced fertility affects both sexes. Large pituitary adenomas may give rise to visual disturbances and headaches. Symptoms of hypopituitarism may be present.

Initial investigations

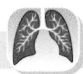

Prolactin levels

Prolactin levels may provide an indication as to the aetiology of hyperprolactinaemia. Values >6000 mU/L are suggestive of a macroprolactinoma, and values up to 3000 mU/L suggest a microadenoma or pituitary stalk compression. Drugs and other pathological conditions mostly cause only a moderate elevation in prolactin levels.

Thyroid function tests

Hypothyroidism must be excluded.

Pregnancy test

A pregnancy test may be indicated to screen for causes of hyperprolactinaemia if there is any doubt.

Further investigations

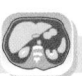

Basal anterior pituitary hormone profile

The anterior pituitary function should be investigated if there is clinical suspicion of hypopituitarism (p. 400).

MRI of the head

MRI of the pituitary is indicated to exclude a pituitary tumour causing stalk compression.

Initial management

Identify and address any underlying cause

In cases of drug-induced hyperprolactinaemia, replacing the offending medication should be attempted but may not always be possible. Neuroleptic drugs may need to be continued and following the exclusion of a pituitary tumour, sex steroid replacement therapy and monitoring may be all that can be offered. Other underlying disorders should be treated as appropriate.

Medical management

Treatment of hyperprolactinaemia is aimed at the restoration of gonadal function and the reversal of galactorrhoea. In macroprolactinomas further goals are tumour size reduction and avoidance of mass effects.

Dopamine agonists

In prolactinomas dopamine agonists are the first-line therapy as they reduce prolactin levels and tumour size. This includes macroprolactinomas with mass effect as long as close monitoring can be provided. Cabergoline is most frequently used as it is more effective and better tolerated than bromocriptine.

Surgical management

Transsphenoidal surgery

Transsphenoidal surgery is reserved for cases with features of tumour compression refractory to medical therapy. Cure is achieved only in around a third of patients and surgery carries the additional risk of hypopituitarism.

Radiation therapy

External pituitary irradiation lowers prolactin levels but leads to hypopituitarism and requires years to take full effect, during which time dopamine agonists are required.

Prognosis

Hyperprolactinaemia without an identifiable cause spontaneously resolves in a third of patients, up to 15% experience a rise in prolactin, and in half there is no change. Untreated microprolactinomas also regress in around a third of cases, enlarge in less than 20%, and remain stable in the remainder. In these patient groups the need for dopamine

Table 6.6	Causes of diabetes insipidus
Central diabetes insipidus	

Trauma (30%)
    Head injury
    Neurosurgery (diabetes insipidus complicates 20% of cases but is often transient)	

Intracranial tumours or infiltration (20%)	
Congenital (5%)	
Idiopathic (30%)	
Nephrogenic diabetes insipidus	

Electrolyte disorders
    Hypokalaemia
    Hypercalcaemia	

Interstitial kidney disease	

Drugs
    Lithium
    Demeclocycline
    Vincristine	

agonist therapy should be reassessed at intervals. Macroprolactinomas may require life-long medical therapy.

i FURTHER INFORMATION

Biller BM, Luciano A, Crosignani PG, et al. Guidelines for the diagnosis and treatment of hyperprolactinemia. Journal of Reproductive Medicine 1999; 44(12 Suppl): 1075–1084.

Diabetes insipidus

Diabetes insipidus is characterized by passing large volumes of dilute or insipid urine due to failure of vasopressin release (central) or failure of the kidneys (nephrogenic) to respond to vasopressin.

Epidemiology

Diabetes insipidus has an estimated prevalence of 4 per 100 000 and affects both sexes equally. Congenital forms of diabetes insipidus occur at a frequency of 1 per 100 000 live births, with an X-linked inheritance in 90%.

Pathology

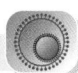

The underlying causes of central (cranial) and nephrogenic diabetes are listed in Table 6.6. Central diabetes insipidus can arise from any hypothalamic disease that interferes with ADH synthesis. Following brain injury a triphasic response is observed. The initial polyuria due to loss of neural control is followed by a transient normalization of urine output due to the release of stored ADH from the damaged neurones. Eventually polyuria recurs due to the absence of further ADH synthesis and depletion of these stores.

In nephrogenic diabetes insipidus the tubules and collecting ducts are resistant to the effects of ADH. Common causes are electrolyte disorders (hypokalaemia or hypercalcaemia), interstitial kidney disease and drugs (e.g. lithium, demeclocycline, vincristine).

Both forms can be transient or permanent and of varying severity. An important differential diagnosis is primary 'psychogenic' polydipsia, where intentional excess water consumption is followed by polyuria, or disease causing dryness of the mouth where excess water is drunk for symptomatic relief. As adequate cortisol levels are necessary for renal water excretion, diabetes insipidus may be unmasked by successful steroid replacement.

Scope of disease

Large, rapid fluid and osmotic shifts can lead to severe dehydration with cardiovascular, renal and central nervous system (CNS) dysfunction. This may be compounded by the loss of thirst sensation associated with hypothalamic disease or reduced consciousness. During pregnancy increased placental breakdown of ADH can aggravate the disorder.

Clinical features

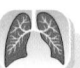

The main symptoms are persistent polyuria, nocturia, thirst and polydipsia. The onset of central diabetes insipidus is usually more abrupt than nephrogenic diabetes insipidus. If access to fluids is denied, dehydration may lead to encephalopathy with irritability, clouding of consciousness, ataxia, hyperthermia, hypotension and coma. Nocturia is uncommon with primary polydipsia.

Initial investigations

24-hour urine collection
Diagnostic polyuria of more than 3 litres in 24 hours should be confirmed and osmotic diuresis due to diabetes mellitus should be excluded. Urine osmolality in complete diabetes insipidus, when water is not drunk, is usually less than 200 mOsm/kg. In partial diabetes insipidus it may be higher but remains inappropriately low for matched serum osmolality.

Urea and electrolytes
Renal function may be impaired with nephrogenic diabetes insipidus. Hypokalaemia and hypercalcaemia should be excluded. Serum sodium and osmolality are at the upper limits of normal with diabetes insipidus, whereas with psychogenic polydipsia dilutional hyponatraemia may be present.

Further investigations

Water deprivation test
A formal water deprivation test (Table 6.7) with response to desmopressin (an ADH analogue) may help in differen-

Table 6.7	The water deprivation test
The patient is allowed fluids during the 12 hours prior to the test, except for caffeine-containing beverages and alcohol, but is not permitted to smoke	
During the test no fluid intake is allowed and the patient must remain supervised at all times. Urine is collected hourly for volume and osmolality, and serum samples 2-hourly for osmolality. After 8 hours 2 μg desmopressin is administered and urine and serum are sampled for a further 2 hours. The patient is weighed hourly and the test terminated if more than 5% of body weight is lost. The test is also stopped if serum osmolality rises to >305 mOsm/kg, with a diagnosis of diabetes insipidus then made	
A normal test results in a rise in urine osmolality to >750 mOsm/kg. In diabetes insipidus the urine osmolality remains inappropriately low (<300 mOsm/kg) despite a rise in serum osmolality. Following desmopressin there is a rise in urine osmolality to >750 mOsm/kg in central but not in nephrogenic diabetes insipidus. Partial diabetes insipidus as well as long-standing primary polydipsia, in which the concentrating ability of the renal medulla may be impaired, often give intermediate results that can be difficult to interpret	

tiating between partial forms of central (desmopressin responsive) and nephrogenic diabetes insipidus (desmopressin unresponsive). Alternatively, ADH release can be measured following the infusion of hypertonic saline.

CT/MRI of the brain
MRI of the brain may be indicated to establish the aetiology in central diabetes insipidus.

Initial management

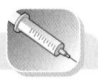

Increase fluid intake
Partial diabetes insipidus with normal thirst sensation may be managed by maintaining appropriate fluid input.

Identify and address any underlying cause
In nephrogenic diabetes insipidus the underlying cause should be corrected and any offending drugs omitted. Psychiatric input may be required in primary polydipsia.

Medical management

Desmopressin
In severe cases of central diabetes insipidus, desmopressin is the drug of choice. It has greater antidiuretic properties and a longer half-life than ADH. It can be administered orally, nasally and parenterally. Urine volume as well as serum sodium and osmolality guides the dosage. Excessive desmopressin leads to hyponatraemia and hypo-osmolality.

In nephrogenic diabetes insipidus, high-dose desmopressin may be useful. Thiazide diuretics may also be used to induce sodium depletion (decreased delivery of sodium to the ascending loop of Henle results in a reduced capacity to dilute urine).

Prognosis

The prognosis depends on the underlying aetiology. The condition is not life-threatening as long as there is access to fluid. Hypertonic encephalopathy has a mortality of up to 50%.

i FURTHER INFORMATION

Baylis PH, Cheetham T. Diabetes insipidus. Archives of Disease in Childhood 1998; 79: 84–89.

Syndrome of inappropriate antidiuretic hormone secretion

Epidemiology

The syndrome of inappropriate ADH secretion (SIADH) is the most common cause of hyponatraemia. It has an incidence of 70 per 100 000 per year that varies widely according to the population studied.

Pathology

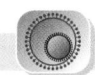

Persistent ADH secretion (or enhanced renal action) causes renal reabsorption of water and results in dilutional hyponatraemia. Fluid retention due to inappropriate ADH secretion is mild and affects the intra- and extracellular space equally, therefore peripheral oedema is absent. The brain is the organ most susceptible to acute changes in serum sodium concentration and osmotic and fluid shifts, but it adapts well to hyponatraemia of gradual onset.

Clinical features

The diagnosis of SIADH can only be made in euvolaemic patients; most of those with mild or chronic SIADH are asymptomatic. Severe acute hyponatraemia can cause irritability, confusion, headache and nausea (serum sodium below 125 mmol/L) progressing to seizures, coma and death (serum sodium below 110 mmol/L) due to the development of cerebral oedema. Abnormalities in renal, liver, adrenal and thyroid function have to be excluded.

Investigations

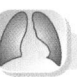

Paired serum and urine osmolality
Simultaneous measurements of serum and urine osmolalities show an inappropriately concentrated urine (>100 mOsm/kg) with serum hypo-osmolality (<270 mOsm/kg). Urinary sodium excretion is inappropriately elevated (>20 mmol/L).

Management

Identify and address underlying cause
Wherever possible the underlying cause (Table 6.8) should be treated.

Fluid restriction
The correction of hyponatraemia should occur gradually to avoid rapid osmotic shifts that might potentially lead to central pontine demyelination. In most cases fluid restriction of 0.5 to 1 L per day is sufficient to normalize hyponatraemia.

Demeclocycline
Demeclocycline induces a reversible state of nephrogenic diabetes insipidus and should be considered in symptomatic patients with severe hyponatraemia (<110 mmol/L) who do not respond to fluid restriction.

Table 6.8	Causes of the syndrome of inappropriate antidiuretic hormone secretion
Pulmonary disease	
Pneumonia	
Tuberculosis	
Lung abscess	
Empyema	
Positive pressure ventilation	
Central nervous system disorders	
Head injuries	
Stroke	
Meningitis	
Encephalitis	
Drugs	
Carbamazepine	
Chlorpropamide	
Psychotropic drugs	
Chemotherapeutic agents	
Ectopic ADH secretion	
Small cell cancer of the lung	
Carcinoma of the pancreas	
Thymoma	
Haematological malignancies	

Hypertonic saline
Severe hyponatraemia with seizures or coma can be corrected by infusion of hypertonic saline. The rate of correction should not exceed 0.5 mmol/L per hour due to the risk of precipitating central pontine demyelination. Serum sodium levels must be monitored frequently.

Prognosis

The outcome is dependent on the underlying disease. Symptomatic hyponatraemia with serum sodium of less than 110 mmol/L carries a mortality risk of more than 25%.

𝒾 FURTHER INFORMATION

Baylis PH. The syndrome of inappropriate antidiuretic hormone secretion. International Journal of Biochemistry and Cell Biology 2003; 35: 1495–1499.

The growth axis

Growth hormone deficiency

Epidemiology

The prevalence of growth hormone deficiency in children is estimated at 27 per 100 000 with up to 50% recovering when linear growth is complete. Idiopathic deficiency is the most common cause, occurring in approximately 1 in 5000 live births. Adult-onset growth hormone deficiency is much less common: the prevalence is estimated at 10 per 100 000. If both adult-onset and persisting childhood disease are included, the prevalence is 30 per 100 000 adults.

Pathology

In most children, the underlying pathology is unknown and the disease is classified as idiopathic growth hormone deficiency. It is not considered to be hereditary and no clear genetic component has been found. A small proportion of children have acquired growth hormone deficiency as a result of damage to the pituitary or hypothalamus, for instance from severe head injury or brain tumours such as craniopharyngioma. Adult-onset growth hormone deficiency is almost invariably due to hypothalamic or pituitary damage as growth hormone deficiency is an early feature (p. 396).

Scope of disease

Children with growth hormone deficiency have a linear growth rate that is a half to a third of normal and end up with a reduced final height. Growth hormone deficiency also has a deleterious effect on muscle mass and bone remodelling.

In adults, growth hormone deficiency may be asymptomatic or lead to non-specific symptoms such as fatigue and poor sense of well-being resulting from derangements of protein, carbohydrate and lipid metabolism. Several epidemiological studies have demonstrated increased risks of cardiovascular mortality in adults with growth hormone deficiency. Muscle mass and bone density are also reduced.

Clinical features
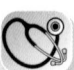

In children, the most prominent feature is 'failure to thrive' or a slow growth rate. Parents might notice that the child is wearing clothes that are smaller than for his or her age. Teachers may comment that the child is the shortest in the class and is unable to keep up with physical activities. Regular measurements of the child's height may reveal lack of progress (less than 5 cm gain per year).

In adults, growth hormone deficiency alone is difficult to diagnose as the signs and symptoms are non-specific. Clinical features include fatigue and lack of energy, changes in body composition with reduced lean mass and increased fat mass, osteopenia, dry skin from reduced sweating, reduced muscle strength, lipid abnormalities and insulin resistance. In view of the non-specific presentation, growth hormone deficiency in adults should be suspected if clinical evaluation uncovers evidence of hypothalamic or pituitary damage or other hormone deficiencies.

Initial investigations

Insulin-like growth factor-1
Measurement of growth hormone is not routinely performed as there is difficulty in establishing a normal range. Single random sampling is unhelpful as growth hormone is secreted intermittently in a pulsatile fashion. Moreover, growth hormone levels in adults are usually low and measurement in normal individuals may yield undetectable levels.

Because of the long half-life of IGF-1, it is often used as a screening test for growth hormone deficiency although levels may remain within the normal reference range in severe GH deficiency in up to 50% of patients. Low levels should prompt further investigations but can also occur in malnutrition, renal disease, hepatic disease and with poorly controlled diabetes mellitus.

Further investigations
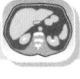

Pharmacological stimulation tests
A well-known pharmacological stimulation test is the insulin tolerance test, which involves administering insulin to provoke hypoglycaemia, and measuring peak growth hormone levels. Growth hormone deficiency is diagnosed with peak levels below 3 µg/L (10 mU/L) in adults and 10 µg/L in children. This test should only be performed under close supervision in expert centres as there is a small risk of death. Other tests use glucagon, arginine or growth hormone releasing hormone (GHRH) as stimulating agents.

MRI of the head
MRI of the brain is performed to elucidate any pathology affecting the hypothalamus or pituitary gland.

Initial management
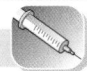

Replacement of other hormone deficiencies
There is usually no urgent need to start growth hormone therapy in adults, and patients should be treated for any other pituitary hormone deficiencies first.

Medical management

Growth hormone replacement
The benefits and harm of growth hormone therapy, plus the inconvenience, can then be weighed up carefully before any decision to commence treatment. Currently, growth hormone is produced by recombinant DNA technology, eliminating the risk of Creutzfeldt–Jakob disease that occurred when cadaver-derived growth hormone was used in the past. As the hormone is a peptide which is digested by stomach acid, the treatment must be given by daily subcutaneous injections.

Treatment of children must be initiated before the epiphyses have fused, and initiation of therapy at a younger age results in increased growth with final height gains of 8–11 cm over children who are untreated. Treatment can be stopped in children who show little improvement (less than 50% increase of growth velocity over the baseline values) in the first year of therapy, when final height is attained, or when the growth velocity has tailed off.

In adults, growth hormone therapy has beneficial effects on bone density and a potentially favourable impact on lipids, but there are no data confirming a survival benefit. Growth hormone therapy is recommended in selected patients[1,2] starting at a low dose and titrated upwards based on symptomatic benefit, normalization of insulin-like growth factor levels, improvement in lipid profile and improvement in waist-to-hip ratio as well as body composition including bone density.

Common adverse effects of growth hormone are fluid retention, carpal tunnel syndrome, arthralgias and myalgia. More serious manifestations include benign intracranial hypertension and the development of insulin resistance. As growth hormone has stimulatory effects, it should not be given to patients with active malignant disease.

Prognosis

Most children respond to growth hormone replacement therapy. Adults receiving growth hormone report improvements to the quality of life, although as yet there is no evidence of a survival benefit.

REFERENCES

(1) American Association of Clinical Endocrinologists. American Association of Clinical Endocrinologists medical guidelines for clinical practice for growth hormone use in adults and children—2003 update. Endocrine Practice 2003; 9(1): 64–76.
(2) National Institute for Clinical Excellence. Guidance on the use of human growth hormone (somatropin) in children with growth failure. Technology Appraisal No. 42. London: NICE, 2002.

Acromegaly

Acromegaly is an insidious disorder usually caused by a pituitary adenoma secreting growth hormone, resulting in bony and soft tissue overgrowth.

Epidemiology

The prevalence of acromegaly is approximately 4–6 per 100 000, with an annual incidence of 0.4 per 100 000 per year.[1] Both sexes are equally affected, typically in the 40–60-year age range with a mean age at presentation of 44 years.

Pathology

A pituitary adenoma is by far the most common cause of acromegaly; rarely, acromegaly can be caused by a hypothalamic or ectopic growth hormone releasing hormone (GHRH) tumour.

Scope of disease

Acromegaly may manifest singly or via a combination of clinical features of growth hormone excess, local tumour effects (p. 398) or hypopituitarism (p. 400).

Acromegaly is a multisystem disease. Elevated growth hormone levels lead to appositional bone growth, most marked in the facial bones, hands and feet, i.e. shoe size, hat size and ring size increase. Cartilage hypertrophy and soft tissue overgrowth can lead to osteoarthritis, kyphoscoliosis and nerve entrapment syndromes. Growth hormone excess can also lead to enlargement of the heart, thyroid, liver and kidney.

Hypertension occurs in approximately 40%, and insulin resistance in 40% (caused by growth hormone excess) can result in 20% developing diabetes mellitus. Acromegaly is also associated with multiple endocrine neoplasia (MEN) type 1 in approximately 5%.

RECENT ADVANCES

An approximately 2-fold increase in the risk of colorectal cancer has recently been reported in patients with acromegaly.[2]

Clinical features

As the onset of symptoms and signs is insidious, the diagnosis of acromegaly is, on average, delayed by 9 years. An index of suspicion is key to the diagnosis, as confirmatory tests are easily performed.

Sweating, seen in >80% patients, and headaches are the main symptoms, and patients may volunteer information such as increasing shoe, glove or hat size. Other complaints include tiredness and paraesthesia of the hand and feet (nerve entrapment) or arthralgia.

Growth hormone deficiency

Acromegaly

On examination there may be coarse features with prominent supraorbital ridges (Fig. 6.3), large ears, nose, tongue (macroglossia) and a large lower jaw causing the lower row of teeth to extend further than the upper row (prognathism). There may be large gaps in the teeth (interdental separation) with laryngeal thickening giving a deep voice. The hands may appear large (spade-like) with thickened and sweaty skin. The thenar eminence may be wasted (carpal tunnel syndrome) and proximal muscle weakness may be present.

In addition, patients may also present with the mass effects of pituitary adenoma or hypopituitarism. Finally, it is important to screen for associated diseases such as hypertension, diabetes mellitus and cardiomegaly. The clinical features are summarized in Table 6.9.

Initial investigations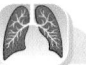

(Growth hormone) glucose suppression test

Due to the pulsatile secretion of growth hormone, random growth hormone levels are of little diagnostic value.

The glucose suppression test is carried out in the same way as an oral glucose tolerance test (therefore the same test also screens for diabetes mellitus). After administration of 75 g of glucose orally, serial plasma levels of growth hormone are taken. An elevated growth hormone level that fails to suppress to less than 2 mU/L with rising glucose levels is diagnostic of autonomic secretion. A normal response is to suppress GH to undetectable levels.

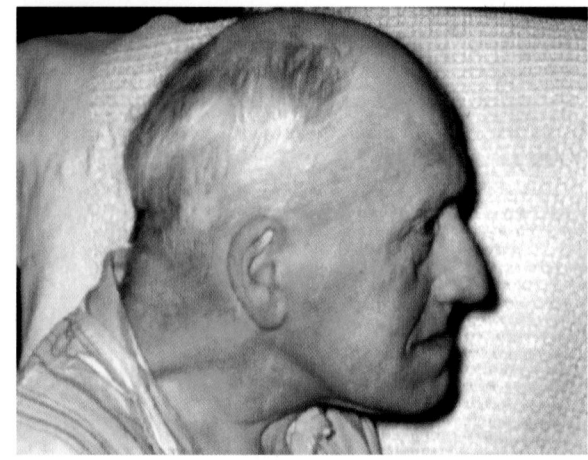

Fig. 6.3 Patient with acromegaly.

Further investigations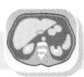

Once the diagnosis is established, further tests are indicated.

Anterior pituitary function tests

Tests of anterior pituitary function are important to screen for hypopituitarism (p. 400). Moreover, prolactin levels are elevated in up to a third of patients due to stalk compression or co-secretion.

Table 6.9	Clinical features of acromegaly	
Location	**Effect of disease**	**Clinical feature**
Hands and heel pad	Skin thickening	Soft, 'doughy' consistency
Wrist	Soft tissue overgrowth, carpal tunnel syndrome	Paraesthesia (Tinel's positive) and thenar wasting
Hands and feet	Enlargement	Spade-like shape, increasing ring, glove and shoe size
Skin (neck/axillae)	Insulin resistance	Acanthosis nigricans
Eyes	Compression of optic chiasm	Bitemporal hemianopia
Fundus	Raised intracranial pressure, degeneration of Bruch's membrane, hypertension, diabetes	Papilloedema, angioid streaks, hypertensive/diabetic retinopathy
Jaw and teeth	Prognathism and interdental spacing	Poor occlusion, overbiting of teeth, arthritis of temporomandibular joint
Tongue	Enlargement	Teeth imprint, snoring, sleep apnoea, difficult intubation
Larynx	Enlargement and vocal cord thickening	Deepening and huskiness of voice
Cardiovascular system	Cardiomegaly, hypertension	Congestive heart failure, atherosclerosis
Thyroid gland	Enlargement	Goitre
Muscle	Proximal weakness	Difficulties climbing stairs
Axial skeleton	Accelerated osteoarthritis	Back pain, kyphosis
Metabolism	Diabetes mellitus/hypercalciuria	Thirst, polyuria, blurred vision, renal stones
Testes or ovaries/other peripheral glands	Hypogonadism/hypopituitarism	Soft, small testes or oligo/amenorrhoea

Goldmann perimetry

Formal visual field assessment is required to screen for bitemporal hemianopia as many adenomas causing acromegaly are relatively large and may compress the optic chiasm.

MRI of head

MRI provides excellent definition of the pituitary and tumour size.

Initial management

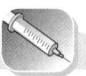

Apart from normalization of growth hormone levels, other therapeutic goals include the reversal of any mass effect of the pituitary tumour and treatment of hypopituitarism.

Concomitant diabetes and hypertension should be treated appropriately, although both usually improve with the correction of growth hormone excess.

Surgical management

Transsphenoidal surgery

Transsphenoidal surgery is the management of choice for patients with acromegaly. However, medical therapy is often administered to normalize growth hormone levels prior to surgery. Under general anaesthesia, and with the assistance of an image intensifier, the sella is approached through the sphenoid. A lumbar subarachnoid drainage catheter may be sited to introduce saline into the subarachnoid space, lowering the pituitary tumour into the operative field. Although complete resection is the aim, the extent of resection that can be achieved depends on the size, shape, location and consistency.

On average, surgery has a 60% success rate of lowering growth hormone to baseline levels, and is more likely to be beneficial in those with microadenomas (40–90% success) than larger, invasive tumours (10–48% success).[3] The rate of major postoperative complications is 8% and includes permanent diabetes insipidus, hypopituitarism, CSF leak and meningitis. The recurrence rate is 7% at a median time interval of 7.9 years.[4]

Medical management

Drug therapy is used in patients with residual disease after transsphenoidal surgery (persistent elevation of IGF-1 and growth hormone, or residual symptoms and signs of acromegaly). At present, somatostatin analogues are the mainstay of medical therapy, while dopamine agonists and growth hormone receptor antagonists are second-line agents. GH receptor antagonists are a newer addition.

Somatostatin analogues

These drugs (e.g. octreotide, lanreotide) inhibit growth hormone secretion by activating somatostatin receptors of pituitary tumours. Suppression of growth hormone and normalization of IGF-1 is achieved in 50–60%, and tumour shrinkage occurs in a third.[5]

Somatostatin analogues are generally well tolerated, although transient gastrointestinal adverse effects such as nausea, abdominal pain and diarrhoea are common during initiation of therapy. The main drawbacks of these agents are cost and the need for monthly intramuscular injections. Gallstones are also a recognized complication.

Dopamine agonists

Bromocriptine was the first drug to show benefit in acromegaly but it is successful only about 10–20% of the time. Newer, long-acting dopamine agonists (e.g. cabergoline) are efficacious in 30–40% of patients and may cause less dopaminergic related adverse effects such as nausea and vomiting.[6] Although dopamine agonists are less effective than somatostatin analogues, they are cheaper and can be administered orally.

> **RECENT ADVANCES**
>
> *Growth hormone receptor antagonism can now be achieved by pegvisomant, a genetically altered growth hormone-like molecule. Although it does not reduce GH secretion, pegvisomant has a success rate of about 90% in normalizing IGF-1.[6] It is currently recommended for patients who are refractory to, or intolerant of, somatostatin analogue therapy.*

Radiotherapy

Radiotherapy is indicated for patients with residual disease after surgery or failure of medical therapy. One disadvantage of radiotherapy is its slow onset of effect (4–6 years to achieve full effect) and concomitant medical therapy is usually required to bridge the latency period. After 10 years of radiotherapy, more than 60% develop hypopituitarism, and other complications include optic neuropathy, secondary intracranial neoplasms and temporal lobe radiation injury.

Prognosis

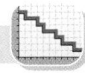

Untreated acromegaly is associated with a 2-fold increased mortality compared to matched population controls. This is mainly due to cardiovascular, cerebrovascular and respiratory disease. However, normalization of growth hormone levels reduces expected mortality back to the population baseline.[7]

i FURTHER INFORMATION

Melmed S, Casanueva FF, Cavagnini F, et al. Acromegaly Treatment Consensus Workshop Participants. Guidelines for acromegaly management. Journal of Clinical Endocrinology and Metabolism 2002; 87: 4054–4058.

Growth hormone deficiency

Acromegaly

409

REFERENCES

(1) *Holdaway IM, Rajasoorya C. Epidemiology of acromegaly. Pituitary 1999; 2: 29–41.*

(2) *Renehan AG, O'Connell J, O'Halloran D, Shanahan F, Potten CS, O'Dwyer ST, Shalet SM. Acromegaly and colorectal cancer: a comprehensive review of epidemiology, biological mechanisms, and clinical implications. Hormone and Metabolic Research 2004; 36: 70–71.*

(3) *Gittoes NJL, Sheppard MC, Johnson AP, Stewart PM. Outcome of surgery for acromegaly—the experience of a dedicated pituitary surgeon. QJM 1999; 92: 741–745.*

(4) *Abosch A, Tyrrell JB, Lamborn KR, Hannegan LT, Applebury CB, Wilson CB. Transsphenoidal microsurgery for growth hormone-secreting pituitary adenomas: initial outcome and long-term results. Journal of Clinical Endocrinology and Metabolism 1998; 83: 3411–3418.*

(5) *Freda PU. Somatostatin analogs in acromegaly. Journal of Clinical Endocrinology and Metabolism 2002; 87: 3013–3018.*

(6) *Paisley AN, Trainer P, Drake W. Medical treatment in acromegaly. Current Opinion in Pharmacology 2003; 3: 672–677.*

(7) *Holdaway IM, Rajasoorya RC, Gamble GD. Factors influencing mortality in acromegaly. Journal of Clinical Endocrinology and Metabolism 2004; 89: 667–674.*

SECTION 6.5 · The thyroid gland

Hypothyroidism

Hypothyroidism is the clinical condition resulting from deficiency of thyroid hormones. Myxoedema is severe hypothyroidism with accumulation of mucopolysaccharides in the tissues. It leads to thickening of the facial features and gives a doughy appearance to the skin.

Epidemiology

Hypothyroidism is much more common in women, with an incidence of approximately 350 per 100 000 per year, as compared to men who have an incidence of 60 per 100 000 per year. The incidence of hypothyroidism increases with age.

Pathology

Primary hypothyroidism accounts for the vast majority of cases and is diagnosed when the abnormality occurs in the thyroid gland (Table 6.10). Destruction of thyroid tissue is often the result of autoimmune thyroiditis (Hashimoto's disease). Thyroid autoantibodies (anti-microsomal, anti-thyroglobulin and anti-peroxidase) are present in the serum, and there is a diffuse lymphocytic infiltrate affecting the thyroid gland. Although there may be a firm goitre initially, the autoimmune destruction subsequently leads to thyroid atrophy. Surgery or radiation to the neck can damage the thyroid gland and cause primary hypothyroidism. Drugs such as amiodarone, lithium and iodine can also interfere with thyroid function.

Transient inflammatory conditions such as subacute (de Quervain's) thyroiditis and lymphocytic thyroiditis can initially cause thyrotoxicosis, which then progresses to hypothyroidism. Subacute thyroiditis is thought to have a viral trigger, while lymphocytic thyroiditis is seen in post-partum women. The hypothyroidism is temporary in both instances, and resolves within 8 weeks.

Rarely, hypothyroidism can occur secondary to pituitary or hypothalamic tumours that disrupt the release of thyroid-stimulating hormone.

Table 6.10	Causes of hypothyroidism
Primary hypothyroidism	
Hashimoto's thyroiditis	
Drugs (amiodarone, iodine)	
De Quervain's thyroiditis	
Lymphocytic thyroiditis	
Complications from treatment of hyperthyroidism (radioiodine, thyroidectomy)	
Secondary hypothyroidism	
Pituitary tumours	
Hypothalamic tumours	

Scope of disease

The severity of hypothyroidism varies from subclinical (detected only by laboratory testing) to clinically overt. Patients with subclinical or compensated hypothyroidism have levels of thyroid-stimulating hormone above the reference range but normal thyroxine levels and no major signs or symptoms of thyroid disease. In contrast, patients with severe disease may present with myxoedema coma, psychosis, heart failure, hypothermia and hypoglycaemia. Untreated hypothyroidism in children leads to cretinism (mental retardation, deafness, short stature and facial deformities).

Clinical features

Hypothyroidism leads to a general slowing down of the body's physiological processes. Early symptoms are insidious and non-specific, as listed in Table 6.11. Patients with long-standing disease may have characteristic facies (Fig. 6.4). It is occasionally difficult to diagnose hypothyroidism with confidence on clinical grounds alone.

Table 6.11	Clinical features of hypothyroidism
General	
Tiredness	
Weight gain	
Cold intolerance	
Constipation	
Cardiovascular	
Angina	
Sinus bradycardia	
Ankle swelling	
Nervous system	
Slowing of mental processes	
Memory impairment	
Sleepiness	
Slow relaxing ankle reflexes	
Skin	
Skin thickening	
Hair loss	
Dry hair and skin	
Periorbital puffiness	
Coarse features	
Metabolic	
Hypercholesterolaemia	
Hyponatraemia	
Macrocytic anaemia	
Raised creatine kinase	

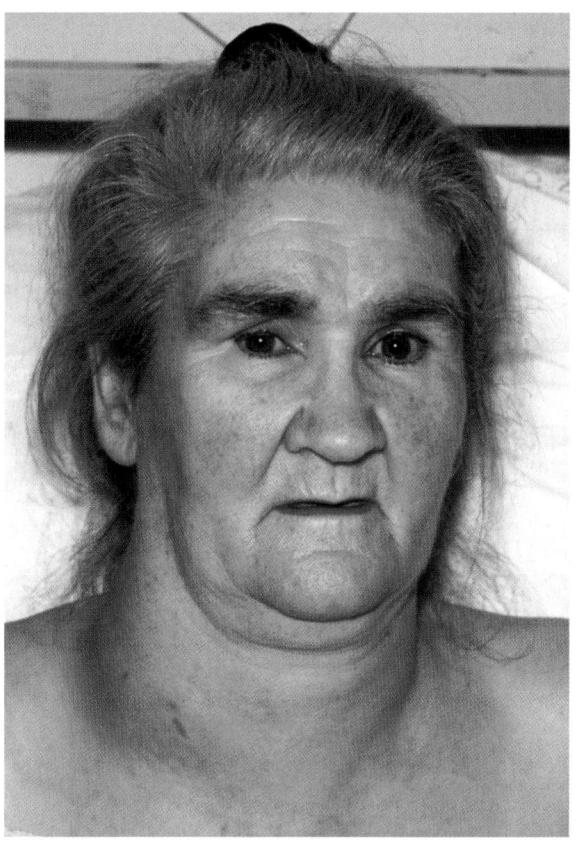

Fig. 6.4 Patient with hypothyroidism.

Initial investigations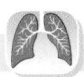

Thyroid-stimulating hormone

The most important diagnostic test is the measurement of serum TSH. Elevated TSH levels are a simple and specific method of diagnosing primary hypothyroidism.

Patients with critical illness from non-thyroid causes may experience derangements in thyroid function, and the test results may be difficult to interpret. In such situations, thyroid testing should be delayed until patient recovery, unless there is substantial clinical suspicion of hypothyroidism.

Further investigations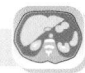

Thyroid-stimulating hormone and free T_4

Patients with suspected secondary hypothyroidism should have both the TSH and the serum thyroxine levels measured. Low thyroxine levels without marked TSH elevation are supportive of this diagnosis, and require further investigations including pituitary function tests and imaging (p. 397).

Thyroid autoantibodies

Measurement of thyroid autoantibodies is not essential but can be used to confirm the aetiology of hypothyroidism if the diagnosis is not clear from the history and clinical examination.

Medical management

Thyroxine

Thyroid hormone deficiency can be treated by a number of synthetic preparations. The most commonly used are those of L-thyroxine (T_4). The average maintenance dose ranges from 75 µg to 200 µg. Treatment should usually be started with 50 µg, except for elderly patients and those with heart disease whose dose should be slowly titrated upwards from an initial 25 µg.

TSH should be monitored at 6–8-weekly intervals to guide dosing, with a target TSH level of about 1.0 mU/L. Patients who are stable need monitoring only once a year. Thyroxine replacement therapy has a narrow therapeutic index and excessive doses can bring on symptoms of thyrotoxicosis such as angina and atrial arrhythmias.

Currently, there is no consensus on the management of patients with subclinical hypothyroidism as it is uncertain whether early therapy will improve the long-term outlook of asymptomatic patients.

Intravenous liothyronine and hydrocortisone

Myxoedema coma is treated with intravenous liothyronine (T_3) 5–20 µg twice daily because liothyronine has a more rapid onset of action. In addition to this, hydrocortisone 100 mg is given intravenously prior to thyroxine therapy (to minimize the risk of acute adrenocortical deficiency induced by thyroxine under these specific circumstances) as it is not possible to rule out secondary hypothyroidism and pituitary failure as a cause of the coma. Supportive care has an important role in the management of myxoedema coma and the patient may need to be treated in the intensive care setting if he or she has respiratory or cardiac failure.

Prognosis

Subclinical hypothyroidism is associated with normal survival in elderly patients.[1] The mortality of patients with myxoedema coma is up to 30%.

FURTHER INFORMATION

American Association of Clinical Endocrinologists. American Association of Clinical Endocrinologists medical guidelines for clinical practice for the evaluation and treatment of hyperthyroidism and hypothyroidism. Endocrine Practice 2002; 8: 457–469.

REFERENCE

(1) Gussekloo J, van Exel E, de Craen AJ, Meinders AE, Frolich M, Westendorp RG. Thyroid status, disability and cognitive function, and survival in old age. JAMA 2004; 292: 2591–2599.

Hyperthyroidism

Hyperthyroidism or thyrotoxicosis consists of the clinical, physiological and biochemical findings resulting from exposure to excessive thyroid hormones.

Epidemiology

Hyperthyroidism occurs predominantly in women (female: male 9:1), with an incidence of approximately 80 per 100 000 per year. Graves' disease tends to present in women in the third and fourth decades.

Pathology

Autoimmune disease and thyroid autonomy are the two most common causes of hyperthyroidism (Table 6.12). In Graves' disease, excessive release of thyroid hormone is due to presence of IgG thyroid-stimulating antibodies (TSI) that bind to the TSH receptor and mimic the action of TSH. Ophthalmopathy (proptosis, exophthalmos, diplopia) and dermopathy (pretibial myxoedema) are specific to Graves' disease, but the aetiology is less well understood. Antigens in the orbit may cross-react with thyroid-stimulating antibodies leading to an inflammatory reaction, proliferation of fibroblasts and orbital oedema.

Toxic multinodular goitre and toxic solitary adenomas are examples of autonomously functioning thyroid tissue that secretes excessive amounts of thyroid hormone. Mutations in the TSH receptor or in the G-protein pathway are thought to lead to clonal expansion of individual cells and autonomous nodule formation.

Lymphocytic thyroiditis (e.g. in post-partum patients) causes excessive T_4 release due to autoimmune destruction of thyroid cells. Choriocarcinoma and hyperemesis gravidarum are uncommon causes of hyperthyroidism. In these conditions, human chorionic gonadotrophin, which has a similar chemical structure to TSH, is present in excessive amounts. The presence of ectopic thyroid tissue is associated with struma ovarii and functioning follicular carcinoma of the thyroid gland. T_3 toxicosis due to elevated T_3 levels occurs rarely in patients with hyperthyroidism. In this

Table 6.12	Causes of hyperthyroidism
Associated with thyroid hyperfunction	
Graves' disease*	
Hyperfunctioning adenoma*	
Toxic multinodular goitre*	
TSH-producing tumour	
Not associated with thyroid hyperfunction	
Subacute thyroiditis	
Struma ovarii	
Functioning follicular thyroid carcinoma	
* Common causes.	

situation, normal serum T_4 levels occur despite clinical evidence of hyperthyroidism.

Scope of disease

Hyperthyroidism occurs as a result of excessive thyroid hormone action. The clinical manifestations stem from a general increase in the cellular metabolic process, as well as greater adrenergic activity. Thyrotoxicosis is a systemic disorder and the effect on each system is summarized in Table 6.13. In addition, Graves' disease is associated with a number of other autoimmune disorders (Table 6.14). Enlargement of the thyroid gland (usually from a multinodular goitre) can result in compression of adjacent structures such as the trachea (stridor, see Fig. 6.6) and the recurrent laryngeal nerve (hoarseness).

Clinical features

The severity of thyrotoxicosis varies from subclinical (detected only by laboratory testing) to clinically overt. Patient may present with classic symptoms of thyrotoxicosis which may be accompanied by specific symptoms of Graves' disease such as ophthalmopathy (Fig. 6.5) and dermopathy.

Table 6.13	Clinical features of hyperthyroidism
General	
Tiredness and muscle weakness	
Weight loss	
Heat intolerance	
Amenorrhoea/infertility	
Cardiovascular	
Palpitations/tachycardia	
Atrial fibrillation	
High-output cardiac failure	
Decreased exercise tolerance	
Nervous system	
Anxiety	
Nervousness	
Personality change	
Poor concentration	
Insomnia	
Gastrointestinal	
Increased appetite	
Frequent bowel movements	
Eyes	
Lid lag	
Lid retraction	
Infiltrative ophthalmopathy (Graves' disease only) 　　Exophthalmos 　　Photophobia 　　Diplopia	

Table 6.14	Other autoimmune diseases associated with Graves' disease
Pernicious anaemia	
Atrophic gastritis	
Diabetes	
Addison's disease	
Idiopathic hypoparathyroidism	

Symptoms of thyrotoxicosis include nervousness, insomnia, tremors, excessive sweating with heat intolerance and weight loss. On examination, the patient may appear thin with sweaty palms and a fine tremor. The pulse rate may be fast and irregular (atrial fibrillation). The thyroid may be diffusely enlarged (Graves' disease) or nodular (toxic multinodular goitre).

Specific clinical features of Graves' disease include a thyroid bruit, ophthalmopathy (exophthalmos, chemosis, diplopia), pretibial myxoedema and thyroid acropachy (resembles clubbing).

> ### ⚡ CLINICAL ALERT
>
> *Patients with severe thyrotoxicosis can present with thyroid storm, a critical illness that includes heart failure, hypotension, fever, marked weakness and muscle wasting, restlessness and confusion. Rapid control of hyperthyroidism in thyroid storm and other emergency situations can be achieved with iodine (potassium iodide or Lugol's solution), β-blockers, propylthiouracil and corticosteroids. Supportive care has an important role in the management of thyroid storm and the patient may need to be treated in the intensive care setting.*

Initial investigations

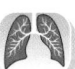

Thyroid-stimulating hormone and free T_4
The simplest initial screening test is the measurement of serum thyroid-stimulating hormone. The diagnosis of hyperthyroidism in patients with suppressed (low) levels of TSH can be confirmed by detection of elevated free T_4 levels.

Hyperthyroidism secondary to pituitary adenomas is rare and results in elevated levels of TSH and serum thyroxine.

Further investigations

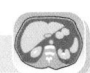

T_3 levels
Measurement of T_3 levels is performed when T_3 toxicosis is suspected in clinically hyperthyroid patients with suppressed TSH but normal T_4 levels.

Hypothyroidism

Hyperthyroidism

Thyroid cancer

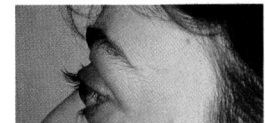

Fig. 6.5 Exophthalmos in a patient with Graves' disease.

Thyroid autoantibodies

Measurement of anti-thyroid peroxidase and anti-thyroglobulin antibodies is not essential, but along with anti-TSH receptor antibodies can be used to confirm Graves' disease or autoimmune thyroid disease as the cause, if the diagnosis is not clear.

Ultrasound of the thyroid

High-resolution ultrasound using a high-frequency trans-ducer provides a comprehensive assessment of thyroid structure and can differentiate between diffuse and focal multinodular disease.

Radioactive iodine uptake test

A ^{131}I radioactive iodine uptake scan measures the absorption of circulating iodine by the thyroid gland. The main indication is elucidating the aetiology of hyperthyroidism when the underlying cause is uncertain. Graves' disease is suggested by high uptake evenly across the gland. Patients with autoimmune destructive thyroiditis show low uptake, while those with toxic nodular goitres show uneven uptake or a 'hot' nodule.

Chest X-ray and CT of the neck and chest

Imaging of the size and position of the thyroid is required when there are symptoms suggestive of compression of adjacent structures and to assess the degree of retrosternal extension. A soft tissue mass may be seen on a plain chest film (Fig. 6.6) and retrosternal extension confirmed on CT (Fig. 6.7).

Initial management

β-Blockers

β-adrenoceptor blockers such as propranolol and metoprolol are able to provide rapid relief of some thyrotoxic symptoms such as tremor, tachycardia and anxiety. β-blockers do not have any effect on thyroxine levels, oxygen consumption, nor do they reduce goitre size or reverse weight loss.

Identify and address the underlying cause

Most patients with symptomatic hyperthyroidism can initially be treated with β-blockers while awaiting planning

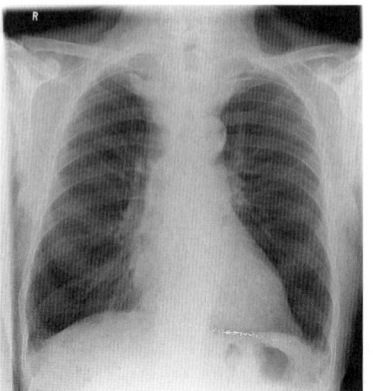

Fig. 6.6 Chest X-ray showing a soft tissue mass in the upper mediastinum.

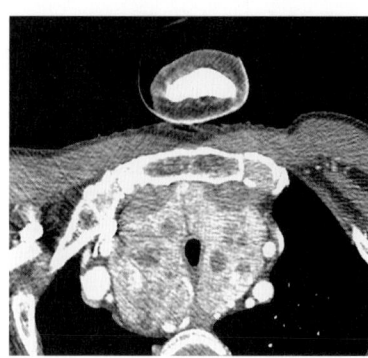

Fig. 6.7 CT scan of the thorax showing a multinodular goitre with retrosternal extension.

surgery, radioactive iodine or pharmacological treatment as the definitive treatment.

Medical management

Antithyroid drugs

Propylthiouracil and methimazole (and its pro-drug carbimazole) are cyclic thiourea derivatives which disrupt the thyroid gland's ability to use iodine. Both agents appear to be equally efficacious, although propylthiouracil may be preferred in thyroid storm because it blocks peripheral conversion of T_4 to T_3. Methimazole (or carbimazole) is more convenient for long-term therapy as it can be given once daily, whereas propylthiouracil requires more frequent dosing.

Dosing is guided by TSH and thyroxine levels, which should be monitored at 4–6-weekly intervals in the first 6 months. There is no consensus on the length of drug therapy but the initial projected duration is about 1–2 years. Up to 40% of patients with Graves' disease are in remission after this time and may be able to come off the drug treatment. Patients who are unable to stop drug therapy or those in whom remission is not achievable (e.g. toxic nodular goitres) should be offered the options of continuing on drugs, surgery or radioactive iodine.

Both propylthiouracil and methimazole agents can cause nausea, loss of taste and allergic reactions, particularly of the skin. The most serious adverse effect is that of agranulo-cytosis, which predisposes the patient to serious infections. As the reaction is uncommon and sporadic, there is no consensus on the value of routine blood count monitoring. Patients are, however, advised to consult their medical practitioner if they develop a fever, sore throat or other signs of infection. Those who develop agranulocytosis should not be exposed to any further antithyroid drug and should instead be offered surgery or radioactive iodine treatment.

Radioactive iodine

Radioactive iodine is widely used in the USA as the definitive therapy for patients with Graves' disease and toxic nodular goitres. The optimal dose is not predictable, and some patients who are initially rendered euthyroid will eventually develop hypothyroidism and require thyroxine replacement therapy. Nevertheless, the treatment appears to be safe, with no increased incidence of tumour, leukaemia and birth defects. Patients receiving radioactive iodine have the advantage of being able to discontinue antithyroid medication.

Surgical management

Thyroidectomy

Thyroidectomy is now reserved for patients who have failed or have intolerance to medical therapy, obstructive symptoms, suspicion of malignancy, in pregnant women with thyrotoxicosis and for cosmesis.

Patients should have their thyroid function stabilized with antithyroid drugs prior to surgery and baseline serum calcium is required preoperatively. In an emergency setting, iodine and β-blockers can be given to restore euthyroidism within hours.

The patient is positioned supine with the neck extended. A horizontal skin incision is undertaken and the thyroid gland identified and mobilized. The gland can be very vascular and ligation of many perforating vessels may be required. The recurrent laryngeal nerve and parathyroid glands are identified and preserved. The amount of thyroid tissue removed depends on the underlying aetiology; bilateral subtotal thyroidectomy is performed for toxic multinodular goitres

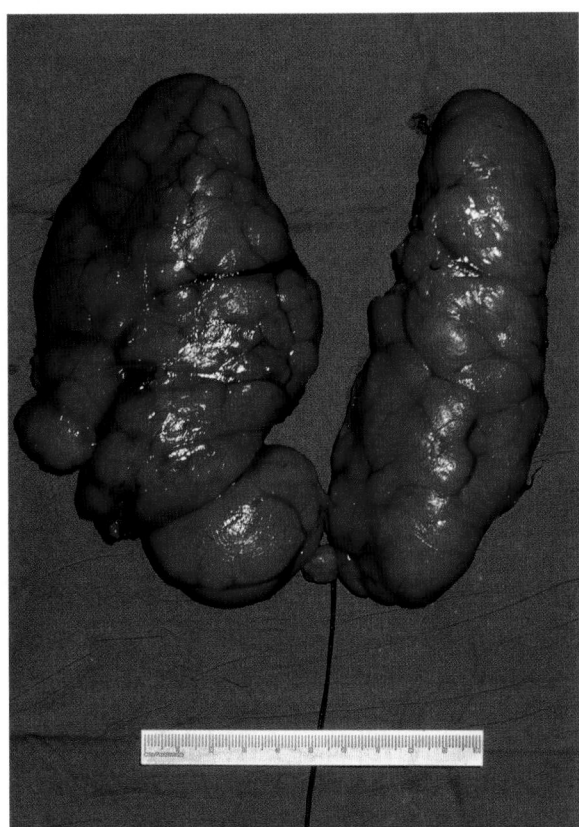

Fig. 6.8 Thyroidectomy. An excised multinodular goitre.

(Fig. 6.8) and Graves' disease, and a unilateral thyroidectomy is performed for patients with solitary adenomas. After meticulous haemostasis the skin is closed.

Successful surgery renders the patient immediately euthyroid. With Graves' disease there is a 5% risk of recurrence at 5 years. Exophthalmos regresses in the majority of patients but progressive eye disease can occur in up to 10%. Complications of surgery include bleeding, hypothyroidism (related to extent of surgical excision), transient hypoparathyroidism (hypocalcaemia) and recurrent laryngeal nerve palsy.

Prognosis

The prognosis is related to the underlying cause. Patients who are cured (e.g. subtotal thyroidectomy for toxic adenoma) will have a normal life expectancy. With Graves' disease, approximately 20% become clinically and biochemically euthyroid on β-blockers alone.[1] The course of ophthalmopathy is largely unpredictable and independent of thyroid status and drug treatment. Typically, it worsens over 18 months, followed by stabilization and spontaneous improvement in patients with mild disease.

> ### *i* FURTHER INFORMATION
>
> American Association of Clinical Endocrinologists. American Association of Clinical Endocrinologists medical guidelines for clinical practice for the evaluation and treatment of hyperthyroidism and hypothyroidism. Endocrine Practice 2002; 8: 457–469.

> **REFERENCE**
>
> **(1)** Weetman AP. Graves' disease. New England Journal of Medicine 2000; 343: 1236–1248.

Thyroid cancer

Epidemiology

Although thyroid cancers are the most common endocrine malignancy, they are generally uncommon, accounting for <1% of all cancers and <0.5% of all cancer deaths, with an annual incidence of approximately 2.3 per 100 000 women and 0.9 per 100 000 men. Papillary carcinoma presents in patients between the second and third decades, follicular carcinoma tends to present in older patients, and anaplastic carcinoma tends to present in patients in the sixth and seventh decades.

Pathology

There are four main types of thyroid cancer: papillary, follicular, anaplastic and medullary thyroid carcinoma.

Exposure to radiation, nuclear fall-out and neck irradiation are considered to be important risk factors in the development of thyroid cancer.

Papillary carcinoma is the most common (70–80%), with a 3:1 female preponderance, and is derived from thyroid follicular cells. The main method of spread is via the lymphatic system, 30% can be multifocal.

Follicular carcinoma also comes from thyroid follicular cells and makes up 10–15% of thyroid cancers, with a 2:1 female preponderance. It is more aggressive than papillary carcinoma and commonly spreads (in 10–15% cases) to lungs and bones via the blood stream. Hürthle cell carcinoma is an aggressive follicular tumour with a worse prognosis.

Anaplastic carcinoma is uncommon, comprising less than 10% of thyroid cancers, with a slight male preponderance, 1.5:1. It is also known as undifferentiated carcinoma because the histological appearance of the cells does not resemble normal thyroid tissue. Anaplastic carcinoma is extremely aggressive and spreads rapidly via local invasion, through the lymph nodes and blood stream.

Medullary carcinoma makes up about 5–10% of thyroid cancers. It arises from the parafollicular C cells that produce calcitonin. It can lead to a wide variety of biochemical derangements. Amyloid is sometimes found in specimens of medullary carcinoma. Most medullary carcinomas are sporadic but some are familial (p. 433) and others are associated with multiple endocrine neoplasia type 2 (p. 433).

Scope of disease

Local
Patients with recent or expanding growth of a thyroid carcinoma may present with a palpable nodule. Infiltration into the recurrent laryngeal nerve leads to hoarseness of voice.

Metastatic
Each tumour type has its own predilection for metastatic spread. Papillary carcinoma tends to spread via the lymphatics to the lymph nodes, follicular carcinomas tend to spread via the blood stream into the lungs and liver, and anaplastic carcinoma can spread via the lymphatics and blood stream.

Paraneoplastic
Patients with medullary carcinoma may develop features related to ectopic production of hormones such as ACTH (Cushing's syndrome), serotonin, vasointestinal peptide (VIP; flushing and diarrhoea) and calcitonin, which can be used as tumour markers.

Clinical features

Thyroid cancer usually presents as a lump (solitary or multinodular) in the neck, in a clinically euthyroid patient with no other symptoms.

When assessing a patient with a thyroid nodule, it must be borne in mind that the vast majority of such nodules are benign. Features that increase the likelihood of malignancy include a family history of cancer, previous neck irradiation, a rapidly growing nodule, hoarseness or change in voice, swollen lymph nodes, difficulty swallowing and stridor. Rarely, patients may present with signs or symptoms of metastatic disease such as pathological fractures from bony metastases.

Initial investigations
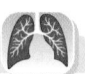

Thyroid-stimulating hormone and free T$_4$
Patients with thyroid cancer usually have normal thyroid function tests.

Fine-needle aspiration
In the majority of patients with a thyroid nodule, fine-needle aspiration is the first and only test required. This involves multiple passes of a needle into the nodule while aspirating into a syringe. The cells are then stained and examined under a microscope, and then classified into categories ranging from benign to suspicious to definitely malignant.

Further investigations
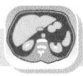

Radionuclide scanning
Fine-needle aspiration has superseded the need for the majority of iodine-131 or technetium-99m labelled pertechnetate scans. Currently radionuclide scans are reserved for patients in whom fine-needle aspiration is non-diagnostic. Classically, malignant nodules are non-functional and appear as cold spots (Fig. 6.9), whereas nodules from toxic adenoma appear as hot spots. Unfortunately, up to 8% of hot and 16% of cold nodules may be malignant.

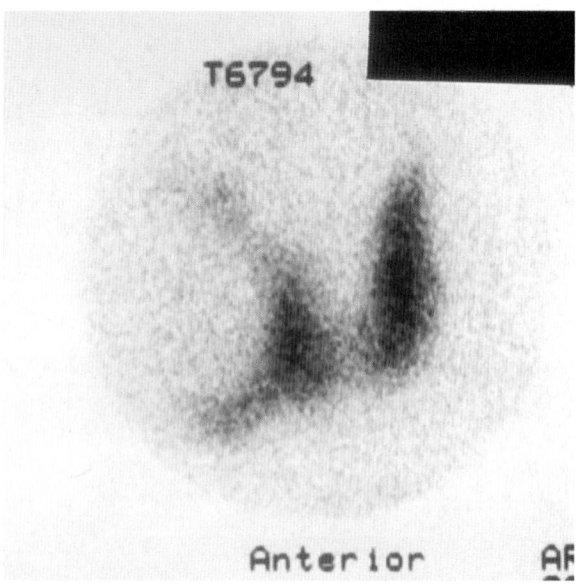

Fig. 6.9 Radioiodine uptake scan. A cold spot can be seen in the right lobe of the thyroid.

Serum calcitonin and carcino-embryonic antigen (CEA)

Calcitonin and CEA are measured if there is clinical suspicion of medullary carcinoma.

Chest X-ray

A screening chest X-ray should be performed to detect lung metastases.

Ultrasound of the thyroid

High-resolution ultrasound of the thyroid can differentiate between diffuse and focal disease, capsular invasion and local lymph node enlargement. It can also be used to direct fine-needle aspiration.

CT or MRI of the neck and chest

Further imaging may be required in patients in whom the borders of the goitre cannot be clearly defined, or where there is a fixed lump.

Surgical management

Thyroidectomy

The extent of surgery ranges from a lobectomy to a total thyroidectomy (p. 415). However, the absence of controlled clinical studies in papillary and follicular carcinoma means that there is no consensus on the exact level of surgical resection and the need and extent of regional lymph node dissection. In general, total or near-total thyroidectomy is recommended for most thyroid carcinomas. Limited surgery in the form of a total lobectomy may be used in papillary or follicular carcinomas in low-risk patients with tumours less than 1 cm.

Treatment of medullary carcinoma is with total thyroidectomy and complete regional neck lymph node dissection. Surgery is not recommended in anaplastic carcinoma unless airway obstruction is imminent.

The debate about extent of surgery arises because the complications of a near-total or total thyroidectomy need to be weighed against the benefits. Advocates of total thyroidectomy cite advantages such as eliminating the possibility of recurrence from a bilateral cancer, facilitating the use of postoperative radio-iodine therapy, which is difficult to administer with the residual thyroid lobe in situ, and monitoring of recurrences. Advocates of less than total thyroidectomy claim that well-differentiated tumours carry a good prognosis in general, that results of a lobectomy are

similar to total thyroidectomy, and that the present use of adjuvant therapy is still undefined.

Medical management

Radioactive iodine

Radioactive iodine (^{131}I) can be used as adjuvant therapy after surgery to ablate residual thyroid tissue in patients with follicular or papillary carcinomas. Thyroid replacement therapy is given to these patients after thyroidectomy. The purpose is to replace any thyroid hormone deficiency and to suppress the TSH so that any remaining cancer cells are not stimulated to grow. Metastatic disease can also be treated with radioactive iodine. There is no role for radioactive iodine in medullary carcinoma because the C cells do not take up iodine.

External beam radiotherapy

Patients with anaplastic carcinoma do not derive substantial benefit from surgery or radioactive iodine; the primary treatment for them is external beam radiotherapy. Metastatic disease can also be treated with external beam radiotherapy.

Prognosis

Mortality of patients depends on the type of cancer, stage and risk category. Patients with a single isolated nodule that responds well to therapy have a 5-year survival probability of more than 90%. In general, the prognosis is better for patients with papillary carcinoma rather than the follicular carcinoma.

In contrast, patients with anaplastic carcinoma and metastasis at presentation have a 5-year survival probability of less than 10%. The overall median survival of patients with anaplastic carcinoma is about 6 months.

Patients with medullary carcinoma have survival rates of about 60% at 10 years.

𝑖 FURTHER INFORMATION

American Association of Clinical Endocrinologists. AACE/AAES medical/surgical guidelines for clinical practice: management of thyroid carcinoma. Endocrine Practice 2001; 7: 203–220.

Udelsman R, Shaha AR. Is total thyroidectomy the best possible surgical management for well-differentiated thyroid cancer? Lancet Oncology 2005; 6: 529–531.

SECTION 6.6   The parathyroid glands

Hyperparathyroidism

Primary hyperparathyroidism is caused by excessive, autonomous secretion of parathyroid hormone (PTH) by the parathyroid gland. Secondary hyperparathyroidism occurs when the parathyroid glands increase in activity in response to low serum calcium.

Epidemiology

Hyperparathyroidism (HPT) is one of the most common causes of hypercalcaemia, accounting for 55% of cases. The incidence is rising due to increased detection rates from the routine evaluation of serum calcium by multi-channel biochemistry analyzers and is estimated to be 25 per 100 000 per year.[1] Hyperparathyroidism is 3 times more common in women than men, and often presents at around 50–60 years of age.

Pathology

Approximately 85% of patients with primary hyperparathyroidism have a single benign parathyroid adenoma and around 5% may have two adenomas (double adenoma). The remaining have gland hyperplasia affecting all four parathyroid glands. A small proportion of patients with hyperplasia have multiple endocrine neoplasia syndrome and this may be suspected in young patients with HPT. Parathyroid cancer itself is very rare.

Chronic renal failure is the most common cause of secondary hyperparathyroidism. In this condition there is a deficit of 1,25-dihydroxyvitamin D production. This, combined with hyperphosphataemia due to decreased renal clearance and the development of a relative bone resistance to PTH, results in hypocalcaemia. This in turn produces a rise in PTH levels, which can be extremely high. These extraordinarily high levels of PTH can raise the serum calcium to normal/low-normal levels.

Scope of disease

Currently, routine evaluation of serum calcium is able to detect patients with early asymptomatic disease. If carefully questioned, patients may complain of symptoms such as fatigue, lassitude, impaired memory, polydipsia, polyuria and constipation. Previously, patients with hyperparathyroidism presented with complications of chronic hypercalcaemia such as renal stones, muscular weakness and bone pain.

Clinical features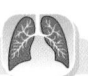

The main features stem from the derangement of serum calcium levels. The principal organs affected are the skeletal, nervous, renal and gastrointestinal systems (Table 6.15), leading to the phrase 'moans, groans, stones and bones'.

Initial investigations

Parathyroid hormone and bone profile

The definitive diagnosis of hyperparathyroidism can be made with the finding of a high parathyroid hormone in the presence of serum calcium levels above or in the upper normal range.

24-Hour urine collection

A 24-hour urine collection for calcium excretion will demonstrate raised or normal levels of urinary calcium to confirm the diagnosis of primary PTH. Low values of calcium excretion suggest the rare condition of familial hypocalciuric hypercalcaemia, for which surgical cervical exploration is contraindicated.

Table 6.15	Clinical features of hyperparathyroidism
Skeletal	
Bone pain	
Osteopenia/osteoporosis	
Fractures	
Renal	
Polyuria	
Renal stones	
Renal failure	
Nervous system	
Tiredness/muscle weakness	
Intellectual or memory impairment	
Confusion	
Gastrointestinal	
Constipation	
Peptic ulcer	
Pancreatitis	

Further investigations

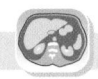

Assessment of target organ damage is useful to assess the severity of the disease.

Urea and electrolytes

Renal function should be assessed as renal impairment is a known complication.

Abdominal film

An abdominal KUB film may detect the presence of renal stones.

Bone densitometry

The deleterious effects of hyperparathyroidism on the bones can be measured using bone densitometry (DEXA) scanning.

Preoperative localization scanning

The parathyroid glands are small and may be difficult to locate during the surgical procedure. Routine parathyroid imaging does not have a diagnostic role but can be helpful in identifying the location of the adenoma and thus facilitating surgical excision. Currently, preoperative ultrasound scanning and use of radioactive sestamibi scintigraphy are the most common methods to preoperatively localize an overactive gland.

Ultrasound scan

Ultrasound scanning is relatively quick and simple but highly operator dependent. Sensitivity and specificity can be up to 85% and 95% respectively in experienced hands.

Sestamibi scan

Sestamibi is a technetium-based radionuclide which is concentrated in both the thyroid gland and in the parathyroid adenoma. It is rapidly washed out of the thyroid but retained in the mitochondria of the overactive parathyroid adenoma. Scintigrams can be taken and will reveal the site of the adenoma with a sensitivity of around 90%. The rare cases of mediastinal ectopic parathyroid adenomas may also be identified by preoperative sestamibi scanning.

CT/MRI scan

CT scans and MRI are also available for localization studies but at present have neither the simplicity of the ultrasound scan nor the accuracy of the sestamibi scan.

Initial management

Address and correct any underlying cause

Patients with secondary hyperparathyroidism should receive treatment for their underlying condition to correct their calcium levels.

Observation

While patients with overt primary hyperparathyroidism are likely to benefit from surgical therapy, there is still considerable controversy about patients with few or no symptoms who are found to have mildly elevated serum calcium and parathyroid hormone levels. Those who elect not to have the operation should have 6-monthly monitoring of serum calcium and annual bone densitometry and creatinine levels.

Surgical management

Bilateral neck exploration and parathyroidectomy

Surgical intervention is the only curative therapy for primary hyperparathyroidism and is successful in more than 90% of patients. The indications for surgery are listed in Table 6.16. The gold standard procedure has been the bilateral neck exploration through a central collar incision identical to that used for thyroid surgery. All four parathyroids are identified and the visibly abnormal one is removed. In cases of parathyroid adenomas (85% of cases of HPT) the abnormal gland is easily recognized as such by visual evaluation. Despite this, excision of parathyroid tissue is always confirmed by frozen section histological evaluation. Adenomas are excised leaving the normal glands in situ. If all four glands are hyperplastic, 3–3½ glands are excised, leaving some functioning parathyroid tissue in situ. Haemostasis is secured and the wound is closed in layers. If all four glands are normal, ectopic parathyroid tissue may be responsible and can be located as low as the thymus gland in the anterior mediastinum.

Postoperative complications are uncommon in experienced hands. Postoperative bleeding may compromise the airway but is rare. Damage to the recurrent laryngeal nerve results in hoarseness of the voice but occurs in less than 1% of cases. Transient postoperative hypocalcaemia can occur due to temporary ongoing postoperative suppression of the non-adenomatous normal parathyroid glands by the preoperative hypercalcaemia or due to movement of calcium into bone in the presence of corrected PTH levels ('hungry bone syndrome'). This can be corrected by short-term calcium administration.

RECENT ADVANCES

In those cases where the preoperative ultrasound scan and sestamibi scan can confidently predict the location of an adenoma (i.e. when there is concordance between the two scans), the incision can be dramatically shortened from the standard collar incision to a 2–2.5 cm incision made directly over the site of the localized adenoma. This allows the adenoma to be excised with the minimum of neck dissection but at the expense of visualizing all four glands. Often these patients can be discharged within 24 hours of their surgery with minimal discomfort.

Medical management

Oestrogen and selective oestrogen receptor modulators

Oestrogen and selective oestrogen receptor modulators (SERMs, such as raloxifene) at present do not have an established role in reversing bone abnormalities.

Bisphosphonates

Bisphosphonates are effective osteoclast inhibitors. They provide an incomplete and temporary calcium lowering effect and may be useful while surgery is being planned. There is no evidence to support their long-term use in hyperparathyroidism.

RECENT ADVANCES

Calcimimetic agents have been developed to interfere with the process of PTH secretion and synthesis. Cinacalcet binds onto the calcium-sensing receptor at the parathyroid gland and makes it more sensitive to external calcium levels. The receptor then provides negative feedback to the parathyroid gland, leading to a lowering of the PTH levels within a few hours. Cinacalcet is currently licensed for use in patients with secondary hyperparathyroidism, but its role in the primary disease has not yet been established.

Prognosis

Patients are being diagnosed earlier in the development of the disease process and there is controversy over the treatment of patients with very mild asymptomatic disease. However, for those patients with symptomatic disease or those who fulfil the criteria for surgery (Table 6.16), surgical intervention significantly reduces the comorbidity induced by hyperparathyroidism as well as having a beneficial effect in reducing morbidity.[2]

Table 6.16	Indications for surgical intervention in primary hyperparathyroidism
Serum calcium >2.85 mmol/L	

Renal manifestations
    Marked hypercalciuria
    Creatinine clearance <30% of normal	

Gastrointestinal manifestations
    Peptic ulcer disease
    Pancreatitis	

Bone manifestation Reduction of bone mineral density by 2 standard deviations from age- and sex-matched mean	
Soft tissue calcification	
Age less than 50 years	
Patient choice or when regular follow-up is difficult or impossible	

 FURTHER INFORMATION

AACE/AAES Task Force on Primary Hyperparathyroidism. Position statement on the diagnosis and management of primary hyperparathyroidism. Endocrine Practice 2005; 11: 49–54.

REFERENCES

(1) *Mundy GR, Cove DH, Fisken R. Primary hyperparathyroidism: changes in the pattern of clinical presentation. Lancet 1980; 1: 1317–1320.*
(2) *Vestergaard P, Mosekilde L. Cohort study on effects of parathyroid surgery on multiple outcomes in primary hyperparathyroidism. BMJ 2003; 327: 530–534.*

SECTION 6.7 The glucocorticoid axis

Cushing's syndrome

Cushing's syndrome arises from chronically elevated glucocorticoid levels. It may be iatrogenic (inhaled, oral or topical steroids), due to adrenal disease, ectopic ACTH production or Cushing's disease, which refers to the specific aetiology of Cushing's syndrome due to a pituitary ACTH-secreting adenoma.

Epidemiology

The incidence of spontaneous Cushing's syndrome is estimated at 50 per 100 000 per year, with Cushing's disease accounting for approximately 0.2–3 per 100 000 per year. Cushing's disease has a female preponderance and most patients are in their third to fourth decade.

Pathology

The most common cause of Cushing's syndrome is iatrogenic, due to the side effects of long-term corticosteroid administration. Cushing's syndrome due to adrenal hypersecretion of cortisol is classified as ACTH dependent (80%), which implies that cortisol excess is due to ACTH hypersecretion, or ACTH independent (20%), which implies a primary pathology of the adrenal glands (Table 6.17).

Table 6.17	Causes of Cushing's syndrome

Iatrogenic
Long-term corticosteroid administration

ACTH-dependent cortisol excess
Pituitary ACTH-producing adenoma (Cushing's disease)

Ectopic ACTH secretion (bronchial, thymic, pancreatic carcinoma)

Ectopic corticotropin-releasing hormone (CRH) secretion

ACTH-independent cortisol excess
Adrenal adenoma

Adrenal nodular hyperplasia

Adrenal carcinoma

Pseudo Cushing's
Alcoholism

Depression

ACTH-dependent hypercortisolaemia caused by a pituitary adenoma (68%) is defined as Cushing's disease; most of these adenomas are microadenomas. 'Ectopic' ACTH is released by other non-endocrine tumours (12%) such as lung, thymic and pancreatic cancer. ACTH-independent hypercortisolaemia is caused by benign (10%) or malignant (8%) adrenal tumours, or by adrenal nodular hyperplasia (1%).

Alcohol and severe depression can give rise to 'pseudo Cushing's syndrome' (1%). In cyclical Cushing's syndrome, clinical features and biochemical abnormalities may wax and wane, posing difficulties in establishing a diagnosis.

Scope of disease

Excess cortisol affects all aspects of substrate metabolism leading to centripetal fat redistribution, muscle wasting and insulin resistance. Bone resorption is increased (osteoporosis), skin and connective tissues become atrophic, and immune function is impaired. Elevated glucocorticoid levels exert effects at the renal mineralocorticoid receptor leading to salt and water retention. Secondary diabetes can occur. Mental well-being is disturbed in over half of patients.

Clinical features

Diagnostic suspicion is often raised by the typical changes in physical appearance: a rounded, plethoric face, thinning of the scalp hair, acne and hirsutism. Truncal obesity with prominent supraclavicular fat pads is characteristic. The skin bruises easily and heals poorly, purple striae may be present, and with ACTH dependence hyperpigmentation can occur. Proximal muscle weakness and back pain are common: osteoporotic vertebral fractures are demonstrable in up to 20%. There is an increased susceptibility to infections. Signs and symptoms of diabetes may be present and hypertension is frequent. Emotional lability, insomnia, depression and psychosis are the most common psychiatric disturbances. A summary of the clinical features is presented in Table 6.18.

Apart from identifying the features of Cushing's syndrome, a detailed clinical assessment will also attempt to detect clinical features that may suggest the underlying cause. A drug history will easily identify any exogenous corticosteroids, patients with a pituitary adenoma may also

Cushing's syndrome

Nelson's syndrome

Adrenocortical insufficiency

Congenital adrenal hyperplasia

Table 6.18	Clinical features of Cushing's syndrome	

Location	Effect of disease	Clinical features
Face	Fat redistribution/connective tissue atrophy	Round plethoric face, telangiectasia
Skin	Atrophy/androgen excess	Thin skin, easy bruising, poor healing
Skin	Melanocyte stimulation by ACTH	Hyperpigmentation, especially of scars
Skin, scalp hair	Adrenal androgen secretion	Male pattern balding, hirsutism, acne
Trunk and limbs	Centripetal fat redistribution	Abdominal obesity with thin arms and legs, interscapular and supraclavicular fat pads, purple striae
Muscle	Proximal weakness	Difficulties climbing stairs
Axial skeleton	Osteoporosis	Back pain, compression fractures
Metabolism	Diabetes mellitus/hypercalciuria	Thirst, polyuria, blurred vision, renal stones
Kidneys	Activation of mineralocorticoid receptor	Hypertension, peripheral oedema
Testes/ovaries	Hypogonadism	Oligo/amenorrhoea
Psyche	Altered mood and mental function	Depression, agitation, psychosis
Other peripheral glands	Hypogonadism/hypopituitarism	Decreased libido, oligo/amenorrhoea
Cushing's disease (in addition to above)		
Pituitary	Compression of optic chiasm	Bitemporal hemianopia
Fundus	Raised intracranial pressure/hypertension and diabetes	Papilloedema/hypertensive and diabetic retinopathy/optic atrophy

have features of a mass effect such as bitemporal hemianopia from pituitary compression of the optic chiasm, and patients with ectopic ACTH production may have symptoms from underlying causes such as stridor with bronchial obstruction from a tumour.

Initial investigations
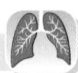

Initial tests aim to establish hypercortisolaemia, and further investigations attempt to identify the aetiology. If initial tests are normal, Cushing's syndrome is unlikely or may be intermittent.

24-Hour urinary free cortisol
24-Hour urinary free cortisol measurements serve as a screening test to establish cortisol excess. They should be repeated as the false-negative rate is 5–10%.

Low-dose dexamethasone suppression test
The low-dose overnight dexamethasone suppression test can be performed in the outpatient setting or as an inpatient. The loss of circadian rhythm in cortisol secretion can be demonstrated in the hospital by a detectable midnight cortisol (>50 nmol/L) taken whilst asleep. Failure to suppress indicates autonomous cortisol secretion.

Further investigations
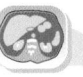

Once excess cortisol is established, further investigations are performed to determine the cause.

Basal ACTH levels
Low or undetectable ACTH levels imply an adrenocortical tumour as the underlying cause or iatrogenic corticosteroid administration. Detectable ACTH levels may arise from a pituitary adenoma or from ectopic sources.

High-dose dexamethasone suppression test
Suppression of cortisol secretion (less than 50% of the baseline value) with high-dose dexamethasone implies a pituitary adenoma or occult ACTH-producing tumour. Failure of suppression with high-dose dexamethasone occurs with adrenocortical tumours, but can also occur with ACTH-secreting tumours that produce a large amount of ACTH.

Urea and electrolytes
Severe hypokalaemic (<3.2 mmol/L) alkalosis in the absence of diuretic therapy occurs with most ectopic ACTH secretion but in less than 10% of those with pituitary-dependent disease.

CT or MRI of the abdomen
Imaging of the adrenal glands is usually performed to screen for tumours in patients with excess serum cortisol and low basal ACTH levels with failure of cortisol suppression on the high-dose dexamethasone suppression test. An adrenal tumour may be identified. Adrenal tumours larger than 6 cm, the presence of irregularities and local invasion are features suggestive of malignancy. Bilateral adrenal enlargement suggests nodular hyperplasia.

CT or MRI of the head
Imaging of the pituitary is performed to screen for adenomas in patients with excess serum cortisol, high basal ACTH levels and evidence of cortisol suppression on the high-dose dexamethasone suppression test. The features of a pituitary adenoma are described on page 396.

Corticotropin-releasing hormone (CRH) stimulation tests
CRH administration causes a >50% rise in ACTH and a >20% rise in cortisol levels in 95% of patients with an ACTH-secreting pituitary adenoma, but occasionally a similar response is seen in ectopic disease. Bilateral inferior petrosal sinus sampling with CRH stimulation is reserved for patients in whom there is continuing diagnostic ambiguity between a hypothalamic or pituitary aetiology. It compares ACTH concentrations obtained in the venous drainage of both sides of the pituitary with peripheral samples.

Further specific imaging
Specific imaging may be required to screen for ectopic ACTH-producing tumours, such as chest X-ray or CT for bronchial tumours.

Initial management

Address any underlying cause
Where possible, substitution of a steroid-sparing immuno-modulation agent should be undertaken for patients with Cushing's syndrome due to exogenous steroid administration for concomitant chronic disease.

Medical management

Metyrapone or ketoconazole
Correction of the glucocorticoid excess is the initial aim of medical therapy irrespective of its aetiology, in particular to reduce subsequent operative risk. Metyrapone or ketoconazole is used, with the dose titrated according to cortisol levels on a day curve (e.g. 9 a.m., 12 p.m., 3 p.m. and 6 p.m. samples)

Surgical management

Surgical management is directed to the underlying diseased organ, which is usually the adrenal or the pituitary gland.

Adrenalectomy
Unilateral adrenalectomy is indicated for Cushing's syndrome due to adrenal adenoma or carcinoma. Bilateral adrenalectomy is usually undertaken for patients with adrenal nodular hyperplasia or as a last resort for patients with refractory ACTH secretion (pituitary or exogenous ACTH secretion).

Prolonged glucocorticoid replacement therapy is required postoperatively until functional recovery of the contralateral gland in patients with unilateral adrenalectomy, and life-long treatment is required when bilateral adrenalectomy is performed. If bilateral, Nelson's syndrome may occur in up to 30% of cases.

Adrenal carcinomas have often metastasized at the time of diagnosis. Surgical resection to reduce tumour mass is usually accompanied by postoperative administration of mitotane, an adrenolytic drug used to reduce cortisol production and possibly improve survival.

Transsphenoidal surgery

Transsphenoidal surgery is performed for patients with an ACTH-secreting pituitary adenoma, possibly followed by external radiotherapy if cortisol levels fail to fall below 50 nmol/L. Until radiotherapy takes full effect, concurrent medical therapy may be required.

Other tumours

ACTH-secreting tumours should be removed and treated according to their aetiology. Medical therapy or adrenalectomy may be indicated if this fails to control cortisol levels.

Prognosis

Untreated Cushing's syndrome has a high mortality due to cardiovascular complications and infections (30–50% at 5 years). Even following successful therapy the initial effects on atherosclerosis persist whilst hypertension and diabetes often resolve. Osteoporosis may require specific therapy.

Recurrence rates for Cushing's disease are low (<20%) if postoperative cortisol levels were undetectable. In ectopic disease the prognosis is dependent on the underlying tumour characteristics. Adrenal adenomas can be cured by adrenalectomy whereas adrenal carcinomas have a poor prognosis.

i **FURTHER INFORMATION**

Arnaldi G, Angeli A, Atkinson AB, et al. Diagnosis and complications of Cushing's syndrome: a consensus statement. Journal of Clinical Endocrinology and Metabolism 2003; 88: 5593–5602.

Nelson's syndrome

Nelson's syndrome is a progressive pituitary tumour that may develop following adrenalectomy for incompletely cured Cushing's disease. It is now very uncommon as adrenalectomy is rarely required to treat Cushing's disease but was previously seen in up to 30% of those treated with bilateral adrenalectomy. It is characterized by marked ACTH hypersecretion leading to skin hyperpigmentation, usually within 2 years of adrenalectomy. Pituitary irradiation reduces this risk.

Adrenocortical insufficiency

Adrenocortical insufficiency can occur primarily due to disease affecting the adrenal glands (Addison's disease) or secondary to diseases affecting the hypothalamic–pituitary axis (Table 6.19).

Epidemiology

The incidence of primary adrenocortical insufficiency (Addison's disease) is 0.6 per 100 000, and the prevalence is estimated at 10 per 100 000. Women are twice as likely as men to suffer from an autoimmune cause of Addison's disease, which is most frequently diagnosed in the fourth decade.

Secondary adrenal insufficiency is more common with a prevalence of 28 per 100 000 due to the use of long-term glucocorticoid therapy. Secondary adrenal insufficiency is more commonly diagnosed in the sixth decade and also has a female preponderance.

Pathology

Addison's disease usually develops after 90% or more of the adrenal cortex has been destroyed, affecting glucocorticoid, mineralocorticoid and sex steroid synthesis. Autoantibody-mediated adrenalitis accounts for more than 70% of cases

Table 6.19	Causes of adrenocortical insufficiency

Primary adrenocortical insufficiency

Autoantibody-mediated adrenalitis (most common cause in developed countries)

Infection (most common cause in non-developed countries)
    Tuberculosis
    Opportunistic pathogens associated with HIV

Adrenal haemorrhage (Waterhouse–Friderichsen syndrome in meningococcal septicaemia)

Adrenal infarction

Adrenal infiltration
    Tumour metastasis
    Amyloidosis

Inborn errors of fatty acid metabolism

Congenital adrenal hyperplasia

Drugs
    Ketoconazole
    Etomidate
    Rifampicin

Trauma
    Traumatic loss of both adrenals
    Surgical resection of both adrenals

Secondary adrenocortical insufficiency

Chronic glucocorticoid therapy

Pituitary or hypothalamic disease
    Tumours
    Infection
    Trauma (previous surgery, radiotherapy)

423

in developed countries, where it often forms part of an autoimmune polyglandular syndrome. In less developed countries, infection is a more common cause. Other causes are listed in Table 6.19.

Secondary adrenal failure is a consequence of central ACTH deficiency, thus only glucocorticoid and sex steroid production is impaired. Mineralocorticoid levels are maintained as they are regulated by the renin–angiotensin system. Secondary adrenal failure can be due to any pituitary or hypothalamic disease. More frequently ACTH deficiency is induced by chronic glucocorticoid therapy. This leads to the atrophy of pituitary corticotroph cells and consequently to a lack of endogenous cortisol response during times of stress. Failure to increase the glucocorticoid dose in such circumstances, reduced absorption due to gastrointestinal disturbances or abrupt withdrawal of long-term therapy are the most common precipitants of secondary adrenal failure.

Both types of adrenal insufficiency usually develop gradually over time, except when a vascular event (haemorrhage or infarction) leads to a sudden loss of the adrenals or the pituitary gland. Often an acute intercurrent illness (infection, myocardial infarction) precipitates the decompensation of an already impaired hypothalamic–pituitary–adrenal (HPA) axis.

Scope of disease

Sudden-onset glucocorticoid deficiency is a life-threatening condition. Water and sodium/potassium balance is mainly caused by mineralocorticoid deficiency in Addison's disease, but is also (in part) due to the lack of cortisol. Hypoglycaemia is only mild and more frequently observed in children. In women, libido and androgen-dependent hair growth is reduced because adrenal dehydroepiandrosterone (DHEA) represents an important precursor molecule for peripheral conversion into androgens. Men are not affected because most androgens derive from the testes. Skin pigmentation is influenced by ACTH levels due to its MSH activity; this can help distinguish between primary and secondary adrenal insufficiency.

Clinical features

Patients with acute adrenal failure present with severe hypotension, nausea and vomiting, non-specific abdominal pain and frequently pyrexia (even in absence of infection). An underlying precipitant illness may be present or a history of compliance problems with prescribed glucocorticoid therapy. Pituitary apoplexy causes headaches and can be associated with visual deterioration.

Chronic adrenal insufficiency leads to lethargy, generalized weakness, anorexia and weight loss. Nausea and vomiting, abdominal pain and postural hypotension are common, whereas salt craving, myalgia and arthralgia are less frequent. Female patients may have reduced axillary and pubic hair as well as lack of libido.

In Addison's disease, hyperpigmentation mainly develops in light-exposed and friction-prone skin areas (bra straps).

The palmar creases, buccal mucosa and recent scars should also be inspected. Features of other associated autoimmune-mediated conditions (e.g. vitiligo, primary hypothyroidism) may be present.

In contrast, chronic secondary adrenal failure leads to generalized pallor. Additional features of pituitary or hypothalamic disease are often present. They include headaches and visual disturbances due to mass effect and those of abnormalities of other endocrine axes.

Initial investigations

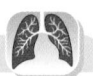

Full blood count

In both primary and secondary adrenal failure mild anaemia and eosinophilia can occur.

Urea and electrolytes

The urea is elevated with dehydration. Hyponatraemia is common, but hyperkalaemia is usually only present if there is also lack of mineralocorticoids.

Serum calcium

Hypercalcaemia can occur due to glucocorticoid deficiency.

Serum cortisol and ACTH

In patients who are not acutely unwell, the adrenal axis should be assessed by cortisol and ACTH levels taken simultaneously at 9 a.m. A cortisol of <150 nmol/L is suggestive of adrenal insufficiency, and a level >550 nmol/L excludes it. ACTH levels help to interpret values in the low normal range as they may be inappropriately elevated (normal range 2–11 pmol/L).

Short Synacthen test

The adrenal reserve can be further assessed by administration of 250 µg corticotropin and sampling of cortisol levels at baseline, 30 min and 60 min ('short Synacthen test'). Peak cortisol levels exceed 550 nmol/L during a normal response. A low-dose test (1 µg corticotropin) has been advocated to have greater sensitivity in subtle adrenal impairment, but is mainly used to assess the HPA axis in pituitary disease.

Long Synacthen test

Secondary adrenal failure is suspected with low levels of both cortisol and ACTH and an insufficient response to 250 µg of corticotropin. This should be investigated with a 'long Synacthen test' whereby 1000 µg corticotropin is administered and cortisol levels are assessed at baseline, and 1, 2, 4, 8, 12, and 24 h later. In a normal response, cortisol rises to above 1000 nmol/L.

Further investigations

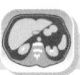

Adrenal autoantibodies

Adrenal autoantibodies (directed against 21-hydroxylase) should be sought to establish the likely aetiology of

Addison's disease. If an autoimmune cause is established, an associated autoimmune polyendocrine syndrome should be excluded.

Plasma renin activity

Plasma renin activity should be measured to assess mineralocorticoid deficiency in suspected Addison's disease.

Thyroid function tests

The measurement of TSH to screen for hypothyroidism is recommended. Thyroid function requires re-evaluation following glucocorticoid replacement as TSH levels are often raised and normalize with glucocorticoid replacement (unless there is coexisting hypothyroidism).

Other specific screening tests

Screening for associated diseases includes a fasting blood glucose (for type 1 diabetes mellitus), hypoparathyroidism, pernicious anaemia and gonadal dysfunction according to clinical suspicion. Investigations for suspected tuberculosis are described on page 123.

MRI of the head

In secondary adrenal failure, the pituitary and hypothalamus should be visualized by MRI and all endocrine axes fully evaluated.

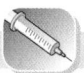

Initial management

Fluid resuscitation

In suspected acute adrenal crisis, baseline blood tests including a cortisol level should be requested and therapy commenced without delay. Fluid resuscitation with 0.9% saline is essential and glucose should be added if hypoglycaemia is present.

Hydrocortisone

A first dose of hydrocortisone 100 mg is given intravenously, followed by 6-hourly intramuscular injections of hydrocortisone 100 mg, or a continuous infusion of 10 mg/h until the patient is well enough to receive oral therapy. A total daily dose of 40 mg (in divided doses of 20, 10 and 10 mg) of hydrocortisone is twice the usual replacement therapy and is tapered once patients are stable.

Fludrocortisone

In Addison's disease fludrocortisone (50–200 µg daily) should be introduced to replace the concomitant mineralocorticoid deficiency. Electrolytes, urea and glucose are used to monitor the initial treatment progress.

Patient education

Patients with adrenal failure must be familiar with their glucocorticoid therapy and educated to avoid risks to their health (Table 6.20). They can be supplied with a supply of hydrocortisone and be taught to self-administer in an emergency.

Table 6.20	Advice for patients on long-term steroid therapy
Do not miss a dose and never stop treatment on your own	
In case of febrile illness double the dose	
In severe illness or prolonged vomiting seek urgent medical help as injections may be necessary	
Keep a steroid emergency card (blue) with you at all times (e.g. in wallet)	
Consider wearing a MedicAlert bracelet	

Medical management

Long-term glucocorticoid replacement

Hydrocortisone tds (10 mg, 5 mg, 5 mg) is given as long-term glucocorticoid replacement therapy. The aim is to mimic the physiological diurnal variations in cortisol as closely as possible, and to provide feedback inhibition of ACTH in Addison's disease. Prednisolone and dexamethasone are sometimes used because of their longer half-lives.

Treatment is monitored clinically (blood pressure, fluid status, features of glucocorticoid excess). Sodium, potassium and renin levels should be within normal range. Results from a cortisol day curve allow adjustments to be made to an individual's replacement therapy. Repeat ACTH levels are indicated if excess pigmentation develops.

Prognosis

Untreated adrenal failure is fatal, and excess mortality and morbidity are associated with delays in diagnosis and management. In autoimmune adrenal failure there is an increased risk of developing other autoimmune disorders, both of endocrine and non-endocrine nature. For adrenal insufficiency due to other aetiologies, the prognosis is related to the underlying disease.

i **FURTHER INFORMATION**

Arlt W, Allolio B. Adrenal insufficiency. Lancet 2003; 361: 1881–1893.

Congenital adrenal hyperplasia

Congenital adrenal hyperplasia is a group of disorders characterized by the deficiency of one of five enzymes required for steroid synthesis due to mutations of the steroidogenic cytochrome p450 (CYP) enzymes.

Epidemiology

In more than 90%, congenital adrenal hyperplasia is due to defects in the 21α-hydroxylase gene (*CYP21A2*). Complete deficiency is estimated to occur in up to 6.6 per 100 000 live births. Incomplete CYP21 deficiency is found in 0.2% of white populations, except in Eastern European Jews where the prevalence reaches 2%. Less than 5% of cases are caused by 11β-hydroxylase deficiency (CYP11B1). Both 17α-hydroxylase (CYP17) and 3β-hydroxysteroid dehydrogenase (3β-HSD) defects are rare. Mutations of an intracellular cholesterol transport protein (StAR) can also lead to CAH.

Pathology

Congenital adrenal hyperplasia is inherited as an autosomal recessive trait. Depending on the enzymatic defect this results in a lack of cortisol and a variable concomitant deficiency of mineralocorticoid or sex steroids. Feedback inhibition on ACTH secretion is lost leading to adrenal hyperplasia in an attempt to overcome the synthetic block. Precursor molecules are metabolized through alternative pathways and can attain androgenic or mineralocorticoid activity.

The presence or absence of glucocorticoids, mineralocorticoids, sex steroids and precursor metabolites determines the features of each type of congenital adrenal hyperplasia. Cortisol deficiency is life threatening and requires prompt diagnosis and therapy shortly after birth. Mineralocorticoid deficiency leads to renal sodium losses and aggravates the symptoms of cortisol deficiency. Excess androgenic activity affects genital development in female patients. In both sexes, excess androgenic activity can affect postnatal growth, trigger central precocious puberty and interfere with fertility. The accumulation of molecules with mineralocorticoid activity causes hypertension and hypokalaemia.

The type of genetic mutation (e.g. gene deletion, frame shift or single point mutation) influences the degree of clinical severity. CYP21A2 activity may range from complete absence (classic CAH), to that required for residual mineralocorticoid synthesis (simple virilizing CAH), to almost half-normal activity (non-classical CAH). Furthermore, symptoms and signs depend on the sex of the patient and the age at diagnosis and intervention.

Clinical features

'Classic' congenital adrenal hyperplasia presents with adrenal crisis and 'salt-wasting'. The newborn develops hypotension, circulatory collapse, hyponatraemia, hyperkalaemia and hypoglycaemia. In addition, females become 'virilized' with clitorimegaly, labial fusion and a penile urethra. Whilst the uterus and ovaries are not affected, the vaginal introitus may be absent. This ambiguous appearance can lead to sex mis-assignment at birth, often requiring reconstructive surgery. Approximately 60% of females are fertile. Male babies have normal genitalia at birth but develop premature pubarche and penile enlargement in early childhood. The testes are small as the androgens are produced in the adrenals. The androgen-induced excess of longitudinal growth in childhood affects both sexes and is offset by premature bone maturation, leading to a reduced final height.

The 'simple virilizing' form of CAH is characterized by a lesser degree of cortisol deficiency and genital abnormalities, and by the absence of sodium loss and hyperkalaemia. Approximately 80% of females are fertile.

'Non-classical' CAH is the mildest form of CYP21A2 deficiency. In women it is often diagnosed around puberty when increased androgenic precursors lead to hirsutism, acne, and oligo/amenorrhoea. One third have polycystic ovaries on ultrasonography and reduced fertility. Most male patients are asymptomatic, but fertility may be affected if androgens suppress pituitary gonadotrophins and thus spermatogenesis.

In CYP11B1 deficiency, additional hypertension and hypokalaemia may develop. This is due to mineralocorticoid activity of the accumulating deoxycorticosterone, with hypertension present in the majority of adult patients.

Mutations of CYP17 cause defects in cortisol and sex steroid synthesis. This may lead to delayed puberty in women and to male pseudohermaphroditism, requiring the therapeutic induction of puberty. Hypertension and hypokalaemia develop due to increased deoxycorticosterone production.

Severe cases of 3β-HSD deficiency demonstrate salt wasting, female virilization and male pseudohermaphroditism.

Investigations
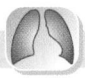

Although cortisol deficiency is central to congenital adrenal hyperplasia, the serum levels of precursor molecules and urinary metabolites are measured to determine the specific enzyme defect. Due to diurnal variations under the influence of ACTH, all blood samples should be collected at 9 a.m. and preferably in the follicular phase of the menstrual cycle in women.

Serum 17-hydroxy-progesterone
17-Hydroxy-progesterone (17-OHP) levels are usually elevated in the classic and simple virilizing forms of CYP21 deficiency, with basal values of >15 nmol/L considered diagnostic and <5 nmol/L normal. In the non-classical form intermediate values should be repeated following tetracosactin (ACTH) stimulation, leading to a substantial rise (>45 nmol/L) when congenital adrenal hyperplasia is present.

Serum testosterone and androstenedione
Testosterone and androstenedione (A4) are elevated, although in non-classical congenital adrenal hyperplasia there is overlap with the levels found in the polycystic ovary syndrome.

Renin levels
Renin levels should be measured to assess mineralocorticoid deficiency and adequacy of fludrocortisone replacement.

ACTH levels
ACTH levels are usually elevated in poorly controlled congenital adrenal hyperplasia but may be normal in the non-classical form.

Urinary steroid profile

A urinary steroid profile is required to diagnose the rarer types of congenital adrenal hyperplasia.

Management

Glucocorticoid replacement

The administration of glucocorticoids prevents adrenal crises and aims to restore feedback inhibition on ACTH to reduce the accumulation of precursors that are responsible for most other features of congenital adrenal hyperplasia.

It can be difficult to avoid glucocorticoid excess from over-replacement, which can stunt growth during childhood. Close monitoring for central obesity, purple striae and hypertension is necessary to detect Cushing's syndrome early. Prednisolone and dexamethasone are the preferred steroids due to their longer half-lives when compared to hydrocortisone.

Mineralocorticoid replacement

For concomitant mineralocorticoid deficiency fludrocortisone (50–200 µg/d) is used and adjusted according to blood pressure and renin levels.

Genetic counselling

Genetic counselling should be offered to prospective parents. Treatment with dexamethasone from 6 weeks post conception aims to prevent virilization of a female fetus in mothers with classic disease.

Prognosis

With appropriate replacement therapy the prognosis is good with normal life expectancy. There is an increased rate of gender identity problems, and in severe cases fertility remains reduced. Frequently a shorter than predicted final height is achieved, due to glucocorticoid therapy in childhood and acceleration of bone maturation. Benign adrenal tumours, and in males testicular adrenal rest tumours, are found more commonly in patients with congenital adrenal hyperplasia, and often respond to appropriate ACTH suppression.

ℹ FURTHER INFORMATION

Speiser PW, White PC. Congenital adrenal hyperplasia. New England Journal of Medicine 2003; 349: 776–788.

Primary aldosteronism

Phaeochromocytoma

SECTION 6.8 The adrenal glands and kidney

Primary aldosteronism

Aldosteronism is the syndrome associated with excessive aldosterone production. Primary aldosteronism (Conn's syndrome) occurs when the cause is due to the adrenal glands, and secondary aldosteronism occurs when the stimulus is extra-adrenal.

Epidemiology

Screening tests and improved diagnostic criteria have led to more patients being diagnosed with primary aldosteronism. Currently, approximately 10% of hypertensive patients are thought to have primary aldosteronism.

Pathology

The causes of aldosteronism are listed in Table 6.21. Adrenal adenoma and adrenal hyperplasia are the two most common causes of primary hyperadrenalism. The adrenal adenoma is small (<2 cm), unilateral and benign. Various adrenal cell types may be found on microscopy of the tumour with cells that resemble those found in the zona glomerulosa, zona fasciculata or zona reticularis. Adrenal hyperplasia (also known as idiopathic aldosteronism) can be micronodular or macronodular, and is usually (but not invariably) bilateral. Rare causes of primary aldosteronism

include adrenal carcinoma and an autosomal dominant form of familial hyperaldosteronism arising from mutations of the 11 β-hydroxylase and aldosterone synthase genes.

The causes of secondary aldosteronism are due to increased levels of aldosterone in response to inappropriate activation of the renin–angiotensin axis (Table 6.21).

Table 6.21	Causes of aldosteronism
Primary aldosteronism (Conn's syndrome)	
Adrenal adenoma	
Adrenal hyperplasia	
Adrenal carcinoma	
Familial hyperaldosteronism	
Secondary aldosteronism	
Physiological	
Pregnancy	
Excess renin production	
Renal artery stenosis	
Cardiac failure	
Renin-secreting tumour	
Bartter's syndrome	

427

Clinical features

The principal manifestation of primary aldosteronism is hypertension and the associated end-organ damage from chronically elevated blood pressure (p. 68). There is no pattern to the blood pressure elevation, and hypertension can range from mild to severe but is seldom malignant. Some patients may be completely asymptomatic. Hypokalaemia may lead to symptoms such as polyuria, nocturia, muscle cramps and weakness.

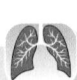

Initial investigations

Urea and electrolytes

Although hypokalaemia has been described as a classical feature, it is present in less than half of the patients. Patients may also have hypernatraemia, hyperchlorhydria and a hypokalaemic alkalosis.

Serum aldosterone and renin levels

The diagnostic criteria for primary aldosteronism are diastolic hypertension without oedema associated with high aldosterone and low serum renin levels. A high plasma aldosterone to renin ratio (more than 30:1) is supportive of primary hyperaldosteronism, although the test results can be influenced by a number of factors. Posture and the time of sampling can affect the results, and blood should be taken in the morning in patients who have been upright for a few hours. A wide variety of medication such as diuretics, β-blockers and non-steroidal anti-inflammatories can also affect the results, and these drugs should be stopped 2–4 weeks before the test. Patients with hypokalaemia should also have this deficiency corrected with potassium supplements prior to testing.

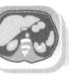

Further investigations

Patients with high aldosterone to renin ratios need to have further tests to confirm (or refute) the diagnosis of primary aldosteronism, including imaging to localize the lesion.

Aldosterone suppression test

Evidence of autonomous secretion (aldosterone-producing tumour) can be assessed by loading the patient with salt, either orally or intravenously (>300 mEq/day). Failure of suppression of aldosterone with urinary excretion of more than 12 μg in 24 hours is suggestive of primary aldosteronism. This test should be performed with caution in patients with poor left ventricular function (secondary aldosteronism) due to the risk of precipitating cardiac failure and is no longer used routinely.

CT of the abdomen

Once the biochemical diagnosis is confirmed, further investigations are directed towards localization of the lesion. CT scanning is capable of detecting some adrenal tumours but may miss lesions smaller than 1 cm. Patients

with adrenal hyperplasia may show normal or bilaterally enlarged glands. MRI scanning can also be used (Fig. 6.10).

Adrenal venous sampling

Adrenal venous blood sampling is invasive but probably provides the most useful information in localizing the source of the excess aldosterone, particularly if imaging is inconclusive. An aldosterone ratio between the two adrenal glands should be more than 10:1 for diagnosis of unilateral adenoma.

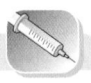

Initial management

Spironolactone

Surgical therapy is recommended for patients with adrenal tumours, while patients with bilateral hyperplasia are best managed with medical therapy. Spironolactone can be used for 3–4 weeks before surgery to minimize hyperaldosteronism preoperatively and to help correct potassium levels.

Surgical management

Laparoscopic adrenalectomy

Laparoscopic adrenalectomy is performed in patients with unilateral adrenal involvement. A pneumoperitoneum is created, a subcostal port is placed for the laparoscope, and three other 10 mm ports are sited.

For right adrenalectomy the liver is mobilized and retracted. The inferior vena cava is displayed and the adrenal gland identified. The main right adrenal vein and any accessory veins are identified and controlled early. Gland dissection is continued and the gland removed via an impervious bag.

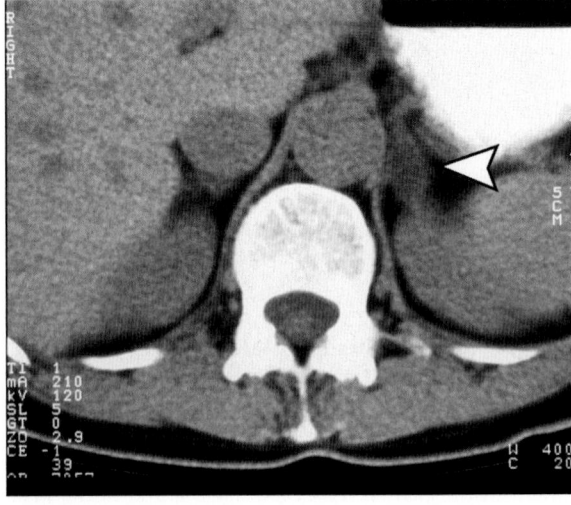

Fig. 6.10 MRI of the abdomen showing an adrenal adenoma (arrow).
Image courtesy of Kevin O'Shaughnessy, Addenbrooke's Hospital, Cambridge, UK.

Left adrenalectomy commences by dissecting the splenorenal ligament to allow retraction of the spleen. The splenic vein is traced laterally, allowing the left adrenal vein and left adrenal gland to be identified. The adrenal vein is divided before the gland is dissected and removed (Fig. 6.11).[1]

Patients with unilateral adrenal hyperplasia derive less benefit from the operation than do patients with adrenal adenomas.

Medical management

Spironolactone or amiloride

Low doses of spironolactone or amiloride are effective in controlling hypertension and hypokalaemia in patients with adrenal hyperplasia. The side effects of spironolactone include impotence, menstrual irregularities and gynaecomastia.

Glucocorticoids

The treatment of familial hyperaldosteronism is with low doses of glucocorticoids.

> **RECENT ADVANCES**
>
> *Eplerenone is a new, more receptor-specific aldosterone antagonist, and may be better tolerated than spironolactone. Clinical trials on the efficacy of this new agent are awaited.*

Prognosis

Surgery is curative in about 50% of patients with primary aldosteronism and reduces the severity in 90%. Antihypertensive therapy can usually be gradually tapered 3–6 months after the operation. Spironolactone is generally effective in controlling the blood pressure in the majority of patients with primary aldosteronism.

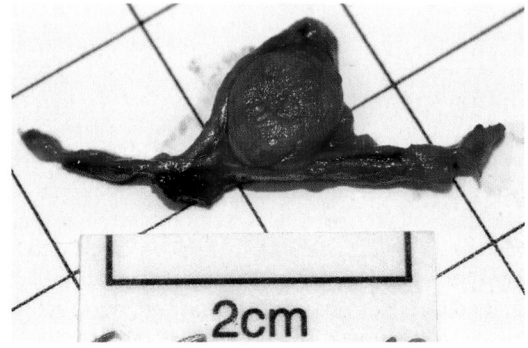

Fig. 6.11 Adrenal adenoma.
Image courtesy of Kevin O'Shaughnessy, Addenbrooke's Hospital, Cambridge, UK.

> **ⅈ FURTHER INFORMATION**
>
> Ganguly A. Primary aldosteronism. New England Journal of Medicine 1998; 339: 1828–1834.

> **REFERENCE**
>
> **(1)** *Harris DA, Au-Yong I, Basnyat PS, Sadler GP, Wheeler MH. Review of surgical management of aldosterone secreting tumours of the adrenal cortex. European Journal of Surgical Oncology 2003; 29: 467–474.*

Phaeochromocytoma

Phaeochromocytomas are tumours arising from the chromaffin cells that produce, store and secrete catecholamines.

Epidemiology

Phaeochromocytoma is a rare tumour, with an incidence of about 0.8 per 100 000 per year. Patients can present at any age but the highest incidence occurs between the ages of 30 and 50 years.

Pathology

Although phaeochromocytomas generally arise from the chromaffin cells of adrenal medulla, they can originate from any extra-adrenal chromaffin cells which lie alongside the sympathetic ganglia of the spinal cord from the neck to the pelvis. Other locations in which phaeochromocytomas have been reported include the carotid body, in the retroperitoneum along the course of the distal aorta, in the ureters and bladder, and in dermoid cysts. Extra-adrenal tumours are more likely to be malignant, and multifocal.

Cytological examination reveals tightly clustered nests of chromaffin cells, some of which may have bizarre shapes. The classification of malignancy is not based on histological appearance but depends on whether the tumour has invaded the capsule or metastasized. The catecholamines secreted by the tumour include noradrenaline, adrenaline and dopamine.

A number of genetic mutations are found in association with phaeochromocytomas: the *RET* oncogene (associated with multiple endocrine neoplasia type 2), the tumour suppressor gene *VHL* (associated with von Hippel–Lindau disease) and succinate dehydrogenase subunits D and B (associated with paragangliomas).

Previously, it was thought that 10% of phaeochromocytomas were malignant, extra-adrenal or bilateral. Currently, the proportions are more accurately defined as 15% malignant, 18% extra-adrenal, and 20% familial respectively.[1]

Scope of disease

The patients have symptoms and signs relating to sympathetic overdrive. In severe cases, malignant hypertension can lead to stroke. Impaired glucose tolerance can occur due to the suppression of insulin by catecholamines. Angina and myocardial infarction have been documented despite the absence of coronary artery disease.

Clinical features

The vast majority of patients present with hypertension. In approximately 60% it is sustained and in 40% it is intermittent. This is accompanied by paroxysmal symptoms related to sympathetic overactivity such as palpitations, anxiety, breathlessness, headache, epigastric pain and a sensation of impending doom. The symptoms lack diagnostic specificity and may be confused with those of a panic attack or anxiety or thyrotoxicosis. In patients with phaeochromocytoma, paroxysmal attacks may be triggered by emotional stress, induction of anaesthesia or abdominal compression.

Physical examination is usually unremarkable.

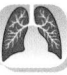

Initial investigations

24-Hour urinary catecholamines and metanephrines

Direct measurement of plasma catecholamines is unhelpful as the levels may be entirely normal in between attacks. Therefore urinary excretion of catecholamines and metabolites is measured over a 24-hour period.[1] The metanephrines, vanillylmandelic acid (VMA) and homovanillic acid (HVA), are the main urinary metabolites, and are only found in small quantities in normal circumstances. Repeated measurement of 24-hour urinary catecholamines and metanephrines may be necessary, given the intermittent nature of secretion by the tumour.

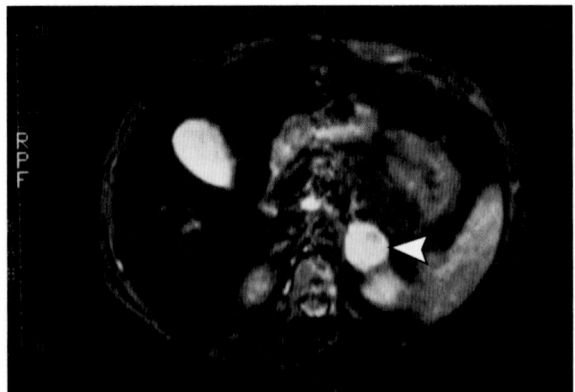

Fig. 6.12 T2-weighted MRI of the abdomen showing a left phaeochromocytoma (arrow).
Image courtesy of Kevin O'Shaughnessy, Addenbrooke's Hospital, Cambridge, UK.

Increased excretion can occur with coma, dehydration, extreme stress and after the consumption of vanilla-containing food, leading to false-positive results. Other drugs that can also interfere with the test results include β-blockers, methyldopa and tricyclic antidepressants.

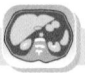

Further investigations

Imaging studies are the next step for patients who have undergone initial biochemical evaluation and are strongly suspected of having a phaeochromocytoma.

CT/MRI of the abdomen

Localizing the site of a phaeochromocytoma can be difficult. A recommended approach is to start with either abdominal CT or MRI (Fig. 6.12, neither modality is demonstrably superior to the other)[2] that can be extended to the chest and neck if no abdominal lesion is identified.

MIBG radioisotope scanning

The next step is functional imaging, using MIBG radioisotope scanning. MIBG is an aralkyl guanidine that has a structural resemblance to noradrenaline. It is taken into sympathomedullary tissues via a noradrenaline transport mechanism. The sensitivity of MIBG scan for phaeochromocytoma is 90% and it is also highly specific at approximately 95% (Fig. 6.13). In rare instances, false-positive results can occur due to uptake by neuroblastomas and carcinoid tumours. The availability of MIBG may be limited, and patients have to be scanned on 3 consecutive days before results become available.

Selective venous sampling

Venous blood sampling is invasive and technically demanding, but is probably the most definitive method if all other imaging tests have failed.

RECENT ADVANCES

There are promising results for studies using PET scanning for the localization of phaechromocytomas.[3]

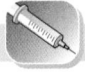

Initial management

Blood pressure control

Surgery is the treatment of choice for patients with phaeochromocytoma, but is seldom required on an urgent basis. It is preferable to achieve blood pressure control and stabilize the patient using α- and β-blocker drug therapy prior to operation. This is commonly achieved by first giving phenoxybenzamine, a non-competitive α-receptor blocker, followed by a β-blocker such as metoprolol. Another treatment option is labetalol, which provides combined α and β blockade.

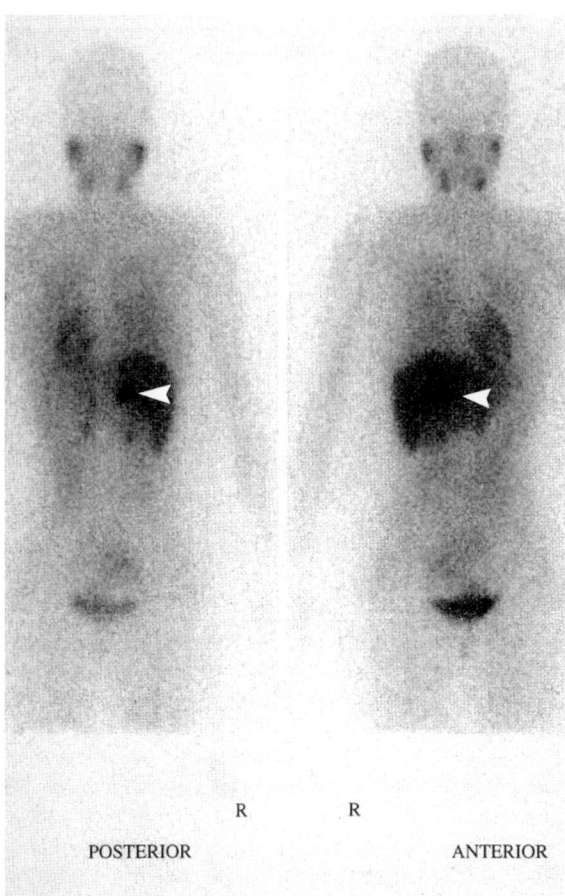

R   R

POSTERIOR   ANTERIOR

Fig. 6.13 An MIBG scan showing high uptake from a phaeochromocytoma (arrows).
Image courtesy of Kevin O'Shaughnessy, Addenbrooke's Hospital, Cambridge, UK.

CLINICAL ALERT

It is not advisable to use β-blockers as the initial or sole agent for the management of patients with phaeochromocytoma. Acute pulmonary oedema has been reported from the suppression of β-mediated cardiac pump activity while the arterioles are still vasoconstricted from α-adrenergic stimulation.

Surgical management

Adrenalectomy
The recommended technique is the open anterior abdominal approach to allow the surgeon to search for other phaeochromocytomas. Laparoscopic adrenalectomy may be an option for small tumours, where imaging processes have localized the lesion with certainty.

Control of blood pressure during surgery can be challenging, especially as surges of catecholamine release can occur with handling of the tumour. A variety of intravenous agents have been used to achieve rapid lowering of blood pressure such as phentolamine (an α-blocker), labetalol and sodium nitroprusside. Arterial line and central venous pressure monitoring is essential, as wide swings in blood pressure can occur.

Medical management

Metyrosine
Patients with metastatic phaeochromocytoma are unsuitable for surgery and best treated with metyrosine, a tyrosine hydroxylase inhibitor which blocks the processes involved in catecholamine synthesis.

> **RECENT ADVANCES**
>
> *Radioactive MIBG is currently being evaluated in the treatment of metastatic disease.*

Prognosis

Patients with benign phaeochromocytoma are cured if the tumour is completely excised. However, there is a 10% risk of recurrence over the next 10 years. The 5-year survival probability for patients with malignant phaeochromocytoma is less than 60%, with a median survival of approximately 16 months.

REFERENCES

(1) Manger WM, Eisenhofer G. Pheochromocytoma: diagnosis and management update. Current Hypertension Reports 2004; 6: 477–484.
(2) Kudva YC, Sawka AM, Young WF Jr. Clinical review 164: The laboratory diagnosis of adrenal pheochromocytoma: the Mayo Clinic experience. Journal of Clinical Endocrinology and Metabolism 2003; 88: 4533–4539.
(3) Ilias I, Pacak K. Current approaches and recommended algorithm for the diagnostic localization of pheochromocytoma. Journal of Clinical Endocrinology and Metabolism 2004; 89: 479–491.

Primary aldosteronism

Phaeochromocytoma

Multiple endocrine disorders

Multiple endocrine neoplasias

The multiple endocrine neoplasias (MEN) are syndromes characterized by the development of tumours in several endocrine tissues. There are two main subtypes: MEN-1 and MEN-2.

Epidemiology

The prevalence of MEN-1 is estimated as 10 per 100 000, and that of MEN-2 as 2 per 100 000.

Pathology

The inheritance of MEN is by autosomal dominant trait. The majority are due to sporadic mutations. MEN syndromes affect a broad range of endocrine tissues, determining the clinical presentation, therapeutic options and prognosis. The genetic penetrance, endocrine glands involved and onset of tumour development differ between the various types and even between affected kindred.

MEN type 1 or Wermer's syndrome is caused by an inactivating mutation of the tumour suppressor gene *MEN1*. The diagnosis is made by the presence of two of the following conditions: parathyroid adenoma, pancreatic endocrine tumour and pituitary adenomas (Table 6.22).

MEN type 2 is caused by an activating mutation in the tumour suppressor gene *ret*. There are three subtypes depending on the genetic mutation. MEN-2A (Sipple's syndrome) comprises 75% of MEN-2 syndromes. MEN-2B does not cause hyperparathyroidism but includes mucosal ganglioneuromas and a marfanoid habitus. Familial medullary thyroid carcinoma (MTC) alone represents the third variant (Table 6.22).

Many of the endocrine tumours remain benign and cause disease through hormone excess (PTH or gastrin in MEN-1 and calcitonin or catecholamines in MEN-2). However, some pancreatic tumours and medullary thyroid carcinoma are malignant and carry significant mortality.

Clinical features

The MEN syndromes present with the symptoms and signs of the respective endocrine tumours. The diagnosis of two characteristic endocrine tumours in the same patient should raise the possibility of a MEN syndrome, in particular in young patients.

In MEN-1, the first abnormality to develop is usually hyperparathyroidism, and such a diagnosis in a patient under 50 years should prompt screening for carrier status. Symptoms of hypercalcaemia (lethargy, thirst and polyuria, constipation and nausea, abdominal pains, renal stones) may develop. Endocrine active pancreatic tumours can cause peptic ulcers due to gastrin excess or hypoglycaemia if an insulinoma is present. Uncontrolled prolactin secretion leads to galactorrhoea, irregular periods and reduced libido, and growth hormone oversecretion to acromegaly. Hypopituitarism can also occur, secondary to any pituitary tumour.

In MEN-2, medullary thyroid carcinoma usually occurs first and presents as anterior neck nodule, or with diarrhoea

Table 6.22	Characteristic features of MEN		
MEN-1	**MEN-2**		
	MEN-2A (75%)	**MEN-2B**	**Familial MTC**
Wermer's syndrome	Sipple's syndrome		
Parathyroid adenoma (more than 90%)	Medullary thyroid carcinoma (90%)	Medullary thyroid carcinoma	Medullary thyroid carcinoma
Pancreatic endocrine tumour (70%)	Phaeochromocytoma (20–50%)	Phaeochromocytoma	
Gastrinomas			
Insulinomas			
Pituitary adenomas (30%)	Parathyroid tumours (10–25%)	Mucosal ganglioneuromas	
Prolactinomas			
GH-secreting tumours		Marfanoid habitus	

MTC, medullary thyroid carcinoma; GH, growth hormone.

if metastatic disease is present. The elevated calcitonin levels rarely lead to features of hypocalcaemia. Catecholamine excess due to phaeochromocytoma causes intermittent headaches, sweating, palpitations and hypertension. The features of hyperparathyroidism in MEN-2A are milder than in MEN-1. In MEN-2B a marfanoid habitus is present and ganglioneuromas develop on the lips, the distal tongue and throughout the gastrointestinal tract. Medullary thyroid carcinoma is clinically more aggressive and occurs earlier than in MEN-2A.

Investigations

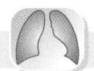

Genetic testing

When MEN is clinically suspected, genetic testing for the mutation is performed to confirm carrier status. In confirmed cases first-degree relatives should subsequently be offered screening. Genetic counselling should be offered to family members undergoing screening and to affected individuals considering conception.

Biochemical screening

Investigations for the individual endocrine abnormalities are the same as for sporadic tumours. An annual biochemical assessment is performed to detect subclinical endocrine manifestations and to monitor therapy. Imaging investigations are required every 3–5 years.

In MEN-1 the biochemical screen should include calcium/PTH, fasting glucose, insulin and gut hormone profile, chromogranin A (a marker for neuroendocrine tumours), PRL and IGF-1. MRI of the pancreas and pituitary is recommended for affected individuals.

In MEN-2 calcitonin (basal or following pentagastrin stimulation), urinary or plasma catecholamines and calcium/ PTH should be measured. Calcitonin also serves as a tumour marker following thyroidectomy for medullary thyroid carcinoma. Adrenal MRI is indicated for carriers.

Management

MEN-1

Parathyroid surgery is performed with the exploration of all four glands as multiple adenomas are common. Following the removal of $3\frac{1}{2}$ glands, half a parathyroid gland is either left in situ or is autotransplanted to the forearm.

Pancreatic tumours are frequently treated with proton pump inhibitors (gastrinoma) or octreotide (other gut hormone excess), but insulinomas require pancreatic resection.

Pituitary adenomas are treated like sporadic tumours, usually with a combination of pituitary surgery, irradiation and medical therapy.

MEN-2

Medullary thyroid carcinoma is multifocal and requires total thyroidectomy and life-long thyroxine replacement. Surgery for medullary thyroid carcinoma in known carriers is advised before the age of 5 years due to its early occurrence and aggressiveness.

Prior to thyroid exploration a phaeochromocytoma must be actively excluded. If present, laparoscopic adrenalectomy following α- and β-adrenergic blockade is commonly performed. The indications for parathyroidectomy in MEN-2A follow the criteria for isolated primary hyperparathyroidism.

Prognosis

Approximately a third of patients die from MEN-1 associated malignant tumours (in particular pancreatic tumours) with reduced overall life expectancy. Affected patients have a 50% risk of death by the age of 50 years.

For MEN-2, the overall 10-year survival probability from diagnosis is approximately 65%. Since genetic testing for carrier status was introduced, mortality from medullary thyroid carcinoma and phaeochromocytoma has been reduced.

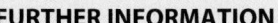

i FURTHER INFORMATION

Brandi ML, Gagel RF, Angeli A, et al. Guidelines for diagnosis and therapy of MEN type 1 and type 2. Journal of Clinical Endocrinology and Metabolism 2001; 86: 5658–5671.

Polyglandular autoimmune syndromes

Polyglandular autoimmune disorders are rare syndromes characterized by the failure of more than two endocrine organs from autoimmune destruction. The pathology consists of chronic lymphocytic infiltrates around the affected organs, as well as the presence of autoantibodies to specific cell components. Non-endocrine tissues may also be affected by the autoimmune pathology, and the polyglandular autoimmune syndromes have been classified into two major subtypes based on age of patient, associated clinical features and mode of inheritance (Table 6.23). Type II syndrome is the more common variant, and measurement of autoantibodies may be helpful in the diagnosis. Specific medical treatment is directed towards the manifestations of the endocrine organ failure.

Table 6.23	Clinical features of polyglandular autoimmune syndromes		
	Type I	**Type II**	**Type III**
Age of onset	Age 3–5 years and early adolescence	Adults aged 30–40 years	Middle-aged
Genetic associations	Mutations in autoimmune regulator gene on chromosome 21	HLA-DR3, HLA-DR4, HLA-B8	HLA-DR1
Main clinical features	Chronic mucocutaneous candidiasis, chronic hypoparathyroidism, adrenal insufficiency	Adrenal insufficiency, hypothyroidism, type 1 diabetes mellitus	Hypothyroidism, type I diabetes mellitus, pernicious anaemia, vitiligo

SECTION 6.10 Disorders of sex and reproduction

Polycystic ovary syndrome

Polycystic ovary syndrome, or Stein–Leventhal syndrome as it was previously known, is a clinical condition with a combination of hyperandrogenism (acne, hirsutism, male pattern baldness but no virilization) and anovulation (menstrual irregularity, infertility) with typical ultrasound changes in the ovaries.

Epidemiology

Polycystic ovary syndrome is the most common endocrine disorder of women of reproductive age, affecting at least 8% of women using clinical criteria alone and 20% using ultrasound findings. It occurs in up to 20% of Caucasians and 50% of Asians. It is thought to be the cause of 95% of cases of hirsutism referred to endocrinology and dermatology outpatient clinics.

Pathology

The characteristic pathological findings are enlarged ovaries with multiple small cysts which are multiple follicles at various stages of development. The ovarian capsule is often thickened or scarred. The follicles fail to mature (possibly due to abnormalities in FSH/LH and androgen levels) and take on the appearance of fluid-filled sacs. Excess androgens are thought to arise from excessive production by the ovaries.

Scope of disease

Patients may have mild symptoms only, with the diagnosis made incidentally on ultrasound scanning. Disruption to the menstrual cycle and lack of ovulation can lead to infertility. Polycystic ovary syndrome has genetic associations with insulin resistance, although obesity and type 2 diabetes mellitus (7-fold increased risk) are common associated features. Polycystic ovary syndrome is also associated with obstructive sleep apnoea, endometrial carcinoma and cardiovascular disease.

Clinical features

Common symptoms are menstrual irregularity, obesity, excessive body and facial hair, acne and male-pattern baldness. Infertility is also an occasional presenting complaint. On examination, hypertension and signs of diabetes may also be evident.

Some patients with the syndrome may have some but not all of the classical findings. The 2003 international criteria are listed in Table 6.24, where two out of three criteria are required for diagnosis.

Initial investigations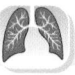

Serum testosterone level

Elevated testosterone levels provide biochemical evidence of hyperandrogenism; however, it is usually within the normal range. Other causes of raised androgen levels include congenital adrenal hyperplasia and androgen-secreting tumours.

Sex hormone binding globulin

Sex hormone binding globulin (SHBG) is low in 50%.

Serum LH and FSH

Raised LH occurs in up to 70%: the higher the LH level, the more likely it is that fertility is affected. There is also an increased LH:FSH ratio.

Table 6.24	Clinical criteria for the diagnosis of polycystic ovary syndrome*
Presence of polycystic ovaries on ultrasound examination	
Oligo-/anovulation	
Clinical or biochemical evidence of androgen excess	

*The internationally agreed definition of polycystic ovary syndrome (2003) relies on the finding of two out of three of the aforementioned criteria.

Pelvic ultrasound scan

Typically (in 90% of cases) there is an increase in ovarian stroma with more than 8 follicular cysts that are <10 mm in size. Transvaginal ultrasound will also detect most solitary virilizing ovarian tumours.

Further investigations

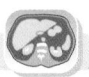

Once the diagnosis is confirmed, further tests are often performed to screen for associated diseases or differential diagnoses associated with androgen excess (based on any associated clinical features).

Screening for associated diseases

Oral glucose tolerance test

An oral glucose tolerance test is recommended in women over the age of 30 because up to 40% can have impaired glucose tolerance associated with this insulin-resistant state and up to 15% develop type 2 diabetes at some time in their lives.

Serum lipid profile

Screening for hyperlipidaemia and hypertriglyceridaemia is undertaken to assess the cardiovascular risk profile.

Screening for endometrial cancer

Patients who have not had a menstrual period for more than a year should be assessed for the risk of endometrial cancer. This may be done through ultrasonic measurement of the endometrial thickness, or through endometrial biopsy.

Screening for differential diagnoses

Screening for adrenal disease

17-OH progesterone levels are performed to exclude late-onset congenital adrenal hyperplasia (p. 426). Dehydro-epiandrosterone and androstenedione can also be significantly raised with adrenal disease.

Screening for prolactinoma

Mild hyperprolactinaemia is seen in 30% of patients but is usually less than 2000 mU/L.

Screening for Cushing's syndrome

Urinary free cortisol and an overnight dexamethasone suppression test should be performed if cortisol excess is suspected.

Initial management

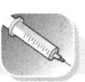

Patient education

Dietary modification to follow a low glycaemic index, low-fat diet can be used and may aid in weight reduction. This may improve insulin resistance and symptoms such as hirsutism.

Medical management

The aims of treatment are symptomatic improvement and reduction of the risk of complications from metabolic and cardiovascular abnormalities.

Suppression of hyperandrogenism

Suppression of hyperandrogenism reduces symptoms such as acne and hirsutism. This can be achieved using oestrogen therapy such as the combined oral contraceptive pill. Oestrogen suppresses LH and the subsequent overproduction of androgens in the ovaries. The progestogen component protects against unopposed oestrogenic stimulation of the endometrium which can cause endometrial cancer. However, synthetic progestogens derived from male hormones should be avoided. In addition to relief of acne and hirsutism, the contraceptive pill restores menstrual regularity. However, the adverse effects include worsening of insulin resistance and increased risk of vascular thrombosis.

Other competitive androgen receptor blockers such as cyproterone acetate (benefits 60%), spironolactone (benefits 45%) and flutamide (benefits 50%) may be used in combination to achieve a greater response. Glucocorticoids have been used but have significant side effects.

Management of infertility

Induction of ovulation is required if the patient wishes to become pregnant. Clomifene is an orally available agent which blocks oestrogen receptors in the hypothalamus, thus triggering additional gonadotrophin release.

Pulsatile gonadotrophin therapy is associated with a 40% conception rate after 4 cycles. Surgical treatment includes laparoscopic diathermy or laser drilling that can restore ovulation in up to 80%. If all these therapies do not help, in vitro fertilization can be successful in up to 80% after 6 cycles.

Management of insulin resistance

Metformin, a biguanide drug used to treat type 2 diabetes mellitus, has been used in treatment of insulin resistance found in polycystic ovary syndrome. Benefits include reduction in fasting insulin levels, blood pressure and low-density lipoprotein cholesterol.[1] In addition, metformin significantly increased the likelihood of ovulation (in up to a third of patients), with an odds ratio of 3.88 (confidence interval (CI) 2.25 to 6.69) compared to placebo. The most common adverse effects of metformin are gastrointestinal disturbance such as nausea and vomiting.

Polycystic ovary syndrome

Hypogonadism

Prognosis

Although polycystic ovary syndrome is associated with cardiovascular risk factors, there is no substantive study evaluating the impact on mortality. Most patients benefit from drug therapy to relieve symptoms, but it is unclear whether any treatment improves survival.

---

i FURTHER INFORMATION

Rotterdam ESHRE/ASRM-Sponsored PCOS Consensus Workshop Group. Revised 2003 consensus on diagnostic criteria and long-term health risks related to polycystic ovary syndrome. Fertility and Sterility 2004; 81: 19–25.

REFERENCE

(1) *Lord JM, Flight IHK, Norman RJ. Insulin-sensitising drugs (metformin, troglitazone, rosiglitazone, pioglitazone, D-chiro-inositol) for polycystic ovary syndrome. Cochrane Database of Systematic Reviews 2003; 3: CD003053.*

Hypogonadism

Hypogonadism is reduced or absent hormone secretion from the gonads (testes or ovaries).

Epidemiology

There is a progressive diminution of gonadal function with ageing in adults. The prevalence of low testosterone levels is less than 5% of men under the age of 40, but approaches 50% in men older than 80 years. The menopause in women occurs on average at the age of 51 years in European populations. Premature ovarian failure is diagnosed in women who become menopausal before the age of 40; it occurs in 1% of women but accounts for 10% of all cases of secondary amenorrhoea.

Pathology

Primary hypogonadism occurs with failure of the testes or ovaries. The underlying disease may be unknown (idiopathic) or due to iatrogenic causes (surgery, radiation or chemotherapy), serious illness (liver or kidney failure), congenital enzyme defects or chromosomal abnormalities (Turner's syndrome, Klinefelter's syndrome). Secondary or central hypogonadism occurs when the pituitary or hypothalamus is affected by intracranial pathology (p. 620).

Scope of disease

Children with hypogonadism fail to develop sexual maturity, and have delayed or absent puberty. Girls may have short stature, while boys have skeletal and muscle abnormalities. Hypogonadism may be unmasked in adults when a childless couple is referred for investigation of infertility. Some men may be completely asymptomatic or regard their symptoms as being part of the normal ageing process. In the long term, hypogonadism has deleterious effects on bone mass in both men and women.

Clinical features

The main features depend on whether the hypogonadism occurs before or after puberty. Hypogonadism delays puberty in children. Short stature and absence of secondary sexual characteristics may be evident. Boys with hypogonadism lack muscle bulk and have little beard development. Girls with hypogonadism may not menstruate and have limited breast growth.

Features of hypogonadism in adults are very different. Women may notice the cessation of their menstrual periods (secondary amenorrhoea), low libido and menopausal symptoms such as hot flushes. Men may be asymptomatic or complain of erectile dysfunction/impotence, loss of body and facial hair, gynaecomastia and decreased muscle bulk. Infertility can be the presenting feature in either instance.

The main features in patients with hypogonadism secondary to hypothalamic or pituitary disorders may be multiple hormone deficiencies, or signs and symptoms of the underlying intracranial pathology.

Initial investigations

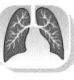

FSH, LH and sex hormone levels
Elevated FSH and LH levels, with low testosterone or oestradiol levels, are indicative of primary hypogonadism.

Further investigations

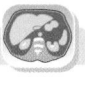

Chromosomal analysis
Chromosomal analysis is used in the investigation of patients suspected of having Klinefelter's or Turner's syndrome.

Anterior pituitary hormone profile and imaging
Low testosterone or oestradiol levels without marked FSH/LH elevation are indicative of secondary hypogonadism. Further investigations of pituitary function and imaging are detailed on page 408.

Pelvic ultrasound scanning
Ultrasound is employed to look at ovarian and uterine morphology in primary amenorrhoea in particular.

Screening for autoimmune disease:
Other associated autoimmune disease such as adrenal insufficiency should also be screened for.

Medical management

Primary hypogonadism itself is rarely reversible; androgen or oestrogen replacement therapy is used to alleviate symptoms and improve quality of life.

Androgen replacement therapy

Testosterone is available in a number of formulations. The most convenient form is oral testosterone undecanoate, but this preparation is expensive, has unpredictable absorption and can give liver problems, so is not recommended. The preferred method is now topical/cutaneous testosterone, either as a patch or a gel. Previously an intramuscular depot of testosterone ester given every 2–3 weeks was the first-line therapy; this, in the form of a newly available 12-weekly depot, is now used as second-line therapy. An implant which delivers testosterone for 4–6 months is also available but needs a skilled person to administer. A new buccal tablet used twice daily with good serum testosterone levels has more recently become available but its place in replacement therapy is not yet clear.

Androgens can hasten epiphyseal fusion in boys and can cause short stature. Other complications include sodium retention and hypertension, and excessive androgenic effects such as acne and hirsutism.

Oestrogen replacement therapy

The most appropriate formulations for use as replacement therapy are the natural oestrogens such as oestradiol, oestrone and oestriol. A small dose of oestrogen, combined with progestogen, is used in women with an intact uterus. The role of the progestogen component is to reduce the risk of endometrial cancer, although this is counterbalanced by the small increase in breast cancer. The principal symptomatic benefits of oestrogen replacement therapy are in development of female sexual features, alleviating hot flushes and vaginal dryness. Risk of fracture from osteoporosis is also reduced by treatment. Adverse effects of oestrogen replacement are uncommon but potentially serious and include increased risk of breast cancer, venous thromboembolism and stroke.[1]

Management of infertility

Patients with secondary hypogonadism can be treated with LH and FSH or pulsed GnRH to restore fertility. These hormones are inconvenient to administer owing to the unavailability of oral formulations. If restoration of fertility is not the primary aim, the same replacement therapy used in primary hypogonadism can be applied.

> **RECENT ADVANCES**
>
> *Raloxifene is a selective oestrogen receptor modulator that improves bone density but does not restore sexual characteristics or provide symptomatic benefit in terms of reducing hot flushes or vaginal atrophy.*

Prognosis

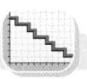

Although hypogonadism is seldom curable, treatment with the appropriate replacement therapy can relieve symptoms and reduce complications.

REFERENCE

(1) *MCA/CSM. HRT—Update on the risk of breast cancer and long-term safety. Current Problems in Pharmacovigilance 2003; 29: 1–3.*

Polycystic ovary syndrome

Hypogonadism

Diabetes and other metabolic diseases

7

Kevin Shotliff

Diabetes

Introduction

Diabetes mellitus is a group of metabolic diseases characterized by hyperglycaemia resulting from defects in insulin secretion, insulin action or both. It causes acute metabolic disturbances, long-term organ damage and reduced life expectancy.

Applied basic sciences of glucose metabolism

Insulin is produced in the pancreas by beta cells of the islets of Langerhans. The proinsulin molecule is split into C-peptide, an inert connecting molecule, and the active insulin molecule. This peptide hormone is predominantly metabolized in the liver where it has its main effects of reducing liver glycogenolysis and gluconeogenesis. It also increases fat and muscle glucose utilization and reduces lipolysis and ketogenesis. The kidney also metabolizes insulin, producing up to 10% of the daily glucose.

439

Diabetes mellitus

Epidemiology

Diabetes mellitus affects up to 6% of the UK population, of whom approximately half are undiagnosed. It occurs equally in both sexes but varies with age and race. The ethnic group at highest risk is the Pina Indians in North America with a 50% prevalence of diabetes. Other high-risk groups include the Afro-Caribbean and Asian population, who have a 4-fold greater risk for diabetes than Caucasians.

Approximately 10% of the population over the age of 65 years, and 16% of Asians in the same age group in the UK, have diabetes. This racial and age effect, along with the potential for a Western lifestyle to generate a more sedentary and obese population, leads to significant differences in the size of the problem in different countries.

Pathology

Diabetes is a heterogeneous disease and has been classified by the American Diabetes Association (ADA) into four groups, summarized in Table 7.1.[1] The characteristics of type 1 and type 2 diabetes are summarized in Table 7.2.

Type 1 diabetes

Previously known as insulin dependent diabetes mellitus (IDDM), or juvenile-onset diabetes, this group of disorders is characterized by an *absolute* deficiency of insulin resulting from cell-mediated autoimmune destruction of the beta cells of the pancreas. Islet cell autoantibodies, auto-antibodies to insulin, anti-GAD (glutamic acid decarboxylase) antibodies and anti-tyrosine phosphatase antibodies (Anti-IA-2 antibodies) are present in 90% of patients. If all four antibodies are present in a non-diabetic individual, he or she will have an 88% chance of developing type 1 diabetes in the next 10 years.

Although a genetic predisposition is suggested, environmental triggers are also important as not all patients with pancreatic autoantibodies develop diabetes. Several

Table 7.1	American Diabetes Association 2003 classification of diabetes

I Type 1 diabetes

Usually results from immune-mediated beta cell destruction leading to absolute insulin deficiency

II Type 2 diabetes

May result from insulin resistance with relative insulin deficiency or be due to a secretory defect with insulin resistance

III Other specific types of diabetes

A. Genetic defects of beta cell function

B. Genetic defects of insulin action

C. Diseases of the exocrine pancreas

D. Endocrinopathies

E. Drug or chemical induced

F. Infection

G. Uncommon forms of immune-mediated diabetes

H. Other genetic syndromes associated with diabetes

IV Gestational diabetes mellitus

regions of the human genome have been linked to the development of type 1 diabetes. The most common are the major histocompatibility complex (MHC) antigens/human leukocyte antigens (HLA), with over 90% of patients in the UK having either HLA-DR3 or DR4 or both.

Type 2 diabetes

Previously known as non-insulin dependent diabetes mellitus (NIDDM), or adult-onset diabetes, this group of patients usually has insulin resistance and *relative* insulin deficiency. Most patients with this form of diabetes are older and obese. In fact, obesity alone produces relative insulin resistance. Blood insulin levels are usually normal or

Table 7.2	Comparison of type 1 and type 2 diabetes	
	Type 1 diabetes	**Type 2 diabetes**
Peak age of onset	12 years	60 years
UK prevalence	0.25%	5–7% (10% of those >65 years of age)
Aetiology	Autoimmune beta cell destruction	Combination of insulin resistance and beta cell dysfunction
Initial presentation	Polyuria, polydipsia and weight loss with ketoacidosis	Hyperglycaemic symptoms but often with complication of diabetes (no ketoacidosis)
Treatment	Insulin from outset	Diet, oral hypoglycaemic agents and/or insulin

elevated. Despite this, serum glucose levels are higher in relation to the level of insulin (compared to normal individuals).

Genetic predisposition to develop type 2 diabetes is much stronger compared to type 1 diabetes. However, the genetics are incompletely understood and type 2 diabetes is not associated with the same HLA-linked genes as type 1 diabetes.

Other specific types of diabetes

A number of forms of diabetes can result from genetic defects of beta cell function (A), often characterized by hyperglycaemia at an early age. This autosomal dominant group of disorders is referred to as maturity-onset diabetes of the young (MODY). They arise from genetic mutations such as a defect on chromosome 20q resulting in altered activity of the hepatic nuclear factor (HNF) 4α gene (*MODY 1*), a defect in the glucokinase gene (*MODY 2*) and gene mutations that alter HNF-1α activity (*MODY 3*).

Genetic defects of insulin action (B) are a rare cause of diabetes. Leprechaunism, with characteristic facial features, is usually fatal in early childhood, and Rabson–Mendenhall syndrome, characterized by abnormalities of teeth and nails and pineal gland hyperplasia, are two examples. Any disease of the exocrine pancreas (C) such as pancreatitis, pancreatic trauma and pancreatic carcinoma can result in diabetes if it is of sufficient severity to destroy the pancreas. Endocrine diseases (D) that result in hormone production antagonistic to insulin may result in diabetes. Examples are Cushing's syndrome (cortisol), acromegaly (growth hormone) and phaeochromocytoma (adrenaline). Drugs (E) such as thiazide diuretics may precipitate diabetes in susceptible individuals, while nicotinic acid and glucocorticoids impair insulin action. Infections (F) such as congenital rubella, Coxsackie B and cytomegalovirus have been implicated in the development of diabetes. An example of an uncommon form of immune-mediated diabetes (G) is characterized by anti-insulin receptor antibodies, occasionally found in patients with autoimmune disorders. Finally, genetic syndromes (H) such as Down's, Turner's and Wolfram's are also associated with diabetes.

Gestational diabetes mellitus

Although deterioration of glucose tolerance occurs normally in pregnancy, gestational diabetes mellitus is defined as any degree of glucose intolerance with the onset or first recognition of pregnancy.

Scope of disease

Complications of diabetes can result from metabolic disturbances associated with acute hyperglycaemia (fasting blood glucose >7.0 mmol/L or post prandial >11.0 mmol/L) such as diabetic ketoacidosis (type 1 diabetes) or hyperosmolar non-ketotic syndrome (type 2 diabetics). Hyperglycaemia also predisposes to impairment of growth and susceptibility to infection.

Chronic hyperglycaemia is associated with increased cerebrovascular disease (stroke, ischaemic heart disease, peripheral vascular disease), kidney disease (diabetic nephropathy), eye disease (diabetic retinopathy), peripheral neuropathy (sensory disorders, foot ulcers) and autonomic neuropathy (gastrointestinal or sexual dysfunction).

Clinical features

Patients with type 1 diabetes usually present with symptoms of marked hyperglycaemia, a classical triad of polyuria, polydipsia and weight loss. In a minority, diabetic ketoacidosis may be the initial presentation. Patients with type 2 diabetes tend to present insidiously with complications of chronic hyperglycaemia. Up to half of new cases may be found on incidental screening.

Apart from establishing a diagnosis, the clinical assessment should be directed to ascertain any underlying cause and screen for potential complications that may result from diabetes.

A careful history may reveal drugs that predispose to diabetes, symptoms of other endocrinopathies associated with diabetes, and evidence of complications such as stroke, angina, myocardial infarction, claudication, foot ulcers and recurrent infections. The history taken for assessment of the newly diagnosed patient should screen for the duration of symptoms (thirst, polyuria, weight loss), possible secondary causes of diabetes (acromegaly), family history, complications of diabetes and risk factors for developing further complications (smoking, hypertension, hyperlipidaemia).

An initial examination should include the estimation of body mass index (BMI), screening for secondary causes of diabetes (the thyroid should be palpated for any abnormality that would suggest concomitant endocrinopathy), cardiovascular complications (blood pressure, peripheral pulses), signs of autonomic or peripheral neuropathy, evidence of retinopathy (p. 454) and acanthosis nigricans (p. 457). The feet should be examined for abnormal sensation and the presence of ulceration.

Initial investigations

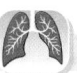

Plasma glucose

Diabetes is a biochemical diagnosis, based on plasma glucose estimations. Two sets of diagnostic criteria are in use, one produced by the World Health Organization (WHO) in 2000 and the other by the ADA in 2003 (Table 7.3).

The revised WHO criteria eliminated the need for an oral glucose tolerance test (OGTT) in all groups except pregnant women. Asymptomatic patients and those with intercurrent illnesses require a further abnormal result before a diagnosis of diabetes can be made. On the ADA criteria, the diagnosis of diabetes needs to be confirmed by repeating any one of the three listed methods on a subsequent day.

Further investigations

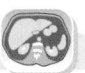

No other specific test is required to diagnose diabetes. Once the diagnosis has been established, further tests are performed to assess glycaemic control and screen for disease-associated complications.

Table 7.3	Diagnostic criteria for diabetes			
		Normal	IFG[a]/ IGT[b]	Diabetes
World Health Organization 2000 criteria				
Symptoms and 2 hr post-prandial glucose (mmol/L)		<7.8	7.8–11.1[b]	>11.1
Fasting plasma glucose (mmol/L)		<6.0	6.0–6.9[a]	>7.0
American Diabetes Association 2003 criteria				
1. Symptoms and casual glucose (mmol/L)		N/A	N/A	>11.1
2. Fasting plasma glucose (mmol/L)		<6.1	6.1–7.0[a]	>7.0
3. Oral glucose tolerance test (mmol/L)		<7.8	7.8–11.1[b]	>11.1

Casual is defined as any time of the day without regard to meals.
Fasting is defined as no calorie intake for at least 8 hours.
The oral glucose tolerance is performed by ingesting 75 g of anhydrous glucose dissolved in water. Plasma glucose levels are estimated 2 hours post ingestion.
[a] Impaired fasting glucose (ADA), impaired fasting hyperglycaemia (WHO).
[b] Impaired glucose tolerance.

Hb_{A1C}

Glycosylated haemoglobin gives an estimation of serum glucose levels over the preceding 2–3 months. In general, good control is reflected by an Hb_{A1C} of less than 7.2%. This test can be repeated 3-monthly, or at least annually to assess glycaemic control.

Fasting lipid profile

Hyperlipidaemia, typically elevated triglycerides and reduced high-density lipoprotein (HDL) cholesterol, in diabetic patients significantly increases the risk of cardiovascular disease.

Urinalysis, 24-hour urine collections and urea and electrolytes

Urine dipstick testing for glucose is an insensitive method to diagnose hyperglycaemia due to variation in renal threshold for glucose but is useful to detect evidence of ketones (ketoacidosis) and proteins (diabetic nephropathy). Examination of the urine for protein is initially for micro-albuminuria/proteinuria (albuminuria >300 mg/24 hours) and, if that is negative, for microalbuminuria (30–299 mg/24hrs) which is the earliest marker of diabetic nephropathy (p. 456). Microalbuminuria is screened with a spot albumin:creatinine ratio and, if positive, a timed urine collection is needed to confirm it.

Elevated plasma urea and creatinine measurements only occur in the later stages of nephropathy.

Thyroid-stimulating hormone (TSH)

In type 1 diabetics and selected type 2 patients with clinical features of thyroid disorders, TSH is a good screening investigation for problems related to autoimmune thyroid disease.

Initial management

Multidisciplinary management

Following the diagnosis of diabetes, patients should see a dietitian and a diabetes nurse specialist. Once an initial assessment has been made, all patients should be put into a formal review system with a primary or secondary care specialist in diabetes for further education, maintenance of good control and complication screening. Patients are taught how to monitor their glucose levels and are educated on self-management of diabetes.

Good glycaemic control reduces microvascular and macrovascular complications.[2] However targets need to be individualized, as less severe glycaemic control may be appropriate for patients with frequent or severe episodes of hypoglycaemia. A summary of targets is listed in Table 7.4.

Patients with impaired glucose tolerance/impaired fasting glycaemia are given the same dietary and lifestyle advice and need their fasting blood glucose levels monitored at least annually.

Physical activity

Regular exercise is associated with improved glucose control, contributes to weight loss and improves well-being.[4]

Dietary advice

For most patients, increased care with the fat and refined carbohydrate content of their diet is needed. If they are overweight a reduction in total calorie intake to help reduce weight is indicated.

Medical management

Type 1 diabetes

Insulin

Insulin is essential for survival in all patients with type 1 diabetes, and for type 2 diabetics who are unable to maintain satisfactory glycaemic or symptomatic control with alternative treatment. Most insulin is manufactured in a biosynthetic human form (from yeast or bacteria) at a standard concentration of 100 units/mL (U100), although a sizable minority of patients still take beef or pork insulins.

Table 7.4	Suggested treatment aims

Fasting blood glucose

<7 mmol/L

Hb$_{A1c}$

<7.2% (or <6.5% in those with significant complications)

Blood pressure

<140/80 mmHg

Lipids

Primary prevention:

Treat if a cardiovascular risk prediction chart[3] gives a >3% risk per year

Secondary prevention:

Following failure of diet treat a:

Total cholesterol <4.5 mmol/L (or <4.0 post coronary artery bypass graft/angioplasty)

LDL cholesterol <2.6 mmol/L

Triglycerides <1.5 mmol/L

Body mass index

20–25

Home monitoring

Capillary blood glucose estimations fasting, pre-meal, 2 hours post prandial and pre bed. These will need to be frequent enough to allow alterations in treatment and assessment of adequate control

Often adequate with 3×/week in stable type 2 patients and daily in stable type 1 patients

Diet

In the overweight patient (e.g. body mass index >25) a reduction in total intake to aid weight reduction is required

<10% of kcals in the form of saturated fat (<8% if hyperlipidaemic)

<30% from all fats

50–60% as carbohydrate which is mostly complex high fibre, and sugar limited to about 25 g/day

Sodium content should be <6 g/day in most people or <3 g/day if hypertensive

Alcohol is a significant source of calories, and a reduction in the overweight or hypertriglyceridaemic patient is advisable

Bovine insulin from cattle pancreas is more antigenic than human or porcine alternatives and gives rise to more lipohypertrophy and lipoatrophy. All insulin regimens result in weight gain and hypoglycaemia.

Insulin is inactivated by gastrointestinal enzymes, therefore it can only be given by intravenous or subcutaneous routes. Intravenous insulin has a half-life of 5 minutes and needs to be given by continuous infusion if a sustained effect is required. Subcutaneous administration of insulin delays absorption and prolongs the duration of activity. The addition of agents such as zinc or modification of the insulin molecule itself (insulin analogues) further alters duration of action and timing of peak effect. An inhaled insulin preparation, for short-acting insulin initially, is being developed which may alter this.

Several types of insulin therapy are available, facilitating individualized treatment regimens (Table 7.5). The dose for initiating insulin therapy can be estimated at 0.5 units per kg per day. However, those who are obese and inactive will require larger doses, while those who are thin and exercise regularly may get by with lower doses.

The regimen of insulin administration depends on the person's level of physical activity, timing and nature of meals, lifestyle requirements and personal preference.

Twice-daily regimen

This is best suited for those with a more stable daily routine who know the level of food intake and exercise they will undertake later. The regimen consists of two injections: two thirds of the daily insulin requirement is given in the morning, and a third is given in the evening. Each injection is made up of two components: a short- and an intermediate-acting insulin. The separate components can be mixed in a syringe by the patient (e.g. 8 units of short-acting and 16 units of intermediate-acting insulin) or may be given as a single pre-mixed formulation (e.g. 24 units of a biphasic insulin comprising 30% short-acting and 70% intermediate-acting).

For example, a 70 kg patient might receive 24 units of insulin before breakfast and 12 units of insulin before the evening meal. The morning short-acting insulin component covers breakfast, and the intermediate-acting component covers lunch. In the evening, the short-acting component covers the evening meal and the intermediate-acting component covers the night.

The disadvantage of the twice-daily regimen is predicting the insulin requirement to cover the subsequent diet and exercise for the day, and often results in fluctuating blood sugar levels with activity.

Basal bolus regimen

The basal bolus regimen is suitable for active patients with unpredictable daily schedules. It consists of short-acting insulin given before meals (three times a day) and an intermediate- or long-acting insulin given before bed.

For example, a 70 kg patient might receive 6 units of short-acting insulin 15–30 minutes before each meal and 18 units of long-acting insulin before bedtime. The pre-meal doses are adjusted in anticipation of planned activity.

Although this regimen allows flexibility with both the timing and size of meals and exercise, the disadvantage is the number of injections and frequent capillary blood glucose measurements that are required to adjust the pre-meal insulin doses.

Continuous subcutaneous insulin infusion (CSII)

In some patients a continuous insulin infusion gives more flexibility to vary the doses of insulin than the basal bolus regimen allows. CSII is a treatment option for patients on multiple dose insulin therapy who, in their efforts to maintain satisfactory glucose control, are troubled by repeated, unexpected hypoglycaemic attacks. In this regimen, insulin is given continuously via a subcutaneous cannula into the anterior abdomen. Whilst popular in Scandinavia and

443

Table 7.5   Types of insulin

Type of insulin	Examples	Peak activity	Duration of action
Short-acting insulin analogue insulin lispro or insulin aspart	Humalog Novorapid	$\frac{1}{2}$–$1\frac{1}{2}$ hours	Up to 6 hours
Short-acting (soluble insulin)	Human Actrapid Humulin S	1–3 hours	Up to 8 hours
Intermediate-acting	Human Insulatard Humulin I Human Monotard Humulin Zn	4–8 hours	Up to 24 hours
Long-acting	Human Ultratard	6–24 hours	Up to 36 hours
Long-acting insulin analogue (insulin glargine)	Lantus	Smooth flat profile with no peak	More than 24 hours
Biphasic isophane insulin (proportion of short-acting varies from 10% to 50%)	Human Mixtard 10 –Mixtard 50 Humulin M1–M5	Varies	Varies

the USA, it is less commonly used in the UK due to cost, potential problems with pump failure, ketoacidosis and cannula site infections. In view of this, patients using CSII should be managed by a specialist team experienced in its use.

Type 2 diabetes

Type 2 diabetics are initially managed by diet and exercise unless they are significantly symptomatic, when a sulphonylurea may be used short term. As the disease worsens, patients may require oral hypoglycaemic agents, if not insulin therapy, to achieve satisfactory symptomatic and glycaemic control.

Oral hypoglycaemic agents

The oral hypoglycaemic agents are classed into sulphonylureas (glibenclamide, tolbutamide), biguanides (metformin), prandial glucose regulators (repaglinide), alpha glucosidase inhibitors (acarbose) and thiazolidinediones (pioglitazone). A summary is provided in Table 7.6.

The oral agents are broadly similar in their ability to lower blood glucose (decrease Hb_{A1C} by $\approx1\%$). Sulphonylureas reduce microvascular complications (principally retinopathy) but not cardiovascular outcomes, and although metformin was no better than other agents in reducing the blood glucose of obese type 2 patients, it is the only drug so far that lowers overall mortality and the incidence of stroke or myocardial infarction. A suggested treatment plan is provided in Figure 7.1.

The side effects of the oral hypoglycaemic agents (except metformin) are weight gain and/or hypoglycaemia. Elderly patients with renal impairment should avoid long-acting sulphonylureas such as glibenclamide in view of the risk of severe hypoglycaemia and, possibly, death.

Table 7.6   Oral hypoglycaemic agents

Class	Examples	Mechanism of action	Important adverse effects
Sulphonylureas	Glibenclamide Tolbutamide Gliclazide Glimepiride	Stimulate pancreatic insulin secretion	Hypoglycaemia, weight gain
Biguanides	Metformin	Decrease hepatic gluconeogenesis Increase muscle glucose uptake and metabolism Reduce peripheral insulin resistance	Anorexia and nausea Lactic acidosis
Prandial glucose regulators	Repaglinide Nateglinide	Stimulate pancreatic insulin secretion	Hypoglycaemia, weight gain
Alpha glucosidase inhibitors	Acarbose	Inhibit intestinal alpha glucosidase Delay digestion and absorption of starch and sucrose	Undigested carbohydrates lead to post-prandial fullness/ bloating, abdominal pain, flatulence and diarrhoea
Thiazolidinediones	Pioglitazone Rosiglitazone	Activate PPAR-gamma receptor Reduce peripheral insulin resistance	Weight gain, gastrointestinal disturbance, anaemia

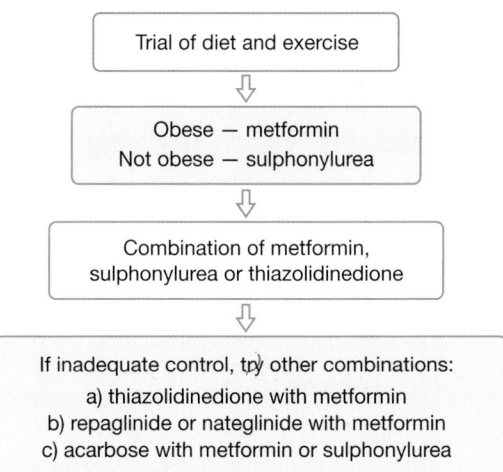

Fig. 7.1 Management of type 2 diabetes. Patients who have contraindications or intolerance to specific drugs will need to have their treatment tailored to their individual requirements.

Lactic acidosis is a serious, rare complication of metformin. Patients at particular risk are those with tissue hypoxia (e.g. uncontrolled heart failure or liver failure) and renal impairment (serum creatinine >150 mmol/L); the drug should be avoided in these instances. Metformin should also be temporarily discontinued in patients who are undergoing radiological studies requiring contrast due to the deleterious effect of contrast media on renal function.

Insulin and oral agent mixtures

After diet, exercise and oral therapy, insulin may be added to the treatment regimen. Oral hypoglycaemic agents can be used for glycaemic control during the day, and pre-bed intermediate-acting insulin for glycaemic control overnight. Metformin is a good oral hypoglycaemic for this combination as it reduces insulin requirements and body weight.

Prevention of complications of diabetes

Guidelines for blood pressure control are provided on page 69, lipid management and targets are dependent on baseline cardiovascular risk. Other important aspects of diabetes care are screening and management of nephropathy, retinopathy and foot care.

Screening

Whilst the value of a formal screening programme is yet to be established, the ADA recommends opportunistic screening of high-risk individuals such as the obese or those with a family history of diabetes. The preferred screening test is a fasting plasma glucose estimation.

Prognosis

Life expectancy in those with diabetes is reduced, depending on the age of diagnosis. Most patients will eventually develop some complications of diabetes. Retinopathy, for example, affects <2% of those with type 1 diabetes at diagnosis and >90% after 20 years, while 25–35% of type 2 patients are affected at diagnosis and up to 80% after 20 years.

FURTHER INFORMATION

American Diabetes Association. Standards of medical care for patients with diabetes mellitus. Diabetes Care 2003; 26: 33S–50.

REFERENCES

(1) *Report of the Expert Committee on the Diagnosis and Classification of Diabetes Mellitus. Diabetes Care 2003; 26: 5S–20.*
(2) *The Diabetes Control and Complications Trial Research Group. The effect of intensive treatment of diabetes on the development and progression of long-term complications in insulin-dependent diabetes mellitus. New England Journal of Medicine 1993; 329: 977–986.*
(3) *Joint Formulary Committee. British National Formulary, 51st edn. London: British Medical Association and Royal Pharmaceutical Society of Great Britain, 2006.*
(4) *American Diabetes Association. Standards of medical care for patients with diabetes mellitus. Diabetes Care 2003; 26: 33S–50.*

Acute complications of diabetes

The complications of diabetes can be split into acute and chronic disorders, the chronic complications being divided into macrovascular and microvascular problems.

Acute disturbances are metabolic: most common are hypoglycaemia from the therapy used and hyperglycaemia from the condition. Metabolic acidosis such as lactic acidosis caused by metformin can also occur. Elevated blood glucose levels in type 1 patients, when associated with insulin deficiency, result in diabetic ketoacidosis; type 2 patients still have a degree of insulin production and develop a non-ketotic hyperosmolar diabetic state.

Diabetic ketoacidosis

Epidemiology

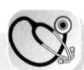

The incidence is 800 per 100 000 diabetic patients per year. Ketoacidosis is the initial presenting feature in up to 30% of patients with diabetes.

Pathology

Insulin deficiency leads to elevated levels of glucagon, catecholamines and cortisol. These counter-regulatory hormones stimulate hepatic glucose production through increased glycogenolysis and enhanced gluconeogenesis. Raised cortisol levels increase proteolysis, providing amino acid precursors for gluconeogenesis. Elevated liver glucose production and decreased peripheral glucose utilization lead to hyperglycaemia, glycosuria, osmotic diuresis and dehydration. With dehydration, glomerular filtration is reduced, causing blood glucose levels to rise and perpetuating a vicious cycle.

In addition, low insulin and elevated catecholamines, cortisol and growth hormone levels activate hormone-sensitive lipase, which causes the breakdown of triglycerides and release of free fatty acids. The free fatty acids are taken up by the liver and converted to ketone bodies that are released into the circulation. Ketones (β-hydroxybutyrate, acetoacetate and acetone) are normally buffered by the blood and excreted by the kidneys, and the effect of ketone accumulation is metabolic acidosis (a potent stimulus for hyperventilation). Precipitating causes are listed in Table 7.7.

Scope of disease

The fluid and electrolyte disturbances at presentation usually amount to a 5 litre deficit of fluid, 300–700 mmol

deficit of sodium, 200–700 mmol deficit of potassium and 350–500 mmol deficit of chloride. Progressive metabolic acidosis with hypovolaemia is fatal if left untreated.

Clinical features

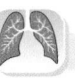

Polyuria, polydipsia and weight loss are the most common features. Often, muscle cramps, abdominal pain and shortness of breath (Kussmaul's breathing from metabolic acidosis) occur. Nausea and vomiting worsen dehydration and electrolyte abnormalities that often precede the onset of coma (10%).

On examination the breath may smell of ketones (like nail varnish remover). Postural hypotension from dehydration, which is exacerbated by peripheral vasodilatation due to acidosis, and hypothermia are frequent clinical findings.

Initial investigations

The diagnosis is based on a collection of biochemical abnormalities.

Blood glucose
Hyperglycaemia—blood glucose >11.1 mmol/L—is present.

Arterial blood gas
A metabolic acidosis is evident. Arterial pH is less than 7.3, and serum bicarbonate less than 15 mmol/L. There is a base excess of less than −10.

Urine dipstick testing
Ketones are present (captopril can give a false positive test for urinary acetone).

Further investigations

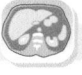

Full blood count
A high white cell count is a non-specific indicator of infection.

Table 7.7	Precipitating conditions for diabetic ketoacidosis	
Infection		30–40%
Non-compliance with treatment		25%
Inappropriate alterations in insulin		13%
Newly diagnosed diabetes		10–20%
Myocardial infarction		1%

Urea and electrolytes (U&Es)

Sodium and potassium levels can be estimated to guide fluid and electrolyte replacement. Renal impairment from dehydration can lead to elevated creatinine levels, but elevated ketones can also lead to artificially high levels of creatinine.

Blood and urine cultures

Infection is the most common precipitating cause.

Chest X-ray

A chest film may reveal pneumonia as a precipitating cause.

Electrocardiogram and serum cardiac markers

In patients over the age of 40, ECG and cardiac enzymes screen for the possibility of myocardial infarction.

Initial management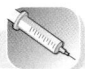

Initial fluid replacement

Intravenous normal saline is administered at a volume of 2 litres in the first 2 hours, then 1 litre over 2 hours, then 2 litres in the next 8 hours, then 4 litres/day thereafter. When the blood glucose is less than 15 mmol/L, 4% dextrose saline or 5% dextrose should be used.

If the patient is profoundly shocked (e.g. systolic BP <80 mmHg with severe dehydration or sepsis) or oliguric, fluids should be given more rapidly and colloids or inotropes may also be needed. In an elderly patient or one with signs of heart failure or cerebral oedema, fluids may need to be given more slowly.

Potassium

Once the serum potassium is known, potassium can be added to the intravenous saline infusion and the dose adjusted based on hourly serum potassium measurements until the serum potassium is stable, when it can be measured on a 4-hourly basis over the next 24 hours.

Insulin

A continuous intravenous infusion of 50 units of soluble insulin in 50 mL of 0.9% saline at 8–10 units/hour is administered. The aim is to lower the serum glucose by 5 mmol/L/hour. The rate is then adjusted to keep blood glucose 10–14 mmol/L until the ketoacidosis has resolved. The maintenance dose of insulin infusion is usually 3–6 units/hour.

Monitoring

Central venous access and urinary catheterization are often necessary to monitor the response to therapy. A nasogastric tube may be useful, especially in the unconscious patient. Continuous ECG monitoring will aid the detection of arrhythmias due to acute derangement in serum potassium levels.

Once treatment has commenced, fluid balance is monitored carefully to avoid fluid overload. Capillary blood glucose is checked hourly. Serum potassium, sodium and glucose are checked 2-hourly and arterial blood gases 2–4-hourly, depending on response. The frequency of the tests can be reduced when the patient is stabilized but electrolytes need to be checked at least daily for the first 3 days.

Magnesium and phosphate levels should also be checked as these can occasionally require replacement therapy.

Medical management

Intravenous bicarbonate

Intravenous bicarbonate is only indicated if the pH is less than 6.9 as it can cause hypokalaemia and paradoxically worsen intracellular acidosis.

Subcutaneous heparin

Prophylactic doses of low molecular weight heparin should be administered to the unconscious or immobile patient.

Antibiotics

Broad-spectrum intravenous antibiotics should be administered if no obvious precipitating cause is found.

Dexamethasone and mannitol

Cerebral oedema typically presents with a declining conscious level 8–24 hours after starting intravenous fluids. If this occurs, dexamethasone (12–16 mg/day) and mannitol (1–2 g/kg body weight) may be given.

Euglycaemic ketoacidosis

In the uncommon condition of euglycaemic ketoacidosis (1–3% of cases at most), ketones are produced early on in patients with a reduced carbohydrate intake. Blood glucose is <17 mmol/L, acidosis is marked and dehydration is not usually severe. Treatment is to initiate oral carbohydrate intake and monitor the need for intravenous insulin and fluids as in full-blown hyperglycaemic ketoacidosis.

Pre-discharge management

Once the blood glucose is stable in the 10–15 mmol/L range, the ketoacidosis has settled and the patient is eating and drinking normally, a subcutaneous insulin regimen is commenced that overlaps with the intravenous infusion by 2 hours.

Blood sugar should be stabilized on subcutaneous insulin prior to discharge. Once the intravenous potassium supplements have stopped, oral supplements should be given for at least 48 hours with regular serum monitoring.

Patient education is important to prevent further occurrences and to encourage earlier presentation to hospital.

Prognosis

Diabetic ketoacidosis has a mortality of approximately 5%, but this can be up to 50% in the elderly. Many deaths

Diabetic ketoacidosis

Hyperosmolar, non-ketotic hyperglycaemia

Hypoglycaemia

occur due to delays in presentation and initiation of treatment.

Hyperosmolar, non-ketotic hyperglycaemia

Epidemiology

Hyperosmolar, non-ketotic hyperglycaemia accounts for approximately 30% of adult hyperglycaemic emergencies. It affects an older population (middle-aged or elderly) compared to ketoacidosis, and two thirds of cases are in patients with previously undiagnosed diabetes.

Pathology

Hyperosmolar, non-ketotic hyperglycaemia occurs from a combination of insulin deficiency and counter-regulatory hormone excess. The circulating levels of insulin are sufficient to prevent ketone production but insufficient to prevent worsening hyperglycaemia, osmotic diuresis and dehydration (approximate 10 litre fluid deficit at presentation). Ingestion of high sugar content drinks, intercurrent infection and myocardial infarction are common precipitants. In addition, drugs such as glucocorticoids, cimetidine, phenytoin, thiazide and loop diuretics have been implicated as precipitating causes.

Hyperosmolar, non-ketotic hyperglycaemia is a state of relative hypercoagulability. Venous thrombosis and stroke can occasionally occur concurrently.

Clinical features

The onset is insidious; ill health and profound dehydration occur over several days. Gastrointestinal symptoms from gastroparesis include vomiting, and gastric erosions can also lead to haematemesis. Seizures occasionally occur when serum osmolality is more than 440, but confusion and coma are uncommon.

Initial investigations

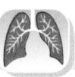

Hyperosmolar, non-ketotic hyperglycaemia is a biochemical diagnosis.

Serum blood glucose
Severe hyperglycaemia occurs with glucose in the range 30–70 mmol/L.

Serum osmolality
The serum osmolality is high, over 350 mmol/kg (normal is 275–295).

Arterial blood gas
The pH is usually in the normal range (7.35–7.45) and the serum bicarbonate more than 18 mmol/L.

Urine dipstick testing
Ketones are usually not present. Occasionally, ketones may be positive because of starvation and vomiting.

Initial management

Initial investigation and treatment is the same as for ketoacidosis, with fluid, electrolyte and insulin replacement, although there are important exceptions as these are older patients.

Intravenous fluid
Fluid administration is less rapid, and central venous access for monitoring is usually required. The rate of infusion should be 1 litre of 0.9% saline over the first hour, 1 litre 2-hourly for the next 2 hours, and then 1 litre 4–6-hourly.

If the patient is hypernatraemic (sodium >155 mmol/L) 0.45% saline rather than 0.9% is used. Half normal saline increases the risk of cerebral oedema if serum sodium or osmolality is altered too rapidly (the mortality can be as high as 70%).

Intravenous insulin
Intravenous insulin is administered at a rate of 3–6 units/hour of soluble insulin, aiming to reduce the blood glucose by a maximum of 5 mmol/L per hour to avoid precipitating cerebral oedema.

Medical management

Subcutaneous heparin
Prophylactic subcutaneous heparin should be considered although recent evidence suggests that more formal anticoagulation carries a high risk of upper gastrointestinal bleeding.

Intravenous antibiotics
More aggressive use of intravenous antibiotics to treat any underlying infection is encouraged.

Pre-discharge management
Intravenous fluids and insulin are continued for at least 24 hours after initial stabilization. Maintenance therapy is initiated with subcutaneous insulin or oral hypoglycaemic agents. Patient education is required to prevent further episodes.

Prognosis

The mortality of hyperosmolar, non-ketotic hyperglycaemia is as high as 50%.

Hypoglycaemia

Hypoglycaemia is an important complication of the treatment of diabetes and should be considered in any patient that is unconscious or having seizures.

Epidemiology

Most patients on insulin experience an episode of hypoglycaemia. Up to 1 in 7 have a severe episode each year, and 3% suffer with recurrent hypoglycaemia.

Pathology

Hypoglycaemia results from an imbalance between glucose supply, glucose utilization and insulin levels.

Reduced glucose supply can occur as a result of missing a meal or as a late effect of alcohol. It can also occur from delayed gastric emptying (autonomic neuropathy), associated coeliac disease, Addison's disease or an acute illness (gastroenteritis).

Increased utilization occurs with exercise and high insulin levels, mostly with sulphonylurea or exogenous insulin therapy. Sulphonylurea therapy can cause hypoglycaemia due to beta cell stimulation, usually with glibenclamide, in the elderly and in those with reduced renal excreting ability. Thiazolidinediones (rosiglitazone and pioglitazone) may also stimulate excessive insulin production.

Nocturnal hypoglycaemia with a hyperglycaemic response in the morning (due to increased counter-regulatory hormones) is known as the Somogyi phenomenon. It tends to occur in younger insulin-treated patients, and may only present with morning headaches or a drunken feeling. Approximately 25% of patients on long-term insulin lose awareness of hypoglycaemia and remain asymptomatic despite low levels of blood glucose.

Clinical features

The features of hypoglycaemia are due to autonomic stimulation and low blood sugar levels in the brain (neuroglycopenia).

Autonomic symptoms usually occur first, when the blood glucose is less than 3.6 mmol/L. Features of autonomic stimulation include sweating, pallor, anxiety, nausea, tremor, shivering, palpitations and tachycardia. Drugs such as non-selective β-blockers and alcohol may mask the symptoms.

Neuroglycopenia symptoms usually occur when the blood glucose is less than 2.6 mmol/L. Features of neuroglycopenia include confusion, tiredness, lack of concentration, headache, dizziness, altered speech, incoordination, drowsiness, aggression and coma.

Initial investigations

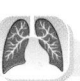

Capillary blood glucose

A rapid fingerprick test can be used to estimate the capillary blood glucose, which is usually less than 3 mmol/L.

Blood glucose, insulin and C-peptide levels

A sample for blood glucose, insulin and C-peptide levels will confirm the diagnosis and may determine the underlying cause.

Initial management

Oral carbohydrate

In the conscious patient, 20–30 g oral carbohydrate (5–6 Dextrosol tablets, a glass of milk or orange juice) is often sufficient to resolve the problem. Once the sugar has been raised rapidly, biscuits can be given to maintain a normal blood glucose level.

In the confused patient, a buccal gel (GlucoGel, a 30% glucose gel) is an alternative but this should not be used in the unconscious patient due to the risk of aspiration.

Intravenous glucose

In the unconscious patient, 50 mL of 50% dextrose is administered intravenously. Alternatively, 250 mL of intravenous 10% dextrose or 1 mg of intramuscular/deep subcutaneous glucagon can be given. Glucagon mobilizes glycogen from the liver but will not work if given repeatedly or in starved patients with no glycogen stores. In this situation or if prolonged treatment is needed intravenous glucose is better: 50% initially then 10%, but care is needed as 50% dextrose into the tissues rather than a vein can cause tissue necrosis.

Medical management

Prevention of recurrence

Having corrected the acute event, it is important to determine the precipitating cause and alter medication or lifestyle to prevent it from recurring. Extreme exercise requires an alteration in insulin doses for 24 hours. Alcohol causes an initial hyperglycaemia but hypoglycaemia 3–6 hours after ingestion and may require alterations in insulin requirements the next morning.

Prognosis

Prolonged and untreated hypoglycaemia can lead to death. Recurrent hypoglycaemic events may herald deterioration in renal or liver function.

Diabetic ketoacidosis

Hyperosmolar, non-ketotic hyperglycaemia

Hypoglycaemia

Chronic complications of diabetes

Macrovascular complications of diabetes

People with diabetes have a significantly greater risk of coronary heart disease, cerebrovascular disease and peripheral vascular disease compared to the non-diabetic population.

Epidemiology

The prevalence of macrovascular disease and outcomes vary with age, sex and ethnicity. Peripheral vascular disease occurs in up to 10%, with a 15-fold greater risk of requiring non-traumatic amputation compared to the non-diabetic population. Thromboembolic cerebrovascular events occur in up to 8%, a 2–4-fold increased risk compared to the non-diabetic population, and account for 15% of deaths in type 2 patients. The risk of having a myocardial infarction is also increased 2–4 times. Women seem particularly at risk of cardiovascular disease compared to the non-diabetic population. It also occurs at an earlier age and affects both sexes equally.

Patients with type 1 diabetes have half the rate of coronary heart disease, a third the rate of cerebrovascular disease and two thirds the rate of peripheral vascular disease compared to type 2 patients.

Pathology

Atherosclerosis has a well-known set of risk factors, all of which apply in the diabetic population. The atheroma is histologically the same as in the non-diabetic population but tends to be more diffuse and progresses more rapidly.

Clinical features

In general, the symptoms and signs of macrovascular complications are similar to those in the non-diabetic population. Exceptions include the increased frequency of silent myocardial infarctions.

Investigations

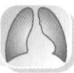

The investigations are specific to the disease complication as listed in the other sections of the text.

Management

The main aim is prevention of macrovascular complications.

Dietary modification

Obesity is an independent risk factor and is more common in type 2 patients. Central obesity (fat stomach rather than fat hips) in particular is more atherogenic. In all patients the first treatment is dietary modification.

Risk factor modification

Advice should also be provided to help patients stop smoking (reduces risk of death by 50% over a 15-year period), reduce weight and increase physical activity.

Hypertension is more common in diabetics. Blood pressure control is a more important individual risk factor for coronary heart disease than glycaemic control.

Hyperinsulinaemia (insulin-resistant type 2 diabetics) results in reduced HDL cholesterol, elevated triglycerides (and VLDL), and smaller, denser, more atherogenic LDL cholesterol. Treatment with a cholesterol-lowering agent is an important aspect of risk factor modification

Glycaemic control

Insulin resistance or elevated circulating insulin/proinsulin-like molecule levels are known to increase the risk of athero-sclerosis in both diabetic and non-diabetic populations. In type 1 patients, worsening hyperglycaemia is related to worsening atherosclerosis. In type 2 patients this association is less clear, but better glycaemic control is associated with a trend of fewer myocardial infarctions.

Prognosis

In general, cardiovascular disease accounts for 75% of deaths in type 2 patients and 35% in type 1.

Microvascular complications of diabetes

There are three main small vessel complications in diabetes, the development of eye disease (retinopathy), kidney disease (nephropathy) and nerve disease (neuropathy).

Diabetic nephropathy

In the UK, 15% of all deaths in diabetic patients less than 50 years old are due to nephropathy. Approximately 1 in 6 patients on dialysis are diabetic; the majority of these have type 2 disease.

Epidemiology

In type 1 diabetics, the prevalence of nephropathy is 35 000 per 100 000 (35%). It is more common in men and in those diagnosed with diabetes before 15 years of age. The incidence is highest 16–20 years after the onset of diabetes, at a rate of 3000 per 100 000 per year.

In type 2 diabetics, the prevalence of nephropathy is 33 000 per 100 000 (33%). There are racial differences: 25% of Caucasians compared to 50% of Asians develop diabetic nephropathy. The duration of diabetes prior to developing nephropathy is shorter in type 2 diabetics and may reflect the initial delay in the diagnosis of diabetes.

Pathology

The risk factors for the development of nephropathy in diabetics are poor glycaemic control, hypertension, smoking and genetic predisposition.

The kidney increases in size, with thickening of the glomerular basement membrane, expansion of glomerular supporting tissues (the mesangium) and fibrotic changes in both efferent and afferent arterioles. It is classified as nodular glomerular sclerosis (Kimmelstiel–Wilson nodules) if it is localized, and diffuse glomerular sclerosis if it is widespread. The thickened basement membrane initially results in an alteration in electrical charge (but not in pore size), allowing increased passage of albumin into the glomerular ultrafiltrate. This is detected as microalbuminuria.

Microalbuminuria
In 20–40% of type 1 diabetics there is an initial period of glomerular hyperfiltration, and microalbuminuria usually occurs 5–15 years after the onset in type 1 diabetics. Microalbuminuria may be present at the time of diagnosis in type 2 diabetics.

Proteinuria/albuminuria
Microalbuminuria may progress to frank proteinuria/albuminuria around 17 years after the diagnosis of type 1 diabetes, marking the start of overt nephropathy. In both type 1 and type 2 patients an approximate 10 mL/min/m^2 reduction in glomerular filtration rate occurs yearly once the albumin excretion rate has reached 300 mg/day.

End-stage renal failure
Once serum creatinine concentration reaches 200 μmol/L, a 1 mL/min/month fall in glomerular filtration rate is expected, leading to end-stage renal failure with uraemia and potentially death, usually 7–10 years after onset of albuminuria. A plot of $^1/_{serum\ creatinine}$ against time demonstrates a relatively straight line, which shows the projected rate of deterioration.

Clinical features

Diabetic nephropathy is defined as albuminuria and declining renal function in a patient with known diabetes who does not have a urinary tract infection, heart failure or any other renal disease. It is usually associated with systemic hypertension, diabetic retinopathy and neuropathy, and in the absence of these the diagnosis needs to be carefully evaluated.

Proteinuria is often picked up at the diabetes clinic as part of annual screening. Patients usually have no symptoms during the early stages. As diabetic nephropathy progresses, patients present with the usual spectrum of symptoms (p. 441) associated with declining glomerular filtration rate. Patients with type II diabetes may present at an advanced stage of renal impairment or even at end-stage. Patients with diabetic nephropathy often have more problems with fluid overload, and as the glomerular filtration rate drops, less insulin is excreted and patients may develop unexplained hypoglycaemia. Nausea may lead to loss of appetite, worsening the severity of hypoglycaemia.

Initial investigations

24-hour urine collection
Proteinuria occurs when urinary protein is more than 0.5 g in 24 hours. Albuminuria is defined as a urinary albumin excretion rate more than 300 mg in 24 hours or more than 200 μg per minute. Microalbuminuria is defined as urinary albumin excretion rate 30–300 mg of albumin in 24 hours or 20–200 μg per minute.

Medical management

Glycaemic control
Tight glycaemic control of type 1 patients has been shown to reduce progression to microalbuminuria by 30% and subsequent progression to albuminuria by 54%, although not all patients with good control may benefit.[1] The current treatment aim is to normalize or reduce Hb$_{A1c}$ (<7.2%) while avoiding weight gain or hypoglycaemia associated with the increased used of both oral hypoglycaemic agents and insulin.

Blood pressure control
Controlling hypertension reduces the progression to microalbuminuria and from this to albuminuria and subsequent progression to end-stage renal failure. Blood pressure should be reduced to 130/80 mmHg (or 120/70 mmHg if there is more than 1 g of proteinuria per day). Weight loss, alcohol restriction and reducing salt intake can help, but drugs are usually needed to achieve this.

Angiotensin-converting enzyme (ACE) inhibitors are currently the preferred first-line agent in both microalbuminuric and albuminuric patients. More than one agent may be required to achieve blood pressure control, and other drugs used singly or in combination are β-blockers, diuretics (furosemide, hydralazine), calcium channel blockers and angiotensin receptor blockers.

Dietary protein restriction
For type 1 patients with microalbuminuria, reducing dietary animal protein intake appears to reduce both hyperfiltra-

tion and microalbuminuria. The benefits are more evident in patients with severe renal impairment. In type 2 patients, dietary modifications are associated with an initial reduction in microalbuminuria. A dietary protein content <0.8 g/kg is suggested.

Lipid lowering

Although lipid lowering has not been shown to reduce the progression of microalbuminuria to albuminuria or renal failure, these patients have a significant dyslipidaemia and a high cardiovascular mortality and require careful lipid monitoring and aggressive treatment. The use of aspirin is also advisable for similar reasons.

Dialysis

The treatment option for end-stage renal failure is dialysis (haemodialysis or ambulatory peritoneal dialysis).

Surgical management

Renal transplantation

Renal transplant improves survival in diabetic patients with end-stage renal disease, but many have contraindications to transplantation. Severe vascular disease can preclude successful anastomoses, and cardiac disease increases perioperative risk. The overall mortality remains higher than with non-diabetics but the long-term survival is better than patients on dialysis. Patients still tend to succumb to cardiovascular deaths.

Prognosis

Of those with type 1 diabetes who develop proteinuria, two thirds will subsequently develop renal failure. The prognosis of patients with diabetes on dialysis is poor. The 5-year survival has been estimated at 30.2%, compared with 62.2% in non-diabetic patients with renal failure.[2]

The increased mortality is due to both atherosclerotic complications and difficulties with dialysis itself. Proteinuria itself is associated with a drop in 10-year survival from 70% to 10%. Type 1 diabetics have a 50-fold mortality once proteinuria develops. Limb amputation in a dialysis-dependent patient is associated with less than 50% survival at 1 year.

REFERENCES

(1) *Effect of intensive therapy on the development and progression of diabetic nephropathy in the Diabetes Control and Complications Trial. The Diabetes Control and Complications (DCCT) Research Group. Kidney International 1995; 47: 1703–1720.*
(2) *Koch M, Thomas B, Tschope W, Ritz E. Survival and predictors of death in dialysed diabetic patients. Diabetologia 1993; 36: 1113–1117.*

Diabetic neuropathy

Diabetic neuropathy can have different manifestations (Table 7.8), but the most common is diffuse, predominantly sensory peripheral neuropathy of the cranial, peripheral or

Table 7.8	Classification of diabetic neuropathies

Sensory neuropathy
    Acute
    Chronic	

Proximal motor neuropathy (diabetic amyotrophy)	

Mononeuropathy
    Entrapment neuropathy
    External pressure palsies
    Spontaneous mononeuropathy	

Autonomic neuropathy	

autonomic nerves. The effects on nerve function can be acute or chronic, transient or permanent. The consequences of neuropathy include neuropathic ulcers (usually on the feet), Charcot arthropathy, altered sensation (both pain and increased sensitivity to normal sensation) and impotence (autonomic neuropathy).

Distal axonal loss occurs with focal demyelination and limited nerve regeneration. Basement membrane thickening is evident in the vasa nervorum of the neurone, with endothelial cell changes and occasionally occlusion of the lumen. The result is delayed nerve conduction velocities or a complete loss of nerve function. Hyperglycaemia is probably the underlying cause of the above histological and functional changes.

Diabetic mononeuropathies

Peripheral mononeuropathies and cranial mononeuropathies may be spontaneous or caused by entrapment or external pressure.

Of the peripheral mononeuropathies, median nerve involvement and carpal tunnel syndrome may be found in up to 10% of patients and require confirmation with nerve conduction studies before surgical decompression. Entrapment of the lateral cutaneous nerve of the thigh is also common in patients with pain over the lateral aspect of the thigh. Common peroneal nerve involvement causing foot drop and tarsal tunnel syndrome is also recognized but less common.

Cranial mononeuropathies usually occur suddenly and have a good prognosis: IIIrd and VIth cranial nerve palsies are most commonly seen. Spontaneous recovery is slow over several months, and no treatment is needed apart from symptomatic help such as an eye patch.

Proximal motor neuropathy (diabetic amyotrophy)

Proximal motor neuropathy is an uncommon but disturbing condition, usually affecting men in their 50s with type 2 diabetes. It presents with severe pain and paraesthesia in the thighs. It is usually a deep aching pain that is burning in nature and of sufficient severity to keep patients awake at night and lead to anorexia. Marked cachexia, proximal muscle weakness and wasting of the quadriceps can be very debilitating.

The lumbar sacral plexus lower motor neurones are affected, and improvement is usually spontaneous over 3–4 months. Before making this diagnosis, however, other causes such as malignancy and lumbar disc disease should be considered.

Oral antidiabetic agents may play a part in the aetiology of this problem, and conversion to insulin therapy is advised, although the anorexia experienced by patients when the pain is severe can make this difficult. Recovery occurs over a few months with only 50% achieving full recovery. No treatment is currently known to be effective.

Diabetic autonomic neuropathy

Epidemiology
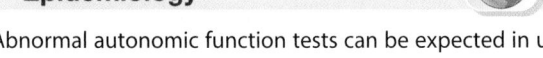

Abnormal autonomic function tests can be expected in up to 40% of the general diabetic population.

Pathology

The pathological features are detailed on page 451.

Clinical features

The most common effect of autonomic neuropathy is erectile dysfunction, which affects 40% of men with diabetes. A small number develop severe gastrointestinal and bladder dysfunction. Other symptoms include postural hypotension (dizziness and syncope in up to 12%), resting tachycardia or fixed heart rate/loss of sinus arrhythmia (in up to 20%), gustatory sweating (sweating after tasting food), dysphagia with delayed gastric emptying, nausea or vomiting, constipation, diarrhoea, urinary retention, overflow incontinence, anhidrosis (absent sweating on the feet is problematic as it increases the risk of ulceration) and abnormal pupillary reflexes.

On examination, lying and standing blood pressure may reveal postural hypotension; the pupillary responses to light may be impaired. Less commonly performed measures include assessment for sinus arrhythmia where the inspiratory and expiratory heart rates after 5 seconds of inspiration or expiration are assessed (<10 beats/minute difference is abnormal, >15 is normal), assessment for the heart rate response to a Valsalva manoeuvre (the ratio of the shortest R-R interval during forced expiration against a closed glottis compared to the longest R-R interval after it, where less than 1.2 s is abnormal) and the blood pressure response to sustained hand grip (diastolic blood pressure prior to the test is compared to diastolic blood pressure after 5 minutes of sustaining a grip; diastolic BP rise >16 mmHg is normal, <10 mmHg is abnormal).

Initial investigations
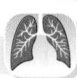

Investigations are usually tailored to specific symptoms; for gastric symptoms a radioisotope test meal may be performed to look for delayed gastric emptying.

Medical management

Management is usually symptomatic. In all patients improvement in diabetic control is advocated despite limited efficacy.

Postural hypotension

Any precipitating cause such as diuretics, vasodilators and tricyclic antidepressants should be excluded. Mechanical measures such as sleeping with the head elevated and wearing support stockings may help. Adequate salt intake should be ensured.

Fludrocortisone, 50 µg od initially and increased as required up to 400 µg, may be helpful but hypertension or oedema may result as a complication. Desmopressin and octreotide have also been used.

Impotence

Libido is not normally affected and pain is also unusual. Autonomic neuropathy is a likely cause but many drugs (thiazides, β-blockers) can also lead to impotence. Other causes include alcohol, tobacco, cannabis and stress.

The main therapies for erectile dysfunction are sildenafil, vardenafil and apomorphine. Intraurethral or intracavernosal therapy such as alprostadil can be used. Mechanical devices include vacuum suction devices

Gastroparesis

Delayed gastric emptying can lead to recurrent hypoglycaemia. Pro-motility agents such as metoclopramide, domperidone or erythromycin may be helpful. Surgical gastric drainage procedures are reserved for severe cases.

Large bowel involvement

Constipation is treated with standard bulking and softening laxatives. Episodic diarrhoea is more troublesome, and treatment for this may include loperamide or codeine phosphate with antibiotics in cases of bacterial overgrowth.

Neuropathic bladder

Sacral nerve involvement can cause bladder abnormalities with reduced sensations of bladder fullness and increased residual volume after micturition. Regular toileting may help but intermittent self-catheterization or a long-term catheter may be required.

Anhidrosis

Dry feet can cause cracks in the skin that act as a site for infection. Emollient creams may help to prevent this.

Prognosis
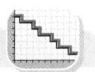

Treatment is usually symptomatic; the underlying disease process is usually permanent.

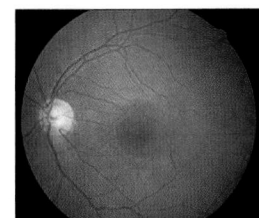

Fig. 7.2 Normal retina. No evidence of diabetic retinopathy.

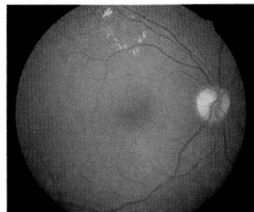

Fig. 7.3 Background diabetic retinopathy. Retinal photograph showing microaneurysms, haemorrhages and exudates.

453

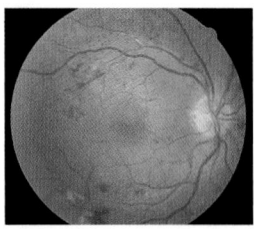

Fig. 7.4 Pre-proliferative diabetic retinopathy. Retinal photograph showing IRMA and multiple blot haemorrhages.

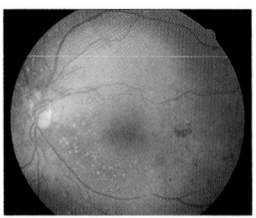

Fig. 7.5 Proliferative diabetic retinopathy. Retinal photograph showing new vessels at the optic disc.

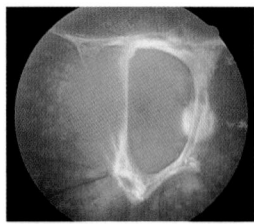

Fig. 7.6 Proliferative diabetic retinopathy. Retinal photograph showing fibrous proliferation.

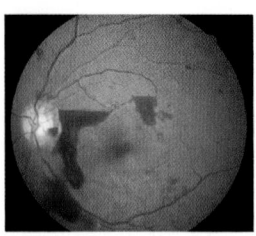

Fig. 7.7 Proliferative diabetic retinopathy. Retinal image showing pre-retinal and vitreous haemorrhages.

Diabetic eye disease

Diabetic retinopathy is the most common cause of blindness in the working population of developed countries. Diabetes is associated with a 10-fold increased risk of blindness. Currently, 2% of the UK diabetic population is thought to be registered blind.

Epidemiology

The prevalence of diabetic retinopathy is approximately 30 000 per 100 000 (30%) patients with diabetes, the figure varies according to the duration of diabetes, glycaemic control, blood pressure control and ethnicity (Table 7.9).

In general, less than 2% of patients with type 1 diabetes have any lesions of diabetic retinopathy at diagnosis but up to 98% have abnormalities 30 years later (30% have proliferative retinopathy). Up to 37% of patients with type 2 diabetes have retinopathy at diagnosis: 85% of those on insulin, and 65% not on insulin develop retinal abnormalities by 15 years.

In the UK, maculopathy is a more common and therefore more significant sight-threatening complication of diabetes. It is suggested that 75% of those with maculopathy have type 2 diabetes.

Cataracts are also more common in people with diabetes and the most common eye abnormality. They occur in up to 60% of 30–54-year-olds.

Pathology

One of the first changes is thickening of the capillary basement membrane and loss of the pericytes embedded in it. In normal retinal capillaries there is a 1:1 relationship between endothelial cells and pericytes. Pericytes may control endothelial cell proliferation, maintain the structural integrity of capillaries and regulate blood flow. Increased blood viscosity, abnormal fibrinolytic activity and reduced red cell deformity in diabetes may lead to capillary occlusion, tissue hypoxia and the stimulus for new vessel formation. The natural progression is from background to

Table 7.9	Risk factors for developing diabetic retinopathy
Duration of diabetes	
Type of diabetes Proliferative disease is more common in type 1 Maculopathy is more common in type 2	
Poor diabetic control	
Hypertension	
Diabetic nephropathy	
Recent cataract surgery	
Pregnancy	
Alcohol	
Smoking	

pre-proliferative/pre-maculopathy then to proliferative retinopathy/maculopathy and ultimately sight-threatening disease (Table 7.10).

Clinical features

The classification of diabetic retinopathy (Table 7.10) is based on ophthalmoscopy but several other changes not seen macroscopically may explain some of the clinical findings.

Background retinopathy

Capillary microaneurysms are the earliest feature, seen clinically as red 'dots'. Small intraretinal haemorrhages or 'blots' also occur, as can haemorrhages into the nerve fibre layers which are often more flame shaped (Fig. 7.3). With increased capillary leakage hard exudates, which are lipid deposits, can also be seen.

Pre-proliferative retinopathy

Cotton wool spots are infarcts in the nerve fibre layer that alter axoplasmic transport in ganglion cell neurones. The oedematous infarct is seen as a pale or grey fuzzy-edged lesion, the appearance giving it its name. Intraretinal microvascular abnormalities (IRMAs) are tortuous, dilated, hypercellular capillaries in the retina that occur in response to retinal ischaemia (Fig. 7.4). Further changes seen include alternating dilatation and constriction of veins (venous beading) and other venous alterations such as duplication and loop formation. Overall there are large areas of capillary non-perfusion in the absence of new vessels.

The Early Treatment of Diabetic Retinopathy Study (ETDRS) suggested four important clinical features: 4 quadrants of severe haemorrhages or 4 quadrants of microaneurysms, 2 quadrants of IRMAs or 1 quadrant with venous beading. A single feature is associated with a 15% risk of developing sight-threatening retinopathy within the next year; with 2 features, the risk rises to 45%.

Proliferative retinopathy

New vessels are formed from the retina and can grow along, into or out from it (Fig. 7.5). Scaffolding for fibrosis (Fig. 7.6) then forms. There are two forms of new vessels: those on the disc or within 1 disc diameter of the disc (NVD), and new vessels elsewhere (NVE). Both are asymptomatic but cause the problems of advanced retinopathy such as haemorrhage (Fig. 7.7), scar tissue formation, traction on the retina and retinal detachment which actually results in loss of vision. That is why panretinal photocoagulation is recommended when they are seen.

Diabetic maculopathy

Oedema in the macula can distort central vision and reduce visual acuity. Changes that can coexist with maculopathy include: oedema (clinically, it may be difficult to focus on the macula with a hand-held ophthalmoscope); exudates (with haemorrhages, hard exudates and circinate exudates); and ischaemia (capillary loss occurs but clinically the macula may look normal on direct ophthalmoscopy although non-perfused areas will show up on fluorescein angiography).

Table 7.10	Classification and features of diabetic retinopathy
Background retinopathy	
Microaneurysms	
Haemorrhages	
Hard exudates	
Pre-proliferative retinopathy	
Soft exudates/cotton wool spots	
Intraretinal microvascular abnormalities (IRMAs)	
Venous abnormalities (e.g. venous beading, looping and reduplication)	
Proliferative retinopathy	
New vessels on the disc or within 1 disc diameter of it (NVD)	
New vessels elsewhere (NVE)	
Rubeosis iridis (± neovascular glaucoma)	
Maculopathy	
Haemorrhages and hard exudates in the macula area	
Reduced visual acuity with no abnormality seen	

Table 7.11	Reasons for and timing of referral to an ophthalmologist
Immediate referral	
Proliferative retinopathy. Untreated NVD carries a 40% risk of blindness in <2 years and laser treatment reduces this	
Rubeosis iridis/neovascular glaucoma	
Vitreous haemorrhage	
Advanced retinopathy with fibrous tissue or retinal detachments	
Early referral (within 6 weeks)	
Preproliferative changes	
Maculopathy. Both for non-proliferative retinopathy involving the macula or for any haemorrhages/hard exudates within 1 disc diameter of the fovea	
Fall of >2 lines on a Snellen chart (whatever fundoscopy shows)	
Routine referral	
Cataracts	
Non-proliferative retinopathy with large circinate exudates not threatening the macula/fovea	

Diabetic nephropathy

Diabetic neuropathy

Diabetic eye disease

Diabetic dermopathy

Diabetic thick skin

Necrobiosis lipoidica

Eruptive xanthoma

Acanthosis nigricans

Acquired perforating dermatosis

Diabetic bullae

A ring or circinate pattern of lipid deposits (Fig. 7.8) suggests a focal defect that may be treated with focal laser therapy, while a more diffuse problem may require more extensive treatment with a macula grid of laser (Fig. 7.9).

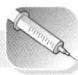

Initial management

Glycaemic control
An initial step is to improve glycaemic control, blood pressure control and lipid control.

Surgical management

Laser treatment
If maculopathy or proliferative disease occurs, surgical interventions may be needed. The timing of these is shown in Table 7.11. Laser treatment is usually the first. In this, 1500–7000 separate burns, of 100–500 µm diameter, each taking about 0.1 seconds to apply, are needed for pan-retinal or 'scatter' laser photocoagulation. For oedematous/exudative maculopathy a macula grid may use only 100–200 burns of 100–200 µm diameter separated by 200–400 µm gaps, avoiding the fovea. The benefits currently outweigh the risks of laser therapy, which include accidental burns to the fovea if the eye moves during therapy, a reduction in night vision and, in a small number, interference with visual field severe enough to affect ability to drive.

Vitrectomy
If the vitreous contains scar tissue, haemorrhage or any opacity, a vitrectomy to remove it may help restore vision. It also allows the chance for intraoperative laser treatment or a better view for postoperative laser therapy. It can also help reduce retinal traction and allows retinal reattachment to be performed.

Prognosis
Prognosis varies with aetiology, stage of disease and treatment received.

Diabetes and the skin

At least 30% of patients have some cutaneous involvement during the course of their disease (Table 7.12). Skin infections occur in up to 50% of patients with poorly controlled disease. Cutaneous changes may result from diabetic complications such as neuropathic ulcers and from treatment reactions such as lipoatrophy with decreased adipose tissue at sites of subcutaneous insulin injection. Rubeosis faciei or the 'flushed face' has been reported in up to 60% of diabetics. It may be caused by microangiopathy or increased photosensitivity. The common skin conditions are detailed in the remaining sections of this chapter.

Less common skin conditions that have a weaker association with diabetes include vitiligo, pseudoxanthoma elasticum and lipoid proteinosis. There are also various other disease processes with cutaneous manifestations that may involve secondary diabetes, including haemochromatosis, hepatic porphyrias and lipodystrophies. The association of granuloma annulare with diabetes mellitus has not been clearly established. Several studies support the view that generalized granuloma annulare, especially in the elderly, is associated with impaired glucose tolerance.

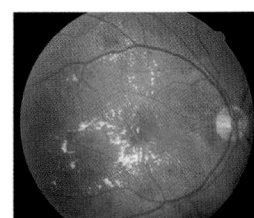

Fig. 7.8 Diabetic maculopathy. Retinal photograph showing haemorrhages and circinate exudates.

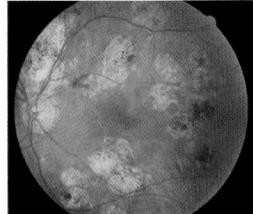

Fig. 7.9 Retinal photograph. Evidence of previous laser therapy.

455

Table 7.12	Skin lesions in diabetes
Conditions specific to diabetes	
Pretibial diabetic dermopathy ('shin spots')	
Diabetic bullae (bullosis diabeticorum, tense blistering on feet/lower legs)	
Diabetic thick skin (scleroderma of diabetes seen in 2.5% with type 2 diabetes)	
Periungual telangiectasia (venous capillary dilatation at the nail fold seen in up to 50% of people with diabetes)	
Conditions seen more commonly in diabetics	
Necrobiosis lipoidica	
Vitiligo (2% with type 1 diabetes)	
Granuloma annulare (this association is not proven conclusively)	
Conditions associated with the other biochemical features seen in diabetes	
Acanthosis nigricans (with insulin resistance)	
Eruptive xanthomata (with hypertriglyceridaemia)	

Diabetic dermopathy

Diabetic dermopathy is considered the most common cutaneous manifestation of diabetes, affecting up to 70% of patients, and is predominantly seen in men over the age of 50. However, diabetic dermopathy is not specific to diabetes because 20% of non-diabetics have similar lesions.

Multiple, bilateral, irregular red papules or plaques appear on the shins. These lesions gradually evolve into atrophic hyperpigmented macules. The pathogenic significance of diabetic angiopathy remains to be established but diabetic dermopathy is often accompanied by micro-angiopathy.

Diabetic thick skin

There are two main forms of diabetic thick skin: diabetic hand syndrome and diabetic scleroderma. The histology often demonstrates abnormally thickened dermal collagen. It is thought that this may be caused by hyperglycaemic accelerated non-enzymatic glycosylation end products which result in increased cross-linking of collagen fibres and resistance to degradation by collagenase. Other theories include insulin acting as a growth factor causing over-production of collagen, or local oxygen reduction secondary to microangiopathy increasing collagen and glycosaminoglycan synthesis by fibroblasts.

Diabetic hand syndrome consists of tight and waxy (scleroderma-like) skin changes over the fingers with limited joint mobility (cheiroarthropathy). Diabetic scleroderma is characterized by poorly demarcated non-pitting induration of the skin over the upper back, neck and shoulders. It is most commonly seen in poorly controlled type 2 diabetic obese men. These changes are often preceded by a respiratory infection or by streptococcal infection. The lesions may become more generalized over trunk and limbs. Topical and intralesional steroids are of limited therapeutic benefit.

Necrobiosis lipoidica

Epidemiology

Necrobiosis lipoidica occurs in about 1% of diabetic patients. The lesions are most often seen on the anterior shins of young and middle-aged adults and are 3 times more common in females.

Pathology

Up to 65% of patients with necrobiosis lipoidica have diabetes at the time of diagnosis; however, approximately 90% eventually develop diabetes or abnormal glucose tolerance. Therefore all patients with necrobiosis should be evaluated and followed for the development of diabetes.

Clinical features

Necrobiosis lipoidica presents as well-demarcated oval plaques of cutaneous atrophy with a shiny surface, yellow waxy centres and brownish red margins surrounded by telangiectasia (Fig. 7.10). The plaques slowly enlarge peripherally and may ulcerate.

Investigations

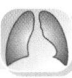

Skin biopsy
Diagnosis is made clinically as the lesions are distinct. Rarely a confirmatory biopsy is required. Histology shows collagen degeneration in the dermis surrounded by histiocytes, and usually epithelioid cell granulomas and giant cells are present.

Management

Immunomodulation
Treatment includes potent topical or intralesional steroids. Oral immunosupression with ciclosporin has also been reported as beneficial.

Aspirin
Low-dose aspirin may help healing.

Wound care
Ulcerated lesions usually heal with local wound care. Attempts at local excision and grafting are usually complicated by recurrences.

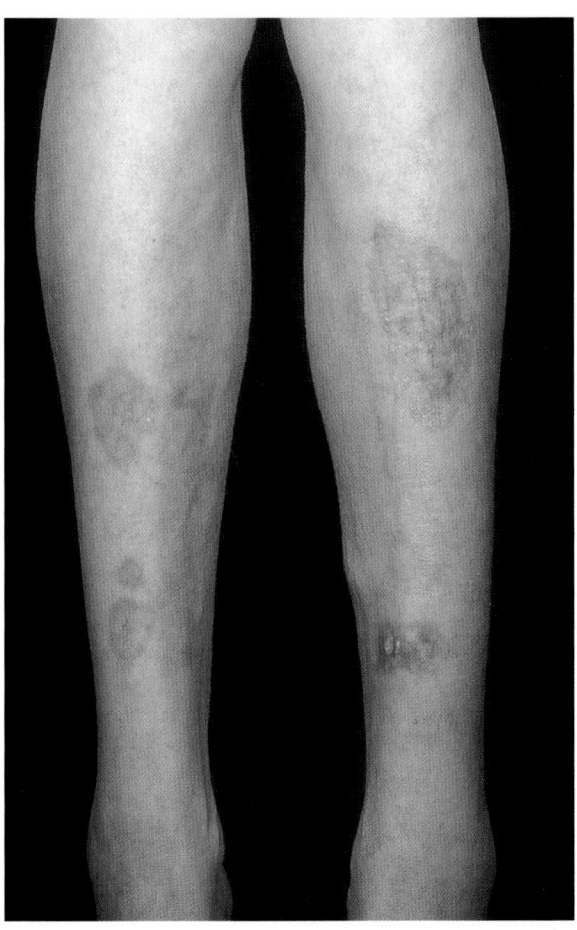

Fig. 7.10 Necrobiosis lipoidica.

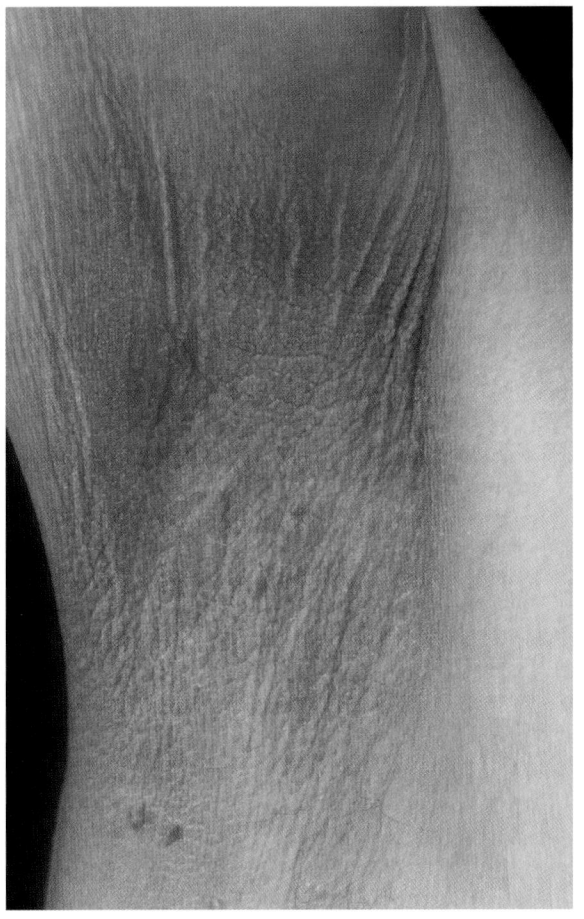

Fig. 7.11 Acanthosis nigricans.

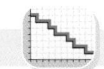

Prognosis

Spontaneous gradual resolution occurs in 15% after 12 years.

Eruptive xanthoma

Eruptive xanthoma may present as sudden crops of yellow papules over buttocks, elbows and knees. The lesions appear in association with elevated levels of triglyceride-rich lipoproteins. The control of diabetes or underlying hyperlipidaemia leads to their resolution.

Acanthosis nigricans

Acanthosis nigricans presents as asymptomatic, hyper-pigmented velvety plaques involving flexural sites, most commonly the axillae (Fig. 7.11) and nape of the neck. It is associated with insulin resistance. The pathogenesis is not known although it is thought that insulin-like epidermal growth factors may result in the epidermal hyperplasia seen in the lesions. The disorder is divided into five subgroups: hereditary (benign autosomal dominant), benign (resulting from endocrine disorders—type 2 diabetes, acromegaly, Cushing's disease), pseudoacanthosis nigricans (obese, Asian or Hispanic adults), drug induced (nicotinic acid, diethylstilbestrol or corticosteroids) and malignant (most commonly adenocarcinoma of the gastrointestinal tract).

Acquired perforating dermatosis

Small, pruritic, umbilicated papules occur, usually on the extensor aspect of limbs and hands. They result from trans-epidermal channels filled with keratin, inflammatory cells, elastin and collagen. Lesions are seen in patients with systemic diseases such as chronic renal failure or diabetes. The lesions are chronic but may heal after months.

Diabetic bullae

Diabetic bullae (bullosis diabeticorum) occur in 0.5% of diabetes. They are more common in men with long-standing diabetes and neuropathy. These painless bullae appear suddenly and may be preceded by trauma. They are most commonly seen on the dorsa and sides of the lower legs and feet and are sometimes associated with similar lesions on the hands. Two different types of bullae have been described. The more frequent lesion is non-scarring, and histologically there is an intraepidermal split. More rarely the bullae are haemorrhagic, healing with scarring, and histologically there is a subepidermal split. The pathogenesis is not well understood. If the bullae are large and symptomatic, they can be aspirated leaving an intact roof. The lesions usually heal spontaneously within 5 weeks but may recur at the same sites.

SECTION 7.5 — Diabetes and surgery

Preoperative assessment

Careful preoperative assessment is essential because of an increased risk of death and complications such as fluid overload from coronary heart disease and diabetic nephropathy. Any preoperative assessment in a patient with known diabetes should therefore include a history of diabetic complications and examination looking for evidence of peripheral vascular disease or peripheral neuropathy and lying/standing blood pressures in case of autonomic neuropathy.

In addition, assessment of current and overall diabetic control is required (blood glucose measurements and glycated haemoglobin, Hb_{A1c}). Any patient whose diabetic control is inadequate, undergoing a procedure that is not needed as an emergency, should have attempts made to improve this either on the ward or in a diabetic clinic. While an Hb_{A1c} <7.2% is considered good control, an acceptable level for most procedures would be <9%. Even with a good Hb_{A1c} level, the preoperative glucose level and, if >11 mmol/L, the urine ketones, should always be measured as the perioperative treatment is based on this and some stabilization prior to administering an anaesthetic may be required, particularly in the emergency situation.

General investigations should include serum urea and electrolytes/creatinine, full blood count, urine dipstick testing for protein, and an ECG in anyone older than 45 years.

Any further investigation will be based upon problems found in the history or examination such as foot ulceration and potential osteomyelitis which may give a source for infection such as methicillin-resistant *Staphylococcus aureus* (MRSA).

Perioperative management

Ideally, patients with diabetes are best operated on in the morning at the start of the list.

Diet-controlled diabetics

Patients normally controlled on diet alone should have their capillary blood glucose levels checked hourly. Intravenous dextrose should be avoided but they often need no other modification to their treatment.

Tablet-controlled diabetics

Patients taking oral agents should stop metformin preoperatively and omit their other antidiabetic medication on the morning of the procedure. If patients are on long-acting agents, such as chlorpropamide, these should be omitted the day before.

Capillary blood glucose levels are monitored regularly (1–2-hourly). If glucose is more than 7.0 mmol/L then a dextrose and insulin regimen should be commenced (Table 7.13) to keep the glucose between 7 and 11 mmol/L.

Insulin-controlled diabetics

Patients on insulin undergoing a morning operation should miss the morning insulin dose and start on a dextrose–insulin regimen. If the operation is to be performed in the afternoon, then half the normal morning dose of soluble insulin with a light breakfast should be given and a dextrose–insulin regimen commenced at midday, aiming to keep the blood glucose between 7 and 11 mmol/L.

Insulin regimen

There are two common regimens: a variable dose sliding scale (Table 7.13) and a fixed dose (per bag) infusion (Table 7.14). Each hospital usually has its own preferred regimen. The sliding scale regimen is popular and consists of a continuous intravenous infusion adjusted on the basis of blood glucose measurements with a fixed dextrose infusion. The continuous fixed dose infusion consists of a single bag containing dextrose, insulin and potassium, known as the 'Alberti regimen' or the 'GIK (glucose insulin potassium) regimen'.

Table 7.13	Sliding scale intravenous insulin infusion regimen

Add 50 units of soluble insulin in 50 mL 0.9% saline (giving 1 unit/mL) in a 50 mL syringe and run through an automated syringe driver. This regimen will need to be tailored to an individual patient, e.g. insulin-resistant patients will need much larger amounts of insulin. A suitable starting regimen is shown below.

Blood glucose (mmol/L)	Insulin infusion rate (units/h)
0–4.0	0.5, recheck in 30 minutes
4.1–7.0	1.0
7.1–11.0	2.0
11.1–17.0	4.0
>17.1	6.0–8.0, review regimen

Hyperlipidaemia

Primary hyperlipidaemia

Secondary hyperlipidaemias

Table 7.14	Glucose–insulin–potassium (GIK) regimen

Although not as popular as the above 'sliding scale' continuous regimen, this method does have the advantage of everything being given together, so reducing the risk of insulin being given on its own.

- Into a 500 mL bag of 5% dextrose add 8 units of soluble insulin and 5 mmol of potassium
- Run this mixture at 100 mL/h and measure capillary blood glucose hourly initially, aiming for levels of 7–11 mmol/L ideally and 5–15 mmol/L at worst
- If >15 mmol/L, swap this infusion for one with 10 units of insulin but also check the serum potassium level to see if that also needs adjusting
- If blood glucose is <5 mmol/L, reduce the insulin to 6 units/ 500 mL of 5% dextrose
- After each alteration, recheck blood glucose levels after 1 hour and adjust further if required. Once stable, reduce the capillary blood glucose levels to 2 hourly
- As with the other intravenous regimen, convert to regular therapy once the patient is eating

Other metabolic diseases

Disorders of lipid metabolism

The two main circulating lipids are triglycerides and cholesterol. They are bound to phospholipid and lipoproteins to make them water soluble for transportation. The surface apoproteins of these soluble masses facilitate the recognition of the different transport complexes.

Chylomicrons

Chylomicrons contain 85% triglycerides and 4% cholesterol. They are produced in the mucosa of the small intestine and broken down in the liver and peripheral tissues by lipoprotein lipase. They initially contain apoprotein B-48 (apo B-48) and acquire apo E and apo C-II from circulating HDL. Following metabolism by lipoprotein lipase in capillary endothelial cells, chylomicron remnants are removed by the liver.

Very low density lipoproteins (VLDL)

VLDL contain 50% triglyceride, 15% cholesterol and 18% phospholipids. They are produced with triglycerides that have been synthesized in the liver. VLDL also contain apo B-100 and apo E. They are broken down by lipoprotein lipase in peripheral tissue to give IDL and other remnants that are removed by the liver.

Intermediate density lipoproteins (IDL)

IDL are VLDL remnants that contain mainly cholesterol and phospholipid. They are removed by the liver or metabolized to LDL.

Low density lipoproteins (LDL)

LDL contain 45% cholesterol, 10% triglyceride and 20% phospholipid. LDL have apo B-100 on their surface and transport most of the cholesterol in circulation. The liver has specific LDL receptors to extract it from the circulation. Half of the body's circulating LDL is removed from the plasma each day, mainly by the liver. Smaller, denser or oxidized LDL (15% of the LDL pool) are removed by a scavenger pathway in macrophages and liver sinusoidal endothelial cells. Accumulation of oxidized LDL in macrophages produces the foam cells that are seen in atheromatous plaques.

High density lipoproteins (HDL)

HDL are produced by the liver and gut. They contain 17% cholesterol, 4% triglyceride and 24% phospholipid. HDL transport 20–50% of circulating cholesterol.

Primary and secondary hyperlipidaemia

Elevated blood lipid levels are a modifiable risk factor for the development of atherosclerosis, a major cause of death from coronary heart disease, peripheral vascular disease and stroke. Hyperlipidaemia occurs due to a combination of genetic factors and dietary intake. Primary hyperlipidaemias are usually genetically determined while secondary hyperlipidaemias occur due to a combination of disease, drugs and diet. In this section, the diseases that give rise to primary and secondary hyperlipidaemias are

459

summarized, and an overall assessment and management of the hyperlipidaemic patient is presented below.

Hyperlipidaemia

Epidemiology

Hyperlipidaemia and hypercholesterolaemia are very common.

Pathology

The causes of hyperlipidaemia are discussed below. The main effect of the disease is the development of atherosclerosis. Subintimal plaques start in medium-sized blood vessel walls when LDL cholesterol accumulates. A cholesterol-rich necrotic core develops and is surrounded by smooth muscle cells and fibrous tissue.

Plaques can result from a combination of diffusion of elevated LDL cholesterol, qualitative abnormalities of LDL cholesterol or endothelial cell damage. The last may be due to physical trauma (hypertension), toxins (tobacco, alcohol), low-grade infection, inflammation, immune complex damage or a combination of these. Plaque ulceration is associated with thrombosis, which can obliterate the lumen of a blood vessel, and distal embolism.

There is a direct linear relationship between hypercholesterolaemia and coronary heart disease. Reductions in total and LDL cholesterol reduce coronary events, cerebrovascular events and mortality. The converse is true of HDL cholesterol, which has an inverse relationship with coronary heart disease (increasing levels are beneficial). The association between isolated hypertriglyceridaemia and vascular disease is still debated, but mixed hyperlipidaemia is clearly associated with coronary heart disease. The Helsinki Heart study showed a 4-fold greater risk of cardiac events if the LDL:HDL ratio was >5.0 and the triglycerides >2.3 mmol/L compared to those with lower levels of triglycerides.

Clinical features

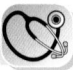

The main presenting features are complications associated with atherosclerosis (coronary heart disease, peripheral vascular disease and stroke). Clinical features directly associated with hyperlipidaemia include xanthomas, xanthelasma and a corneal arcus.

Initial investigations

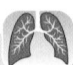

Serum lipid profile

In practice, patients are managed by their levels of cholesterol (total cholesterol, LDL, HDL) and triglycerides. A lipid profile needs to be a fasting sample (preferably after a 12-hour overnight fast). In non-fasting samples, only total and HDL cholesterol measurements are accurate.

Triglycerides rise post-prandially and LDL is usually calculated.

Measurements should not be taken during an acute illness or during periods of rapid weight loss as these lead to artificially low results. This is particularly important from 24 hours after a myocardial infarction for up to 6 weeks (less if thrombolysis was undertaken). During this time, the levels of total and LDL cholesterol may be artificially reduced. Pregnancy or recent weight gain is associated with increased lipid levels. After rapid weight gain or weight loss, at least 1 month should elapse once the patient is stable before lipid levels are reassessed.

Hypercholesterolaemia is defined as elevated total or LDL cholesterol with normal triglyceride levels. Hypertriglyceridaemia is an isolated elevation of triglyceride levels. An elevation of both cholesterol and triglycerides is termed mixed hyperlipidaemia.

Total cholesterol measurements alone can be misleading as isolated HDL elevations will elevate the total serum cholesterol level. Use of total cholesterol to HDL ratio or a LDL:HDL ratio is preferred, especially in women and in diabetics.

Initial management

The emphasis will depend on the cause of the hyperlipidaemia and is aimed at reducing cardiovascular and cerebrovascular risk. There are now recommended target values when treating patients (Table 7.15). If these optimal levels are not achievable, at least a 30% fall from pre-treatment serum cholesterol concentration is acceptable.

Dietary advice

In general, fat should constitute less than 30% of consumed calories, and saturated fats must be less than 30% of the total fat content. The total dietary cholesterol should not exceed 300 mg per day.

Three to four months should be allowed to elapse to see if dietary manipulation works. It is unusual to see more than a 25% fall in cholesterol from dietary measures.

Weight control

A 10 kg weight loss in an obese subject reduces LDL cholesterol by 7% and increases HDL cholesterol by 13%.

Table 7.15	Target lipid levels
Patients without complications of atherosclerosis	
Total cholesterol <5.2 mmol/L	
LDL cholesterol <4.0 mmol/L	
HDL cholesterol >1.0 mmol/L	
Patients with coronary heart disease	
Total cholesterol of <4.0 mmol/L	
LDL cholesterol <2.5 mmol/L	
Triglycerides <1.5 mmol/L	

Physical activity

Acute exercise transiently changes lipoprotein levels and increases lipoprotein lipase activity. These effects are more lasting with regular exercise. Triglyceride levels fall, HDL cholesterol levels rise, especially the HDL2 subfraction with more vigorous exercise, and LDL cholesterol is less dense and atherogenic. The alteration seen is dose dependent with increasing exercise, and a 20% alteration in each variable is achievable after 6 weeks.

Other vascular risk factor modification

Other risk factors such as hypertension, smoking and diabetes blood glucose control should be addressed.

Medical management

HMG CoA reductase inhibitors (statins)

Statins lower cholesterol by 25–40% and triglycerides by 10–20%. Complications include hepatitis and myositis (rare), therefore liver function tests and creatine kinase should be measured before they are prescribed. Statins should be discontinued if the liver enzymes aspartate (AST) and alanine (ALT) aminotransferase show more than a 2–3-fold elevation above the upper limit of normal.

Fibrates

These medications are less effective than the statins at lowering cholesterol but better at increasing HDL cholesterol and more effective in lowering triglycerides. They should not be prescribed to patients with severe liver disease or renal dysfunction. Fibrates reduce triglyceride levels by about 50% and increase HDL cholesterol by 15–20%.

Anion exchange resins (bile acid sequestrants)

Colestyramine and colestipol are effective in lowering cholesterol, but compliance can be poor due to gastrointestinal side effects. These medications can exacerbate hypertriglyceridaemia. Under optimum conditions, LDL cholesterol can be reduced by 20–30%. HDL cholesterol is slightly increased. Bile acid binding resins can affect uptake of other medications, which need to be taken at least an hour before or 4–6 hours after the resins.

Nicotinic acid and acipimox

Nicotinic acid is the most effective medication to increase HDL cholesterol. It can lower triglycerides as well as total and LDL cholesterol. However, it is severely limited by its side effects, especially vasodilatation (facial flushing). Nicotinic acid can adversely affect glucose control in diabetes mellitus. Acipimox, a nicotinic acid analogue, is currently under evaluation.

Omega 3 fatty acids

These fish oils are useful in reducing hypertriglyceridaemia but are ineffective in lowering cholesterol.

Prognosis

In general, statin therapy for hypercholesterolaemia reduces major coronary events by 27%, stroke by 18%, and all-cause mortality by 15%.[1]

> **REFERENCE**
>
> (1) Cheung BM, Lauder IJ, Lau CP, Kumana CR. Meta-analysis of large randomized controlled trials to evaluate the impact of statins on cardiovascular outcomes. British Journal of Clinical Pharmacology 2004; 57: 640–651.

Primary hyperlipidaemia

Familial hypercholesterolaemia

Familial hypercholesterolaemia is an autosomal dominant disorder, with a gene frequency of 1 in 500 in Western Europe and North America. The genetic defects are mutations in the LDL receptor gene, the apolipoprotein B-100 gene and the recently identified proprotein convertase subtilisin/kexin type 9 gene (PCSK9).[1] The result is high serum LDL levels due to prolonged LDL clearance, from 2.5 days to 4.5 days in heterozygotes and longer in homozygotes.

Patients with familial hypercholesterolaemia have early-onset coronary disease and a standardized mortality ratio 9 times greater than normal. Homozygotes typically present in childhood. Heterozygotes usually present after 30 years of age. Lipid deposits occur around the eyes (xanthelasma) and tendons (xanthomas of the fingers, hands, elbow, knee and Achilles tendon). Achilles tendinitis may be the first clue to the presence of this condition in childhood, and the corneal arcus occurs early in life (30–40 years old).

Biochemically, familial hypercholesterolaemia (FH) is characterized by high total cholesterol (>7.8 mmol/L heterozygotes, >15 mmol/L homozygotes) and high LDL (from birth).

> **REFERENCE**
>
> (1) Austin MA, Hutter CM, Zimmern RL, Humphries SE. Genetic causes of monogenic heterozygous familial hypercholesterolemia: a HuGE prevalence review. American Journal of Epidemiology 2004; 160: 407–420.

Familial hypertriglyceridaemia

Familial hypertriglyceridaemia affects 1 in 300 people, often as an autosomal dominant disorder. The biochemical disorder is elevated VLDL levels and frequently hypercholesterolaemia. It is characterized by eruptive xanthomata, which are red and painful, and lipaemia retinalis. Exacerbating factors include alcohol and medications (thiazide diuretics, glucocorticoids, oral contraceptive pill). Adherence to a low-fat, alcohol-free diet with weight reduction usually helps.

Two rare but important familial causes of gross hypertriglyceridaemia are lipoprotein lipase deficiency and apolipoprotein C-II deficiency. Both are autosomal recessive conditions that present in childhood. Lipoprotein lipase is required to metabolize chylomicrons, and a defect or absence of this enzyme results in hyperchylomicronaemia. Apo C-II is required for the activation of lipoprotein lipase, and deficiency gives the same clinical picture. Patients do not have premature coronary disease but can develop recurrent abdominal pain from pancreatitis.

Polygenic hypercholesterolaemia

Polygenic hypercholesterolaemia is the most common cause of hypercholesterolaemia. It arises due to a combination of genetic and environmental (dietary) factors. LDL clearance appears to be reduced by a variety of mechanisms and hepatic VLDL production is increased.

This disease is often linked with a high fat intake and obesity. Patients do not have xanthelasmata or extensor tendon deposits as seen in familial hyperlipidaemia. It is often diagnosed during primary cholesterol screening programmes or when investigating manifestations of atherosclerosis.

Familial combined hyperlipidaemia

Familial combined hyperlipidaemia occurs in 1 in 250 individuals. It is the most common type of inherited dyslipidaemia and associated with 10% of patients with premature coronary disease. The aetiology is not yet known, and the condition has no unique clinical manifestations that distinguish it from the other inherited hyperlipidaemic syndromes. The diagnosis is based on raised lipids (greater than 95th centile for age) and a family history of premature coronary disease in first-degree relatives.

Familial defective apolipoprotein B-100

Familial defective apolipoprotein B-100 affects 1 in 500 individuals. All lipids originating from the liver are bound to apo B-100. The genetic defect of apo B-100 results in the delayed clearance of cholesterol due to the production of an oxidation-prone LDL that overloads the scavenger pathways.

Familial dysbetalipoproteinaemia

Familial dysbetalipoproteinaemia is also known as type III hyperlipidaemia or broad beta disease. It is an uncommon disorder affecting 0.04% of people with elevated IDL and chylomicron remnants. This condition is characterized by accumulation of IDL. A characteristic clinical feature is the presence of palmar striae and tuberous xanthomata over the tuberosities of the elbows and knees. The xanthomata can also be found on pressure areas such as the heels.

Rare familial mixed dyslipidaemias

Familial lecithin cholesterol acyltransferase (LCAT) deficiency

LCAT is the enzyme required for intravascular lipoprotein metabolism. The deficiency is a recessively inherited disorder that results in elevated serum cholesterol and triglyceride levels. Clinically, corneal lipid deposits result in

Table 7.16	Causes of secondary hyperlipidaemia		
Elevated LDL cholesterol	**Elevated triglycerides**	**Reduced HDL cholesterol**
Diet (high saturated fats, high calories, anorexia)	Diet (weight gain + excess alcohol)	Diet (some low-fat diets)
Drugs (glucocorticoids, thiazide + loop diuretics, ciclosporin)	Drugs (glucocorticoids, β-adrenergic blockers, oestrogen, isotretinoin)	Drugs (anabolic steroids, tobacco, β-adrenergic blockers)
Hypothyroidism	Hypothyroidism	Type 2 diabetes
Nephrotic syndrome	Type 2 diabetes	Insulin resistance syndromes/obesity
Chronic liver disease	Insulin resistance syndromes	Chronic renal failure
Cholestasis + biliary obstruction	Cushing's syndrome	
Pregnancy	Chronic renal failure Peritoneal dialysis Pregnancy	

visual disturbances, and renal deposits result in glomerular damage, proteinuria and renal failure.

Tangier disease

Tangier disease is also known as analphalipoproteinaemia or familial alpha lipoprotein deficiency. It is an autosomal recessive condition that results in the deficiency of apo A-I. The result is low levels of HDL and cholesterol with normal to high levels of triglycerides. Cholesterol accumulation results in enlarged orange-coloured tonsils, hepatosplenomegaly, polyneuropathy and corneal opacities. It is not associated with premature coronary disease.

Fish eye disease

Fish eye disease is a rare disorder from northern Sweden characterized by high VLDL, low HDL levels and triglyceride-rich LDL. Hypertriglyceridaemia and dense corneal opacities can occur, giving rise to visual impairment.

Abetalipoproteinaemia

Abetalipoproteinaemia is a rare condition that results in fat accumulation in the intestine due to failure of apo B-100 production. It results in neurological abnormalities, retinitis pigmentosa and acanthocytosis. Vitamin E injections may prevent the onset of some of the neurological abnormalities.

Secondary hyperlipidaemias

Secondary dyslipidaemias are relatively common, accounting for up to 20% of patients with hyperlipidaemia. Biochemically, there can be a mixed hyperlipidaemia, lone increase in serum cholesterol or triglyceride levels. The causes are listed in Table 7.16, and management is based upon identifying and treating the underlying disease before treatment of the raised lipid levels. Often, more than one cause is apparent.

SECTION 7.7 # Inborn errors of carbohydrate metabolism

Glucose is the main sugar utilized by the body. It is stored in liver and muscle as glycogen, a polymer structure with glycogenin holding together the numerous D-glucose molecules. In this form, glucose is osmotically inert and does not damage the cell that contains it. Dietary sugars are broken down in the gut and absorbed (fructose and galactose), these are then broken down further into more usable components such as glucose.

Glycogen storage disorders are a series of rare, usually autosomal recessive inherited enzyme defects resulting in the excessive accumulation of glycogen and tissue damage. These glycogen storage diseases are classified by the enzyme defect. They usually present in childhood with growth retardation, hepatosplenomegaly and hypoglycaemia. The glycogen storage diseases are often fatal, with the exception of McArdle's disease that presents in adults.

Disorders of fructose metabolism

Fructose is an important intermediary in glycolytic and gluconeogenesis pathways. Hereditary fructose intolerance is an autosomal recessive condition affecting 1 in 20 000 births. It causes vomiting, diarrhoea, abdominal pain and hypoglycaemia when fructose, sucrose or sorbitol is ingested. Symptoms manifest in early infancy or from the time of weaning onto a solid diet. Long-term organ damage can be avoided by an exclusion diet.

Essential or benign fructosuria is an autosomal recessive condition characterized by fructokinase deficiency. It occurs in 1 in 130 000. Fructose is found in urine, and patients used to be mistaken for type 2 diabetics until glucose detection was improved.

Fructose-1-phosphate aldolase deficiency results in the accumulation of fructose-1-phosphate causing hepatosplenomegaly, hypoglycaemia and renal tubular defects unless the condition is diagnosed and a fructose-free diet followed from birth.

Hepatosplenomegaly is also seen in fructose-1,6-diphosphatase deficiency which causes failure of gluconeogenesis. This is an extremely rare autosomal recessive inherited condition causing acidosis with starvation, or fatal infection in the first year of life.

Disorders of galactose metabolism

Dietary lactose is broken down into galactose by gut mucosal enzymes and is further metabolized to glucose or complexed with protein or lipid complexes (e.g. galactosylated lipids).

Galactokinase deficiency occurs in 1 in 100 000 live births. It results in galactosaemia, often with cataract formation in childhood or by the age of 40 years in heterozygotes.

An autosomal recessive deficiency of the enzyme galactose-1-phosphate uridyl transferase is more lethal and affects 1 in 62 000 live births. Unless treated with a galactose-free diet it can lead to accumulation of galactose-1-phosphate in the blood causing neonatal hypoglycaemia and acidosis. The disease leads to mental retardation, liver and proximal renal tubule damage, and cataract development. It is often fatal.

463

Uridine diphosphate 4-epimerase deficiency is a rare autosomal recessive inherited disorder that is usually of no clinical significance apart from galactosuria which may be mistaken for diabetes mellitus.

Disorders of mucopolysaccharide metabolism

As with simple sugar metabolism there are also inherited disorders of complex carbohydrate metabolism that result in the inability of exo glycosidases to remove individual carbohydrate groups from glycosaminoglycans or muco-polysaccharides. This leads to the accumulation of partially degraded glycosaminoglycans or carbohydrate polymers in organs such as the central nervous system, skeleton and connective tissue.

Mucopolysaccharidosis I

Hurler's syndrome (type IH) affects the skin, soft tissues and subcutaneous cartilage. Affected patients have a gargoyle-like appearance with a flattened nasal bridge, large tongue, hyperplastic gums and widely spaced poorly formed teeth. Corneal clouding also occurs. The facial appearance develops over time with physical and mental deterioration from a few months of age. Deposits in the meninges can lead to hydrocephalus, and deposits in the joints and soft tissues lead to stiffness and contractures. By 6–12 months of age the diagnosis is usually established and death occurs before 10 years of age.

Scheie disease (type IS) is a milder mutation of the iduronidase locus that causes Hurler's disease. Arthropathy and cardiac valvular disease occur, but this form of disease has a better prognosis.

Hurler–Scheie disease (type I/S) is of intermediate severity between IH and IS.

Mucopolysaccharidosis II

Mucopolysaccharidosis II is an X-linked condition with similar features to Hunter's syndrome. Corneal clouding is absent and it follows a slower course with death occurring in late childhood or teenage years.

Mucopolysaccharidosis III

There are four distinct biochemical subtypes of Sanfilippo disease, which are clinically identical. Accelerated growth and abundant coarse scalp hair in children with severe mental retardation and hyperkinetic behaviour is seen. Death usually occurs by 20 years of age.

Mucopolysaccharidosis IV

Morquio syndrome is not as severe as types I and II but affected individuals have severe skeletal deformities with growth virtually stopping from 6 years onwards. Although deformed and dwarfed, they may be mentally unaffected.

Mucopolysaccharidosis VI

Patients with Maroteaux–Lamy disease have a similar facial appearance to that of Hurler's disease (type IH) with hepatosplenomegaly, skeletal, corneal and cardiac changes.

Mucopolysaccharidosis VII

Individuals with β-glucuronidase deficiency have clinical features similar to Hurler's disease (type IH) but much less mucopolysacchariduria.

SECTION 7.8 Inborn errors of amino acid metabolism

Dietary protein provides us with amino acids, many of which are not synthesized by the body. Excess dietary amino acids are metabolized rather than stored. The amino group is removed and converted to urea or ammonia while the carbon skeleton is converted to metabolites such as acetyl coenzyme A and pyruvate. Defects can occur with enzyme pathways (urea cycle and carbon chain metabolism), or during the processing and transport of amino acids. Most of the inborn errors of amino acid metabolism are inherited as an autosomal recessive trait.

Aminoaciduria

Aminoaciduria can occur as a result of high circulating levels of amino acids (e.g. phenylketonuria) or with transport defects in the renal tubules. These transporter defects can be generalized (Fanconi syndrome), specific (cystinosis, Hartnup's) or occur due to secondary tubule damage (galactosaemia).

Fanconi's syndrome

Generalized aminoaciduria (Fanconi syndrome) can occur as a juvenile form starting at 6–9 months of age or as an adult form starting in the second to fourth decade. This syndrome can be caused by specific transporter problems or by nephrotoxins. The components of the Fanconi syndrome are low molecular weight proteinuria (including loss of immunoglobulins), tubular transport defects (for most amino acids, glucose, bicarbonate, potassium and urate), metabolic bone disease (osteomalacia, rickets due to urinary phosphate loss) and slow loss of glomerular function. Treatment is of the underlying disorder if possible and supplementation with vitamin D, potassium, sodium bicarbonate and phosphate.

Lowe's syndrome

Other causes of generalized transport problems include the X-linked Lowe's syndrome (oculocerebrorenal dystrophy) in which generalized aminoaciduria occurs with dwarfism, severe mental retardation, hypotonia, microphthalmos, congenital cataracts and glaucoma.

Cystinosis

Cystinosis is an autosomal recessive condition with abnormal cystine transport across the lysosomal membrane causing cystine accumulation and proximal renal tubule damage leading to Fanconi syndrome.

Hartnup's disease

In Hartnup's disease there is defective jejunal and renal tubular absorption of most neutral amino acids, but not of their peptides. This results in malabsorption or urinary losses of amino acids such as tryptophan which gives nicotinamide deficiency (pellagra). Isolated tryptophan malabsorption causes babies to excrete tryptophan, which oxidizes and turns their nappies blue (blue diaper syndrome).

Disorders of tyrosine metabolism

Tyrosine is important in the production of catecholamines, dopamine and some pigments in hair and skin. Tyrosinaemia type 1 (fumarylacetoacetate hydrolase deficiency) and type 2 (tyrosine aminotransferase deficiency) are severe conditions with mental retardation, kidney and liver damage. Type 2 is the milder; type 1 is usually fatal within the first year of life. Dietary modification, avoiding tyrosine and phenylalanine, along with liver transplantation and renal replacement therapy may improve survival.

Albinism occurs in 1 in 13 000 infants and is due to tyrosinase deficiency in melanocytes. Currently more than 10 subtypes have been identified. Clinical features are absent pigmentation in skin (pink-white skin), hair (whitish hair), iris (grey-blue eyes), fundi and the inner ear (this pigment is said to protect against noise trauma). Structural eye problems can be seen in some forms (e.g. oculocutaneous albinism) and with a bleeding tendency in Hermansky–Pudlak syndrome and a leukocyte killing defect in Chediak–Higashi syndrome.

Disorders of phenylalanine metabolism (phenylketonuria)

Phenylalanine metabolism defects are common. Phenylketonuria is an autosomal recessive condition due to phenylalanine-4-hydroxylase deficiency and has a frequency of 1 in 12 000 live births in a Western population. All newborn infants in the UK are tested for this by the Guthrie bacteria inhibition assay, using a heel prick blood sample taken on about the seventh day of life.

Phenylalanine is hydroxylated to form tyrosine, and defects in this pathway lead to excessive serum levels (20–60 times normal) that accumulate and cause impaired brain growth and lower neurotransmitter levels with fewer nerve cells. Microcephaly, mental retardation and epilepsy are common. If untreated, 1 in 20 adults with this condition develop neurological defects, usually a spastic paraparesis.

Treatment is with dietary protein restriction to keep phenylalanine levels low, without inhibiting normal growth and development. Low serum levels allow normal IQ development. It is not certain if tight control is required after the teenage years.

Disorders of urea metabolism

These include rare conditions such as carbamyl phosphate synthetase deficiency, ornithine transcarbamylase deficiency, arginosuccinic acid synthetase deficiency and arginosuccinic acid lyase deficiency. All cause poor feeding, lethargy and a hyperammonaemic coma, typically starting within 72 hours of commencing feeding after birth. Delayed presentations can occur with poor growth, epilepsy and neurological problems.

Disorders of carbon chain metabolism

Branched chain ketoaciduria occurs as an autosomal recessive defect in mitochondrial enzymes that metabolize leucine, isoleucine and valine. Several defects occur, all of which are rare. The incidence is 0.83 per 100 000 per year in Europe and 0.5 per 100 000 in the USA. Typically, infants are well at birth but feed poorly after 2–3 days, then become sleepy, comatose and apnoeic. This often leads to death. Hypoglycaemia, hyperammonaemia, mild metabolic acidosis and ketonuria occur. The urine has a sweet smell like maple syrup (maple syrup disease). If infants survive, neurological abnormalities and mental retardation are usual. Acute treatment is with a high-dextrose feed and an amino acid mixture excluding leucine, isoleucine and valine. In the long term, dietary exclusion of these amino acids to keep serum levels as low as possible is attempted.

Disorders of sulphur amino acid metabolism

A sulphur molecule is removed from methionine and added to serine to give cysteine. In homocystinuria problems with re-methylation of methionine occur due to autosomal recessive defects in several enzyme pathways. Methylene tetrahydrofolate reductase deficiency can present in early to late childhood with neurological problems including psychomotor retardation, epilepsy and a thrombotic tendency. Treatment with folinic acid, vitamin B_{12} (hydroxycobalamin), B_6 (pyridoxine) and methionine has been advocated.

Methionine synthetase deficiency presents with developmental delay and a megaloblastic anaemia in childhood. If diagnosis is delayed, it can present in late childhood with dementia, spasticity or cardiac defects. Treatment with high-dose vitamin B_{12} and folinic acid is advocated.

SECTION 7.9 Lysosomal storage diseases

Large molecules that are ingested by cells are degraded in subcellular organelles called lysosomes. These cellular vesicles contain acid hydrolases, a family of glycoprotein enzymes that have their protein component made in the endoplasmic reticulum. The oligosaccharide side chains added in the Golgi apparatus and the terminal mannose-6-phosphate residue mark them for packing into the lysosome.

In patients with inborn errors of lysosomal function, these specific enzymes are faulty, such that undegraded or partially degraded macromolecules accumulate inside the lysosome and damage the cell. Occasionally excretion of the degradation product or efflux from the lysosome is affected (cystinosis) and the macromolecules accumulate outside the lysosome. Any part of the formation or uptake into the lysosome can be affected, usually by an autosomal recessive defect. These diseases are classified by the product that accumulates, and increasingly by molecular characteristics of the enzyme or lysosomal membrane defects.

Cystinosis

Cystinosis is an autosomal recessive condition occurring in 1 in 200 000 live births. It occurs due to abnormal cystine transport across the lysosomal membrane leading to cystine accumulation in reticuloendothelial cells. In the proximal renal tubule, the damage leads to Fanconi syndrome. Poor feeding and failure to thrive are seen in the infantile form with death by 10 years of age due to renal failure and a proximal renal tubular acidosis. Hypothyroidism, retinopathy, photophobia and corneal cystine deposits are also seen. An intermediate form may present with renal impairment later, and the adult form is relatively benign. Altered vitamin metabolism can lead to rickets but responds to vitamin D replacement. Cystine-associated damage may be reduced by cysteamine therapy. Phosphocysteamine and cysteamine barbitrate are alternatives but ultimately dialysis or renal transplantation may be needed.

Gaucher's disease

Gaucher's disease occurs due to glucocerebrosidase deficiency. Glucocerebroside accumulation leads to hepatosplenomegaly, and large Gaucher's cells (glucocerebroside-containing reticuloendothelial histiocytes) are present in the bone marrow. The frequency of Gaucher's disease is highest in Ashkenazi Jews (1 in 3000 births), and presents in adults with insidious onset of thrombocytopenia, anaemia (due to hypersplenism), hepatosplenomegaly and characteristic skin pigmentation in exposed areas such as the forehead and hands. Patients may develop pathological fractures. In general, the lifespan is normal. The less common acute form in infancy or childhood has a worse outlook, often with neurological involvement.

Fabry's disease

Fabry's disease is an X-linked recessive condition characterized by α-galactosyl-lactosylceramide accumulation due to α-galactosidase deficiency. Affected males develop the full clinical syndrome, while females are usually asymptomatic or mildly affected carriers. Angiokeratomas (bright red to blue-black telangiectasia) develop on the skin in childhood or around puberty. Accumulation of the undigested compound in endothelial and smooth muscle cells in blood vessels leads to vascular disease of the liver, kidney, heart and brain. Painful crises are often the most debilitating symptom. Corneal opacities, cataracts and a peripheral neuropathy are also common. Affected men die in their 40s or 50s with renal failure, heart or cerebrovascular disease. α-Galactosidase enzyme replacement therapy may benefit some patients.

Niemann–Pick disease

Niemann–Pick disease is due to sphingomyelinase deficiency. It results in lipid (sphingomyelin) accumulation within reticuloendothelial macrophages of the liver, spleen, bone marrow and lymph nodes. It presents by 6 months of age with hepatosplenomegaly, lymphadenopathy and mental retardation. On examining the fundi, half of cases show a cherry red spot in the macula, and typical foam cells or sea-blue histiocytes are seen on histological examination. Death usually occurs by 2 years.

Tay–Sachs and Sandhoff's disease

The GM$_2$ gangliosidoses include Tay–Sachs and Sandhoff's disease. The defect is a deficiency of one or both isoenzymes of hexosaminidase (A and B). Isolated hexosaminidase A deficiency leads to Tay–Sachs disease, an autosomal recessive condition affecting 1 in 2000 Ashkenazi Jews, characterized by GM$_2$ ganglioside accumulation in the central and peripheral nervous system. Deficiency of both isoenzymes (A and B) is Sandhoff's disease, characterized by accumulation of GM$_1$ gangliosides. Both diseases have a juvenile and an adult form. The juvenile form usually leads to death by 10 years of age, whilst the adult form manifests with cerebellar dysarthria and ataxia.

In Tay–Sachs disease, neuronal accumulation of GM$_2$ ganglioside causes progressive generalized motor weakness from 6 months of age. By 18 months deafness, blindness, psychomotor regression and epilepsy occur. A cherry red spot on the macula, a large head and a typical startle reaction to sudden noise are often seen early on in the disease. Death usually occurs by 3 years of age with multiple fits and a vegetative state with decerebrate rigidity.

Amyloidosis

Amyloidosis results from the extracellular accumulation of insoluble, fibrous amyloid protein. It often occurs as a complication of disease.

Epidemiology

The incidence of amyloidosis has been reported to be 1.2 per 100 000 per year.[1] The epidemiology varies with the underlying disease.

Pathology

There are numerous precursors of amyloid that form the basis of classification of this disease, however they all share an identical secondary structure—a β-pleated sheet. Localized amyloidosis without evidence of systemic involvement is associated with ageing and normally occurs in the brain, heart, prostate, seminal vesicles and joints. Systemic amyloidosis has neoplastic, inflammatory or genetic origins.

AA amyloidosis

Serum amyloid A (AA) is produced as an acute phase reactant, and AA amyloidosis is associated with chronic inflammation, chronic infection and malignancy. It is seen in up to 10% of patients with rheumatoid disease, systemic lupus erythematosus and Crohn's disease (but not ulcerative colitis). Worldwide, tuberculosis and leprosy are also common underlying causes. It can also occur in association with Hodgkin's disease and renal cell carcinoma.

AL amyloidosis

Immunocyte-related or AL amyloidosis is caused by immunoglobulin light chain accumulation in B-cell lymphoproliferative disorders such as myeloma, non-Hodgkin's lymphomas, Waldenström's macroglobulinaemia and 'benign' monoclonal gammopathy.

Dialysis-associated amyloidosis

Amyloidosis can be a cause of renal impairment, and is also associated with the treatment in patients receiving dialysis. β$_2$-Microglobulin (amyloid protein) deposition is associated with chronic haemodialysis, usually after 5 years, and less frequently with peritoneal dialysis.

Cerebral amyloidosis

Prion diseases such as Creutzfeldt–Jakob disease and kuru are associated with amyloid deposition in the brain, although the significance is uncertain. In Alzheimer's disease, a 4 kD peptide, B-amyloid (A4 protein), is present in cerebral vessel walls and mature white matter plaques. The amyloid precursor protein, APP or Pro A4, is coded on chromosome 21, and in Down's syndrome (trisomy 21) early dementia occurs (at the age of 40).

Hereditary amyloidosis

Hereditary systemic amyloidosis includes familial amyloid polyneuropathy, an autosomal dominant condition characterized by defects of prealbumin or transthyretin metabolism. Familial Mediterranean fever is an autosomal recessive condition seen in non-Ashkenazi Jews, Armenians, Anatolian Turks and Levantine Arabs. A high rate of systemic AA amyloidosis is associated with recurrent episodes of fever, abdominal pain, pleurisy and arthritis.

Clinical features

Amyloidosis is a multisystem disorder. The history is usually a combination of fatigue, weight loss, easy bruising, weight loss, breathlessness, peripheral oedema and sensory symptoms (carpal tunnel syndrome). Amyloidosis can also present with renal impairment, cardiac failure (restrictive cardiomyopathy) and sensory glove and stocking polyneuropathy. Autonomic disturbances can lead to symptoms of postural hypotension and change in bowel habit.

On examination, there may be evidence of macroglossia, subcutaneous amyloid deposits and nail dystrophy. The liver or spleen may be enlarged.

In addition there may be symptoms and signs of the underlying disease process that leads to amyloidosis.

Initial investigations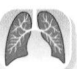

Full blood count
An anaemia may be present due to myeloma. The platelet count may be elevated from splenic dysfunction.

Markers of inflammation
The erythrocyte sedimentation rate (ESR) may be elevated as a non-specific indicator of inflammation.

Urea and electrolytes
The creatinine may be raised with nephropathy (p. 699).

Serum electrophoresis
Electrophoresis should be performed to screen for monoclonal bands, to identify diseases associated with AL amyloidosis.

Urinalysis
Proteinuria occurs with nephrotic syndrome. Immunoglobulin light chains may be evident with plasma cell myeloma.

Electrocardiogram
Low amplitude voltages and heart block can occur with cardiac amyloidosis.

Further investigations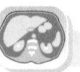

Tissue diagnosis
A tissue biopsy is required to obtain histological confirmation of the diagnosis. Ideally this should be a biopsy of the affected organ. Less invasive alternatives include subcutaneous fat biopsies and rectal biopsies.

Amyloid stains pink with haematoxylin and eosin, and red with Congo red dye. Typically, it demonstrates a green birefringence/fluorescence with polarized light. Immunohistochemical staining can determine the composition of the fibrils, and radio-labelled serum amyloid P component (SAP) studies can also identify the deposits.

Initial management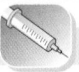

Treatment of the underlying condition
An important aspect is to identify and treat the underlying condition that has led to amyloidosis.

Supportive measures
The mainstay of management is supportive treatment, with measures such as the use of specialized stockings for postural hypotension, diuretics for heart failure and dialysis for renal failure.

Medical management

Chemotherapy
The use of melphalan has been associated with improved survival in patients with AL amyloidosis. Other chemotherapeutic agents include vincristine, doxorubicin and dexamethasone.

Surgical management

Organ transplantation
Cardiac transplantation and chemotherapy have been used selectively in patients with end-stage cardiac amyloidosis. Liver transplantation is potentially curative in patients with familial amyloidotic polyneuropathy: circulating levels of mutant transthyretin have been known to disappear after transplantation, as it is exclusively produced by hepatocytes.

Prognosis

The prognosis depends on the subtype of amyloid, the underlying disease process and the organs involved. The worst prognosis is AL amyloidosis, with an untreated survival of approximately 2 years.

i FURTHER INFORMATION

Khan MF, Falk RH. Amyloidosis. Postgraduate Medical Journal 2001; 77: 686–693.

REFERENCE

(1) *Khan MF, Falk RH. Amyloidosis. Postgraduate Medical Journal 2001; 77: 686–693.*

SECTION 7.11 | Porphyria

Porphyrin is a component of haem, and the porphyrias are a group of disorders of specific enzymes in the haem biosynthetic pathway. Nine enzymes are involved in the conversion of glycine and succinyl CoA to haem, and abnormalities may cause the accumulation and increased excretion of haem precursors.

Clinically, porphyrias are classified into acute and non-acute. The acute porphyrias present with severe neuro-psychiatric problems due to excess porphyrin precursors (δ-amino-laevulinic acid and porphobilinogen) while the non-acute porphyrias accumulate porphyrins (but not their precursors) and present with cutaneous photo-sensitivity alone.

There is marked geographical variation. The prevalence of acute intermittent porphyria and porphyria cutanea tarda (Fig. 7.12) is highest in Scotland at 2 per 100 000. The prevalence of variegate porphyria is highest in South African whites at 100 per 100 000.

Acute porphyrias

Acute intermittent porphyria

Epidemiology

Acute intermittent porphyria is the most common and severe of the acute porphyrias. The onset is typically between puberty and 30 years of age. The female prepon-derance (5:1 ratio) may be related to oestrogen and the use of the combined oral contraceptive pill.

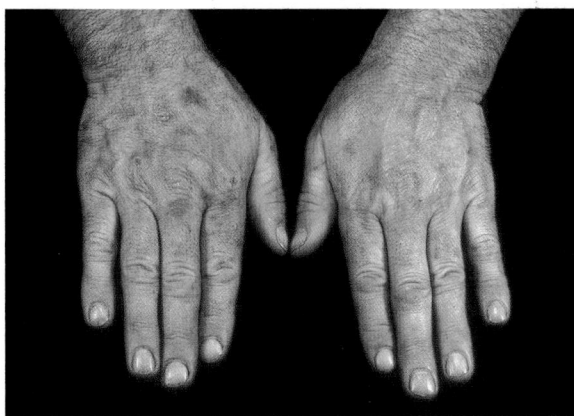

Fig. 7.12 Skin lesions of porphyria cutanea tarda.

Pathology

Acute intermittent porphyria is an autosomal dominant condition, due to porphobilinogen deaminase deficiency. Known precipitants of an acute attack include barbiturates, fasting or reduced calorie intake, infection and alcohol. Pregnancy and the week prior to menstruation are also associated with an increased risk of attacks that become less frequent after the menopause.

Clinical features

Gastrointestinal symptoms are present in 95% with diffuse abdominal pain, anorexia, vomiting and constipation (probably related to the haem precursors causing autonomic dysfunction). In 70%, hypertension, tachycardia, sweating and pallor occur. A peripheral polyneuropathy is also seen in up to 70%, and is more often motor than sensory. Careful monitoring is required as it may progress to compromise respiratory function. Neuropsychiatric symptoms including depression, anxiety and frank psychosis with hallucinations and a schizophrenia-like illness are seen in 50%, and these may persist between acute episodes.

Initial investigations

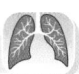

Urinary protoporphyrins
Urine that turns a red-brown colour on standing (Fig. 7.13) is typical due to excessive porphobilinogen. Porphobilinogen

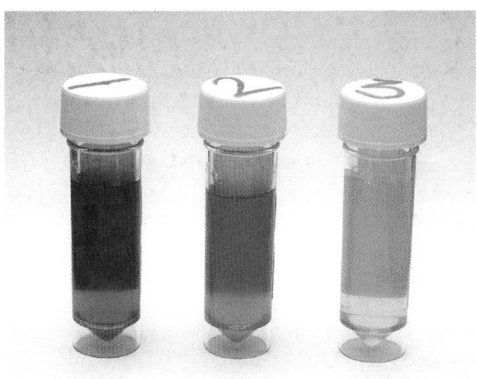

Fig. 7.13 Urine changes in acute intermittent porphyria. The urine has changed to a red-brown colour on standing for 8 hours. Bottle 3, immediate sample; bottle 2 after 4 hours; bottle 1 after 8 hours. Courtesy of Dr Christine Burness, Royal Hallamshire Hospital, Sheffield, UK.

469

can be detected by adding Ehrlich's aldehyde reagent, when the urine turns red-pink.

Erythrocyte PBG deaminase and ALA synthetase
Measuring erythrocyte porphobilinogen deaminase and δ-amino-laevulinic acid synthetase is also extremely sensitive in between attacks.

Initial management

Analgesia
Initial treatment is supportive and includes adequate pain relief. Opioids may be required.

Carbohydrate intake
Increased carbohydrate intake and intravenous dextrose supplementation is administered.

Patient education
Educating patients and the medical staff looking after them to avoid known precipitating factors is important to avoid further episodes.

Medical management

Beta-blocker
Sympathetic overactivity can be controlled with propranolol if required.

Haem arginate
Intravenous haem supplements may reduce porphyrin precursor excretion and lead to a faster recovery.

Luteinizing hormone releasing hormone
Luteinizing hormone releasing hormone analogues may help if there is a menstrual-related problem.

Prognosis

Acute gastrointestinal symptoms may resolve over hours, and the acute attack often resolves over several days.

Variegate porphyria

Variegate porphyria is an autosomal dominant condition due to deficiency of protoporphyrin oxidase. It presents with attacks identical to those seen with acute intermittent porphyria, and the management of acute episodes is the same. Although there is amino-laevulinic acid and porphobilinogen deaminase excess, there is also porphyrin overproduction resulting in cutaneous photosensitivity. The bullous rash is due to activation of porphyrins deposited in the skin and is treated with barrier creams.

Hereditary coproporphyria

An autosomal dominant condition with coproporphyria oxidase deficiency, hereditary coproporphyria is clinically similar to variegate porphyria in signs, symptoms and treatment.

Non-acute porphyrias

Porphyria cutanea tarda

Porphyria cutanea tarda can be inherited as an autosomal dominant condition with hepatic uroporphyrinogen decarboxylase deficiency (or dysfunction) leading to increased urinary uroporphyrin and a bullous skin eruption on exposure to sunlight that scars as it heals. Pruritus, increased skin fragility, hyperpigmentation and hirsutism can also occur. The most common precipitant is alcohol but oestrogenic steroids and hexachlorobenzene (fungicide) have also been implicated.

Clinical and biochemical evidence of liver disease is often present. Biochemically, increased urinary uroporphyrin and abnormal liver function tests are usual. Serum iron and transferrin levels are often elevated.

Treatment is to avoid the offending agent, in particular alcohol, while venesection may help iron overload. A rising urinary uroporphyrin level suggests that further venesection is required to keep the haemoglobin below 12 g/dL. Chloroquine has also been used to promote urinary uroporphyrin excretion.

Congenital porphyria

Congenital porphyria is a rare autosomal recessive condition due to a defect of uroporphyrinogen co-synthetase. It is also known as Gunther's disease or erythropoietic porphyria. Clinical features include severe photosensitive skin eruptions with vesicles and bullae forming ulcers that leave disfiguring scars as they heal. Blindness can occur due to lenticular scarring. Curved dystrophic nails with a claw-shaped scarred hand and brownish discolouration of the teeth (erythrodontia) are also seen. Ineffective erythropoiesis may lead to anaemia. Treatment with chloroquine may help, as can bone marrow transplantation in some cases.

Erythropoietic protoporphyria

Erythropoietic protoporphyria is an autosomal dominant condition resulting in reduced ferrochelatase activity in the peripheral blood, liver, bone marrow and skin.

It is more common than congenital porphyria and gives a red, painful photosensitive rash. It is diagnosed by fluorescence of peripheral red blood cells and increased protoporphyrin levels in the red blood cell and faeces.

It is treated with oral β-carotene supplementation, which gives protection against the sun. A common side effect is a yellow tint to the skin (carotenaemia) after prolonged treatment. This can be reduced with canth xanthin.

Diseases of the bones and joints

8

Andrew Östör, Nick Carrington, Brian Hazleman, Nick Harris

SECTION 8.1   Introduction

Disorder of the musculoskeletal system, in one form or another, is part of the human experience whether it be soft tissue disease, arthritis or bony fracture. The economic impact this has on society is enormous with treatment and lost productivity accounting for up to 2% of the gross national product. As a result it is paramount that the clinician be familiar with the fundamentals of assessing and managing this varied group of conditions. Although rheumatology and orthopaedics are often seen as separate disciplines, the nexus between them is crucial, symbiotic and synergistic. The following chapter aims to give a broad overview of the diseases of bones and joints with an emphasis on the integration of medicine and surgery where appropriate.

Applied basic sciences of the musculoskeletal system

Anatomy

The synovial joint is a complex structure composed of several specialized tissues (Fig. 8.1). The non-weight-bearing area of the joint cavity is lined by a synovial membrane comprised of type A synoviocytes (macrophage-like cells), type B synoviocytes (fibroblast-like cells), a matrix of proteoglycans and glycosaminoglycans, and a vascular connective tissue stroma. A viscous synovial fluid containing a high concentration of hyaluronic acid is produced by the membrane and acts as a lubricant and nourishing agent.

Articular cartilage covers the surface of subchondral bone and consists of chondrocytes resting in a matrix of collagen, proteoglycans and other proteins. Articular cartilage is very well hydrated, with water making up 70% of its weight. Chondrocytes, comprising 5–10% of normal articular cartilage by volume, synthesize collagen and proteoglycans which are pivotal in maintaining the biomechanical properties of the joint. Type II collagen is predominant in articular cartilage and the triple helical structure provides tensile strength. Proteoglycans, consisting of a polypeptide core with glycosaminoglycan side-chains, are responsible for water trapping and provide the compressibility and malleability of cartilage. Synovial fluid is paramount in providing nutrients to this avascular structure which also lacks lymphatics. Turnover of collagen is tightly controlled; however, degeneration of cartilage results from excessive loading, disuse and inflammation.

Subchondral bone is predominantly comprised of type I collagen which provides tensile and compressive strength. The remainder of the bone matrix is comprised of proteoglycans, glycoproteins, glycosaminoglycans (hyaluronic acid) and other proteins. The two major cell types found in bone are osteoclasts and osteoblasts. Compressive force leads to bone remodelling to optimize load-bearing. The remodelling process is also important for calcium, phosphate and magnesium homeostasis.

Immunology

A deeper understanding of the immunology of inflammatory arthritis has grown immensely over the last two decades. Using rheumatoid arthritis as an example, destruction of cartilage and bone is mediated by inflammatory cells which elaborate cytokines. In brief, the principal cells infiltrating the synovial membrane are macrophages, monocytes, B

473

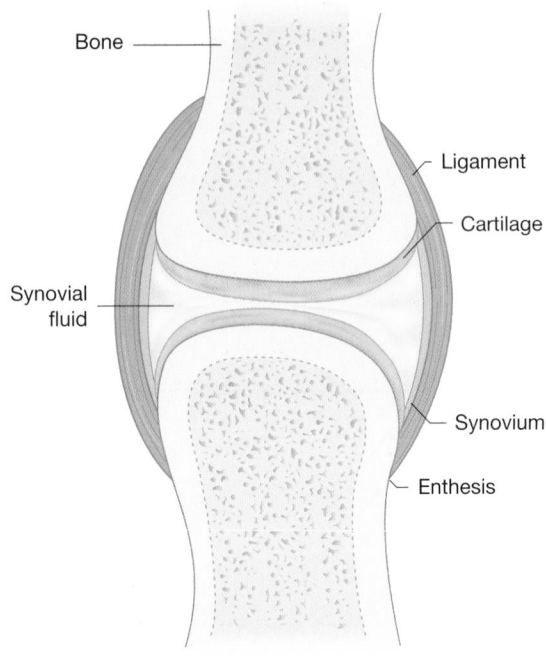

Fig. 8.1 A normal synovial joint.

and T lymphocytes (especially CD4+ T cells), plasma cells and dendritic cells. The predominant cytokines involved in the inflammation are tumour necrosis factor-α (TNF-α), interleukin-1 (IL-1) and IL-6; however, many others are involved including IL-12, IL-15, IL-18 and interferon-γ (INF-γ).

Anti-inflammatory cytokines are also present in the diseased joint such as IL-4, IL-10, IL-13 and transforming growth factor-β as well as neutralizing factors such as TNF-α receptors and IL-1 receptor antagonist (IL-1 ra). A T helper type 1 cell (Th1) cytokine profile (pro-inflammatory in autoimmunity) predominates over the T helper 2 (Th2) type (anti-inflammatory). In addition, destructive enzymes are produced during the inflammatory response such as collagenases, stromelysins and gelatinases (the matrix metalloproteinases). Neovascularization also plays a role in promoting ongoing inflammation.

RECENT ADVANCES

Current data suggest that the pathogenesis of rheumatoid disease is an imbalance of pro-inflammatory over anti-inflammatory cytokines. This realization has spurred interest in the development of cytokine blocking agents as therapeutic tools.

Symptoms of bone and joint disease

The medical history is pivotal and its role cannot be overemphasized. The chance of obtaining the correct diagnosis is greatly improved if patients are allowed time to explain their symptoms in their own words. The history commences with an exploration of the patient's presenting complaint. Pain is the cardinal symptom with varying degrees of stiffness, swelling, weakness, crepitus, clicking and loss of function. Certain aspects of the past social, family, sporting, occupational, drug, allergy and treatment history are pertinent. Demographic information, including the age, sex and race of a patient, also has diagnostic significance.

It is during the history that the doctor–patient relationship develops, and recognition of both verbal and nonverbal cues is important. The history concludes with an enquiry into the expectations of patients regarding the diagnosis and treatment and their attitude to their illness.

Pain

Pain is the cardinal symptom in musculoskeletal medicine and may arise from multiple sources. Certain patients have difficulty characterizing their symptoms and use terms such as ache, soreness, burning or discomfort. Many conditions are localized and an appropriate starting point is to ask the patient exactly where the pain is. Pain severity may be volunteered by the patient but is heavily reliant on psychological factors. The radiation of pain may give important diagnostic clues.

When and what the patient was doing at the time the pain started, what has happened subsequently and whether the pain is constant or remitting and relapsing allows the clinician to narrow the diagnostic possibilities. Inflammatory pain often develops insidiously over weeks to months whereas pain usually develops immediately following sporting injury. Symptoms may fluctuate depending upon posture, movement, activity, rest and time of the day. Resting an affected limb usually ameliorates discomfort in degenerative joint disease and ligamentous and tendinous injuries.

Stiffness

A subjective complaint of prolonged stiffness is the hallmark of inflammatory disease such as rheumatoid arthritis. The stiffness is usually worse in the morning and after rest (gelling phenomenon) and improves with activity. Stiffness exacerbated by movement and ameliorated by inactivity suggests degenerative disease such as osteoarthritis. Associated swelling of an affected area is a highly significant finding as part of the inflammatory response, however this may be quite subjective. Patients may describe weakness of an affected area that may be constant or present only when performing particular tasks. It is important to ascertain whether the weakness is due to pain or to structural damage, this being apparent on examination.

Clicks

Clicks are produced when a soft tissue moves over a bony prominence and may be due to inflammation, instability, a previous tear or scarring of soft tissues. It may also arise from soft tissues within the joint, such as in meniscal damage of the knee and from changes in bony contour following a fracture. The grating of irregular surfaces may produce crepitus, which is frequently heard, particularly in arthritides. Clicks and crepitus in the absence of other symptoms are of little consequence.

Triggering

A feature of tendon pathology is triggering, which is most commonly due to tendon scarring. It manifests as locking, usually of the digits, which may be overcome by effort or by passively moving the joint.

Colour changes

Colour change such as erythema is a significant feature of inflammatory disease and may be diagnostic, such as in Raynaud's phenomenon.

Other aspects of the history

The World Health Organization has developed an international classification for the terms disease, impairment, disability and handicap, which are the main consequences of musculoskeletal disease. Disease or disorder is the medical diagnosis from which the patient suffers. Impairment is the manifestation of disease or more simply the symptoms and signs that develop. Disability is the functional limitation imposed by the impairment. Handicap is the impact the disability has on the patient functioning in society and encompasses the effect on interpersonal relationships. Severe disability, however, may not necessarily cause equally profound handicap; for example, many public amenities have wheelchair access.

Patients may describe difficulties with personal hygiene, ambulation, performance of household chores and sexual function. The impact of disease on a patient's work commitments and responsibilities may be dire.

Attitudes, expectations and responses to illness may vary enormously between patients. Pride or embarrassment may limit patients volunteering information, therefore delicate direct questioning is required. An understanding of the effect of disease on marriage is crucial as support supplied by a spouse may be invaluable.

Systems review

Various systemic symptoms are common to diverse musculoskeletal diseases such as fatigue, lethargy and malaise. Others are more sinister such as fever, anorexia and loss of weight. Involvement of a specific organ system, such as dermatological, gastrointestinal, ophthalmological or mucous membrane, warrants further investigation.

Family history

Family history of rheumatic disease is important with the focus placed on the possibility of hereditary conditions leading to illness such as HLA-B27 associated spondyloarthropathies, gout, psoriasis and hypermobility. The true hereditary disorders of connective tissue such as Marfan's and Ehlers–Danlos syndromes and osteogenesis imperfecta are generally diagnosed in infancy or childhood. However, patients may occasionally display milder phenotypes and present later in life.

Occupational history

Musculoskeletal disease accounts for a significant amount of sick leave from work. The economic burden for the community is immense. Certain types of labour may lead to chronic low-grade trauma resulting in occupational repetitive strain injuries. Ergonomic assessment of the work area may be required to assess contributing factors to soft tissue injury.

A sporting history is important as connective tissues are prone to damage during these pursuits. A review of the frequency, intensity and duration of participation in sporting endeavour will aid diagnosis and help identify precipitating and perpetuating causes. Truly hypermobile patients or those at the upper end of normality are frequently selected for dance schools and gymnastics and are predisposed to injury.

Medication history

Certain drugs have been implicated in the development of musculoskeletal disorders. Enquiry regarding the use of glucocorticoids, fluoroquinolone antibiotics and anabolic steroids may shed light on an underlying cause for dysfunction or fracture.

Past and present treatment

Various treatments are available to ease musculoskeletal disease. Inquiry should be made into which therapies have been utilized, both prescription and over the counter, including doses, efficacy, side effects and possible reasons for discontinuation. Physical therapies including exercise, splints, mobility aids and orthosis as well as any surgical intervention require documentation. Treatment administered by paramedical health-care workers such as chiropractors, osteopaths, myotherapists, naturopaths and alternative therapies may alter the clinical expression of disease and influence patient expectation.

Past medical history

Associated medical conditions that may complicate the disease or the management of musculoskeletal disorders include chronic suppurative disease, peptic ulcer disease, bronchospasm and medication allergy. Patients frequently believe they have an allergy to aspirin or aspirin-like compounds; however, often no clear history of an allergic reaction is found with patients describing rather well-known side effects of the medication.

Examination of the locomotor system

The examination of the musculoskeletal system stems directly from the information obtained during the history. The examination aids in confirming a diagnosis and provides information regarding disease activity, functional capacity, asymptomatic pathology and coexistent disease. In addition the examination gives meaning to the patient's symptoms. A sound knowledge of the anatomy is essential, especially for localized disease. Features suggestive of

Applied basic sciences of the musculoskeletal system

Symptoms of bone and joint disease

Examination of the locomotor system

475

systemic disease warrant more extensive examination. The diagnosis is rarely reliant solely on the examination findings.

A fundamental rule in examination is to expose the patient adequately. The examination should occur in a warm, well-lit, private area with a chaperone if required. Comparing and contrasting signs on one side with the contralateral side is fundamental.

The musculoskeletal examination follows the sequence: look (inspection), feel (palpation), move (active, passive, resisted), measure (where appropriate) and functional assessment. Special tests and a general and/or neurological examination are required depending upon the disease process. It should be noted that strict adherence to the above protocol is not necessary in all situations. The examination, both consciously and subconsciously, commences at the beginning of the review when the patient rises from the waiting room chair and walks into the doctor's office. Vital information may be gleaned by observation at this early stage and whilst taking the history.

Inspection

General features of the examination include inspection of body habitus, posture, mobility and gait. Specific features include asymmetry, muscle wasting, swelling (localized or diffuse) and structural abnormality including malalignment and deformity. Further aspects include discolouration, noting particularly any pallor, erythema, mottling, cyanosis or bruising. Note should be made of any nodulosis, nail changes, rashes, excess adipose tissue and features of a peripheral neuropathy or endocrinopathy.

Palpation

Palpation should be prefaced by enquiry into any tender areas. Tenderness is a significant feature and may be localized or diffuse. When it is localized, a search for the site of maximal tenderness may identify the involved anatomical structure. Care should be employed as certain conditions cause exquisite tenderness.

Temperature change is of paramount importance being suggestive of inflammation. Infection in this case requires exclusion forthwith. Swelling may be soft tissue or bony in consistency. Frequently crepitus is easier to palpate than to hear. An increase or decrease in moisture of a limb may indicate neurovascular compromise, for example in complex regional pain syndromes. Deeper palpation may detect muscle knots, spasm, guarding and tenderness. Peripheral pulses should be documented.

Movement

Three specific types of movements are assessed: active, passive and resisted. Muscle strength can be quantified using Medical Research Council (MRC) guidelines (Table 8.1).

Active movement testing

This is performed by asking the patient to move the affected area through its full range of movement without examiner intervention. This assesses the integrity of

Table 8.1	Medical Research Council grades of muscle power
Grade	**Definition**
0	No movement
1	Visible or palpable flicker of contraction
2	Active movement with gravity eliminated
3	Active movement against gravity
4	Active movement against gravity and resistance but which is weaker than normal
5	Normal power

muscles, tendons, ligaments and bones. Quality as well as the quantity of movement may also be assessed. Information regarding flexibility, mobility and strength is gathered by observation of the rhythm, symmetry and rate of movement.

Passive movement testing

Passive movement is assessed by asking the patient to relax and allow the examiner to move the affected limb without patient effort. Some patients however find it quite difficult to relax. Passive movement assesses ligaments, joint capsule, fascia and bursae, nerve roots and dura mater. Passive movement also gives information regarding the integrity of muscles and tendons.

Resisted movement testing

Isometric (same length) contraction of muscle is assessed with resisted movement. The purpose of this is to isolate the pathology to a musculotendinous unit. The affected limb is placed in a neutral position and the patient is instructed to contract the muscle against resistance. Weakness without pain implies neurological deficit; weakness with pain implies musculotendinous inflammation or degeneration. Interpretation may be difficult when weakness is due to pain without inherent weakness, for example in polymyalgia rheumatica.

Goniometry

In practice, 'eyeball' estimation is usually sufficient for assessment of range of movement of a joint; however, formal measurement is possible with a goniometer.

Neurological examination

A thorough neurological examination may be required depending upon the history and musculoskeletal examination findings. The sequence of neurological examination commences with tone followed by power, coordination, reflexes and sensation. Light touch and pinprick are used to assess sensation.

Special tests

Many conditions display features that are detected by special tests. These will be covered in detail in the individual sections.

Functional assessment

This is the most important part of the physical examination and is actually being appraised throughout the interview. Overall function is assessed as the patient rises from the waiting room chair and walks into the office. Subtle deficiencies may be apparent when an attempt is made to undress or to lie on the examination couch. Performance of specific tasks such as removing glasses or reaching for a wallet assesses upper limb function. Manual dexterity may be assessed by attempts to do up buttons and write. Formal assessment by an occupational therapist is frequently necessary and enlightening.

GALS (gait, arms, legs, spine)

The GALS assessment, developed in the UK, is a screening system for significant musculoskeletal disease. The usefulness lies in its application to any patient who presents with a medical condition. Clinicians tend to be very well versed in examination of the cardiovascular, respiratory and abdominal examination and to lesser extent the neurological system; however, the rheumatologic/orthopaedic examination has been largely ignored. GALS is not universally accepted but is recommended as a screening tool (Table 8.2).

Applied basic sciences of the musculoskeletal system

Symptoms of bone and joint disease

Examination of the locomotor system

Table 8.2	Main features of the GALS screening musculoskeletal examination*
Activity	**Observation**
Gait	Symmetry and smoothness of movement Normal stride length Ability to turn normally
Spine (standing)	
Inspection from behind	Scoliosis Symmetrical muscle bulk Level iliac crests No popliteal swelling Normal hindfoot alignment
Trigger point tenderness	Pressure over mid supraspinatus
Inspection from the side	Kyphosis Normal flexion ('touch your toes')
Inspection from in front	Normal cervical lateral flexion ('touch your ear on your shoulder')
Arms (sitting on couch)	
Hands	Wrist/finger swelling/deformity Squeeze across 2nd to 5th metacarpals (tenderness indicates synovitis of metacarpophalangeal joints) Turn hands over (inspect for muscle wasting, assess normal pronation/supination of forearm)
Grip strength	Power grip ('make a tight fist') Precision grip ('put fingers on thumb')
Elbows	Full extension ('arms out straight')
Shoulders	Abduction and external rotation of the shoulders ('hands behind your head')
Legs (lying on couch)	
Knees	Knee swelling/deformity Quadriceps muscle bulk Check for knee effusion Crepitus during passive knee flexion
Hips	Check internal rotation of hips
Feet	Squeeze across metatarsals (tenderness indicates synovitis of metatarsophalangeal joints) Check for callouses

* From Doherty M, Dacre J, Dieppe P, Snaith M. The 'GALS' locomotor screen. Annals of the Rheumatic Diseases 1992; 51: 1165–1169.

SECTION 8.2 | Investigations of the locomotor system

Laboratory investigation is crucial in defining musculo-skeletal disorder. This is especially important in connective tissue disease and other inflammatory arthritides. As many of these conditions have systemic features, blood test changes are frequent and are imperative to monitor disease progress and medication toxicity.

Blood tests

Full blood count

Inflammatory disorder may lead to anaemia of chronic disease, leukopenia or leukocytosis in the case of infection. Thrombocytosis occurs during an acute phase response; however, systemic lupus erythematosus (SLE) is associated with thrombocytopenia.

Markers of inflammation

The erythrocyte sedimentation rate (ESR) and C-reactive protein (CRP) are very useful as general markers of inflammation but are non-specific.

Serum uric acid

Uric acid level estimation is helpful in suspected cases of gout. The higher the value the greater the risk of an acute attack of uric acid disease; however, this may occur with a normal or even low serum uric acid level.

Bone profile

Calcium, phosphate and alkaline phosphatase levels are important to aid in the diagnosis of several conditions including secondary osteoporosis, Paget's disease and metabolic bone disease.

Autoimmune studies

Rheumatoid factors are immunoglobulins directed against the Fc portion of immunoglobulin G (IgG). IgM rheumatoid factor is the predominant type. Rheumatoid factors are most commonly detected by latex agglutination. In this test, latex particles coated with IgG are agglutinated by addition of rheumatoid factors from the patient's serum.

Anti-nuclear antibodies (ANAs) are frequently elevated in connective tissue disease and are detected by immuno-fluorescence. Test serum is incubated with tissue to allow fixation of antibodies; unfixed antibodies are washed away and the specimen is then stained with a fluorescent antibody to human globulin which binds to any fixed antibody. Ultraviolet microscopy is then used to identify the antibodies. Various staining patterns are described (peripheral, speckled, homogenous, centromere, nucleolar). However, these are less useful than extractable nuclear antigen antibodies, which are subclasses of ANAs. Anti-double-stranded antibodies are specific for SLE and are detected by enzyme-linked immunosorbent assay (ELISA). The various autoantibodies are described in the relevant sections.

Anti-neutrophil cytoplasmic antibodies are specific for vasculitis and are described in the relevant section of the text.

Diagnostic imaging

Plain radiology

Radiology of the musculoskeletal system may be considered an extension of the examination. X-rays of the involved areas may be invaluable in helping to define the aetiology of the symptoms as different arthritides often display characteristic changes. Each of these will be detailed in the individual sections. X-rays are best for bony changes. X-rays do not display soft tissue disease, therefore other radiological modalities such as ultrasound, computed tomography (CT) or magnetic resonance imaging (MRI) are required for their imaging.

Ultrasound

Ultrasound examination is an excellent modality for demonstrating predominantly soft tissue disease (i.e. muscles, tendons, ligaments, bursae). It has also been found to be sensitive in detecting early joint changes in inflammatory arthritis. Ultrasound is dependent, however, upon the expertise of the operator.

CT

With the advent of MRI and ultrasound, CT has a limited role in musculoskeletal disorders. It is most beneficial at demonstrating changes in the spine including the intervertebral discs and spinal cord.

MRI

MRI is the most sensitive and specific imaging modality used to demonstrate changes in the joints and soft tissues. Image enhancement with gadolinium-DPTA allows early detection of inflammatory changes. MRI is predominantly used to image the spine, large joints and soft tissues.

Bone scintigraphy

Bone scanning with radionucleotide-labelled blood cells is helpful in demonstrating areas of inflammation. Although non-specific, changes may help diagnose disease when the history and examination are unclear.

SECTION 8.3 Diagnostic procedures

Joint aspiration

Synovial fluid examination is invaluable in defining inflammatory arthritis and helps differentiate infection, rheumatoid and crystal disease. This section focuses on aspiration of the knee, the joint that is most commonly aspirated.

Indications

Aspiration is indicated whenever a patient presents with a painful swollen knee joint. Synovial fluid obtained can then be sent for Gram stain and culture as well as for white cell count and crystal analysis in order to differentiate infection from other causes of joint disease.

Patient preparation

Knee aspiration can be done as an outpatient procedure. The patient sits comfortably with the knee slightly flexed. Careful preparation with antiseptic solution is required.

Procedure

With strict aseptic precautions, a 10 mL syringe and an 18–21 gauge needle can be introduced into the knee joint via a lateral or medial approach. The landmark is the centre of the triangle formed by the condyle of the femur, the tibial plateau and the junction of the lower third with the upper two thirds of the patella.

Complications

When performed correctly, the risk of introducing infection into a sterile knee is extremely small (estimated to be 1 in 50 000).

Post procedure care

If infection has been excluded, the patient can be discharged soon after the procedure and told to rest the limb for 48 hours.

SECTION 8.4 General locomotor disease

Osteoarthritis

Osteoarthritis is by far the most common condition affecting synovial joints and is associated with significant morbidity and health service utilization. A precise definition of osteoarthritis however remains elusive. Pathologically, it represents focal cartilage loss in synovial joints with associated bony destruction manifesting radiologically as joint space narrowing, sclerosis of subchondral bone and osteophyte formation. Both primary and secondary forms of the disease are recognized.

Osteoarthritis is a part of a metabolically active, physiological response of degeneration and subsequent repair and may be reversible. Uncoupling of this equilibrium leads to inexorable joint damage.

Epidemiology

Osteoarthritis is identified in all races and geographical locations, and the incidence increases progressively with age. Symptomatic osteoarthritis of the knee affects up to 15% of people over 55 years of age, but in many cases it is clinically silent (radiological evidence of osteoarthritis is found in more than 70% of those over 65 years).

Symptomatic osteoarthritis and severe radiographic changes seen in the hand and knee are more common in females. Caucasians are more frequently affected than blacks or Asians, which may reflect a genetic predisposition rather than a cultural difference.

Pathology

The pathogenesis of osteoarthritis is multifactorial and primary osteoarthritis is said to be present when an underlying cause is unidentifiable. Secondary osteoarthritis occurs when an associated condition predisposes to degenerative change (Table 8.3). Individual risk factors are divided into those that are generalized and/or localized. Generalized factors include genetic predisposition, gender, age and obesity. Localized factors include those which result in abnormal mechanical loading on a joint such as meniscectomy, instability and bony dysplasia.

Factors which have been implicated in the aetiology include failure of bone and cartilage remodelling,

479

Table 8.3	Causes of secondary osteoarthritis
Inflammatory arthritis	
Septic arthritis	
Avascular necrosis	
Intra-articular fracture	
Joint dysplasias	
Congenital dislocation of the hip	
Legg–Calvé–Perthes disease	
Acromegaly	
Ochronosis	
Haemochromatosis	

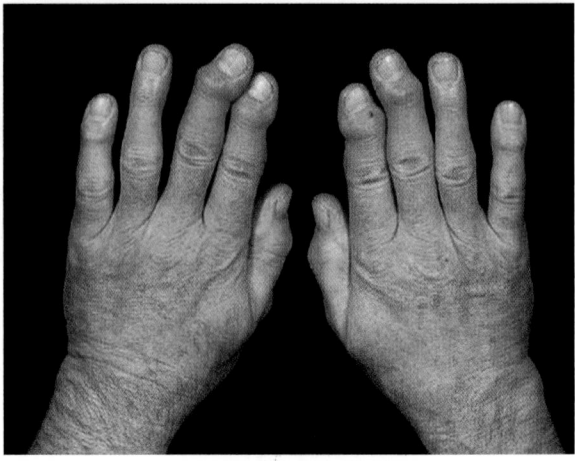

Fig. 8.2 Osteoarthritis of the hands. Nodal osteoarthritis of the distal interphalangeal joints (Heberden's nodes).

inflammation with enzymatic destruction of cartilage, ageing, abnormal joint loading, deposits of calcium apatite and calcium pyrophosphate, and abnormalities of neuro-muscular function around a joint.

Genetic factors are important; a family history is present in 20% of patients with primary generalized disease. Genetic defects in type II collagen have been described in a rare familial form of osteoarthritis, and there is some evidence of an association with HLA factors.

At the molecular level, early disease leads to increased proteoglycan turnover and alteration in proteoglycan composition with an increase in type II collagen production. Histologically, the cartilage shows thinning, fibrillation, cleft formation, erosion and eventual loss of joint surface congruity.

Scope of disease

The predominant complication of osteoarthritis is progressive joint destruction. Lower limb osteoarthritis may lead to reduced mobility, and osteoarthritis of the hand may result in difficulty with manual tasks. This can be especially disabling in younger individuals who rely on normal joint function for employment.

Clinical features

Joint pain is the predominant symptom, being exacerbated by activity and relieved with rest. The commonly affected joints are the knees, hips, first carpo-metacarpal, distal and proximal interphalangeal (DIP and PIP; Fig. 8.2) and cervical and lumbar spine apophysial (facet) joints. Other symptoms include swelling, stiffness, reduced function and joint deformity.

On examination, crepitus, instability, muscle weakness or wasting and occasionally synovitis may be evident. Knee and hip osteoarthritis may lead to limitation of mobility. It is noteworthy that there may be significant discordance between symptoms and signs. In addition, pain (a subjec-tive experience) and functional impairment may be greatly affected by personality, anxiety, affect and daily activity.

Certain subtypes of osteoarthritis have been described, however the distinctions are arbitrary. Nodal generalized osteoarthritis (menopausal osteoarthritis) is commonly familial and is characterized by Heberden's nodes (DIP joint) and Bouchard's nodes (PIP joint) as seen in Figure 8.2.

Osteoarthritis with calcium pyrophosphate deposition usually affects elderly women, especially the knees, and is associated with inflammation and hypertrophic X-ray changes. Calcium hydroxyapatite associated destructive arthritis is confined to the shoulders (Milwaukee shoulder) and knees. It is associated with a poor outcome (p. 509).

Osteoarthritis of premature onset commonly occurs after trauma or following procedures such as meniscectomy. Multiple joint involvement in patients less than 50 years should prompt investigation for systemic conditions which may present with arthritis such as haemochromatosis, ochronosis, acromegaly and hereditary defects (Table 8.3). Comorbid conditions require exclusion as a cause of symptoms such as soft tissue lesions (bursitis, enthesitis), fibromyalgia, crystal deposition disease, inflammatory arthritis and joint sepsis.

Initial investigations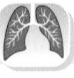

Radiography of the affected joints
The diagnosis of osteoarthritis is heavily reliant upon typical changes on the plain radiographs. Classic changes include joint space narrowing (due to cartilage loss), bony sclerosis, osteophytosis (the bony response to injury) and bone cysts (Fig. 8.3). These changes may not be detected by X-rays in patients with early disease. Usually, the plain X-ray is sufficient to confirm the diagnosis but there may be large discrepancies between symptoms and radiological change.

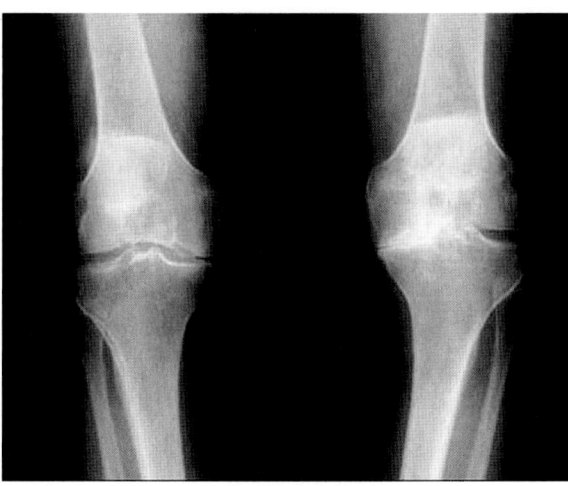

Fig. 8.3 Osteoarthritis of the knees. Plain film showing obliteration of the medial joint space of the left knee. Courtesy of the Univadis database.

Further investigations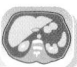

MRI
MRI is sensitive for early changes of osteoarthritis. It is not routinely indicated but may be helpful when the plain X-ray is normal to screen for synovitis.

Investigating other causes of arthritis
The differential diagnosis of hydroxyapatite associated destructive arthritis includes Charcot arthropathy, avascular necrosis and joint sepsis, which require exclusion with appropriate investigation.

Joint aspiration
If an effusion is present, aspiration of the joint is paramount to exclude the presence of an inflammatory disorder, crystal disease and sepsis.

Initial management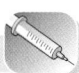

Patient education
Patient education on the natural history of the disease is an important aspect of management. Self-management programmes and regular telephone contact with a professional have been shown to significantly ameliorate patient anxiety and to reduce the need for more intensive medical intervention.

Physiotherapy and occupational therapy
Assessment by physiotherapists and occupational therapists is important for joint protection, strengthening of the supporting muscle structures, appropriate footwear (orthoses, insoles), knee bracing and walking aids.

Weight control and exercise
Other modalities include weight control and general exercise programmes.

Medical management

Analgesia
Pain control is the principal reason for patient presentation. Initial pharmacological therapy involves the use of paracetamol (acetaminophen) followed by escalating use of non-steroidal anti-inflammatory drugs (NSAIDs, oral and topical), codeine derivatives, tramadol and stronger opioids. As symptoms are often episodic, intermittent use of analgesics may suffice. Topical analgesic and anti-inflammatory creams include capsaicin and methyl salicylate. Despite being recommended, the efficacy of paracetamol in osteoarthritis has been questioned.[1,2]

Corticosteroids
Intra-articular corticosteroids are indicated for those with an inflammatory component, however the effect is usually short-lived (weeks).

> **RECENT ADVANCES**
>
> *Viscosupplementation with intra-articular hyaluronic acid injections has been found to be effective in mild to moderate osteoarthritis of the knee.[3] Symptomatic slow-acting drugs for osteoarthritis (SYSADOA) such as glucosamine sulphate[4] have been demonstrated to reduce the progression of osteoarthritis in the lower limbs. Preliminary results obtained in patients with osteoarthritis of the hands suggest that chondroitin sulphate may also have disease-modulating effects[5] although further studies are required to truly determine the usefulness of these agents. Studies so far with these chemical entities (nutripharmaceuticals) have utilized prescription formulations, not over-the-counter compounds or food supplements.*

Surgical management
Arthroscopy, synovectomy/debridement, arthroplasty, osteotomy, arthrodesis, tendon repair and nerve decompression are some of the surgical procedures available. Patients with persistent synovitis of large joints may benefit from either surgical or chemical synovectomy with yttrium-90.

Prognosis
The natural history of osteoarthritis is poorly documented. There is evidence that the process may stop or even improve. Progressive disease causes weight-bearing joint failure in only a minority.

With appropriate therapy the prognosis of osteoarthritis is favourable, especially in patients with generalized nodal disease. Patients with mild disease can be effectively managed with simple analgesics and education whereas severely damaged joints can be renewed with joint arthroplasty. Hydroxyapatite associated joint disease has a poor prognosis in terms of joint function.

FURTHER INFORMATION

American College of Rheumatology Subcommittee on Osteoarthritis Guidelines. Recommendations for the medical management of osteoarthritis of the hip and knee. 2000 Update. Arthritis and Rheumatism 2000; 43: 1905–1915.

Jordan KM, Arden NK, Doherty M, et al. EULAR Recommendations 2003: an evidence based approach to the management of knee osteoarthritis: Report of a Task Force of the Standing Committee for International Clinical Studies Including Therapeutic Trials (ESCISIT). Annals of the Rheumatic Diseases 2003; 62: 1145–1155.

REFERENCES

(1) Miceli-Richard C, Le Bars M, Schmidely N, Dougados M. Paracetamol in osteoarthritis of the knee. Annals of the Rheumatic Diseases 2004; 63: 923–930.

(2) Case JP, Baliunas AJ, Block JA. Lack of efficacy of acetaminophen in treating symptomatic knee osteoarthritis: a randomized, double-blind, placebo-controlled comparison trial with diclofenac sodium. Archives of Internal Medicine 2003; 163: 169–178.

(3) Petrella RJ, DiSilvestro MD, Hildebrand C. Effects of hyaluronate sodium on pain and physical functioning in osteoarthritis of the knee: a randomized, double-blind, placebo-controlled clinical trial. Archives of Internal Medicine 2002; 162: 292–298.

(4) Pavelka K, Gatterova J, Olejarova M, Machacek S, Giacovelli G, Rovati LC. Glucosamine sulfate use and delay of progression of knee osteoarthritis: a 3-year, randomized, placebo-controlled, double-blind study. Archives of Internal Medicine 2002; 162: 2113–2123.

(5) Richy F, Bruyere O, Ethgen O, Cucherat M, Henrotin Y, Reginster JY. Structural and symptomatic efficacy of glucosamine and chondroitin in knee osteoarthritis: a comprehensive meta-analysis. Archives of Internal Medicine 2003; 163: 1514–1522.

Rheumatoid disease (arthritis)

Rheumatoid disease is the most common chronic inflammatory condition affecting synovial joints and is associated with significant disability, morbidity and healthcare utilization. A persistent symmetrical polyarthritis is the usual presentation; however, extra-articular disease is common. Due to its systemic nature rheumatoid arthritis should more correctly be termed rheumatoid disease.

Epidemiology

Rheumatoid disease is common, affecting 1–3% of the population. The illness may commence at any age but predominantly affects individuals in the fifth decade of life with a 3:1 female preponderance. In older age groups the incidence is approximately equal in both sexes.

Pathology

The aetiology of rheumatoid disease is unknown; however, it is likely to be multifactorial. The disease may be triggered by an environmental agent (possibly infection) acting in a genetically predisposed individual. Family and twin studies have revealed a genetic susceptibility in up to 30%. The disease is polygenic with different genes (genotype) leading to a similar clinical picture (phenotype). Caucasian patients who express the MHC class II tissue type HLA-DRB1 are particularly susceptible. No causative environmental agent has been definitively identified. It is possible that a transient infection may trigger a chronic inflammatory response in synovial joints.

Hormones may play a role as rheumatoid disease is more common in women, often improves during pregnancy and relapses in the puerperium. The incidence of rheumatoid disease appears to be falling, and this may in part be due to exogenous oestrogens in the contraceptive pill.

No consistent dietary intervention has been shown to precipitate the disease. Fish oils, especially omega-3 polyunsaturated fatty acids, may have a therapeutic effect. Smoking has been implicated as a risk and severity factor.

The pathological hallmark of rheumatoid disease is destruction of articular cartilage and subchondral bone by synovial hyperplasia. This ectopic, inflamed and invading synovium is referred to as pannus. The normal synovial lining is 2–3 cell layers thick. In the diseased state it may be 10 cells thick with an infiltrate of macrophages, B lymphocytes, Th1 CD4+ lymphocytes, plasma cells and dendritic cells. As the synovium thickens, secretion of cytokines (the immunological signal peptides) and proteolytic enzymes such as the matrix metalloproteinases leads to the degradation of cartilage and bone.

The predominant cytokines mediating the inflammation in rheumatoid disease are TNF-α, IL-1 and IL-6, however many others are present. A cytokine imbalance in favour of the pro-inflammatory factors may be the pivotal pathogenic mechanism in rheumatoid disease (Table 8.4).

Rheumatoid disease has a variety of extra-articular manifestations, but less is known about the pathogenesis of these features. Rheumatoid nodules contain a core of fibrinoid necrosis surrounded by palisading macrophages and lymphocytes. Rheumatoid factors (immunoglobulins to the Fc portion of IgG) may be responsible for the extra-articular features.

Table 8.4	Pro- and anti-inflammatory cytokines in rheumatoid disease	
Pro-inflammatory	**Anti-inflammatory**	
TNF-α	sTNFR	
IL-1	IL-1Ra	
IL-6	sIL-1R	
LT-α	IL-4	
Chemokines	IL-10 TGF-β	

Scope of disease

Both inflammation and joint destruction are the characteristic features of rheumatoid disease and can progress independently. Approximately 75% of patients have two or more extra-articular features at some stage. Complications, varying in frequency and severity, include visual impairment including blindness, vocal cord dysfunction secondary to inflammation of the arytenoid cartilage, quadriparesis secondary to atlanto-axial subluxation, pleural and pericardial effusions, pulmonary fibrosis, rheumatoid nodule formation and rheumatoid vasculitis. Secondary Sjögren's syndrome, cardiovascular disease, carpal tunnel syndrome and Baker's cysts frequently occur. All these can result in substantial disability and handicap.

Clinical features

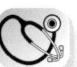

The most common presentation is symmetrical polyarthritis affecting the small joints of the hands (metacarpophalangeal, proximal interphalangeal joints) and wrists (Fig. 8.4). The feet (subtalar and metatarsophalangeal joints) are frequently involved early in the disease. Other features at presentation include diffuse joint stiffness, worse upon rising in the morning and after rest (gelling phenomenon). The onset may be explosive or insidious and may lead to reduced manual dexterity and mobility.

Any synovial joint may be affected in rheumatoid disease, with the knees, shoulders and elbows being frequently involved. Crico-arytenoid joint involvement in the larynx may lead to hoarseness and vocal cord collapse. Any synovium-lined structure may be involved such as tendon sheaths and bursae.

The well-described palindromic onset involves synovitis that flits from joint to joint. Occasionally rheumatoid disease may present with a polymyalgia rheumatica type onset, especially in older patients where myalgia is prominent.

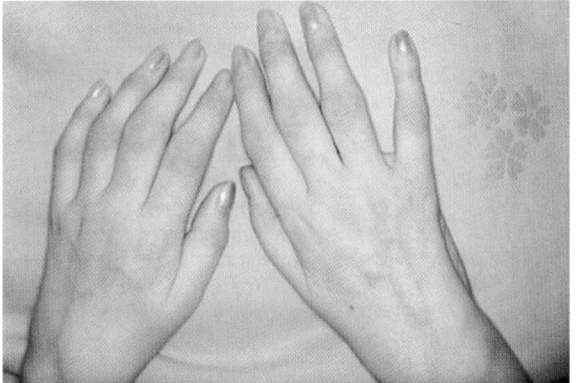

Fig. 8.4 Symmetrical small joint polyarthritis of early rheumatoid disease.

With the advent of early, more aggressive effective therapies, classic features of rheumatoid disease may become less prevalent. Swan-neck and boutonnière deformities of the fingers and Z deformity of the thumb result from joint destruction and altered axis of tendon tracking. Other typical features include ulnar deviation and subluxation of the metacarpo-phalangeal (MCP, Fig. 8.5) and wrist joints. 'Triggering' of the fingers may result from tenosynovitis. Similar changes may occur in the feet with loss of the longitudinal arch and pes planus due to valgus deformity at the subtalar joints. The feeling of 'walking on pebbles' results from the excessive pressure on the metatarsal heads due to a cock-up deformity of the toes.

Muscle wasting is common in rheumatoid disease and is secondary to disuse atrophy. Compressive neuropathies may also occur, the most common being carpal tunnel syndrome with an equivalent syndrome occurring in the feet, tarsal tunnel syndrome.

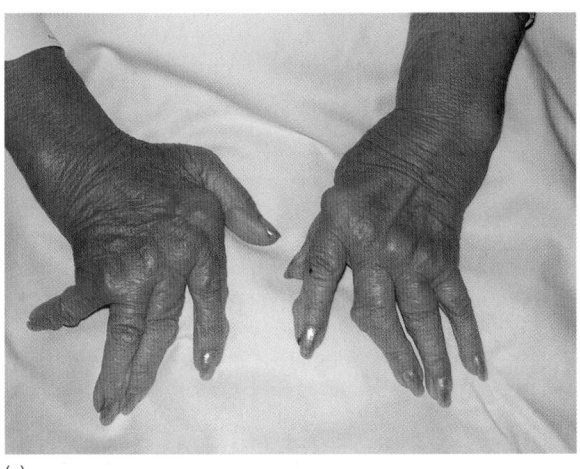

(a)

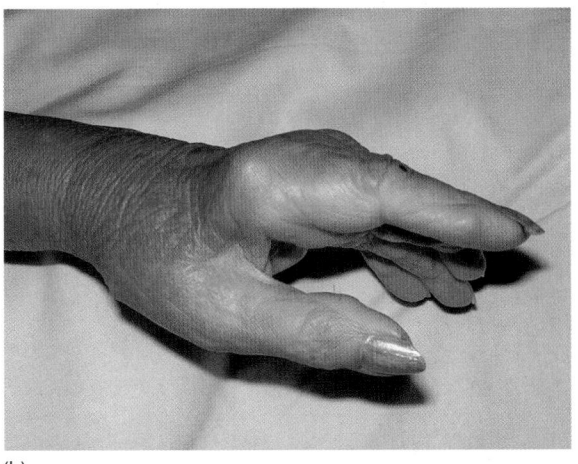

(b)

Fig. 8.5a, b Advanced rheumatoid disease. Patient with severe disease, ulnar deviation of the metacarpo-phalangeal joints, rheumatoid nodules and a vasculitic lesion on the index finger of the left hand.

One of the most significant complications of rheumatoid disease is involvement of the articulation between the posterior aspect of the odontoid peg of C2 (the axis) and the transverse ligament of the atlas resulting in atlanto-axial subluxation. The dire outcome of this complication is spinal cord compression. Care is required during intubation and the anaesthetist must be aware of this complication. A distance greater than 4 mm from the anterior aspect of the peg to the posterior aspect of the anterior arch of C1 is abnormal. However, neurological complications are less common than might be expected as 25% of patients requiring joint replacement have some degree of C1/C2 subluxation.

Extra-articular features usually occur in severe, seropositive (rheumatoid factor positive) disease but may occur at any time in the course of the condition (Table 8.5). The rheumatoid nodule is the most common extra-articular manifestation, occurring in up to 25% of patients. The

Table 8.5	Extra-articular features of rheumatoid arthritis
Common	
Anaemia	
Fever, weight loss, malaise	
Nodules	
Tendinitis and bursitis	
Ophthalmological complications (scleritis, scleromalacia perforans, sicca symptoms)	
Carpal tunnel syndrome	
Nail fold vasculitis	
Peripheral neuropathy	
Pleural effusion	
Pulmonary fibrosis	
Muscle wasting	
Depression	
Infection	
Peripheral oedema	
Lymphadenopathy	
Osteoporosis	
Cardiovascular disease	
Rare	
Hearing impairment	
Myositis	
Episcleritis	
Systemic vasculitis	
Pericarditis	
Pulmonary nodules	
Splenomegaly	
Amyloidosis	

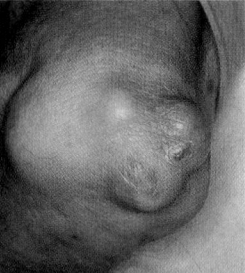

Fig. 8.6 Rheumatoid nodules over the elbow. Courtesy of Drs A Doria and R Rondinone and the EULAR image database.

nodules are usually located subcutaneously adjacent to pressure points such as extensor surfaces of the forearms and elbows (Fig. 8.6). Nodules may vary in diameter from millimetres to centimetres and may be solitary or multiple. A single rheumatoid nodule in the lung can mimic malignancy or an infective process such as tuberculosis. Multiple pulmonary rheumatoid nodules occur in association with coal-worker's pneumoconiosis (Caplan's syndrome).

Raynaud's phenomenon is common in rheumatoid disease and other connective tissue diseases. Upon exposure to cold the extremities characteristically turn white, blue and red during the reactive hyperaemic phase, however many patients describe 'incomplete' forms. If severe digital ulceration occurs, cryoglobulinaemia, rheumatoid vasculitis or systemic sclerosis requires exclusion.

Systemic symptoms such as fever, malaise, anorexia and weight loss frequently occur. Presence of these features increases the likelihood of premature death. Pulmonary involvement is common with pleurisy, pleural effusions, interstitial pneumonitis, pulmonary fibrosis and obliterative bronchiolitis. Nervous system involvement may manifest as neural entrapment, sensory neuropathy, sensorimotor peripheral neuropathy or mononeuritis multiplex (the latter two resulting from vasculitis of the vasa nervorum). The heart is less commonly involved but there may be pericardial chest pain and effusion. There is an increased risk of cardiovascular disease in these patients.

Rarer associations include lymphadenopathy and amyloidosis with deposition of serum amyloid A protein manifesting as proteinuria or malabsorption (p. 241). Rheumatoid vasculitis may lead to nail fold infarcts in the periphery and leg ulceration. Renal involvement in rheumatoid disease is rare. Osteoporosis may occur as a result of the disease, immobility or corticosteroid therapy. There is an increased incidence of infections in patients with rheumatoid disease. Felty's syndrome (rheumatoid factor positive rheumatoid arthritis, splenomegaly and pancytopenia, most frequently neutropenia) may lead to recurrent bacterial infections, chronic leg ulcers and increased mortality.

Avascular necrosis of the femoral head and other sites occurs, especially in those treated with corticosteroids, and leads to severe pain and bone collapse.

Rheumatoid systemic vasculitis requires aggressive therapy with high-dose immunosuppression.

The diagnosis of rheumatoid disease may be difficult and several other conditions should be considered. The American College of Rheumatology devised diagnostic criteria for rheumatoid arthritis (Table 8.6), however these were originally designed to classify patients with established disease and are therefore less sensitive and specific for early arthritis.

Table 8.6	American College of Rheumatology diagnostic criteria for rheumatoid arthritis* (1987)

Four of the seven criteria must be met. Criteria 1–4 must have been present for at least 6 weeks:

1. Morning stiffness in and around joints lasting 1 hour or more before maximal improvement
2. Soft tissue swelling (arthritis) of three or more joint areas
3. Swelling (arthritis) of the proximal interphalangeal, metacarpo-phalangeal or wrist joints
4. Symmetrical arthritis
5. Subcutaneous nodules
6. Positive test for rheumatoid factor
7. Radiographic erosions and/or periarticular osteopenia in hand and/or wrist joints

* Arnett FC, Edworthy SM, Bloch DA, et al. The American Rheumatism Association 1987 revised criteria for the classification of rheumatoid arthritis. Arthritis and Rheumatism 1998; 31: 15–24.

Initial investigations

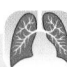

Laboratory and radiological investigations are supportive of a clinical diagnosis; however, there is no pathognomonic test for rheumatoid disease. At presentation, the investigation of polyarthritis is guided by clinical suspicion.

Full blood count
Anaemia is common and can occur as a result of chronic disease, blood loss (iron deficiency anaemia from NSAID-induced stomach ulceration), Felty's syndrome (pancytopenia) or bone marrow suppression (methotrexate treatment). Thrombocytosis develops as part of the acute phase response.

Erythrocyte sedimentation rate/C-reactive protein
The erythrocyte sedimentation rate and C-reactive protein levels are often elevated as part of the acute phase response.

Urea and electrolytes/liver profile
Baseline liver and renal function tests are performed prior to therapy. Mild alterations of liver function tests are a frequent finding but are usually not associated with significant liver disease.

Serum autoantibodies
Rheumatoid factor is present in 80% of patients but may be elevated in many other conditions (Table 8.7). Anti-nuclear antibodies are indicators of connective tissue disease but may be present in rheumatoid arthritis. Anti-cyclic citrullinated peptide antibodies may be more sensitive and specific than rheumatoid factor.

X-rays of hands and feet
Classical features include soft tissue swelling, loss of joint space, periarticular osteopenia and juxta-articular erosions. However, radiographs are frequently normal at presentation as bone changes take at least 3 months to appear (Fig. 8.7).

Table 8.7	Causes of a raised rheumatoid factor

Inflammatory disease

Rheumatoid disease

Connective tissue diseases, e.g. systemic lupus erythematosus, Sjögren's syndrome

Cryptogenic fibrosing alveolitis

Chronic active hepatitis

Cryoglobulinaemia

Infection

Infectious mononucleosis

Subacute bacterial endocarditis

Tuberculosis

Malaria

Schistosomiasis

Post vaccination

Malignancy

Lymphoma

Leukaemia

Myeloma

Solid tumours

Normal variant

Up to 15% of the healthy population have positive rheumatoid factor

Joint aspiration
Aspiration of joint fluid is extremely useful to exclude infection or inflammation due to uric acid or pyrophosphate crystals.

>  **CLINICAL ALERT**
>
> *Monitoring of drug toxicity involves regular blood investigations such as FBC, liver function tests, renal function, ESR, CRP and urinalysis (Table 8.8).*

Further investigations

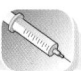

Investigations for other causes of polyarthritis
If the diagnosis is in question, investigation for other causes of a polyarthritis is mandatory including uric acid level, thyroid function tests, creatine kinase, vasculitis and infection screens.

Initial management

The principles of management of rheumatoid disease aim at symptom relief, preservation of function, retarding the erosive process and maintaining quality of life. The current focus is on early and more aggressive treatment as such intervention results in maximum long-term benefit with minimum risk.[1]

Connective tissue disorders

Vasculitis

Crystal deposition disorders

Arthritis and infection

Osteoporosis and metabolic bone disease

Polymyalgia rheumatica and giant cell arteritis

Miscellaneous rheumatological disease

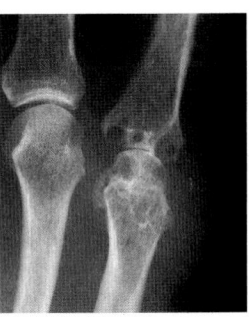

Fig. 8.7 Plain film of rheumatoid arthritis showing joint space narrowing, erosions, periarticular osteopenia and soft tissue swelling of the fifth metacarpo-phalangeal joint.

485

Table 8.8 Principal disease-modifying antirheumatic medications (DMARDs)

DMARD	Dose	Time until effect	Side effects	Cautions and contraindications	Monitoring
Methotrexate	7.5–25 mg/week orally or i.m. or s.c.	6–12 weeks	Dyspepsia, stomatitis, cough, diarrhoea, anorexia, alopecia, bleeding or bruising, fever, pneumonitis, increased nodulosis	Bone marrow suppression, hepatic and pulmonary disease, alcoholism, immunodeficiency, active infection, pregnancy, concomitant trimethoprim	FBC, LFTs second weekly. Once stable dose, 4–6 weekly
Sulfasalazine	2–3 g/day orally in 2–3 divided doses	2–3 months	Gastrointestinal upset, diarrhoea, dizziness, headache, rash including photosensitivity, anorexia, abnormal liver function, neutropenia	Allergy to sulpha drugs, renal or hepatic disease, blood dyscrasias	Monthly FBC, LFTs until stable dose then 3 monthly
Hydroxychloroquine	200–400 mg/day orally (<7 mg/kg body weight)	2–3 months	Diarrhoea, anorexia, alopecia, nausea, rash, retinopathy, neuromyopathy	Allergy to antimalarials, retinal abnormality, G6PD deficiency, pregnancy	Yearly optometrist review of vision
Gold salts (aurothiomalate)	10 mg test dose then 25–50 mg weekly–monthly (i.m.)	2–3 months	Photosensitivity, taste dysgeusia, rash, painful gums, bleeding or bruising, mouth ulcers, proteinuria, bone marrow suppression	Renal disease, bone marrow suppression, colitis	FBC, LFTs, U&Es, Urinalysis monthly prior to dose
Leflunomide	100 mg daily for 3 days loading dose (frequently omitted due to side effects). 10–20 mg maintenance dose	6–8 weeks	Gastrointestinal upset, bone marrow suppression, rash, liver test abnormalities, alopecia, diarrhoea, hypertension	Leukopenia, thrombocytopenia	FBC, LFTs second weekly. Once stable dose, 4–6 weekly
Azathioprine	50–150 mg in divided dose, based on body weight	6–12 weeks	Anorexia, nausea, vomiting, rash, bone marrow suppression, infection, malignancy, pancreatitis	Renal or hepatic disease, pregnancy, concomitant use of allopurinol	FBC, LFTs second weekly until stable dose then monthly
Ciclosporin	2.5–5 mg/kg/day in divided dose	6–12 weeks	Bleeding, gum hypertrophy, fluid retention, hypertension, hirsutism, renal impairment, anorexia, tremor	Hepatic and renal disease, active infection, hypertension	FBC, LFTs, creatinine and BP second weekly until stable dose then 3 monthly, serum lipids 6 monthly
Cyclophosphamide	50–150 mg orally daily or 1 g/m² 1–3 monthly infusions	2–8 weeks	Infertility, anorexia, bone marrow suppression, infection, haemorrhagic cystitis, malignancy	Renal and hepatic disease, active infection, pregnancy	FBC, LFTs, renal function 2–4 weekly
Penicillamine	125–250 mg/day initially up to maximum of 1500 mg/day in divided dose	3–6 months	Diarrhoea, arthralgia, taste dysgeusia, fever, allergic reactions, oral ulceration, nausea and vomiting, rash, bone marrow suppression, weakness, autoimmune phenomena	Penicillin allergy, blood dyscrasia, renal disease	FBC and urinalysis second weekly until stable dose then 1–2 monthly

FBC, full blood count; LFTs, liver function tests; G6PD, glucose-6-phosphate dehydrogenase; U&Es, urea and electrolytes; BP, blood pressure.

Patient education

Patient education is a very important aspect of management. Patients should be informed of the chronic nature of rheumatoid disease and the importance of controlling the illness in order to improve prognosis.

Physiotherapy and occupational therapy

These disciplines have multiple beneficial aspects including optimization of joint movement and function and muscle strengthening by relieving pain and stiffness. Modalities utilized include heat, ice, wax baths and hydrotherapy. The use of splints, where appropriate, may be required for joint protection to avoid deformity and improve power and function of limbs.

An adequate programme of rest with graded exercise improves outcome. Orthoses are frequently required for deformed feet. Occupational therapists assess patients' disability and handicap and administer aids for daily living such as handles for cutlery and taps and long-handled combs.

Medical management

As the primary concern of the patient is pain relief, adequate analgesia is paramount. Simple analgesics such as paracetamol with or without codeine may be required (side effects are common in the elderly).

Non-steroidal anti-inflammatory drugs

NSAIDs form one of the cornerstones of medical therapy. By decreasing prostaglandin production they have analgesic, antipyretic and anti-inflammatory effects. They do not, however, alter the natural history of the disease. Traditional NSAIDs are frequently used and a large variation in response exists, therefore trials of different medications are necessary to optimize treatment. NSAIDs account for up to 20% of all cases of peptic ulcer haemorrhage and perforation, with many being fatal.

> **RECENT ADVANCES**
>
> *Cyclo-oxygenase-2 (COX-2) inhibitors, drugs which specifically target the COX-2 isoenzyme, were developed as an alternative to traditional NSAIDs due to their potential for less gastrointestinal toxicity. However, as an increase in cardiovascular disease was seen with certain agents, rofecoxib was withdrawn from the worldwide market in September 2004. The other COX-2 inhibitors and traditional NSAIDs are currently under close scrutiny for the emergence of data suggesting similar effects.*[2]

Corticosteroids

Corticosteroids are extremely effective in reducing the inflammatory response. Unfortunately their long-term toxicity (Table 8.6) limits their use to the minimum dosage required to stabilize the arthritis. Higher doses are occasionally required for severe exacerbations of arthritis or extra-articular manifestations. Guidelines have been developed for the prevention of steroid-induced osteoporosis.

Intra-articular corticosteroid injections, following joint aspiration, are frequently used with excellent response and minimal side effects. Sepsis must be excluded prior to injection, with urgent Gram stain and culture of synovial fluid if infection is considered a possibility.

Disease-modifying antirheumatic medications (DMARDs) (see Table 8.10)

These medications are now introduced much earlier in the treatment of rheumatoid disease due to their efficacy in preventing progression of disease. The two main reasons for discontinuation of DMARDs are inefficacy and toxicity. The challenge is to identify patients most likely to suffer from aggressive disease and institute treatment expediently.

Methotrexate

Due to its efficacy and tolerability, the folic acid antagonist methotrexate has emerged as the benchmark against which all other therapies for rheumatoid disease are tested. Methotrexate inhibits dihydrofolate reductase in cell metabolism. The mechanism of action in rheumatoid disease is believed to include inhibition of trafficking of white cells from blood vessels into synovium and suppression of pro-inflammatory cytokines.

Hydroxychloroquine

The antimalarial hydroxychloroquine is effective in milder forms of rheumatoid disease. Its disease-modifying capacity is weaker than the other DMARDS and it does not appear to retard erosive disease. Monitoring for the rare event of retinal toxicity is necessary.

Sulfasalazine

Sulfasalazine is a compound of sulphapyridine and 5-aminosalicylic acid. Like hydroxychloroquine, sulfasalazine is effective in mild to moderate rheumatoid disease. Serious side effects are rare but blood dyscrasias, hepatotoxicity and skin reactions may occur.

Gold salts (sodium aurothiomalate)

Gold salts have been used for over 50 years in the treatment of rheumatoid disease. Unfortunately over a third of patients develop serious side effects requiring cessation of therapy. Gold is now being used less frequently.

Leflunomide

Leflunomide inhibits pyrimidine synthesis in T cells and has effects comparable to methotrexate. Leflunomide was designed specifically for rheumatoid disease. It has a long half-life, and if toxicity occurs, clearance of the drug is aided by the administration of colestyramine.

Other agents

Currently, ciclosporin, azathioprine and penicillamine are rarely used for rheumatoid disease due to the availability of more efficacious and less toxic compounds. Cyclophosphamide is employed for systemic rheumatoid vasculitis.

Combination therapy

Many patients are not adequately controlled on mono-therapy and so combinations of DMARDs have been utilized with synergistic effect without a concomitant rise in toxicity. Various combinations have been studied, the best described being that of methotrexate, sulfasalazine and hydroxychloroquine. In practice, rheumatologists use various combinations of antirheumatic drugs in order to achieve the optimal response.

RECENT ADVANCES

Biological response modifiers herald a new era in the treatment of rheumatic disorders.

TNF-α inhibitors have been the most extensively studied and produce rapid and sustained amelioration of the signs and symptoms of rheumatoid disease. In addition, these agents retard the radiological progression of rheumatoid disease more effectively than traditional DMARDs. In addition, 30–40% of patients do not respond to biological agents. The currently available compounds include infliximab[3] and adalimumab (anti-TNF antibodies), etanercept (TNF receptor fusion protein) and anakinra (IL-1 receptor blocker). Many more biological agents such as rituximab (a β-cell antibody),[4] are in development and are being investigated in clinical trials with promising results.

Surgical management

Synovectomy

A surgical synovectomy and debridement/arthroplasty procedure involves excision of excess synovial tissue and rough surfaces of the joint. An alternative to surgical syno-vectomy is the use of the radioactive compound yttrium which, when injected intra-articularly, induces a chemical synovectomy. Details of surgical procedures are presented in the section on regional joint disease.

Prognosis

Not all patients with rheumatoid disease have a uniform outcome. There is good evidence that early intervention gives the maximum long-term benefit for the minimum risk. The use of suppressive drugs within 6 months of disease onset improves prognosis as it is at this stage that inflam-mation is present with little joint destruction. Severe joint damage and many of the extra-articular manifestations may be avoided with appropriate management.

Currently, only 50% of patients are employed after 10 years, and 40% have ceased work after 2 years from diagnosis. Approximately 75% develop at least moderate impairment of function. Factors associated with a poor prognosis include extra-articular manifestations, insidious onset, high rheumatoid factor titres, functional disability at 1 year, HLA-DR4 genotype and early erosive disease on X-ray.

In general, life expectancy is reduced by 3 years in females and 7 years in males.

i FURTHER INFORMATION

American College of Rheumatology Subcommittee on Rheumatoid Arthritis Guidelines. Guidelines for the Management of Rheumatoid Arthritis, 2002 Update. Arthritis and Rheumatism 2002; 46: 328–346.

Arthritis Research Campaign: www.arc.org.uk

REFERENCES

(1) Keen HI, Emery P. How should we manage early rheumatoid arthritis? From imaging to intervention. Current Opinion in Rheumatology 2005;17: 280–285.
(2) Ostor AJK, Hazleman BL. The murky waters of the coxibs: a review of the current state of play. Inflammopharmacology 2005; 13: 371–380.
(3) Maini RN, Breedveld FC, Kalden JR, et al. Sustained improvement over two years in physical function, structural damage, and signs and symptoms among patients with rheumatoid arthritis treated with infliximab and methotrexate. Arthritis and Rheumatism 2004; 50: 1051–1065.
(4) Edwards JC, Szczepanski L, Szechinski J, et al. Efficacy of B-cell-targeted therapy with rituximab in patients with rheumatoid arthritis. New England Journal of Medicine 2004 ; 350: 2572–2581.

Seronegative spondyloarthropathies

The seronegative spondyloarthropathies are a collection of inflammatory arthritides with common clinical manifes-tations distinct from rheumatoid disease. The term 'seronegative' denotes the absence of rheumatoid factor in the serum.

There are five subgroups of spondyloarthropathies, see Table 8.9.

Epidemiology

Seronegative spondyloarthropathies tend to affect young adults, although the initial presentation may occur at any age.

Ankylosing spondylitis principally affects young males with an incidence of approximately 100 per 100 000 per year. It is common in North American Haida Indians, but uncom-mon in African blacks, Aborigines and Japanese populations.

Table 8.9	Subgroups of spondyloarthropathies
Ankylosing spondylitis	
Psoriatic arthritis	
Reactive arthritis	
Enteropathic arthritis (arthritis associated with inflammatory bowel disease)	
Undifferentiated spondyloarthropathy	

Psoriasis affects 3% of the general population; 10% of people with psoriasis will develop an associated arthritis.

Reactive arthritis (previously known as Reiter's disease) is a non-septic arthritis following a gastrointestinal, urinary tract, or other infection. It has an incidence of approximately 30 per 100 000 per year.

Arthritis occurring with inflammatory bowel disease is termed enteropathic arthritis and occurs in over 10% of those with ulcerative colitis and 20% of those with Crohn's disease.

In addition, there is a group of incomplete or undifferentiated spondyloarthropathies which are less common and account for a small minority of cases. Juvenile spondyloarthropathy is rare.

Pathology

The predominant site of inflammation is the enthesis (the insertion site of ligaments and tendons into bone). There is a predilection for the spine, especially the sacroiliac joints.

Although the aetiology is unknown, advances have helped define the genetics and inflammatory mediators in seronegative spondyloarthropathies. As in many other connective tissue diseases, the spondyloarthropathies are probably triggered by an environmental agent in a genetically predisposed individual. Of paramount importance is the increased frequency of HLA-B27 in this group. The pathogenesis remains unclear, as HLA-B27 is not present in all patients and is found in up to 8% of the unaffected general population.

The molecular mimicry model hypothesizes that antigens identified on microorganisms have a homologous appearance to normal cell markers. During the inflammatory response these native cell markers are identified as foreign and are attacked leading to the clinical manifestations. Another possible mechanism of disease is leakage of bowel bacteria into the circulation causing an immune reaction. Regardless of the mechanism, CD4+ T cells are central to the pathogenesis. Other inflammatory cells and cytokines, especially TNF-α, are pivotal to the disease process. Interestingly, the synovitis is indistinguishable from rheumatoid disease on immunohistochemistry and histology.

Scope of disease

Pain, deformity and disability are the major sequelae of unbridled inflammation. Other complications, predominantly occurring in ankylosing spondylitis, include bony ankylosis, cardiac valvular disease, aortitis and pulmonary fibrosis. Osteoporosis is more prevalent in these patients as a consequence of active disease. Conjunctivitis and anterior uveitis can occur, requiring urgent ophthalmological review and slit-lamp examination to differentiate the two.

Clinical features

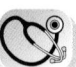

The most widely used diagnostic classification criteria for the seronegative spondyloarthropathies are those of the European Spondyloarthropathy Study Group (Table 8.10).

Table 8.10	European Spondyloarthropathy Study Group (ESSG) diagnostic criteria
Inflammatory spinal pain or synovitis (asymmetrical* or predominantly in the lower limbs*) and one or more of the following:	
Positive family history	
Psoriasis	
Inflammatory bowel disease	
Alternate buttock pain	
Enthesopathy	
Sacroiliitis*	

* Without sacroiliitis, sensitivity = 77%, specificity = 89%; with sacroiliitis, sensitivity = 86%, specificity = 87%.

The sensitivity and specificity for the diagnosis of seronegative spondyloarthropathies of these criteria exceed 85%. There is significant clinical overlap between the seronegative spondyloarthropathy subgroups. Systemic symptoms are common to all and may include mild fever, myalgia, fatigue, lethargy and loss of weight.

Ankylosing spondylitis

Ankylosing spondylitis commonly presents with lower back pain and stiffness with unilateral or bilateral radiation of pain into the buttocks. Symptoms may last for hours and are worse upon rising in the morning and after inactivity. Back pain at night is highly suggestive of inflammation and fatigue is a common complaint. Other manifestations include red, painful, gritty eyes from iritis, and enthesopathy such as Achilles tendonitis and plantar fasciitis. Peripheral joint synovitis has a characteristic distribution with only one or a few weight-bearing joints affected. The combination of synovitis and tenosynovitis results in dactylitis. Anterior chest pain results from involvement of the costochondral joints. Later manifestations include symptoms of cardiac valvular dysfunction and pulmonary compromise. Aortitis is a cause of death in some patients (Table 8.11).

Table 8.11	Extra-articular features of ankylosing spondylitis
Systemic symptoms (lethargy, malaise, fever, loss of weight)	
Acute iritis	
Apical pulmonary fibrosis	
Cardiac disease	
Aortic and mitral valve incompetence	
Heart conduction defects	
Neurological disease	
Cauda equina syndrome	
Atlanto-axial subluxation	
Spinal fractures	
Amyloidosis	

489

The Schober test, used to identify patients with ankylosing spondylitis, assesses the degree of distraction of the lumbar spine after forward flexion.

Psoriatic arthritis

Dermatological lesions (plaque, guttate or pustular psoriasis) with or without nail involvement (Fig. 8.8) generally precede psoriatic arthritis by some years. Occasionally, the skin changes may develop after the onset of arthritis. Arthritis without skin manifestations is termed psoriatic arthritis sine psoriasis. Five main categories of psoriatic arthritis have been described, see Table 8.12. Lower limb large joints are most frequently affected. Skin lesions may be scarce; a search for these should include the scalp, natal cleft, feet, genitalia and tongue.

Reactive/Reiter's syndrome

The original description of Reiter's syndrome was a triad of arthritis, conjunctivitis and urethritis following an episode of bloody dysentery. It has now been defined by the American College of Rheumatology as a month of peripheral arthritis associated with urethritis or cervicitis or both. The classic triad is present in approximately a third of patients.

Reactive arthritis develops a few weeks after a bacterial infection, usually of the gastrointestinal or lower genital tract. Other features may include cervicitis, prostatitis and salpingitis. Conjunctivitis occurs synchronously in one third of patients with reactive arthritis. Acute anterior uveitis runs an independent course compared with the joint manifestations. The typical skin lesion of reactive arthritis is keratoderma blennorrhagica, which occurs most commonly on the palms and soles (Fig. 8.9). The arthritis tends to involve the large weight-bearing joints with intermittent recurrences. Many infections have been implicated in reactive arthritis, however viable microorganisms are not present in the inflamed joint (Table 8.13).

Enteropathic arthritis

Enteropathic arthritis predominantly affects lower limb large joints in association with symptoms of inflammatory bowel disease (p. 272). Other features include erythema nodosum, pyoderma gangrenosum, aphthous mouth ulcers and acute anterior uveitis. Even in the absence of HLA-B27, inflammatory changes in the gut have been described in all the spondyloarthropathies and are frequently asymptomatic. Gut diseases associated with spondyloarthropathies are listed in Table 8.14.

Initial investigations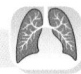

Full blood count

Anaemia, thrombocytosis and leukocytosis (possible infection) may be present.

Table 8.12	Subtypes of psoriatic arthritis
Mono- or oligo-arthritis (usually lower limb large joints)	
Symmetrical polyarthritis (similar to rheumatoid arthritis)	
DIP joint inflammation with nail involvement	
Arthritis mutilans (the most severe form)	
Spondylitis (with radiological sacroiliitis in 20%)	

Table 8.13	Organisms associated with reactive arthritis
Genitourinary	
Chlamydia trachomatis	
Ureaplasma urealyticum	
Neisseria gonorrhoeae	
Gastrointestinal	
Shigella spp.	
Salmonella spp.	
Yersinia spp.	
Campylobacter jejuni	
Clostridium difficile	
Giardia lamblia	
Escherichia coli (enterotoxigenic strains)	
Entamoeba histolytica	
Other	
Borrelia burgdorferi	
Chlamydia pneumoniae	
Streptococcus pyogenes	
Blastocystis hominis	

Fig. 8.9 Keratoderma blennorrhagica on the soles in reactive arthritis.

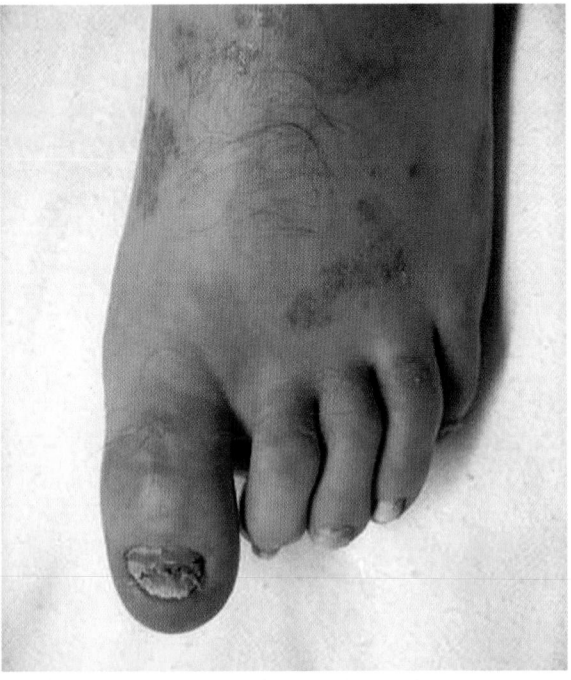

Fig. 8.8 Psoriasis with onychodystrophy of toenails.
Courtesy of Dr G Wright and the EULAR image database.

Table 8.14	Gastrointestinal diseases associated with spondyloarthropathies
Acute bacterial infection	
Giardiasis and amoebiasis	
Inflammatory bowel disease	
Whipple's disease	
Coeliac disease	
Jejunoileal bypass syndrome	
Subclinical lesions	

Markers of inflammation

An acute phase response is reflected by an elevated ESR and CRP.

Urea and electrolytes/liver function tests

Renal and liver function require testing prior to drug therapy. Hypoalbuminaemia can result from an acute phase response.

Rheumatoid factor

Rheumatoid factor is absent in the serum.

Plain X-rays of affected joints

Plain radiology is necessary to assess joint and enthesis involvement, which may appear as erosions or bony spurs. X-rays of the sacroiliac joints (Fig. 8.10) are especially useful as these are frequently involved (Table 8.15). Early changes occur at the lower, anterior synovial portion of the joint and include juxta-articular osteoporosis, widening of the sacroiliac joint and marginal sclerosis. More advanced changes include juxta-articular sclerosis and joint space obliteration from ankylosis. Early changes in the spine include erosions of the vertebral bodies and squaring of the vertebrae. In established disease bridging syndesmophytes develop and may lead to the classic 'bamboo spine' seen in ankylosing spondylitis (Fig. 8.11).

Radiological features of psoriatic arthritis include erosions of the DIP joints with ankylosis, resorption of the terminal tufts and marginal bone overgrowth at tendon insertions. Bony overgrowth with osteolysis of the middle phalanx leads to the 'pencil in cup' deformity (Fig. 8.12). Asymmetrical sacroiliitis occurs in up to 30%.

Periostitis is the most characteristic radiological finding in reactive arthritis. Peripheral joint destruction does not occur in enteropathic arthritis.

Further investigations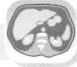

MRI of the sacroiliac joints

The most sensitive technique for demonstrating early disease, especially of the sacroiliac joints, is MRI. This is reserved for selected cases when the diagnosis remains in doubt after initial investigations.

HLA-B27 testing

Routine testing of HLA-B27 does not add to the diagnosis but helps identify those with a genetic predisposition and lends weight to the diagnosis in those with an unclear clinical picture.

HIV test

Patients with extensive or severe psoriatic arthritis and those with reactive arthritis should be tested for HIV.

Initial management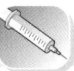

Management is directed at relieving pain, halting the destructive process and maintaining joint function. The focus is on non-pharmacological measures.

Patient education and support

Patient education is essential to ensure compliance and to aid in accepting the life-long nature of the disease. Several support groups exist for patients with spondyloarthropathies. HLA-B27 is present in virtually all patients with ankylosing spondylitis and 50% of their progeny will carry this antigen. If positive, the child has a one in three

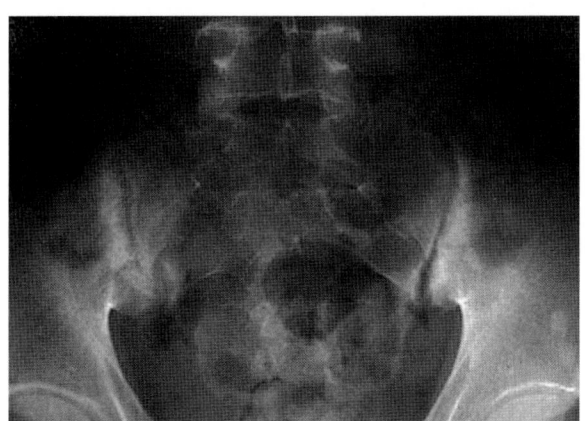

Fig. 8.10 Plain radiograph of the pelvis showing bilateral sacroiliitis in a patient with ankylosing spondylitis.

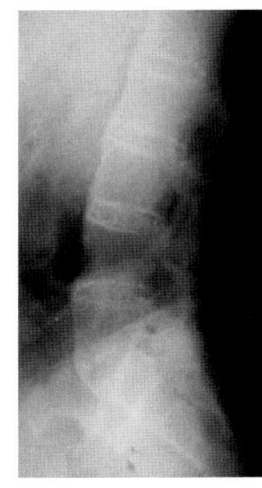

Fig. 8.11 Bamboo spine. Lateral radiograph of the lumbosacral spine in a patient with ankylosing spondylitis showing syndesmophytes with bamboo appearance. Courtesy of Drs A Iagnocco and G Valesini and the EULAR image database.

Connective tissue disorders

Vasculitis

Crystal deposition disorders

Arthritis and infection

Osteoporosis and metabolic bone disease

Polymyalgia rheumatica and giant cell arteritis

Miscellaneous rheumatological disease

Table 8.15	Frequency and symmetry of sacroiliitis in spondyloarthropathies			
Characteristic	Ankylosing spondylitis	Reactive arthritis	Psoriatic arthritis	Enteropathic arthritis
Sacroiliitis or spondylitis	Virtually 100%	<50%	<30%	<20%
Symmetry of sacroiliitis	Symmetric	Asymmetric	Variable	Symmetric

chance of developing ankylosing spondylitis therefore genetic counselling is important in patients wishing to conceive.

Physiotherapy

Physiotherapy is crucial for exercise programmes and stretching regimens. General mobility can also be preserved and many patients benefit from hydrotherapy.

Medical management

Non-steroidal anti-inflammatory agents

Pharmacotherapy revolves around the use of NSAIDs, which may suffice for symptomatic relief to allow adequate physiotherapy.

Disease-modifying antirheumatic drugs

Sulfasalazine has traditionally been used for spondyloarthropathies, especially ankylosing spondylitis and psoriatic arthritis; however, neither this DMARD nor methotrexate alters the natural history of axial disease.

Immunomodulation

Intermittent intra-articular corticosteroids are very effective for symptom relief. Systemic steroids are best avoided as they are not particularly effective and have significant side effects. They are occasionally required for severe symptoms and complications such as uveitis. Psoriatic skin disease may flare on weaning corticosteroids.

Antibiotics

Tetracycline is useful in the treatment of non-specific urethritis but is not beneficial for the other manifestations of reactive arthritis.

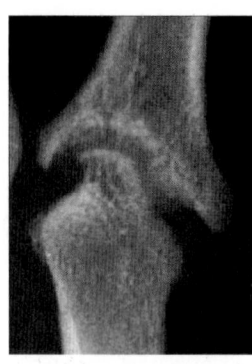

Fig. 8.12 Plain film of pencil-in-cup deformity of psoriatic arthritis. Courtesy of Drs W Grassi and E Filippucci and the EULAR image database.

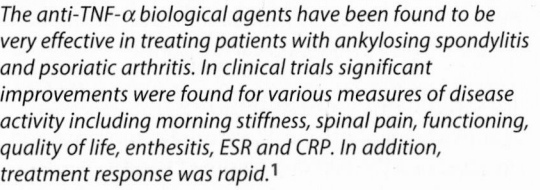

RECENT ADVANCES

The anti-TNF-α biological agents have been found to be very effective in treating patients with ankylosing spondylitis and psoriatic arthritis. In clinical trials significant improvements were found for various measures of disease activity including morning stiffness, spinal pain, functioning, quality of life, enthesitis, ESR and CRP. In addition, treatment response was rapid.[1]

⚡ **CLINICAL ALERT**

Any patient who presents with either reactive arthritis or severe and/or extensive psoriatic arthritis should be investigated for HIV infection. Despite the association, however, there is no clear evidence that HIV is a risk factor for spondyloarthropathies. Atlanto-axial subluxation and cauda equina syndrome may occur in ankylosing spondylitis.

Surgical management

Hip replacement

Hip replacement is frequently required for hip involvement.

Spinal osteotomy

Occasionally spinal osteotomy is necessary for severe spinal deformity.

Prognosis

Maintenance of joint function is excellent with early identification of disease and appropriate management. Five per cent of patients with ankylosing spondylitis have an unfavourable course from the onset. Up to 80% of patients with reactive arthritis have some evidence of disease activity after 5 years. Vigilance is required to intervene when complications develop. Tissue typing for HLA-B27 is unreliable as a guide to prognosis.

i **FURTHER INFORMATION**

Dougados M, van der Linden S, Juhlin R, et al. The European Spondylarthropathy Study Group preliminary criteria for the classification of spondylarthropathy. Arthritis and Rheumatism 1991; 34: 1228–1230.

REFERENCE

(1) *Gorman JD, Sack KE, Davis JC Jr. Treatment of ankylosing spondylitis by inhibition of tumor necrosis factor alpha. New England Journal of Medicine 2002; 346: 1349–1356.*

Connective tissue disorders

Systemic lupus erythematosus

Systemic lupus erythematosus (SLE) is the quintessential autoimmune connective tissue disease. The manifestations are varied, any organ system may be involved and the disease is characterised by relapses and remissions.

Epidemiology

The incidence of SLE varies with geographical location. It has been estimated to be 2 per 100 000 per year in New York (USA) to 4 per 100 000 per year in the UK and up to 8.7 per 100 000 per year in Brazil.[1] Women are affected 9 times more frequently than males and the disease is much more common in Black and Chinese populations. The mean age at presentation is 33 years, and the disease has a predilection for women of child-bearing age. Genetic factors play an important role as there is a 60% concordance of SLE in monozygotic twins.

Pathology

The aetiology of SLE is unknown. In common with other connective tissue diseases, lupus may be triggered by an environmental agent, possibly a virus, acting in a genetically susceptible individual. The disease has been associated with HLA-B8, DR2 and DR3. Patients with a genetic deficiency of the C2 complement component have an increased incidence of SLE.

Well-known triggers and exacerbating factors include infections, medications and ultraviolet (sunlight) exposure. In contradistinction to rheumatoid disease, women with lupus may experience an exacerbation of disease during pregnancy with resolution following delivery.

The key serological abnormality is development of antinuclear antibodies (ANAs) underscoring SLE as an immune-complex mediated condition. The clinical manifestations result from antigen–antibody complex deposition in tissues. Autoantibodies, detected by immunofluorescence (Fig. 8.13), are directed against nuclear antigens. Anti-double stranded DNA identified by enzyme-linked immunoadsorbent assay (ELISA) and anti-Sm (Smith) antibodies are highly specific for SLE (Table 8.16).

Diffuse small and medium vessel vasculitis contributes to the pathogenesis.

Scope of disease

The major complications of lupus involve damage to the kidney and central nervous system. The various types of renal damage have been classified by the World Health Organization (Table 8.17). Renal lesions may not progress from one form to another and a variety of changes may coexist. Central nervous system disease is common and may present in a multitude of ways (Table 8.18).

Avascular necrosis affecting weight-bearing joints occurs more frequently in SLE patients, especially those

Table 8.16	Autoantibodies in SLE
Anti-nuclear antibodies	
Anti-dsDNA	
Anti-ssDNA	
Anti-centromere	

Extractable nuclear antigens (subclassification of ANAs)
  Anti Ro (SS-A)
  Anti La (SS-B)
  Anti Sm
  Anti U1 RNP
  Anti Scl 70
  Anti Jo1
  Anti Histone	

Table 8.17	WHO classification of lupus nephritis on renal biopsy
I	Normal glomeruli
II	Pure mesangial alterations
III A	Focal segmental glomerulonephritis
III B	Focal proliferative glomerulonephritis
IV	Diffuse glomerulonephritis
V	Diffuse membranous glomerulonephritis
VI	Advanced sclerosing glomerulonephritis

Table 8.18	Neuropsychiatric manifestations of lupus
Headache/migraine
Seizures
Chorea
Tremor
Stroke
Cranial nerve palsies
Mononeuritis multiplex
Peripheral neuropathy
Organic brain syndrome/cognitive disorder
Psychosis

who have received corticosteroids. There is an increased incidence of pericarditis and myocarditis. Rarely, non-infective endocarditis can occur (Libman–Sacks endocarditis). In the lungs SLE can lead to pleurisy and interstitial pneumonia. Patients with lupus are more susceptible to infections and should receive prophylactic vaccinations.

 CLINICAL ALERT

The anti-phospholipid syndrome (p. 830) may occur in isolation or in the presence of connective tissue disease. It is characterized by arterial and venous thrombosis, recurrent miscarriages, thrombocytopenia and anti-phospholipid antibodies (anti-cardiolipin antibodies and/or the lupus anticoagulant). The lupus anticoagulant is a double misnomer as it may be present with or without the features of SLE (primary anti-phospholipid syndrome) and leads to in vitro anticoagulation (prolonged activated partial thromboplastin time, APTT) but in vivo thrombophilia.

Clinical features

The name lupus (Latin, meaning 'wolf') was first used to describe the rash of cutaneous disease that made the patient appear to have been ravaged by a wild dog. Lupus

Connective tissue disorders

Vasculitis

Crystal deposition disorders

Arthritis and infection

Osteoporosis and metabolic bone disease

Polymyalgia rheumatica and giant cell arteritis

Miscellaneous rheumatological disease

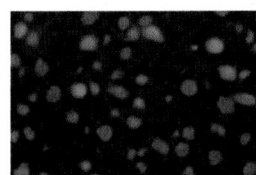

Fig. 8.13
Immunofluorescence testing for anti-nuclear antibodies. Courtesy of the Univadis database.

commonly presents with the characteristic photosensitive malar or 'butterfly' rash sparing the nasolabial folds (Fig. 8.14) and a symmetrical small joint polyarthralgia or arthritis (Table 8.19). Other initial features include mouth ulcers, alopecia and systemic symptoms. Renal disease occurs in up to 60%. Central nervous system involvement is common and may be difficult to diagnose and treat (Table 8.18). Bacterial infection is common, as is the development of the features of immune thrombocytopenic purpura (p. 819).

SLE can mimic a number of conditions, and the diagnosis can be elusive. The American College of Rheumatology classification criteria developed for SLE have now become surrogate diagnostic criteria, in which the presence of 4 out of 11 features is considered to be indicative of SLE (Table 8.20).

Initial investigations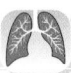

Screening blood investigations aid in diagnosis and help to assess disease activity.

Full blood count

Frequent abnormalities include anaemia, neutropenia and/or absolute lymphocytopenia, thrombocytopenia and autoimmune haemolytic anaemia.

Table 8.19	Clinical features of SLE
Skin rash	
Arthralgia, arthritis	
Mouth ulceration	
Alopecia (may be scarring)	
Myalgia	
Malaise	
Fever	
Fatigue	
Weight loss	
Livido reticularis	
Vasculitis lesions	
Lymphadenopathy	
Immune thrombocytopenic purpura (ITP)-like disease	
Pericarditis	
Pleurisy, pneumonitis	
Nephritic syndrome	
Hypertension	
Renal failure	
Neuropsychiatric disease (Table 8.21)	
Non-infective endocarditis (Libman–Sacks endocarditis)	
Raynaud's phenomenon	
Infections	

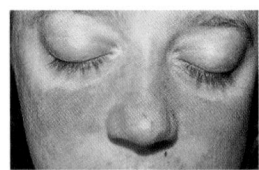

Fig. 8.14 Typical malar or butterfly rash of systemic lupus erythematosus with sparing of nasolabial folds. Courtesy of Drs A Doria and R Rondinone and the EULAR image database.

Table 8.20	American College of Rheumatology classification criteria for SLE (1982 Revised Criteria)
Malar rash	
Discoid rash	
Photosensitivity	
Oral ulcers	
Arthritis	
Serositis	
Renal disorder	
Neurologic disorder	
Haematologic disorder	
Immunologic disorder	
Antinuclear antibodies	

* Four out of the 11 criteria must be present during the course of disease to be classified as having SLE.

Markers of inflammation

The ESR is often elevated without a commensurate rise in the CRP level. CRP elevation may indicate intercurrent infection.

Urea and electrolytes

Elevated serum creatinine indicates renal impairment.

Liver profile

Hypoalbuminaemia can occur.

Serum autoantibodies

Anti-nuclear antibodies are present in almost 100% of patients. These may be further subdivided into antibodies directed at extractable nuclear antigens (Table 8.19). The presence of IgG anti-cardiolipin antibodies and/or the lupus anticoagulant is serological evidence of the anti-phospholipid syndrome.

Complement levels

Complement levels (C3, C4 and CH50) are reduced during flares of lupus due to consumption. They are tested serially to monitor disease activity.

Urinalysis

Proteinuria and haematuria (an active urinary sediment) may be an early indicator of renal disease.

Further investigations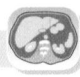

Coagulation screen

A clotting profile is indicated to screen for anti-phospholipid syndrome where the APTT is prolonged.

CT of the head

These are useful investigations for patients with central nervous system manifestations of SLE. MRI is far more sensitive.

Renal biopsy

A renal biopsy is often required for patients with renal impairment to obtain a histopathological diagnosis.

Serum lipid profile

Lipid levels should be checked as cardiovascular disease is more common in SLE.

Initial management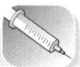

Patient education and support

A multidisciplinary team approach is required for patient education and to develop support networks. The importance of this cannot be overemphasized as lupus is a chronic, relapsing and remitting disorder with life-threatening complications.

Avoid precipitating factors

Prophylactic measures include avoidance of exposure to UV radiation with appropriate attire (e.g. sun hats) and sun-blocking creams.

Medical management

Pharmacological therapy essentially involves symptom relief as the aetiology is unknown and there is no cure for lupus.

Non-steroidal anti-inflammatory agents

NSAIDs are beneficial for joint manifestations.

Antimalarial agents

Antimalarial agents such as hydroxychloroquine and chloroquine are effective for skin and joint symptoms and to maintain disease remission.[2]

Immunomodulation

Topical steroid creams for facial lesions are beneficial but should not have a high corticosteroid concentration.

Corticosteroids are frequently required for severe joint disease. High doses should be reserved for severe disease as side effects are common. A maintenance dose of 5–10 mg of prednisolone is usually adequate. Severe manifestations, especially renal and CNS disease, require intravenous pulses of corticosteroids with the addition of a steroid-sparing agent such as azathioprine or methotrexate. In organ- or life-threatening disease cyclophosphamide is required.

Psychiatric input

A formal neurocognitive and psychiatric assessment can be invaluable in patients with CNS involvement.

Surgical management

Joint replacement

Joint replacement may be required for arthritic complications, such as hip replacement for avascular necrosis of the femoral head.

Renal transplantation

In appropriate patients, renal transplantation is an effective treatment for end-stage renal failure.

Prognosis

The prognosis of SLE improves if a multidisciplinary team approach is used. The worst outcome is seen in patients with lupus nephritis who have a 15-year mortality of 40%. CNS involvement is frequent in well-established cases and 50% of patients with renal involvement also have some CNS abnormality. In the absence of severe CNS or renal disease the 15-year survival is 80%. Regular follow-up is required to monitor for relapse of disease, for the development of associated conditions and for side effects of treatment.

---

i **FURTHER INFORMATION**

Ioannou Y, Isenberg DA. Current concepts for the management of systemic lupus erythematosus in adults: a therapeutic challenge. Postgraduate Medical Journal 2002; 78: 599–606.

REFERENCES

(1) Petri M. Epidemiology of systemic lupus erythematosus. Best Practice and Research Clinical Rheumatology 2002; 16: 847–858.
(2) A randomized study of the effect of withdrawing hydroxychloroquine sulfate in systemic lupus erythematosus. The Canadian Hydroxychloroquine Study Group. New England Journal of Medicine 1991; 324: 150–154.

Systemic sclerosis

Systemic sclerosis, also known as scleroderma, is a multi-system disorder characterized by progressive fibrosis of connective tissues throughout the body. There are two main subsets of systemic sclerosis: limited cutaneous systemic sclerosis and diffuse cutaneous systemic sclerosis (depending upon the extent of skin involvement). Other forms of the disease are listed in Table 8.21.

Epidemiology

The prevalence of systemic sclerosis is approximately 1 per 100 000 in the fifth decade of life. It is three times more common in females.

Pathology

The relative risk of developing systemic sclerosis is increased 25-fold with a history of exposure to silica dust and 110-fold with frank silicosis. The potential role of infectious agents is suggested by homology between viral

Connective tissue disorders

Vasculitis

Crystal deposition disorders

Arthritis and infection

Osteoporosis and metabolic bone disease

Polymyalgia rheumatica and giant cell arteritis

Miscellaneous rheumatological disease

Table 8.21	Classification of systemic sclerosis
Localized	
Morphoea	
Linear scleroderma	
En coup de sabre	
Systemic	
Limited cutaneous systemic sclerosis (previously CREST syndrome)	
Diffuse cutaneous systemic sclerosis	
Scleroderma sine scleroderma	
Chemical or drug induced	
Bleomycin	
Polyvinylchloride	
Silicon dioxide	
L-tryptophan (eosinophilia–myalgia syndrome)	
Adulterated rapeseed oil (toxic oil syndrome)	
Overlap syndromes	
Mixed connective tissue disease	
Scleroderma mimics	
Sclerederma of Buschke	
Eosinophilic fasciitis	

antigens and autoantigens in systemic sclerosis. Genetic factors appear to influence the clinical course of the disease.

The hallmark of systemic sclerosis is diffuse small vessel vasculopathy and fibrosis. Small arteries, arterioles and capillaries are involved and display proliferative and obliterative changes. In addition there is activation of endothelial cells and platelets.

The vascular disease is not considered a vasculitis. Fibrosis is caused by activation of fibroblasts which deposit collagen, fibronectin and glycosaminoglycans in the skin, internal organs and blood vessels. Cytokine stimulation of extracellular membrane production and higher basal amounts of extracellular matrix produced by outgrowth of fibroblasts lead to fibrosis.

Although the aetiology is unknown, the pathogenesis must account for the triad of small vessel vasculopathy, autoimmunity and fibrosis. Activation of T cells is crucial in the pathogenesis, and expression of different cytokines varies with the stage of the disease. Anti-nuclear antibodies are present in 95% of patients, suggesting dysregulation of the immune system.

Scope of disease

Digital infarction secondary to severe Raynaud's phenomenon and larger artery occlusive disease may occur. Pulmonary hypertension with or without pulmonary fibrosis and biliary cirrhosis occurs, especially in limited disease. Renal crisis is a life-threatening complication of diffuse disease characterized by hypertension and rapidly progressive renal impairment, however this may occur in normotensive patients. Interstitial alveolitis is another potentially fatal complication of diffuse disease.

Clinical features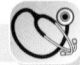

Most commonly patients describe tightening of skin of the hands (Fig. 8.15), arms and legs, and Raynaud's phenomenon.

Limited disease was previously known as CREST syndrome (calcinosis, Raynaud's phenomenon, oesophageal dysmotility, sclerodactyly and telangiectasia).

Diffuse disease may be preceded by an oedematous phase of the legs and arms with skin involvement being more extensive and involving the trunk, face and neck. Early end-organ involvement such as renal failure and pulmonary fibrosis can also occur. Renal crisis manifests as increasing renal impairment, proteinuria and hypertension. Acute disease presents with intractable hypertension, rapid renal failure and microangiopathic haemolytic anaemia.

A small subset of patients have systemic sclerosis without skin involvement but suffer from Raynaud's phenomenon and internal organ disease.

The gastrointestinal tract is commonly affected, manifesting as dysphagia and reflux oesophagitis. Other features depend upon organ involvement and may manifest as pulmonary, cardiac, small and large gut and

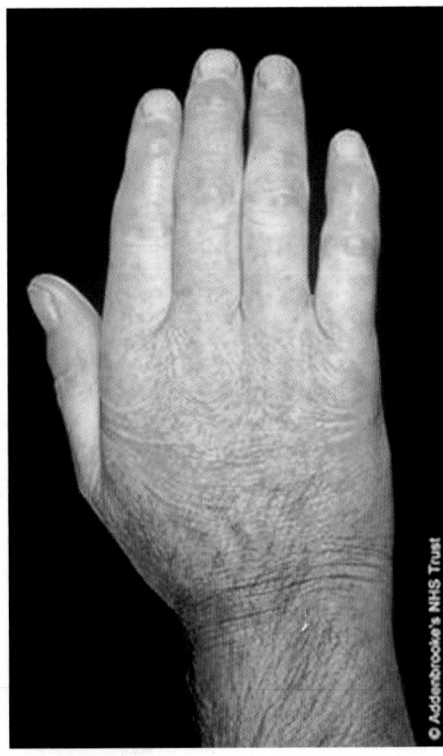

Fig. 8.15 Sclerodactyly. Tightening of the skin and a mottled appearance of the fingers in a patient with diffuse cutaneous systemic sclerosis.

renal disease. Polyarthritis or arthralgia is common. In the later stages, myopathy and muscle atrophy are common and limb contractures may occur. Ischaemic changes with gangrene of the fingertips may result from the vasculopathy.

The diagnosis of systemic sclerosis may be aided by applying the American College of Rheumatology classification criteria (Table 8.22).

Several scleroderma-like syndromes exist, such as sclerederma of Buschke (thickening of the skin, particularly of the upper back in diabetics), eosinophilic fasciitis (Schulman's syndrome, a rare disorder with swelling and thickening of forearms and legs, peripheral blood eosinophilia and an eosinophilic infiltrate of the involved areas) and scleroderma-like disease (drug or chemically induced by agents such as bleomycin and polyvinyl-chloride).

Initial investigations
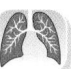

Full blood count, markers of inflammation
Screening blood investigations include assessment for anaemia and inflammatory markers (ESR and CRP); however, these are usually normal.

Table 8.22	American College of Rheumatology criteria for the classification of systemic sclerosis (scleroderma)*

Major criterion

Proximal scleroderma

Symmetric thickening, tightening, and induration of the skin of the fingers and the skin proximal to the metacarpo-phalangeal or metatarsophalangeal joints. The changes may affect the entire extremity, face, neck, and trunk (thorax and abdomen)

Minor criteria

Sclerodactyly

Above-indicated skin changes limited to the fingers

Digital pitting scars or loss of substance from the finger pad

Depressed areas at tips of fingers or loss of digital pad tissue as a result of ischaemia

Bibasilar pulmonary fibrosis

Bilateral pattern of linear or lineonodular densities most pronounced in basilar portions of the lungs on standard chest X-ray; may assume appearance of diffuse mottling or 'honeycomb lung'. These changes should not be attributable to primary lung disease

*For the purposes of classifying patients in clinical trials, population surveys and other studies, a person shall be said to have systemic sclerosis (scleroderma) if the one major or two more minor criteria are present. Localized forms of scleroderma, eosinophilic fasciitis, and the various forms of pseudoscleroderma are excluded from these criteria. Adapted from the Subcommittee for Scleroderma Criteria of the American Rheumatism Association Diagnostic and Therapeutic Criteria Committee: Preliminary criteria for the classification of systemic sclerosis (scleroderma). Arthritis and Rheumatism 1980; 23: 581–590.

Urea and electrolytes
Serum creatinine is usually assessed as a screening investigation for renal impairment.

Serum autoantibodies
Autoimmune studies are paramount and a variety of autoantibodies may occur in scleroderma (Table 8.23). Anti-centromere antibodies are specific for limited disease and anti-Scl-70 antibodies (directed against the topoisomerase enzyme) are present in 20% of patients with diffuse disease.

Urinalysis
Urinalysis for proteinuria aids in assessing renal involvement.

Further investigations
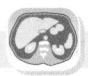

Chest X-ray
A plain chest film is useful in patients with a diagnosis of systemic sclerosis to screen for asymptomatic lung disease.

Pulmonary function tests
Early interstitial lung disease may be detected with a reduced transfer factor (p. 103).

CT chest
High-resolution CT of the chest is performed when initial investigations suggest pulmonary involvement. Pulmonary fibrosis and alveolitis are detected as linear-reticular shadows.

Transthoracic echocardiography
A transthoracic echocardiogram can assess the degree of pulmonary hypertension.

Barium swallow
A barium swallow is indicated for patients with dysphagia.

Oesophageal manometry
Oesophageal manometry is a useful investigation to characterize any motility disorders identified on the barium swallow.

Table 8.23	Predominant autoantibodies in systemic sclerosis

Anti-centromere antibodies

Anti-nuclear antibodies

Anti-nucleolar antibodies

Anti-polymyositis/systemic sclerosis overlay (Pm/Scl)

Anti-topoisomerase I (formerly Scl-70)

Anti-ribonucleoprotein (RNP)

Anti Jo-1 (anti-histidyl-transfer RNA synthetase)

Anti-Ro, anti-La antibodies

Connective tissue disorders

Vasculitis

Crystal deposition disorders

Arthritis and infection

Osteoporosis and metabolic bone disease

Polymyalgia rheumatica and giant cell arteritis

Miscellaneous rheumatological disease

Initial management

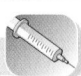

There is no specific treatment for the sclerodermatous process. Management is therefore aimed at patient education, alleviation of symptoms and prevention of end-organ damage.

Patient education and support

Patients should be informed about the variable course of the disease. Avoidance of cold environments, abstinence from smoking and heated gloves are simple measures to minimise recurrent attacks of Raynaud's phenomenon.

Medical management

Arthropathy and myositis

NSAIDs are used for arthropathy and corticosteroids for associated myositis. High-dose penicillamine, previously prescribed for scleroderma, is no longer recommended as it does not appear to have any advantage over low-dose regimens.[1]

> **CLINICAL ALERT**
>
> *Avoidance of high doses of corticosteroids is important as precipitation of renal crisis may develop.*

Digital ulceration and Raynaud's

Infusions of prostacyclin analogues (iloprost, alprostadil) are effective for digital lesions such as ulceration, infection and severe vasospasm. Sympathectomy may also be effective.

Reflux oesophagitis

Proton pump inhibitors are used for reflux oesophagitis and oesophageal dysmotility.

Small bowel overgrowth

Small bowel bacterial overgrowth is treated with rotating courses of antibiotics.

Alveolitis

Lung disease is now the leading cause of death in systemic sclerosis due to pulmonary hypertension and alveolitis. Inflammatory alveolitis may be reversible with immunomodulation (corticosteroids and cyclophosphamide).

Pulmonary hypertension

Isolated pulmonary hypertension, in the absence of interstitial fibrosis, has the worst prognosis of all visceral problems in systemic sclerosis. The prognosis of pulmonary hypertension has been improved with prostacyclin analogues and bosentan, an endothelin receptor antagonist. Bosentan improves cardiopulmonary haemodynamics and exercise capacity in patients with pulmonary hypertension. Benefits are seen in patients with primary pulmonary hypertension and pulmonary hypertension secondary to connective tissue disease.[2]

Renal crises

Scleroderma renal crisis and progressive renal failure are major causes of death in systemic sclerosis. Treatment with ACE inhibitors has resulted in avoidance of permanent dialysis in 61%, and a survival similar to scleroderma patients without renal crises.[3]

Surgical management

Thoracoscopic sympathectomy

Sympathectomy for severe Raynaud's phenomenon can be undertaken. A minimal access approach to the sympathetic chain can be achieved with video-assisted thoracoscopy. Diathermy ablation of the sympathetic chain (T1 to T4) results in symptomatic improvement in 93% but is associated with a high recurrence rate (82% by 5 years).[4]

Renal transplantation

Renal transplantation is an option for patients with end-stage renal disease.

Lung transplantation

Lung transplantation is reserved for patients with end-stage pulmonary fibrosis and quiescent disease.[5]

Prognosis

The overall course is highly variable and disease activity is difficult to measure; however, once remission occurs, relapse is uncommon. Spontaneous improvement, particularly of skin disease, does occur. Patients with anti-centromere antibodies have a relatively good prognosis but may develop digital amputation, pulmonary hypertension and biliary cirrhosis. Following the effective treatment of renal disease with ACE inhibitors, the predominant cause for premature mortality is pulmonary involvement. The prognosis even for lung disease has improved with early and aggressive therapy.

> *i* **FURTHER INFORMATION**
>
> Systemic sclerosis. Rheumatic Disease Clinics of North America 2003; 29: 211–426.

REFERENCES

(1) Clements PJ, Furst DE, Wong WK, et al. High-dose versus low-dose D-penicillamine in early diffuse systemic sclerosis: analysis of a two-year, double-blind, randomized, controlled clinical trial. Arthritis and Rheumatism 1999; 42: 1194–1203.

(2) Rubin LJ, Badesch DB, Barst RJ, et al. Bosentan therapy for pulmonary arterial hypertension. New England Journal of Medicine 2002; 346: 896–903.

(3) Steen VD, Medsger TA Jr. Long-term outcomes of scleroderma renal crisis. Annals of Internal Medicine 2000; 133: 600–603.

(4) Matsumoto Y, Ueyama T, Endo M, et al. Endoscopic thoracic sympathicotomy for Raynaud's phenomenon. Journal of Vascular Surgery 2002; 36: 57–61.

(5) International guidelines for the selection of lung transplant candidates. The American Society for Transplant Physicians (ASTP)/American Thoracic Society(ATS)/European Respiratory Society(ERS)/International Society for Heart and Lung Transplantation (ISHLT). American Journal of Respiratory Critical Care Medicine 1998; 158: 335–339.

Polymyositis and dermatomyositis

Polymyositis and dermatomyositis are rare autoimmune conditions resulting in muscle inflammation. They are characterized by proximal muscle weakness and in the case of dermatomyositis, skin involvement.

Epidemiology

Due to the rarity of these conditions, accurate epidemiological data are difficult to obtain. The incidence has been estimated to be 0.1 per 100 000 per year. The myositides may occur at any age with peaks in childhood and in the fifth and sixth decades of life.

Pathology

The myositides may be primary, or secondary to connective tissue disorders. The aetiology of primary disease has been attributed to viral infection since many viridae are able to produce an acute myositic picture, although this is unproven. Many other infections, however, also produce a myopathic picture. The role of genetics is unclear but a weak association with HLA-B8 and DR3 has been found.

Scope of disease

The main complication of myositis is profound muscle weakness and respiratory embarrassment with diaphragmatic involvement. As both striated and smooth muscles are affected, dysphagia may occur with resultant poor nutrition and aspiration. Pulmonary fibrosis occurs in a proportion, and cardiac involvement can lead to arrhythmia and heart failure.

 CLINICAL ALERT

Dermatomyositis can also be a paraneoplastic syndrome in up to 20% of patients. Therefore the clinician should screen for clinical features of breast, bowel, lung or ovarian cancer. This association is less prominent with polymyositis.

Clinical features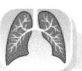

Patients tend to present with an insidious onset of symmetrical proximal muscle weakness resulting in difficulties climbing stairs, rising from low chairs and getting out of automobiles. Muscle pain may occur but is infrequent.

The lilac (heliotrope) rash of dermatomyositis (Fig. 8.16) classically affects the skin overlying the proximal interphalangeal and metacarpo-phalangeal joints (Gottron's papules, Fig. 8.17) and eyelids with associated periorbital oedema.

Shortness of breath may occur with diaphragm involvement and cardiac disease may lead to arrhythmias or symptoms of heart failure. Swallowing difficulties and reflux oesophagitis develop due to loss of peristalsis. Progressive disease may lead to muscle wasting and contractures. A mild arthralgia occurs in up to 25%. Calcinosis is common in children and may be recalcitrant to therapy.

Initial investigations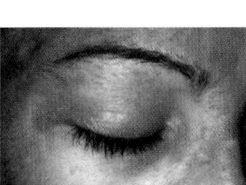

Creatine phosphokinase

Creatine phosphokinase is usually elevated secondary to muscle inflammation. It is also a useful marker to monitor disease activity.

Serum autoantibodies

Anti-Jo1 antibodies are specific for associated pulmonary fibrosis in polymyositis.

Connective tissue disorders

Vasculitis

Crystal deposition disorders

Arthritis and infection

Osteoporosis and metabolic bone disease

Polymyalgia rheumatica and giant cell arteritis

Miscellaneous rheumatological disease

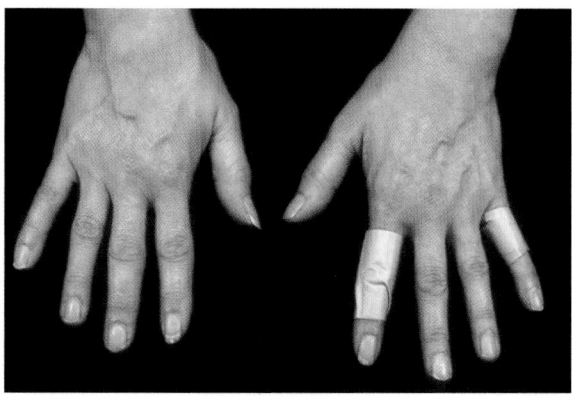

Fig. 8.17 Gottron's papules.

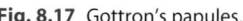

Fig. 8.16 Heliotrope facial rash of dermatomyositis. Courtesy of Dr W Grassi and the EULAR database.

Nerve conduction studies and electromyography

Nerve conduction studies are usually normal whilst electromyography reveals brief duration and low-amplitude waveforms.

Muscle biopsy

Inflammatory changes may be seen on muscle biopsy. A normal biopsy does not exclude the disease, as the inflammation occurs in a patchy distribution.

Further investigations

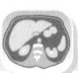

Chest X-ray

A plain chest film should be performed for patients with dyspnoea to screen for pulmonary fibrosis and neoplasms. If pulmonary fibrosis is present a high-resolution CT scan of the chest should be arranged.

Pulmonary function tests

Deteriorating FEV_1 indicates progressive disease.

MRI

MRI may detect subtle or early changes. As myositis may be patchy, MRI is the best imaging modality to localize disease prior to muscle biopsy.

Initial management

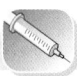

Patient education

Education regarding the disease is paramount as therapy is often required long term.

Medical management

Immunomodulation

The mainstay of pharmacological therapy is corticosteroids. Frequently, high doses (prednisolone 40–60 mg per day) are required for prolonged periods therefore bone prophylaxis measures should be instituted. Steroid-sparing agents include azathioprine and methotrexate. Severe disease requires more intensive therapy with cyclophosphamide or intravenous gamma globulin. Plasmapheresis has not been found to be effective.

Prognosis

The prognosis is improved with the early institution of corticosteroids. Pulmonary disease is a major cause of prolonged morbidity.

i FURTHER INFORMATION

Mastaglia FL, Garlepp MJ, Phillips BA, Zilko PJ. Inflammatory myopathies: clinical, diagnostic and therapeutic aspects. Muscle and Nerve 2003; 27: 407–425.

Sjögren's syndrome

Sjögren's syndrome is an autoimmune condition characterized by inflammation of the exocrine glands. The disease may be primary or secondary to other connective tissue diseases, especially rheumatoid disease, systemic lupus erythematosus and systemic sclerosis. The salivary glands are most commonly affected.

Epidemiology

Determination of the prevalence of Sjögren's syndrome is problematic due to classification difficulties and poor identification of mild cases. It has been estimated, however, to be 100 per 100 000 individuals. It is 9 times more common in women compared to men and tends to present in the fourth decade.

Pathology

The aetiology of Sjögren's syndrome is unknown. Biopsy of involved salivary glands displays focal lymphoid infiltrates predominantly comprised of CD4-positive T cells. HLA-DR antigens are expressed on glandular epithelial cells; these antigens are absent in normal specimens. Cell-mediated immune mechanisms are chiefly responsible for glandular destruction.

Scope of disease

Severe dryness of the eyes (keratoconjunctivitis sicca) and mouth (xerostomia) may lead to pain and ulceration. There is an increased incidence of chronic pancreatitis in patients with Sjögren's syndrome, and the occurrence of B-cell lymphoma is significantly greater than in the general population.

Clinical features

Ocular and oral dryness (sicca symptoms) are the predominant manifestations of Sjögren's syndrome. Difficulty swallowing occurs as a consequence of xerostomia. Fatigue is common and may be profound. Central nervous system lesions and peripheral neuropathy may develop. Mild interstitial nephritis may occur, usually without clinical consequence. Sinusitis results from upper airway dryness. Pulmonary involvement manifests as a lymphocytic interstitial pneumonitis with associated pleural effusions. Dyspareunia secondary to vaginal dryness is not uncommon. Swelling of the salivary glands occurs and may herald lymphoma development. The differential diagnosis includes infiltrative and infectious processes and neuropathic disorders including autonomic dysfunction. Medications such as antihypertensives, antidepressants and anticholinergics may produce oral and ocular dryness. Arthralgia is a common accompaniment.

Connective tissue disorders

Vasculitis

Crystal deposition disorders

Arthritis and infection

Osteoporosis and metabolic bone disease

Polymyalgia rheumatica and giant cell arteritis

Miscellaneous rheumatological disease

CLINICAL ALERT

The incidence of lymphoma is more than 30 times greater in patients with Sjögren's syndrome than in the normal population. The development of a mass, particularly in the head and neck, requires urgent biopsy to exclude this complication.

Initial investigations

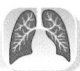

Serum autoantibodies

Autoimmune studies are frequently positive, especially anti-nuclear antibodies and anti-Ro (SS-A) and anti-La (SS-B) antibodies.

Schirmer's test

Schirmer's test assesses ocular dryness. Filter paper is placed in the lower eyelid and tear production is measured by how far the 'wetness' travels along the paper. Less than 5 mm in 5 minutes is abnormal.

Further investigations

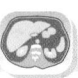

Salivary gland biopsy

Confirmation of the diagnosis may be made histologically following cone biopsy surgical excision of a salivary gland.

Initial management

Patient education

Patients should be informed about the chronicity of the condition. Symptomatic relief is the mainstay of treatment for Sjögren's syndrome. Avoidance of anticholinergic medications helps to reduce mucosal dryness. Frequent sips of fluid aid the xerostomia and patients are instructed to carry around a water bottle and have fluid next to their bed.

Artificial tears

Artificial tears for dry eyes should be applied liberally.

Medical management

Non-steroidal anti-inflammatory drugs and hydroxychloroquine

NSAIDs and hydroxychloroquine are effective for arthralgia, myalgia and fatigue.

Immunomodulation

Corticosteroids are reserved for more severe symptoms. Cholinergic agents, such as pilocarpine, are beneficial.

Prognosis

Patients with Sjögren's syndrome require long-term follow-up. The prognosis is favourable with vigilance for the development of lymphoma.

i FURTHER INFORMATION

Mariette X. Current and potential treatment for primary Sjögren's syndrome. Joint Bone Spine 2002; 69: 363–366.

Vasculitis

Vasculitis is a heterogeneous group of diseases characterized by inflammation and necrosis of blood vessel walls. The Chapel Hill consensus and the American College of Rheumatology Criteria are used to classify the vasculitides. A simplified approach categorizing the vasculitides by the size of the vessels involved is presented in this section as vessel size usually determines the treatment approach.

Vasculitis may be primary or secondary to systemic illness, especially connective tissue disease (Table 8.24). Early diagnosis and treatment is paramount as life-threatening complications may ensue. Several conditions mimic vasculitis and require exclusion.

i FURTHER INFORMATION

American College of Rheumatology Subcommittee on Classification of Vasculitis: The American College of Rheumatology 1990 Criteria for the Classification of Vasculitis. Arthritis and Rheumatism 1990; 33: 1065–1144.

Small vessel vasculitis

Epidemiology

Small vessel vasculitis (leukocytoclastic vasculitis) confined to the skin is usually a secondary disease, with an incidence of 2 per 100 000 per year. Henoch–Schönlein purpura predominantly affects children and young adults with an incidence of 10 per 100 000 per year in the under-14 age group. Cryoglobulinaemic vasculitis is rare (hepatitis C serology is positive in over 90% of cases). Hypersensitivity vasculitis most commonly occurs as a consequence of drug reactions.

Table 8.24 Classification of vasculitis

Vessels affected	Primary	Secondary
Large arteries	Giant cell arteritis Takayasu's arteritis Isolated CNS angiitis	Aortitis associated with rheumatoid arthritis Infection (syphilis)
Medium arteries	Classic polyarteritis nodosa Kawasaki's disease	Infection (i.e. hepatitis B) Hairy cell leukaemia
Medium arteries and small vessels	Wegener's granulomatosis Churg–Strauss syndrome Microscopic polyangiitis	Rheumatoid arthritis SLE Sjögren's syndrome Drugs Infection (e.g. HIV)
Small vessels (leukocytoclastic)	Henoch–Schönlein purpura Essential mixed cryoglobulinaemia Cutaneous leukocytoclastic angiitis	Drugs (i.e. sulphonamides, penicillins, thiazide diuretics) Infection (e.g. hepatitis B, C)

Pathology

Henoch–Schönlein purpura and cryoglobulinaemia are immune complex deposition diseases. Biopsy of cutaneous lesions reveals a small vessel cellular infiltrate, fibrinoid necrosis of vessel walls, fragmented polymorphonuclear cells and nuclear fragments (leukocytoclasis). The presence of IgA and C3 in vasculitic lesions points to a diagnosis of Henoch–Schönlein purpura. Cryoglobulinaemia results from precipitation of immunoglobulins in the cold, resulting in complement activation and subsequent vasculitis.

Scope of disease

The predominant complication of Henoch–Schönlein purpura is gastrointestinal ischaemia and infarction. This may present as an acute abdomen; however, surgery should be avoided unless bowel necrosis has occurred. Renal impairment may develop if the mesangium is involved. Cryoglobulinaemia may lead to glomerulonephritis, peripheral neuropathy and digital gangrene.

Clinical features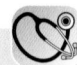

Leukocytoclastic vasculitis often presents with a palpable purpuric rash due to inflammation of cutaneous capillaries. Dependent areas are most commonly affected with a predilection for the anterior aspect of the lower limbs (Fig. 8.18). Henoch–Schönlein purpura presents with abdominal pain, arthritis, rash and occasionally symptoms of renal impairment. Nail fold infarction may occur and bullous skin lesions may ulcerate. Cryoglobulinaemia classically presents with palpable purpura in the extremities, arthralgia and muscle weakness. Other skin lesions include petechiae, urticaria and acrocyanosis.

Initial investigations

Full blood count
Leukocytosis suggests primary vasculitis or infection. Leukopenia is more likely in secondary vasculitis. Thrombocytosis occurs as an acute phase response. Eosinophilia is common following a drug reaction.

Markers of inflammation
An acute phase response is common with a raised ESR and CRP.

Urea and electrolytes
Renal involvement is suggested by an elevated urea or creatinine.

Urinalysis
Urinalysis may reveal haematuria, proteinuria and red and white cell casts (active urinary sediment).

Liver profile
Non-specific changes may be found or elevated transaminases may develop secondary to hepatitis.

Serum autoantibodies
The presence of rheumatoid factors or anti-nuclear antibodies suggests vasculitis secondary to connective tissue disease. Complement levels are usually low in SLE and in infectious causes but are elevated in the primary vasculitides.

Further investigations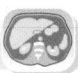

Skin biopsy
Biopsy of affected organs, especially the skin, can help to confirm the diagnosis (Fig. 8.18).

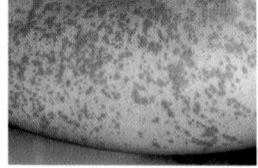

Fig. 8.18 Small vessel vasculitis. Rash of Henoch–Schönlein purpura.

Serum cryoglobulins

Investigation for cryoglobulins requires blood to be kept warm prior to laboratory analysis.

Hepatitis screen

Screening for hepatitis C and malignancy is required in patients who present with cryoglobulinaemia.

Initial management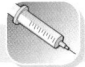

Identification and treatment of underlying cause

An important aspect is the identification and treatment of any underlying or precipitating cause.

Medical management

Immunomodulation

The treatment of small vessel vasculitis, including Henoch–Schönlein purpura, is expectant. Corticosteroids are infrequently required. Systemic involvement of disease responds well to short courses of prednisolone (20–40 mg tapering over 3 months).

Prognosis

Small vessel disease without systemic involvement, including Henoch–Schönlein purpura, has an excellent prognosis.

Medium vessel vasculitis

This group comprises the major necrotizing vasculitides such as classic polyarteritis nodosa, microscopic polyangiitis (microscopic polyarteritis), Wegener's granulomatosis, Churg–Strauss syndrome (allergic granulomatosis and angiitis) and Kawasaki's disease (mucocutaneous lymph node syndrome).

Epidemiology

The onset of these uncommon conditions peaks in the fifth decade of life (except Kawasaki's disease) with an overall annual incidence of approximately 1.5 per 100 000 per year. Specifically, Wegener's granulomatosis is the most common small–medium vessel vasculitis with an annual incidence of 1 per 100 000 per year. Churg–Strauss syndrome is rare and presents more commonly in women and asthmatics. Kawasaki's disease is most common in Japan and principally affects children less than 5 years of age. Medium vessel vasculitis may occur secondary to other illness, especially connective tissue disease.

Pathology

The aetiology of the vasculitides is unknown; however, immune system dysfunction has been well described. Autoantibodies, endothelial cells, T lymphocytes and cytokines all play a role in the pathogenesis. Wegener's granulomatosis, Churg–Strauss and microscopic polyangiitis are also known as anti-neutrophil cytoplasmic antibody (ANCA) associated primary systemic vasculitides. The role of ANCAs in the pathogenesis of these disorders remains unclear.

Wegener's granulomatosis is characterized by the triad of necrotizing granulomata of the upper and lower respiratory tracts and focal necrotizing glomerulonephritis; however, limited forms exist.

Biopsies in Churg–Strauss syndrome reveal the unique feature of eosinophilic granulomas.

In polyarteritis nodosa and microscopic polyangiitis, immune complex deposition leads to a panarteritis. In the acute phase, polymorphonuclear infiltration and fibrinoid necrosis occur. Multiple aneurysm formation is common in polyarteritis nodosa due to disruption of the elastic lamina and arterial dilatation. In the chronic phase of polyarteritis nodosa, narrowing of the vessel lumen occurs due to fibrosis and ensuing thrombosis.

Due to seasonal variation and epidemics of disease, an infective cause for Kawasaki's disease has been sought, however no consistent aetiological agent has been identified.

The entire vessel wall is infiltrated with inflammatory cells with associated thrombosis, aneurysm formation and endothelial proliferation.

Scope of disease

The main complication of small–medium vessel vasculitis is end-organ dysfunction. Wegener's granulomatosis may lead to deafness, severe epistaxis, respiratory compromise, renal failure, saddle-nose deformity, tracheal stenosis and visual disturbance. Churg–Strauss syndrome may lead to severe respiratory illness and neuropathy. Microscopic polyangiitis chiefly affects the kidneys and may lead to renal failure. The complications of polyarteritis nodosa include multiple mononeuropathies, orchitis and renal failure.

In vasculitis secondary to systemic disease, complications of the underlying condition may occur such as hepatitis-associated liver failure. Cardiac involvement in Kawasaki's disease may lead to arrhythmias, myocardial ischaemia and infarction.

Clinical features

General symptoms of systemic vasculitis include fever, malaise, myalgia, arthralgia, weight loss and fatigue.

Specific symptoms of Wegener's granulomatosis include chronic rhinitis, sinusitis, nasal crusting, chest pain, cough, shortness of breath and haemoptysis. Wegener's granulomatosis may be confined to the upper respiratory tract with oral and nasal ulcerations being early findings. The organs affected by Wegener's granulomatosis are the ear, nose (Fig. 8.19), throat, lungs and kidneys.

Patients with Churg–Strauss syndrome may complain of atopy and late-onset asthma as well as shortness of breath

Connective tissue disorders

Vasculitis

Crystal deposition disorders

Arthritis and infection

Osteoporosis and metabolic bone disease

Polymyalgia rheumatica and giant cell arteritis

Miscellaneous rheumatological disease

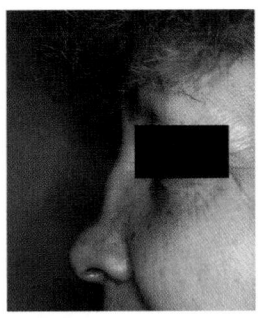

Fig. 8.19 Saddle nose deformity. This deformity is due to cartilage destruction in Wegener's granulomatosis. Courtesy of the Univadis database.

503

and cough. Lung involvement helps to differentiate Churg–Strauss syndrome from polyarteritis nodosa.

Polyarteritis nodosa usually presents with constitutional symptoms, rash, mononeuritis multiplex, arthralgia, hypertension, gastrointestinal upset and orchitis, although any organ may be affected.

Microscopic polyangiitis may present with any of these features, however renal impairment is more common and is usually present at the time of diagnosis. It is distinguished from polyarteritis nodosa mainly by the predominant involvement of small vessels, prominent glomerulonephritis, pulmonary manifestations and presence of p-ANCA.

Kawasaki's disease presents acutely with fever, rash, lymphadenopathy and palmoplantar erythema. Coronary artery disease may occur in any of the small–medium vessel vasculitides, however it is especially common in Kawasaki's disease.

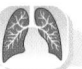

Initial investigations

Full blood count
The presence of leukocytosis suggests primary vasculitis or infection. Leukopenia is more likely in secondary vasculitis. Eosinophilia is common in Churg–Strauss syndrome or following a drug reaction.

Markers of inflammation
An acute phase response is common with a raised ESR and CRP.

Urea and electrolytes
Renal involvement is suggested by an elevated urea or creatinine.

Urinalysis
Microscopy may reveal haematuria, proteinuria and red and white cell casts (active urinary sediment).

Liver profile
Non-specific changes may be found or elevated transaminases may develop secondary to hepatitis.

Serum autoantibodies
Anti-neutrophil cytoplasmic antibodies (ANCAs), identified by immunofluorescence, are directed at antigens in the cytoplasm of neutrophils. Antibodies with cytoplasmic specificity (c-ANCA) are directed at the serine proteinase III (PR3) antigen. c-ANCA is strongly associated with Wegener's granulomatosis and is present in 80% of patients. Antibodies with a perinuclear specificity (p-ANCA) are directed at the myeloperoxidase (MPO) antigen. p-ANCA may be elevated in any of the vasculitides but most commonly in microscopic polyarteritis.

The presence of rheumatoid factors or anti-nuclear antibodies suggests vasculitis secondary to connective tissue disease. Hepatitis B serology is positive in 15% of patients with polyarteritis nodosa.

Chest X-ray
A plain chest film may reveal patchy or nodular infiltrates or extensive interstitial disease, particularly in Wegener's granulomatosis and Churg–Strauss syndrome. Pulmonary lesions may cavitate.

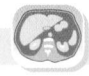

Further investigations

Sinus X-rays
Sinus films may be helpful when upper respiratory tract symptoms exist.

Mesenteric angiogram
A mesenteric angiogram in polyarteritis nodosa may reveal multiple arterial aneurysms and tapered narrowings, however the changes are non-specific.

Initial management

Identification and treatment of underlying cause
An important aspect is the identification and treatment of any primary condition such as hepatitis B or C.

Multidisciplinary approach
A multidisciplinary approach is required in the treatment of patients with small–medium sized vasculitis as multisystem complications can develop in diseases such as Wegener's granulomatosis. Input from various specialists, including ENT, thoracic and ophthalmic surgeons, is required.

Medical management

Immunomodulation
High-dose intravenous or oral corticosteroids are the mainstay of treatment. The addition of cyclophosphamide for patients with small–medium necrotizing vasculitis has greatly improved their prognosis.[1,2]

Cyclophosphamide is usually given as an intravenous pulse monthly for at least 6 months after remission induction with co-administration of corticosteroids. Oral cyclophosphamide is an alternative but is associated with greater toxicity. A course of cyclophosphamide is usually replaced by weekly methotrexate or azathioprine once remission has been achieved. The main side effects of cyclophosphamide are haemorrhagic cystitis and bladder tumours; these are reduced by simultaneous administration of MESNA, an acrolein binding agent. Gonad toxicity is a particular problem for males and women of child-bearing age. Sperm and egg storage should be offered to patients prior to treatment although the success of egg storage is unknown.

In any intensive immunosuppressive protocol, prophylactic treatment against *Pneumocystis carinii* pneumonia should be instituted with co-trimoxazole.

Co-trimoxazole

Limited Wegener's granulomatosis may be treated with co-trimoxazole (trimethoprim and sulfamethoxazole) alone.

Plasmapheresis

Plasmapheresis may be required for patients with Wegener's granulomatosis complicated by pulmonary haemorrhage and severe renal disease.

Intravenous immunoglobulin

Patients with Kawasaki's disease respond very well to intravenous immunoglobulin treatment.

Prognosis

The 5-year survival of polyarteritis nodosa is over 60%. Most deaths are due to uncontrolled vasculitis or complications of therapy. Regular follow-up is required indefinitely as relapse of vasculitis may occur at any time.

i FURTHER INFORMATION

Weyand CM, Goronzy JJ. Medium- and large-vessel vasculitis. New England Journal of Medicine 2003; 349: 160–169.

REFERENCES

(1) Haubitz M, Schellong S, Gobel U, Schurek HJ, Schaumann D, Koch KM, Brunkhorst R. Intravenous pulse administration of cyclophosphamide versus daily oral treatment in patients with antineutrophil cytoplasmic antibody-associated vasculitis and renal involvement: a prospective, randomized study. Arthritis and Rheumatism 1998; 41: 1835–1844.

(2) Guillevin L, Cordier JF, Lhote F, et al. A prospective, multicenter, randomized trial comparing steroids and pulse cyclophosphamide versus steroids and oral cyclophosphamide in the treatment of generalized Wegener's granulomatosis. Arthritis and Rheumatism 1997; 40: 2187–2198.

Large vessel vasculitis

Large vessel vasculitis consists of giant cell arteritis and Takayasu's arteritis (pulseless disease).

Takayasu's arteritis

Epidemiology

The incidence of Takayasu's arteritis is 0.2 per 100 000 per year. The disease predominantly affects Asian women less than 40 years of age.

Pathology

Large vessel granulomatous panarteritis is the hallmark of Takayasu's arteritis, however the aetiology is unknown. The vasculitis principally affects the aorta and its branches.

Clinical features

Takayasu's arteritis commonly presents with non-specific symptoms such as fever and weight loss. Weak or absent peripheral pulses and limb claudication are common due to large vessel occlusion, especially of the upper limbs, which may lead to necrosis and gangrene of the periphery. Other features include hypertension, headache, dizziness, amaurosis, diplopia, exertional dyspnoea and angina.

Investigations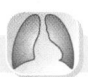

Angiography

Angiography may reveal smooth tapered narrowing, stenosis and aneurysm formation in Takayasu's arteritis.

CT/MRI

These modalities may demonstrate vessel wall inflammation and vessel shape.

Positron emission tomography (PET)

PET is a very sensitive investigation to demonstrate vasculitis and can be indispensable in cases of diagnostic confusion.

Medical management

Immunomodulation

Corticosteroids are the treatment of choice for Takayasu's arteritis; however, high doses are usually required for prolonged periods (40–60 mg of prednisolone) with tapering over 12 months or more. Dose reduction should follow clinical and laboratory response.

Antihypertensive therapy

Antihypertensive therapy (p. 70) is mandatory in Takayasu's arteritis as it is associated with increased morbidity and mortality.

Prognosis

The overall 15-year survival of Takayasu's arteritis is 80%.

Buerger's disease

Buerger's disease (thromboangiitis obliterans) affects medium and small sized arteries of the extremities. The condition almost exclusively affects smokers and may lead to digital gangrene. The mainstay of therapy is abstinence from tobacco inhalation.

Behçet's disease

Behçet's disease is a multisystem inflammatory disorder that is most prevalent in Middle Eastern populations. The disease is characterized by recurrent oral and genital ulceration. Treatment includes the use of corticosteroids, colchicine, thalidomide and other immunosuppressive agents.

Crystal deposition disorders

Crystalline disease is a significant cause of pain and disability. Acute monoarthritis is the chief presentation of this group of disorders, of which uric acid deposition (gout) is the most common variant.

Gout

Gout is an inflammatory arthritis that results from the deposition of urate crystals in or around the joints. Although urate crystal deposition is associated with hyperuricaemia, only one quarter of people with hyperuricaemia progress to develop symptomatic gout (the likelihood is directly related to the duration and degree of hyperuricaemia).

Epidemiology

Gout is a disease principally of middle-aged men in developed countries. The prevalence of gout in the USA and UK is 300 per 100 000 and is increasing. Males are affected 10 times more frequently than women. The incidence in women increases after the menopause as oestrogen has a uricosuric effect.

Pathology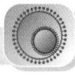

The end product of purine nucleotide breakdown is uric acid. Seventy-five per cent of uric acid is excreted in the kidneys; the rest is lost in the faeces. Uric acid is effectively filtered at the glomerulus, however 90% is subsequently reabsorbed.

Primary hyperuricaemia

Hyperuricaemia is defined as a uric acid level greater than 0.42 mmol/L in men and 0.36 mmol/L in women, and develops as a consequence of under-excretion (80%) of uric acid by the kidney, overproduction (20%) of uric acid, or both. An elevated uric acid level is present in up to 5% of the general population at any one point during adult life

and is related to age, sex, body habitus and genetic constitution. Under-excretion of uric acid accounts for by far the majority of patients with hyperuricaemia, however the reason for this is unclear.

Up to 20% of affected individuals report a family history of the condition. Lesch–Nyhan syndrome is a rare X-linked genetic disorder resulting from the absence of an enzyme responsible for purine metabolism and is characterized by early-onset gout, spasticity, choreoathetosis, mental retardation and compulsive self mutilation.

Secondary hyperuricaemia

Overproduction of uric acid occurs in acquired disorders leading to an excessive rate of cell, and therefore nucleic acid, turnover. These include myeloproliferative and lympho-proliferative disorders, haemolytic anaemias, Paget's disease of bone and psoriasis. Certain medications such as low-dose aspirin, diuretics and ciclosporin alter renal tubular handling of uric acid and can contribute to the development of gout. Diuretics are the main cause of hyperuricaemia but clinical gout is an uncommon association.

Arthritis

Acute attacks of gout occur when monosodium urate crystals are deposited in oversaturated joint tissues. Inflammation occurs as a consequence of ingestion of crystals by polymorphonuclear leukocytes with subsequent release of inflammatory mediators. In a minority of patients gouty tophi develop following multiple episodes of acute gout. Urate crystals in synovial fluid may precipitate de novo or result from rupture of preformed synovial deposits (Fig. 8.20). The histopathology of the gouty tophus reveals a core of monosodium urate crystals surrounded by a chronic foreign body granuloma.

Scope of disease

An acute attack of gouty arthritis may cause significant morbidity as a result of severe pain and subsequent immobility. Tophi may cause joint destruction and neural impingement if the spine is involved.

Renal impairment from unchecked hyperuricaemia may occur, however renal failure is a rare complication. Acute uric acid nephropathy is now exceedingly uncommon with hyperhydration and the prophylactic use of allopurinol prior to chemotherapy. Other renal complications include chronic urate nephropathy and uric acid stones.

Uric acid calculi may develop in up to 10% of gout sufferers, especially in hotter climates. The stones may be

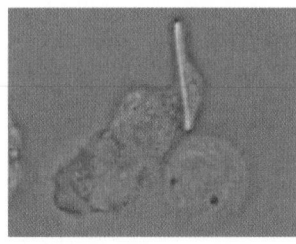

Fig. 8.20 Gouty crystal phagocytosis. An image from high-resolution (×3000) digital videomicroscopy. Courtesy of W Grassi, R De Angelis, A Farina, P Del Medico and the EULAR image database.

radiolucent (uric acid alone) or radio-opaque (combined with calcium salts). Most commonly they are due to overindulgence of purine-rich foods and dehydration. Gout is also associated with several medical conditions and screening for these should be undertaken (Table 8.25).

Clinical features

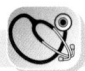

The most common presentation of gout is podagra, i.e. monoarthritis of the great toe (1st metatarsophalangeal joint). However, any joint may be affected—the more frequently affected areas are the feet, ankles, knees, wrists and fingers, and 1 in 10 attacks affects more than one joint.

The pain of gout is excruciating, likened to a vice being maximally twisted around the affected joint. Even the weight of the bedclothes resting on the joint may be unbearable. Without treatment, the attack settles spontaneously in 2–3 weeks. This may be the first and only manifestation of the disorder. In others, multiple attacks are followed by an intercritical phase where the paroxysms are less severe but prolonged. Subsequently chronic tophaceous gout may develop (Fig. 8.21) with tophi being deposited in any joint or bone. Most commonly these occur at the elbow (olecranon bursa), tragus of the ear and extensor surfaces of the limbs.

A detailed clinical assessment includes assessment of the frequency of attacks, precipitating factors (Table 8.26) and screening for associated diseases such as hypertension, hyperlipidaemia, ischaemic heart disease and diabetes.

Fever may develop during an attack, mimicking sepsis, and appropriate investigations are mandatory to exclude the possibility of septic arthritis. Other conditions that may present in a similar way to gout are listed in Table 8.27.

Initial investigations

Full blood count, markers of inflammation

A leukocytosis with raised inflammatory markers (CRP, ESR) frequently develops.

Serum uric acid levels

The blood uric acid level may be raised, normal or even low in an acute attack and cannot be relied upon to help diagnostically. The greater the hyperuricaemia, however, the more likely gout is to develop.

Joint aspiration

Many cases of gout are presumed due to the classic presentation of podagra, however a definitive diagnosis can only be made by demonstrating gouty crystals in joint aspirates.

Table 8.25	Classification of hyperuricaemia
Uric acid overproduction	
Primary hyperuricaemia	
Idiopathic	
Hypoxanthine guanine phosphoribosyl transferase deficiency (Lesch–Nyhan syndrome)	
Phosphoribosyl pyrophosphate synthetase superactivity	
Secondary hyperuricaemia	
Excessive dietary intake of purine-rich foods	
Increased nucleotide turnover (e.g. myeloproliferative and lymphoproliferative disorders, haemolytic anaemias, psoriasis)	
Accelerated ATP degradation: Glycogen storage diseases Severe muscle exertion	
Uric acid under-excretion	
Primary hyperuricaemia	
Idiopathic	
Secondary hyperuricaemia	
Renal impairment Inhibition of urate secretion (e.g. ketoacidosis, lactic acidosis) Enhanced urate reabsorption Drugs (ciclosporin, pyrazinamide, ethambutol, low-dose salicylates) Lead nephropathy Hypertension Hypothyroidism Hyperparathyroidism	
Combined overproduction and under-excretion	
Ethanol abuse	
Hypoxaemia and tissue underperfusion	
G6PD deficiency	

Table 8.26	Precipitants of acute gout
Joint injury/trauma	
Excessive physical exercise	
Alcohol	
Diet rich in purine nucleotides	
Starvation	
Surgery	
Medications: diuretics, initiation of uricosuric agents or allopurinol	
Severe intercurrent illness	

Table 8.27	Differential diagnosis of gout
Acute arthritis	
Septic arthritis	
Other crystalline arthritis	
Traumatic arthritis	
Rheumatoid arthritis	
Seronegative spondylarthritis	
Chronic arthritis	
Nodular rheumatoid arthritis	
Osteoarthritis with Heberden's and Bouchard's nodes	
Xanthomatosis	

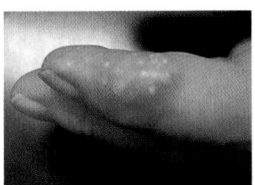

Fig. 8.21 Subcutaneous tophi in chronic gout of the hand.
Courtesy of A Taggart and the EULAR database.

The uric acid crystals are needle-like when viewed under polarized light microscopy and are strongly negatively birefringent (yellow when aligned with the compensator and blue when perpendicular to the polarizer; Fig. 8.20).

Further investigations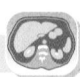

Investigating hyperuricaemia

As gout is associated with other medical conditions, screening for these is appropriate with blood glucose level, lipid profile and blood pressure estimation.

X-ray of the joints

Radiography is helpful in chronic cases as the changes of gouty arthropathy are characteristic with 'punched-out' erosions having sclerotic margins and overhanging edges (Fig. 8.22).

Initial management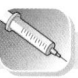

Non-steroidal anti-inflammatory agents

An acute attack of gout is best treated with NSAIDs. Traditionally indometacin (50 mg 4-hourly until the attack resolves) has been the treatment of choice, however any NSAID may be used. A course should last for 1–2 weeks in full therapeutic doses.

Colchicine

If NSAIDs are contraindicated, colchicine is appropriate starting at 0.5 mg 6-hourly followed by dose reduction depending upon response. The use of this medication is limited by its side effect profile. Diarrhoea, which may be explosive, is the most untoward effect; however, this settles upon withdrawal of the drug.

Diet and patient education

Long-term therapy is aimed at reducing hyperuricaemia by decreasing the intake of purine-rich foods (Table 8.28). A high fluid intake is recommended for patients who develop uric acid stones.

Medical management

Other treatments include oral corticosteroids or intramuscular or intra-articular corticosteroid injections.

Table 8.28	Purine-rich foods
Meats	Beef, liver, kidney, sweetbreads, meat extracts, gravy
Seafood	Crustaceans
Vegetables	Peas, beans, spinach, lentils, alfalfa, citrus fruits, tomatoes
Beverages	Beer and beer products

Allopurinol

Preventative treatment with allopurinol is reserved for patients who have multiple attacks of gout (more than 3 per year), for those with tophi and those with renal impairment.

Allopurinol inhibits the enzyme xanthine oxidase, the final enzyme required for the production of uric acid, and is extremely effective at preventing attacks. Successful lowering of plasma urate abolishes the risk of gout and tophi will eventually disappear. The aim is to lower the uric acid as far as possible. Allopurinol is not given in the acute setting as it may precipitate or prolong an attack. It is commenced several weeks following an acute episode concurrently with an NSAID or colchicine for 3 months and then continued indefinitely.

Uricosuric agents

Sulfinpyrazone and probenecid act by blocking renal tubular transport of uric acid, allowing the filtered load to be excreted. They are not as effective as allopurinol and do not help in patients with renal failure. They are rarely used these days.

Treatment of any underlying condition

The treatment of associated and any underlying conditions that would predispose to hyperuricaemia is an important aspect in the management of patients with gout. Obese patients should lose weight, alcohol should be reduced and the need for diuretics be reconsidered.

> **RECENT ADVANCES**
>
> *Etoricoxib, a COX-2 inhibitor, has been found to have comparable efficacy to indometacin in the treatment of acute gouty arthritis and is generally safe and well tolerated.[1]*

Prognosis

With effective treatment the prognosis is excellent and recurrences are limited. Complications such as urate calculi are rare. The main cause of mortality in patients with gout is associated disease such as hypertension, ischaemic heart disease and diabetes.

i FURTHER INFORMATION

Rott KT, Agudelo CA. Gout. JAMA 2003; 289: 2857–2860.

REFERENCE

(1) *Schumacher HR Jr, Boice JA, Daikh DI, et al. Randomised double blind trial of etoricoxib and indometacin in treatment of acute gouty arthritis. BMJ 2002; 324: 1488–1492.*

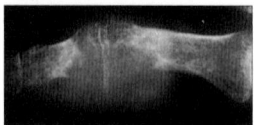

Fig. 8.22 Tophaceous gout. A plain film showing destruction of the second proximal interphalangeal joint. Courtesy of B Manger, Department of Medicine III, and the EULAR database.

Calcium pyrophosphate dihydrate deposition disease and other crystal diseases

There are diseases in which crystals other than uric acid may precipitate in joints and cause arthritis (Table 8.29). The most common of these is pseudogout resulting from deposition of calcium pyrophosphate dihydrate (CPPD) crystals (Fig. 8.23).

Epidemiology

Little has been documented about the epidemiology of CPPD disease. It is estimated to be a third as common as gout, affects men more than women and occurs usually after the sixth decade. Up to 7% of the elderly have radiological change of chondrocalcinosis (calcification of the cartilage, a manifestation of CPPD).

Pathology

The idiopathic form of CPPD is thought to be a localized disease that originates from cartilage. In a minority of patients, CPPD disease is hereditary or associated with metabolic disease (Table 8.30).

A particularly destructive arthritis is 'Milwaukee shoulder' resulting from predominantly calcium hydroxyapatite deposition. This is associated with rotator cuff rupture and glenohumeral arthritis.

Table 8.29	Crystals associated with arthritis
Monosodium urate monohydrate crystals (gout)	
Calcium pyrophosphate dehydrate crystals (pseudogout)	
Basic calcium phosphates, e.g. calcium hydroxyapatite crystals	
Calcium oxalates	
Cholesterol crystals	
Protein crystals	
Steroid crystals	

Table 8.30	Conditions associated with calcium pyrophosphate dehydrate (CPPD) disease (pseudogout)
Hyperparathyroidism	
Haemochromatosis	
Hypophosphatasia	
Hypomagnesaemia	
Wilson's disease	
Gout	
Ochronosis	

Intra-articular corticosteroid injections rarely lead to acute arthritis secondary to steroid crystal precipitation. Less crystalline formulations such as hydrocortisone may be associated with a decreased incidence of this complication.

Clinical features

Pseudogout more commonly affects the knees, wrists and shoulders and occurs in an older age group compared with its uric acid counterpart. Attacks are usually not as acute or severe as gout although the presentation may be identical. Joint sepsis requires exclusion, especially when systemic features such as fever and malaise are present. The presentation of CPPD may be chronic and may mimic non-erosive inflammatory arthritis or inflammatory osteoarthritis.

The features of calcium hydroxyapatite deposition disease are painful, grossly swollen, tender joints with large cool effusions. The shoulder joint is most commonly affected. The management of this disorder is challenging as no therapy has been found to be particularly effective.

Investigations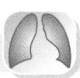

X-ray of the joint

Radiology may be very helpful in demonstrating chondrocalcinosis. The X-ray appearance of calcium pyrophosphate crystal deposition in articular and fibrocartilage is demonstrated in Figure 8.24. This does not confirm acute pseudogout but is rather a marker for the disease. The appearance is best demonstrated in the menisci of the knee, the symphysis pubis and the triangular cartilage of the wrist.

Aspiration of the joint

Definitive diagnosis of pseudogout can only be made by demonstrating rhomboid-shaped crystals in a synovial fluid aspirate. The crystals have a characteristic weakly positive birefringence (blue when aligned and yellow when perpendicular compared with gouty crystals) when viewed under polarized light microscopy.

Screening for underlying disease

Screening for conditions associated with pseudogout with appropriate tests is essential (Table 8.30).

Management

Non-steroidal anti-inflammatory agents

NSAIDs are used as first-line treatment for an acute attack of pseudogout.

Immunomodulation

Intra-articular, intramuscular or oral corticosteroids are effective in most patients.

Prognosis

The prognosis depends on the underlying cause.

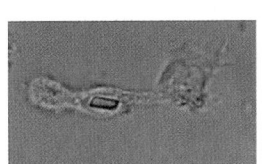

Fig. 8.23 Intracellular crystal of calcium pyrophosphate dihydrate. Courtesy of W Grassi, R De Angelis, A Farina, P Del Medico and the EULAR image database.

ℹ️ FURTHER INFORMATION

Agudelo CA, Wise CM. Crystal-associated arthritis in the elderly. Rheumatic Diseases Clinics of North America 2000; 26: 527–546.

Arthritis and infection

Infection is a common cause of arthralgia and arthritis. Microorganisms may invade joints directly or arthritis may develop following preceding infection at a distant site. A variety of contagions have been implicated in causing arthritis, however the most worrisome is acute bacterial septic arthritis. Irrevocable joint damage and septicaemia may develop if treatment is delayed.

Epidemiology

The incidence of septic arthritis is approximately 10 per 100 000 per year in Western countries. Children under 3 years and adults over 60 years are most susceptible. Both sexes are equally affected.

Pathology

The majority of bacterial arthritis occurs as a result of haematogenous spread. The other main source is contiguous spread from osteomyelitis. Direct inoculation of a joint is very uncommon. The risk of septic arthritis following joint injection is around 4 per 100 000.

Patients with underlying joint disease (e.g. osteoarthritis or rheumatoid arthritis) have an increased incidence of septic arthritis and up to 2% of joint prosthesis become infected over 10 years. The risk factors for septic arthritis are listed in Table 8.31. The most common site for septic arthritis is the knee in adults and hip in children.

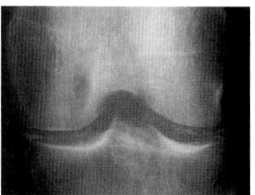

Fig. 8.24 A plain film of the knee showing marked calcifications of menisci due to chondrocalcinosis. Courtesy of B Manger, Department of Medicine III, and the EULAR image database.

510

Table 8.31	Risk factors for septic arthritis
Underlying joint disease (e.g. rheumatoid disease, osteoarthritis)	
Prosthetic joints	
Age <3 years or >60 years	
Diabetes mellitus	
Sickle-cell disease	
Malignancy	
Immunosuppressive disease or therapy	
HIV positivity	
Intravenous drug use	
Joint trauma	
Previous septic arthritis	
Socially disadvantaged	

Staphylococcus aureus and *Streptococcus pyogenes* account for the vast majority of cases. Gram-negative bacterial septic arthritis more commonly affects young children, those with chronic illness and intravenous drug users. *Haemophilus* infection was a common cause in children but has now been overtaken by *Staphylococcus aureus*. Although infrequent, *Neisseria gonorrhoeae* requires exclusion in those who are sexually active. Anaerobic infection is uncommon, however it does occur in diabetics and those with prosthetic joints.

Arthritis develops in up to 10% of patients with meningococcal septicaemia.

Infective endocarditis results in joint manifestations in around 50% of patients. Large joints are most frequently involved.

Fungal infections of joints are rare, however they must be excluded in patients who are immunocompromised.

A number of viridae may lead to arthritis or arthralgia (Table 8.32). Mild polyarticular disease is most common and may occur concurrently with, following or even preceding other clinical features of viral infection. The arthritis tends to resolve spontaneously over days to weeks. Infection with parvovirus B19, responsible for fifth or slapped cheek disease (exanthema erythema infectiosum) in children, requires special mention as it may produce an inflammatory arthritis indistinguishable from rheumatoid arthritis in adults. Evidence of recent infection with development of IgM antibodies to parvovirus may help differentiate the two conditions.

Septic arthritis should be distinguished from reactive arthritis (where an immune-mediated arthritis develops due to an infection that does not involve a joint).

Scope of disease

Failure to treat septic arthritis expediently may result in permanent joint damage or destruction. Unchecked infection eventually causes bony ankylosis.

Clinical features

Septic arthritis most commonly presents as a painful, swollen, tender, red, immobile joint. The features are more

Table 8.32	Viridae causing arthritis
Rubella and rubella vaccination	
Hepatitis A, B, C	
Mumps	
Epstein–Barr virus (infectious mononucleosis)	
Adenovirus	
Arbovirus	
Varicella zoster (chickenpox)	
Parvovirus B19	
HIV	
Alphaviridae	

subtle in patients who are immunocompromised. The only sign an infant may display is refusal to move a limb or general irritability. Fever with rigors may accompany the arthritis. Less than 20% of staphylococcal infections involve more than one joint.

Gonococcal arthritis usually develops within 3 weeks of initial infection and more than one joint is affected in 85% of cases. The small joints of the hand and knees are frequently involved and tenosynovitis is common. An erythematous rash, which may be macular, vesicular or pustular, accompanies the arthritis in one third of patients.

Features of Lyme disease include fever, headache, regional lymphadenopathy, myalgia, meningeal irritation and cardiac involvement.

A flare of inflammatory arthritis (rheumatoid disease, spondyloarthropathy) or crystal disease (gout) can be difficult to differentiate from sepsis, and appropriate investigation is required. Low-grade infection of prosthetic joints may be notoriously difficult to diagnose. *Mycobacterium tuberculosis* must always be considered in chronic disease, especially of the sacroiliac, hip and knee joints. The differential diagnosis of acute septic arthritis is listed in Table 8.35.

 CLINICAL ALERT

Gonococcal arthritis most commonly affects females and homosexual males. The primary infection is frequently asymptomatic. Neisseria gonorrhoeae may be difficult to isolate and special media are required to culture the organism. Repeated joint and blood cultures may be necessary. Once detected, investigation for other sexually transmitted diseases and contact tracing should be implemented.

Initial investigations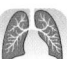

Full blood count
A leukocytosis is present in 50% of cases.

Markers of inflammation
Inflammatory markers (ESR, CRP) are usually elevated.

Table 8.33	Differential diagnosis of acute septic arthritis
Crystal disease (e.g. gout, pseudogout)	
Lyme arthritis	
Haemarthrosis	
Inflammatory arthritis (e.g. rheumatoid arthritis, spondyloarthropathy)	
Joint trauma	
Rheumatic fever	

Synovial fluid aspiration
When there is concern about septic arthritis, immediate synovial fluid aspiration (arthrocentesis) is compulsory. Confirmation of infection depends upon isolation of the organism in joint fluid. Urgent Gram stain may identify a pathogen rapidly as cultures may take days to become positive. The causative organism is identified in synovial fluid in around 60%, if no prior antibiotics have been administered. In addition to microbiological assessment, synovial fluid is sent for crystal analysis and cell count.

Other cultures
Blood cultures should also be procured. Specimens from possible sources of infection should be obtained and cultured (e.g. skin and wound swabs, sputum, throat swab and urine). Special media (Thayer Martin media or chocolate agar) are required for gonococcal detection and sputum, urine and urethral and cervical swabs should also be collected.

Plain X-rays
Plain films of affected joints may show features of pre-existing joint disease and soft tissue swelling.

Ultrasound of the hip
Ultrasound is beneficial for assessment of the hip, revealing joint effusion and capsule thickening, especially in infants and children.

Further investigations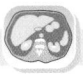

Serology for Lyme disease
If positive for *Borrelia burgdorferi* antibodies, the diagnosis of Lyme disease is confirmed.

Bone scan
Isotope bone scans are required to identify associated osteomyelitis.

Arthroscopy
If the index of suspicion is high, arthroscopic joint washout in theatre is beneficial.

Initial management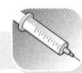

Analgesia
Analgesia is important and the affected joint may require splinting.

Medical management

Antibiotics
Treatment is initiated immediately after arthrocentesis. Intravenous antibiotics are usually given for 2–6 weeks followed by up to 12 weeks of oral therapy (Table 8.34). The

Table 8.34	Initial antibiotic regimens for bacterial septic arthritis
Staphylococcal or streptococcal infection	
Flucloxacillin (up to 2 g 6-hourly) or, if penicillin allergic,	
Clindamycin (0.6–2.7 g daily in 2–4 divided doses. Up to 4.8 g daily for life-threatening infection) plus	
Gentamicin (3–5 mg/kg/day once daily or in divided doses)	
MRSA or *Staphylococcus epidermidis*	
Vancomycin (500 mg 6-hourly) or teicoplanin (three loading doses of 400 mg 12-hourly, then maintenance dose of 400 mg daily)	
In children (*Haemophilus* species)	
Cefotaxime (100–150 mg/kg/day in 2–4 divided doses, up to 200 mg/kg/day in very severe infections)	
Antibiotic therapy is changed according to the sensitivity of the isolated organism and regional differences in bacterial resistance	

usual practice is 2 weeks of intravenous followed by 4 weeks of oral antibiotics. Empirical antibiotics are administered initially (flucloxacillin and gentamicin) and may be changed depending upon organism culture and sensitivity. Microbiological advice is essential as regional variations in bacterial resistance exist. The treatment of Lyme disease is with high-dose penicillin or tetracycline.

Physiotherapy
Once inflammation has subsided, physiotherapy should begin with passive followed by active joint mobilization.

Surgical management

Arthroscopy and washout
Joint washout may be required in the management of joint infection.

Management of infected prosthetic joints
Frequent re-accumulation of synovial fluid, joint damage, associated osteomyelitis and failure to respond to antibiotics within 72 hours are indications for surgical intervention. This may include repeat joint washout, use of antibiotic-impregnated cement and continuous joint irrigation.

Prognosis

Untreated septic arthritis leads to fibrous or bony ankylosis. Up to 50% of patients suffer from some degree of joint dysfunction following infection, however long-term damage is reduced by early therapeutic intervention. The mortality from septic arthritis may be as high as 22%. The poorest outcomes are seen in the elderly, those with severe underlying disease and those whose treatment has been delayed.

FURTHER INFORMATION

Garcia-De La Torre I. Advances in the management of septic arthritis. Rheumatic Diseases Clinics of North America 2003; 29: 61075.

Osteoporosis and metabolic bone disease

Osteoporosis

Osteoporosis is a generalized skeletal disorder characterized by the combination of low bone mass and micro-architectural deterioration of bone tissue. The World Health Organization has defined osteoporosis as bone mineral density (BMD) at least 2.5 standard deviations below the mean for young adult women (Table 8.35).

The consequence of osteoporosis is increased bone fragility with resultant fractures of the vertebrae, femur and forearm most commonly. With an ageing population, the resources required for the management and rehabilitation of the complications of osteoporosis have made this disease an increasingly important public health and economic concern.

Epidemiology

Osteoporosis is a worldwide problem, however the fracture rate varies greatly between different ethnic groups. The incidence of fractures is greatest in whites and Asians and least in black populations. It is estimated that 20% of men and 45% of postmenopausal women have osteoporosis.[1] Hip fracture incidence increases exponentially in older age groups.

Pathology

The skeleton is comprised of cortical (80%) and trabecular (20%) bone and is constantly being remodelled. The process of resorption and formation is necessary to maintain bony integrity and calcium homeostasis. Bone loss results from a predominance of resorption by osteoclasts over formation by osteoblasts. Osteoporosis predominantly affects the more metabolically active trabecular bone (found in vertebrae and metaphysis of long bones) leading to loss of the normal architecture and strength.

Type 1 osteoporosis results from oestrogen deficiency following the menopause or gonadal failure in males. The bone homeostatic balance is disturbed resulting in increased trabecular bone resorption.

Type 2 or age-associated osteoporosis chiefly affects cortical bone. This occurs as bone formation normally decreases during each remodelling cycle. Peak bone mass is achieved by age 30 and thereafter bone is lost at a rate

Table 8.35	WHO definition of osteopenia and osteoporosis*
Disease category	**Bone mineral density**
Normal	Not less than 1 SD below young adult mean value
Low bone mass (osteopenia)	>1 SD below the young adult mean value but <2.5 SD below young adult mean value
Osteoporosis	>2.5 SD below young adult mean value
Severe osteoporosis (established osteoporosis)	>2.5 SD below young adult mean value in the presence of one or more low-trauma or fragility fractures

SD, standard deviation.

* Kanis JA. Assessment of fracture risk and its application to screening for postmenopausal osteoporosis: report of a WHO study group (WHO Technical Report Series 843). Geneva: WHO, 1994.

of about 1% per year with a sharp decline after the menopause. Osteoporosis can also be secondary to medical illness (Table 8.36).

The risk factors for osteoporotic fractures are listed in Table 8.37. The two major determinants are low bone mineral density (as assessed by dual emission X-ray absorptiometry (DEXA) scan) and a previous fragility fracture. Corticosteroid use is the main iatrogenic risk factor for osteoporosis.

Transient regional osteoporosis is a rare condition presenting as monoarticular (especially hip joint) pain and reduced mobility in young to middle-aged patients. Florid osteopenia of the involved joint occurs, and usually settles spontaneously over several months.

Osteoporosis can also occur transiently during pregnancy. The left hip is typically affected. The cause is unknown, however complete recovery usually ensues within 6 months of onset.

Scope of disease

Pain following fracture may be excruciating (although 30% of vertebral crush fractures are asymptomatic). Deformity is common with height loss, increased thoracic kyphosis and abdominal protrusion. A restrictive lung disease picture may develop secondary to a pronounced kyphosis.

Clinical features

Osteoporosis has been described as a silent disease as insufficiency fractures are the only clinical manifestation of the condition. By this time osteoporosis is well established. Vertebral fractures lead to pain, loss of height, abdominal protrusion, and even shortness of breath if restrictive lung disease develops. Neck of femur and Colles' fractures usually result from falls, which are frequent in the elderly.

Table 8.36	Classification of osteoporosis

Primary

Type 1 (postmenopausal)

Type 2 (age-associated)

Idiopathic (at ages <50 years)

Secondary

Endocrine
  Thyrotoxicosis
  Primary hyperparathyroidism
  Cushing's syndrome
  Hypogonadism

Gastrointestinal
  Malabsorption syndrome (i.e. coeliac disease)
  Partial gastrectomy
  Liver disease (i.e. primary biliary cirrhosis)

Rheumatological
  Rheumatoid disease
  Ankylosing spondylitis
  Connective tissue disease (i.e. SLE)

Malignancy
  Multiple myeloma
  Metastatic carcinoma

Drugs
  Corticosteroids
  Heparin

Table 8.37	Risk factors for osteoporosis

Previous fragility fracture

Low bone mineral density

Female

Elderly

Early menopause (age <45 years), nulliparity

Hypogonadism

Smoking

Heavy alcohol intake

Physical inactivity

Thin body habitus

Poor diet

Balance and gait impairment

Hereditary factors (e.g. white or Asian)

Other insufficiency fractures may occur such as pelvic fractures which lead to pain and reduced mobility.

Initial investigations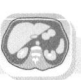

Lateral spine X-rays

Lateral X-rays of the thoracic and lumbar spine, to demonstrate crush fractures, are simple and extremely useful (Fig. 8.25).

DEXA

DEXA has revolutionized bone mass estimation. The indications for bone mineral density testing are listed in Table 8.38. Osteoporosis is defined as bone mineral density of at least 2.5 standard deviations below the mean for young adult women (Fig. 8.26).

Further investigations

Screening for secondary causes

Screening tests for secondary osteoporosis include serum calcium, phosphate, alkaline phosphatase levels, protein electrophoresis, parathyroid and thyroid hormone levels. Estimation of sex hormone levels (testosterone, LH, FSH) is indicated if hypogonadism is suspected.

Initial management

Identify and treat any underlying cause

Apart from the treatment of established osteoporosis and fractures, management should be directed towards any

Table 8.38	Indications for bone mineral density testing
Definite indications	
Oestrogen deficiency states	
Vertebral deformity or radiographic evidence of osteopenia	
Monitoring response to treatment	
Long-term glucocorticoid therapy	
Certain forms of secondary osteoporosis	
Relative indications	
Asymptomatic primary hyperparathyroidism	
Screening for osteoporosis	
Identifying patients with rapid bone loss	

underlying cause. Corticosteroid-induced osteoporosis is a major concern and clinicians should always use the lowest possible steroid dose.

Patient education

Patients should be informed that the condition is 'silent' prior to fracture and life-long therapy is required. A multidisciplinary approach is essential. Physiotherapy is important to maintain muscle tone and bulk, and prevention of falls is an important aspect of the management. Many hospitals have multidisciplinary 'falls in the elderly' clinics.

Medical management

Slowing the disease progression and prevention of fractures are key aspects of the management of osteoporosis.

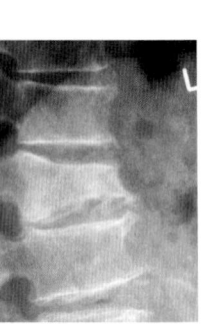

Fig. 8.25 Compression fracture of a vertebral body secondary to osteoporosis.

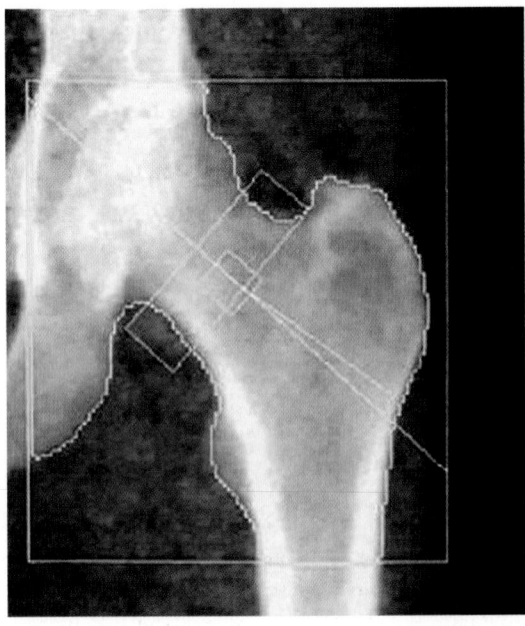
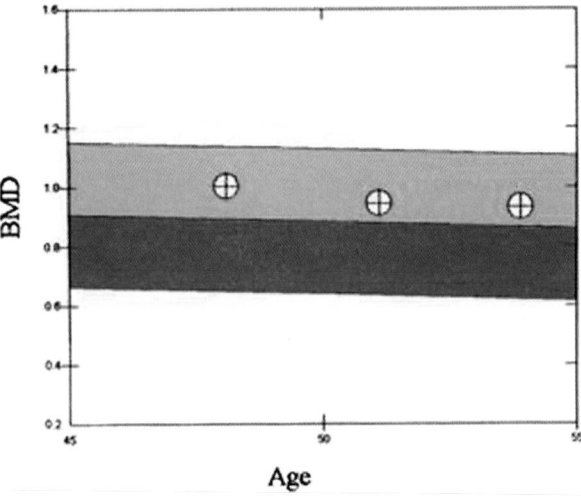

Fig. 8.26 Bone mineral density as determined by DEXA scan: X-ray on left; change in bone mineral density over time on right.

Currently, the approach to the diagnosis and management of osteoporosis is moving away from bone mineral density alone towards early treatment of patients with a significant risk of fracture.[2]

Bisphosphonates

Bisphosphonates (i.e. alendronate, risedronate) are currently the most effective readily available agents for retarding bone turnover. They decrease fracture incidence and increase bone mineral density.[3, 4] Erosive oesophagitis is the main side effect and may be reduced by once-weekly dosing.

Calcium and vitamin D

Calcium and vitamin D supplements are often required, especially in the elderly or housebound.

Hormone replacement therapy

Hormone replacement therapy and selective oestrogen receptor modulators (SERMs) have some benefit in preventing fractures in postmenopausal women.

Calcitonin

Calcitonin has also been shown to be effective in osteoporosis.

RECENT ADVANCES

Recombinant human parathyroid hormone (teriparatide) has been shown to increase spinal and femoral neck bone mineral density and to reduce the risk of vertebral and non-vertebral osteoporotic fractures by 65% and 53% respectively in postmenopausal women when administered subcutaneously once daily.[5] Strontium ranelate has also shown great promise as the first dual action agent for osteoporosis retarding bone resorption and increasing bone formation. This medication significantly reduces fracture risk.[6]

Surgical management

Osteoporotic fractures

Surgical management may be required for patients with established fractures.

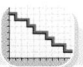

Prognosis

Osteoporotic fractures are associated with increased mortality and significantly reduced quality of life. After 12 months the death rate following hip fracture is 20%. Elderly patients with intercurrent illness have a particularly poor outcome. Loss of independence requires intensive monitoring or long-term care in nursing home facilities.

REFERENCES

(1) *Melton LJ III. The prevalence of osteoporosis: gender and racial comparison. Calcified Tissue International 2001; 69: 179–181.*
(2) *Melton LJ III, Johnell O, Lau E, Mautalen CA, Seeman E. Osteoporosis and the global competition for health care resources. Journal of Bone and Mineral Research 2004; 19: 1055–1058.*
(3) *Cummings SR, Black DM, Thompson DE, et al. Effect of alendronate on risk of fracture in women with low bone density but without vertebral fractures: results from the Fracture Intervention Trial. JAMA 1998; 280: 2077–2082.*
(4) *Harris ST, Watts NB, Genant HK, et al. Effects of risedronate treatment on vertebral and nonvertebral fractures in women with postmenopausal osteoporosis: a randomized controlled trial. Vertebral Efficacy With Risedronate Therapy (VERT) Study Group. JAMA 1999; 282: 1344–1352.*
(5) *Neer RM, Arnaud CD, Zanchetta JR, et al. Effect of parathyroid hormone (1-34) on fractures and bone mineral density in postmenopausal women with osteoporosis. New England Journal of Medicine 2001; 344: 1434–1441.*
(6) *Reginster JY, Seeman E, De Vernejoul MC, Adami S, Compston J, Phenekos C. Strontium ranelate reduces the risk of nonvertebral fractures in postmenopausal women with osteoporosis: Treatment of Peripheral Osteoporosis (TROPOS) study. Journal of Clinical*

Osteomalacia

Osteomalacia (meaning soft bones) is characterized by defective bone mineralization, most commonly due to vitamin D deficiency. In children osteomalacia manifests as rickets.

Epidemiology

Osteomalacia has become uncommon since the realization that exposure to sunlight or vitamin D replacement cured the disorder. Currently those most at risk are Asian women and the housebound elderly.

Pathology

The pathogenesis involves deficiency of vitamin D, altered vitamin D metabolism or disorders of phosphate homeostasis (Table 8.39). Exposure to ultraviolet light (sunlight) results in formation of vitamin D from cholesterol

---

Table 8.39	Aetiology of osteomalacia
Abnormal vitamin D metabolism	

Reduced bioavailability
   Nutritional deficiency
   Lack of sunlight exposure
   Malabsorptive states	

Defective metabolism (hereditary and acquired causes)	
Receptor defects	
Altered phosphate homeostasis	
Chronic phosphate malabsorption	
Renal phosphate loss (e.g. X-linked hypophosphataemia, Fanconi syndromes, oncogenic hypophosphataemic osteomalacia)	
Defective mineralization	

precursors. This is subsequently hydroxylated in the liver and kidney, resulting in the active metabolite 1,25-dihydroxyvitamin D. Calcium and phosphate metabolism is disturbed in the absence of vitamin D.

The result is the accumulation of un-mineralized bone matrix (osteoid), which normally comprises less than 5% of the skeleton, to levels as high as 50%. Osteomalacia is differentiated from osteoporosis by a reduction in the ratio of mineralized bone to matrix.

Scope of disease

Skeletal deformities in children include reduced linear growth, bowing of the legs and the 'rickety rosary' of costochondral junction involvement. In adults bone pain, muscle weakness and stress fractures occur in characteristic locations (Looser's zones).

Clinical features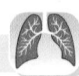

In children, poor skeletal growth, bony deformity and bone pain are the main features. In adults proximal muscle weakness and bone pain also occur and may be severe. This may lead to profound difficulty with mobilization. Incomplete fractures compound the problem.

Initial investigations

Serum calcium, phosphate and vitamin D levels

In nutritional deficiency, calcium, phosphate and vitamin D levels (25-D and 1-25-D) are low.

Liver profile

ALP is usually elevated, being of bony origin.

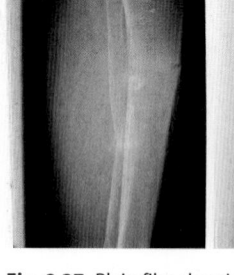

Fig. 8.27 Plain film showing Looser's zone in the anterior tibia with healing pseudo-fractures in posterior tibia and fibula.

Parathyroid hormone levels

In nutritional deficiency, PTH levels are elevated.

24-hour urine collection

Twenty-four hour urine collection reveals reduced calcium excretion and increased phosphate excretion.

X-ray of the tibia and fibula

Plain radiology may reveal Looser's zones which are pathognomonic for osteomalacia (Fig. 8.27).

Further investigations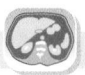

Bone biopsy

If the diagnosis is still in doubt after initial investigations, bone biopsy may be required, with a non-decalcified specimen required for analysis.

Medical management

Calcium, phosphate and vitamin D supplementation

Vitamin D (either calcitriol or alfacalcidol) replacement is essential and is often administered with calcium and phosphate supplements.

Physiotherapy

Initial physiotherapy to improve mobility is important as the response to replacement therapy may take months.

Prognosis

The prognosis is excellent once replacement therapy has been instituted. The deformity in children, however, is irreversible.

Paget's disease of bone

Paget's disease of the bone is a result of the uncoupling of bone resorption and formation, leading to bony overgrowth.

Epidemiology

There is marked geographical variation of Paget's disease. In the USA, Paget's disease has been estimated to affect 3% of the population over 45 years and 10% of those over 80 years of age. It is much rarer in Asian populations, and the disease has only occasionally been reported in Japan. True estimation of the prevalence is difficult as the disease is asymptomatic in many.

Pathology

The cause of Paget's disease is unknown. Hereditary factors play a role as up to 30% of patients have a family history of the disease. Viral infection has been implicated in the aetiology: a virus (resembling the paramyxovirus) has been identified in osteoclasts at Pagetic sites. Infection early in life may lead to the development of hyperactive multi-nucleated osteoclasts. Increased activity of these cells leads to excess bone formation. Histopathology reveals a mosaic pattern as a result of abnormal deposition of cortical bone.

Scope of disease

The manifestation of Paget's disease depends upon the site involved. Neural compression, spinal cord impinge-ment, pathological fractures, secondary osteoarthritis and deafness can occur. High-output cardiac failure may develop due to excessive perfusion of the hyper-vascular bone. Osteosarcoma develops in less than 0.1% of patients.

Clinical features

In the majority the disease is asymptomatic and is identi-fied incidentally on X-rays for unrelated causes. When symptomatic, the clinical features are bone pain and defor-mity, which may be severe. The spine, pelvis, skull, femur and tibia are commonly involved. In the past, when hat wearing was fashionable, patients could be identified by an increase in their hat size. A 'sabre' tibia deformity may develop (Fig. 8.28). The typical leonine facies may occur with Pagetic involvement of the facial bones. Disease of the ossicles or the temporal bone may lead to deafness. Peripheral neuropathies may develop with bony over-growth at the elbow or in the spine. Ataxia, limb weakness and respiratory compromise may occur with base of skull involvement.

Initial investigations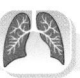

Liver profile

The alkaline phosphatase level (of bony origin) is often elevated and a massive rise in this enzyme may portend the development of osteosarcoma.

Plain X-rays

Plain films are important to identify the characteristic abnor-mality in patients who complain of bone pain. Radiology frequently uncovers asymptomatic disease.

Further investigations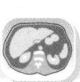

Bone biopsy

Bone biopsy is performed if the diagnosis is in doubt or if osteosarcoma is suspected.

Technetium bone scan

A technetium bone scan may be helpful in estimating extent of the disease.

Medical management

Bisphosphonates

Bisphosphonates such as alendronate decrease bone turnover and have analgesic properties. They are the treat-ment of choice for symptomatic Paget's disease.[1]

Simple analgesics

Simple analgesics such as paracetamol and NSAIDs may be required for bone pain.

Prognosis

The prognosis of Paget's disease is excellent with the intro-duction of bisphosphonate therapy. The risk of osteosar-comatous transformation is exceedingly small.

---

i FURTHER INFORMATION

Drake WM, Kendler DL, Brown JP. Consensus statement on the modern therapy of Paget's disease of bone from a Western Osteoporosis Alliance symposium. Clinical Therapeutics 2001; 23: 620–626.

REFERENCE

(1) *Lombardi A. Treatment of Paget's disease of bone with alendronate. Bone 1999; 24: 59S–61S.*

Renal osteodystrophy

Bone disease is very common in patients with end-stage kidney disease and in those on dialysis. Poor production of calcitriol (1,25 vitamin D) frequently results in secondary hyperparathyroidism and subsequently the bone condition osteitis fibrosa et cystica. Osteomalacia may also compli-cate renal failure. Several other bony abnormalities may occur and bone biopsy is only way to establish a definitive diagnosis.

Polymyalgia rheumatica and giant cell arteritis

Polymyalgia rheumatica occurs almost exclusively in elderly Caucasians and manifests as severe pain and stiffness in the shoulder and hip girdles with a raised ESR. Giant cell arteritis (also known as temporal arteritis) usually occurs in a similar patient population to polymyalgia rheumatica and has a characteristic presentation caused by large vessel vasculitis. It is possible that each represents a polar extreme of the same condition as significant clinical overlap exists.

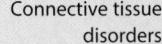

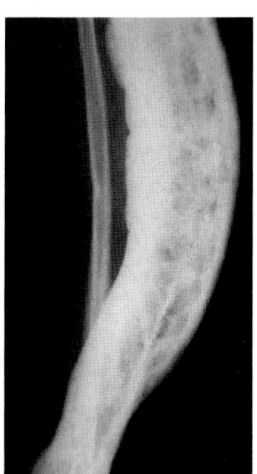

Fig. 8.28 Plain film of Paget's disease with severe sabre deformity of the tibia. Courtesy of W Grassi and the EULAR image database.

517

Epidemiology

The incidence of polymyalgia rheumatica and biopsy-confirmed giant cell arteritis is 50 per 100 000 per year and 18 per 100 000 per year respectively in those over 50 years old. The majority of cases of both polymyalgia rheumatica and giant cell arteritis occur in white females over the age of 60 years. The disease spectrum is exceedingly rare in those less than 50 years, and it is 3 times more common in women as compared to men.

Pathology

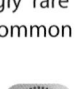

The aetiology of polymyalgia rheumatica and giant cell arteritis is unknown, however the pathological changes are well described. Vasculitis of medium sized arteries and synovitis has been demonstrated in polymyalgia rheumatica. Although the disease often commences with a viral-like prodromal illness, no infectious agent has been isolated.

Giant cell arteritis is a large vessel vasculitis with an inflammatory cell infiltrate, most commonly affecting the temporal arteries. Other vessels that may be involved include the carotid, vertebral, meningeal and rarely the intracerebral arteries and aorta. The principal inflammatory cell present in vasculitic lesions is the CD4+ T lymphocyte. The histological appearance is characteristic with a giant cell infiltrate and disruption of the media and internal elastic lamina. The intima is oedematous and thickened with encroachment on the lumen (Fig. 8.29).

The presence of the MHC class I molecule HLA-DR4 is increased in both giant cell arteritis and polymyalgia rheumatica.

Scope of disease

The main complication of polymyalgia rheumatica is reduced mobility due to pain and stiffness. The most feared and catastrophic complication of giant cell arteritis is sudden-onset irreversible blindness.

Clinical features

Polymyalgia rheumatica usually commences insidiously with bilateral and symmetrical pain and stiffness in the shoulder and pelvic girdles. Stiffness may be pronounced, especially in the morning and after rest. Patients complain of weakness of the arms and legs and difficulty with tasks such as getting out of low chairs and automobiles. On examination, objective signs of reduced power are usually absent.

The classical features of giant cell arteritis are scalp tenderness, jaw claudication (jaw pain whilst chewing food), temporal headache and visual disturbance. The last feature may manifest as blurriness, diplopia, amaurosis fugax and partial or complete blindness. Systemic symptoms such as low-grade fever, lethargy and myalgia are common. Muscles and other soft tissues may be tender and the temporal arteries are often thickened, tender and nodular with reduced or absent pulsation.

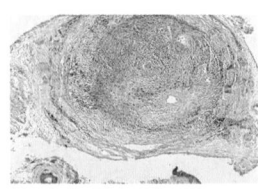

Fig. 8.29 Temporal arteritis. Biopsy of temporal artery showing an inflammatory cell infiltrate and narrowing of the lumen.

Approximately 50% of patients with giant cell arteritis complain of symptoms of polymyalgia rheumatica and up to 15% of patients with polymyalgia rheumatica have evidence of giant cell arteritis on temporal artery biopsy. Classification criteria have been developed for the diagnosis of polymyalgia rheumatica and giant cell arteritis (Tables 8.41 and 8.42). A differential diagnosis of other conditions that present similarly is listed in Table 8.43.

> ### CLINICAL ALERT
>
> *Visual disturbance in giant cell arteritis requires immediate investigation and expedient treatment with corticosteroids. Irreversible blindness is the result of progressive disease and may occur very soon after symptoms develop.*

Initial investigations

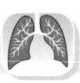

Markers of inflammation

An elevated ESR or CRP is crucial to the diagnosis. However, these may not be elevated in all cases.

Table 8.40	Diagnostic criteria for polymyalgia rheumatica*
Shoulder and pelvic girdle pain which is primarily muscular in the absence of true muscle weakness	
Morning stiffness	
Duration of at least 2 months unless treated	
ESR over 30 mm/hr or C-reactive protein over 6 µg/mL	
Absence of rheumatoid or inflammatory arthritis or malignant disease	
Absence of objective signs of muscle disease	
Prompt and dramatic response to systemic corticosteroids	

*Jones JG, Hazleman BL. The prognosis and management of polymyalgia rheumatica. Annals of the Rheumatic Diseases 1981; 40: 1–5.

Table 8.41	American College of Rheumatology 1990 criteria for the classification of giant cell arteritis (traditional format)*
Age at disease onset ≥50 years	
New headache	
Temporal artery tenderness or decreased pulsation	
Elevation of ESR ≥50 mm/hr	
Abnormal artery biopsies showing necrotizing arteritis with mononuclear infiltrate or granulomatous inflammation usually with multinucleated giant cells	

Diagnosis of giant cell arteritis requires that three of five criteria are present
* Hunder GG, Bloch DA, Michel BA, et al. The American College of Rheumatology 1990 criteria for the classification of giant cell arteritis. Arthritis and Rheumatism 1990; 33: 1122–1128.

Table 8.42	Differential diagnosis of polymyalgia rheumatica
Osteoarthritis, cervical spondylosis	
Rheumatoid and other inflammatory arthritis	
Hypothyroidism	
Fibromyalgia/regional pain syndromes	
Malignancy	
Lymphoproliferative disease	
Multiple myeloma	
Connective tissue disease	
Myopathy/myositis	
Infection	
Parkinsonism	
Bone disease, e.g. osteomalacia, osteomyelitis	
Amyloidosis	
Functional	

Full blood count

Other features of polymyalgia and giant cell arteritis include a normocytic anaemia.

Temporal artery biopsy

Temporal artery biopsy is extremely helpful in patients with symptoms of giant cell arteritis, especially when visual disturbance exists. A specimen greater than 2 cm is required because skip lesions occur. However, therapy should never be delayed whilst awaiting surgery. Positive biopsies not only confirm the diagnosis but are reassuring when recalcitrant cases require prolonged, high doses of corticosteroids and possibly disease-modifying antirheumatic drugs.

Further investigations

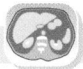

MRI of the shoulder

In difficult cases, MRI of the shoulder girdle displays synovitis of bursal sacs with high sensitivity in polymyalgia rheumatica.

Medical management

Immunomodulation

Corticosteroids are the mainstay of therapy. Polymyalgia rheumatica can be successfully treated with low to medium doses (starting dose 15 mg/day) weaning over 1–2 years depending upon clinical response and ESR, although this may remain elevated in some patients despite adequate treatment. Patients with giant cell arteritis require higher doses (starting dose 40 mg/day) but those with visual symptoms require even higher doses (60 mg/day or intravenous corticosteroids) weaning over months to a maintenance dose.

Patients who require high doses for prolonged periods should have prophylaxis against steroid-induced osteo-

porosis (p. 513). Methotrexate and azathioprine have been used as steroid-sparing agents with disappointing results.

Prognosis

The prognosis is excellent with early and adequate therapy. Prior to corticosteroid use, the prevalence of blindness was 30–60% in patients with giant cell arteritis. Patients should be informed that they may require treatment for 2–4 years or longer. Relapse occurs most commonly in the first 18 months of treatment. About 50% of patients discontinue treatment by 2 years.

i FURTHER INFORMATION

Salvarani C, Catini F, Boiardi L, Hunder GG. Polymyalgia rheumatica and giant-cell arteritis. New England Journal of Medicine 2002; 347: 261–271.

Miscellaneous rheumatological disease

Complex regional pain syndrome

Complex regional pain syndrome, also known as reflex sympathetic dystrophy, Sudeck's atrophy, algodystrophy, causalgia and shoulder–hand syndrome, is an unusual disorder characterized by severe limb pain, oedema and autonomic dysfunction. The syndrome often commences after minor trauma. The pain does not follow a dermatomal distribution and patients complain of allodynia and hyperalgesia. Three recognized phases occur—the acute, dystrophic and atrophic phases—however, not all patients follow this pattern. The mechanism behind complex regional pain syndrome is considered to be abnormal neurotransmission in the central nervous system and local inflammation. Diagnosis of this condition may be difficult and is generally made on clinical grounds. Plain radiographs may show patchy osteopenia. Triple phase bone scanning is specific for complex regional pain syndrome, however its sensitivity varies from 50% to 90%. Treatment involves adequate analgesia and physiotherapy. In more crippling cases, sympathetic nerve blocks and intravenous pamidronate (a bisphosphonate) are useful. Corticosteroids are not beneficial. The condition may last for years.

i FURTHER INFORMATION

Wasner G, Schattschneider J, Binder A, Baron R. Complex regional pain syndrome: diagnostic, mechanisms, CNS involvement and therapy. Spinal Cord 2003; 41: 61–75.

Diffuse pain syndromes

Diffuse pain syndromes including fibromyalgia are a group of conditions manifesting as chronic diffuse pain. The majority of sufferers are female. The hallmarks of fibromyalgia are non-restorative sleep and a lowered pain threshold on palpation. The presence of tender points is part of the diagnostic criteria, however many patients are diffusely tender (Fig. 8.30). Fibromyalgia may be primary or associated with other conditions, especially connective tissue disease such as SLE. Pharmacological therapy involves the use of simple analgesics, NSAIDs and low doses of tricyclic antidepressants (i.e. amitriptyline). Low-grade aerobic exercise including hydrotherapy has been found to be effective.

Table 8.43	The 9-point Beighton scoring system for joint hypermobility*
Scoring 1 point on each side	
Passive dorsiflexion of the fifth MCP joint to 90°	
Apposition of the thumb to the flexor aspect of the forearm	
Hyperextension of the elbow beyond 90°	
Hyperextension of the knee beyond 90°	
Scoring 1 point	
Forward trunk flexion placing hands flat on the floor with knees extended	
Maximum score = 9	

* From Beighton P, Solomon L, Soskolne C. Articular mobility in an African population. Annals of the Rheumatic Diseases 1973; 32: 413–418.

> ### *i* FURTHER INFORMATION
>
> Wolfe F, Smythe HA, Yunus MB, et al. The American College of Rheumatology 1990 criteria for the classification of fibromyalgia. Report of the Multicentre Criteria Committee. Arthritis and Rheumatism 1990; 33: 160–172.

Hypermobility

Hypermobility usually results from excessive ligamentous laxity. Criteria have been developed to aid diagnosis of this condition (Table 8.43). Affected individuals are predisposed to soft tissue injury, especially ligamentous and tendon damage. Hypermobility is seen more frequently in ballet dancers and gymnasts as suppleness is a prerequisite for these professions. The predisposition may be compounded by stretching exercises. Hypermobility is also a feature of the heritable disorders of connective tissue such as Ehlers–Danlos syndrome. Treatment involves avoiding exacerbating activities and physiotherapy for muscle-strengthening exercises.

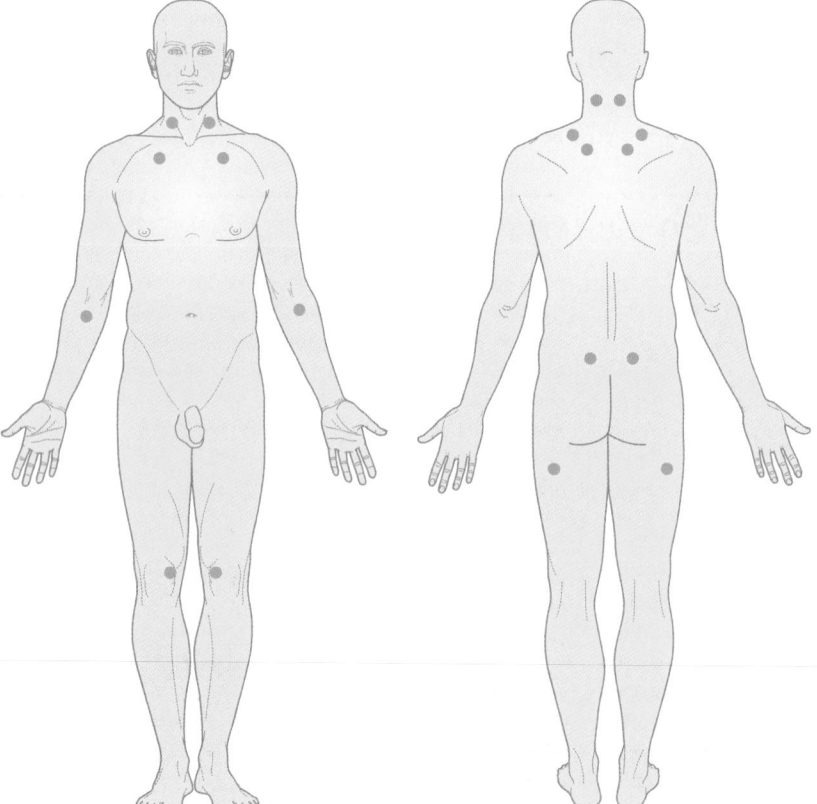

Fig. 8.30 Fibromyalgia tender points.

Osteonecrosis

Osteonecrosis, also known as avascular necrosis of bone, most commonly affects the epiphysis of long bones. The femoral head is particularly susceptible due to its limited blood supply. Several conditions predispose to this disastrous condition and it is a feared complication of prolonged therapy with high doses of corticosteroids. The disease usually presents with severe pain in the affected area. Severe functional loss develops months to years after initial presentation. Characteristic subchondral lucency (crescent sign) is seen on plain radiographs. MRI is much more sensitive than plain radiology and is even able to detect preclinical disease. Treatment of early disease involves analgesia, physiotherapy to maintain muscle strength, and devices to assist ambulation. Core decompression or the use of bone grafts is possible in select patients, however more significant disease requires total joint arthroplasty.

Adult onset Still's disease

Adult onset Still's disease is a rare condition characterized by arthralgia, myalgia, a salmon-pink macular evanescent rash (Fig. 8.31) and high spiking fever. Inflammatory markers such as the ESR and white blood count are invariably raised. A significantly elevated ferritin level is highly suggestive of adult onset Still's disease. The diagnosis is often elusive as patients rarely have the full hand of clinical features and other disorders require exclusion such as infection, vasculitis, granulomatous disease, malignancy and connective tissue disease. Criteria have been developed to aid diagnosis (Table 8.44). Treatment is with full dose NSAIDs initially. Corticosteroids are reserved for more severe disease. The prognosis is favourable; however, some develop a chronic course and require DMARD therapy such as methotrexate.

Table 8.44	Criteria for the diagnosis of adult onset Still's disease*

A diagnosis of adult Still's disease requires the presence of all of the following:
  Fever ≥39°C (102.2°F)
  Arthralgia or arthritis
  Rheumatoid factor <1:80
  Antinuclear antibody <1:100

In addition, any of the following are required:
  White blood cell count ≥15 000 cells/mm³
  Still's rash
  Pleuritis or pericarditis
  Hepatomegaly or splenomegaly or generalized lymphadenopathy

* From Cush JJ, Medsger TA Jr, Christy WC, Herbert D, Cooperstein LA. Adult-onset Still's disease: clinical course and outcome. Arthritis and Rheumatism 1987; 30: 186–194.

Regional joint disease

The shoulder

Disorders of the shoulder may affect the shoulder joint (glenohumeral joint), joints of the shoulder girdle (acromio-clavicular and sternoclavicular joints) or the rotator cuff muscles and their tendons (supraspinatus, infraspinatus, subscapularis and teres minor).

Epidemiology

Many shoulder conditions have an age and sex predilection (Table 8.45). Instability is an important problem: primary anterior dislocation has an incidence of 12.3 per 100 000 per year and a lifetime prevalence of 2%. Epidemiology for other shoulder conditions is lacking as many conditions such as cuff tears may be asymptomatic. Cadaveric studies have shown a prevalence of up to 37 000 per 100 000 for partial thickness and 27 000 per 100 000 for full thickness cuff tears.

Pathology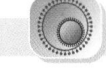

Inflammation

There are three potential locations for inflammation: the joints, the rotator cuff tendons and the bursae (particularly subacromial).

Degenerative arthritis of the shoulder joint may be primary or (more commonly) secondary to injury or disease. Cartilage wear, sclerosis (hardening of the bone), osteophyte formation and the development of bone cysts are characteristics of osteoarthritis, and a thickened contracted joint capsule leads to loss of function (Fig. 8.32). Rotator

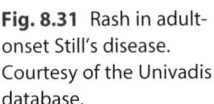

Fig. 8.31 Rash in adult-onset Still's disease. Courtesy of the Univadis database.

Table 8.45	Shoulder diseases by age group			
Infants	**Young adults**	**Middle age**		**Elderly**
Infection	Shoulder instability, particularly males	Impingement and cuff tears in males, frozen shoulder in females		Degenerative arthritis

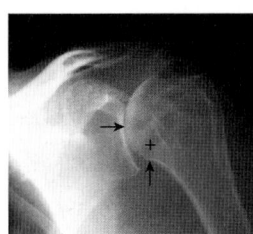

Fig. 8.32 Anterior–posterior (AP) view of the osteoarthritic shoulder. The plain film shows a narrowed joint space and sclerosis (solid arrow), cysts (cross) and superior migration suggesting massive rotator cuff tear (hollow arrow).

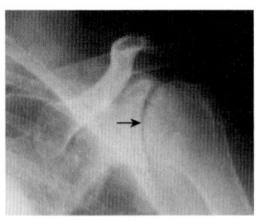

Fig. 8.33 AP view of the rheumatoid shoulder. The plain film shows a narrowed joint space and glenoid (arrow).

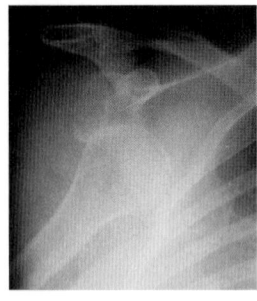

Fig. 8.35 AP view of the shoulder. The plain film shows an anterior dislocation.

cuff arthropathy follows massive cuff tear and leads to superior subluxation of the head with sclerosis of the acromion.[1] The shoulder is affected in up to 90% of rheumatoid patients, with varying degrees of synovitis, erosion and destruction. If severe, there may be medial migration of the humeral head due to destruction of the glenoid (Fig. 8.33).

Acute calcific tendonitis results in deposition of hydroxyapatite crystals (p. 509) in the supraspinatus tendon near its insertion on the greater tuberosity of the humerus (Fig. 8.34). It is thought that the inflammation associated with the resorption of the deposit is responsible for causing the severe pain. There may also be inflammation of the tendon in relation to subacromial impingement. Recently the role of an hypoxic degenerate area near the cuff insertion has been recognized as a factor in the development of cuff tears.[2] These tears may extend and retract causing weakness of the shoulder and rotator cuff arthropathy.

With impingement, the subacromial bursa can become thickened, inflamed and scarred. It has been recognized that the tip of the acromion is often more hooked and prominent in these patients, provoking impingement with abduction of the arm.[3]

Trauma

Anterior dislocation of the glenohumeral joint (98%) occurs following forced abduction, external rotation and extension of the shoulder (Fig. 8.35). The anteroinferior capsule

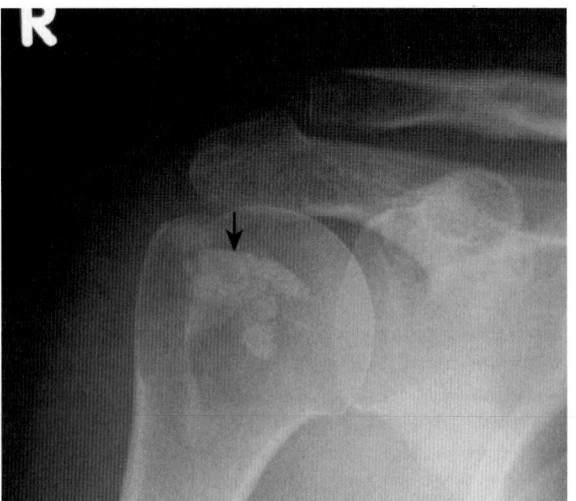

Fig. 8.34 AP view of the shoulder. The plain film shows a large calcific deposition projected over the humeral head (arrow).

and labrum are usually torn off the glenoid, sometimes with a bony fragment (Bankart lesion). There is often an associated rotator cuff tear in middle age.[4] Posterior dislocation is rare (2%) and is associated with epilepsy or electric shock. The forces that cause posterior dislocation often result in damage to the posterior capsule and labrum. Multi-directional instability is usually seen with generalized ligamentous laxity leading to redundant stretched inferior joint capsule. Dislocation may damage the surface of the humeral head and this increases the risk of future instability and arthritis.

Infection

Septic arthritis of the shoulder is rare and is more likely to occur in neonates, the elderly and immunosuppressed patients. Joint destruction and fibrosis can occur without prompt diagnosis and treatment. Sternoclavicular infection may spread to the mediastinum.

Osteomyelitis is also rare, but is most often seen in neonates. Infection can spread from the metaphysis across the growth plate (via vessels that can remain patent for 12 months) and cause damage to both this and the joint. This can result in partial or complete growth arrest as well as destruction of the joint.

Endocrine and metabolic disorders

Diabetes mellitus predisposes to neuropathic arthropathy (a destructive arthritis) probably due to a neuropathy. There is resorption, destruction and fragmentation of the humeral head with soft tissue calcification. This may be painless. Repetitive microtrauma (fragmentation) or hyperaemia (resorption) secondary to autonomic neuropathy may be the underlying cause. Other causes of autonomic neuropathy in the shoulder are syringomyelia and cervical spine injury. Patients with diabetes or thyroid disorders are predisposed to adhesive capsulitis (frozen shoulder), a disorder of unknown aetiology, characterized by contractile fibrosis and adhesions of the anterior capsule.[6]

Vascular

The shoulder is a common site for non-traumatic avascular necrosis. The majority (70%) of cases occur secondary to steroid use. Avascular necrosis is usually bilateral and can manifest as mild resolving necrosis, through to fracture and collapse of the humeral head and ultimately secondary arthritic change.

Neoplastic

The unicameral bone cyst is the most common benign bone neoplasm (20%), of which 67% are located in the proximal humerus. These are fluid-filled cysts with thin sclerotic walls. Approximately 65% of these lesions will fracture and resolve by skeletal maturity, although spontaneous healing can occur. Other primary neoplasms are rare, but secondary metastatic deposits in the proximal humerus are common, often presenting as pathological fractures.

Scope of disease

The shoulder joint is important in positioning the hand about the body for function, working in tandem with the joints of the elbow and wrist. The shoulder girdle provides attachment for powerful muscles. The symptoms of shoulder disease can lead to loss of strength and movement, resulting in difficulties with daily activities such as washing and lifting.

Clinical features

Pain

True shoulder pain is usually experienced anterolaterally over the deltoid. The pain may be localized, diffuse or referred. Localized (point specific) pain usually occurs with trauma or rotator cuff damage. Diffuse pain is usually experienced with arthritis and bursitis. Shoulder pain may be referred down the arm (particularly with rotator cuff pathology). Acute onset of pain may be due to calcific tendonitis or shoulder injury. Precipitating factors are important, in particular the position of the arm (e.g. the painful arc in impingement syndrome).

It is important to remember that shoulder pain may be extrinsic, referred from the cervical spine, diaphragm or apex of the lung, or occur as a result of thoracic outlet syndrome and brachial neuritis.

Stiffness

Some loss of movement occurs with most shoulder disorders, but particularly with adhesive capsulitis.

Weakness

Weakness at the shoulder joint may be muscular (rotator cuff tears) or neural (axillary, suprascapular nerve palsy and brachial neuritis).

Instability

With shoulder instability, patients may feel that their shoulder starts to dislocate in certain provocative positions, usually abduction and external rotation (anterior instability) or across the chest (posterior instability). Minimal trauma causing the first dislocation suggests pre-existing lax shoulder ligaments.

Medical history

As with all upper limb problems, the dominant limb must be established. A detailed history is required to screen for a previous history of trauma and any coexistent disease (rheumatoid arthritis, diabetes). Occupation is important (overhead workers are predisposed to the symptoms of impingement or instability).

An orthopaedic examination is performed as follows:

Examination

Look

The patient should be undressed to the waist. Inspection provides a lot of information. Surgical scars are usually anterior, and wasting of the deltoid is also best appreciated anteriorly. Wasting of the rotator cuff muscles is seen posteriorly. Swelling is unusual, but may be seen anteriorly with an inflamed bursa or arthritis. Medial migration of the rheumatoid shoulder and anterior dislocations cause a 'squared-shoulder' appearance with marked prominence of the acromion.

Feel

Warmth over the shoulder joint may be indicative of infection or inflammation. Tenderness over an arthritic glenohumeral joint is best elicited posteriorly. Tenderness beneath the anterolateral acromion occurs with impingement and cuff tears. Acromioclavicular joint pathology will cause localized tenderness over this joint.

Move

Movement in both shoulders should be compared, both active and passive. Careful assessment will provide the diagnosis in a majority of cases. When assessing elevation of the arm, the scapula must be observed or palpated to determine its 'rhythm' (approximately one third of the movement should occur between the scapula and the thoracic wall). Crepitus with movement is common with an arthritic joint. If active and passive movements are equally reduced, particularly external rotation, then a diagnosis of frozen shoulder is likely. Greater passive than active motion is common with rotator cuff pathology and the arm will usually fall when released with a massive cuff tear ('drop sign'). A painful arc with active elevation (usually 60–120°) is the classic finding with impingement, and this pain can be eradicated by injecting the subacromial space with local anaesthetic.[5] Strength of the rotator cuff muscles should be tested as weakness could signify a tear. Weakness from nerve palsy can be difficult to distinguish but suprascapular nerve palsy will leave subscapularis unaffected (internal rotation) and axillary nerve palsy will affect only deltoid (wasting) and often give numbness over the regimental badge area. Pseudoparalysis (reluctance to use the limb) may be the only clue to the diagnosis of septic arthritis in an infant.

Special tests

These are mainly designed to diagnose instability. Apprehension can be induced by placing the shoulder in abduction and external rotation for anterior instability, and in flexion and adduction for posterior instability. The apprehension or discomfort can be reduced by pushing the humeral head posteriorly or anteriorly respectively, reducing the provoked subluxation. In multidirectional instability the shoulder will sublux inferiorly with traction on the arm (sulcus sign) and can usually be pushed both anteriorly and posteriorly with respect to the glenoid (drawer test). Generalized joint laxity should also be assessed as it is commonly found with multidirectional instability: hyper-extension of elbows, knees and metacarpophalangeal joints of fingers, opposing the thumb to the ipsilateral forearm and placing palms of hands on the floor with knees extended.

Initial investigations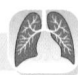

Shoulder X-rays

The standard views are anterior–posterior (AP) and axillary. The AP view will demonstrate calcific deposits in the supraspinatus tendon and the pathological changes in arthritis (subchondral sclerosis, marginal osteophytes and cysts for osteoarthritis; periarticular osteoporosis, erosions and subluxation for rheumatoid arthritis). Superior head migration occurs with massive rotator cuff tear, and associated osteoarthritic changes affecting the acromion and superior head suggest cuff arthropathy (Fig. 8.36). The axillary view can demonstrate subluxation or dislocation not appreciated on the AP view (particularly posterior dislocation) and may demonstrate a glenoid or tuberosity fracture.

Further investigations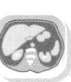

Full blood count, erythrocyte sedimentation rate/C-reactive protein

Inflammatory markers and white cell count are usually raised in the presence of infection.

Ultrasound of the shoulder

This is the first line of investigation in most units if a cuff tear is suspected. There is good sensitivity and specificity for full thickness tears but not for partial tears. Effusions and synovitis can also be identified. Ultrasound can be useful for accurate placement of injections in calcific tendonitis and can guide joint aspiration with suspected infection.

MRI of the shoulder

MRI is the first choice in suspected capsulolabral injury following a dislocation but has similar accuracy to ultrasound for cuff tears. MRI is the most accurate investigation for bone marrow abnormalities such as avascular necrosis.

Nerve conduction studies

Nerve conduction studies may be useful in cases of suspected axillary or suprascapular nerve palsy, or for distinguishing pain referred from the neck.

Initial management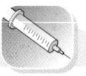

Patient education

Many shoulder conditions will respond to a period of rest, and inflammatory problems may benefit from the application of heat or ice.

Analgesia

Standard analgesics including NSAIDs can prove useful for most painful shoulder conditions.

Corticosteroids

Targeted injections of steroid can improve symptoms of impingement, rheumatoid arthritis and adhesive capsulitis.

Physiotherapy

Physiotherapy is used in the treatment of frozen shoulder and can also help with impingement. It can help preserve motion and strength in the arthritic shoulder. Specific strengthening and proprioceptive retraining of the rotator cuff is the first line of treatment after dislocation.

Surgical management

Arthrodesis (shoulder fusion)

Arthrodesis is an uncommon operation but can still be of value as a salvage procedure following septic arthritis with joint destruction or severe cuff arthropathy.

Shoulder replacement

This involves replacement of the humeral head and often the glenoid (Fig. 8.37). It is an option for patients with severe shoulder arthritis except those due to neuropathic or post-infective causes and those with massive cuff tears. Best results have been obtained in patients with osteoarthritis and low-grade rheumatoid arthritis, up to 95% reporting satisfactory or excellent results.[7] The worst results occurred when treating advanced rheumatoid or cuff tear arthropathy, and in revision replacement surgery.

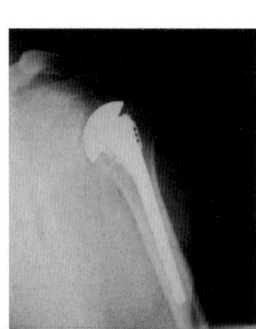

Fig. 8.37 AP view of a total shoulder replacement.

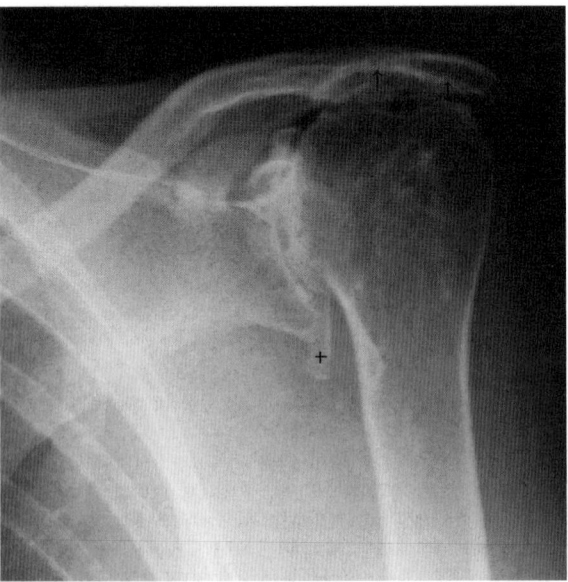

Fig. 8.36 AP view of the shoulder. The plain film shows a mixed picture of osteoarthritis and rheumatoid disease, demonstrating an inferior osteophyte (cross), a narrowed gleno-humeral space due to cuff tear (longer arrow) and acromial erosion (shorter arrow).

Specific conditions

Osteoarthritis/avascular necrosis

Once symptoms of pain are severe, shoulder replacement can be considered but whilst pain is relieved, restoration of range of movement is more unpredictable.

Rheumatoid arthritis

If general rheumatoid treatment is failing, surgical synovectomy of the shoulder joint and subacromial bursa can be performed. This should be done in early disease, and whilst good pain relief and functional improvement are seen, disease progression is not halted. Ultimately shoulder replacement is often required.

Calcific tendonitis

Extracorporeal shockwave therapy has been advocated by some to be beneficial for calcific tendonitis.[8] 'Needling' the deposit and injecting local anaesthetic can also speed up recovery.

Impingement and cuff tears

Following the general measures above, steroid injections can be beneficial when there is an element of inflammation (subacromial). Recalcitrant symptoms warrant surgical decompression and cuff repair. The former can be performed arthroscopically but the latter usually requires an open procedure. Decompression alone gives a 95% chance of relieving the pain of impingement. Small cuff tears require symptomatic treatment only. Larger tears warrant surgical repair but a re-rupture rate of up to 50% exists. If treated early (particularly in younger groups) satisfaction is usually high.

Shoulder instability

Following primary dislocation and reduction, an initial period of 3 weeks rest in a sling is followed by physiotherapy aimed at strengthening the rotator cuff and the scapular stabilizers (dynamic stability). There is a recurrence rate of up to 80% for anterior dislocation in patients less than 20 years. Patients in this group (in particular overhead athletes or workers) may require surgical stabilization. Repair of the torn capsule and labrum can be performed open (with up to 11% recurrence) or arthroscopically (up to 50% recurrence) with the latter preserving more external rotation.[9] Posterior and multidirectional instability rarely require surgical intervention.

Adhesive capsulitis

The natural history of this condition is of resolution but this can take over 3 years. Physiotherapy is the initial treatment and may be more effective following an injection of steroid to the shoulder joint. Manipulation of the joint under general anaesthetic can break the adhesions restricting movement. More recently there is a trend towards arthroscopic division of these adhesions, however there have been no randomized trials comparing this to the natural history of the condition.[10]

Septic arthritis

Urgent washout of the joint is required. This may be performed arthroscopically and often needs repeating. Once a sample of fluid for culture is obtained, broad-spectrum intravenous antibiotics are commenced. These are converted to oral once clinical improvement is noted. Specific antibiotics are commenced following the culture report and a total course of 6 weeks is required.

REFERENCES

(1) *Neer CS, Craig EV, Fukada H. Cuff tear arthropathy. Journal of Bone and Joint Surgery 1983; 65A: 1232–1244.*
(2) *Uhthoff HK, Sarkar K. Calcifying tendonitis. In: Rockwood CA, Matsen FA (eds) The shoulder. Philadelphia: WB Saunders, 1990.*
(3) *Bigliani LU, Ticker JB, Flatow EL, et al. The relationship of acromial architecture to rotator cuff disease. Clinics in Sports Medicine 1991; 10: 823–838.*
(4) *Neviaser RJ, Neviaser TS, Neviaser JS. Concurrent rupture of the rotator cuff and anterior dislocation of the shoulder in the older patient. Journal of Bone and Joint Surgery 1988; 70A: 1308–1311.*
(5) *Bunker TD, Anthony PP. The pathology of frozen shoulder. Journal of Bone and Joint Surgery 1995; 77B: 677–683.*
(6) *Neer CS, Welsh RP. The shoulder in sports. Orthopaedic Clinics of North America 1977; 8: 583–591.*
(7) *Neer CS. Glenohumeral arthroplasty. In: Neer CS (ed.) Shoulder reconstruction. Philadelphia, WB Saunders, 1990: pp. 143–271.*
(8) *Rompe J D, Zoellner J, Nafe B, Shock wave therapy versus conventional surgery in the treatment of calcifying tendinitis of the shoulder. Clinical Orthopaedics and Related Research 2001; 387: 72–82.*
(9) *Conboy VB. Instability of the glenohumeral joint. In: Bulstrode C et al (eds) Oxford Textbook of orthopaedics and trauma. Oxford: Oxford University Press, 2002: pp. 704–721.*
(10) *Chabler AFW, Carr AJ. The role of surgery in frozen shoulder. Journal of Bone and Joint Surgery 2003; 85B: 6, 789–795.*

The elbow

The elbow joint is a common site of injury. Chronic symptoms including pain, stiffness and instability can follow. A range of inflammatory conditions affect the elbow joint and surrounding structures. Nerve entrapment about the elbow is also a common cause of disability.

Epidemiology

The age-related diseases of the elbow are listed in Table 8.46. Many elbow conditions are associated with repetitive occupational and sporting activities.

Lateral epicondylitis (tennis elbow) has a prevalence of 1–3% in the general population but has a peak in the fourth decade with 10% of women and 19% of men affected. Approximately 50% of tennis players over 30 years are affected. Men in heavy manual work with impact loading are more likely to suffer with elbow osteoarthritis. The prevalence in the general population is 3.5%.[1]

Table 8.46	Diseases of the elbow by age group			
Children		**Young adults**	**Middle age**	**Elderly**
Fractures, which may lead to subsequent deformity with growth		Instability	Epicondylitis Arthritis Bursitis	Arthritis Nerve entrapment

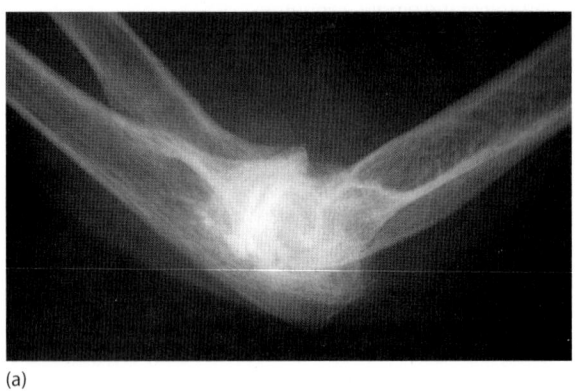 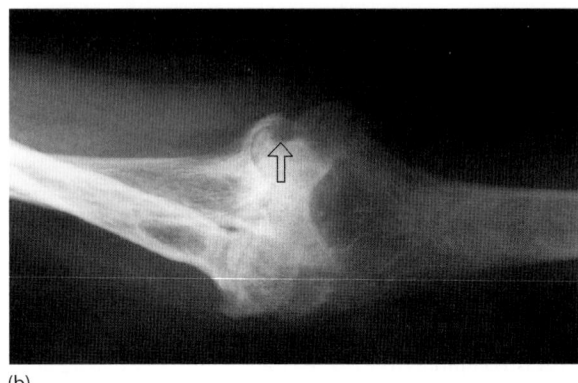

(a)   (b)

Fig. 8.38a, b (a) A lateral view of the rheumatoid elbow showing complete loss of joint space; (b) an AP view showing a large medial erosion.

Pathology

Infection
Osteomyelitis and septic arthritis of the elbow are rare. Inadvertent placement of intravenous needles in drug addicts may provoke a septic arthritis and prompt diagnosis and treatment are required to prevent joint damage and fibrosis. Infection of the olecranon bursa is common. Approximately 30% of all inflamed olecranon bursae are septic and there is an association with diabetes and alcoholism.[2]

Inflammation
Non-septic olecranon bursitis can be either traumatic (repetitive occupational trauma) or inflammatory. The latter group includes rheumatoid and the crystal arthropathies (gout and pseudogout). There is generally less inflammation and pain than in the septic cases.

Epicondylitis can be either medial (golfer's elbow) or lateral (tennis elbow). The pathological changes are the same and result from angiofibroblastic hyperplasia.[3] Normal tendon fibres are disrupted and torn: most commonly extensor carpi radialis brevis (lateral) and pronator teres/flexor carpi radialis (medial) are involved.

Osteoarthritis is frequently seen in the radio-capitellar joint. There is often a history of trauma to the elbow. Osteophytes may cause elbow impingement or detach and end up as a loose body in the joint.

Rheumatoid disease has many pathological manifestations about the elbow. Synovitis may spread from the joint to communicate with the olecranon bursa or can form cysts within the bone or the anterior soft tissues. The ulnar nerve can become compressed. There is both erosion of bone (Fig. 8.38a and b) and soft tissue calcification (particularly the medial collateral ligament). Ultimately the elbow may become a flail joint with fracture or dislocation. Rheumatoid nodules are also common over the olecranon.

After the knee, the elbow is the most common joint to develop arthropathy from haemophilia. Recurrent haemarthroses lead to synovitis and arthritis.

Trauma
Chronic instability of the elbow joint may follow acute dislocation, repetitive activity (overhead throwing in particular) or rheumatoid arthritis. The elbow is the second most common joint in adults to dislocate and up to 35% of patients suffer long-term instability.[4]

An important complication following elbow trauma is heterotopic ossification. Trabecular bone forms in haematoma, ligament, capsule or striated muscle (myositis ossificans), resulting in significant loss of movement. This can occur after burns, major trauma and head injury.

Loose bodies
Fragments of the joint surface can detach following trauma or local ischaemia (osteochondritis dissecans). The latter usually affects the capitellum in male adolescents. Degenerative arthritis will frequently lead to loose fragments in the joint. Synovial chondromatosis is a condition characterized by benign synovial metaplasia and hundreds of loose cartilaginous or bony loose bodies. These often return after removal.

Scope of disease

The elbow controls both the distance (flexion/extension) of the hand from the body and the position (supination/pronation). Combined with wrist and shoulder movement, normal function is essential for feeding and personal hygiene. The functional range required for most daily tasks has been measured as 30–130° of flexion and 100° of rotation (split equally between pronation and supination). Loss of flexion and supination are most disabling, although pronation is essential for keyboard operators.

Clinical features

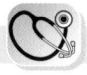

Pain

The location of pain about the elbow can help with differential diagnosis (Table 8.47), but pain can also be referred to the elbow from the neck, shoulder or wrist.

Stiffness

This is commonly seen after trauma and degenerative or inflammatory arthropathies.

Instability

Instability may follow acute injury or arise insidiously from sports or occupational injuries (particularly throwing and overhead activity). It can also occur with an inflammatory arthropathy.

Locking

Intermittent restriction of movement is suggestive of a loose body, and this can occur with or without pain.

Medical history

It is important to establish dominance, occupation, history of injury and presence of coexistent disease, particularly an arthropathy. There may be a family history of inflammatory arthropathy.

Examination

Look

Both upper limbs should be fully exposed. The carrying angle of the elbow is assessed in full extension, with supination of the forearm. This should approximate to 10° in men and 13° in women. Measurement may be inaccurate with fixed flexion deformity or loss of supination. Abnormal attitude or deformity may be due to trauma, arthropathy or rarely congenital. Rheumatoid nodules or a swollen olecranon bursa may be seen on the extensor aspect. An elbow effusion is best appreciated on the lateral side in the triangular area bounded by the lateral epicondyle, radial head and the olecranon tip.

Feel

Careful palpation is performed following the surface anatomy of the elbow. Tenderness of the lateral and medial epicondyles or the adjacent common extensors/flexors is suggestive of epicondylitis. The radial head is palpated just distal to the lateral epicondyle while rotating the forearm to detect its movement. Tenderness here would suggest an arthropathy. The olecranon bursa is palpated posteriorly and may be tender without much swelling. Finally the ulnar nerve is palpated in its groove. Tinel's tap over the nerve may demonstrate compression with replication of symptoms in the forearm and hand.

Move

The normal flexion arc ranges from 15° of hyperextension to 145° of flexion. The limit of supination is 85° and that of pronation is 75°. Feel for crepitus in the joint with movement as this may suggest an arthropathy.

Test for lateral epicondylitis

Causes of lateral elbow pain may be determined by location of tenderness. Resisted wrist extension with the wrist flexed and pronated and the elbow extended can reproduce pain with lateral epicondylitis.

Test for medial epicondylitis

Medial epicondylitis symptoms can be reproduced by resisting wrist flexion with the wrist pronated and extended and the elbow extended.

Assessment of the radial nerve

Weakness of wrist and finger (at MCP joint) extension may be present with radial nerve entrapment, and pain may be provoked while resisting supination with the elbow extended.

Tinel's test

A positive Tinel's test with wasting and weakness of the small muscles of the hand may be present with ulnar nerve entrapment.

Table 8.47	The location of pain associated with elbow pathology	
Medial	**Lateral**	**General/combination**
Medial epicondylitis	Lateral epicondylitis	Osteoarthritis
Ulnar nerve entrapment (± neurological symptoms distally)	Radial nerve entrapment (± neurological symptoms distally)	Rheumatoid disease
Medial chronic instability (particularly throwers)	Radiocapitellar arthritis	Infection

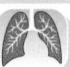

Initial investigations

Plain X-rays

The standard views are AP and lateral. Plain films may demonstrate the presence of arthropathy in the joint. This may be localized to either the radiocapitellar or the humeroulnar compartments. Loose bodies may be apparent if calcified. Rheumatoid changes can be classified according to Larsen (Table 8.48).

Calcification around the epicondyles can be seen in up to 20% of patients undergoing surgery for epicondylitis. The lateral X-ray may demonstrate an elbow effusion with the anterior or posterior fat pads lifting away from the coronoid and olecranon fossae respectively (Fig. 8.39).

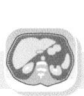

Further investigations

Full blood count/markers of inflammation

If infection is suspected, inflammatory markers (CRP/plasma viscosity) and white count should be obtained. These may also be deranged with active inflammation.

Ultrasound of the elbow

The uses of ultrasound are limited about the elbow, but it can help if effusion is difficult to detect clinically and may allow aspiration under guidance. An aspirate may help diagnose a crystal arthropathy or infection.

CT of the elbow

CT is generally reserved for fractures. An arthrogram can also be performed with CT/MRI if loose bodies are suspected.

MRI of the elbow

MRI may demonstrate the location of osteochondritis and any inflammation within the common extensor or flexor muscle origins in epicondylitis.

Nerve conduction studies

Neurophysiology studies may prove invaluable in the diagnosis of nerve entrapment about the elbow or suspected referred pain from the neck or brachial plexus. However, radial nerve entrapment can be present despite normal neurophysiology results.

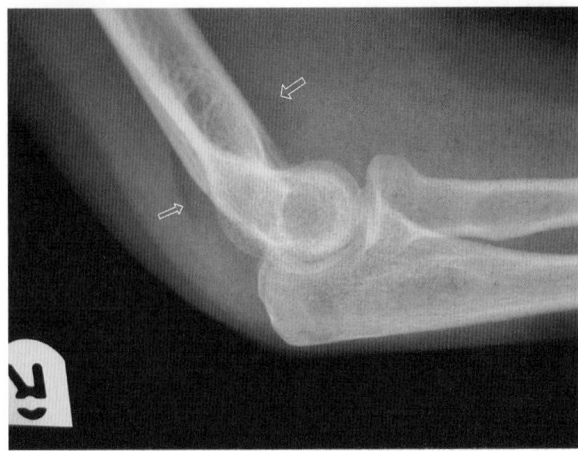

Fig. 8.39 A lateral view of the elbow showing displaced anterior and posterior fat pads, pathognomic of an elbow effusion (synovial fluid, blood, pus, etc.).

Initial management

Patient education

Many elbow problems can be helped by rest and modification of activities. This may require an occupational change.

Simple analgesia

Most elbow pathology produces pain, and analgesia should be considered. NSAIDs can be particularly helpful for the inflammation associated with bursitis, epicondylitis and arthropathy. Steroid injection can also be considered for these conditions.

Physiotherapy

This has a role to play in most elbow conditions although its effectiveness varies.

Surgical management

General
Arthrodesis

This is rarely performed because of subsequent functional limitations. Good movement of the ipsilateral shoulder and contralateral elbow are vital. The usual position of fusion is in flexion, allowing the hand to reach the mouth. Severe destruction as seen with tuberculosis or haemophilia may be an indication.

Arthroplasty

Joint replacement is an option for advanced degenerative or inflammatory arthropathy (Fig. 8.40a and b). The results are poorer for post-traumatic arthritis than for rheumatoid with 5-year implant survival rates of 53% and 84% respectively. This reflects the level of physical activity and demand in these patient groups.

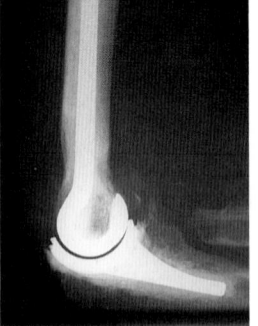

(a)

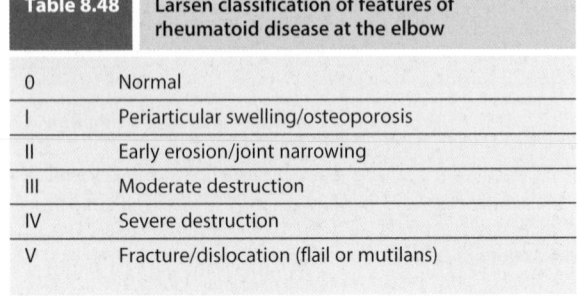

(b)

Fig. 8.40a, b (a) AP and (b) lateral views of an elbow replacement.

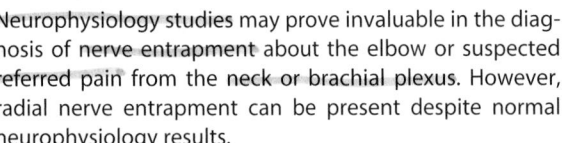

Table 8.48	Larsen classification of features of rheumatoid disease at the elbow
0	Normal
I	Periarticular swelling/osteoporosis
II	Early erosion/joint narrowing
III	Moderate destruction
IV	Severe destruction
V	Fracture/dislocation (flail or mutilans)

Specific

Epicondylitis

Approximately 90% of the symptoms from lateral epicondylitis resolve within 2 years following non-surgical measures. Frictional physiotherapy, counterforce braces (which prevent full muscular contraction force reaching the epicondyles), NSAIDs and steroid injections all play a part. Extracorporeal shockwave therapy was initially heralded as beneficial but more recent evidence suggests no benefit over placebo.[5] Refractory cases may require surgical release of the common extensors/flexors with a predicted satisfactory outcome of 80–100%.

Osteoarthritis

Analgesia, steroid injections, splints and physiotherapy are initial options for management. Surgical debridement of impinging osteophytes and loose bodies usually provides symptomatic improvement. For patients with severe symptoms, joint replacement can be considered with caution, as up to 50% may have problems such as loosening or implant failure by 5 years.[6]

Rheumatoid disease

Medical management of the rheumatoid arthritis, steroid injections and braces should all be considered before surgical options. The three main symptoms are stiffness, instability and pain. The latter is the strongest indication for surgery. Synovectomy and radial head excision can give initial pain relief in 70–90% of cases, but deterioration occurs with time. Joint replacement can offer good results in 80–90% of cases at up to 5 years but there is less information about the longer term.[7] Infection remains a problem with many patients receiving immunosuppressants. Revision of joint replacement for loosening or infection is still regarded as highly challenging.

Non-infective bursitis

Aspiration followed by protective padding and bandaging to the elbow is the initial management. NSAIDs can hasten resolution but steroid injection carries a high complication rate with 12% developing infection and 20% subdermal atrophy. Excision is reserved for chronic cases because of the risk of wound breakdown.

Infection

The principles of management have already been laid out in the section on the shoulder (p. 524). It is possible to wash out the elbow joint arthroscopically. Infective olecranon bursitis requires aspiration, elevation and antibiotics, and if not resolving may need incising and draining. With chronic infection the bursa may need to be completely excised.

REFERENCES

(1) Stanley D. Prevalence and etiology of symptomatic elbow osteoarthritis. Journal of Shoulder and Elbow Surgery 1994; 3: 386–389.
(2) McNab ISH. Bursitis of the elbow. In: Bulstrode C et al (eds) The Oxford Textbook of orthopaedics and trauma. Oxford: Oxford University Press, 2002, pp. 810–814.
(3) Nirschl RP, Pettrone F. Tennis elbow—the surgical treatment of lateral epicondylitis. Journal of Bone and Joint Surgery 1979; 61A: 832–839.
(4) Mehlhoff TL, Noble PC, Bennett JB, Tullos HS. Simple dislocation of the elbow in the adult. Journal of Bone and Joint Surgery 1988; 70A: 244–249.
(5) Melikyan EY, Shahin E, Miles J, Bainbridge L C. Extracorporeal shockwave treatment for tennis elbow. Journal of Bone and Joint Surgery 2003; 85B: 6, 852–855.
(6) Kraay MJ, Figgie MP, Inglis AE, Wolfe SW, Ranawat CS. Primary semiconstrained total elbow arthroplasty. Journal of Bone and Joint Surgery 1994; 76B: 636–640.
(7) Rymaszewski LA. Rheumatoid arthritis of the elbow. In: Bulstrode C et al (eds) The Oxford Textbook of orthopaedics and trauma. Oxford: Oxford University Press, 2002, pp. 781–798.

The wrist

The wrist joint plays a crucial role in the normal function of the upper limb. It works in harmony with the shoulder, elbow and hand for most daily tasks. Pathological processes may influence all the joints (rheumatoid arthritis) or the wrist alone (Kienböck's disease). In addition, the wrist is composed of a number of joints that can be affected individually (e.g. distal radio-ulnar joint, radio-carpal joint, midcarpal joint).

Epidemiology

The age-related diseases of the wrist are listed in Table 8.49. Kienböck's disease affects men twice as commonly as women whilst ganglia are seen more commonly in women. The incidence of ganglia of the wrist is 43 per 100 000 per year in women and 25 per 100 000 per year in men.[1]

Table 8.49	Diseases of the wrist by age group	
Young adults	**Middle age**	**Elderly**
Ganglia	De Quervain's tenosynovitis	Degenerative arthritis
De Quervain's tenosynovitis	Degenerative and rheumatoid arthritis	
Instability	Kienböck's disease Triangular fibrocartilage complex (TFCC) tears	

Pathology

Infection

Infections of the wrist are rare. As the various components of the joint lie superficially, they are prone to puncture, and septic arthritis of the wrist may occasionally be seen in intravenous drug users. The synovial flexor sheaths to the thumb and little finger pass across the wrist joint within the carpal tunnel as the radial and ulnar bursae respectively. This allows infection within these tendon sheaths to spread proximally from the hand.

Inflammation

Degenerative arthritis of the wrist most frequently affects the radio-carpal joint, particularly the scaphoid fossa (55%). It is uncommon as a primary disease and there is usually a history of fracture, ligament damage (instability) or avascular necrosis.

Calcium pyrophosphate deposition disease affecting the wrist is common: deposits build up on the joint surfaces and the triangular fibrocartilage. Degeneration between the carpal bones occurs, with the scapho-trapezoid-trapezial joint being affected in 26%. The distal radio-ulnar joint is rarely affected in isolation but may become so with advanced radio-carpal disease.

The wrist is involved in 90% of patients with severe rheumatoid disease. The spectrum ranges from synovitis and minor erosions, through capsular attrition with volar subluxation and ulnar translocation, to severe destruction and loss of a recognizable carpus (Fig. 8.41). The distal radio-ulnar joint commonly shows a pattern of gross synovitis, capsular damage and erosion leading to dorsal subluxation of the ulnar head remnant. The extensor carpi ulnaris tendon often subluxes in a volar direction and the overlying extensors to the little and ring fingers may rupture (Vaughan–Jackson lesion).

De Quervain's tenosynovitis is inflammation of the contents of the first extensor compartment of the wrist. The abductor pollicis longus (APL) and extensor pollicis brevis (EPB) tendons become inflamed and thickened, with resulting loss of movement. Abductor pollicis longus may trigger within the stenosed compartment.

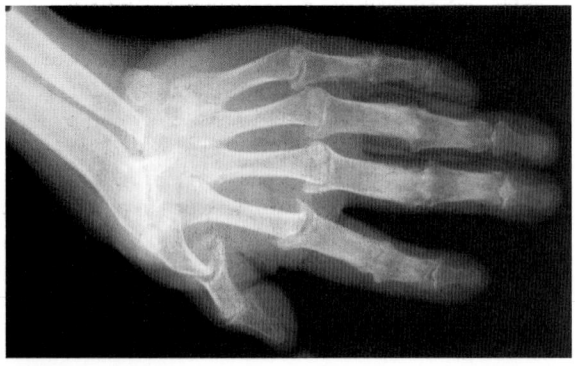

Fig. 8.41 Plain film of a rheumatoid wrist. AP view showing severe destruction of the wrist joint/carpus and the MCPJs and PIPJs, but sparing of the DIPJs.

Ganglia are believed to be part of a degenerative process affecting the capsule of a joint. Fissures develop in the capsule, which often acts as a one-way valve. The mucinous contents of ganglia are similar in constitution to synovial fluid (but they are not the same). There is no synovial lining to these cysts; their walls are composed of compressed collagen and scanty flat cells. The most common site of a wrist ganglion is dorsal arising from the scapholunate ligament. The pedicle can pass some distance beneath the extensor retinaculum and there may be a number of loculi. Palmar wrist ganglions can be traced to the radio-carpal joint in 66%, and may extend in to the carpal tunnel or along the sheath of flexor carpi radialis. They are in close proximity to the radial artery, which can become stretched over a large ganglion.

Degeneration may affect the triangular fibrocartilage complex causing wear, perforation and even detachment. Distal radio-ulnar joint arthritis can result. Often the ulna is relatively long (ulna plus variance) and the ulnar head abuts against the carpus. The intervening triangular fibrocartilage complex becomes trapped with ulnar deviation and pronation of the wrist.

Vascular

Avascular necrosis of the lunate may occur spontaneously (Kienböck's disease). The surface of this bone is largely hyaline cartilage, and it is only the small volar and dorsal areas that receive a blood supply. Although the aetiology is multifactorial, the contribution of tenuous vascularity may be important. Repetitive microtrauma may lead to necrosis of the lunate. Kienböck's disease is three times more common in patients with a short ulna (ulna minus variance). The lunate may progress from necrosis and fragmentation to collapse and remodelling. Secondary osteoarthritis is common with severe collapse.

Scope of disease

A range of flexion/extension, pronation/supination and radial/ulnar deviation at the wrist is required for accurate placement of the hand. The movements occur in harmony with the other joints of the upper limb. Composite synergistic movement also occurs such as the dorsiflexion at the wrist (wrist extensors) required when performing maximal power grip (finger flexors). Approximately 80% of daily activities can be achieved with 30° of extension and flexion and 25° of combined radial and ulnar deviation (1:4), but almost complete pronation/supination is required.

Clinical features

Pain

Isolating the site of tenderness about the wrist may be useful in indicating the aetiology of the disease (Table 8.50). However, pain can also be referred from the neck, elbow or back of the hand. Pain with pronation is common with

Table 8.50	Site of tenderness of the associated diseases	
Radial	**Central**	**Ulnar**
Radio-carpal, scapho-trapezo-trapezoidal or basal thumb arthritis	Osteoarthritis Rheumatoid disease	Distal radio-ulnar joint arthritis or instability
		Triangular fibrocartilage complex tear
De Quervain's tenosynovitis	Kienböck's disease	Ulno-carpal abutment
Radial neuritis	Ganglion	Piso-triquetral arthritis
Scapholunate instability	Carpal tunnel syndrome	Luno-triquetral instability

distal radio-ulnar joint and triangular fibrocartilage complex pathology. Pain on the radial aspect when using the thumb (particularly when lifting) suggests de Quervain's tenosynovitis. Pain at night occurs with nerve compression, infection and tumours.

Stiffness

Stiffness occurs with a number of pathologies but is particularly common with rheumatoid disease and complex regional pain syndrome.

Instability

Patients often describe a 'clunk' or 'click' that may be painful and lead to loss of power.

Swelling

Diffuse swelling can occur with arthritis, tendonitis or chronic regional pain syndrome. Localized swelling may be due to a ganglion, particularly if the size varies over time.

Medical history

It is important to establish dominance, occupation, history of injury and coexistent disease, particularly an arthropathy. There may be a family history of inflammatory arthropathy.

Examination

An orthopaedic examination is performed as follows:

Look

Both upper limbs should be fully exposed, and the resting position of the forearm, wrist and hand should be inspected. The classic rheumatoid deformity at the wrist is volar subluxation, supination and ulnar translocation of the carpus relative to the forearm. The ulnar head is often dorsally subluxed. Dorsal diffuse swelling can occur with tenosynovitis, or the whole wrist may appear swollen with arthritis or chronic regional pain syndrome. The fingers may be swollen and discoloured with chronic regional pain syndrome. Swelling due to a ganglion can be very subtle, particularly on the dorsal aspect of the wrist; therefore both sides should be compared.

Feel

Systematic palpation is performed. Tenderness over the radial styloid (first extensor compartment) may suggest de Quervain's tenosynovitis. The superficial radial nerve emerges immediately proximal to this (from beneath brachioradialis) and may become trapped causing tenderness (Wartenberg's syndrome). Distal to the styloid is the anatomical snuffbox bounded by extensor pollicis longus dorsally and abductor pollicis longus/extensor pollicis brevis on the volar aspect. Scaphoid tenderness is detected here. Lister's tubercle can be felt over the dorsum of the radius and just distal in line with this is the scapho-lunate joint. The distal radio-ulnar joint can be palpated by rolling the examining finger radially off the dorsal ulna. When palpating a suspected ganglion, remember that these may feel bony hard when tense and may transilluminate if sufficiently enlarged.

Move

The range of motion should be compared to the opposite wrist. Thumb movement should also be assessed as there is often marked reduction with de Quervain's tenosynovitis.

Finkelstein's test

This is a test for de Quervain's tenosynovitis. The thumb is adducted into the palm; if this does not reproduce pain then subsequent ulnar deviation of the wrist should. Look for swelling and crepitus over the abductor pollicis longus/extensor pollicis brevis tendons.

Ulno-carpal stress test

Axial load to an ulnar-deviated wrist with subsequent pronation/supination may provoke pain with distal radio-ulnar joint or triangular fibrocartilage complex disease. Compressing the ulna against the radius distally may identify pain from the distal radio-ulnar joint alone.

Kirk Watson's test

This is a test for scapho-lunate instability. The examiner sits facing the patient and takes the hand to be examined, applying thumb pressure over the scaphoid tubercle and counterpressure over the dorsum of the wrist. The wrist is then moved from ulnar to radial deviation, with the thumb pressure causing the scaphoid to sublux dorsally as it is unable to adopt its usual flexed position. A click is often felt, but pain is not specific to instability.

Piso-triquetral grind test

The pisiform can be grasped between thumb and index finger and ground against the triquetral beneath, provoking pain with an arthritic joint.

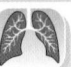

Initial investigations

Plain X-rays

The standard views of the wrist are the PA and lateral. Most pathology is visible on the PA film. The sclerosis and loss of joint space with degenerative arthritis may be seen. Look at the radio-scaphoid, scapho-trapezoid-trapezial and trapezio-metacarpal joints in particular. Patchy sclerosis, fragmentation and collapse of the lunate are seen with severe Kienböck's disease. Separation of the lunate from the scaphoid by more than 3 mm suggests ligament rupture and possible instability. This can be provoked by an X-ray taken with the fist clenched. An oblique view is required to identify piso-triquetral arthritis, and a scaphoid view is required for scaphoid injuries. Stress views may also be requested to assess for ligamentous injuries.

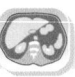

Further investigations

Full blood count/markers of inflammation

The white cell count and ESR may be elevated with both inflammation and infection.

Ultrasound of the wrist

Ultrasound is a useful investigation for identifying ganglia, tenosynovitis and tendon rupture.

Isotope bone scan

An isotope bone scan is a useful screening test for patients with chronic wrist pain. Increased activity is seen with occult avascular necrosis and early arthritis.

CT of the wrist

A CT scan is best reserved for identifying occult fractures, but if performed as a CT arthrogram it can also aid diagnosis of ligament rupture. The distal radio-ulnar joint, radio-carpal joint and midcarpal joint are anatomically separate and passage of contrast between them suggests a tear.

MRI of the wrist

MRI allows better visualization of the soft tissues and has 90% accuracy for diagnosing triangular fibrocartilage complex tears. Tendon pathology and ganglia are also well seen. Early stages of avascular necrosis can be identified before the onset of changes on plain X-rays. MRI arthrography can also be performed.

Nerve conduction studies

Neurophysiological studies are performed when nerve entrapment is suspected.

Arthroscopy

Wrist arthroscopy is reserved for patients with chronic pain and when simple investigations fail to provide a diagnosis. Localized degeneration, ligament damage and triangular fibrocartilage complex tears are well visualized.

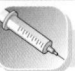

Initial management

Patient education

Many causes of wrist pain can be improved with rest or adjustment of activity. A change of occupation may be required.

Simple analgesia

NSAIDs or steroid injections may help in a number of conditions in which inflammation plays a part. Adequate analgesia is required when aggressive physiotherapy is planned.

Physiotherapy

Physiotherapy can help preserve or restore movement and strength, particularly in the arthritic conditions. Splints can be provided for support and relief, particularly in rheumatoid disease. A wrist splint with a thumb extension is useful for de Quervain's tenosynovitis.

Surgical management

General management

Arthrodesis

There are a number of options for arthrodesis about the wrist because of the complexity of the joint. These can be simplified by considering them as limited (e.g. scapho-trapezoid-trapezial) or complete (wrist fusion). A complete wrist fusion incorporates the radio-carpal, midcarpal and carpo-metacarpal joints (Fig. 8.42). This is an option for end-stage arthritic joints, both primary (rheumatoid disease, osteoarthritis) and secondary (Kienböck's disease), but has high success rates for all groups. The wrist is fused in about 15–25° extension and 0–15° ulnar deviation. A dorsal plate is best with degenerative arthritis but a Steinman pin can be used in patients with rheumatoid disease, passed down the third metacarpal, across the wrist and into the radius.

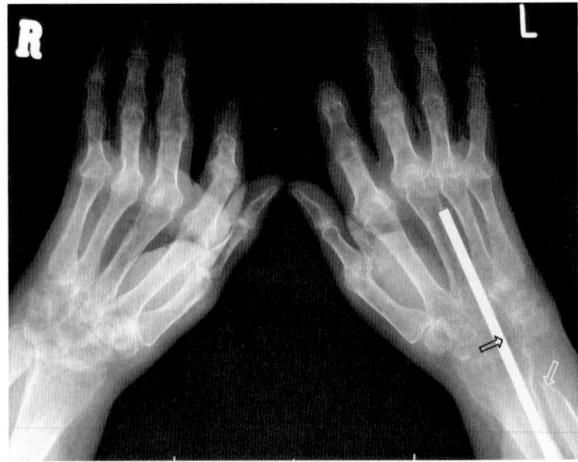

Fig. 8.42 AP view of both wrists showing early rheumatoid changes on the left, and a wrist fusion using an intramedullary rod (black arrow) on the right. The ulnar head has been excised (open arrow).

Arthroplasty

Replacement of the wrist joint is generally reserved for patients with rheumatoid disease. Poor results are seen with degenerative arthritis due to implant loosening or failure.

Specific management

Infection

The usual procedure of joint washout applies for septic arthritis. Six weeks of antibiotics are then required. Infection of the radial or ulnar bursae may require carpal tunnel decompression to allow adequate debridement and washout. Tuberculous infection, whilst rare, must be appreciated and adequate antibiotics prescribed for 6–9 months.

Rheumatoid disease

When simple non-operative measures mentioned above are inadequate, a series of surgical options are available. Synovectomy may be of benefit when the joint is still well preserved with reconstruction of the attenuated dorsal capsule using the extensor retinaculum. The distal radio-ulnar joint is often the source of symptoms early in the disease process. Excision of the distal ulna and capsular reconstruction (Darrach procedure), distal radio-ulnar fusion with excision of a small segment of distal ulna to allow pronosupination (Sauve Kapandji procedure), or ulnar head replacement are all options with good early results.

More severe radio-carpal joint involvement may require a limited fusion (radio-lunate or radio-scapho-lunate). This requires a healthy midcarpal joint and allows some preserved movement. Finally, severe disease leaves the options of wrist fusion or replacement. If both wrists are to be treated then it is usual to consider replacement of the dominant wrist and fusion of the other to allow greater independence. Replacement remains experimental and no one technique is problem free. Silastic replacements give good results in the low demand patient. Higher demand patients need good quality bone stock to allow cemented fixation of metallic/polyethylene designs, but high satisfaction with a well-functioning implant can still be expected for as long as 8 years.[2] Wrist fusion gives more predictable success but sacrifices function as a result.

Osteoarthritis

When the simple non-operative measures mentioned above are inadequate a series of surgical options are available. Degeneration is usually progressive involving the radio-scaphoid articulation first. Excision of the radial styloid may ease pain and impingement. More extensive disease but with a well-preserved lunate fossa and capitate can be treated by excision of the whole of the proximal carpal row, which will still allow a functional range of motion. Alternatively a limited fusion can be performed, such as scapho-trapezoid-trapezial or 'four corner' (lunate–capitate–hamate–triquetral). The latter is often combined with scaphoid excision. All of the above can be combined with a wrist denervation in which the terminal pain fibres of the posterior and anterior interosseous nerves

are divided. This can give 70% patients relief from 70% of their pain for 7 years.[3] Pisiform excision can reduce the pain from piso-hamate arthritis. End-stage wrist degeneration is best treated by formal wrist fusion. Replacement can give success in up to 85% at 10 years[3] but these patients are often young and salvage options are limited for a failed replacement.

Kienböck's disease

In Kienböck's disease, the symptoms do not always tally with the radiological appearance. In early stages, the wrist can be rested in a splint. Once fragmentation occurs, a joint levelling procedure (for patients with an ulna minus variant) is warranted, which lengthens the ulna or shortens the radius by 2 mm. When bone collapse occurs, a limited fusion may be necessary such as a scapho-capitate to bypass loads away from the lunate. Finally, severe secondary arthritis may require wrist fusion or occasionally replacement.

De Quervain's tenosynovitis

If the regimen of rest, analgesia and splinting fails, 60% may recover following an injection of steroid.[4] Persistent symptoms warrant surgical release of the first extensor compartment.

Triangular fibrocartilage complex degeneration

If medical treatment fails, arthroscopic assessment of the wrist may be useful and debridement of the triangular fibrocartilage complex can be carried out. If ulna plus variance is the cause of the symptoms (abutment), then the ulna may be surgically shortened.

Instability

Instability of the wrist joint is a complex subject, and specific management of the different patterns of instability is beyond the scope of this section. However, there are basic principles that can be applied. First, chronic instability will often provoke secondary osteoarthritis and the principles outlined above for management of degenerative arthritis can be applied. Before degenerative changes ensue, there may be options for ligament repair and soft tissue reconstruction. These patients are often young and active and movement must be preserved where possible. The objective is to relieve the symptoms of pain and instability and reduce the risk of subsequent arthritic change.

REFERENCES

(1) Janzon L, Niechajev IA. Wrist ganglia. Incidence and recurrence rate after operation. Scandinavian Journal of Plastic and Reconstructive Surgery 1981; 15: 53–56.
(2) Takwale VJ, Nuttal D, Trail IA, Stanley JK. Biaxial total wrist replacement in patients with rheumatoid arthritis. Clinical review, survivorship and radiological analysis. Journal of Bone and Joint Surgery 2002; 83B: 692–699.
(3) Stanley JK. Degenerative arthritis of the wrist. Current Orthopaedics 1999; 13: 4, 290–296.
(4) Harvey FJ, Harvey PM, Horsley MW. De Quervain's disease—surgical or non-surgical treatment. Journal of Hand Surgery 1990; 15A: 83–87.

The hand

The hand is involved in many local and systemic disease processes that may have a significant impact on function. It is always important to consider the hand when assessing disease of the other upper limb joints.

Epidemiology

The relationship between age and diseases of the hand is presented in Table 8.51. There is a strong racial influence on the incidence of Dupuytren's disease. Above the age of 60, 30% of Norwegian and 15% of British men have the disease. It is rare in African nations.

Osteoarthritis is more common in women. Approximately 62% of those aged 55–65 years suffer with distal interphalangeal joint (DIPJ) arthritis and 33% with trapezio-metacarpal arthritis (basal thumb).

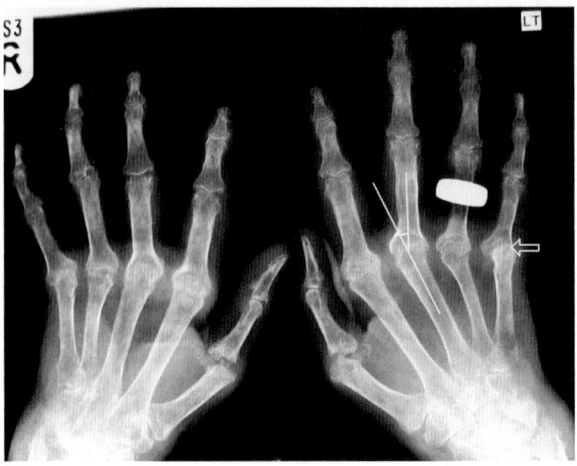

Fig. 8.43 Plain film of rheumatoid disease of the hands. X-ray showing moderate disease with destruction of the MCPJs (arrow) and PIPJs. There is early ulnar deviation of the MCPJs. DIPJs are spared, but the thumb is diseased.

Pathology

Inflammation

Inflammation can involve the joints, soft tissues or both. Rheumatoid disease of the hand leads to synovitis, joint destruction (erosion) and instability with subluxation or dislocation. The bulky synovitis distends and stretches the capsule and collaterals, leading to instability.

The metacarpophalangeal joints deviate in an ulnar direction, possibly due to pressure from the thumb when pinching (Fig. 8.43). Palmar subluxation of the proximal phalanges is caused by the powerful flexors and can lead to further ulnar deviation of the joints.

The proximal interphalangeal joints (PIPJ) follow one of two patterns, the swan-neck and the boutonnière deformity. The swan-neck deformity is hyperextension of the PIPJ and flexion of the distal interphalangeal joint (DIPJ), usually with rupture of the PIPJ volar plate and the flexor superficialis tendon insertion. A boutonnière deformity is a flexed PIPJ and hyperextended DIPJ due to rupture of the central slip of the extensor complex and subluxation of the lateral bands. These deformities are initially flexible but may become fixed.

The thumb may adopt a number of patterns depending on the joints involved. Rheumatoid nodules are often found over the PIPJ or the finger pulps. Tenosynovitis affects both the flexors and extensors. The swelling is most noticeable dorsally. Extensor tendons may rupture, usually due to attrition on rough eroded bone, and this may lead to

a dropped metacarpo-phalangeal joint (MCPJ)—extensor lag. Synovitis can also lead to increased bulk of the flexor tendon complex, which may provoke triggering. Fibrous adhesions can form leading to reduced excursion and subsequent rupture due to synovial destruction or tendon attrition.

Osteoarthritis tends to favour the distal interphalangeal joints and thumb (trapezio-metacarpal joint). It is usually idiopathic but may be secondary to trauma or infection. There is local joint swelling with osteophytic nodes and small cystic swellings (mucous cysts) that resemble ganglions. Heberden's nodes occur at the DIPJ and Bouchard's nodes at the PIPJ. Joint destruction leads to loss of flexion, and an adduction deformity of the thumb, resulting in limitation of extension and abduction.

Inflammation of the tendon sheath (tenosynovitis) can be acute (usually due to infection or crystals) or chronic (rheumatoid disease). The 'blackthorn' foreign body gives a classic subacute aseptic tenosynovitis. Common to all is pain, swelling, crepitus and reduced excursion due to adhesions. Triggering of the flexor tendons is a chronic form usually provoked by a nodular thickening of the tendon (calcific deposits in areas of degeneration). It is most commonly seen in the ring finger. There is secondary stenosis of the pulley with tenosynovitis and the finger may become locked in flexion. This can be secondary to rheumatoid disease or diabetes.

Table 8.51	Diseases of the hand by age group	
Young adult	**Middle age**	**Elderly**
Ganglia	Dupuytren's in men	Dupuytren's (men) and arthritis (RA and OA in women)
Enchondromas	Rheumatoid arthritis (RA), osteoarthritis (OA) and triggering in women Giant cell tumours	

Degenerative changes in tendons may lead to rupture; however, in the majority of cases there is pre-existing rheumatoid disease, osteoarthritis or a history of trauma or steroid use. Rupture of the finger extensors and flexors is often multiple and sequential if the underlying cause is not identified and treated.

Nerve entrapment

The locations of compression in the upper limb are grouped to aid understanding and differential diagnosis. Pathological changes are secondary to compression and symptoms are usually localized to the hand. Impaired microcirculation to the nerve can lead to reduced axonal transport, demyelination, and eventual axonal death with Wallerian degeneration. Pregnancy, diabetes and thyroid disorders can lower the threshold at which symptoms are noted, and tethering by fibrosis can exacerbate ischaemia. Distal muscle atrophy may be irreversible after 2 years.

Ulnar nerve compression is usually due to compression in the cubital tunnel posterior to the medial epicondyle, but it can also occur as a complication of a fracture or arthritis with a valgus deformity at the elbow joint. More proximally the nerve can be trapped at the medial intermuscular septum and distally between the two heads of flexor carpi ulnaris. At the wrist it can be trapped within Guyon's canal, formed by the piso-hamate ligament, the transverse carpal ligament and the hook of the hamate. Alternatively compression of the nerve can be due to increased volume in the canal from ganglia or ulnar artery aneurysms.

The median nerve is rarely compressed about the elbow. From proximal to distal the following sites are recognized, below the ligament of Struthers from a supracondylar process, between the two heads of pronator teres and below the fibrous arch of flexor digitorum superficialis. Compression in the carpal tunnel at the wrist is the most common site (the roof is formed by the transverse carpal ligament, passing from the scaphoid tubercle and trapezium to the pisiform and hook of hamate). Compression is often idiopathic, but can occur as a complication of wrist fracture, arthritis, tenosynovitis, ganglia and oedema with pregnancy.

The posterior interosseous branch of the radial nerve, which supplies most of the extensor muscles of the forearm, can be trapped at the fibrous edge of extensor carpi radialis brevis or within supinator muscle (arcade of Frohse). The superficial branch of the radial nerve may become trapped distally as it emerges from beneath the tendon of brachioradialis (Wartenberg's syndrome).

Infection

Infection is usually seen after bites, puncture wounds or open fractures. It may involve any tissue but certain patterns are recognized and outlined below.

Osteomyelitis is rare and usually develops as a consequence of infection in adjacent tissue or joints. Septic arthritis is also uncommon, but may follow a puncture wound of the second MCPJ sustained with a punch to the mouth ('fight bite'). Rapid joint destruction and fibrosis can occur if infection is not recognized and treated early.

The flexor sheaths (enclosed synovial spaces surrounding the flexor tendons) can become infected, usually following puncture. The ring finger is most commonly affected and infection may discharge into the midpalmar space. The sheaths to the little finger and thumb extend through the carpal tunnel as the ulnar and radial bursae of the wrist respectively. Infection of these sheaths can spread proximal to the wrist. Fibrosis can develop within the sheath leading to loss of tendon excursion, and raised pressure within the sheath may lead to tendon necrosis and rupture with significant loss of function.

The pulp of the fingertips is anchored between skin and bone by strong fibrous trabeculae. This allows pus within this space (felon) to reach very high pressures causing tissue necrosis. It usually follows puncture wounds in manual workers and gardeners.

An abscess alongside the nail (paronychia) usually occurs after local trauma and may damage the nail fold germinal cells, affecting further growth when severe. The palmar fascia complex helps to anchor the skin to deeper structures, aiding grip. Infection may collect in these spaces and abscesses can communicate between them through a small channel, particularly in the first ray (collar-stud abscess).

The above infections are usually a result of staphylococci or streptococci. Anaerobic organisms can be found following bites. Mycobacterial infection (tuberculosis or atypical) can occur in all of the above locations and is most likely to be seen in farm or animal workers.

Endocrine

The bony changes of hyperparathyroidism (osteitis fibrosa cystica) occur mainly with primary disease. Features include subperiosteal erosions of the proximal phalanges and brown tumours within the bones (fibrous tissue).

Dupuytren's disease is commonly found in association with endocrine disease (particularly diabetes mellitus), alcoholism and smoking. There are strong familial and racial tendencies highlighting the genetic influence. Early disease leads to palmar pitting and nodules, with subsequent thickening of the palmar and digital fascia and cords leading to fixed flexion deformity of the digits. It is most common in the ulnar side of the hand, supporting a traumatic aetiology, as the ring and little fingers experience heavy loads and shear with gripping. Histologically there is fibroblast and collagen proliferation with subsequent contraction due to myofibroblasts. These are similar to the changes with wound healing and contraction (inflammatory theory). Flexion deformity of the MCPJ usually precedes that of the PIPJ. The latter is often irreversible due to shortening of the collateral ligaments. A spiral cord may develop in the finger and tends to pull the neurovascular bundle medially and superficially, endangering it during surgery. More aggressive disease (Dupuytren's diathesis) is identified by the presence of Garrod's dorsal knuckle pads over the PIPJs, nodules in the plantar fascia of the foot (Ledderhose's) and penile fibrosis (Peyronie's).

535

Neoplasia

Cancers involving the hand are rare. They can be soft tissue or bony. Giant cell tumours involve areas with a synovial lining and are part of the spectrum of pigmented villo-nodular synovitis. Middle-aged women are most often affected. The tumour lies within the flexor sheath as a lobulated mass consisting of fibroblasts, giant cells and histiocytes. Although benign, giant cell tumours have a high recurrence rate with incomplete excision.

The glomus tumour is a benign dermal lesion of epithelioid glomus cells (thermoregulatory). Up to 50% occur in the hand, often beneath the nail (subungual). There is a red–blue skin discolouration and the classic triad of pain, tenderness and temperature sensitivity.

Enchondromas constitute up to 24% of all benign bone tumours and are most commonly found in the phalanges of the hands and feet. They consist of hyaline cartilage with areas of calcification. The histological appearance overlaps with low-grade chondrosarcoma, occasionally posing diagnostic difficulty. Lesions may fracture with minor trauma. There is a less than 1% lifetime risk of malignant transformation.

Scope of disease

Satisfactory function of the hand is required for most activities of daily living such as washing and eating. Severe loss of function can occur with minor disease, particularly when it involves the thumb. Opposition of the thumb is a function unique to primates and allows complex tasks to be performed. When function of the thumb is lost completely, the overall impact is loss of 50% of the function of the hand.

Clinical features

Pain

A throbbing severe pain, disturbing sleep, is common with deep infection. Pain causing waking from sleep may be due to nerve entrapment and is often associated with paraesthesia and numbness. Pain radiating proximally or distally from the flexor surface of the wrist also occurs with nerve entrapment. Arthritic pain is localized to the arthritic joints and is worse with activity, particularly with basal thumb osteoarthritis, which is classically painful when wringing out a cloth.

Swelling

Swelling about the hand is non-specific but when localized and distinct may be due to a ganglion or mucous cyst.

Paraesthesia/numbness

This is poorly localized subjectively, but may suggest nerve entrapment or diabetes.

Weakness

Weakness may be due to nerve, muscle, tendon or joint disease and may be associated with pain in many cases.

Deformity

Deformity may be a chronic process with arthropathy and Dupuytren's, or more acute with trauma, tendon rupture and triggering.

Instability

Instability is commonly associated with rheumatoid and ligamentous ruptures due to trauma. Ulnar collateral rupture in the thumb MCPJ will cause instability of the thumb when pinching.

Stiffness

Stiffness may be localized or diffuse. Trauma, arthritis, infection and complex regional pain syndrome are common causes.

Functional impact

It is important to establish the impact of the disease on function of the hand. Dominance, occupation and hobbies are all important when assessing functional impact.

Medical history

Enquiries should be undertaken about systemic and polyarticular joint disease.

Examination

Look

Both upper limbs should be fully exposed to allow comparison. Inspection of the resting position of the hands is important. The classic deformities in rheumatoid disease may be instantly recognized as palmar deviation, supination and ulnar translocation of the carpus at the wrist, ulnar deviation and palmar subluxation of the second to fifth MCPJ, boutonnière deformity of the digits (PIPJ flexion and DIPJ hyperextension), swan-neck deformities of the digits (PIPJ hyperextension and DIPJ flexion). The thumb may adopt a boutonnière or swan-neck deformity but is commonly described as a Z-thumb deformity.

Wrist drop is associated with high radial nerve palsy. Dropped digits at the MCPJ (lag) may be due to extensor tendon rupture, extensor tendon subluxation in rheumatoid disease or posterior interosseous nerve compression. This must be distinguished from a flexion contracture of the MCPJ with Dupuytren's and triggering. Examination of the palm should reveal the pitting, nodules and cords of Dupuytren's. The nodule of a triggering digit may be detected on palpation. Flexion contracture of the ring and little interphalangeal joints (IPJ) may be seen with ulnar nerve palsy but the metacarpo-phalangeal joints (MCPJ) are usually hyperextended.

Localized swelling is seen with ganglia or giant cell tumours. Large ganglia may transilluminate. Diffuse swelling is most noticeable dorsally or when it involves the digits. Swelling confined to the dorsum of the hand and wrist may indicate tenosynovitis. The pattern of joint swelling may aid in diagnosis of an arthropathy. Symmetrical bilateral involvement of the MCPJ and PIPJ would suggest rheumatoid disease whereas distal joint involvement occurs with osteoarthritis and psoriatic arthropathy. There may be skin changes with the latter, and pitting/ ridging of the nails. Mucous cysts and nodular enlargement of the IPJs suggest osteoarthritis. Patterns of muscle wasting in the hand are informative; thenar wasting is seen with carpal tunnel syndrome, basal thumb arthritis and compression of the T1 nerve root. Hypothenar wasting is most often seen with ulnar nerve entrapment along with wasting of the first dorsal interosseous muscle in the first web space. Chronic disease of the hand such as rheumatoid arthritis can lead to a mixed pattern of wasting.

Feel

Palpation must be systematic but can be targeted based on the findings on inspection. Individual joint tenderness is sought. Palpation of tendons may reveal tenderness and thickening, with crepitus on movement suggesting tenosynovitis. There may be a palpable nodule in a flexor tendon in the distal palm which can be felt to move distally with extension of the digit, with an accompanying flick of the finger if triggering. The nodules or cords of Dupuytren's are felt more superficially, often with adherent overlying skin, and do not move with the tendon. A swelling must be assessed for anatomical location and attachments. Lesions originating from the tendon sheath such as ganglia and giant cell tumours usually remain static with finger movement. A ganglion may feel bony hard but should transilluminate. Giant cell tumours feel firm and lobular.

Sensation in the hand should be assessed. The minimal zones represent the most exclusive area of innervation, least influenced by crossover or overlap. These are the palmar surface of the index finger (median nerve) and little finger (ulnar nerve) and the dorsal first web space (radial nerve).

Move

Power and passive and active range of motion should be examined. Specific tests for active movement are required. Because of the common muscle belly of flexor digitorum profundus the other digits must be immobilized in extension when testing the flexor superficialis (PIPJ flexion). The control of DIPJ flexion (profundus) is assessed by fixing the PIPJ in extension. Flexion of the MCPJ and extension of the IPJ is a function of the intrinsic muscles of the hand. Extension of the MCPJ is by the long extensors. Extension of the index and little fingers is usually possible independently because of the additional extensor indicis and digiti minimi tendons. Loss of movement may be due to a number of causes such as skin scar contraction (particularly palmar, preventing extension), flexor tendon or sheath pathology such as adhesions and triggering preventing extension or flexion, muscle contracture or paralysis and tightness of capsule or collateral ligaments, usually causing loss of IPJ extension and MCPJ flexion.

The fixed length phenomenon can be used to study this further. Muscle contracture (such as intrinsic muscles) leads to loss of movement that varies depending on the position of adjacent joints. Therefore the restricted flexion of the PIPJ with tight intrinsic muscles can be improved by flexing the MCPJ but only if the capsule/ligaments are not also tight. Greater passive than active movement may occur when tendon adhesions prevent normal active excursion.

Huston's tabletop test

This is used to diagnose Dupuytren's contractures of the hand, where flexion contracture prevents placement of the hand flat on a table.

Allen's test of the digital arteries

Allen's test on the digits to check for two functioning digital arteries is important when considering surgery to the hand for Dupuytren's disease. The finger is emptied of blood and pressure applied to the digital arteries at the base. Release of each vessel separately should show return of the pink colour of the finger if the artery is patent. This is particularly important when considering revision surgery, as there may have been previous damage to a digital vessel.

Assessment of the median nerve

Compression of the median nerve commonly occurs at the wrist (carpal tunnel). Power of thumb abduction (abductor pollicis brevis) may be reduced with associated thenar wasting. Phalen's test involves provocation by maximal palmar flexion of the wrists and is usually positive within 30–60 seconds. Thenar sensation should be preserved as the superficial palmar branch arises proximal to the carpal tunnel. Numbness of the thenar eminence may indicate more proximal compression such as pronator syndrome. This rarely results in motor deficit but symptoms of pain and paraesthesia can be reproduced by resisting pronation of the forearm with the elbow flexed.

Assessment of the ulnar nerve

Compression of the ulnar nerve commonly occurs at the elbow. Compression in Guyon's canal at the wrist will preserve the sensation on the dorsum of the ulnar side of the hand as this branch comes off more proximally. Innervation of the interossei muscles can be checked by attempting active crossing of the fingers. The adductor pollicis muscle may be weak and this is demonstrated by Froment's test, which consists of withdrawing a sheet of paper that is grasped by the thumb against the index finger. Flexion of the IPJ is a positive Froment's sign suggesting weakness of the adductor pollicis muscle. The degree of ring and little finger clawing is important. Mild clawing suggests more proximal compression, as the flexor digitorum profundus to these fingers is also weakened, reducing the driving force of the deformity (ulna paradox).

Assessment of the radial nerve

Compression of the radial nerve can result in a pure sensory deficit. Classically the superficial branch is trapped beneath the tendon of brachioradialis proximal to the wrist (Wartenberg's syndrome). The posterior interosseous nerve may be trapped as it passes through supinator muscle,

537

resulting in weakness of finger and wrist extension. Some preservation of wrist extension occurs as the extensor carpi radialis longus and brevis are supplied more proximally. The wrist classically extends into a position of radial deviation. There is no wrist extension with a high radial nerve lesion. Entrapment in supinator can be provoked by resisting supination with the elbow extended.

Functional tests of the hand
It is useful to objectively assess and document functions of the hand, particularly in patients with rheumatoid disease. When observing the use of a key ('key grip'), pen ('pulp pinch') and picking up a coin ('precision pinch'), the function of the radial side of the hand is being studied, the thumb in particular. When observing the power grip and hook grip (holding the handle of a bag), the ulnar side of the hand is being assessed, as flexion of the little and ring fingers is dominant. Asking the patient to pick up a glass looks at the span grip incorporating both sides of the hand.

Initial investigations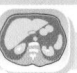

Plain X-rays
The standard views of the hand are the AP, lateral and oblique. The oblique views allow better visualization of the finger joints and metacarpals, which are superimposed on a pure lateral film. Most abnormalities are observed on the AP film. The classic radiological features of osteoarthritis (p. 480) and rheumatoid disease (p. 534) have been mentioned previously. The erosions of rheumatoid disease are often noticeable about the small joints of the hand and significant subluxation of the joints can occur (Fig. 8.44). Enchondromas appear as lytic lesions with a thin cortical periphery, and the bone often appears expanded with speckles of calcification within the lesion.

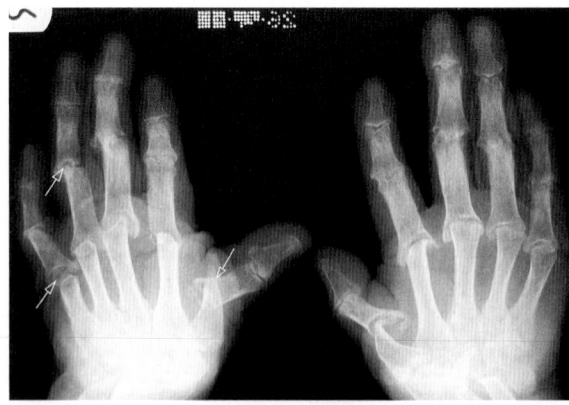

Fig. 8.44 Plain film of severe rheumatoid disease of the hands. X-ray showing severe mutilating joint destruction with frank dislocation of MCPJs and PIPJs (arrows).

Further investigations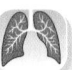

Full blood count/markers of inflammation
The white cell count and ESR may be elevated with infection and inflammation.

Ultrasound of the hand
This is a useful investigation for tendon sheath pathology such as tenosynovitis or tendon rupture. Dynamic assessment with movement of the digit allows greater understanding of tendon behaviour when adhesions may be affecting function. Ganglia should be distinguishable from giant cell tumours if the diagnosis is in doubt. High-resolution ultrasound can be used to look for the synovitis and early erosions seen in rheumatoid disease and influence management.[1]

MRI of the hand
MRI is the investigation of choice for complex soft tissue masses. Giant cell tumours can be seen tracking large distances within the flexor sheath. MRI can also demonstrate the extent of soft tissue or bony infection.

Nerve conduction studies
Nerve conduction studies are invaluable when the diagnosis of nerve compression is suspected. It can also assess the severity, anatomical level and degree of recovery after surgery. It is usually required prior to surgical decompression.

Initial management

Patient education
Rest and adjustment of activities may be required.

Analgesia
Simple analgesia or NSAIDs can be used as appropriate.

Steroid injections
Steroid injections can be of use with arthropathies, tenosynovitis, triggering and carpal tunnel syndrome.

Physiotherapy, occupational therapy
Physiotherapy is useful to restore and maintain the range of motion in arthritic joints, and plays a vital role in re-establishing movement after surgery for Dupuytren's.

Surgical management

General
Arthrodesis
Arthrodesis is a useful procedure for painful arthritic joints. Most joints in the hand can be successfully fused but the loss of movement results in sacrifice of function. Generally the joints of the thumb are better fused than replaced as stability of the thumb when pinching is important. Similarly the index and middle fingers must be stable for pinching, and arthrodesis will sacrifice little

function. The ring and little fingers are involved in grip, and replacement may be more appropriate, preserving power. MCPJ fusions do lead to functional limitations and are uncommonly performed. The position of finger fusion ensures a closer position of the little and ring fingers to the palm for gripping, preserving power, whilst still allowing a relatively extended position in the index finger for pinching.

Arthroplasty

Joint replacement is reserved for painful arthritic joints when it is preferable to preserve movement. It is particularly suitable for the finger MCPJs and ring and little finger PIPJs. Generally it is more successful in lower demand patient groups such as patients with rheumatoid disease and in the elderly. Most implants are flexible Silastic hinges but some cemented metallic or polyethylene designs are available. Silicon synovitis can complicate Silastic replacements but causes less problems than the loosening often seen with the cemented varieties.

Specific

Osteoarthritis

If symptomatic treatment is insufficient, surgery can play a role in management. However, patients are often young, physically active and still working, and these demands must be considered when planning treatment. For these reasons, arthrodesis is most commonly chosen because of the lower risk of long-term failure. The procedure may lead to loss of function and the patient must be aware of this. The loss of function with PIPJ fusion may lead to patients accepting the risks involved with PIPJ replacement, but activity modification must be encouraged and if this is not possible then fusion is still preferable. DIPJ fusion is a dependable procedure.

Basal thumb arthritis has a high prevalence and can be disabling. Steroid injection and splinting may help early on. Early disease is often associated with laxity and subluxation of the trapezio-metacarpal joint and soft tissue stabilization can reduce pain and disease progression. More severe disease requires arthrodesis (manual workers) or excision of the trapezium and soft tissue reconstruction. Thumb pinch is less strong in the latter group but greater movement is preserved.

Painful arthritis affecting the thumb MCPJ or IPJ can also be treated with arthrodeses, but a general rule is that one of the three thumb joints should be preserved to allow some flexion when pinching.

Rheumatoid disease

A large amount of skill is required in management of the rheumatoid hand, as indications for surgical intervention are not clear cut. Overall, the goals are control of pain and preservation of function. Surgery to the elbow and shoulder is often required prior to the hand as a well-functioning hand that cannot be positioned in space remains useless. Similarly, surgery to the proximal joints in the hand and wrist usually takes priority. The options for the wrist have already been discussed. Flexor tenosynovectomy and carpal tunnel decompression offer therapeutic and prophylactic treatment, as tendon rupture should hopefully be prevented.

MCPJ replacement is a well-established and successful treatment for pain and severe deformity.[2] It is combined with a soft tissue reconstruction about the joints. A small increase in range of motion can be expected, but functional improvement is only slight. In the long term the implants can fail and deformity returns.

Surgery to the fingers may be to address deformity (swan-neck or boutonnière) or pain from arthritic destruction. Soft tissue reconstructions are often unrewarding, particularly for boutonnière deformities, and dynamic finger splints may give adequate functional gains. Once painful, the joints may be fused or replaced as outlined above. Fusion of the thumb MCPJ with or without the IPJ is often required to address the instability that commonly develops.

Trigger finger

The tenosynovitis associated with a triggering digit tends to exacerbate the stenosis, causing further inflammation. This cycle needs to be broken. Resting splints for the finger prevent the triggering and allow swelling to settle. Steroid injections are successful in up to 70% cases.[3] If this fails then surgical release of the first flexor pulley in the distal palm removes the stenotic lesion which caused the nodular tendon to trigger. However, this is not recommended in rheumatoid cases, when tenosynovectomy is the most appropriate treatment.

Nerve compression

With mild to moderate compression the use of resting or night splints can be helpful for both carpal tunnel syndrome and compression of the ulnar nerve in the cubital tunnel. The idiopathic nature of many nerve compressions may allow spontaneous recovery, preventing the need for surgery. Where functional impact is severe surgical decompression is warranted. Good results can be expected in 85–90% of cubital tunnel and more than 95% of carpal tunnel releases. When muscle atrophy has been present for 1–2 years, it may not recover, leaving permanent weakness. The ulnar nerve at the elbow may require translocation anteriorly if taut (e.g. the valgus elbow) and can be placed below muscle or fat. Compression of the ulnar nerve in Guyon's canal is rare but is usually due to a space-occupying lesion and therefore surgical treatment is generally required. Similarly, compression of the radial nerve and its branches is uncommon and notoriously difficult to diagnose. Symptoms can settle with rest and splintage but decompression may ultimately be necessary, although results are not generally as good.

Dupuytren's contracture

Neither splints nor physiotherapy can halt the progression of a Dupuytren's contracture. Steroid injection to painful palmar nodules can reduce tenderness. Once

539

functional disturbance occurs, surgical treatment is indicated, particularly when there is flexion contracture of the PIPJ, as this can become permanent if not tackled early. The aim is to straighten the finger. Recurrence of up to 50% at 10 years is likely, regardless of the technique chosen, although not all will require surgery.[4]

Fasciectomy is most commonly performed and the majority of the visible diseased tissue is excised. There is some evidence that excision of diseased overlying skin with subsequent full thickness skin grafting can reduce the rate of recurrence.[5] There is the potential for greater morbidity with this technique and it is generally reserved for cases of aggressive disease, severe deformity with a shortage of skin on straightening the digit, or recurrent disease. For all techniques the closure must follow a zigzag pattern to reduce the risk of skin contracture. This can be achieved by creating a zigzag incision (Bruner's) or using a straight incision and creating Z-plasty releases along the length of the wound. The latter is more successful when the deformity is severe. On occasions the skin defect in the palm is left open and allowed to heal by secondary intention. Post-operatively, splinting and physiotherapy are essential to guarantee good outcome. Occasionally when deformity is severe it may be necessary to consider amputation of the finger.

Infection

Abscesses of the hand can reach high pressure causing necrosis of surrounding tissues and should be incised and fully drained early. Infective tenosynovitis is particularly disabling when not recognized and treated early. Kanavel criteria for the diagnosis of infective tenosynovitis are a flexed posture of the finger, sausage-like swelling, tenderness over the flexor sheath extending into the palm and pain with passive extension. There should be a low threshold to drain the flexor tendon sheath as an emergency procedure. This requires a distal incision in the finger and one in the palm giving access to each end of the sheath, allowing thorough irrigation.

Giant cell tumour of the tendon sheath

This is a benign and slow-growing tumour but it often causes functional disturbance and complete excision is recommended. However, there is a 10% recurrence rate and persistent recurrence occasionally requires amputation.

Enchondroma

In general, surgery is required when deformity or pathological fracture develops. Curettage and bone grafting of the lesion is usually curative. The rare occurrence of malignant transformation may be heralded by a rapid increase in lesion size, pain without obvious fracture and more aggressive radiological features such as cortical breach. In these cases, amputation of the digit may be required.

REFERENCES

(1) *Wakefield RJ, Gibbon WW, Conaghan PG, et al. The value of sonography in the detection of bone erosions in patients with rheumatoid arthritis: A comparison with conventional radiography. Arthritis and Rheumatism* 2000; 43: 2762–2770.
(2) *Kirschenaum D, Schneider LH, Adams DC, Cody RP. Arthroplasty of the metacarpophalangeal joints with use of silicone-rubber implants in patients who have rheumatoid arthritis. Long-term results. Journal of Bone and Joint Surgery (Am)* 1993; 75A: 3–12.
(3) *Newport ML, Lane LB, Stuchin SA. Treatment of trigger finger by steroid injection. Journal of Hand Surgery* 1990; 15A: 748–750.
(4) *Burge P. Dupuytren's disease. In: Bulstrode C et al (eds) Oxford Textbook of orthopaedics and trauma. Oxford: Oxford University Press,* 2002: pp. 877–886.
(5) *Brotherston TM, Balakrishnan C, Milner RH, Brown HG. Long-term follow-up of dermofasciectomy for dupuytren's contracture. British Journal of Plastic Surgery* 1994; 47: 440–443.

The cervical spine

The cervical spine is a complex system of vertebral bodies, intervertebral discs, facet joints and ligaments. The seven vertebrae connect the thoracic spine to the skull and cumulatively allow flexion, extension, rotation and lateral flexion of the neck. This mobility enables fine positioning of the head.

Epidemiology

Age-related diseases of the cervical spine are summarized in Table 8.52. The neck is a frequent site of injury and the consequence of chronic pain and stiffness is loss of function and productivity. The 'whiplash' culture of injury and litigation for financial compensation has made this condition increasingly common.

Cervical spine involvement is common in rheumatoid disease; up to 65% get atlanto-axial instability and up to 34% have secondary neurological change.

Infection is rare in the cervical spine but is more likely to occur in the elderly, alcoholics, diabetics, intravenous drug users and rheumatoid patients.

Pathology

Degeneration

Degenerative disease of the cervical spine is also described as cervical spondylosis. The discs become dehydrated and

Table 8.52	Diseases of the cervical spine by age group	
Young adults	**Middle age**	**Elderly**
Trauma	Rheumatoid arthritis	Spondylosis
Infection	Spondylosis	Infection
	(degenerative disease)	Tumours
	Ankylosing spondylitis	
	Tumour	

fissures develop posteriorly. The central nucleus pulposus may then prolapse through these fissures causing a localized fibrotic response. A large prolapse may compress nerve roots or the spinal cord if it occupies a central position. Osteophytes may develop about the disc space and cause compression of the nerve roots. Facet joint degeneration may lead to hypertrophy with osteophyte formation, further reducing space for passage of nerve roots through the neural foramina. Compression of nerve roots leads to radiculopathy with pain radiating to the distribution of the nerve root, whereas cord compression causes myelopathy with effects on both the upper and lower limbs and possibly bladder and bowel function.

Inflammation

Rheumatoid arthritis can affect the synovial joints of the cervical spine. Synovitis, pannus formation, erosions and destruction can lead to significant instability. Atlanto-axial instability is common, with the first cervical vertebra (atlas) usually slipping forwards relative to the second (axis). The spinal canal is large at this level but a significant slip may lead to myelopathy. Damage to the joints between the occiput and atlas may lead to cranial settling, where the atlas migrates through the foramen magnum, compressing the brain stem or upper spinal cord. Instability may also occur below the axis, with myelopathy being more likely due to the progressively narrowing spinal canal.

There is an important genetic contribution in ankylosing spondylitis, with a strong association with HLA-B27 (p. 491). Sacroiliitis develops initially with progressive involvement of the spine in a caudal (sacral) to cranial (cervical) direction. There is inflammation of paraspinal ligaments and facet joints, followed by fibrosis and ossification. There is a tendency for the spine to become kyphotic and rigid. This increased stiffness predisposes to unstable fractures with a low rate of healing. Neurological compromise is common. Isolated areas of the spine may develop pseudarthrosis, an abnormal mobile fibrotic joint that may be secondary to a fracture. There may also be involvement of large synovial joints such as the hip.

Malignancy

The malignancies that most commonly affect the cervical spine are metastatic carcinoma from breast, bronchus, kidney, prostate and thyroid. Lesions may be lytic with loss of bone structure, or blastic with abnormal bone formation. In both cases structural strength is abnormal and fracture or collapse can follow. Such carcinomas may invade the surrounding soft tissues and cavities leading to nerve root or cord compression.

Plasma cell myeloma (p. 810) is the most common primary tumour of bone, though more specifically there is neoplastic proliferation of plasma cells, occupants of the marrow cavity. The effects on the bone are secondary with lytic, destructive lesions developing due to increased osteoclast activation. The lesions are usually multiple and, whilst favouring the axial skeleton, they may exist elsewhere. The weakened bone is prone to fracture and collapse, predisposing to cord compression.

Infection

Whilst the lumbar and thoracic spine is more frequently involved in pyogenic, granulomatous (tubercular) and parasitic infections, complications in the cervical spine infection may have devastating consequences. The intervertebral disc provides a relatively avascular area for colonization and is rapidly destroyed. Infection spreads to the adjacent vertebral bodies and may cross to further disc spaces. The posterior elements can also be involved, and abscesses may form in the spinal canal (epidural) or in surrounding tissues. Bony destruction occurs with time leading to vertebral collapse. This may provoke spinal cord compression, although it is possible for this to occur with an epidural abscess alone. The spinal cord may also be compromised by thrombosis of spinal arteries or veins secondary to the infection. Paralysis or death may follow depending on the level affected.

Scope of disease

The importance of the cervical spine in positioning the head for function means that the impact of disease (pain and stiffness) can have a significant effect on quality of life. It is difficult to rest the cervical spine when painful and many days of work may be lost. The consequences of nerve root or spinal cord compression are also severe with the possibility of permanent loss of limb, bladder or bowel function, leading to greater dependence on others in the long term.

Clinical features

Pain

Pain from neck pathology may be felt in the neck or may radiate to the shoulder and arm (Table 8.53). There may be associated neurological symptoms in the upper limb.

Stiffness

Most cervical spine pathology leads to some stiffness, either from disease of the joints or from secondary muscle spasm. Complete ankylosis in a flexed position is suggestive of ankylosing spondylitis.

Neurological symptoms

Paraesthesia, numbness, spasticity, weakness, gait abnormality and bladder or bowel disturbance are all manifestations of radiculopathy and myelopathy and must be queried.

Medical history

General conditions such as rheumatoid disease and diabetes mellitus should be noted. A family history of ankylosing spondylitis may exist, and any past history of malignancy must be identified.

Examination
Look

The whole spine should be inspected. There may be general evidence of rheumatoid disease on inspection. A flexion deformity of the cervical spine with loss of forward vision

541

Table 8.53 The location of pain and underlying disease process

Posterior neck	Shoulder girdle with neurological symptoms	Arm with neurological symptoms
Cervical spondylosis	Disc protrusion above C5	Disc protrusion C5 and below
Muscle spasm post injury	Brachial neuritis	Thoracic outlet syndrome Tumours abutting the brachial plexus (Pancoast tumour)

suggests ankylosing spondylitis. There may be wasting of muscles of the shoulder girdle and upper limb with cervical root compression. Finally the gait should be examined. A broad unsteady gait is seen with cervical myelopathy.

Feel
Palpation of the posterior elements of the cervical spine and adjacent muscles may reveal tenderness but this is non-specific.

Move
Flexion, extension, lateral flexion and rotation are the composite movements performed by the cervical spine. Greater loss of flexion and extension are noted with spondylosis (degeneration). Approximately 60% of rotation occurs at the atlanto-axial joint, and rotational movements are most affected by disease at this level (e.g. rheumatoid disease).

Neurological examination
A full neurological examination should be performed including upper and lower limbs and a rectal examination (to assess rectal tone). Lower limb neurology is covered in the thoraco-lumbar spine section (p. 545). Peripheral nerves must also be assessed to rule out entrapment in the upper limb. Table 8.54 describes clinical findings with specific root entrapment.

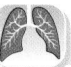

Initial investigations

Plain X-rays
The standard radiographic views of the cervical spine are AP and lateral. The lateral view is most useful for assessing the disc spaces, facet joints, spinal alignment and any bony abnormalities (collapse or lytic lesions). A good lateral view should show the whole cervical spine down to the first thoracic vertebrae. It is sometimes necessary to pull down on the shoulders to see the C7–T1 junction. If the junction cannot be clearly seen, a 'swimmer's' view may be taken in which one arm is placed above the head. The effect of neck position on instability is revealed with lateral views taken in flexion (Fig. 8.45a) and extension (Fig. 8.45b). Subluxation may only be noticeable in one position (usually flexion).

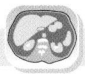

Further investigations

Full blood count/erythrocyte sedimentation rate
White count and inflammatory markers may be raised with infection, inflammatory arthropathy or even some tumours.

Malignancy screen
If malignancy is suspected, plasma electrophoresis (for myeloma), tumour markers (including prostate specific antigen in men), liver function tests and bone biochemistry should be performed.

CT of the cervical spine
CT is a useful investigation to assess bony alignment, destruction and the cervico-thoracic junction that is difficult to identify on plain X-rays.

MRI of the neck
With MRI, information can be obtained on all aspects of spinal pathology, the spinal cord and the nerve roots. It is

Table 8.54 Clinical features with root entrapment

Root	Disc level	Pain/numbness	Weakness/wasting	Reflex loss
C3	C2–3	Back of neck and ear	Nil	Nil
C4	C3–4	Back of neck and upper anterior chest	Nil	Nil
C5	C4–5	To shoulder tip and over deltoid	Deltoid (shoulder abduction)	Nil
C6	C5–6	Thumb and first web space	Biceps (elbow flexion)	Biceps jerk
C7	C6–7	Middle finger	Triceps (elbow extension)	Triceps jerk
C8	C7–T1	Little finger	Intrinsic muscles (MCPJ flexion and IPJ extension)	Nil

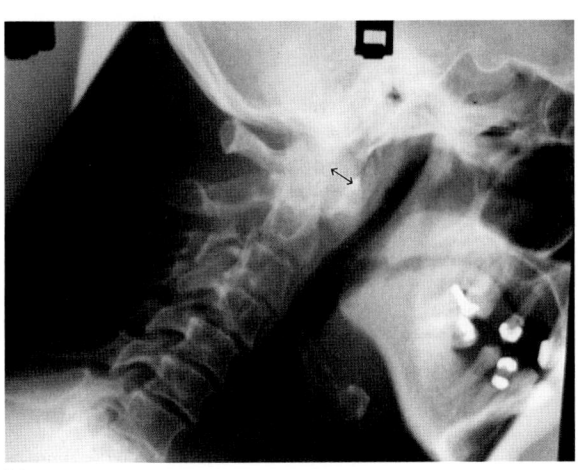

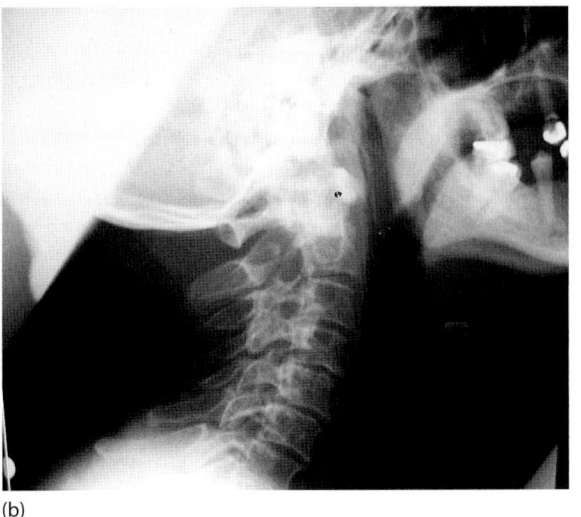

(a)

(b)

Fig. 8.45a, b Plain film of rheumatoid disease of the cervical spine. (a) 'Flexion' lateral view of the rheumatoid cervical spine showing atlanto-axial instability. The skull and atlas (first cervical vertebra) are allowed to slip forwards relative to the axis (second cervical vertebra). (b) The 'extension' lateral view allows the atlas to return to its normal position relative to the axis.

the investigation of choice when tumour or infection is suspected.

Cervical myelography (injection of radio-opaque dye into the spinal canal allowing visualization of the spinal cord, its exiting nerve roots, and any compressive lesion) has been largely replaced by MRI.

Nerve conduction studies

This may be a useful investigation when neurological symptoms could be arising from more peripheral pathology (brachial plexus and distal nerves).

Initial management

Patient education

The impact of heavy manual work on the symptoms of neck pathology necessitates periods of rest. A soft or hard cervical collar may help to provide rest and support but can also increase stiffness and muscle weakness with prolonged use.

Simple analgesia

Simple analgesics and NSAIDs should be prescribed to patients in pain. Spasm of the paraspinal muscles may be a contributing source of pain and is relieved by low doses of diazepam.

Physiotherapy

Work on range of motion and strength of the neck can be complemented by massage, traction and manipulation.

Surgical management

General
Arthrodesis

Arthrodesis can relieve pain from severe degeneration or instability with fusion at the offending level. Arthrodesis is also used where significant excision of vertebral bodies is performed for infection or tumour. The rates of union are generally good. Currently, joint replacement is not available for the cervical spine.

Specific
Spondylosis/disc prolapse

Initial measures are analgesia, the use of a collar and physiotherapy. Surgical intervention is indicated when pain is unresponsive to the above measures or worsening neurological deficit occurs (particularly myelopathy). Stenosis of the spinal canal requires decompression and fusion. This is usually performed from the front of the neck via the disc spaces. Compression of the nerve roots laterally can be decompressed via posterior lamino-foraminotomies, preserving the disc space and adjacent facet joints.

Rheumatoid disease

Cervical instability that is not prevented by use of a collar will require fusion (Fig. 8.46). If neurological changes have developed, surgical decompression may also be necessary. There is a tendency for short fusions (2 or 3 vertebrae) to fail early in the rheumatoid spine with instability developing above and below the fused segment. It is therefore often better to fuse the vertebrae from the thorax to the occiput.[1]

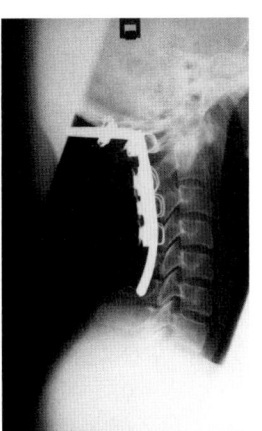

Fig. 8.46 Occipito-cervical fusion in a patient with rheumatoid atlanto-axial instability.

Malignancy

A percutaneous biopsy may be necessary for tissue diagnosis. Many tumours respond well to radiotherapy, chemotherapy or hormone therapy.

Surgical decompression and stabilization is required for acute cord compression, which may be the initial presentation. High doses of intravenous steroid (dexamethasone) may reduce the effects of acute cord compression.

Surgery is also indicated for patients with persistent pain despite tumour-directed medical therapy, although the risk of complications is high with advanced malignant disease (multiple spinal metastases and visceral involvement). Patients should therefore be fully staged prior to any surgical intervention when possible. Neurological compromise following cord compression does not always fully recover despite adequate decompression.

Infection

The spine is generally less accessible than many peripheral joints and there is greater reliance on percutaneous needle aspiration to obtain samples for culture. Drains may also be placed percutaneously into large paraspinal abscesses. The neck can be supported in a collar if instability from destructive infection is a concern. Antibiotics are chosen based on culture results.

Surgery is only considered with acute cord compression, worsening neurological symptoms, gross instability or poor response to medical treatment. The infected tissue and abscess requires debridement from the front or back of the neck and the spine must then be stabilized with bone graft and/or instrumentation (plates, rods, cages and screws).

REFERENCE

(1) Fairbank J. *Inflammatory disorders of the cervical spine*. In: Bulstrode C et al (eds) *Oxford Textbook of orthopaedics and trauma*. Oxford: Oxford University Press, 2002: pp. 492–494.

The thoraco-lumbar spine

The thoraco-lumbar spine consists of 17 vertebral bodies, intervening intervertebral discs, facet joints, ligaments and muscles. It forms the appendicular framework for the skeleton and normal function is vital for daily tasks. Rotation, flexion, extension and lateral flexion allow alteration of posture and position.

Epidemiology

Table 8.55 outlines the age and sex predilection of thoraco-lumbar diseases. Back pain is very common. The incidence is 6000 per 100 000 per year with a lifetime prevalence of up to 80%.[1] The condition accounts for 13% of sick leave from work.

Approximately 20 000 per 100 000 people under 60 years have an asymptomatic disc prolapse,[2] although the exact prevalence of symptomatic disc disease is difficult to quantify.

Mild scoliosis (curvature of less than 10°) occurs in up to 10% of adolescents. Severe progressive adolescent curvatures are seen more frequently in girls. By comparison, the prevalence of Scheuermann's kyphosis is approximately 1000 per 100 000 with a male predominance. Ankylosing spondylitis is also more common in men, but with a lower prevalence.

The prevalence of identifiable spondylolysis in the adult population is estimated to be 7000 per 100 000; however, the prevalence of symptomatic disease is much lower. There is an undeniable genetic influence on susceptibility, and high rates (41%) are seen in some ethnic groups such as the Japanese Aino.

Pathology

Degeneration

Spondylosis is a general term that encapsulates the various degenerative processes of the spine. The symptoms and effects depend on the region of the spine involved. With advancing age the intervertebral discs become dehydrated, and fissuring of the posterior annulus fibrosus occurs. Chemical changes occur in the nucleus pulposus, and the overall effect is a reduced load-bearing ability. This results in rupture of the posterior annulus allowing extrusion of the nucleus pulposus (prolapse). This material tends to provoke an inflammatory response causing fibrosis, adhesions and tethering of nerve roots. Large prolapses may compress the nerve roots causing sciatica. Severe

Table 8.55	Diseases of the thoraco-lumbar spine by age group		
Children	**Young adults**	**Middle age**	**Elderly**
Infection	Infection	Rheumatoid arthritis (women)	Spinal stenosis (degeneration)
Congenital scoliosis	Adolescent idiopathic scoliosis (women)	Degenerative disease	Infection
Congenital kyphosis	Ankylosing spondylitis (men)	Ankylosing spondylitis (men)	Tumours
Spondylolysis	Scheuermann's disease (men) Spondylolysis Disc prolapse	Tumours Disc prolapse	Kyphosis with osteoporotic collapse (women)

prolonged compression may irreversibly damage the root. Large central prolapses may compress the spinal cord (above L1) or the cauda equina (S2–S4 roots). The cauda equina is essential for normal function of the bladder and bowels. Over 95% of disc prolapses are lumbar and usually involve L4–5 or L5–S1. Thoracic disc prolapse is less common but the effects are often more marked due to the reduced volume of the spinal canal at this level.

Degenerative changes of the facet joints result in hypertrophic osteophyte formation and capsular thickening. Loss of disc height from dehydration and prolapse (Fig. 8.47) leads to buckling of both the ligamentum flavum and posterior longitudinal ligament (Fig. 8.48). Instability may lead to spondylolisthesis. All these processes can narrow the spinal canal and reduced blood flow can lead to ischaemia of the local neural structures causing neurogenic claudication.

Spondylolisthesis describes the pathological process of anterior slippage of one vertebral body on another. The erect human posture and lumbar lordosis may predispose. The majority of cases are due to degeneration of facet joints and disc spaces, or spondylolysis (see trauma/instability). Degenerative slips are rarely severe in magnitude but the narrowing of the spinal canal has implications as outlined above.

Trauma/instability

Isthmic spondylolisthesis (the most common subtype) is due to bilateral fractures of the pars interarticularis (bony bridge between the facet joints) and results in a forward slip of the anterior spinal elements. In most cases, this is due to stress fractures, which chronically displace or elongate the pars as it heals. Approximately 90% involve the L5 pars, allowing L5 to slip anterior to S1. In general slips are usually mild and often asymptomatic, but large slips may lead to pain or adjacent nerve root entrapment. Because the posterior elements remain undisplaced the spinal canal is enlarged rather than narrowed.

Inflammation

Rheumatoid disease has greatest pathological effects in the cervical spine, but the synovial facet joints of the thoraco-lumbar spine may also be involved. Destruction of these joints can destabilize the spine, giving rise to a collapsing secondary deformity. Osteoporotic crush fractures are common and scoliosis or kyphosis may develop.

Ankylosing spondylitis (p. 488) proceeds from the sacrum upwards, therefore thoraco-lumbar disease presents early. The kyphotic deformity occurs because pain is less severe when this position is adopted.

Malignancy

The thoraco-lumbar spine is a common site for metastatic carcinoma due to its high vascularity and proximity to the viscera. The prevertebral venous plexus of Batson in the pelvis allows retrograde flow of blood from the pelvic viscera to the spine, which can be a haematogenous route for metastatic seeding. Deposits can lead to vertebral collapse, instability and spondylolisthesis. Compression of the spinal cord or nerve roots can occur.

The thoraco-lumbar spine is the most common primary site of plasma cell myeloma (p. 810). Hypercalcaemia can result from osteoclasis, and deposition of monoclonal proteins in the kidneys may lead to renal failure.

Metabolic

The development of kyphosis of the thoraco-lumbar spine with age is usually due to spontaneous vertebral body crush fractures (Fig. 8.49). Osteoporosis leads to loss of trabeculae in the vertebral bodies, while osteomalacia results in defective mineralization. Both conditions weaken the bone and predispose to collapse. Decreased bone mineral density can be well demonstrated in the elderly spine.[3]

Infection

Infection may be pyogenic, granulomatous or parasitic. There is usually haematogenous spread from a distant focus (e.g. tuberculosis of the lung). *Staphylococcus aureus* is the most common pyogenic organism and the lumbar spine is most often affected. The relatively avascular disc space is rapidly colonized due to poor host defence, with subsequent destruction of the disc and adjacent vertebral bodies. Abscess formation can occur in the epidural space adjacent to the disc. A combination of pus and granulation tissue can lead to spinal cord compression. Alternatively this can also arise following vertebral destruction and collapse.

Approximately 3% of patients with tuberculosis develop skeletal system infection. Of these, 50% are spinal with the thoraco-lumbar junction as the most commonly infected site. There may be skip lesions (in the spine) in 5%. Large paravertebral 'cold' abscesses form in 50% and these may spread posteriorly to the skin or anteriorly to within the psoas muscle. There is a high rate of spontaneous fusion of the spine with successful medical treatment.

Congenital/developmental

Kyphosis is a relative shortening of the anterior spine, allowing a flexed posture to develop. Lordosis is a relative shortening of the posterior spine, allowing an extended posture to develop. Scoliosis describes a lateral curvature of the spine.

Congenital curves develop due to abnormal embryology of the spine with failure of separation or formation of vertebral bodies. Idiopathic scoliosis usually involves the thoracic spine or thoraco-lumbar junction. The pathogenesis is thought to be a relative overgrowth of the anterior vertebral bodies (due to posterior avascularity) forcing the spine to twist and buckle laterally as growth proceeds. The main curve becomes stiff and compensatory flexible curves develop above and below to maintain normal posture. Curves over 30° at their apex are more likely to progress in adulthood, at up to 1° per year. Scheuermann's kyphosis is thought to occur from anterior spinal avascularity which may be lumbar or thoracic and gives rise to a deformity that becomes fixed with time. Abnormalities of the vertebral end plate allow discs to prolapse into the vertebral bodies (Schmorl's nodes).

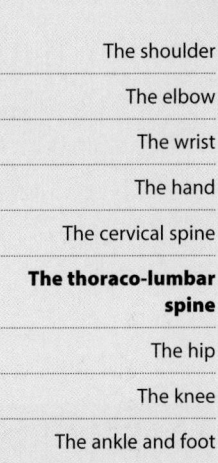

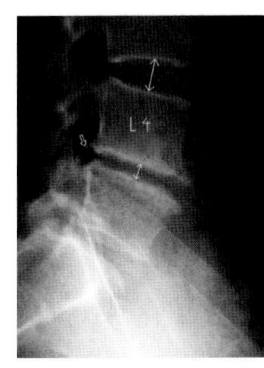

Fig. 8.47 The lumbar spine. A coned lateral view at the L4 level showing a well-preserved disc space at L3/4, but loss of height and osteophyte formation at L4/5. There is ossification of the posterior longitudinal ligament at this level (open arrow), which overlies a posterior disc protrusion, narrowing the spinal canal.

Scope of disease

Most thoraco-lumbar pathology results in pain and stiffness, and can lead to incapacity and depression (often influenced by socioeconomic conditions). Many symptoms are chronic and can be difficult to control. Following recovery there remains a risk of exacerbation, particularly in patients whose occupation involves heavy labour. The modern compensation culture has been blamed for delayed recovery from spinal pathology, possibly due to altered incentives and motivation.

Clinical features

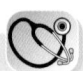

Pain

Pain from thoraco-lumbar disease may be felt in the back or radiate to the buttocks and legs. The pattern of this radiation can give information about the source of the pain, in particular when nerve root compression exists (Table 8.56). There may be associated neurological symptoms in the perineum or lower limbs.

Shooting, severe leg pain exacerbated by coughing or sneezing suggests nerve root compression. The leg pain is usually more severe than the associated back pain. A chronic aching pain in the legs that is worse when walking, particularly downhill, is characteristic of spinal stenosis. This is frequently bilateral, though not always with equal severity. Back pain at rest or at night may be due to sinister pathology such as infection or tumour.

Stiffness

Stiffness is a non-specific symptom. Early ankylosing spondylitis commonly gives morning stiffness, whilst later disease leads to permanent stiffness due to ankylosis.

Neurological symptoms

Paraesthesia, numbness, spasticity, weakness, gait abnormality and bladder or bowel disturbance suggest nerve root or spinal cord compression. Pain and numbness from root compression is frequently located in the dermatomal distribution.

Medical history

General conditions such as rheumatoid disease and diabetes mellitus should be noted. A family history of ankylosing spondylitis may be present, and any history of malignancy is relevant.

Examination

Look

The entire spine should be inspected. There may be general evidence of rheumatoid disease on inspection. In a slim patient the spinal alignment can be assessed. Scoliosis often worsens with forward flexion. A kyphotic deformity is best appreciated from the side. Loss of the lumbar lordosis is a feature of disc prolapse with associated muscle spasm, whilst an exaggerated lordosis is a common finding with spondylolisthesis.

Feel

Palpation of the posterior elements of the thoraco-lumbar spine may identify a spinal deformity that is not appreciable on inspection. Tenderness is a non-specific finding. A spondylolisthesis will cause a sudden step in the spinous processes at the diseased level, due to the upper spine sliding forwards relative to the lower spine. However, with spondylolysis the step is felt at the level above, as the posterior elements are left in place by the displacing vertebral body. Percussion of the posterior spine may elicit deep pain due to infection or tumour.

Move

Flexion, extension, lateral flexion and rotation are assessed. Painful and limited extension is a classical finding with spondylolisthesis, and this movement is often painful with ankylosing spondylitis leading to the flexed or kyphotic posture. Lateral flexion may give clues to the flexibility of a scoliotic curve, with the upper and lower portions often correcting with this movement.

Neurological examination

A full neurological examination should be performed including rectal examination (for anal tone) and assessment of perineal sensation. Peripheral nerve entrapment in the lower limb is uncommon but must be considered. Table 8.57 describes the clinical findings with specific root entrapment.

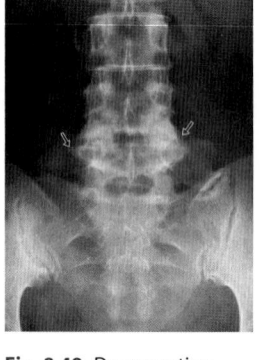

Fig. 8.48 Degenerative disease of the spine. An AP view showing the prolific osteophyte formation (arrows) that can occur at degenerative levels of the spine.

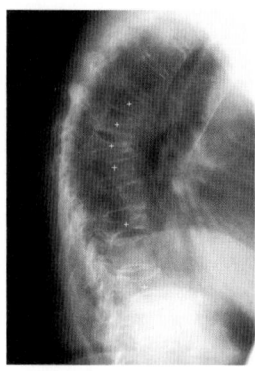

Fig. 8.49 Lateral view of the thoraco-lumbar spine in a patient with osteoporosis showing multilevel vertebral collapse (crosses), leading to a kyphotic deformity.

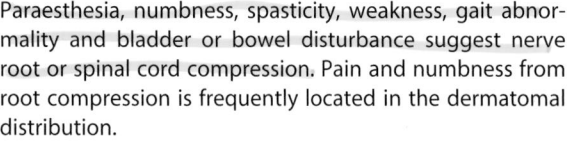

Table 8.56	Location and radiation of back pain		
Back pain	**Buttock pain**	**Anterior thigh pain**	**Posterior leg pain below knee**
Degenerative disease	Sacroiliitis	Spondylolisthesis	L4, L5 or S1 root compression
Rheumatoid disease	Spinal stenosis	Spondylolysis	
Scoliosis/kyphosis	Degenerative lumbar disease	L2 or L3 root compression	
Tumour		High lumbar spinal stenosis (often bilateral)	
Spondylolisthesis		Hip arthritis	
Infection			

Table 8.57	Symptoms of nerve root entrapment			
Root	**Disc level**	**Pain/numbness**	**Weakness/wasting**	**Reflex loss**
L2	L1–2	Proximal anterior thigh	Hip flexors	Nil
L3	L2–3	Distal anterior thigh	Hip flexors	Nil
L4	L3–4	Medial calf	Quadriceps (knee extension)	Knee jerk
L5	L4–5	Lateral calf, dorsal foot, big toe	Extensor hallucis longus (hallux dorsiflexion)	Nil
S1	L5–S1	Posterior calf, sole of foot, little toe	Gastrocsoleus (ankle plantarflexion)	Ankle jerk
Cauda equina (S2–4)	Any of above	Perianal and perineal	Bladder and bowel sphincters	Cremasteric

Assessment for L5/S1 nerve root compression

Lifting the heel up with the leg straight will stretch the sciatic nerve, and pain from L5 and S1 root compression is classically reproduced before significant hip flexion is achieved.

Assessment for L3/L4 nerve root compression

The femoral stretch test involves placing the patient supine or on the side and then extending the hip followed by gradual flexion of the knee. L3 or L4 root compression pain may be reproduced.

Initial investigations

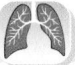

Plain X-rays

The standard views of the thoraco-lumbar spine are the AP and lateral. Spinal deformity may be appreciated on both views. Spondylolisthesis can be identified and measured on the lateral film. Associated spondylolysis may be noted. The pars interarticularis is better seen with oblique lateral X-rays. When clear definition of the vertebrae is needed, X-rays must be 'coned' at that level. This can be important if tumour or infection is suspected. The upper thoracic spine is always poorly visualized on lateral X-rays due to the overlying shoulder girdles, and CT or MRI may be necessary.

Further investigations

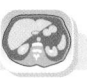

Full blood count/markers of inflammation

The white count and ESR may be elevated with infection and inflammation.

Tumour markers

Tumour markers may be indicated depending on the suspected pathology.

Bone biochemistry

Serum calcium, phosphate and alkaline phosphatase may be abnormal with metabolic disease or malignancy.

CT of the spine

CT is a sensitive means of detecting bony destruction and deformity. It is also used to identify disc prolapse, particularly when performed as a CT myelogram.

MRI of the spine

MRI is now the gold standard for intervertebral disc pathology, infection and tumours.

Percutaneous needle biopsy

Needle biopsy can be performed under X-ray or CT control and allows access to deep areas of infection or tumour, enabling samples to be taken for histology and microbiology.

Nerve conduction studies

Tests of neurophysiology alone are not reliable as a means of identifying the levels of nerve root compression but may be helpful with conflicting clinical and radiological findings. It is an important technique when more peripheral nerve compression is suspected.

Initial management

Patient education

Rest has historically been advised in most cases of back pain, but recently the importance of active mobilization has been appreciated. Bed rest should be minimized and must be followed by a combination of exercise and education.[4]

Simple analgesia

Simple analgesics and NSAIDs may be prescribed for symptomatic relief. Paraspinal muscle spasm can account for a lot of the pain, and low doses of diazepam may relieve this. Epidural steroid injections are more effective than placebo for pain relief in cases of root compression but do not reduce the need for surgery.[5]

Physiotherapy

Muscle strengthening, massage, manipulation, posture education and psychological support and motivation have

547

important contributions to patient management. Graduated return to activity can be encouraged. The use of a corset is not advisable in most cases of back pain due to restriction of movement and muscle use.

Surgical management

General

Arthrodesis

As for the cervical spine, there is no current role for arthroplasty but arthrodesis remains an important technique. The indications are infection, tumour, instability, fracture, following spinal decompression and when correcting spinal deformity. The rates of union are generally good. Anterior surgery may be performed via the abdomen or thorax when access to the vertebral bodies is required.

Specific

Disc prolapse

Initial measures involve analgesia, diazepam for spasm, mobilization exercises, concentration on posture and epidural steroid injection. Rest from exertion is important but bed rest should be minimal. Physiotherapy can be helpful. Most cases resolve spontaneously.[6]

Urgent discectomy is required for progressive neurological deficits, cauda equina syndrome, when conservative treatment does not lead to symptom improvement after 6–12 weeks, or when recurrent sciatica develops. Lumbar discectomy is now frequently performed with the assistance of an operating microscope through short incisions, with probable reduction in hospital stay and less postoperative pain. There is a 90% rate of initial success. There is a higher threshold to operate on thoracic disc prolapses. The main indication is significant neurological deficit, as access to the discs is difficult and may require removal of the head of a rib or use of video-assisted thoracoscopy.

Spinal stenosis

The associated spinal degenerative disease may account for significant back pain. Surgery is indicated for severe neurological symptoms and pain in the legs. Decompression of the spinal canal is undertaken both posteriorly and laterally over the exiting nerve roots (Fig. 8.50). This may lead to destabilization of the spine and concomitant spinal fusion may be necessary. The use of spinal instrumentation can increase the rate of fusion and allow earlier mobilization.

Rheumatoid arthritis

Rheumatoid disease of the thoraco-lumbar spine may lead to deformity, instability and canal stenosis. Most cases can be treated symptomatically with analgesia and bracing. When there is uncontrollable pain or cord compression, surgical decompression and fusion may be required.

The natural history in ankylosing spondylitis is kyphosis and ankylosis of the spine from the lumbar to the cervical

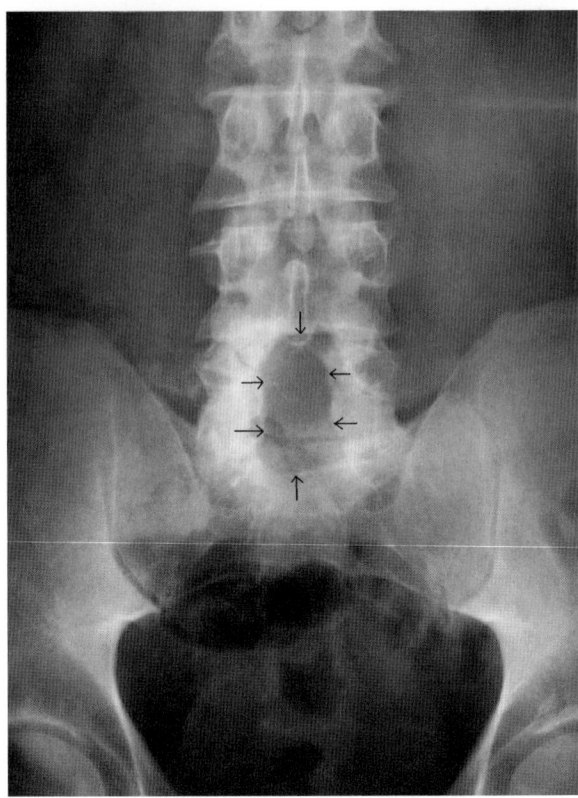

Fig. 8.50 AP view of the lumbosacral spine showing the defect created during spinal decompression (arrows). This defect is created by removing the posterior spinous process, the laminae and often part of the facet joint.

region. This progression cannot be prevented but the position of ankylosis may be controlled. Bracing the spine to prevent flexion may ensure a more upright gait, and NSAIDs can reduce pain and stiffness. When kyphosis is severe, osteotomy can be performed in the lumbar or cervical spine with correction of the deformity, but there is a risk of paralysis with such surgery.

Spondylolysis/spondylolisthesis

Spondylolysis is generally a benign disease. Treatment is focused on load reduction, strengthening abdominal and back muscles, bracing and steroid injections. Surgery is indicated for severe pain, significant spondylolisthesis or the development of neurological symptoms. In young adults with minor slips, the spondylolysis can be directly stabilized with screws. More severe slips require fusion and fixation. Reduction of the slip is not recommended due to a risk of neurological damage.

The treatment principles are similar for degenerative spondylolisthesis, but neurological compromise is more common and posterior decompression is often necessary.

Infection

Percutaneous aspiration, biopsy and drain placement are frequently utilized for thoraco-lumbar spine infection. Corsets or plaster jackets can help with cases of instability. High-dose antibiotics are required for 6 weeks or more depending on response. Surgery is indicated for acute cord compression, worsening neurological symptoms, gross instability or poor response to medical treatment. Debridement of the infected tissue and abscess is performed. Infection can be accessed from the front or back of the spine, with bony stabilization being performed as necessary for significant bone or joint damage.

Malignancy

The management of tumour involving the thoraco-lumbar spine requires a multidisciplinary approach. Initial diagnosis can be achieved with percutaneous needle biopsies. Myeloma and metastatic disease may respond well to radiotherapy, chemotherapy or hormonal therapy. Significant visceral (lung and liver) or diffuse spinal involvement usually denotes a poor prognosis and surgery may not be appropriate. Pain from diseased vertebrae can be improved by bracing.

The indications for surgical intervention are cord compression or uncontrollable pain from collapse or instability. Metastases may be isolated (e.g. renal) and excision of the lesion and surrounding vertebrae may be curative. Anterior surgery is usually performed via the chest or abdomen, removing diseased bone and tumour and replacing this with large bone grafts or metal cages. Radiotherapy can be useful as an alternative to or following surgery. There is an appreciable risk of paralysis and morbidity with such surgery on the spine and the risks/benefits must be assessed in each case. As for cervical spine compression, paralysis from cord compression may not always fully recover following decompression.

Congenital/developmental deformity

In the majority of cases the patient's main concern is the deformity. It is possible to function normally with significant scoliosis or kyphosis, however some spinal curvatures can progress and lead to disability in later life. The role of bracing to counter the curve progression remains controversial. It is only considered of use in the growing skeleton.

Back pain ('fatigue pain') can be a difficult problem with scoliosis but usually responds to physiotherapy and massage. The indications for surgery are severe curvature, prevention of progressive curvature, or when marked psychological effects of the deformity are present. Long spinal fusions are performed around the apex of the curve with correction of the deformity through the removed disc spaces. The fusion is held with long metal rods and supplemented with bone graft. Surgery through the chest is often required and there is a small risk of paralysis (<1%), although intraoperative cord monitoring can virtually eliminate this risk.

REFERENCES

(1) Klaber Moffett J, Richardson G, Sheldon T, Maynard A. Back pain: its management and cost to society. York: Centre for Health Economics, 1995.
(2) Boden SD, Davis DO, Dian TS. Abnormal magnetic resonance scans of the lumbar spine in asymptomatic subjects. A prospective investigation. Journal of Bone and Joint Surgery 1990; 72: 403–408.
(3) Porter RW, Johnson K, McCutchan JDS. Wrist fracture, heel bone density and thoracic kyphosis: a case control study. Bone 1990; 11: 211–214.
(4) Waddell G, Feder G, Lewis M. Systematic reviews of bedrest and advice to stay active for acute low back pain. British Journal of General Practice 1997; 47: 647–652.
(5) Watts R, Sillagy C. A meta-analysis on the efficacy of epidural corticosteroids in the treatment of sciatica. Anaesthesia and Intensive Care 1995; 23: 564–569.
(6) Weber H. Lumbar disc herniation: a controlled prospective study with 30 years of observation. Spine 1983; 18: 24–27.

The hip

Hip pathology represents a large proportion of the orthopaedic workload and its socioeconomic impact can be great.

Epidemiology

Diseases of the hip are common. Approximately 5% of the population over 65 years has degenerative arthritis of the hip,[1] and up to 50% of patients with rheumatoid disease have hip involvement. The age and sex predilection of other hip conditions are listed in Table 8.58.

Pathology

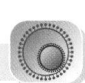

Inflammation

Inflammation can involve the joint (arthropathies) or adjacent tendons and bursae. Rheumatoid disease can lead to the usual pathological changes of synovitis, pannus formation, cartilage loss and erosions. There is osteoporosis of the periarticular bone and on the acetabular side this can result in medial migration of the head (protrusio).

Degenerative arthritis leads to fibrillation and eburnation of the joint surface, subchondral sclerosis, peripheral osteophytes and subchondral cysts. Thickening and contracture of the capsule leads to a reduction in movement. The hip often adopts a position of flexion, adduction and external rotation. Cysts can collapse causing flattening of the femoral head and shortening of the limb (Fig. 8.51). Protrusio may develop and in some cases there can be almost complete destruction of the head (erosive osteoarthritis).

In ankylosing spondylitis similar changes to degenerative arthritis occur. There is usually gross stiffness and fixed flexion deformity. The latter is due in part to the hyperlordosis of the lumbar spine, which is an attempt to compensate for the thoracic hyperkyphosis.

549

Table 8.58	Diseases of the hip by age group			
Children	**Young adults**	**Middle aged**	**Elderly**
Perthes' disease in boys	Degenerative arthritis (secondary)	Rheumatoid and degenerative arthritis	Degenerative arthritis
Developmental dysplasia in girls	Avascular necrosis in men	Avascular necrosis in men	Metastatic disease
Slipped capital femoral epiphysis (SCFE)		Metastatic disease	Osteoporosis
Irritable hip		Myeloma	Myeloma
Infection		Paget's disease	Paget's disease

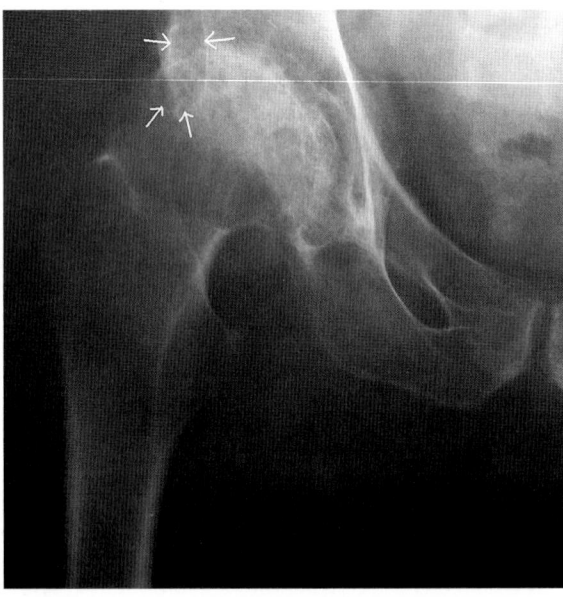

Fig. 8.51 Plain film of an osteoarthritic hip showing loss of joint space, osteophytes, sclerosis and 'kissing' cysts (arrows) in the femoral head and acetabulum. These may collapse suddenly, giving severe pain and shortening of the limb.

Vascular

Avascular necrosis (osteonecrosis) is frequently encountered in the hip and its effects on this joint are perhaps more catastrophic than in any other joint affected. The cause is identified in the majority (66%); these causes are listed in Table 8.59. In the remainder, there is no identifiable cause (idiopathic).

Vascular obstruction usually follows from a single ischaemic event. Initial bone marrow oedema is followed by cell death after 12–48 hours of ischaemia. The location and degree of this osteonecrosis is variable. A peripheral inflammatory response develops with ingrowth of granulation tissue bringing new capillaries and bone formation ('creeping substitution'). Full recovery of the lesion can take 2 or more years. During this time the weakened area of bone may collapse secondary to microfractures (Fig. 8.52). Flattening of the head and incongruence of the joint can lead to secondary arthritis. Large lesions in the superior weight-bearing dome carry the worst prognosis because of the greater risk of collapse.

Perthes' disease is a particular form of osteonecrosis of the hip seen in childhood with significant implications in the adult. The incidence is thought to be about 11 per 100 000 per year, with boys aged 4–9 years being most prone to develop Perthes' disease. It is thought that a genetic susceptibility exists. Unlike adult osteonecrosis,

Haemophiliac arthropathy frequently affects the hip but is not always recognized. Recurrent bleeds increase the pressure within the hip causing areas of osteonecrosis and subsequent arthritis. Protrusio of the hip is common.

Bursitis most often affects the trochanteric bursa and is usually mechanical or frictional (irritation from the fascia lata over the greater trochanter). It can also occur with rheumatoid disease, crystal arthropathies or trauma. Thickening and fibrosis of the bursa may result. Similar changes can occur with the iliopsoas bursa adjacent to the insertion of this tendon on the lesser trochanter.

Tears of the acetabular labrum are thought to be degenerative in 50%.[2] There is usually an element of acetabular dysplasia, leading to abnormally high loads on the labrum.

Table 8.59	Causes of avascular necrosis of the hip
Alcoholism
Steroids
Sickle cell disease (most common cause worldwide)
Trauma (femoral neck fracture, hip dislocation)
Radiotherapy
Chemotherapy
Renal transplant
Decompression sickness following diving (Caisson's disease)
Hyperlipidaemia
Systemic lupus erythematosus

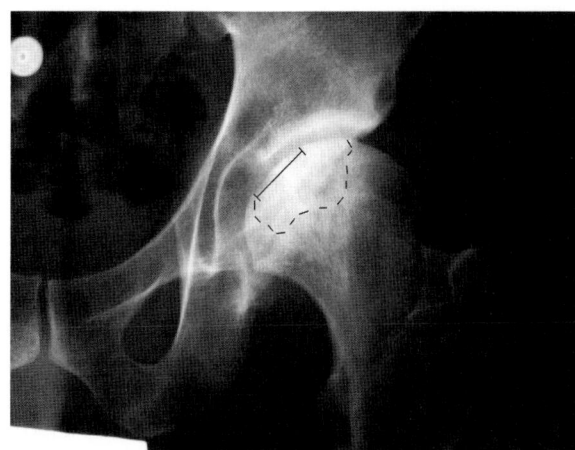

Fig. 8.52 Osteonecrosis of the femoral head showing the segmental nature of the disease. An area of flattening centrally indicates collapse.

multiple small infarcts occur, but the subsequent pathological process is identical. Repair of the femoral head consists of bone and fibrocartilage formation, giving a fragmented appearance on X-ray. With collapse and repair the head often becomes flattened and partly extruded from the acetabulum. Growth plate damage is common and secondary degeneration of a deformed hip occurs, particularly laterally due to impingement ('hinge abduction'). Arthritis in early adulthood is to be expected with severe cases.

Infection

Septic arthritis of the hip tends to occur in infants and intravenous drug users. The deep location of the joint makes diagnosis difficult and this can lead to delayed presentation with joint destruction and fibrosis.

Osteomyelitis about the hip is rare, but again is most likely to be seen in infants. Damage to the growth plate may affect subsequent growth leading to secondary deformity or a short limb. In neonates there may be persisting vascular channels across the growth plate and infection may enter the joint via these channels causing septic arthritis and further damage.

After the spine, the hip is the most common location for articular tuberculosis. Infection spreads from primary sites in the lungs or viscera. It is more common in children and involvement is initially bony, with subsequent synovitis and effusion. Joint destruction and arthritis follow and the hip may sublux. Once infection has resolved, it often leaves a fibrous ankylosis.

Infection involving joint replacement is an increasing problem. Deep infection rates of 1% are widely quoted and resistant organisms are on the increase. These rates are higher with surgery on patients with rheumatoid disease who are taking immunosuppressants, in diabetics and in revision hip surgery. Following implantation, bacteria may contaminate the prosthesis, lying dormant for many years. Once they become active and replicate, the adjacent host response can lead to activation of osteoclasts causing net bone resorption, loosening of the prosthesis and occasionally periprosthetic fracture. Infection may also present as a septic arthritis, due to bacterial colonization at the time of implantation or to haematogenous spread from elsewhere. Instrumentation of contaminated areas such as the oral cavity and urinary tract is frequently implicated.

Neoplasia

The most common malignancy in bone is secondary metastatic deposits. The femur and acetabulum are frequently involved, particularly the subtrochanteric region of the femur (Fig. 8.53a and b). Breast, lung, prostate, kidney and thyroid malignancies form the majority of primary malignancies. Deposits can be lytic (any primary tumour) or blastic (usually prostate or breast). In the latter group abnormal bone production is stimulated by the lesion. Both types cause structural weakness of the bone with the risk of fracture. Plasma cell myeloma can be regarded as the most common primary bone malignancy, although strictly speaking it is the plasma cells of the marrow that are involved. The hip and pelvis are affected in 20% of cases with osteopenia and lysis. Fracture is a common complication.

Congenital/developmental

Acetabular and femoral dysplasias are important causes of early degenerative arthritis of the hip. Now known as developmental dysplasia of the hip (DDH), it is thought to affect 400 per 100 000 live births. Late in pregnancy, as free space within the uterine cavity reduces and gestational hormone levels alter, the hips are thought to be prone to transient instability and can sublux or dislocate. This instability often corrects within days of birth. If it persists, abnormal development of the acetabulum occurs. The hip remains shallow, allowing persistent subluxation. The risk is greater in female babies (×4), those lying in breech position (×10), those with oligohydramnios (×10) and those with a positive family history. Most cases are detected early by the clinical screening programme. Approximately 20 per 100 000 newborns present late with more severe dysplasia or frank dislocation. A spectrum of persistent dysplasia is seen in adult hips, ranging from slight shallowness of the acetabulum to frank dislocation of the hip which sits in a false or pseudo-acetabulum (superior to the true acetabulum). Secondary degeneration occasionally occurs in adolescents and frank arthritis can present as early as the third decade.

Endocrine

Paget's disease (p. 517) frequently involves the hip. The bone is abnormal and secondary deformities (coxa vara and protrusio) and pathological fractures occur. Secondary degeneration of the hip occurs in up to 50% of affected joints. There is a risk of developing an osteosarcoma in the affected bone of up to 1%.

Osteoporosis (p. 512) affects the whole skeleton, but 'fragility' hip fractures are the most common fracture requiring hospital admission. Significant morbidity can

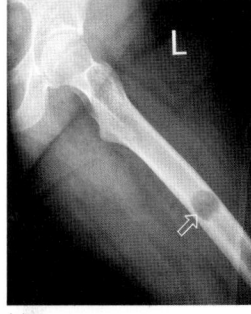

(a)

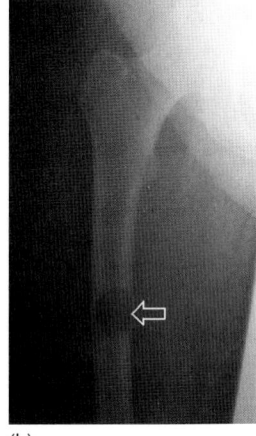

(b)

Fig. 8.53a, b (a) AP and (b) lateral views of metastatic adenocarcinoma deposit in the subtrochanteric femur. The severe cortical thinning warns that fracture is imminent.

551

arise. There is a reduction in bone mass but normal bone mineralization. Macroscopically there is thinning of the trabeculae and some are lost altogether giving enlarged haversian canals and marrow spaces.

Trauma

Periprosthetic hip fractures are part of the bigger problem of aseptic loosening of hip replacement prostheses. High fluid pressure and micromotion are thought to be responsible for wear debris reaching the bone–cement interface via cracks in the cement mantle, stimulating an inflammatory response. Osteoclast activity is increased and lytic cavities develop causing weakening of the bone. This can lead to loosening of the hip prosthesis or even fracture of the bone around it (periprosthetic).

Scope of disease

Disease affecting the hip joint can have a significant effect on function and quality of life. Loss of mobility can threaten independence. Pain from arthritis can be present at rest and at night, causing low mood. Many disease processes lead to a fixed deformity and this may result in compensatory deformities elsewhere. For example, a fixed flexion deformity of the hip can lead to hyperlordosis of the lumbar spine, an adduction deformity of the hip can lead to valgus deformity of the knee, and a short leg (>2 cm) can cause scoliosis and back pain.

Clinical features

Pain

The location and nature of pain in relation to diseases of the hip is presented in Table 8.60. Pain can be referred from the hip to the anterior thigh or knee. Pain at rest and at night is often seen with arthritis, but tumour and infection may be the cause. Arthritic pain is typically worse with mobility. Sudden worsening of pain with degenerative arthritis or osteonecrosis may herald collapse of a cyst in the femoral head or acetabulum.

Stiffness

Stiffness is a common symptom of hip disease. Many activities are affected, such as the ability to put on socks and shoes. Stiffness in the morning that improves over the day is characteristic of rheumatoid disease. Severe limita-

tion of movement occurs with ankylosing spondylitis and gross heterotopic ossification.

Limp

A limp is a common complaint that may be attributable to pain, deformity (stiffness), weakness or leg length inequality.

Snapping/clicking

Snapping and clicking about the hip most likely arise from the iliopsoas tendon, fascia lata, or intra-articular pathology such as a torn labrum. The patient may be able to localize the sensation or demonstrate provoking movements.

Medical history

Relevant family history and past medical history are important. Degenerative arthritis presenting in early adulthood is highly likely to be secondary to childhood pathology such as dysplasia, Perthes' disease, slipped capital femoral epiphysis or infection. Should osteonecrosis be suspected it is important to eliminate possible causes from Table 8.59. A history of malignancy is important in cases of unexplained hip pain.

Examination

Look

An assessment of leg length is performed. Real length is the distance from a fixed pelvic landmark such as the anterior superior iliac spine (ASIS) to a fixed point on the leg distally (medial malleolus). Any fixed flexion deformity of the hip or knee must be matched on the other leg for measurements to be compared. Apparent length is measured from a point in the midline (xiphisternum) and is dictated by pelvic tilt and deformities in the hip and knee joints. General features of rheumatoid disease or ankylosing spondylitis should be recognized.

Deformity may be apparent with the patient supine. The pelvis may be tilted to compensate for an adducted hip and hyperlordosis of the lumbar spine may allow a hip with fixed flexion to rest flat on the couch. Thomas' test demonstrates this fixed flexion. Both hips should be flexed up, the contralateral hip maximally with the patient pulling the knee towards the chest. This flattens the lumbar lordosis, confirmed by a hand placed under the lumbar spine. The hip being examined is then slowly extended and should reach the couch. The angle above the couch that is reached is the degree of fixed flexion (although the first 20° accounts for hip extension). When the leg lies in excessive

Table 8.60	Location of pain in relation to diseases of the hip		
Groin	**Lateral**	**Buttock**
Hip joint	Trochanteric bursitis	Lumbosacral disease
Iliopsoas pathology	Sciatica	Sciatica
Acetabular labrum	Meralgia paraesthetica (lateral femoral cutaneous nerve entrapment).	Loose acetabular component in total hip replacement
Inguinal pathology (hernia, etc.)		

external rotation, slipped capital femoral epiphysis may be the cause.

Feel

A deep joint such as the hip does not lend itself to palpation. Tenderness in the groin is non-specific. The greater trochanter should be palpated and may be diffusely tender with bursitis. If this has not already been done, the pelvis should be squared.

Move

The usual range of hip movements is flexion 130° (including pelvic flexion by flattening lordosis), extension 20°, adduction 30°, abduction 45°, internal rotation 30°, external rotation 50° (hip extended) and internal rotation 40°, external rotation 45° (hip flexed)

A reduction in movement does not help to distinguish hip pathologies. However, some patterns do exist. Degenerative arthritis tends to restrict abduction, extension and internal rotation. Attempts to internally rotate the hip passively are usually painful as the hip capsule tightens. In cases of developmental dysplasia there is often excessive anteversion of the femoral neck on the shaft. This gives a much larger proportion of internal rotation, particularly in flexion. When slipped capital femoral epiphysis has led to hip degeneration the altered anatomy affects movement. The hip tends to abduct with flexion due to impingement of the neck on the anterior acetabulum.

Gait

The patient should be asked to walk and the gait studied. An antalgic gait suggests pain, and classically the stance phase, during which the leg bears weight, is shortened, as is the length of stride. A Trendelenburg gait is caused by hip abductor weakness, with the contralateral side of the pelvis dropping rather than rising when the affected leg is in stance. With a short leg the pelvis and shoulder can be seen to drop as the heel strikes the ground and rise as the leg swings.

Trendelenburg test

The Trendelenburg test examines for abductor weakness. The patient stands facing the examiner, who places his or her hands on the anterior superior iliac spines. The patient is then asked to stand on one leg, flexing the other knee behind him/her. The abductor muscles should contract, causing the contralateral side of the pelvis to rise, but weakness causes it to fall and the patient has to lean his or her shoulders to the side of the stance leg to remain balanced, or bear weight through the examiner's arms.

Provocation tests

If labral instability is suspected, provocation tests can be carried out. Anterior labral pathology will give pain if the hip is extended and externally rotated, while flexion, adduction and internal rotation will provoke posterior labral pathology. It must be remembered that associated hip degeneration may cause pain with all of these movements.

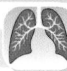

Initial investigations

Plain X-rays

The standard views of the hip are the AP and lateral. The AP film provides most information and it is often helpful to get an AP film of the pelvis showing both hips to allow comparison.

The standard changes of osteoarthritis (p. 479) and rheumatoid disease (p. 482) will be seen. Cysts in the head or acetabulum should be recognized as these may collapse, accelerating the degenerative process. The medial wall of the acetabulum may migrate into the pelvis (protrusio), particularly in rheumatoid or Paget's disease and after hip surgery.

Osteonecrosis leads to a classic sequence of changes. Early changes are only detectable on MRI. Later changes detectable on plain radiographs are an initial mixture of sclerosis (reduced remodelling) and osteopenia (increased vascularity and resorption), followed by subchondral fracture and collapse ('crescent sign'). Ultimately there may be fragmentation and gross collapse of the head, with secondary degenerative arthritis.

Dysplasia of the hip is recognized by a shallow acetabulum, subluxing femoral head, extreme valgus of the neck and a very narrow femoral canal. There may even be a pseudo-acetabulum with the hip articulating with the side of the pelvis above the true acetabulum.

Loosening and infection of a hip replacement may be heralded by a lytic line greater than 2 mm in thickness at the implant–bone interface. Lytic cavities may also develop, and the implant may migrate from its initial position. Periosteal new bone formation is suggestive of infection.

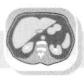

Further investigations

Full blood count/markers of inflammation

The usual tests for infection and inflammation may be appropriate. Monitoring the CRP assesses the response of infection to treatment.

Bone biochemistry

Bone biochemistry (serum calcium, phosphate, alkaline phosphatase) is useful when investigating malignancy and metabolic bone disease.

Tumour markers

Selected tumour markers, where appropriate, and plasma electrophoresis to detect plasma cell myeloma (p. 541) are necessary when malignancy is suspected.

Ultrasound of the hip

Ultrasound of the hip is most useful in children. Before 4 months of age the only means of visualizing the femoral head is by ultrasound. Following this the ossific nucleus appears on X-ray. Hip effusion and synovitis is also readily seen, and can be more easily tapped under ultrasound control.

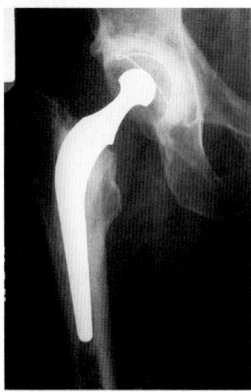

Fig. 8.54 Cemented Charnley total hip replacement.

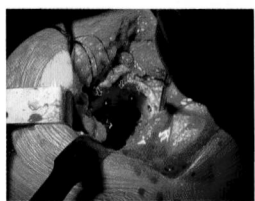

(a)

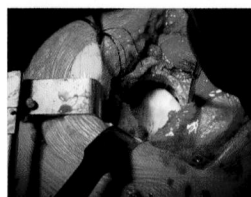

(b)

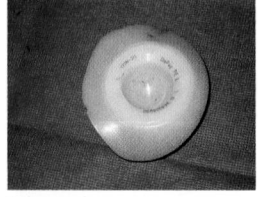

(c)

Fig. 8.55a–e Operative photos of a hip replacement. (a) The exposed acetabulum, following removal of the diseased femoral head. The rim of the acetabulum is highlighted (arrows) as are the 'keyholes' created in the bone for the cement to fill (crosses). (b) The acetabulum has been filled with cement, which will act as a 'grout' to hold the polyethylene cup in place. (c) The polyethylene cup, with a rim to help compress the cement into the bone.

Isotope bone scan

Infection, tumour, loose prostheses and osteonecrosis may all show as 'hot spots' on a bone scan. Early osteonecrosis (1–2 weeks) may appear as a cold spot due to lack of blood supply and isotope uptake. Labelled white cell scans can be useful when investigating a hip replacement for infection, but there is a high false negative rate (poor specificity).

CT of the hip

A CT scan is only useful for investigating fractures or complex hip anatomy prior to surgery (developmental dysplasia of the hip or slipped capital femoral epiphysis).

MRI of the hip

MRI is the most sensitive investigation for osteonecrosis, with changes preceding those on X-rays. The degree of involvement of the femoral head can be estimated. It is also more specific when investigating tumour and infection. It can demonstrate labral tears and loose bodies when the joint is distended with fluid prior to MRI (MR arthrography).

Initial management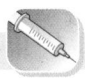

Patient education

Simple measures such as weight loss, rest and increased social support can dramatically improve symptoms of hip disease. The use of a stick in the contralateral hand reduces the force across the affected hip by 40% and can consequently reduce pain.

Simple analgesia

Simple analgesia and NSAIDs can both give relief. Steroid injection of the hip is best performed under X-ray or ultrasound guidance. However, it has poor efficacy as a therapeutic procedure and is best reserved as a diagnostic test when there is uncertainty that pain is arising from the hip joint.

Physiotherapy

Stretching of the hip muscles can overcome the spasm that may account for hip pain. Home exercises and hydrotherapy are both beneficial for hip arthritis.[3]

Surgical management

General

Arthrodesis

This was frequently the operation of choice in the young adult with severe hip pain but is now used less commonly as techniques of osteotomy and arthroplasty have improved. Currently, the main indication is post-infective arthritis. The ipsilateral knee, spine and contralateral hip must be normal as these take increased strain. The hip is fused in 20° of flexion and neutral rotation and abduction. The leg will be shorter and lumbar spine hyperlordosis must occur to allow an upright posture. Running is not possible but heavy labour may be. Approximately 60% of patients will have back pain 30 years post-fusion and 50% develop ipsilateral knee arthritis.

Arthroplasty

Hip replacement is one of the most successful and cost-effective surgical operations of recent years.[4] Replacements can be cemented (Figs 8.54 and 8.55) or uncemented (encouraging bone ingrowth). Resurfacing hip replacement aims to preserve the proximal femur and is targeted at the young active population. It remains experimental with only 8 years results so far.

All replacements give good relief of pain in most cases (>95%) and an early improvement in quality of life. Standard hip replacements have results past 20 years, with 95% prosthetic joint survival at 10 years and 85% at 20 years.[5] However, this can vary depending on the surgeon, type of replacement, reason for replacement, and age and sex of the patient. Worse results are seen in younger male patients, with osteonecrosis and Paget's disease, and when revision surgery is being performed. Replacement is generally contraindicated when there is active or recent sepsis, neuropathic arthritis and severe dementia or psychiatric illness. Despite such good results there is a 5% risk of major complications such as deep infection (1%), dislocation (3%) and cardiorespiratory arrest (1%). The latter may be due to massive pulmonary embolism, which is thought to occur in 0.2%, whilst asymptomatic deep vein thrombosis may occur in up to 50%.

Specific
Osteoarthritis

Non-operative measures listed above can be more successful in this group than in patients with rheumatoid disease. In young patients there may be a role for osteotomy. This is usually performed around the acetabulum in dysplastic hips to restore anatomical cover to the femoral head. It also acts to position more normal cartilage in the weight-bearing portion of the joint. This can give many years of pain relief and delay the need for a total hip replacement. There is a recent trend towards hip resurfacing in the young adult, as femoral bone stock is preserved and high levels of physical activity are possible following surgery. Long-term results are awaited but survival of 99.8% out to 8 years (mean 3 years) has been achieved.[6] Young active males are a difficult group to treat and standard total hip replacement has shown disappointing survival of only 85% at 10 years.[5] However, total hip replacement remains the gold standard for most patients with osteoarthritis and prosthetic joint survival greater than 90% at 10 years is expected following recent recommendations by the National Institute of Clinical Excellence.[7]

Rheumatoid disease

Due to multiple joint disease, the management of patients with rheumatoid disease of the hip is difficult. Patients may have difficulty using walking aids due to upper limb disease, and the specific contribution of the hip joint to loss of mobility may be difficult to ascertain in the presence of knee, ankle and foot disease. However, total hip replacement can give good results, although the infection rate is higher (5%). The presence of foot ulceration must be noted and treated first to reduce the risk of infection. It is generally recommended that the hip be replaced before the knee.

Osteonecrosis

The most important aspect in the management of osteonecrosis is to identify and correct any underlying risk factor or disease. Weight should be kept off the hip to reduce the risk of collapse. In early cases before collapse occurs, core decompression can give good pain relief and improve prognosis.[8] A 6 mm core of bone is removed from the greater trochanter up to a point 5 mm from the joint surface within the necrotic lesion. Some centres describe augmenting this channel with a vascularized fibular autograft. Once collapse has occurred the options are rotational osteotomy to move healthy bone into the weight-bearing dome, or hip replacement. Results of hip replacement are worse in this group, probably because of the younger age of patients and associated disease.

Bursitis

The majority of cases involve the trochanteric bursa. Tightness of the abductors and fascia lata is common and stretching exercises may help. Local heat or therapeutic ultrasound can also be of value. NSAIDs can reduce the inflammation and steroid injections are often necessary. Most cases will settle with time; surgical treatment is rarely required. It is not uncommon to see bursitis following total hip replacement and these cases may be more resistant to the above measures because of scar tissue.

Infection

Septic arthritis is the most common form of infection seen about the hip. Difficulty arises with diagnosis as the joint is deep and difficult to palpate and patients are often very young. There should be a high level of suspicion, and diagnostic aspiration under ultrasound guidance should be performed if there is doubt. Urgent washout of the joint is warranted to minimize the risk of cartilage damage. Six weeks of the appropriate antibiotics should follow. Tuberculosis should be treated medically with the recommended 6–9 months of triple or quadruple therapy. In a few cases, gross destruction and instability necessitate hip fusion. Secondary arthritic change can be treated with a total hip replacement but a disease-free interval of 10 years is recommended.

Infection of a hip replacement can present acutely as a septic arthritis, and washout with debridement may cure up to 50% if treated within 2 weeks. When infection is chronic there are two options. In the frail or elderly patient with a low-grade infection and no gross loosening of the prosthesis, suppression of the infection with long-term low-dose antibiotics may suffice. However, most cases require removal of the prosthesis and debridement as a first stage. Appropriate oral antibiotics are given for several months with monitoring of the CRP until it is considered safe to insert a new prosthesis (rarely before 8 weeks). There is an 85% chance of successful eradication of infection. Some surgeons advocate a one-stage revision for low-grade infections with similar success rates.[9]

Neoplasia

There is a risk of pathological fracture with metastatic deposits and myeloma. This may present acutely, however in most cases it is heralded by worsening pain prior to fracture, when prophylactic surgical treatment is possible. Oncologists should be involved at the outset as adjuvant radiotherapy or chemotherapy may be required. Femoral lesions require intramedullary nailing to protect the whole length of the femur and femoral neck in case further lesions occur. With gross bony destruction the nail can be augmented with cement. If there is acetabular involvement and a good prognosis it may be possible to perform a cemented total hip replacement. In both cases good pain relief can be expected.

Labral degeneration

Labral degeneration is an underdiagnosed condition. Controversy surrounds the optimum management. The symptoms settle with rest and NSAIDs in the majority. Advocates of hip arthroscopy describe good results following arthroscopic debridement, but few centres perform this surgery regularly.

Paget's disease

Treatment with bisphosphonates should be instituted (p. 517). When secondary hip degeneration has occurred, total hip replacement can be considered but the complication rate is higher. There is a risk of bleeding when Paget's is active and fracture may occur due to the hard and brittle bone. There is often deformity of the hip due to varus neck, femoral bowing and acetabular protrusio. A course of bisphosphonate prior to surgery is recommended to reduce the bleeding risk. In the long term, there is a higher rate of prosthetic loosening.

Aseptic loosening and periprosthetic fracture

As more hips are being replaced, the number of patients with prosthetic joint failure increases. Approximately 75% of revision joint replacements are performed for aseptic loosening (loosening without an infective cause). Once loose, there is a risk of fracture about the prosthesis. In both cases there may be significant bone loss. Revision surgery may require the use of bone graft, either as chips packed firmly into the cavities or as bulky structural grafts applied to the femur or acetabulum. It may take many years for this graft to become incorporated by the host. Fractures about a loose prosthesis can be treated by replacement with a longer prosthesis that bypasses the fracture, or by a standard prosthesis with a plate and graft to the outside of the femur.

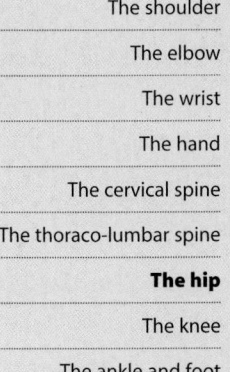

(d)

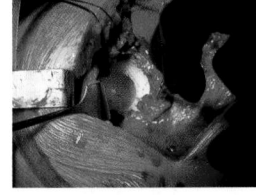

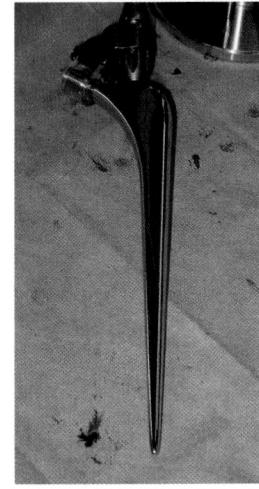

(e)

Fig. 8.55a–e—cont'd (d) The cup is cemented in place and finally (e) the femoral component is mounted on its holder prior to implantation.

REFERENCES

(1) Wilcock G. *The prevalence of osteoarthritis of the hip requiring total hip replacement in the elderly. International Journal of Epidemiology 1979; 8: 247–250.*

(2) Lage LA, Patel JV, Villar RN. *The acetabular labral tear: an arthroscopic classification. Arthroscopy 1996; 12: 269–272.*

(3) Green J, McKenna F, Redfern EJ, Chamberlain MA. *Home exercises are as effective as outpatient hydrotherapy for osteoarthritis of the hip. British Journal of Rheumatology 1993; 32: 812–815.*

(4) Jonsson B, Larsson S. *Functional improvements and costs of hip and knee arthroplasty in destructive rheumatoid arthritis. Scandinavian Journal of Rheumatology 1991; 20: 351–357.*

(5) Herberts P, Malchau H. *Long-term registration has improved the quality of hip replacement: a review of the Swedish THR register comparing 160,000 cases. Acta Orthopaedica Scandinavica 2000; 71: 111–121.*

(6) Daniel J, Pynsent PB, McMinn DJ. *Metal-on-metal resurfacing of the hip in patients under the age of 55 years with osteoarthritis. Journal of Bone and Joint Surgery (Br) 2004; 86-B: 177–184.*

(7) NICE. *Guidance on the selection of prostheses for primary total hip replacement. London: National Institute of Clinical Excellence, 2000.*

(8) Ficat RP. *Idiopathic bone necrosis of the femoral head. Journal of Bone and Joint Surgery (Br) 1985; 67B: 3–9.*

(9) Raut VV, Siney PD, Wroblewski BM. *One stage revision of infected total hip replacement with discharging sinus. Journal of Bone and Joint Surgery (Br) 1994; 76B: 721–724.*

The knee

The knee is a complex joint that can be affected by a number of diseases. Knee disease accounts for a large proportion of the orthopaedic workload from arthroscopic surgery and knee replacement.

Epidemiology

The age-related diseases of the knee are summarized in Table 8.61.

Primary osteoarthritis is common. The prevalence in the 64–74-year-old population is 2000 per 100 000 men and 6600 per 100 000 women.

The incidence of anterior cruciate ligament (ACL) rupture is 20 per 100 000 per year. Approximately 25% of severe sports injuries affect the knee and one third of these involve the ACL.

Pathology

Inflammation

The knee joint is frequently involved in rheumatoid arthritis. The large size of the joint predisposes to extensive synovitis and effusion. Erosions and damage to important ligamentous structures may lead to instability and subluxation of the knee. Involvement of adjacent bursae is common. With time a mixed pattern of rheumatoid and degenerative changes is often found.

Gout (sodium urate crystals) and pseudogout (calcium pyrophosphate crystals) can both affect the knee. Acute attacks cause severe synovitis and effusion. Over time, crystals deposit on the articular, meniscal and synovial surfaces and may lead to secondary degeneration.

Inflammation about the patella tendon is commonly encountered in young adults. Most often associated with repetitive loading of the extensor mechanism during jumping and running, it may be described as patellar tendinosis, peritendinitis, insertional tendinopathy or even 'jumper's knee'. There is usually degeneration and necrosis of the central fibres near the insertion on the distal patellar pole, with surrounding inflammation of the paratenon. Patellar tendon rupture may occur in the long term.

Pre-patellar bursitis (housemaid's knee) and infra-patellar bursitis (clergyman's knee) are often seen following excessive periods of kneeling. Traumatic irritation is the likely cause. Inflammation of these bursae can also be seen in association with rheumatoid disease and gout. The bursa can become grossly distended with a risk of secondary infection.

The knee is frequently involved in haemophilia, with recurrent haemarthroses leading to adhesions, fibrosis, stiffness and ultimately degeneration.

Synovial chondromatosis is a metaplastic monoarticular condition that usually affects young adult females. Cartilaginous bodies develop on the synovium and subsequently detach. The loose bodies may eventually mineralize. There

Table 8.61	Diseases of the knee by age group		
Children	**Young adults**	**Middle age**	**Elderly**
Osteochondritis	Osteochondritis	Rheumatoid and degenerative arthritis	Degenerative arthritis
Osteochondroma	Osteochondromas	Gout/pseudogout	Avascular necrosis
Infection	Giant cell tumours	Meniscal tears (degenerative)	Paget's disease
'Anterior knee pain'	'Anterior knee pain'		Infection
	Tendonitis		
	Meniscal tears (traumatic)		
	Cruciate ligament rupture		
	Pigmented villonodular synovitis		
	Synovial chondromatosis		

is irritation within the joint with effusion, locking and grinding. Cartilage damage is common and may lead to secondary degeneration.

Degenerative

Chondromalacia patellae is a condition that usually affects young women. The medial facet of the patella is most commonly affected, with softening, fibrillation and eburnation of the articular cartilage. Progression to frank arthritis is rare. The risk is greater with lateral facet involvement, which is thought to occur in association with tightness of the lateral patellar retinaculum, causing high pressures in the patello-femoral joint with flexion.

Degenerative arthritis (Fig. 8.56 a and b) follows classic pathological stages: initially softening of the hyaline cartilage, then fibrillation, ulcer formation or flap tears and eburnation (exposure of subchondral bone) occurs. There may be mild synovitis, widespread osteophytes, and secondary deformity with capsular and ligamentous contractures (commonly fixed flexion and varus). A distended popliteal (Baker's) cyst is a common finding. With time, the cruciate ligaments may rupture due to osteophytic impingement.

The patello-femoral joint is involved in isolation in 8% of women and 2% of men with symptomatic degenerative arthritis over the age of 55. There is often a history of patello-femoral instability and injury. In 92% the medial compartment is affected first and the disease usually remains limited to this compartment.

The meniscus may also develop areas of degeneration, weakening the structure and predisposing to complex tears. These tears can provoke the development of meniscal cysts and the lateral side is more commonly involved.

Trauma/instability

Anterior cruciate ligament rupture is a common problem that may not be recognized at presentation. The usual functions of the ligament are lost allowing anterolateral subluxation of the tibia on the femur. This instability is known to predispose to chondral damage and meniscal tears. The ligament may heal following rupture, but this is never in the original position and laxity is inevitable. Posterior cruciate ligament tears are uncommon in isolation. Meniscal damage and posterolateral corner rupture (capsule, popliteus tendon and lateral collateral ligament) are often found in association. However, if other damage does not prove symptomatic, chronic instability is uncommon.

Patellar instability usually manifests as a tendency for the patella to sublux laterally in early flexion, and frank dislocation can also occur. This occurs most commonly in females in their second decade. There may be a history of initial dislocation with tearing of the stabilizing restraints

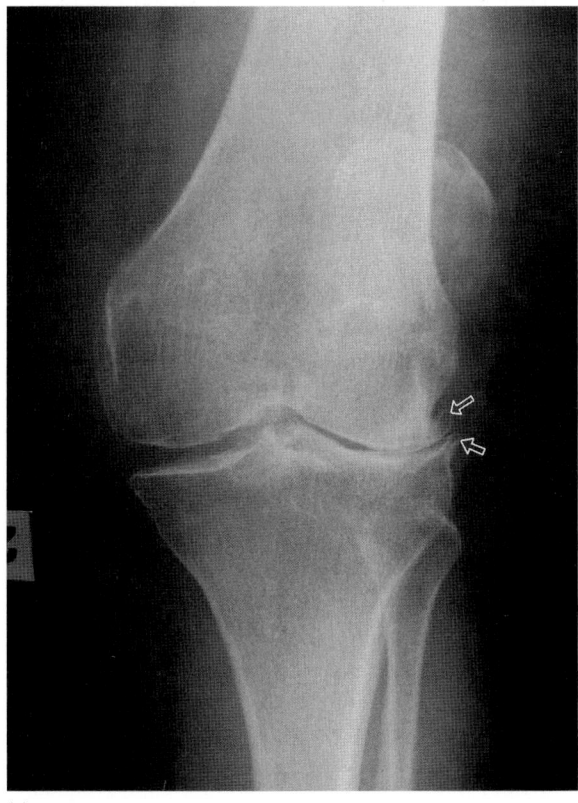

(a)

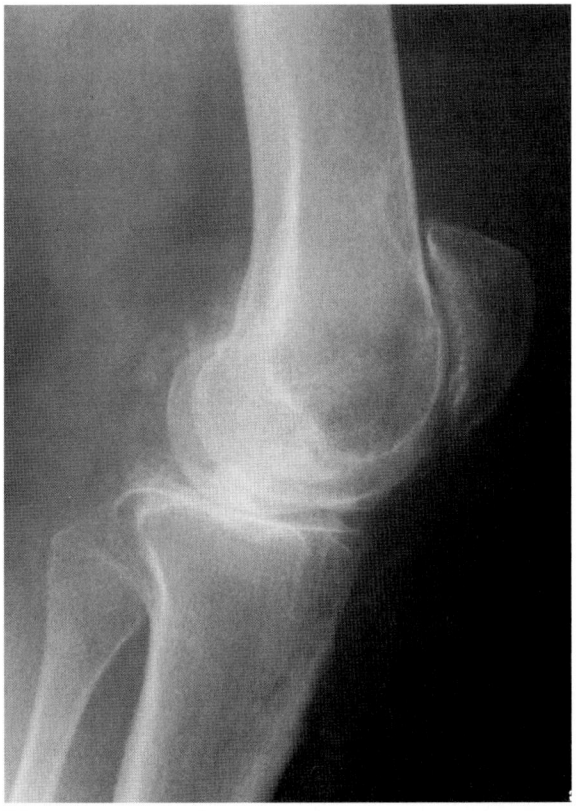

(b)

Fig. 8.56a, b Osteoarthritis of the knee. (a) AP and (b) lateral plain films of the knee showing primarily lateral and patello-femoral compartment osteoarthritis. There is narrowed joint space and peripheral osteophyte formation (arrows).

557

(medial patello-femoral ligament, retinaculum and vastus medialis). With these restraints damaged, patellar tracking can be altered. In some cases generalized ligamentous laxity can lead to instability. Rarely, abnormal anatomical development of the patella, trochlear groove or malrotation of the limb (persistent femoral anteversion or external tibial torsion) can cause instability through abnormal tracking. Chronic instability and maltracking may lead to degenerative changes in the patello-femoral joint.

Periprosthetic fractures about knee arthroplasties are less common than about the hip. However, loosening of the prosthesis can occur and this is usually tibial.

Vascular

Osteonecrosis most often affects the weight-bearing portions of the knee in women aged over 60 years. The medial femoral condyle is involved in 98% of cases. It is uncertain whether the initial insult is ischaemic or traumatic (osteoporosis predisposes). Most cases are idiopathic but it may follow steroid use, renal transplantation and systemic lupus erythematosus. The pathological changes in the hip are mirrored (p. 549–552) with necrosis followed by fracture and collapse, fragmentation, remodelling and finally arthrosis (Fig. 8.57).

Osteochondritis is a more localized condition seen in adolescents. Most commonly, necrosis of a portion of the weight-bearing zone of the medial femoral condyle occurs. Trauma is thought to be the most likely cause. This area can fissure and detach (osteochondritis dissecans) causing irritation and locking of the knee. If attachments remain it may heal back over a period of up to 2 years.

Infection

Infection may involve the knee joint, adjacent bone, bursae or an implant such as a knee replacement. The knee is the joint most commonly affected by septic arthritis in childhood. The relatively superficial knee capsule makes it prone to puncture from the needles of intravenous drug abusers. Infection leads to synovial proliferation and adhesions. The large volume of the knee joint and compartmentalization can lead to loculi of pus within the joint. Without prompt treatment, destruction of the articular surface occurs and a fixed flexion deformity is common with chronic infection due to thickening and contracture of the posterior capsule.

Approximately 10% of osteoarticular tuberculosis affects the knee, and it is usually of the synovial type. The synovium becomes thickened and tubercles develop within it. There is gradual articular erosion, destruction and instability.

Deep infection occurs in up to 2% of total knee replacements, with a higher frequency in patients with rheumatoid disease (4%). There may be sinus formation and chronic induration of the anterior soft tissues. The pathological features are identical to those of hip arthroplasty infection.

The subcutaneous pre-patellar and infra-patellar bursae are prone to chronic repetitive injury through kneeling, and infection can occur from puncture or abrasion injuries. The bursa fills with a tense abscess and can discharge to adjacent subcutaneous tissues or to the skin's surface.

Neoplasia

Approximately 36% of solitary osteochondromas occur about the knee. Osteochondroma is the most common benign bone tumour, accounting for 41% of new referrals. The lesion consists of a bony stalk in continuity with normal bone. There is an overlying hyaline cartilage cap, ranging from 0.5 to 1.5 cm in thickness, which becomes thinner following skeletal maturity. The lesions are believed to develop as a result of aberrant physeal cartilage separating from the growth plate. Growth continues perpendicular to the longitudinal axis of the bone and ceases with skeletal maturity. Over the lifetime of an osteochondroma there is a risk of malignant transformation, but this is less than 1% per lesion.

Giant cell tumours make up 20% of benign bone tumours. The most common location is about the knee. These lesions are metaphyseal extending to subchondral bone. Macroscopically they are soft friable lesions with cystic and haemorrhagic areas. The cortex may be breached and the lesions may fracture. Giant cells are characteristically seen microscopically. Though benign, giant cell tumours may metastasize to the lungs in up to 9%. There is a lifetime risk of malignant transformation to osteosarcoma in 5% of cases.

Osteosarcoma is the most common primary malignant bone tumour and is usually seen in the second decade. The most common locations are the distal femur and proximal tibia. Malignant osteoblasts produce osteoid and bone, but there can also be fibroblastic or chondroblastic elements. They may metastasize (usually to the lungs). The 5-year survival is 80% with localized disease and 40% with lung metastases.

Pigmented villonodular synovitis (PVNS) is a benign neoplastic condition causing synovial proliferation, most commonly affecting the knee. This process can be localized to one part of the knee or may be diffuse and aggressive, causing extra-articular invasion and destruction. Haemosiderin deposits develop, accounting for the pigmented appearance.

Endocrine

Paget's disease may lead to bowing of the femur or tibia adjacent to the knee. This most often leads to a varus deformity, and secondary arthrosis of the medial compartment is common due to the altered mechanical axis of the knee.

Scope of disease

The knee has an important role in ambulation. Flexion allows the foot to clear the ground during the swing phase of gait, and enables stairs and slopes to be tackled. The joint and surrounding muscles act as a shock absorber when running and jumping. Further flexion is necessary for sitting, kneeling and squatting. Loss of deep flexion may have important cultural implications if prayer and worship are affected. Chronic knee conditions may restrict manual work, sport and recreation. The young age of many patients with knee pathology exaggerates these problems. Pathology often presents during the third to sixth decades and there is therefore an impact on activity, quality of life and employment in this active group.

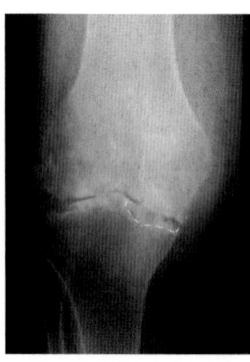

Fig. 8.57 Medial tibial osteonecrosis. Plain film showing collapse (dashed line) and secondary arthritis.

Clinical features

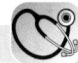

Pain

The site of pain and associated diseases of the knee are listed in Table 8.62. Aggravating factors are important as many diseases become more symptomatic with activity (mechanical pain). Tears of the posterior horns of the menisci are characteristically more painful in deep flexion (e.g. squatting). Activities involving twisting or sudden change in direction are likely to exacerbate meniscal symptoms. Patello-femoral pathology classically causes pain when rising from a seat and descending a flight of stairs. Pain associated with catching or locking could be due to meniscal tears or loose bodies. Pain at rest or at night should raise the suspicion of infection, tumour or osteonecrosis.

Stiffness

Stiffness is a frequent symptom of rheumatoid, haemophiliac and degenerative arthritis.

Instability

It is important to distinguish whether 'giving way' of the knee is as a result of laxity or pain. Many diseases cause the knee to 'give way' due to pain. This occurs as a result of reflex quadriceps inhibition. The classic painless giving way of anterior cruciate ligament insufficiency occurs whilst twisting the leg over a planted foot. This may occur with walking or vigorous exertion. Posterior cruciate ligament instability may cause the knee to give way whilst descending stairs.

Locking

The inability to fully extend the knee actively may be due to meniscal tears, chondral flaps, the prolapsed stump of a ruptured anterior cruciate ligament, loose bodies and patello-femoral arthritis.

Medical history

Occupation and hobbies have an important bearing on management of a number of knee conditions, and may even provide clues to the diagnosis. The mechanism of injury can be particularly helpful when ligamentous injury is suspected.

Examination

Look

The lower limbs should be fully exposed and inspected for any features of polyarticular disease. With the patient supine and the knee fully extended, abnormal swellings may be noted. Localized swelling over the anterior knee is likely to represent disease of the bursae. The swelling of synovitis or knee effusion is seen as an inverted horseshoe shape lateral, proximal (supra-patellar pouch) and medial to the patella. Varus and valgus deformity can be noted; 6° of valgus is physiological (anatomical axis). If the knee will not extend flat on the couch, then it can be assumed that there is either fixed flexion contracture of the capsule (arthritis), tight hamstring tendons following injury or that the knee is locked. Erythema should raise the suspicion of infection.

Feel

Warmth of the knee may suggest inflammation or infection. Swelling of the joint must be assessed. Synovial thickening should be obvious and does not allow a fluid thrill, whereas an effusion can be swept about the knee if small and allows a fluid thrill if large. An effusion is non-specific. Loose bodies may be felt if large and lying in the supra-patellar pouch or medial and lateral gutters. Careful movement of the patella within the trochlear groove may elicit pain with patello-femoral disease. Tenderness of the tibio-femoral joint line may indicate meniscal disease. Tenderness and thickening over the patellar tendon or anterior bursae would suggest inflammation.

Move

The range of motion is from 0 to 140° of flexion with up to 10° of hyperextension. Flexion usually continues until the calf meets the thigh. It is useful to place a hand over the knee joint to detect crepitus with movement, most commonly as a result of degenerative disease.

Gait

It is important to observe the gait of the patient: any deformity of the knee is usually maximized when weight-bearing.

Assessment of the lateral collateral ligament

With the knee in 20° of flexion a varus stress is applied to detect laxity of the lateral collateral ligament complex. This

Table 8.62	Location of pain and diseases of the knee		
Medial		**Anterior**	**Lateral**
Medial arthritis		Patello-femoral arthritis	Lateral arthritis
Medial meniscal tears		Chondromalacia patellae	Lateral meniscal tears
Pes anserinus bursitis (hamstring insertion)		Patellar tendonitis Patellar maltracking Posterior cruciate ligament rupture Pre-patellar/infra-patellar bursitis Hip pathology	Iliotibial band friction syndrome

can also detect whether the valgus deformity of lateral compartment arthritis is correctable.

Assessment of the medial collateral ligament

With the knee in 20° of flexion a valgus stress is applied to detect laxity of the medial collateral ligament. Again this will also allow correction of the varus deformity of medial compartment arthritis if the medial collateral ligament has not contracted and shortened.

Assessment of the anterior cruciate ligament

With the knee flexed to 90° abnormal anterior displacement of the tibia on the femur can be detected with the anterior drawer test, suggesting anterior cruciate ligament laxity. A more sensitive test is the Lachman test, with the same anterior displacement occurring at 30° of flexion. With gross instability a pivot shift may occur; the foot is held internally rotated by the examiner with a valgus strain to the knee, causing subluxation in extension, which reduces with a visible clunk as the knee is flexed.

Assessment of the posterior cruciate ligament

With the knees flexed to 90° a posterior sag of the tibia on the femur may be noticeable from the side if posterior cruciate ligament laxity is present. In the same position it may be possible to push the tibia posteriorly (posterior drawer). With the knee flexed to 90° over the edge of a couch the patient is asked to actively extend the knee, and any posterior subluxation noticeably reduces as the quadriceps contraction pulls the tibia forwards on the femur ('quads active test').

McMurray's test

Meniscal tears may produce pain or a palpable click if a force is applied up the tibia with the knee flexed, and the tibia is rotated internally and externally.

Assessment of patella tracking

Patellar maltracking is best appreciated by sitting the patient on the edge of the couch with the knee flexed to 90°, and then asking him or her to actively extend the knee fully. As full extension approaches the patella may skip laterally as engagement with the trochlea is lost (J-sign). There may also be apprehension if lateral pressure is applied to the patella in extension and the patient is asked to flex the knee.

Initial investigations

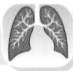

Plain X-rays

The standard views are AP and lateral. Medial and lateral compartment arthritis, osteonecrosis and tumours will all be most obvious on an AP view. The lateral view demonstrates patello-femoral joint arthritis, but for more information on this joint a skyline view is recommended. This view also allows assessment of tilt or subluxation of the patella. Bony loose bodies in the knee may be seen on these standard views, but a 'notch view' allows better visualization of loose bodies in the intercondylar notch (AP taken at 40° of flexion).

Further investigations

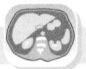

Full blood count/markers of inflammation

The white cell count and ESR may be elevated with infection or inflammation. The CRP can be used to assess the response of infection to treatment.

Bone biochemistry

Serum calcium, phosphate and alkaline phosphatase are useful when investigating malignancy and metabolic bone disease.

Serum uric acid

The serum uric acid levels may be high with gout (p. 507).

Ultrasound of the knee

Superficial structures are well appreciated on ultrasound, and it can give diagnostic information when cysts or tendonitis are being investigated.

Isotope bone scan

Infection, tumour, loose prostheses and osteonecrosis may all show as 'hot spots' due to increased tracer uptake on a bone scan. Early osteonecrosis (1–2 weeks) may appear as a 'cold' or photopenic area that reflects the lack of blood supply and isotope uptake. As with the hip, labelled white cell scans have high sensitivity when investigating prosthetic infection, however the high false negative rate remains a problem (poor specificity).

CT of the knee

This is usually reserved for the investigation of knee fractures. However, with modern 3D reconstructions useful information can be obtained regarding the geometry of the distal femur, particularly when studying the maltracking patella.

MRI of the knee

High degrees of accuracy have been reported when assessing soft tissue injuries of the knee involving the medial meniscus 89%, lateral meniscus 90% and anterior cruciate ligament 93% using arthroscopy as the gold standard.[1] However, lesions of the articular cartilage are less well seen. MRI has been shown to reduce the rate of arthroscopic treatment of the knee. Infection and osteonecrosis can be clearly identified. Loose bodies may be identified on conventional MRI with improved detection on MR arthrography.

Initial management

Patient education

Weight loss, rest and adjustment of activity can all help improve the symptoms of knee pathology. Walking aids may also be useful.

Simple analgesia

Simple analgesia and NSAIDs can both give relief. Steroid injection of the knee can be performed in the clinic, and is most effective when there is an element of synovitis. The response to injection with degenerative arthritis is usually short-lived and unpredictable. More recently, injections of hyaluronic acid have been advocated for early degeneration, but efficacy is no better than NSAIDs or steroid injection.[2]

Physiotherapy

Many knee conditions can be dramatically improved with effective physiotherapy. Strengthening the vastus medialis obliquus can help with maltracking and patello-femoral joint degeneration. Strong hamstrings may compensate for anterior cruciate ligament deficiency and quadriceps can compensate for posterior cruciate ligament deficiency.

Surgical management

General

Arthrodesis

With the high success rates in modern knee replacement, arthrodesis is rarely performed. To allow a stable limb for walking, the knee must be fused in about 10° of flexion, but this prevents easy stowage of the leg when sitting in confined areas, such as planes or cars. Whilst pain relief can be guaranteed in over 90%, it remains the less popular option. Knee fusion is indicated in situations when knee replacement is not advisable, such as post-infective arthritis, salvage for failed total knee replacement and post-traumatic arthritis in a young adult. The ipsilateral hip and ankle and the contralateral knee must be free from disease. Greatest rates of union have been achieved using modern long intramedullary nails that pass from the femur to the tibia.

Arthroplasty

Having followed hip replacements in development, knee replacements are now proving more successful. Over 90% prosthetic joint survival at 15 years can be expected[3] with similar levels of patient satisfaction. Several options exist when considering replacement. In certain cases, isolated areas of the joint can be replaced, such as medial unicompartmental and patello-femoral replacements. A standard knee replacement resurfaces the whole of the femur and tibia with the option to replace the patellar surface also (Fig. 8.58). Most implants are cemented in place (Fig. 8.59). The major complications of infection, pulmonary embolus, stiffness and persistent pain are uncommon (less than 5%).

Specific

Degenerative arthritis

The treatment of disorders of the patello-femoral joint relies heavily on non-operative measures such as physiotherapy. Quadriceps strengthening can improve control of patellar tracking, particularly when vastus medialis is targeted. This may reduce pain from chondromalacia patellae or frank arthritis.

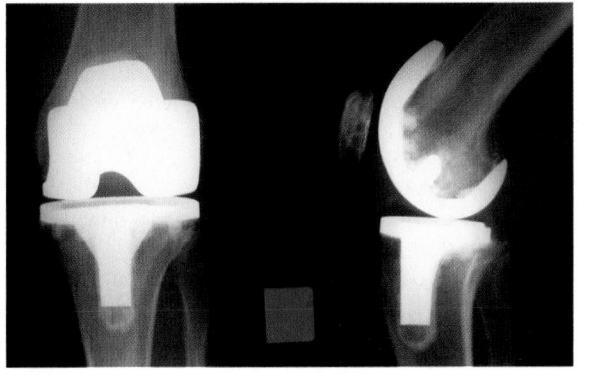

Fig. 8.58 AP (left of figure) and lateral (right of figure) views of a cemented left knee replacement. The patellar surface has also been replaced.

Persistent discomfort may be improved with an arthroscopic debridement, but this is only likely with large unstable cartilage flaps. When the lateral retinaculum is tight, surgical release of this structure may reduce the pressure in the joint and improve tracking, both leading to reduced pain. Severe isolated patello-femoral arthritis can now be treated by replacement, but this remains experimental.

Degenerative disease of the knee joint proper responds well to general measures such as rest, weight loss, walking aids and orthoses. Physiotherapy may help preserve strength and movement. Steroid injections give unpredictable benefit, as do hyaluronic acid injections. When there are distinctive mechanical symptoms such as locking, arthroscopic debridement will offer some relief, but it has no place as a general measure for all arthritic knees. When the disease is isolated to one tibiofemoral compartment the surgical options are osteotomy, unicompartmental and total knee replacement.

Osteotomy aims to correct malalignment of the limb secondary to the arthritis, shifting a greater proportion of load through the unaffected compartment of the knee. With medial compartment arthritis a high tibial osteotomy is performed, and with lateral compartment arthritis a distal femoral osteotomy is usually required. This technique is generally reserved for young, active patients where joint replacement is not ideal. Survival without conversion to joint replacement is 89% at 5 years and 75% at 10 years.[4]

Unicompartmental replacement replaces only the affected part of the knee. It is dependent on an intact anterior cruciate ligament and a correctable deformity. The 10-year prosthetic joint survival rate is 98% for medial unicompartmental replacement, and it can be used in young adults.[5]

Total knee replacement is preferred when the lateral compartment is affected or the criteria for unicompartmental replacement are not met. More extensive involvement of the joint is best treated with total knee replacement. Modern total knee replacements have a prosthetic joint survival of 95% at 10 years with early complication rates less than 5%.[6]

There is ongoing debate regarding replacement of the patella. Persistent anterior knee pain may occur in up to 10% of knees that are not replaced, but complication rates of up to 10% exist with replacement such as fracture, maltracking or loosening.[7]

Inflammatory arthritis

Standard medical treatment for rheumatoid disease may prevent or delay the need for surgical intervention. Gross synovitis can be improved with open or arthroscopic synovectomy. Good results can be expected with knee replacement in over 90% of cases at 10 years.[6] However, the infection rate is higher (5%) due to the relative immunosuppression of patients with rheumatoid disease. Synovectomy and replacement both have a role in cases of haemophiliac arthropathy, but results are slightly less favourable than those for degenerative disease.

Patellar tendonitis

General measures such as rest, ice, NSAIDs and physiotherapy should be employed. Refractory cases may require excision of the thickened paratenon or occasionally part of the tendon if an isolated necrotic area exists.

Osteochondritis

Osteochondritis must be allowed to follow its natural course. The leg should be rested and sports avoided. Stable lesions may take up to 2 years to heal. Unstable lesions may require exploration and fixation with screws or absorbable pins. If detached, replacement and fixation is preferable as lesions may be large and affect weight-bearing portions of the joint.

Meniscal tears

Small degenerative tears may settle spontaneously. Arthroscopy and excision of the damaged meniscus is indicated for persistent symptoms or locking of the knee. Excision of the whole meniscus results in degenerative changes to the joint surface that develop within 20–30 years on the medial aspect and within 10 years on the lateral aspect.

Anterior cruciate ligament rupture

The treatment of acute rupture is not covered here. However, patients may be seen many years after anterior cruciate ligament rupture with instability or meniscal tears. Instability can be managed by adjusting activity, physiotherapy or occasionally with use of a brace. If these measures are ineffective, the ligament may be reconstructed. Most current techniques are performed arthroscopically, with use of the central third of the patellar tendon or doubled-up hamstring tendons as graft. Approximately 95% of patients will return to similar levels of pre-injury activity. The rate of meniscal tears is reduced but it is not clear if subsequent degeneration of the knee can be prevented or slowed.

Posterior cruciate ligament rupture

Isolated posterior cruciate ligament rupture rarely causes problems. Physiotherapy and braces can be employed. Reconstruction is indicated when combined ligamentous injury occurs, most often with torn lateral collateral and posterolateral structures. This rarely presents as a chronic condition. Injuries to all these structures are much more significant and usually obvious in the early stage of the disease.

Osteonecrosis

Osteonecrosis may be treated with protected weight bearing in the early stages of the disease to prevent collapse of the lesion. Osteonecrosis may also occur with preexisting arthritis. If symptoms are severe, unicompartmental or total knee replacement may be appropriate with similar results to degenerative arthritis.

Aseptic loosening and periprosthetic fracture

Total knee replacements usually fail by loosening or destruction of the polyethylene tray. There may be significant loss of bone, particularly if subsidence has occurred. Revision implants allow the use of stems and wedges to bypass this bone loss and achieve stable fixation. However, prosthetic joint survival of less than 90% at 10 years, with a 10% early complication rate can be expected. On occasions revision is impossible and fusion or amputation may have to be considered. Fracture about a prosthesis that is loose requires revision to long-stemmed implants, possibly in conjunction with internal fixation.

Infection

Septic arthritis requires prompt diagnosis, assisted by the ease of joint aspiration. The joint can be successfully washed out arthroscopically. This may need to be repeated on two or three occasions. Antibiotics are required for up to 6 weeks. Osteomyelitis should be treated by antibiotics; surgical intervention is rarely necessary. Infective bursitis may be treated by initial aspiration and antibiotics, but formal incision and drainage may be required if it does not resolve. Tuberculous infection of the knee joint is mainly treated medically with prolonged courses of antitubercular chemotherapy. If chronic pain and instability develops, fusion of the knee may be required.

Acutely infected prosthetic joints should be treated aggressively. Early washout, debridement and antibiotics may eradicate the infection. In chronic infection, a number of options are available. In the elderly and infirm with low-grade infection, long-term suppression with antibiotics can be successful. With gross loosening of the prosthesis and bone loss, conversion to knee fusion may be the only viable option. In the majority of cases, it is possible to perform a two-stage revision, allowing several months between removal and reimplantation of prostheses to let the infection settle. Eradication can be expected in about 85% of cases, but overall patient satisfaction is lower than with primary replacement. Persistent infection may necessitate above-knee amputation in a small number of cases.

Pigmented villonodular synovitis/synovial chondromatosis

Both of these conditions usually require synovectomy, but numerous washouts may stem the mechanical symptoms caused by loose bodies in synovial chondromatosis.

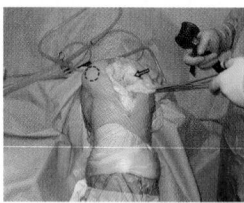
(a)

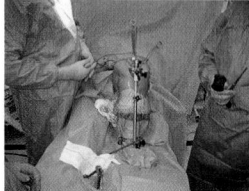
(b)

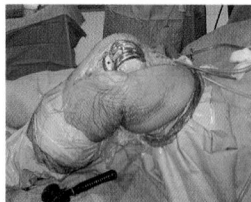
(c)

(d)

Fig. 8.59a–e Total knee replacement. (a) A lot of equipment is required to perform the operation. (b) The knee joint is opened and the patella pushed to one side (hashed line). The bare bone over the femoral condyles is evidence of severe arthritis (arrow). (c) A jig is applied to the lower leg to guide the bony resection from the tibia and the knee replacement has been cemented in place (d). The polyethylene tibial insert is seen between the two metal components (cross).

Neoplasia

Osteochondromas are usually amenable to simple excision when symptomatic. Recurrence rates are usually very low. Giant cell tumours are more difficult to deal with as they often occupy a large percentage of the joint surface. Complete excision is difficult and requires a combination of curettage, high-speed burrs, chemical (phenol) and thermal (liquid nitrogen) ablation. The large defect is then filled with bone graft and/or cement. Recurrence occurs in up to 20% of cases and may occur many years later.

REFERENCES

(1) *Mackensie R, Palmer CR, Lomas DJ, Dixon AK. Magnetic resonance imaging of the knee: performance statistics. Clinical Radiology 1996: 51: 251–257.*
(2) *Leopold SS, Redd BB, Warme WJ, Wehrle PA, Pettis PD, Shott S. Corticosteroid compared with hyaluronic acid injections for the treatment of osteoarthritis of the knee: a prospective, randomized trial. Journal of Bone and Joint Surgery (Am) 2003; 85: 1197–1203.*
(3) *Ranawat CS, Flynn WF, Saddler S. Long-term results of the total condylar knee arthroplasty. A 15 year survivorship analysis. Clinical Orthopaedics and Related Research 1993: 286: 94–102.*
(4) *Coventry MB, Ilstrup DM, Wallrichs SL. Proximal tibial osteotomy. A critical long-term study of eighty-seven cases. Journal of Bone and Joint Surgery (Am) 1993; 75: 196–201.*
(5) *Murray DW, Goodfellow JW, O'Connor JJ. The Oxford medial unicompartmental arthroplasty: A ten-year survival study. Journal of Bone and Joint Surgery (Br) 1998; 80-B: 983–989.*
(6) *Swedish Knee Arthroplasty Register Report. 2004. Available on line from Swedish Knee Arthroplasty Register at http://www.ort.lu.se/knee/indexeng.html*
(7) *Wood DJ, Smith AJ, Collopy D, White B, Brankov B, Bulsara MK. Patellar resurfacing in total knee arthroplasty: a prospective, randomized trial. Journal of Bone and Joint Surgery (Am) 2002; 84: 187–193.*

The ankle and foot

The foot and ankle are composed of a complex collection of joints, ligaments and musculotendinous units that interact for normal function. Large loads must be taken by this unit, particularly when running or jumping. The foot can be stiff for stable and powerful propulsion or flexible to absorb the forces of the heel and foot striking the ground. The vital role of the ankle and foot during ambulation results in a significant impact on productivity and independence of the person when it is affected by disease.

Epidemiology

The age predilection of foot and ankle conditions is listed in Table 8.63. The prevalence of arthritis tends to be lower in the ankle than in other large joints.

Although hallux valgus has a multifactorial aetiology, the very low rates in populations that do not wear shoes highlight the influence of footwear in the development of this disease.

It is thought that over 2000 per 100 000 adults over 60 years have first metatarso-phalangeal joint (MTPJ) arthritis. Rheumatoid arthritis is thought to affect 1000 per 100 000 worldwide, with up to 92% having foot or ankle involvement. Foot or ankle arthritis is the presenting symptom in 17%.

Approximately 20% of diabetic hospital admissions are for problems relating to the feet (p. 565), and 20% of diabetics have a clinically significant neuropathy after 10 years of disease, rising to 50% at 20 years.

Approximately 25% of all sport injuries involve the foot and ankle, but chronic problems such as instability are uncommon.

Pathology

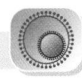

Congenital/developmental

Hallux valgus has a multifactorial aetiology with strong environmental and social influences. There is a genetic association in patients who present in the second decade, usually with a primary varus deformity of the first metatarsal and secondary distal hallux valgus deformity.

Regardless of the aetiology, the pathological changes around the first MTPJ are similar. There is gradual deviation of the metatarsal into varus and the hallux into valgus, stretching the medial capsule and collateral ligament with contracture of the lateral structures. The hallux may eventually dislocate laterally from the metatarsal head (incongruence). The plantar sesamoids sublux laterally, rolling around the metatarsal head.

The medial bunion consists of a bony prominence with thickening of the overlying bursa. The skin is thinned and ischaemic over the bunion and may ulcerate allowing deep infection. With time, the altered anatomy of the MTPJ may lead to secondary degenerative change. As a result of the

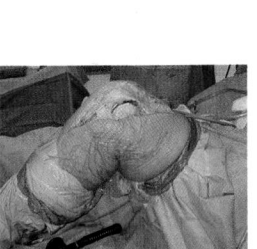

(e)

Fig. 8.59a–e—cont'd
(e) Finally, the patella is replaced over the femur, showing how it tracks over the new joint.

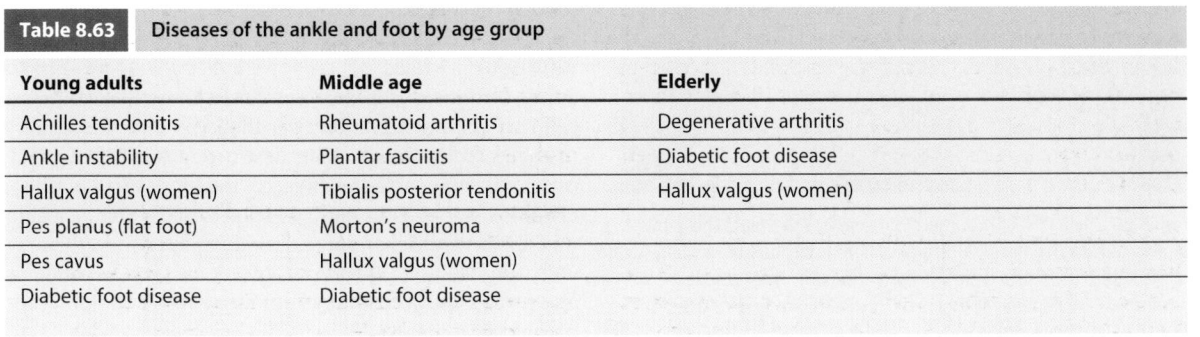

Table 8.63	Diseases of the ankle and foot by age group	
Young adults	**Middle age**	**Elderly**
Achilles tendonitis	Rheumatoid arthritis	Degenerative arthritis
Ankle instability	Plantar fasciitis	Diabetic foot disease
Hallux valgus (women)	Tibialis posterior tendonitis	Hallux valgus (women)
Pes planus (flat foot)	Morton's neuroma	
Pes cavus	Hallux valgus (women)	
Diabetic foot disease	Diabetic foot disease	

hallux valgus, the second and occasionally third toes may become clawed, over-riding the hallux.

Tarsal coalition (peroneal spastic flat foot) is characterized by reduced hindfoot movement and pain. It usually presents in childhood or adolescence. In all cases there is an abnormal bar of tissue connecting two separate tarsal bones. The most common forms of tarsal coalition are calcaneo-navicular and talo-calcaneal. Approximately 50% occur bilaterally. This condition is thought to have an autosomal dominant transmission with variable penetrance. The bar between the bones may be fibrous, cartilaginous or bony, when ossification develops (8–12 years for calcaneo-navicular and 12–16 years for talo-calcaneal). Stiffness worsens following ossification and secondary degeneration of the joints may follow.

Inflammation

Foot and ankle disease are common in rheumatoid arthritis. Early synovitis may become bulky and cause capsular distension and erosions, resulting in joint instability, subluxation and secondary deformities. Planovalgus deformity of the hindfoot is common with rupture of the tibialis posterior tendon. In the forefoot there is usually hallux valgus (80%) (Fig. 8.60) and clawing of the lesser toes. Clawing occurs when attenuation of the volar MTPJ structures allows the toes to dislocate dorsally, forcing the metatarsal heads in a plantar direction. As the toes sublux, the plantar skin with its protective fat pad is pulled distally from the metatarsal heads. These two factors lead to increased pressure in the sole and predispose to ulceration. Involvement of the midfoot is rare.

Plantar fasciitis is an inflammatory condition affecting the attachment of the plantar fascia to the medial calcaneal tuberosity in the sole. The fascia can become contracted. There is often a bony spur present at this site but plantar fasciitis can exist without a spur.

Inflammation about the Achilles tendon insertion follows a spectrum of pathology. Early para-tenonitis is inflammation of the paratenon, usually with thickening, fibrosis and

adhesions to the tendon. Tendinosis follows with nodular thickening of the tendon. Microscopically the area is hypocellular with mucoid degeneration and occasional areas of necrosis. The tendon becomes weak and rupture may eventually occur.

Degenerative

Degenerative arthritis tends to occur in the ankle joint, subtalar joint, talo-navicular joint and the first MTPJ. Arthritis in other ankle and foot joints is uncommon and is usually due to trauma or infection. In most cases of symptomatic ankle and subtalar arthritis, there is a history of injury, which can be minor. Severe ankle, talar or calcaneal fractures lead to accelerated degenerative change. Avascular necrosis of the talus (usually following trauma) will also lead to degenerative change in the adjacent joints. Primary osteoarthritis is rare in the foot and ankle. Alteration of the mechanical axis may predispose to arthritis, with severe knee and hindfoot deformities causing particular problems.

Early osteophyte formation usually occurs in the anterior aspect of the ankle and causes impingement with dorsiflexion. Synovitis may occur locally. The cartilage is gradually worn and stiffness develops, usually with a secondary (varus) deformity.

Degenerative arthritis of the first MTPJ, also known as hallux rigidus, may follow trauma or osteochondritis or develop secondary to hypermobility. In many cases no obvious cause is identified. Initially degeneration occurs in the dorsum of the joint and osteophyte formation can restrict dorsiflexion. With time, degeneration becomes more generalized and the joint may become ankylosed in slight plantarflexion. The dorsal osteophyte becomes prominent, leading to rubbing and ulceration.

The tibialis posterior tendon may develop degenerative changes, the most common of which results in an acquired 'flat foot' deformity (pes planus). The normal function of the tendon is to maintain the medial longitudinal plantar arch, and tendon rupture leads to collapse of the arch giving a valgus hindfoot and a planus midfoot. With time, the hindfoot deformities may become fixed and secondary degeneration develops in the subtalar joint. The change in the tendon varies from a longitudinal split to attenuation and complete rupture. This is often associated with tenosynovitis. A vascular watershed with relative local ischaemia of the tibialis posterior tendon is believed to exist approximately 1.5 cm distal to the medial malleolus, predisposing to the above pathological changes.

Infection

Septic arthritis of the foot and ankle joints is uncommon but may follow ulceration over the joint with neuropathy or rheumatoid disease. Joint destruction and fibrosis may occur, as may osteomyelitis of the periarticular bone. Chronic osteomyelitis can spread across the foot, causing destruction and secondary deformities, as is often the case with tuberculosis. Superficial infections such as cellulitis and abscesses are common but rarely result in significant pathological changes.

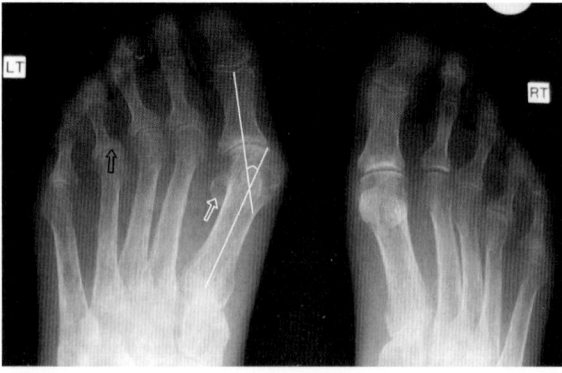

Fig. 8.60 Plain film of rheumatoid disease of the feet. The X-ray shows some asymmetry of disease. There is left hallux valgus with some subluxation and destruction of the joint. The subluxed sesamoids are shown (white arrow) and early disease of the fourth MTPJ (black arrow).

Vascular

Osteonecrosis of the talus most commonly occurs following trauma, particularly displaced talar neck fractures and talar dislocations when the tenuous blood supply is disturbed. Rarely, osteonecrosis may occur spontaneously in high-risk groups (p. 521). Standard changes of osteonecrosis follow, with risk of talar collapse due to the high loads through the ankle joint. The process of revascularization and remodelling can take up to 2 years. Deformity and secondary arthritis can occur in the ankle and subtalar joints.

Freiberg's disease usually affects the second metatarsal head and is characterized by osteonecrosis, rarefaction and collapse. There is often fragmentation, degeneration with capsular thickening and joint stiffness.

Endocrine

Long-standing diabetes mellitus has significant implications for the feet and ankles. The development of sensory neuropathy and vasculopathy may lead to unrecognized injury, secondary ulceration and infection. Deformity of the foot can occur with a motor neuropathy, exacerbating the pressure areas. Neuropathic osteoarthropathy (Charcot) may develop, with a prevalence of approximately 500 per 100 000. Although the exact cause is uncertain, sensory neuropathy may result in the loss of protective joint sensation and repetitive microtrauma can lead to gradual damage. Autonomic neuropathy may also lead to higher levels of blood flow, resulting in greater bony resorption and increased fragility. The midfoot is most commonly affected followed by the hindfoot and the ankle. Initially there is swelling, warmth and erythema that mimics infection. Pain is experienced in 50% despite neuropathy. There is loss of joint space, resorption of bone, and joints may become unstable leading to dislocation and deformity. Later, as inflammation reduces, there is new bone formation in the soft tissues around the joints. Finally, the healing process takes place, with reduction in swelling and stabilization of joints. However, significant deformities may persist, and secondary ulceration is common.

Neurological

Neurological pathology may be localized to the foot (peripheral) or secondary to more proximal neurological disease (central).

Morton's neuroma is thickening of a branch of the interdigital nerve, most commonly in the third web space, possibly due to a combination of the greater mobility of the fourth and fifth rays (relative to the third), and reduced mobility of this nerve branch as it is formed from the confluence of the medial and lateral plantar nerves. Localized swelling and fibrosis develops, reducing the space available for the nerve between the metatarsal heads and the intermetatarsal ligament and leading to pain and tenderness.

The posterior tibial nerve can become compressed within the tarsal tunnel (formed by the flexor retinaculum below the medial malleolus), usually due to a lesion within the tunnel itself, such as a ganglion, lipoma or synovitis. The compressed nerve eventually becomes atrophic.

Proximal neurological disease commonly affecting the foot includes cerebral palsy, polio and hereditary sensory and motor neuropathy (HSMN) type 1. HSMN type 1 is an autosomal dominant condition, causing a hypertrophic demyelinating neuropathy, with the development of cavovarus hindfoot and midfoot deformities (pes cavus) and plantarflexion of the first ray. The toes tend to claw, causing various pressure points and pain. A similar picture may develop in rarer diseases such as Friedreich's ataxia or tethered cord syndrome.

Trauma/instability

Lateral ankle ligament sprains are common and long-term symptoms may occur in up to 50%. Although instability accounts for a large proportion, most cases are thought to be 'functional' and due to poor muscle coordination (proprioception). True mechanical instability refers to laxity in the ligaments, and may affect part or the entirety of the lateral ligament complex. With time there is damage to the ankle joint due to recurrent subluxation.

Miscellaneous conditions

Toe deformities are frequent but are often due to other pathological processes such as hallux valgus or pes cavus. When other diseases and congenital conditions have been excluded, shoe wear should be considered as an underlying cause.

Claw toes involve a flexion deformity of the interphalangeal joints (IPJs) with hyperextension of the MTPJs. This may occur with compartment syndrome, stroke or in cerebral palsy. With time the deformity becomes fixed.

Mallet toe describes a flexion deformity at the distal IPJ, often due to contracture of a flexor tendon. Hammer toe flexion deformity occurs at the proximal IPJ. All of these deformities cause pressure areas, with callosity of the overlying skin, and neuropathy or vasculopathy will predispose to ulceration.

Scope of disease

The foot and ankle are important for balance and ambulation. They must tolerate high loads and be adaptable to changes in terrain for all phases of the gait cycle. When the gait cycle is altered by pathological changes, it can jeopardize the patient's independence or employment.

Clinical features

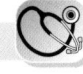

A detailed history should be taken about the duration of the disease, symptoms of pain and to screen for any coexisting medical diseases such as diabetes, rheumatoid disease and gout. A history of previous injury is also important.

Pain

Pain from the ankle joint is usually felt anteriorly, particularly when impingement occurs. Subtalar joint pain is felt below the malleoli, usually laterally. Diseases of the midfoot and forefoot tend to produce pain localized to these joints.

Pain beneath the heel is likely to be due to plantar fasciitis; when behind the heel, Achilles tendonitis is more likely. Pain in the sole of the forefoot is often described as metatarsalgia and can be due to a number of causes. The cause can be narrowed down by the presence or absence of plantar callosities (Table 8.64).

Instability

Patients with instability usually complain of recurrent sprains or episodes of giving way. Lateral ankle pain may also be a feature.

Deformity/shoe wear problems

Patients may report a progressive deformity and this may cause rubbing and difficulty with footwear.

Examination

Look

The patient should be standing and the foot and ankle observed from behind. The normal hindfoot forms an angle of 5° valgus. Varus deformity may be evident in the ankle joint and/or the subtalar joint (arthropathy, cavovarus foot or persistent clubfoot deformity). Excessive valgus may be evident in the ankle (arthropathy) or the subtalar joint (e.g. ruptured tibialis posterior tendon). The patient is asked to rise onto tiptoes and the valgus hindfoot should move into varus if a mobile subtalar joint and functioning tibialis posterior exist. Flat foot deformity is observed by a flattened longitudinal medial arch such as the planovalgus deformity of tibialis posterior rupture. There are often 'too many toes' visible from behind the patient. Swelling may be seen about the inflamed Achilles tendon. From the front ankle swelling may be noticeable, as may the high arch of pes cavus. Deformity of the toes and hallux is maximized with the patient standing. The sole of the foot should be studied for callosity or ulcers, and inspection of the shoe may reveal abnormal areas of wear due to abnormal gait.

Feel

Systematic palpation is undertaken over the anatomical landmarks. Starting on the medial side of the tibialis anterior tendon in front of the medial malleolus the ankle joint can be palpated (notch of Harty). The lateral side of the ankle joint is then palpated; just proximal to this is the distal tibio-fibular joint. The lateral ankle collateral ligaments are palpated in front of and below the lateral malleolus and the peroneal tendons posterior to it. Below the lateral malleolus is the sinus tarsi where tenderness of the subtalar joint may be detected. Posteriorly, thickening of the Achilles tendon or paratenon is felt. Passing back medially round the hindfoot, the medial ankle collateral ligament is felt and the tibialis posterior tendon. Moving down to the sole, the medial calcaneal tuberosity may be tender with plantar fasciitis. More distally in the sole the metatarsal heads can be felt (metatarsalgia) and finally the joints of the hallux and toes may be palpated if indicated.

Move

Movement should be studied actively and passively and comparison of both sides should be performed. Normal ankle movement ranges from 20° dorsiflexion to 40° plantarflexion. Inversion of the hindfoot is usually twice that of eversion (20° vs 10°). Limited hindfoot movement may occur with arthropathy, spasticity or tarsal coalition. The MTPJ of the hallux should dorsiflex 80° relative to the metatarsal shaft and this may be reduced with hallux rigidus. Dorsiflexion of the hallux also acts to tighten the plantar fascia, causing heightening of the medial longitudinal arch when flat foot deformity remains mobile ('windlass effect').

Tinel's test

Patients with tarsal tunnel syndrome may experience pins and needles when the examiner taps over the nerve below the medial malleolus (positive Tinel's test). There may be reduced sensation in the sole with severe cases.

Assessment of the anterior talofibular ligament

The anterior drawer test is performed with the foot flat on the couch and the knee flexed. Posterior pressure on the tibia causes the foot to sublux anteriorly, indicating a lax anterior talofibular ligament.

Assessment of the calcaneo-fibular ligament

The varus stress test involves pushing the hindfoot into varus with a neutral ankle to assess for excessive laxity.

Assessment of the tibialis posterior tendon

Resisted foot inversion may detect weakness of tibialis posterior, suggesting rupture.

Mulder's test

A Morton's neuroma may be felt to 'clunk' in the sole if pressure is applied in the sole over the lesion while the metatarsals are squeezed together (Mulder's sign).

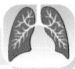

Initial investigations

Plain X-rays

Standard ankle views include AP and lateral; standard views of the foot are AP, oblique and lateral. These views allow most joints to be visualized, but the subtalar joint and its

Table 8.64	Causes of pain in the sole of the foot
With callosity	**No callosity**
Hallux valgus	Morton's neuroma
Claw, hammer or mallet toes	Tarsal tunnel syndrome
Intractable plantar keratoses	Prolapsed intervertebral disc (neurological symptoms present) MTPJ instability or capsulitis Stress fractures (no neurological symptoms)

three facets are sometimes poorly seen. Broden's oblique views allow each facet to be seen, which may help to identify localized arthritis.

Instability of the lateral ligaments is identified by stress X-rays (e.g. pushing the hindfoot into varus and taking an AP film). Alternatively a lateral X-ray can be taken with the heel pulled forwards relative to the ankle joint. Deformity of the hindfoot joints is often best appreciated by a weight-bearing AP X-ray.

Further investigations

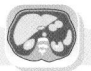

Full blood count/markers of inflammation
White cell count and ESR may be elevated with infection and inflammation.

Serum autoantibodies
As rheumatoid arthritis may present in the foot or ankle, it may be appropriate to measure autoantibody and rheumatoid factor levels.

Ultrasound of the ankle
This can be used to detect an effusion in an ankle joint, soft tissue abscesses and large Morton's neuromas. It is also possible to visualize the individual flexor and extensor tendons as well as the Achilles tendon for tenosynovitis, attenuation and tears.

Isotope bone scan
Joints that are arthritic and inflamed are likely to show as areas of increased tracer uptake on bone scans. This may help to localize the joint responsible for pain if symptoms are diffuse and several joints are diseased.

CT of the ankle
CT provides information about subtalar joint anatomy, which is often poorly seen on plain X-ray, and is particularly helpful for planning arthrodesis, detecting tarsal coalition and assessing complex fractures.

MRI of the ankle
MRI is a sensitive means of detecting soft tissue or bony infection and assessing the ankle ligaments and tendons. MRI has 96% accuracy in detecting tibialis posterior tears[1] and can also detect areas of osteochondral damage to the talus and large Morton's neuromas.

Diagnostic injections
Injection of local anaesthetic and steroid can be directed using X-ray, ultrasound or CT, and may help to localize the joint responsible for the symptoms.

Initial management

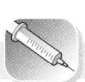

Patient education
Many foot and ankle conditions can be improved by adjusting work, activity, sports, etc. Unsuitable choice of footwear can exacerbate problems. Soft-soled shoes may help absorb shock, and inbuilt arch supports may offer support if there is collapse of the longitudinal arch. A wide toe box is important when deformity of the toes exists. Chiropody can be important when thickened callosities develop over prominent areas, particularly when neuropathy exists.

Simple analgesia
Simple analgesics and NSAIDs can all play a role, particularly with the inflammatory and arthritic conditions. Targeted injections of steroid and anaesthetic may also be useful.

Physiotherapy
Gait abnormalities may improve with education, restoring normal foot alignment. Proprioceptive training can be helpful when there is instability.

Orthotics
Insoles, custom shoes, splints and braces may help to correct minor underlying deformities of the foot.

Surgical management

General
Arthrodesis
Arthrodesis remains the gold standard surgical treatment in many cases of painful arthritis of the ankle, subtalar, talo-navicular, calcaneo-cuboid and first MTPJ. Fusion relieves pain, corrects deformities and has a high rate of union (95%). With loss of movement, however, there is inevitably some loss of function. Also, there is an increased load through adjacent joints, which may accelerate degeneration.

Arthroplasty
Modern ankle replacements are offering encouraging long-term results. Patients generally prefer the option of replacement because movement and function are better preserved. A more normal gait can be expected. Eighty eight per cent survival at 8 years for rheumatoid and osteoarthritis has been achieved.[2] Failure of ankle replacements can be difficult to manage, often requiring fusion of both the ankle and subtalar joints.

Specific
Hallux valgus
Accommodation is key to non-operative treatment: the wider forefoot and secondary deformities of the lesser toes require a larger toe box on shoes to prevent cramping and pressure. Custom shoes can be fashioned and orthotists can provide pads and spacers to sit between toes.

When the above measures are unsuccessful and persistent pain remains, surgical treatment options should be considered. The principles behind most procedures are corrective osteotomy of the first metatarsal and occasionally the proximal phalanx of the great toe, combined with a lateral soft tissue release and medial soft tissue tightening. Good or excellent results can be achieved in 90%.[3] Where there is mild arthritis of the MTPJ and the patient is elderly, a Keller's excision arthroplasty can be considered, excising the proximal third of the proximal phalanx. Unsatisfactory results are seen in more active patients.

Hallux rigidus

An initial measure is the adjustment of shoe wear with a rocker-bottom sole to avoid dorsiflexion forces on the first MTPJ during toe-off. Surgery involves cheilectomy in well-preserved joints, where the dorsal 20–30% of the metatarsal head and all osteophytes are excised to restore dorsiflexion of the big toe. Severe arthritis is best treated with fusion: rates of union are over 90%. MTPJ replacement remains experimental.

Inflammatory arthritis

Consideration must be given to deformity, pressure areas and callosities. Shoes must accommodate deformity, and instability requires support with splints such as an ankle–foot orthosis (AFO). Surgical treatment should be considered for patients with persistent symptoms despite optimum medical management. Synovectomy is rarely effective as the disease progresses rapidly and the window of opportunity is small.

Good results can be achieved with arthrodesis of the ankle, hindfoot (Fig. 8.61) and first MTPJ although there is a greater risk of infection and soft tissue healing problems. When deformity of the ankle is minor, replacement can be considered over arthrodesis. Plantar pressure symptoms caused by dorsal dislocation of the lesser MTPJs can be improved by excision of the metatarsal heads (forefoot arthroplasty) and fusion of the great toe.

Plantar fasciitis

NSAIDs, shock-absorbing heel pads and resting night splints may be helpful. There is only limited evidence to support steroid injection,[4] and surgical release is rarely required.

Achilles tendonitis

Rest, NSAIDs, physiotherapy and stretching exercises are successful in most cases. Steroid injection is not recommended due to the risk of tendon rupture. Recalcitrant cases may improve with excision of the inflamed paratenon and degenerate tendon.

Degenerative arthritis

Restriction of activity, NSAIDs, custom boots and shock-absorbing silicone heel pads can help. Surgical options include debridement of anterior ankle osteophytes; this can give some relief and improve dorsiflexion in early cases. Severe ankle arthritis (Fig. 8.62) is better treated by arthrodesis or arthroplasty. Ankle replacement is favoured where preservation of movement is preferred and the underlying deformity is not too severe (Fig. 8.63). With severe deformity, ankle fusion allows repositioning of the heel below the leg in neutral or slight valgus. The joint is fused in neutral flexion with slight external rotation of the talus on the tibia.

If pain from subtalar joint arthritis cannot be managed by the above non-operative means, arthrodesis is the only option. It may be necessary to fuse the calcaneo-cuboid and talo-navicular joints simultaneously, if diseased ('triple fusion') (Fig. 8.61).

Diabetic foot disease

Optimum glycaemic control is the first priority, with regular attention to the feet, particularly when neuropathy exists. Chiropody, orthotics and good footwear are recommended. Infection requires aggressive early treatment. Injuries

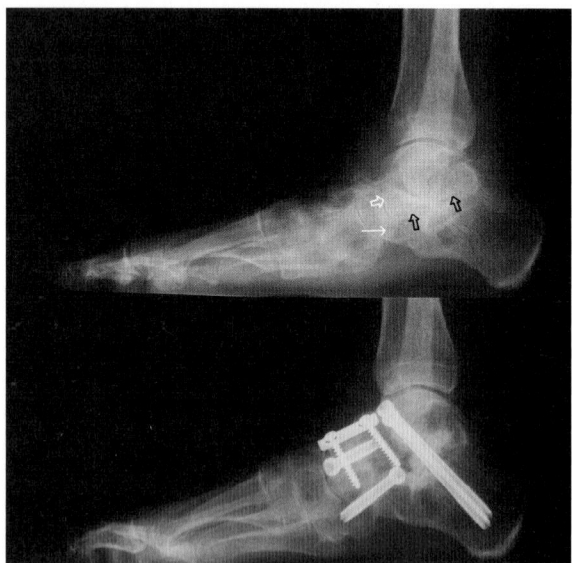

Fig. 8.61 Triple fusion. Preoperative (upper panel) and postoperative films showing subtalar (black arrows), talo-navicular (white open arrow) and calcaneo-cuboid (white arrow) destruction due to rheumatoid arthritis, with subsequent triple fusion procedure. The planus deformity has been corrected.

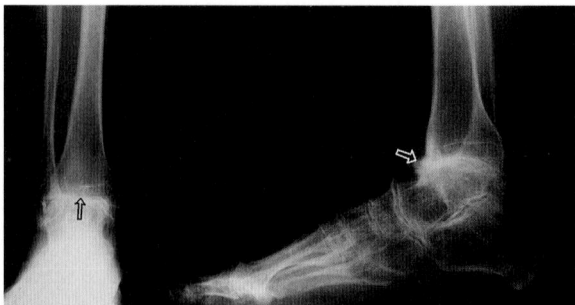

Fig. 8.62 Ankle osteoarthritis. Plain films showing loss of joint space with sclerosis (black arrow) and anterior osteophyte (white arrow).

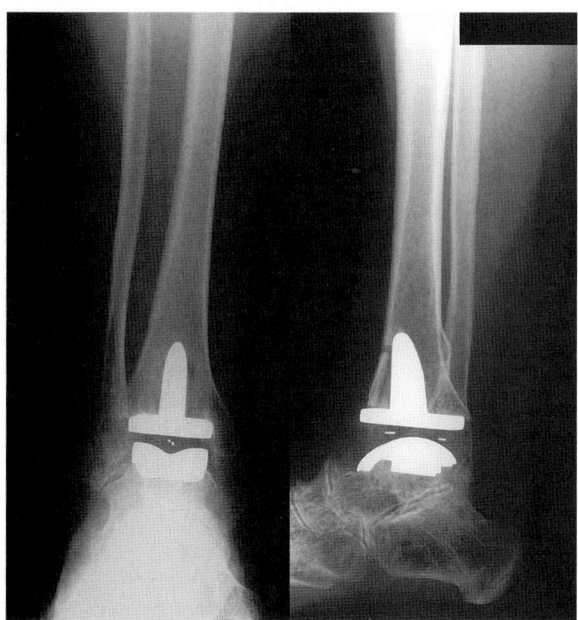

Fig. 8.63 Total right ankle replacement. AP (left panel) and lateral views.

require longer periods in cast, due to loss of protective sensation. Charcot neuroarthropathy must be recognized early, before deformity occurs. Casts or braces can help to shift loads away from the affected joints and may be necessary for up to 2 years. Once deformity is present, other means of supporting the foot can be used, such as an Ilizarov frame, allowing some correction of deformity. Burnt out disease may leave deformity and irregular bony prominences. The risk of ulceration may necessitate excision of these prominent areas.

Morton's neuroma

Foot pads and accommodating shoes can improve symptoms. Steroid injection may reduce the need for surgical intervention. Persistent symptoms may require surgical excision, which is best performed through the dorsum of the foot to prevent a tender scar on the sole.

Infection

The majority of soft tissue infections without abscess formation respond well to intravenous antibiotics and elevation. Abscess or septic effusions require formal surgical drainage, and samples for microbiological analysis. Septic arthritis of the ankle is amenable to arthroscopic washout, but other joints of the foot that are smaller and less accessible require formal arthrotomy for debridement and washout. Once antibiotics have been commenced it is often useful to splint the foot and ankle in a cast to restrict movement and prevent secondary deformity. Standard bacterial joint or bone sepsis requires 6 weeks of anti-

biotics. Infection with tuberculosis requires more lengthy chemotherapy.

Tibialis posterior tendonitis

In early cases where tenosynovitis predominates, rest, NSAIDs, longitudinal arch supports, ankle–foot orthoses and steroid injections may be helpful. Surgical treatment consists initially of decompression of the tendon. If the patient develops a mobile flat foot deformity, one option is a tendon transfer combined with a calcaneal osteotomy. Fixed valgus and secondary arthritis may necessitate subtalar or triple fusion.

Tarsal coalition

Splinting and rest is successful in a third of cases. Surgery is appropriate for patients with persistent symptoms. The abnormal bar is excised with interposition of adjacent fat or muscle. Results are less favourable for talo-calcaneal bars and secondary degeneration may occur.

Osteonecrosis

Talar osteonecrosis may lead to catastrophic collapse of the ankle joint surface. Deformity and loss of bone make joint reconstruction difficult.

Freiberg's disease can be managed with analgesia, pads and careful shoe choice. Where symptoms persist, debridement of the irregular joint surface may remove irritability. A shortening osteotomy of the metatarsal may ultimately be necessary, reducing forces across the joint. Excision of the joint is not recommended.

Tarsal tunnel syndrome

Steroid injection and splints may help, but persistent cases may require surgical decompression with excision of associated lesions.

Pes cavus

This condition is usually progressive and when recognized early should be managed with physiotherapy to maintain flexibility. Orthotics may be helpful. Once severe deformity occurs, a standard surgical procedure includes division of the shortened plantar fascia, calcaneal osteotomy with dorsal and lateral displacement of the heel, dorsal closing wedge osteotomy of the first metatarsal, fusion of the hallux IPJ and tendon transfers. When arthritis occurs or deformity and neurological disease are severe, triple fusion is required.

Lateral instability

The distinction must be made between functional and mechanical instability, although both may be improved with physiotherapy working on lateral stabilizers (peronei) and proprioception. In persistent cases of mechanical instability, surgical stabilization may be attempted. Anatomical techniques involve tightening of the lax ligamentous structures (Broström procedure). When this tissue is deficient, peroneus brevis can be used to augment

569

ligamentous stabilization but in return sacrifices part of the dynamic lateral stability. Alternatively a hamstring tendon graft can be used. Results are generally good with all techniques.

REFERENCES

(1) *Rosenberg ZS, Cheung Y, Jahss MH, Noto AM, Norman A, Leeds NE. Rupture of the posterior tibial tendon: CT and MRI imaging with surgical correlation. Radiology 1988; 169: 229–235.*
(2) *Wood PLR, Deakin S. Total ankle replacement: The results in 200 ankles. Journal of Bone and Joint Surgery (Br) 2003; 85B: 334–341.*
(3) *Mann RA, Rudicel S, Graves SC. Repair of hallux valgus with a distal soft tissue and proximal metatarsal osteotomy. Journal of Bone and Joint Surgery (Am) 1992; 74A: 124–129.*
(4) *Crawford F, Thomson C. Interventions for treating plantar heel pain. The Cochrane Database of Systematic Reviews, 2005, Issue 2.*

Diseases of the nervous system and voluntary muscle

9

Fiona McKevitt, Jeremy Rowe, Marios Hadjivassiliou

Introduction

The study of the nervous system is fascinating. A systematic and logical approach is required to localize the site and cause of a lesion for appropriate investigation, diagnosis and management. An understanding of the anatomy of the nervous system therefore is essential to diagnose the potential causes of neurological symptoms and signs.

Applied basic sciences of the nervous system

Anatomy and physiology

The nervous system comprises the central nervous system (brain and spinal cord) and the peripheral nervous system (peripheral nerves and neuromuscular junction).

The brain (or encephalon) incorporates the forebrain, midbrain and hindbrain. The forebrain consists of the diencephalon (thalamus and hypothalamus) and the telencephalon (the two cerebral hemispheres). The latter comprises the cerebral cortex and basal ganglia. The midbrain (or mesencephalon) and hindbrain (medulla oblongata, pons and cerebellum) form the brainstem.

The central nervous system (CNS) is surrounded by three meninges: the dura mater (adherent to the cranial bones within the skull), the arachnoid mater and the pia mater, which is tightly bound to the CNS.

The cerebral hemispheres

There is a dominant and a non-dominant cerebral hemisphere. In the majority of right-handed people, and in 70–75% of left-handed people, this is on the left. Each cerebral cortex is divided into four lobes, each with differing functions (Fig. 9.1).

Lesions of the frontal lobe lead to hemiparesis, personality change (apathy, disinhibition), urinary incontinence, expressive dysphasia (Broca's area is located in the inferior lateral frontal lobe), cognitive decline, the emergence of primitive reflexes (ipsilateral palmo-mental, contralateral grasp) and motor seizures.

Lesions of the parietal lobe lead to contralateral hemisensory loss, contralateral sensory inattention, visual field defect (homonymous quadrantanopia), dysgraphaesthesia (inability to recognize patterns drawn on the palm), astereognosis (inability to recognize objects placed in the hand) and sensory seizures. In addition, lesions of the dominant parietal lobe lead to receptive dysphasia (Wernicke's area is located in the parieto-temporal lobe), motor dyspraxia (inability to perform a series of movements despite normal power, sensation and coordination) and acalculia, whilst lesions of the non-dominant parietal lobe lead to dressing apraxia and constructional apraxia.

Lesions of the temporal lobe lead to receptive dysphasia, visual field defects (homonymous quadrantanopia), hallucinations of smell, taste and sound, memory defects and complex partial seizures.

Lesions of the occipital lobe lead to contralateral homonymous hemianopia, cortical blindness (if bilateral) and visual seizures (e.g. balls of light).

The basal ganglia

The basal ganglia (extrapyramidal system) comprise the caudate nucleus, putamen, globus pallidus (collectively

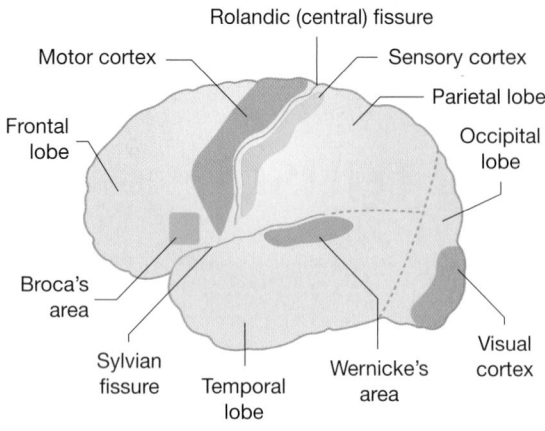

Motor cortex

Rolandic (central) fissure

Sensory cortex

Parietal lobe

Frontal lobe

Occipital lobe

Broca's area

Sylvian fissure

Temporal lobe

Wernicke's area

Visual cortex

Fig. 9.1 Lobes of the brain.

Table 9.1	Clinical differences between pseudo-bulbar palsy and bulbar palsy	
	Pseudo-bulbar palsy	**Bulbar palsy**
Signs	Tongue—stiff, slow	Tongue—wasted, fasciculations
	Speech—slow, spastic	Speech—nasal
	Gag reflex—intact	Gag reflex—absent
	Jaw jerk—brisk	
	Emotional lability	
Causes	Motor neurone disease	Motor neurone disease
	Bilateral strokes	Poliomyelitis
	Multiple sclerosis	Brainstem infarction/ tumour
		Syringobulbia
		Polyneuritis cranialis (variant of Guillain– Barré)

called the corpus striatum), substantia nigra, subthalamic nucleus, claustrum and amygdala. This region is responsible for modifying and initiating voluntary muscle movement through its connections with the thalamus and cerebral cortex.

The brainstem

The midbrain connects the diencephalon to the pons and the cerebellum. It contains the cerebral peduncles and the IIIrd and IVth nuclei. Lesions here can result in diplopia, pupil dilatation, vertical gaze defects and contralateral weakness or sensory loss of the face and limbs.

The pons lies between the midbrain and the medulla and has connections with the cerebellum. It contains the Vth to VIIIth nuclei, the sympathetic chain, the fourth ventricle and the medial longitudinal fasciculus, which connects the IIIrd and VIth nerve nuclei. Lesions here can result in facial sensory loss, diplopia, ipsilateral facial weakness and deafness. There may be a Horner's syndrome or, if the lesion is bilateral, bilateral pinpoint pupils. There may be an abnormality of conjugate gaze such as an internuclear ophthalmoplegia.

The medulla connects the pons to the spinal cord at the foramen magnum. It also has connections to the cerebellum. It contains the IXth to XIIth nerve nuclei, the sympathetic chain and connections to the cerebellum. In the medulla at the level of the pyramids the corticospinal tracts cross and the dorsal column nuclei cross to form the medial lemniscus. Lesions at this level can result in dysphagia, dysarthria, Horner's syndrome, vertigo and nystagmus, contralateral limb weakness and contralateral limb sensory loss, but ipsilateral sensory loss to the face.

A bulbar palsy refers to a lower motor neurone lesion of these lower cranial nerves whereas weakness of the bulbar muscles (tongue, palate and pharynx) due to an upper motor neurone lesion is called a pseudobulbar palsy; the clinical differences are outlined in Table 9.1.

The cerebellum

The cerebellum coordinates ipsilateral limb movement. It comprises two hemispheres joined by the vermis, which is concerned with midline posture and balance. Cerebellar lesions result in nystagmus, vertigo, dysarthria, impaired finger–nose pointing with intention tremor and past-pointing, dysdiadochokinesis and impaired heel–shin testing. The gait is ataxic and wide based. There is impaired tandem walking and loss of balance. If the vermis is involved there is truncal ataxia.

The spinal cord

The spinal cord extends from the foramen magnum to the filum terminale at L1/2. Below this the nerve roots form the cauda equina. At each level of the spinal cord a pair of nerve roots emerges on each side. The posterior root carries afferent sensory fibres to the posterior column of the spinal cord and the anterior root carries efferent motor fibres arising from the anterior horn cell of the spinal cord.

Blood supply

The brain has an anterior blood supply, which supplies approximately 80% of the brain (internal carotid arteries), and a posterior blood supply (vertebral arteries). The internal carotid artery supplies the majority of the cerebral hemispheres and the eye. Its terminal branches are the anterior and middle cerebral artery. The vertebral arteries join to form the basilar artery, the branches of which supply the medulla, pons and cerebellum, terminating as the posterior cerebral artery which supplies the midbrain, the posterior hemisphere and the diencephalon.

The internal carotid and vertebrobasilar systems are linked together to form the circle of Willis by the anterior and posterior communicating arteries (Fig. 9.2). The dura contains venous sinuses that drain the brain.

The spinal cord is supplied by the anterior spinal arteries (anterior two thirds) and the posterior spinal arteries.

Cerebrospinal fluid (CSF)

The total volume of CSF is 100–150 mL, although the choroid plexus (situated in the lateral ventricles) produces

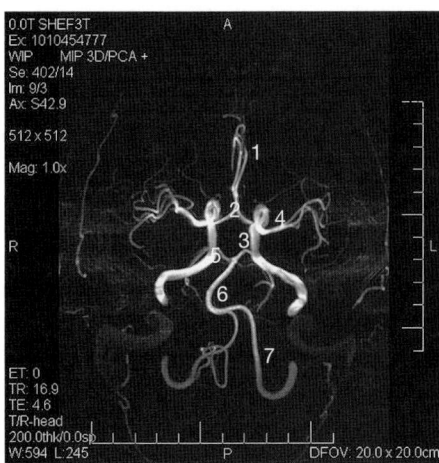

Fig. 9.2 Magnetic resonance angiography of the circle of Willis: 1, anterior cerebral artery; 2, anterior communicating artery; 3, internal carotid artery; 4, middle cerebral artery; 5, posterior cerebral artery; 6, basilar artery; 7, vertebral artery. Courtesy of Mr John Wattam, Royal Hallamshire Hospital, Sheffield, UK.

Table 9.2	Causes of autonomic failure
Primary pure autonomic failure	
Multisystem atrophy	
Diabetes mellitus	
Porphyria	
Amyloidosis	
Guillain–Barré syndrome	
HIV infection	
Drugs—tricyclic antidepressants	

lation. Common symptoms of autonomic failure include postural hypotension, resting tachycardia, impaired heart rate response to the Valsalva manoeuvre, impotence, dry eyes and mouth, Horner's syndrome and abnormal bowel and bladder function. The causes of autonomic failure are listed in Table 9.2.

Motor pathways

One very important distinction that needs to be made in the nervous system is the difference between an upper motor neurone lesion (UMN) and a lower motor neurone lesion (LMN).

An **upper motor neurone** begins with the motor neurones in the frontal cerebral cortex. These pass back through the internal capsule (where they are tightly packed) and pass through the brainstem as the corticospinal tract. They cross at the pyramids in the medulla, and this is where the tract receives its alternative name (the pyramidal tract). The tract continues in the lateral portion of the spinal cord and terminates either on the motor nuclei of the cranial nerves or on the anterior horn cells of the spinal cord.

The pathway from the motor nuclei of the cranial nerves, or from the anterior horn cells via a peripheral nerve to the motor end-plate, is the **lower motor neurone**. The clinical differences between upper and lower motor neurone lesions are listed in Table 9.3.

0.5 litres daily. The CSF passes from the lateral ventricles through the interventricular foramina (of Monro) into the third ventricle, down the cerebral aqueduct through the brainstem and into the fourth ventricle in the posterior fossa. It then exits into the subarachnoid space, via the foramina of Magendie and Luschka, to circulate around the surface of the brain before being reabsorbed by the arachnoid villi into the venous sinuses. The subarachnoid space containing the CSF over the surface of the brain is continuous with that around the spinal cord, which ends in the lumbar cistern.

The autonomic nervous system

The autonomic nervous system (parasympathetic and sympathetic) innervates all the internal organs. It is responsible for blood pressure, heart rate, pupillary response, lacrimation, sweating, bronchial constriction and dilatation, sphincter control, bowels, erection and ejacu-

Table 9.3	Clinical differences between an upper motor neurone and a lower motor neurone lesion	
	Upper motor neurone	**Lower motor neurone**
Inspection	No wasting (only after prolonged disuse)	Wasted, fasciculations
Tone	Increased	Decreased
Reflexes	Exaggerated Plantar response extensor Abdominal reflexes absent	Absent
Clonus	Present	Absent
Power	Weak in a characteristic pattern (extensors weaker than flexors in upper limb, flexors weaker than extensors in lower limb)	
Facial weakness	Sparing of the upper facial muscles	Total unilateral facial weakness

Sensory pathways

The afferent fibres within the peripheral nerve enter the spinal cord via the posterior root. Pain and temperature sensation fibres synapse in the posterior horn and secondary axons cross over to the contralateral spinal cord (a few levels higher) and run in the lateral part of the spinal cord as the spinothalamic tract. They join the medial lemniscus in the medulla and enter the thalamus. They then continue to the sensory cortex in the parietal lobe. Light touch, proprioception and vibration run in the posterior columns of the spinal cord ipsilaterally. They continue as the dorsal column nuclei in the medulla. Secondary axons then cross in the medulla to continue as the medial lemniscus with the pain and temperature fibres.

Cells of the nervous system

The neurone is the communicating cell of the nervous system. It has a cell body, many short projections (dendrites) and a long projection, the axon. The central nervous system is comprised of grey matter (the cell bodies) and white matter (the axons). Myelination greatly increases the conduction velocity of the neurone. Pain fibres or autonomic nerves are unmyelinated and are therefore slow conductors. Glial cells (*glia* is Greek for glue) support the neurones in the nervous system. They consist of macroglia, both astrocytes (form part of the blood–brain barrier) and oligodendrocytes (produce myelin), ependymal cells (line the ventricles and spinal canal) and microglia (tissue macrophages). In the peripheral nervous system, Schwann cells are responsible for producing myelin for the peripheral nerves.

Communication between nerves occurs at the synapse of one neurone with the next and is dependent on the release of a neurotransmitter. These may be excitatory (glutamate, aspartate, acetylcholine, noradrenaline, adrenaline, substance P) or inhibitory (dopamine, glycine, γ-aminobutyric acid—GABA). Neurotransmitters are also released at the neuromuscular junction (p. 629).

Symptoms of neurological disease

Speed of onset

For all neurological symptoms, information regarding the speed of onset is crucial to aid diagnosis. Symptoms can commence suddenly or over minutes, hours, days, weeks, months or even years. Events that occur instantaneously are usually due to a vascular event such as stroke or subarachnoid haemorrhage. Symptoms that occur over minutes are characteristic of migraine or partial seizures. Infective (e.g. meningitis or encephalitis) or inflammatory processes (e.g. multiple sclerosis or Guillain–Barré syndrome) usually develop over hours or days, and symptoms that develop over weeks are characteristic of malignancy or muscle disorders (e.g. polymyalgia rheumatica). Neurodegenerative disorders such as Parkinson's disease, motor neurone disease or Alzheimer's disease tend to present after months or years.

Supplementary information

The past medical, drug and social histories may yield important additional information. A history of smoking, hypertension and hypercholesterolaemia, for example, are risk factors for stroke and numerous neurological diseases have a hereditary component that may be evident in the family history.

Headache

Headache is a very common symptom. It is important to enquire about the character of the headache, its speed of onset, duration and site. Exacerbating symptoms such as cough, straining or posture, or headache that is worse at a particular time of day should be sought. Any additional features such as nausea or photophobia may give more clues regarding the aetiology.

Blackouts

An eyewitness account is vital to obtain an accurate description of the episode of loss of consciousness. Prodromal symptoms such as rising sensation from the stomach (suggestive of a seizure), blurred vision, nausea, light-headedness (suggestive of vasovagal syncope) or palpitations (cardiac arrhythmia) may give clues to the underlying cause. Preceding events, the position at the time of the attack and recovery time may give additional information.

Dizziness

Dizziness may refer to vertigo (sensation of oneself or the room spinning around), light-headedness or loss of balance, therefore it is important to define exactly what is meant by this symptom.

Loss of balance

The speed of onset is important and additional features such as dysarthria and incoordination (cerebellar/brainstem lesion) or cognitive decline and incontinence (normal pressure hydrocephalus) may give clues to the site of the underlying problem. Balance problems also occur in Parkinsonism and labyrinthine disturbances.

Difficulty walking

Difficulty with walking can be due to diseases of the vasculature, bones or joints, muscles, peripheral or central nervous system. A detailed history should ascertain if the primary reason is leg weakness, loss of balance, impaired sensation or gait apraxia.

Arm or leg weakness

Weakness in the arm or legs can be due to muscle, peripheral or central nervous disorders. Associated features, pain, wasting, brisk reflexes, proximal or distal weakness can aid in diagnosis. Bilateral generalized weakness may be due to a muscle or generalized peripheral nerve disorder. Proximal muscle weakness can occur with Cushing's disease and polymyalgia rheumatica. Associated bladder or bowel dysfunction can occur with diseases of the spinal cord.

Sensory disturbance

The site and nature of the disturbance is important to ascertain: pain and temperature loss indicates spinothalamic tract involvement; proprioception and vibration loss indicates dorsal column involvement. Sensory disturbances include pins and needles (paraesthesia), numbness, increased pain sensation (hyperalgesia) or dysaesthesia (touch that feels painful). The sensory disturbance can originate from peripheral nerves, nerve roots, spinal cord or the central nervous system.

Visual disturbance

Sudden onset of unilateral visual loss is often due to a vascular cause (amaurosis fugax). This is often described 'as if a curtain has come down'. Gradual onset visual loss with pain may be due to optic neuritis. Double vision (diplopia) can be due to a lesion of the cranial nerves or ocular muscles. Zigzag lines can be seen in association with the aura symptoms of migraine.

Speech disturbance

Dysarthria is the inability to articulate clearly, resulting in slurring of words. It may be due to a lesion in the cerebral hemisphere (stroke), lesions in the cerebellum (distinctive staccato quality), extrapyramidal lesions (Parkinson's disease) or disorders of the muscles of articulation (myasthenia gravis or muscular dystrophy).

Expressive dysphasia is the inability to express speech. The patient typically knows what he or she wants to say but is unable to say it. Nominal aphasia is the inability to name objects, for example, a watch is described as 'something to tell the time with'.

Receptive dysphasia is an inability to comprehend the spoken word.

Dysphonia is hoarse speech or speech of low volume. It is seen in vocal cord lesions (Xth nerve palsies) or weakness of chest muscles (myasthenia gravis).

Dysphagia

Dysphagia is difficulty in swallowing (p. 213). Neurological causes include bulbar palsy (Guillain–Barré syndrome, poliomyelitis, myasthenia gravis) and pseudobulbar palsy (motor neurone disease, bilateral hemisphere strokes). Other causes of dysphagia include tonsillitis, external compression of the oesophagus (bronchial carcinoma), intrinsic disorders of the oesophagus (stricture or malignancy, pharyngeal pouch, systemic sclerosis) and psychological causes (globus hystericus).

Examination of the nervous system

Examination of the nervous system begins with a general inspection. Abnormal posture, fasciculations (fine movements of the muscles) and abnormal movements (chorea, myoclonic jerks, tremor) should be observed for. The examination should then focus on the cranial nerves, the upper and lower limbs (including gait), speech and cognition.

Cranial nerves

I. Olfactory nerve

The olfactory nerve is a sensory nerve that arises from the olfactory receptors of the nose. The fibres pass through the cribriform plate of the ethmoid bone to the olfactory bulb (inferior surface of the frontal lobe). The tract passes back to the olfactory cortex situated in the temporal lobe.

Testing of olfactory function (sense of smell) is performed by individually assessing each nostril using a distinctive strong-smelling substance such as coffee or vanilla. Causes of the loss of sense of smell include cold, sinusitis and head injury. Unilateral anosmia can be due to a frontal lobe tumour (e.g. olfactory groove meningioma).

II. Optic nerve

The optic nerve is a sensory nerve. Fibres pass back from the retina as the optic nerve and join the contralateral nerve to form the optic chiasm. Fibres in the nasal portion of the optic nerve cross to the opposite side of the chiasm to join the uncrossed temporal fibres. They then pass back as the optic tract to the lateral geniculate body in the thalamus. From this they continue as the optic radiation (the upper fibres in the parietal lobe, the lower in the temporal lobe). They then join again and pass into the occipital visual cortex.

There are several components to test the second cranial nerve: visual acuity, pupils (though the IIIrd nerve carries the parasympathetic supply of the pupil and is responsible for the efferent limb of the light reflex and accommodation), visual field testing, colour vision and fundoscopy.

Visual acuity

Visual acuity is examined using the Snellen chart (p. 639). The patient is tested, each eye separately, at a distance of 6 metres from the eye chart. The number of the smallest line read is recorded. Visual acuity is documented as the distance away from the chart over the smallest line read. Normal vision is recorded as 6/6 as the distance away from the chart is usually 6 m (but less if visual acuity is poor). A 6/60 result would imply poor visual acuity since the 60 denotes what a normally sighted person could read at 60 metres. If vision is poor, the test is repeated through a pinhole. If glasses are worn this must be documented.

Examination of the pupils

The pupils are inspected and the size assessed. Normal pupils are round, regular and equal. Reaction to light and accommodation is then tested. A bright light is shone into one eye. This and the contralateral pupil should react by constricting briskly to this stimulus. Constriction of the pupil illuminated is the direct light response, and constriction of the contralateral pupil is the consensual light response. An optic nerve lesion results in an abnormal *afferent* pupillary response: the direct light response is absent and the contralateral eye has no consensual light response. A IIIrd nerve lesion, however, will cause an abnormal *efferent* pupillary response: there is no direct light reflex but the contralateral eye has a consensual light response. The accommodation response (IIIrd nerve) is tested by first asking the patient to look into the distance and then to look at a near object. Both pupils should constrict.

Horner's syndrome consists of unilateral pupil miosis (pupil constriction), unilateral ptosis, enophthalmos (sunken eye) and unilateral impaired facial sweating (Fig. 9.3). It is due to a lesion of the cervical sympathetic fibres. These originate in the hypothalamus, pass through the brainstem into the cervical spinal cord, and exit at T1 root. The fibres then enter the cervical sympathetic chain via the cervical sympathetic ganglia and travel upwards with the internal carotid artery through the neck to the eye. The causes of a Horner's syndrome are presented in Table 9.4; other pupil abnormalities are listed in Table 9.5.

Visual fields

Visual field testing is performed by the examiner sitting directly opposite the patient and comparing his or her visual field with that of the patient's. Each eye is tested in turn. Using first a red then a white pin (red colour vision's visual field is smaller than that of white), the examiner brings the pin from the periphery inwards at a 45° angle. Upper and lower temporal and nasal field quadrants are all tested in turn. The blind spot is also mapped out. An enlarged blind spot indicates papilloedema.

Any defect is recorded as a hemianopia if it involves half a field, or as a quadrantanopia if it involves a quarter of a field. Homonymous refers to a defect in corresponding sections, e.g. the temporal field on the right and the nasal field on the left (Fig. 9.4). A scotoma is a discrete area of visual field loss. Figure 9.4 demonstrates the visual defects

Table 9.5	Pupil abnormalities
Abnormality	**Cause**
Small pupils	
Bilateral small and irregular	Argyll Robertson pupil due to syphilis and diabetes
Bilateral pinpoint	Drugs (morphine) or pontine lesion
Unilateral small	Horner's syndrome if accompanied by partial ptosis, enophthalmos and impaired facial sweating
Large pupils	
Unilateral dilated	Holmes–Adie pupil, unreactive to light but slowly reactive to accommodation. May be associated with depressed ankle jerks
Unilateral dilated and deviated down and out	IIIrd nerve lesion. No reaction to light or accommodation and associated with ptosis and impaired eye movements
Loss of direct light reflex	Optic nerve lesion (optic neuritis, retro-orbital tumour)

that result as a consequence of lesions at different points in the visual pathway.

Colour vision

Colour vision is tested by Ishihara charts (dots of various colours form numbers within a page of many dots). Red colour desaturation is an early sign of optic nerve

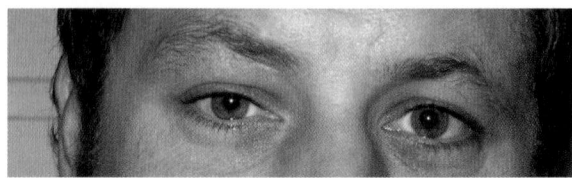

Fig. 9.3 Right Horner's syndrome. Note the right-sided ptosis, enophthalmos and meiosis.

Table 9.4	Causes of a Horner's syndrome

Brainstem
  Demyelination
  Tumour
  Infarction (lateral medullary syndrome)

Cervical cord and T1 root lesion
  Syringomyelia
  Cervical rib
  Bronchial carcinoma

Neck
  Neck surgery
  Carotid artery dissection

Miscellaneous
  Cluster headache

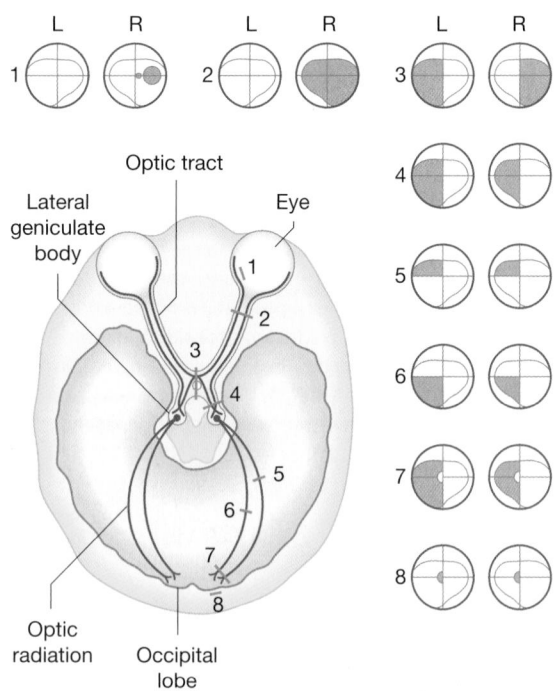

Fig. 9.4 The main figure depicts the visual pathway. Visual defects associated with lesions at each part of the pathway are shown.

pathology. Colour blindness is an X-linked recessive disorder.

Fundoscopy

Fundoscopy is an important aspect of the neurological examination. Signs of diabetes and hypertension may be noted, suggesting the underlying pathology. In addition, abnormalities such as retinal pigmentation (retinitis pigmentosus) and subhyaloid haemorrhages (seen in subarachnoid haemorrhage) may be detected. Optic nerve pathology can result in papilloedema (oedema of the optic disc resulting in absent venous pulsation, swelling of the disc and blurring of the disc margins) or optic atrophy (pallor of the optic disc). The causes are presented in Tables 9.6 and 9.7 respectively.

III, IV and VI. Oculomotor, trochlear and abducens nerves

These cranial nerves supply the external eye muscles. They are almost exclusively motor nerves but the oculomotor

Table 9.6	Causes of papilloedema

Raised intracranial pressure
   Idiopathic intracranial pressure
   Cerebral tumour
   Venous sinus thrombosis

Hypertension

Optic nerve inflammation/infiltration
   Optic neuritis
   Optic nerve tumour

Retinal venous occlusion
   Central retinal vein occlusion
   Cavernous sinus thrombosis

Miscellaneous
   Hypercapnia
   Hypocalcaemia
   Guillain–Barré syndrome
   Hypervitaminosis A

Table 9.7	Causes of optic atrophy

Optic neuritis

Long-standing papilloedema

Ischaemia (ischaemic optic atrophy)

Optic nerve compression
   Frontal lobe tumour
   Pituitary tumour

Toxins
   Tobacco
   Quinine

Degenerative disorders
   Leber's optic atrophy
   Friedreich's ataxia

B_{12} deficiency

nerve is also responsible for the parasympathetic supply of the eye. The IIIrd nerve supplies all the external eye muscles except for the superior oblique (IVth) and the lateral rectus muscles (VIth). With the IVth nerve it is situated in the midbrain. The VIth nerve is situated in the pons. All three nerves pass through the cavernous sinus and through the superior orbital fissure into the orbit.

The eyes are first inspected. Pupil size and any ptosis are noted. Eye movements are then assessed by asking patients to keep their head still but follow the examiner's finger with their eyes. They are asked to report if double vision is experienced. The examiner's finger is then moved in a horizontal plane and in a vertical plane at extremes of gaze and in the midline position. Conjugate gaze is therefore tested. Range of eye movement and nystagmus is observed. If the patient experiences diplopia, the direction in which it is maximal is asked for.

A lesion of the oculomotor nerve results in ptosis, a deviated eye which looks down and out, and a dilated pupil unreactive to light and accommodation (Fig. 9.5). The causes include diabetes (pupil often spared), posterior communicating artery aneurysm and a midbrain stroke (with contralateral hemiplegia).

An isolated trochlear nerve lesion is rare. Diplopia is experienced during walking down a flight of stairs or reading. The head may be tilted to compensate. The causes include diabetes and head injuries.

Due to its long course, damage to the abducens nerve is common. It may occur due to raised intracranial pressure causing compression of the nerve against the petrous temporal bone. This incorrectly localizes the lesion to the pons (a false localizing sign). There is an inability to abduct the eye, and diplopia is experienced looking laterally on the side of the lesion. Causes of a VIth nerve lesion include raised intracranial pressure, head injury, diabetes and demyelination.

Lesions of all three nerves may result from cavernous sinus pathology (cavernous sinus thrombosis, pituitary adenoma or internal carotid artery aneurysm) or a superior orbital fissure lesion (meningioma).

Abnormalities of lateral gaze

Lateral gaze may be impaired due to a frontal lobe lesion. If the lesion is due to a stroke or tumour (a destructive lesion) the eyes will be deviated to the side of the lesion. However, if the lesion is due to seizure activity (an irritative lesion) the eyes will deviate away from the abnormal side.

A lesion of the medial longitudinal fasciculus results in failure of adduction of the ipsilateral eye and nystagmus of the contralateral abducting eye. This is called an internuclear ophthalmoplegia (INO) and may be due to demyelination or brainstem infarction or tumour.

'Doll's eye' movements are absent in brainstem lesions. Conjugate eye movements can be tested in the unconscious patient by moving the head from side to side. The eyes should not move with the head but if they do there is said to be an absence of doll's eye movements. This is one of the tests of brainstem function.

Applied basic sciences of the nervous system

Symptoms of neurological disease

Examination of the nervous system

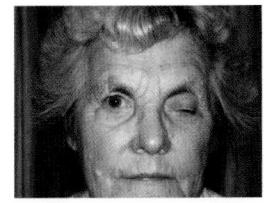
(a)

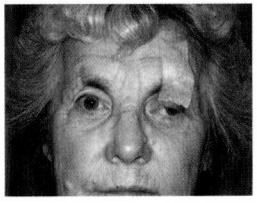
(b)

Fig. 9.5a, b Left III(rd) nerve palsy. Note the left ptosis and an eye that is deviated down and out.

Abnormalities of upward gaze

These may be due to a midbrain lesion, e.g. pineal tumour. Parinaud's syndrome is a combination of failed upgaze with an absent light reflex. However, impaired upgaze is also seen in progressive supranuclear gaze palsy.

V. Trigeminal nerve

The Vth cranial nerve has motor, sensory and reflex components. It is the largest cranial nerve and the motor nucleus is situated in the pons. The sensory fibres arise from three divisions: the ophthalmic (V_1), maxillary (V_2) and mandibular (V_3). V_1 runs with the IIIrd, IVth and VIth nerves through the cavernous sinus and superior orbital fissure. The cranial exits for V_2 and V_3 are the foramen rotundum and foramen ovale respectively.

The motor component is tested by asking the patient to clench the teeth and feeling the masseter muscle bulk. The patient is then asked to open the jaw against resistance. If weak, the jaw will deviate towards the side of the lesion.

The sensory component is tested by assessing pain (pinprick) and light touch (cotton wool testing) in all three divisions (forehead, cheek and chin).

The corneal response is assessed by gently touching the cornea with a wisp of cotton wool. The patient should blink briskly. It should be done from the side so as to avoid a blink response to the visual threat. The absence of the corneal response is an early indicator of a lesion of the first division of the trigeminal nerve.

The jaw jerk is assessed by the examiner placing his or her finger or thumb on the patient's chin. The patient is asked to slightly open the mouth, and the overlying finger or thumb is then gently tapped with a tendon hammer. A brisk jerk is a sign of a bilateral upper motor neurone lesion above the level of the pons (e.g. motor neurone disease, multiple sclerosis).

The causes of a Vth nerve lesion are listed in Table 9.8.

VII. Facial nerve

The facial nerve has sensory, motor and parasympathetic components. The VIIth nucleus is situated in the pons, where it receives fibres from both cerebral hemispheres. The facial nerve crosses the cerebello-pontine angle and with the VIIIth nerve passes through the facial canal in the petrous temporal bone. It gives off branches—the greater petrosal nerve, the nerve to the stapedius and the chorda tympani (taste to anterior two thirds of tongue) nerve—

and then leaves through the stylomastoid foramen. It enters the substance of the parotid gland and then divides into five terminal branches.

The face is first inspected for signs of asymmetry. The patient is then asked to raise the eyebrows, close the eyes tight shut, blow out the cheeks and then show the teeth (do not ask the patient to smile as this is an emotional response and may be preserved in upper motor neurone lesions). An upper motor neurone lesion causes sparing of the upper facial muscles; however, the nasolabial fold is flattened, the corner of the mouth will droop and saliva may drool.

A lower motor neurone lesion causes unilateral facial weakness; therefore, in addition to the above findings, forehead wrinkles are lost, there is incomplete eye closure and Bell's phenomenon may be seen (on attempted eye closure the eye rolls up, but since eye closure is incomplete the white of the eye is seen, Fig. 9.6b). Taste is also impaired and hyperacusis may be noticed. The causes of a VIIth nerve lesion and bilateral facial weakness are listed in Tables 9.9 and 9.10 respectively.

VIII. Vestibulocochlear nerve

The vestibulocochlear nerve has two components, the cochlear and the vestibular nerves. The cochlear nerve arises from the spiral organ of Corti in the cochlea. The vestibular fibres arise from the three semicircular canals, the utricle and saccule. Both components pass to the nucleus in the pons via the internal acoustic meatus.

Cochlear nerve

Patients should be asked about hearing impairment, and an estimate of hearing loss is gained by whispering

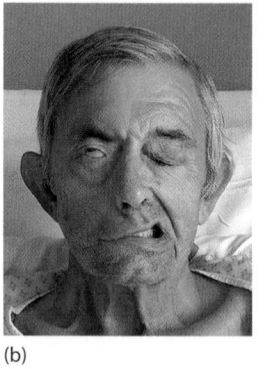

(a)

(b)

Fig. 9.6a, b Right VIIth nerve palsy. (a) Note the drooping right lip. (b) When the patient attempts to shut his eye and show his teeth, the eye rolls up (Bell's sign), and the asymmetry in lip raising is evident.

Table 9.8	Causes of a Vth nerve lesion

Pons
  Demyelination
  Infarction
  Tumour

Cerebellar pontine angle (often with VIIth and VIIIth nerve)
  Acoustic neuroma
  Meningioma
  Cavernous sinus lesion (V_1 with IIIrd, IVth and VIth nerve involvement)

Table 9.9	Causes of a VIIth nerve lesion

Upper motor neurone lesions

Infarction

Haemorrhage

Tumour

Demyelination

Lower motor neurone lesions

Pons
  Infarction
  Tumour
  Demyelination

Cerebello-pontine angle
  Acoustic neuroma
  Meningioma

Facial canal (in addition, taste impairment and hyperacusis)
  Bell's palsy (most common)
  Herpes zoster
  Skull base tumour
  Paget's disease
  Middle ear infection

Parotid
  Tumour
  Mumps
  Sarcoidosis

Applied basic sciences
of the nervous system

Symptoms of
neurological disease

**Examination of the
nervous system**

Table 9.10   Causes of bilateral facial weakness

Guillain–Barré syndrome
Sarcoidosis
Lyme disease
Myasthenia gravis
Motor neurone disease

Myopathies
   Myotonic dystrophy
   Facio-scapulo-humeral dystrophy

Table 9.11   Causes of hearing loss

Conductive
Ear wax
Glue ear (serous otitis media)
Otosclerosis
Sensorineural

Internal ear
   Drugs (gentamicin, aspirin)
   Infection (mumps, syphilis, rubella)
   Ménière's disease

Cochlear nerve
   Presbyacusis
   Cerebello-pontine angle lesion
   Paget's disease
   Meningitis
   Sarcoidosis

numbers into each ear. A tuning fork (256 or 512 Hz) test of hearing is performed if there is suspicion of hearing loss.

Firstly Rinne's test is performed. A tuning fork is struck and placed behind and then beside the ear on the mastoid process. Air conduction (AC) should be louder than bone conduction (BC) and this is termed Rinne's positive. Weber's test is then performed. The tuning fork is struck and placed in the middle of the forehead. The patient is asked where it is heard loudest. It should normally be heard in the midline. If the patient has sensorineural deafness, AC is greater than BC but during Weber's test the sound is heard loudest on the unaffected side. If BC is greater than AC, the patient is said to have conductive deafness. During Weber's test the sound will be localized to the affected side. Formal testing of hearing is performed by audiometry. The causes of hearing loss are listed in Table 9.11.

Vestibular nerve

Disturbance of vestibular function results in vertigo. This is the sensation of rotation of self or the environment and is often associated with nausea and vomiting. It may be accompanied by nystagmus (observed on earlier testing when assessing eye movements). Nystagmus is a rhythmical involuntary movement of the eyes. A vestibular lesion may be central (brainstem and cerebellar connections) or peripheral (labyrinthine). The nystagmus is usually hori-

zontal, though it may also be rotatory in labyrinthine disorders. It is described as jerk nystagmus, which has a fast and slow phase. On lateral gaze the eye drifts back to the midline position but then is jerked back rapidly to the direction of the attempted gaze. The direction of the nystagmus is said to be that of the fast phase, and nystagmus is often more marked by gaze in that direction. In labyrinthine disorders the fast phase is away from the side of the lesion, whereas in disorders of the cerebellum it is to the side of the lesion. Nystagmus can also occur in lesions of the foramen magnum, resulting in downbeat nystagmus. The causes of nystagmus are listed in Table 9.12.

Vertigo can be further assessed by the Hallpike manoeuvre. From a sitting position the patient is lowered to a lying position, with the head turned to one side and below the horizontal plane of the bed or couch. The eyes are examined (for 30 seconds) for the presence of nystagmus. The patient is returned to sitting and the test is repeated in the opposite direction. If there is a labyrinth or vestibular connection disorder, rotatory nystagmus will be seen—this is a positive test.

IX, X. Glossopharyngeal and vagus nerves

These nerves are examined together. The glossopharyngeal nerve is mostly sensory, whereas the vagus nerve is mainly motor. The nuclei are located in the medulla and the cranial exit is the jugular foramen.

The patient is asked to open the mouth and say 'aah'. Movement of the soft palate and uvula is observed. Asymmetry of the soft palate and deviation of the uvula away from the lesion indicates a Xth nerve lesion. Pharyngeal sensation is tested. Reduced sensation indicates a IXth nerve lesion. The gag reflex (touching the pharynx or base of the tonsillar fossa with an orange stick) comprises an afferent limb (IXth) and an efferent limb (Xth).

Disorders of the IXth and Xth nerves result in dysphagia and dysphonia. A hoarse voice is suggestive of recurrent laryngeal nerve palsy (a branch of the Xth nerve) and nasal speech is suggestive of a Xth nerve palsy. Palatal weakness is also suggested if there is nasal regurgitation of fluids. The causes of IXth and Xth nerve weakness are listed in Table 9.13 and the causes of laryngeal nerve palsy are listed in Table 9.14.

Table 9.12   Causes of nystagmus

Brainstem
   Wernicke's encephalopathy
   Demyelination
   Infarction
   Drugs (phenytoin)

Cerebellum
   Demyelination
   Tumour
   Infarction

Labyrinthine
   Ménière's disease
   Vestibular neuronitis
   Benign paroxysmal positional vertigo (BPPV)

579

Table 9.13	Causes of ninth and tenth nerve weakness
Bilateral stroke	
Motor neurone disease	
Brainstem infarction (lateral medullary syndrome)	
Polyneuritis cranialis (variant of Guillain–Barré syndrome)	
Diphtheria	
Jugular foramen lesion (carcinoma of nasopharynx, glomus tumour)	

Table 9.14	Causes of recurrent laryngeal nerve palsy
Mediastinal tumour (thymoma)	
Bronchial carcinoma	
Aortic arch aneurysm	
Neck trauma or surgery	

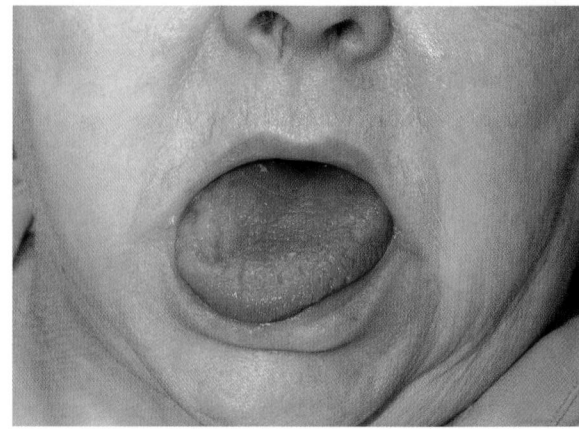

Fig. 9.7 Right hypoglossal XIIth nerve palsy. Note the tongue deviated to the right (side of the lesion) with atrophy of the right side of the tongue.

XI. Accessory nerve

This is a motor nerve that has a spinal and a cranial component. The nucleus is located in the medulla and the cranial exit is the jugular foramen.

The accessory nerve is tested by examining the trapezius and sternomastoid muscles. Asking the patient to shrug the shoulders against resistance tests the trapezius muscle. The sternomastoid is tested by asking the patient to turn the head whilst applying resistance to the chin, and the opposite sternomastoid muscle bulk is assessed. Isolated XIth nerve lesions are rare and can be due to jugular foramen lesions and neck trauma or surgery.

XII. Hypoglossal nerve

The hypoglossal nerve is a motor nerve. The nucleus is in the medulla and the hypoglossal canal is the cranial exit.

Hypoglossal nerve function is assessed by examination of the tongue. A lower motor neurone lesion is associated with atrophy and fasciculations. A bilateral upper motor neurone lesion results in a small, conical tongue that is slow to move. The patient is asked to protrude the tongue and then move it from side to side. The tongue is then retracted and strength tested by asking the patient to press the tongue into the side of each cheek. If there is a lesion of the hypoglossal nerve the tongue deviates towards the side of the lesion (Fig. 9.7). The causes of tongue weakness are listed in Table 9.15.

Upper and lower limb examination

Examination of the limbs comprises assessment of tone, reflexes, motor function, sensation and coordination. The examination begins with inspection looking for muscle wasting, scars, fasciculations or abnormal posture.

Tone

Tone is examined by means of passive limb movements. Increased tone may be due to an upper motor neurone

lesion. This is termed 'clasp-knife rigidity' as it is initially difficult to overcome then suddenly the tone reduces. Increased tone may also be due to an extrapyramidal lesion. This is termed 'lead-pipe rigidity' as the increased tone is uniform throughout. Decreased tone is produced by a lower motor neurone or spinal shock. Clonus is tested for in the lower limb at the knee or ankle. It is a rhythmical involuntary contraction of a muscle placed under tension, and pathological clonus (sustained) indicates an upper motor neurone lesion.

Reflexes

Reflexes (Table 9.16) are tested with a tendon hammer. The patient should be relaxed and in a comfortable position. Increased reflexes indicate an upper motor neurone lesion. Absent reflexes indicate a lower motor neurone lesion. Before reflexes are documented as absent, reinforcement should be employed. This is achieved by asking the patient to relax and then clench the jaw as the reflex is tested. In the lower limb the same is achieved by asking the patient to clench the hands together tightly. Abdominal reflexes are obtained by gently scratching each quadrant of the abdomen in a diagonal fashion with an orange stick. The underlying muscle should contract unless

Table 9.15	Causes of tongue weakness

Bilateral upper motor neurone XIIth nerve lesion
    Motor neurone disease
    Bilateral strokes	

Unilateral lower motor neurone XIIth nerve lesion
    Skull base tumour
    Neck trauma or surgery	

Bilateral lower motor neurone XIIth nerve lesion
    Motor neurone disease
    Syringobulbia	

Myasthenia gravis	

Table 9.16	Reflexes
Tendon jerk	**Root value**
Ankle	S1/2
Knee	L3/4
Abdominal	T8–12
Biceps	C5/6
Supinator	C6
Triceps	C7/8

there is an upper motor neurone lesion. This reflex may also be absent in the elderly or in multiparous women. The plantar reflex is obtained by drawing an orange stick along the lateral border of the foot from the heel to the little toe, then over to the big toe. A normal response is plantarflexion of the big toe. A pathological response is extension of the big toe. This signifies an upper motor neurone lesion, though bilateral extensor responses may be seen after a seizure.

Motor function
Motor function is first tested by asking the patient to extend both arms forward and then close the eyes. If the arm drifts downwards this indicates weakness of that limb. Lower limb motor function is tested by asking the patient to lift each leg separately off the bed, watching for downward drift. Each muscle group is then tested individually, e.g. shoulder abduction and adduction, elbow flexion and extension. Power is graded on a scale of 0–5 (Table 9.17), and the motor root values are listed in Table 9.18.

Sensation
Sensation requires testing of five separate components: pain (by pinprick), temperature (with hot and cold water-filled test tubes), light touch (by cotton wool), vibration (with a 128 Hz tuning fork) and proprioception (by assessing fine movements of the toes and fingers).

Sensation should be tested by dermatome (Fig. 9.8) and also distally from the feet and hands upwards as this will reveal glove and stocking sensory loss (seen in

peripheral neuropathy). It is important when assessing joint position sense (proprioception) that the sides of the finger or toe are held and small movements are made. This ensures that the sensory modality of light touch is not employed.

Coordination
Coordination is assessed in the upper limb by asking the patient to touch their nose then the examiner's extended finger (finger–nose pointing) and also by rapid alternating hand movements (dysdiadochokinesis is slow and uncoordinated alternating hand movements). In the lower limb the patient is asked to place the ankle on the contralateral knee, slide it down the leg and then return it to the knee (heel–shin testing). If the leg is weak, coordination may be tested by asking the patient to tap the foot in time. Tandem walking (heel–toe walking) also tests lower limb coordination.

Assessing gait and performing the Romberg's test completes the examination of the limbs. Romberg's test assesses proprioception. Patients are asked to stand still with feet together. Once steady, they are asked to close their eyes. If they fall, Romberg's test is positive.

Speech
This is examined by asking the patient some simple questions. The quality of speech is observed. Mild dysarthria is made more pronounced by asking the patient to repeat 'West Register Street' and 'baby hippopotamus'. Cerebellar speech is often described as 'staccato' or 'scanning' whereas pseudobulbar speech is described as 'hot potato'. The causes of dysarthria are listed in Table 9.19.

Dysphonia occurs in lesions of the recurrent laryngeal nerve, in vocal cord lesions and in Parkinsonism.

Table 9.17	Medical Research Council scale for muscle power	
Normal power		5
Movement weaker than normal but possible against resistance		4
Movement not possible against resistance but possible against gravity		3
Movement not possible against gravity		2
Visible contraction but no movement		1
No active contraction		0

Table 9.18	Motor root values
Shoulder	
Abduction	C5/6
Adduction	C6/7/8
Elbow	
Flexion	C5/6
Extension	C7/8
Wrist	
Flexion	C6/7/8
Extension	C7/8
Finger	
Flexion	C8
Extension	C7
Abduction	T1
Hip	
Flexion	L1/2/3
Extension	L5, S1
Knee	
Flexion	L5, S1/2
Extension	L3/4
Ankle	
Dorsiflexion	L4/L5
Plantarflexion	S1/2

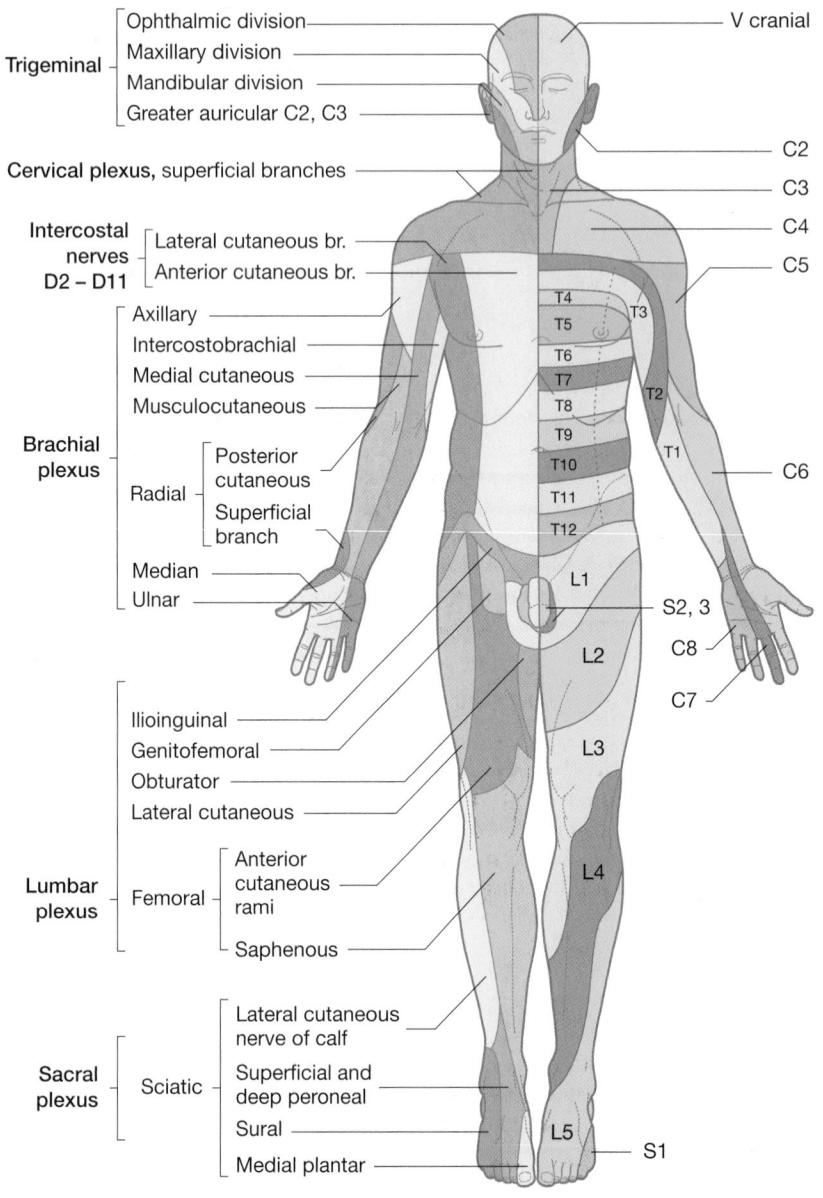

Fig. 9.8 The chart illustrates the approximate sensory distributions of the dermatomes and individual nerves.

If no meaningful responses are made the patient may have an expressive or receptive dysphasia. To distinguish between them, ask the patient to follow a command ('close your eyes'). A patient with expressive dysphasia will be able to do this. Two- or three-stage commands should also be assessed for to detect more subtle abnormalities. Nominal dysphasia is tested by asking the patient to name objects (ring, glasses, pen) and parts of an object (watch winder, watch-face, watch-

strap). Finally the patient should be asked to read to assess for dyslexia, and to write a sentence to assess for dysgraphia.

Cognition

This is covered in more depth in the section on disorders of consciousness (p. 590). Part of the assessment of cognition, however, is the mini-mental state examination listed in Table 9.20.

Table 9.19	Causes of dysarthria

Pseudobulbar palsy
   Motor neurone disease
   Bilateral strokes
   Demyelination

Bulbar palsy
   Motor neurone disease
   Syringobulbia
   Poliomyelitis
   Guillain–Barré syndrome

Cerebellar lesions
   Infarction
   Tumour
   Demyelination
   Toxins (alcohol)

Extrapyramidal
   Parkinsonism

Facial myopathy
   Myasthenia gravis
   Myotonic dystrophy

Oral lesions
   Ill-fitting dentures

Table 9.20	Mini-mental state examination

Orientation

Year	Score 5 points
Month	
Day	
Date	
Season (1 point for each correct answer)	

Country	Score 5 points
County	
Town	
Hospital	
Ward (1 point for each correct answer)	

Registration

| Name three objects (hat, cup, ball) and ask to repeat (1 point for each correct answer) | Score 3 points |

Attention

| Subtract 7 from 100 five times down to 65 *or* Spell WORLD backwards (1 point for each correct answer) | Score 5 points |

Recall

| Ask the patient to recall the three objects from previously (1 point for each correct answer) | Score 3 points |

Language

Name two objects pointed to (1 point for each correct answer)	Score 2 points
Repeat 'No ifs, ands or buts'	Score 1 point
Perform a three stage command, e.g. 'take this piece of paper, fold it in two and place it on your lap' (1 point for each correct command performed)	Score 3 points
Follow a written command ('close your eyes')	Score 1 point
Write a sentence (this must contain a subject and verb and be meaningful)	Score 1 point

Visuospatial

| Copy intersecting pentagons (draw this first for the patient) | Score 1 point |
| | Total score/30 |

Applied basic sciences of the nervous system

Symptoms of neurological disease

Examination of the nervous system

Investigations for nervous system disease

Diagnostic imaging

Computed tomography (CT)

CT is advantageous in that it is readily available and a rapid form of brain imaging. It is excellent at detecting haemorrhage and calcification, both of which are seen as hyperdense areas on CT. Cerebral infarction is detected as a hypodense area but may be isodense with brain within the first 24 hours. The sensitivity of CT can be improved by using an iodine-based contrast agent. Abscesses and tumours enhance following intravenous injection with contrast.

Magnetic resonance imaging (MRI)

MRI examination allows excellent definition of central nervous system structures (brain and spinal cord). It is far more sensitive than CT though it is not the ideal imaging tool to detect early intracranial haemorrhage. It is more time consuming than CT and patients may suffer from claustrophobia during the procedure. The images obtained however are highly detailed and brain stem and posterior fossa anatomy is far better demonstrated than on CT. Examination of both arterial supply and venous drainage of the brain is also possible (MRA and MRV) allowing diagnosis of aneurysms, artery dissections and venous sinus thrombosis.

Angiography

Imaging the vascular anatomy can be obtained by angiography. This is currently the gold standard for assessing the arterial circulation though there is a small risk of stroke attached to this invasive procedure.

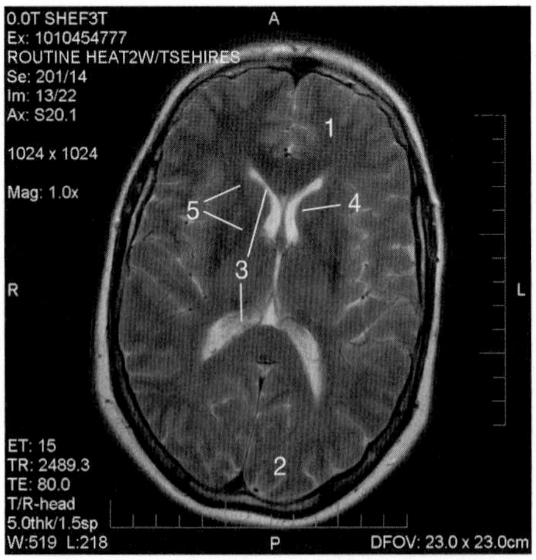

Neurophysiology

Electroencephalography (EEG)

EEG assesses cerebral function by recording the electrical potential of the brain through a large number of electrodes attached to the scalp (Fig. 9.10). It is useful in the investigation of epilepsy.

Alpha rhythms can normally be seen in healthy individuals. Abnormal rhythmic activity such as delta waves can be seen with intracranial tumours.

Spikes, spike–wave complexes or sharp waves may be detected between seizures (interictal), though an EEG recording during seizure activity has more diagnostic value. Hyperventilation, photic stimulation, sleep or sleep deprivation may induce abnormalities that were previously undetected during the interictal EEG. Ambulatory EEG with video monitoring can record for 24 hours or longer and is useful if patients are experiencing frequent attacks of an uncertain nature.

EEG is also of benefit in encephalitis and may have a characteristic pattern, especially in herpes simplex encephalitis. Characteristic patterns are also seen in Creutzfeldt–Jakob disease. The EEG can also be used both diagnostically and prognostically in coma.

Electromyography (EMG)

This is used for the investigation of disease of the muscle, neuromuscular junction, plexus, nerve root and anterior horn cells. A needle is inserted into a muscle and a recording is taken at rest and during contraction (Fig. 9.11).

The EMG can differentiate between denervated (due to disease of the supplying nerve, producing high amplitude long-duration potentials) and myopathic muscle (intrinsic muscle disorder producing small-amplitude, short-duration potentials). Single fibre EMG is a more sensitive test to examine for 'jitter', revealing a disorder of the neuromuscular junction.

Nerve conduction studies

During nerve conduction studies the nerve is stimulated and the response of the muscle it supplies is recorded. The motor velocity and the compound muscle action potential are measured. The former is decreased in demyelination, whereas the latter is decreased in both demyelination and axonal degeneration. Nerve conduction studies are useful for diagnosing conditions such as carpal tunnel syndrome

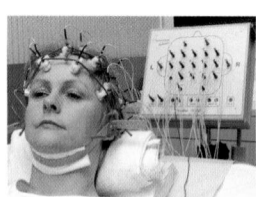

Fig. 9.10 An EEG being recorded.
Courtesy of the Neurophysiology Department, Royal Hallamshire Hospital, Sheffield, UK.

Fig. 9.9 A normal axial, T2 weighted MRI of the head. 1, Frontal lobe; 2, occipital lobe; 3, lateral ventricles; 4, head of caudate nucleus; 5, internal capsule.
Courtesy of Mr John Wattam, Royal Hallamshire Hospital, Sheffield, UK.

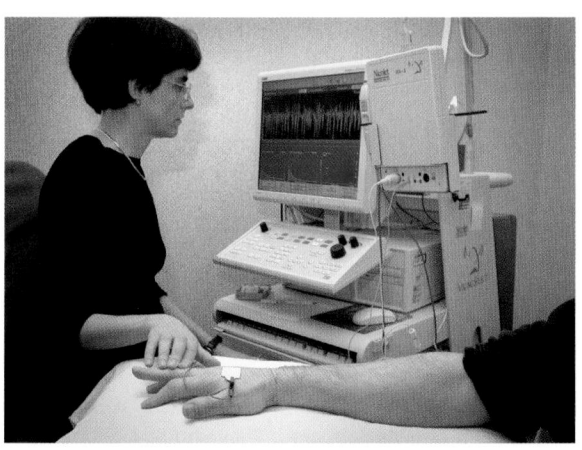

Fig. 9.11 A patient undergoing EMG. Note the needle inserted in the forearm.
Courtesy of the Neurophysiology Department, Royal Hallamshire Hospital, Sheffield, UK.

and Guillain–Barré syndrome. Sensory action potentials are recorded by applying an electrical stimulation distally (e.g. the index finger) and measuring the response more proximally (e.g. the wrist). This technique can aid in the diagnosis of a polyneuropathy.

Visual evoked potentials (VEPs)

These are of value in the diagnosis of multiple sclerosis. A single flash of light will generate a response in the occipital cortex. The normal latency in the detection of a response (principal positive deflection) is 100 ms and a delay suggests a lesion of the optic nerve such as demyelination.

Lumbar puncture

Edrophonium (Tensilon) test

SECTION 9.3
Diagnostic procedures

Lumbar puncture

Indications
This investigation allows examination of the constituents of the cerebrospinal fluid (CSF) and measurement of the CSF pressure. It is contraindicated in the presence of a space-occupying lesion, and brain imaging should always be performed if there is focal neurology or evidence of raised intracranial pressure. Other contraindications include infection of the skin on the overlying spine and thrombocytopenia.

Patient preparation
Patients are admitted to hospital, and consent is required. Patients are positioned in a lateral position with the legs curled up against the chest and the neck flexed.

Procedure
The skin is prepared with antiseptic solution. The L3/4 or L4/5 intervertebral space is identified (the fourth lumbar spine lies level with the superior iliac crest, Fig. 9.12). Local anaesthetic (lidocaine 1–2%) is infiltrated into the skin and the targeted interspace. A spinal needle is introduced in the midline between the spinous processes of the vertebrae at the chosen interspace, perpendicular to the skin and in the direction of the umbilicus. The needle is slowly advanced until the dura mater is pierced (a 'giving' or 'popping' sensation is felt). At this point the stylet of the spinal needle is withdrawn and CSF should be observed. The CSF pressure is measured with a manometer and then CSF is collected into at least three sterile containers. A paired blood glucose sample is also obtained.

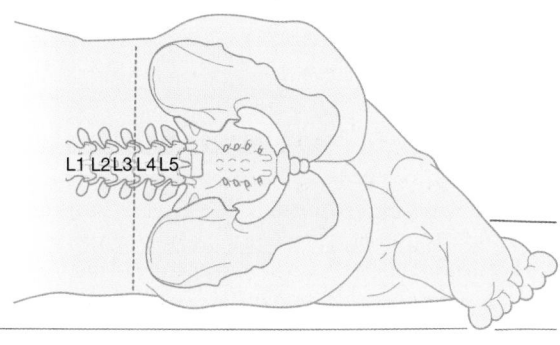

Fig. 9.12 Anatomical landmarks for a lumbar puncture. The level of the iliac crest corresponds to the 4th lumbar spine.

L1 L2 L3 L4 L5

Microscopy, culture, protein and glucose levels of the CSF are routinely performed. Additional tests are listed in Table 9.21.

The risks of this procedure include headache, which becomes worse in the upright position. This is due to low CSF pressure secondary to CSF leakage through the hole in the dura. This complication, which is typically encountered within the first 48 hours, is reduced if atraumatic and smaller gauge needles are used. Backache may also be experienced but the most serious complication is brain herniation. This may result due to the presence of raised intracranial pressure, particularly if there is a space-occupying lesion within the posterior fossa.

Post procedure care

Patients are kept lying down for an hour after the procedure, to reduce the pressure in the spinal cord and minimize a CSF leak.

Edrophonium (Tensilon) test

Edrophonium is a rapid-acting, short-duration, parenteral cholinesterase inhibitor that can be used to reverse the muscle weakness associated with myasthenia gravis and hence assist in the diagnosis of the disease.

Indications

The main indication for the edrophonium test is suspicion of myasthenia gravis.

Patient preparation

Patients should be informed about the procedure and possible side effects. The patient is placed on a cardiac monitor with resuscitation equipment and atropine (to counteract the edrophonium) available.

Procedure

Decide which muscle to assess. An independent person should dilute 10 mg edrophonium (Tensilon) with saline into 10 mL syringe. A second syringe with 10 mL saline only should also be prepared. They should be labelled A and B.

The test should be performed in a double-blind fashion, that is neither the clinician performing the test nor the patient should be aware of which syringe contains edrophonium. Patients are given 300 μg atropine intravenously to prevent muscarinic side effects.

Exactly 2 mL from syringe A is administered intravenously; if there are no adverse effects, the remainder is administered. Monitor the effects on the strength of the chosen muscle. After 5 minutes the test is repeated in the same manner with syringe B. The test is positive if there has

Table 9.21	CSF findings and possible diagnoses
Pressure (10–20 cmH$_2$O)	>20 cmH$_2$O (or >25 cmH$_2$O in obese) indicates raised intracranial pressure
Appearance (clear and colourless)	If turbid, suggests infection (bacterial meningitis) Xanthochromia (yellow discolouration) indicates a subarachnoid haemorrhage
White cell count (<5 lymphocytes)	Increased neutrophil count indicates infection (bacterial meningitis) Increased lymphocyte count may indicate viral meningitis, TB meningitis, sarcoidosis, malignancy (lymphoma), cryptococcus, encephalitis
Red cell count (0)	Raised RCC indicates either a traumatic tap as a result of the lumbar puncture or, if uniform throughout 3 collecting bottles, a subarachnoid haemorrhage
Protein (1.5–4.0 g/L)	Protein can be slightly raised in many conditions such as encephalitis and sarcoidosis but is greatly raised in spinal block, Guillain–Barré syndrome and chronic demyelinating peripheral neuropathy (CIDP)
Glucose (2.8–4.4 mmol/L, usually 2/3 blood glucose)	This is low in infection (bacterial, fungal or TB meningitis), malignant infiltration and sarcoidosis
Microscopy	May reveal bacteria in bacterial meningitis
Virology	Can detect herpes simplex virus
Ziehl–Neelsen stain	Positive in TB
TB PCR	Positive in TB
Indian ink stain	Positive in cryptococcus infection
Oligoclonal bands	If oligoclonal bands are present in the CSF but absent in the serum this indicates CNS inflammation such as multiple sclerosis
Cytology	May reveal malignant cells
ACE	Elevated in neurosarcoidosis
Protein 14-3-3 and S-100b	Abnormal in Creutzfeldt–Jakob disease

Normal values in parentheses.
ACE, angiotensin-converting enzyme; TB, tuberculosis.

been an improvement in muscle strength following injection with edrophonium.

Cholinergic effects include bradycardia, abdominal cramps, diarrhoea and syncope.

Post procedure care

The effects of edrophonium are short and last for approximately 5 minutes, after which complications are uncommon.

SECTION 9.4

Manifestations of nervous system disease

Headache

Headache is the most common neurological problem presenting to both the general practitioner and neurology outpatient clinic. In addition, it commonly presents as an acute neurological emergency. This section focuses on migraine and lists an overview of other common causes (Table 9.22).

Migraine

Migraine is a common cause of headache, characterized by paroxysmal severe headache, nausea, photophobia (dislike of light) and/or phonophobia (dislike of noise). It may or may not be associated with an aura.

Epidemiology

Migraine affects 10% of the population, and is more common in women. The age of onset is usually after puberty and before 50 years.

Pathology

The aetiology of migraine is genetic and environmental although a rare variant, familial hemiplegic migraine, has been mapped to a single gene on chromosome 19, a gene that codes for calcium channels.[1]

The mechanism for migraine aura is currently thought to be a slowly spreading wave of decreased neuronal activity across the cerebral cortex (cortical spreading depression).

Table 9.22	Common causes of headache
Cause	**Clinical features**
Migraine	Episodic, often unilateral, moderate to severe, lasts 4–72 hours, associated with nausea, photophobia or phonophobia
Tension-type headache	Daily mild–moderate headache, lasting over 4 hours, bilateral, sensation of a tight band across the head
Cluster headache	Severe, unilateral headaches, lasting 15–45 minutes. Conjunctival injection can occur and the patient often paces the room
Idiopathic intracranial hypertension	Headache with papilloedema, visual obscurations
Trigeminal neuralgia	Severe stabbing facial pain, lasts a few seconds, occurs in the trigeminal distribution
Low CSF volume headache	Persistent headache, usually after a lumbar puncture but can also occur with spontaneous CSF leak, relieved by lying down
Subarachnoid haemorrhage	Sudden-onset severe occipital headache, may be associated with loss of consciousness and coma
Brain tumour	Early morning headache, worse on waking, aggravated by coughing or straining
Giant cell arteritis	Pain over the superficial temporal artery. Usually occurs in patients over 50 years. The erythrocyte sedimentation rate is usually elevated
Meningitis	Headache associated with fever, neck stiffness and petechial skin rash
Analgesic abuse headache	Daily headache associated with the ingestion of large quantities of codeine-based products

Table 9.23	Migraine triggers
Menstruation	
Dietary factors (cheese, red wine, chocolate)	
Excessive sleep or lack of sleep	
Irregular meals	
Exercise	
Emotional stress	
Strong smells	

The headache is thought to originate from activation of meningeal and blood vessel pain receptors by the trigeminovascular system, combined with a change in central pain modulation.[2] Migraine can be precipitated by certain triggers (Table 9.23) and the frequency is often reduced during pregnancy.

Scope of disease

Ischaemic stroke is a rare complication that may occur during an attack of migraine with aura. This is one of the reasons why the oral contraceptive pill is contraindicated in patients with migraine with aura.

Clinical features

The classical migraine attack consists of four phases—premonition, aura, headache and resolution—but two types of migraine exist, migraine with aura and migraine without aura. The latter is more common, accounting for approximately 75% of cases.

The premonition phase may consist of symptoms of lethargy, yawning or hunger hours to days before the onset of the headache.

The migraine aura consists of neurological symptoms that precede or accompany the attack. Symptoms are usually visual with zigzag lines, teichopsia (glittering coloured images) or visual field defects. Sensory symp-toms include slow spreading paraesthesia up the leg, arm or face. Aphasia or, less commonly, a transient hemi-paresis may also occur. Aura symptoms usually last for 4–60 minutes before the onset of the headache and can occur on alternating sides during different attacks. Aura without headache can occur, particularly with increasing age, leading to a misdiagnosis of focal seizures or transient ischaemic attacks.

Migraine headache is moderate to severe, often unilateral and pulsating in nature. It can however spread bilaterally or be bilateral from onset. The pain is aggravated by movement and can be associated with nausea, vomiting, photophobia or phonophobia. The headache usually occurs during waking hours and can last 4–72 hours. The patient often retreats to a quiet darkened room as rest often relieves the symptoms.

During the resolution phase, patients may feel tired, irritable or listless.

The clinical features and other causes of headache are presented in Table 9.22.

Initial investigations
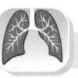

The diagnosis can often be made on history alone and further investigations are not usually required.

Further investigations
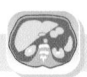

CT/MRI of the head
CT of the head or MRI of the brain is recommended to screen for structural abnormalities if new-onset migraine occurs after the age of 50 years, if there is an abnormal neurological examination, if aura is not associated with headache or if the aura is always on the same side.

Initial management

Analgesia
Simple analgesics (paracetamol, ibuprofen or high-dose aspirin 600–900 mg) with an antiemetic are effective for many patients with mild to moderate migraine.

Antiemetics
Metoclopramide or domperidone can be used. In addition to improving nausea they also increase analgesic absorption as gastric stasis often occurs during migraine.

Triptans
5-Hydroxytryptamine agonists (sumatriptan or rizatriptan) are effective agents for treating migraine, reserved for moderate to severe attacks.

Medical management

Prophylactic agents
Regular treatment, aimed at reducing the frequency of attacks, is recommended when attacks are occurring at a frequency of more than 2 per month. Beta-blockers (propranolol), low-dose amitriptyline, sodium valproate, pizotifen and methysergide are commonly prescribed agents.

Prognosis
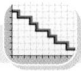

Migraine often decreases in frequency with increasing age and in pregnancy. On average a migraine sufferer can expect 2 attacks per month, although the frequency of attack are very variable.

i FURTHER INFORMATION

Headache Classification Committee. The international classification of headache disorders, 2nd edn. Cephalalgia 2004; 24(suppl 1): 8–160.

REFERENCES

(1) *Joutel A, Bousser MG, Biousse V, et al. A gene for familial hemiplegic migraine maps to chromosome 19. Nature Genetics 1993; 5: 40–45.*
(2) *Silberstein SD. Migraine. Lancet 2004; 363: 381–391.*

Chronic tension-type headache

This is a common daily headache of mild to moderate severity that occurs on more than 15 days per month, lasts more than 4 hours, and is not relieved by analgesia. It is bilateral and band-like in quality and is often described as if the patient's head is in a vice, or wearing a hat that is too tight. It is not associated with vomiting and, if present, nausea is mild. There is no photophobia or phonophobia and daily activities can be continued. It does tend to get worse as the day progresses.

Relaxation techniques and reassurance that the underlying pathology is not a brain tumour are often sufficient to treat this condition but occasionally medication (low-dose amitriptyline) is required.

Cluster headache

Cluster headaches are less common than migraine and occur more frequently in men. The patient is usually aged 20–40 years. The attacks often occur at the same time of day and occur in clusters for 1–3 months at a time. The headache is always unilateral and very severe. It lasts 15 minutes to 3 hours, occurs more commonly at night and is often focused around the eye. In addition there may be lacrimation, conjunctival injection, nasal congestion, rhinorrhoea, ptosis or miosis. A persistent Horner's syndrome can occur. During the attack the patient is restless and often paces around the room.

Acute treatment includes high-flow oxygen or subcutaneous sumatriptan. Verapamil, steroids or methysergide are used as preventative agents.

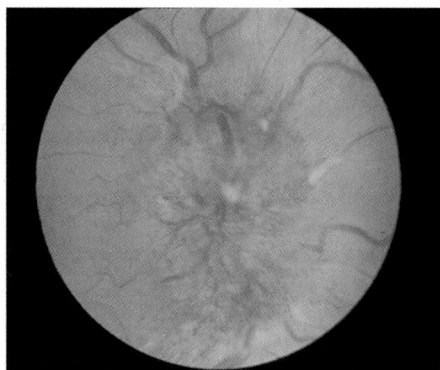

Fig. 9.13 Papilloedema.

Idiopathic intracranial headache

Idiopathic intracranial hypertension (synonyms: benign intracranial hypertension, pseudotumour cerebri) is a disorder characterized by elevated CSF pressure in the absence of a space-occupying lesion and with normal-sized ventricles.

Epidemiology

The condition tends to present in young females, particularly those with an increased body mass index.

Pathology

The cause is often not identified but known associated risk factors are pregnancy, coagulopathies, the oral contraceptive pill, tetracycline, retinoids and vitamin A poisoning.

Clinical features

Patients present with headache and papilloedema (Fig. 9.13). Nausea, visual obscurations (vision going grey, particularly on bending over), decreased visual acuity, diplopia (due to VIth nerve palsy), visual field defects or an enlarged blind spot may also be present.

Investigations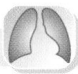

CT/MRI

It is crucial that venous sinus thrombosis is excluded (Fig. 9.14) as it presents with similar symptoms. Brain imaging with MRI and magnetic resonance venography (MRV) is therefore required.

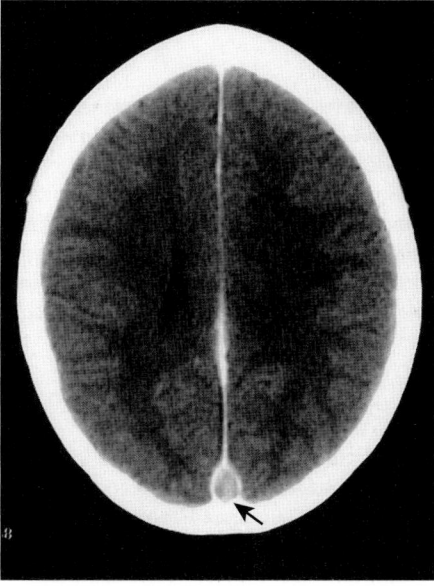

Fig. 9.14 CT scan of sagittal sinus thrombosis. There is a low-attenuating thrombus within the superior sagittal sinus (arrow), surrounded by an area of enhancement.

Headache

Migraine

Lumbar puncture

The diagnosis is confirmed with documented elevated CSF pressure. Lumbar puncture should only be performed following a normal CT or MRI scan.

Management

Treatment includes weight loss and acetazolamide (a diuretic). Severe cases may require the insertion of a ventriculo-peritoneal or lumbo-peritoneal shunt.

Prognosis

Idiopathic intracranial hypertension can lead to permanent visual loss, therefore visual fields and acuity should be closely monitored and appropriate treatment instigated.

Trigeminal neuralgia

Trigeminal neuralgia is a severely painful condition causing a brief (lasting seconds to less than 2 minutes) stabbing unilateral pain in the distribution of one or more divisions of the trigeminal nerve. It is often triggered by shaving, chewing or talking. The cause may be compression of the trigeminal nerve by blood vessels. Carbamazepine is the drug of choice, and other agents include phenytoin or gabapentin. If patients are not controlled pharmacologically, more invasive measures—injection techniques of the nerve, stereotactic radiosurgery or microvascular decompression surgery—may be tried.

SECTION 9.5   Disorders of consciousness

Consciousness is a state of awareness of self and the surrounding environment. Disorders of consciousness can be separated into disorders of arousal (coma) or disorders of cognition or the content of consciousness (dementia or delirium).

Coma

Coma is a state of unarousable unresponsiveness. This is defined as an absence of awareness of self and the environment with no evidence of arousal. The eyes are closed and there is no sleep–wake cycle.

Pathology

The ascending reticular activating system (located in the brainstem) and its connections to the cerebral cortex are responsible for the state of arousal. Lesions of the brainstem (reticular activating system) or cerebral cortex—diffuse bilateral damage or severe unilateral cerebral hemisphere damage with brain shift—can result in coma. Other causes are listed in Table 9.24 and include structural brain lesions (tumours), intracranial bleeding (subarachnoid haemorrhage) and metabolic abnormalities.

Scope of disease

Complications arising from immobility, including deep vein thrombosis, pulmonary embolism and respiratory tract infection, may occur. Prolonged coma can develop into a persistent vegetative state. This state is characterized by recovery of wakefulness but awareness of self and the surroundings remains absent. Spontaneous eye opening occurs, the sleep–wake cycle is present, there is an ability to breathe spontaneously and the circulation is stable.

Clinical features

A rapid thorough assessment of the patient is essential to ascertain both the underlying cause of the coma and to prevent further clinical deterioration. Initially assessment of general appearance is performed. Features such as cyanosis, jaundice, rash or abnormal posture should be documented. Pulse, blood pressure, temperature, respiration and oxygen saturation are checked. As well as aiding in stabilizing the patient, clues to the underlying diagnosis may be given.

The Glasgow coma scale is a scoring system used to assess the depth of coma (Table 9.25). Points are awarded for motor response, eye opening and verbal response; the best response is recorded. Coma is defined as a motor score of 4 or less, an eye opening score of 2 or less, and a verbal score of 2 or less.

Focal neurological signs such as asymmetrical reflexes, an extensor planter response, facial weakness or increased tone may be present indicating an underlying structural cause for the coma. It is important to remember that hypoglycaemia may also cause focal neurological signs. The presence of meningism (neck stiffness, Kernig's sign) may indicate subarachnoid haemorrhage or meningitis as the underlying cause.

The examination of the eyes is important. Pupil size and reactivity may reveal pinpoint pupils (pontine lesion or opiate overdose), a small pupil (Horner's syndrome) or a deviated dilated pupil (IIIrd nerve palsy). A unilateral fixed and dilated pupil may indicate raised intracranial pressure and coning (herniation of the brain). If eye movements are purposeful in an unresponsive patient, alternative diagnoses should be considered (Table 9.26). Absent doll's eye movements and absent corneal response indicate a brainstem lesion. Fundoscopy may reveal papilloedema (raised intracranial pressure) or subhyaloid haemorrhage (subarachnoid haemorrhage, Fig. 9.15).

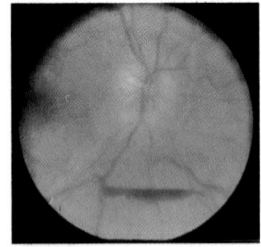

Fig. 9.15 Subhyaloid haemorrhage.

Table 9.24	Causes of coma and further investigations	
	Cause	**Investigations/clues to diagnosis**
Structural	Cerebral infarction/haemorrhage Subarachnoid haemorrhage (SAH) Tumour Hydrocephalus Cerebral abscess Subdural/extradural haematoma	CT head (± lumbar puncture for subarachnoid haemorrhage)
Metabolic	Hypoxia/hypercapnia Hypo/hypernatraemia Hypo/hyperglycaemia Hypo/hypercalcaemia Hypothyroidism Hypo/hyperthermia Hypermagnesaemia Liver/renal failure Addison's disease	Arterial blood gas Urea and electrolytes (U&Es) Random blood glucose Calcium level, ECG Thyroid function tests Temperature Magnesium level Liver function tests and U&Es Cortisol level
Infective	Meningitis Encephalitis Sepsis	Lumbar puncture Lumbar puncture Blood cultures
Toxins and drugs	Lead Cyanide Carbon monoxide Alcohol Sedatives Opiates Barbiturates	Lead levels, full blood count Almond odour, metabolic acidosis and hypoxia Pink skin colour Blood alcohol levels Urine toxicology Urine toxicology Urine toxicology
Other	Postictal Hypertensive encephalopathy Cardiac arrhythmia Hypotension	EEG ECG

Table 9.25	Glasgow coma score	
Eye opening		
Spontaneous		4
To verbal command		3
To painful stimuli		2
Nil		1
Verbal response		
Oriented		5
Confused speech		4
Inappropriate words		3
Incomprehensible sounds		2
Nil		1
Motor response		
Obeys command		6
Localizes to pain		5
Withdraws to pain		4
Abnormal flexion to pain		3
Extends to pain		2
Nil		1

Table 9.26	Differential diagnosis of coma	
Locked-in syndrome		Awareness is preserved but there is total paralysis except for eye opening and vertical eye movement. The lesion is below the IIIrd nucleus in the midbrain
Catatonia		This is usually a psychiatric condition. There are no spontaneous movements but eyes are open and unblinking. An EEG may help with the diagnosis
Pseudo-coma		Eyes are closed and resist opening. An EEG will help with diagnosis

General examination is also indicated and may reveal non-neurological causes for coma, for example liver failure.

Initial investigations

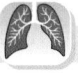

Full blood count

A raised white cell count may indicate infection. A reduced platelet count may indicate disseminated intravascular coagulation or a cause for intracerebral haemorrhage.

Urea and electrolytes
Renal failure can lead to coma.

Liver profile
Liver failure can lead to coma.

Serum calcium
Calcium abnormalities can lead to coma.

Thyroid function tests
Thyroid function abnormalities can lead to coma.

Random blood glucose
Assessment of blood glucose can be made initially with a finger prick test. Both hyperglycaemia and hypoglycaemia may cause coma.

Arterial blood gas
Hypercapnia and hypoxia can cause coma. In addition acidotic or alkalotic states can be diagnosed.

Blood and urine toxicology screen
This may reveal the underlying cause of the coma.

ECG
Abnormalities associated with coma include myocardial infarction, arrhythmia, abnormal QT interval (seen in hypo- or hypercalcaemia) and conduction block.

CT of the head
CT of the head may demonstrate a structural lesion such as tumour, haemorrhage or subdural haematoma. This is crucial, particularly when considering a lumbar puncture in a comatose patient.

Further investigations
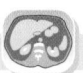

Lumbar puncture
This would be abnormal in meningitis, encephalitis and subarachnoid haemorrhage.

Blood cultures
Blood cultures should be performed in pyrexial patients to screen for septicaemia.

Cortisol level
Levels are low in Addison's disease.

EEG
EEG may reveal non-convulsive status epilepticus or encephalitis. It is also a prognostic tool for assessing coma.

Initial management

Airway, breathing and circulation
The airway should be protected and breathing and cardio-vascular status appropriately managed. Oxygen is given.

Medical management

Medical management is directed principally to the underlying cause.

Trial of naloxone
In patients with suspected opiate overdose, naloxone will rapidly reverse the effects of any opiate.

Intravenous glucose
Intravenous glucose (25–50 mL of 50% glucose) is administered to all patients with hypoglycaemia.

Prognosis

Traumatic and non-traumatic comas are considered separately with respect to prognosis. The prognosis of traumatic coma is worse with increasing age and depth of coma in the first week.

The prognosis of non-traumatic coma depends on the cause. Cerebrovascular causes of coma (stroke and subarachnoid haemorrhage) and hypoxic/ischaemic causes of coma (cardiac arrest) are associated with a worse prognosis than coma due to a metabolic cause or drug overdose. In addition the depth of coma after 6 hours and the duration of the coma are also prognostic indicators. A lower Glasgow coma score and a longer duration of coma are associated with a worse outcome. The presence of brainstem signs is also associated with a worse outcome.[1]

> ### FURTHER INFORMATION
>
> The vegetative state: guidance on diagnosis and management. A report of a working party of the Royal College of Physicians. Clinical Medicine 2003; 3: 249–254.

REFERENCE

(1) *Levy DE, Bates D, Caronna JJ, et al. Prognosis in nontraumatic coma. Annals of Internal Medicine 1981; 94: 293–301.*

Acute confusional state (delirium)

Delirium is a disorder of consciousness characterized by an acute onset and fluctuating course. There is often marked behavioural disturbance, agitation and poor attention span; patients are easily distractible. Frequently patients are disorientated to time, person and place. Thinking is disorganized and speech is often rambling.

Common causes are infection, drugs, alcohol withdrawal (delirium tremens) and metabolic disturbances. Other causes are similar to those for coma and dementia.

Dementias

Dementia

Dementia is a syndrome and not a diagnosis. It is defined as an acquired impairment of intellectual function and other cognitive skills leading to inability to perform daily activities as well as behavioural changes. Causes are listed in Table 9.27.

Epidemiology

About 5% of the population over the age of 65 and 20% after the age of 80 are estimated to have dementia. Alzheimer's disease accounts for approximately 60% of cases of dementia in Europe and North America. Vascular dementia (multi-infarct dementia) is the second most common (15%–20%).

Pathology

The aetiology of dementia remains unclear. The major pathological features in Alzheimer's disease are brain atrophy with neurofibrillary tangles, senile plaques and cerebrovascular deposition of amyloid and neuronal loss. Many of these changes may simply reflect increased deposi-

Table 9.27	Causes of dementia or neurocognitive decline

Degenerative disease

Alzheimer's disease
Dementia with Lewy bodies
Multi-system atrophy
Progressive supranuclear palsy
Huntington's disease
Frontotemporal dementia

Vascular

Multi-infarct dementia
Cerebral amyloid angiopathy

Metabolic and deficiency states

Hypoglycaemia
Hypothyroidism
B_{12}/folate deficiencies
Renal/liver failure
Hyponatraemia
Hypo/hypercalcaemia
Wilson's disease

Infective

AIDS dementia
Syphilis
Whipple's disease
Creutzfeldt–Jakob disease

Other causes

Chronic subdural haematoma
Normal pressure hydrocephalus
Chronic alcoholism

tion of amyloid due to abnormal amyloid precursor protein (APP) metabolism. Neurofibrillary tangles are formed from abnormally phosphorylated tau protein, which disrupts intracellular architecture and cell functioning. Insight into the pathogenesis has largely been derived from familial cases (less than 5% of Alzheimer's disease are autosomal dominant). Such cases are associated with mutations in three genes: amyloid precursor protein (APP), presenilin 1 and presenilin 2 and tend to present earlier, between the ages of 40 and 60. The apolipoprotein E_4 gene increases susceptibility to Alzheimer's disease and is associated with late onset sporadic disease. Furthermore mutations in the tau gene are also thought to play a role in Alzheimer's disease, as well as other neurodegenerative diseases (e.g. frontotemporal dementia).

> ### ⚡ CLINICAL ALERT
>
> *A small proportion of patients with clinical dementia have a reversible or treatable cause such as vitamin deficiency, endocrine disturbance or infection.*

Scope of disease

Alzheimer's disease is associated with increased mortality and is the fourth leading cause of death in patients over 65. Survival has increased with improved supportive care. The cause of death is usually pneumonia.

Clinical features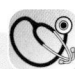

Initial assessment of dementia is aided by the relatives of the patient, who are usually the ones to notice a problem. Patients may lack recognition of their illness. Social history in relation to work performance and ability to deal with everyday family affairs is very useful.

Alzheimer's disease usually presents with mild progressive memory impairment. Language disturbance, anomia (inability to name objects) and progressive aphasia and visual-spatial impairments follow. Problems with apraxia (impaired motor activities despite intact motor function) and agnosia (impaired recognition or identification of objects despite intact sensory function) are also seen. Neuropsychiatric symptoms are common, particularly as the disease progresses. These include mood disturbances, personality change, disorders of behavior, hallucinations and delusions.

A useful bedside assessment of cognitive function is the Folstein Mini-Mental State Examination which consists of 30 questions. For subjects with more than 8 years of education, a score of 23 or less out of 30 usually indicates cognitive impairment.

Detailed neuropsychological testing can be undertaken, particularly in borderline cases or where depression may be contributing to the apparent cognitive decline (pseudo-dementia).

Coma

Acute confusional state (delirium)

Dementia

Dementia with Lewy bodies

Vascular dementia

Frontotemporal dementias

Mixed dementia

Creutzfeldt–Jakob disease

Examination in the early stages is usually normal apart from the identified cognitive deficits. In the later stages increased muscle tone can be common, extrapyramidal abnormalities may be found, myoclonic jerks may develop and primitive developmental reflexes (grasping, pouting and palmomental) may be present. Late in the disease the patient becomes mute, incontinent and bedridden with impaired swallowing. Weight loss is common at this stage.

Initial investigations

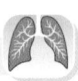

Full blood count
High mean corpuscular volume may indicate excessive alcohol intake, low vitamin B$_{12}$ or hypothyroidism: all of which can be associated with cognitive decline.

Markers of inflammation
Elevated erythrocyte sedimentation rate (ESR) may suggest an inflammatory cause such as CNS vasculitis.

Liver profile
Elevated gamma-glutamyltransferase may also indicate excessive alcohol intake, abnormal transaminases and low albumin may be seen in cirrhosis.

Calcium
Hypercalcaemia can cause confusion and cognitive impairment.

Random blood sugar
Ketoacidosis, recurrent hypoglycaemic events may cause confusion and cognitive impairment.

Syphilis serology
End stage neurosyphilis may present with dementia.

Thyroid function tests
Both hyper and hypo-thyroidism may be associated with cognitive deficits.

CT/MRI
This will exclude structural pathology such as brain tumour as the cause of cognitive decline. It will also establish other causes of dementia such as multi-infarct dementia. The pattern of brain atrophy may indicate the type of dementia for example medial temporal lobe and hippocampus in Alzheimer's or frontotemporal in frontotemporal dementia.

Further investigations

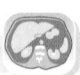

EEG
The information from an electroencephalogram is usually nonspecific but diffuse slowing may be in support of dementia as opposed to pseudodementia. Periodic complexes can be seen in prion disease (Creutzfeldt–Jacob disease). Poorly controlled epilepsy may cause cognitive decline.

Neuropsychological assessment
This is usually done over a period of several days and takes several hours to be completed. Tests specific to different parts of the brain may help in the classification of the type of dementia. Repeat assessment over a period of a year can also clarify between true dementia, pseudo-dementia and non-progressive cognitive decline due to any brain insult.

CSF examination
Normal CSF will exclude an inflammatory process and infection (such as TB or HIV, both of which can be associated with dementia). Improvement of mobility (apraxia) and cognition following draining of CSF may suggest normal pressure hydrocephalus. If CJD is suspected protein 14-3-3 and S100b should be requested.

PET/SPECT scan
This may reveal decreased perfusion or metabolism in a characteristic distribution.

Initial management

Patient and family support
The mainstay of treatment is providing supportive measures, particularly for the carers, for example offering contact with caregiver associations, giving advice regarding safety for driving and legal advice regarding enduring power of attorney.

Medical management

Acetylcholinesterase inhibitors
Acetylcholinesterase inhibitors should be limited to those patients with a Mini-Mental score of 12 or above, however, they do not have an impact on prognosis, and the clinical efficacy is small.[1] The effects need to be assessed on a 3-monthly basis.

Anti-depressants and anti-psychotics
Anti-depressants and anti-psychotics may be required for patients with disruptive features of Alzheimer's disease and other dementias. Anti-cholinergic drugs should be avoided in these circumstances as they may worsen cognitive function. Anti-psychotic drugs in general should only be used as a last resort and should be avoided in patients with dementia from Lewy body disease.

Prognosis

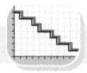

Death usually occurs 7–10 years after diagnosis with bronchopneumonia as the most common cause.

REFERENCE

(1) *Courtney C, Farrell D, Gray R, et al. Long-term donepezil treatment in 565 patients with Alzheimer's disease (AD2000): randomised double-blind trial. Lancet 2004; 363:2105–15.*

Dementia with Lewy bodies

The clinical picture is dementia with mild Parkinsonian features. Cognitive impairment is similar to that of Alzheimer's but with the addition of fluctuating cognition and early prominent visual hallucinations. These patients have marked neuroleptic sensitivity, which can be fatal.

Vascular dementia

This is not a homogeneous group. Vascular dementia can result from a single brain lesion, multiple cortical infarcts or multiple subcortical infarcts (also known as subcortical arteriosclerotic encephalopathy). The patients may have a history of transient ischaemic attacks (TIAs) or strokes and often have evidence of generalized vascular disease. Addressing the risk factors for cerebrovascular disease may be helpful in arresting or slowing progression.

Frontotemporal dementias

This is a heterogeneous group of disorders (previous names include Pick's disease) that have a strong genetic component and are characterised by focal atrophy of the frontal lobe, temporal lobe or both. Clinical features depend on the site of onset. Profound alteration in personality and social conduct with lack of insight occurs with frontal lobe involvement. Language disturbances also occur with dominant frontal lobe involvement (progressive aphasia). Loss of knowledge of words (semantic dementia) occurs with dominant temporal lobe onset.

Mixed dementia

There is increasing evidence that coexistent cerebrovascular disease increases the clinical expression and rate of cognitive decline in patients with Alzheimer's disease. Addressing the risk factors for cerebrovascular disease may be helpful in slowing progression.

Creutzfeldt–Jakob disease

Creutzfeldt–Jakob disease (CJD) is characterized by the deposition of an abnormal prion protein within the brain. It exists in four different forms: sporadic, genetic, iatrogenic and variant.

Sporadic CJD (no known cause) presents as a rare rapidly progressive dementia associated with cerebellar ataxia and early myoclonus. EEG reveals periodic sharp complexes (Fig. 9.16), and CSF protein 14-3-3 and S-100b is present in the CSF. Characteristic hyperintensities may be evident on MRI (Fig. 9.17).

Variant CJD is due to dietary exposure to bovine spongiform encephalopathy (BSE) infected beef. A total of 164 cases of definite or probable variant CJD have been reported in the UK to date. Variant CJD tends to affect a much younger age group (average age of onset 27 years) with psychiatric or behavioural symptoms followed several months later by progressive neurological symptoms (ataxia, abnormal sensations, involuntary movements). EEG is not helpful but MRI may show characteristic features.

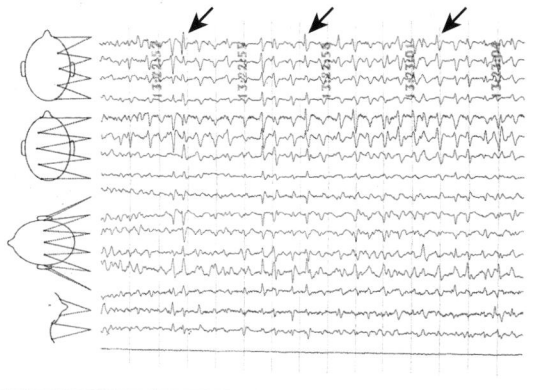

Fig. 9.16 EEG in a patient with sporadic CJD. Periodic sharp waves are seen (arrows).

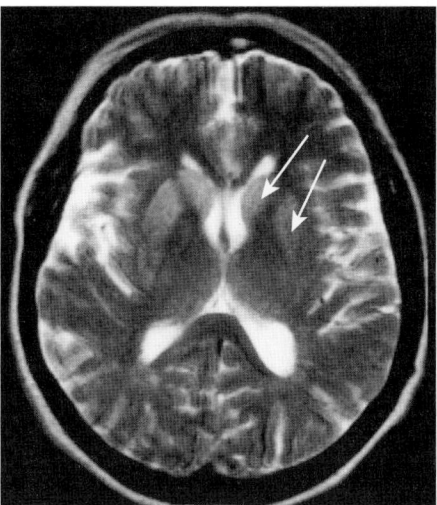

Fig. 9.17 MRI of sporadic CJD. Bilateral hyperintensities are seen in the basal ganglia (caudate and putamen).

Definite diagnosis is achieved on clinical examination supplemented by EEG, imaging and CSF examination. Brain biopsy is required if a different diagnosis (e.g. vasculitis) needs to be excluded. Post mortem is suggested to confirm the diagnosis and vCJD may be diagnosed on tonsil biopsy as the lymphoid system is involved.

There is currently no treatment. The median time to death for sporadic CJD is 4 months; for variant CJD it is 14 months.

FURTHER INFORMATION

National Creutzfeldt–Jakob Disease Surveillance Unit
www.cjd.ed.ac.uk

SECTION 9.6 — Cerebrovascular disease

Stroke

Stroke is a sudden onset of a focal neurological deficit that persists for more than 24 hours. It is defined by the World Health Organization (WHO) as rapidly developing clinical signs of focal (or global) disturbance of cerebral function, with symptoms lasting for 24 hours or longer, or leading to death, with no apparent cause other than that of vascular origin. This definition includes non-haemorrhagic stroke, intracerebral haemorrhage and subarachnoid haemorrhage (p. 603).

A transient ischaemic attack (TIA) is an acute loss of focal cerebral or monocular function with symptoms lasting less than 24 hours. It is usually ischaemic in origin.

Epidemiology

Stroke is the third most common cause of death in the Western world and a major cause of disability. It has a male preponderance and an incidence of 200 per 100 000 per year, although this rises rapidly with age.[1] Risk factors for stroke are summarized in Table 9.28.

Pathology

The pathogenesis of stroke is heterogeneous: 80% are of ischaemic origin, 10% are due to primary intracerebral haemorrhage and 10% are due to subarachnoid haemorrhage.

Ischaemia

Ischaemia and infarction result from impairment of the blood supply to the brain. Within seconds of the onset of ischaemia, the brain will not meet its metabolic demands for oxidative metabolism (glucose and oxygen). Glutamate (an excitatory neurotransmitter) is released, intracellular calcium increases and cell death ensues. Ischaemia usually results from thrombosis, for example when thrombus is superimposed on an atherosclerotic plaque (which may cause occlusion or embolize) or embolism (e.g. from a cardiac source such as atrial fibrillation). It may rarely result from low flow distal to a severely stenosed or occluded artery during a period of decreased global cerebral perfusion (e.g. secondary to reduced cardiac output).

Table 9.28	Risk factors for stroke
Increasing age	
Male sex	
Hypertension	
Smoking	
Hypercholesterolaemia	
Diabetes mellitus	
Ischaemic heart disease	
Peripheral vascular disease	

Cardiogenic
    Atrial fibrillation
    Valvular heart disease
    Left ventricular thrombus	

Coagulopathies
    Protein C and protein S deficiency
    Antithrombin III deficiency
    Anti-phospholipid antibody syndrome	

Oral contraceptive pill	

Vasculitis
    Systemic lupus erythematosus
    Rheumatoid disease
    Giant cell arteritis
    Takayasu's disease
    Behçet's disease	

Cervical artery dissection (consider if young with neck pain)	
Sickle cell disease	
Polycythaemia	
Essential thrombocytosis	
Hyperviscosity syndrome—Waldenström's disease, multiple myeloma	

Haemorrhage

By far the most common cause is systemic arterial hypertension. Intracerebral haemorrhage can also occur from rupture of a vascular malformation (arteriovenous or cavernous). Other risk factors include drug abuse with cocaine or amphetamines, anticoagulation therapy, blood dyscrasias or amyloid angiopathy. Rupture of capillaries or arterioles leads to extravasation of blood into the cerebral parenchyma.

Scope of disease

Oedema or haemorrhagic transformation can lead to clinical deterioration and death. Seizures can occur at the time of presentation (3%) or later as a consequence of the stroke (3%). Almost 45% of all stroke patients will have a degree of dysphagia, and aspiration may therefore occur. Complications of immobility may lead to deep vein thrombosis, pulmonary embolism and pressure sores. Infection (pneumonia) is a common cause of death.

Clinical features

Stroke is a clinical diagnosis. Patients usually present with a history of sudden-onset focal neurological symptoms that conform to the affected vascular territory.

Anterior circulation strokes may present with a combination of higher cortical dysfunction (dysphasia, apraxia, visuo-spatial neglect), contralateral hemiparesis, hemisensory loss or homonymous hemianopia.

Posterior circulation strokes may present with vertigo, nausea, imbalance, double vision, dysarthria or isolated homonymous hemianopia.

Symptoms of headache, meningism or decreased consciousness may indicate intracranial haemorrhage.

Examination should be systematic and include evaluation of higher cortical function (p. 571) and general examination to elicit a possible cause for the stroke. Care should be taken to assess swallowing. Loss of power may be detected in the face, arms or legs. Sensory loss occurs in a cortical distribution; reflexes are brisk with increased tone and up-going plantar responses.

Specific clinical syndromes can result from infarction of particular anatomical territories (Table 9.29).

The history and physical examination are essential to ascertain the underlying risk or precipitating factors and to evaluate the aetiology, site and severity of the stroke. Classification of the subtype of stroke according to the

Table 9.29	Clinical syndromes

Weber's syndrome

IIIrd nerve palsy with contralateral hemiplegia. This is due to infarction of the cerebral peduncle where the IIIrd nerve leaves the midbrain

Lateral medullary syndrome (Wallenberg's syndrome)

This is due to thrombosis of the posterior inferior cerebellar artery (PICA) which supplies the lateral medulla. The structures involved include the nucleus ambiguus, vestibular nucleus, inferior cerebellar peduncle, spinothalamic tract, Vth nucleus and sympathetic chain. This results in dysphagia, dysarthria, vertigo, ipsilateral ataxia, pain, temperature and sensory loss in the contralateral limb, sensory loss in the ipsilateral face, and ipsilateral Horner's syndrome respectively

Oxford Community Stroke Project (Table 9.30) is essential for management, to guide further investigations and determine prognosis.

Initial investigations

Full blood count
FBC is useful to assess for polycythaemia and thrombocytosis.

Markers of inflammation
The ESR may be raised in patients with vasculitis (especially giant cell arteritis).

Random blood sugar
It is important to exclude hypoglycaemia as it mimics stroke. Ideally, a rapid assessment of blood glucose should be made using a finger prick test. Diabetes mellitus is also a risk factor for stroke but in addition hyperglycaemia at presentation is associated with a worse prognosis.

Stroke

Traumatic intracranial haematoma

Subarachnoid haemorrhage

Table 9.30	Oxford Community Stroke Project classification*		
	Clinical features	Risk of recurrent stroke at one year	Risk of mortality at 30 days
Total anterior circulation syndrome (TACS)	Hemiparesis, hemianopia and higher cortical dysfunction, e.g. dysphasia	6%	39%
Partial anterior circulation syndrome (PACS)	Any two of hemiparesis, hemianopia or higher cortical dysfunction, e.g. dysphasia	17%	4%
	Or isolated higher cortical dysfunction alone		
Lacunar syndrome (LACS)	Pure motor stroke Pure sensory stroke Sensorimotor stroke Ataxic hemiparesis No higher cortical dysfunction and involving at least two out of three body parts (face/arm/leg).	2%	9%
Posterior circulation syndrome (POCS)	Brainstem signs or cerebellar signs or isolated hemianopia.	20%	7%

* From Bamford J, Sandercock P, Dennis M, Burn J, Warlow C. Classification and natural history of clinically identifiable subtypes of cerebral infarction. Lancet 1991; 337:1521–6.

Serum cholesterol

Hypercholesterolaemia is a risk factor for ischaemic stroke.

ECG

ECG may confirm atrial fibrillation or reveal a recent myocardial infarction.

CT of the head

In the acute setting, CT of the head is mandatory to distinguish between infarction (Fig. 9.18) and haemorrhage (Fig. 9.19) and should be performed within 48 hours of the onset of symptoms.[2] It is also useful to screen for other conditions that may mimic an infarct such as tumour or subdural haemorrhage (p. 601). However, infarcts may not be visible on a CT scan within the first 24 hours and up to 50% are never visible.

Further investigations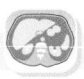

Thrombophilia screen

A thrombophilia screen is recommended for younger patients (<50 years) to assess for antithrombin III deficiency, protein C deficiency, protein S deficiency, lupus anticoagulant and anticardiolipin antibody.

Vasculitic screen

This should be performed in the younger patient or if there is a raised ESR.

Homocysteine level

If elevated, this is a risk factor for stroke and again should be performed in the young stroke patient.

Carotid duplex

This should be performed for patients with anterior circulation stroke to screen for carotid artery stenosis.

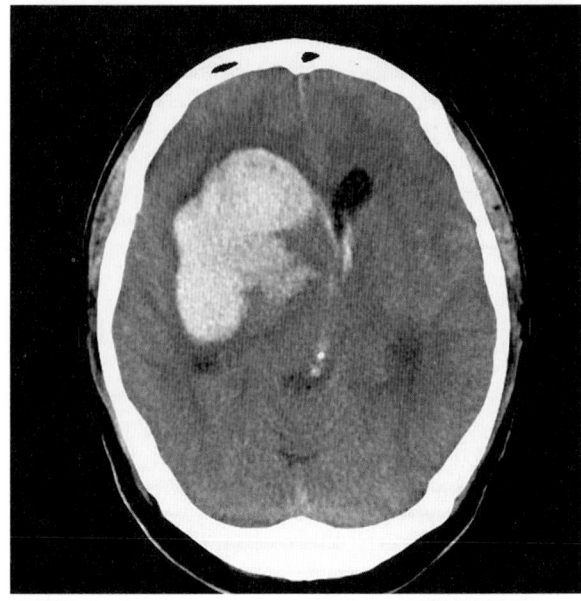

Fig. 9.19 CT scan demonstrating a right intracranial haemorrhage with midline shift.
Courtesy of Dr Stuart Coley, Royal Hallamshire Hospital, Sheffield, UK.

Echocardiogram—transthoracic/transoesophageal

This should be performed in patients less than 50 years old, in patients with multiple territory strokes, or if there is a suggestion of a heart murmur or an irregular pulse (atrial thrombus in atrial fibrillation).

MRI/MRA

MRI is an excellent imaging tool and has high sensitivity for detecting ischaemia even in the acute period. It is better than CT at defining the structures of the posterior fossa and is therefore useful in patients with features of posterior circulation or brainstem infarction. It is, however, less reliable at detecting acute haemorrhage and is time consuming and more expensive.

Magnetic resonance angiography (MRA) can assess for carotid artery stenosis and carotid or vertebral artery dissection and therefore is a less invasive alternative to angiography.

Cerebral/carotid angiogram

Angiography is performed to assess the extra- or intracranial vasculature. Cerebral angiography may be performed following an intracerebral haemorrhage when there is no obvious underlying cause and to assess for an aneurysm (p. 604) or vascular malformation (p. 603).

Carotid angiography is performed when cervical artery dissection is suspected. It is also used prior to carotid artery stenting (Fig. 9.20) and in some centres prior to carotid endarterectomy (Fig. 9.21) to further assess the degree of carotid artery stenosis.

Initial management

Swallowing

Swallowing should be formally assessed to estimate the risk of aspiration.

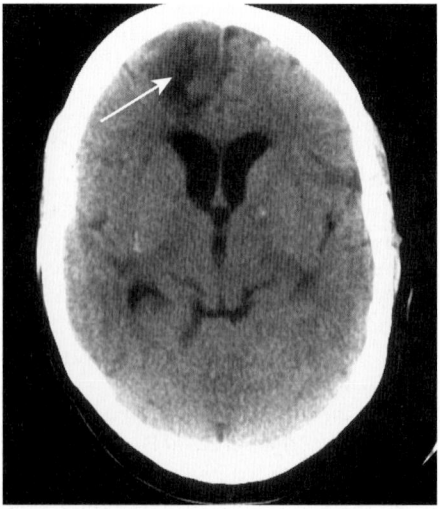

Fig. 9.18 A CT scan demonstrating a right anterior circulation infarct (arrow).

Aspirin

Aspirin 300 mg is given as soon as possible after the onset of stroke symptoms if a diagnosis of haemorrhage is considered unlikely and if thrombolytic agents (rTPA) are not being given.

Compression stockings

Compression stockings are used to prevent the complication of deep vein thrombosis.

Prevention of pressure sores

Regular turning is required to prevent pressure sores, and adequate nutrition should be maintained.

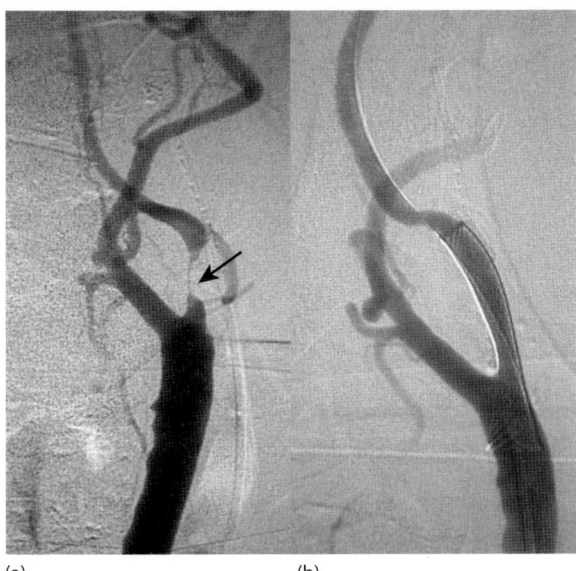

(a)   (b)

Fig. 9.20a, b Carotid artery stenting. (a) An angiogram demonstrating a 99% stenosis of the left carotid artery; (b) image of the same area after carotid angioplasty and stenting. Courtesy of Prof Peter Gaines, Sheffield Vascular Institute, Sheffield, UK.

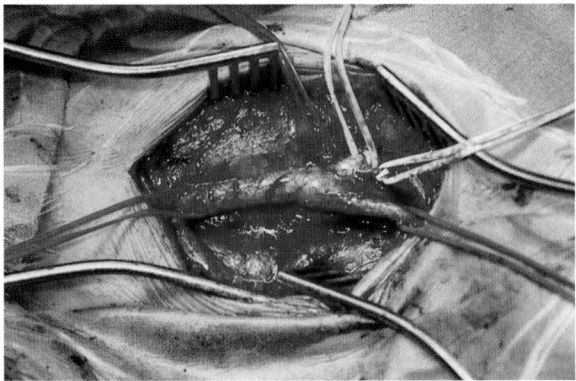

Fig. 9.21 Carotid endarterectomy. Surgical exposure to the common carotid artery.

Nutrition

Malnutrition is associated with a worse outcome. Adequate nutrition is therefore essential, especially if swallowing is impaired. Nasogastric or even percutaneous endoscopic gastrostomy (PEG) feeding may need to be considered.

Admission to a stroke unit

Admission to a stroke unit with specialized facilities for comprehensive rehabilitation results in lower morbidity and mortality, and referral to a specialist rehabilitation team is therefore recommended within 7 days of admission.

RECENT ADVANCES

Intravenous recombinant tissue plasminogen activator (rTPA) is recommended treatment within 3 hours of onset of ischaemic stroke in carefully selected patients at experienced centres. The benefit beyond 3 hours from onset of symptoms is not yet established.

Medical management

The aims of medical management are correction of any underlying risk factors and secondary prevention of further stroke.

Antiplatelet therapy

Aspirin 75 mg–150 mg in combination with dipyridamole modified release (200 mg twice daily) is recommenced for secondary prevention. In aspirin-intolerant patients clopidogrel 75 mg daily should be considered. The addition of clopidogrel to aspirin does not result in significant reduction in stroke, and is associated with increased bleeding complications.[2]

Aspirin 75 mg–150 mg in combination with dipyridamole modified release (200 mg twice daily) is recommended for secondary prevention.*

*www.nice.org.uk Vascular disease—clopidogrel and dipyridamole. May 2005

*ESPRIT study group; Halkes PH, van Gijn J, Kappelle LJ, Koudstall PJ, Algra A. Aspirin plus dipyridamole versus aspirin alone after cerebral ischaemia of arterial origin (ESPRIT): randomised controlled trial. Lancet. 2006;367: 1665–73.

Antihypertensive treatment

Blood pressure should be monitored and treated according to the British Hypertension Society guidelines (p. 70). Furthermore there is evidence that lowering blood pressure, irrespective of baseline levels of blood pressure, has beneficial effects on reducing the risk of further stroke.[3]

Anticoagulation

Anticoagulation with warfarin is recommended to decrease the risk of recurrent stroke in patients with atrial fibrillation. This should be commenced 2 weeks after the stroke in the absence of any contraindications to reduce the risk of haemorrhagic transformation.

599

Statin therapy

Statin therapy reduces the risk of further stroke irrespective of baseline cholesterol levels.[4]

Smoking cessation

Patients should be strongly advised to stop smoking.

Surgical management

Carotid endarterectomy

Carotid endarterectomy should be performed for patients with more than 70% ipsilateral carotid artery stenosis within 6 months of an anterior circulation stroke (p. 85).

Carotid artery stenting

This is an alternative to carotid endarterectomy at selected centres.

Prognosis

For patients with transient ischaemic attacks, the risk of stroke at 7 days is 8.0% and at 1 month 11.5%.[5] The outcome of stroke depends on the stroke type and age of the patient (Table 9.30). Overall stroke mortality is 19% at 1 month and 31% at 1 year though this differs for cerebral infarction (10%, 23%) and primary intracranial haemorrhage (52%, 62%).[6]

The risk of recurrence is 13% by 1 year and 4% thereafter. Of those who survive, 50–66% will be independent at 1 year.[7]

---

i FURTHER INFORMATION

Warlow CP, Dennis MS, van Gijn J, Hankey GJ, Sandercock PAG, Bamford JM, Wardlaw J. Stroke: a practical guide to management. Oxford: Blackwell Science, 2000.

REFERENCES

(1) *Bonita R. Epidemiology of stroke. Lancet 1992; 339: 342–344.*
(2) *Diener HC, Bogousslavsky J, Brass LM, et al. Aspirin and clopidogrel compared with clopidogrel alone after recent ischaemic stroke or transient ischaemic attack in high-risk patients (MATCH): Randomised, double-blind, placebo-controlled trial. Lancet 2004; 364: 331–337.*
(3) *Randomised trial of a perindopril-based blood-pressure-lowering regimen among 6,105 individuals with previous stroke or transient ischaemic attack. Lancet 2001; 358: 1033–1041.*
(4) *MRC/BHF heart protection study of cholesterol lowering with simvastatin in 20,536 high-risk individuals: A randomised placebo-controlled trial. Lancet 2002; 360: 7–22.*
(5) *Coull AJ, Lovett JK, Rothwell PM. Oxford Vascular Study. Population based study of early risk of stroke after transient ischaemic attack or minor stroke: implications for public education and organisation of services. BMJ 2004; 328: 326.*
(6) *Dennis MS, Burn JP, Sandercock PA, Bamford JM, Wade DT, Warlow CP. Long-term survival after first-ever stroke: The Oxfordshire community stroke project. Stroke 1993; 24: 796–800.*
(7) *Burn J, Dennis M, Bamford J, Sandercock P, Wade D, Warlow C. Long-term risk of recurrent stroke after a first-ever stroke. The Oxfordshire community stroke project. Stroke 1994; 25: 333–337.*

Traumatic intracranial haematoma

Traumatic intracranial haematoma is a potentially avoidable cause of death and major disability following a head injury. Haematomas are classified anatomically into extradural, subdural and intracerebral (Fig. 9.22), although it is possible for a haematoma to occupy more than one intracranial site.

Epidemiology

Acute intracranial haematomas occur in up to 5% of closed head injuries, usually as a result of road traffic accidents, falls, assaults or work-related injuries. Reflecting the patterns of activity, injuries are most common in young males and frequently involve alcohol.

Chronic subdural haematoma, however, is more common in the elderly, as cerebral atrophy contributes to the pathogenesis. Frequently there is no clear history of trauma.

Pathology

Acute intracranial haematomas

The dura is the periosteum of the inside of the skull. An extradural haematoma forms between the skull and the dura due to bone and associated blood vessel bleeding. As such, extradural haematomas are associated (at least in adults) with skull fractures. The most common site is the temporal region where the bone is thin, and where a fracture may tear the middle meningeal vessels. As the injury is essentially of the skull, there may be little or no primary brain injury.

Acute subdural haematoma generally results from severe trauma and cortical lacerations resulting in contusions of the frontal or temporal lobe. This is a more severe injury and is accompanied by primary brain damage and cerebral oedema.

As part of the primary brain injury, there may be areas of haemorrhage or contusions in the brain substance itself. These may be under the site of the impact, or opposite the result of the brain being shunted and moving within the cranial cavity (contrecoup injury). These areas of contusion are frequently multiple, but may enlarge and coalesce, forming an intracerebral haematoma admixed with necrotic brain.

Chronic subdural haematoma

Chronic subdural haematomata may be a complication of an acute head injury, or occur without a preceding history of trauma (in elderly people with cortical atrophy) by tearing of the bridging veins running from the cortical surface to the venous sinuses resulting in a low (venous) pressure haemorrhage. The bleeding may not be apparent immediately, but clot haemolysis may exert osmotic pressure, accumulating fluid to expand, and result in a delayed subacute (4–21 days) or chronic (more than 21 days) presentation.

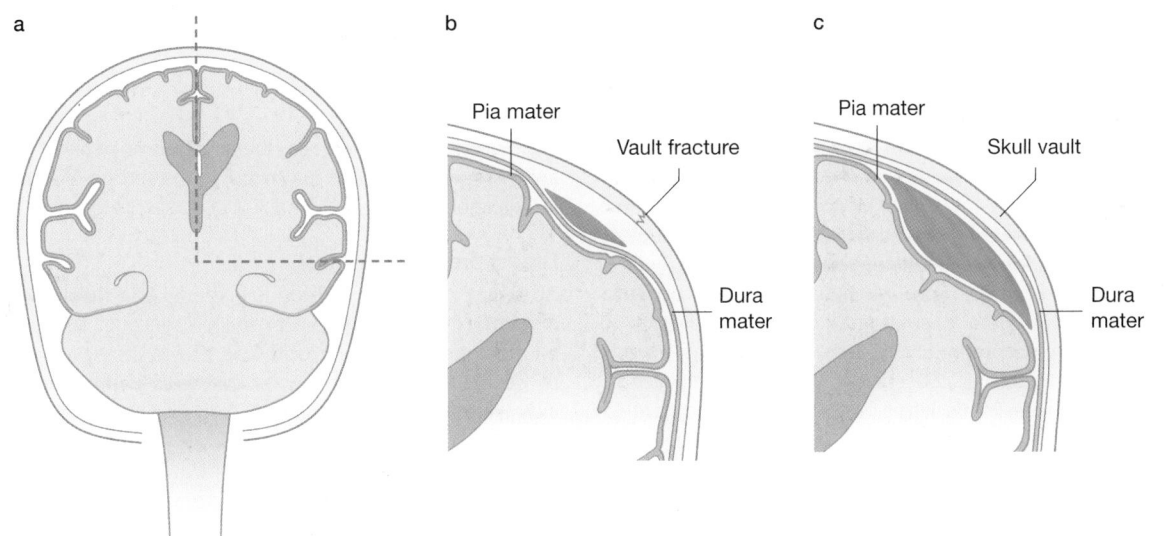

Fig. 9.22 Traumatic intracranial haematomas. Diagram illustrating the site of accumulation of blood with (b) extradural and (c) subdural haematoma.

Scope of disease

Primary injury

With any head injury, there is a component of primary damage at the time of impact and shearing forces causing diffuse axonal injury, about which nothing can be done.

Secondary injury

Importantly, however, there may also be secondary damage, which is treatable. This secondary damage includes the pressure effects of blood clots or brain swelling, which may raise intracranial pressure and compromise cerebral perfusion, adding secondary ischaemic insult. This may be worsened by cardiovascular instability, hypoventilation, seizures and pyrexia (by increasing the cerebral metabolic rate).

Clinical features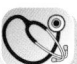

Whilst the nature of trauma may be self evident, additional history may be available from attendant ambulance and medical staff. The mechanism of injury can be important in identifying other associated injuries.

The classical presentation of extradural haematoma is that of head injury with transient or no loss of consciousness, the patient initially being alert and well but deteriorating over several hours due to clot formation. The most important features are headache, deteriorating conscious state, focal neurological signs and, later, evidence of raised intracranial pressure (bradycardia, hypotension).

Patients with acute subdural and intracranial haematomas tend to present with severe head injuries and a neurological state that fails to improve or deteriorates.

Patients with chronic subdural haematomas may present in three classical ways: with features of raised intracranial

pressure (headache, vomiting, drowsiness) without focal neurological signs, with fluctuating drowsiness or with progressive dementia.

On examination, an important feature is the level of consciousness and any change in it. This is formally assessed by the Glasgow coma score (GCS, Table 9.25). A patient who has been unresponsive since the time of the injury may have sustained a significant primary injury, with a correspondingly poor prognosis. In contrast, a patient who has recovered consciousness to some degree has demonstrated a capacity for recovery; if there is any later deterioration, this must be due to secondary events, which may be treatable.

Examination of the patient includes the pupillary responses; the motor, verbal and eye opening responses that make up the GCS; and signs of injury over the head itself. A fixed dilated pupil may be an indication of an expanding haematoma, causing uncal herniation and compression of the IIIrd cranial nerve on that side (NB, a pupil may also appear fixed from direct trauma to the eye). The GCS has to be interpreted in the context of anaesthetic agents administered if the patient is intubated and ventilated. Lacerations and injuries to the head are examined for evidence of underlying skull fractures.

> ### ⚡ CLINICAL ALERT
>
> Depending on the severity of the injury and the patient's conscious state, assessment of the patient may be combined with resuscitation. This aims to establish an airway, adequate ventilation, and a stable blood pressure, always considering the possibility of additional injuries, including those to the cervical spine.

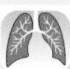

Initial investigations

CT of the head (without contrast)

This is the key investigation in the management of head injury (Fig. 9.23). CT scanning is indicated if there is a decreased level of consciousness, focal neurological deficit, evidence of a skull fracture, if the patient is difficult to assess (most commonly due to alcohol), or if there are other grounds for being concerned about intracranial haemorrhage such as the use of anticoagulants.

Care needs to be taken when screening for subacute and chronic subdural haematomas, as the radiodensity of the haematoma progressively decreases from high (fresh blood) to low (chronic collection). Therefore, the collection may be the same radiodensity with the brain and hard to visualize.

Plain skull film

The role of plain skull radiographs is limited and they are not indicated if the patient warrants a CT scan because of other criteria. A plain radiograph may reveal a skull fracture, but all fractures, particularly those involving the skull base, may not be apparent, hence a normal examination is of limited use.

Initial management

The aims of management are to prevent the deleterious effects of secondary injury by ensuring adequate cerebral metabolic requirements, and to prevent or control intracranial hypertension.

Oxygen

It is important to maintain cerebral metabolic needs in the presence of a head injury; hypoxic patients should receive supplementary oxygen. Endotracheal intubation is required for patients who are not sufficiently conscious to protect their airway, or in the setting of extreme restlessness.

Glucose

Supplementary glucose may be required in patients who are hypoglycaemic. This may occur in the setting of alcohol intoxication.

Blood pressure control

Adequate cerebral perfusion is essential and replacement of blood may be required in the presence of secondary injuries and extensive blood loss. Fluids, however, need to be managed judiciously as overzealous infusion may exacerbate cerebral oedema.

Medical therapy

Diuretics

Diuretics such as mannitol are used, usually as a temporary measure to reduce cerebral oedema prior to emergency surgery.

Anticonvulsants

Diazepam is the first-line treatment for seizures, followed by phenytoin. Adequate seizure control is important to prevent further hypoxia.

> **RECENT ADVANCES**
>
> *The use of steroids in head injury is highly controversial. A small survival advantage has been suggested by meta-analysis.[1] A multicentre randomized trial has recently confirmed that the use of steroids is actually associated with an increase in early mortality, and should be avoided.[2]*

Surgical management

In general, the medical treatment of haematomas is limited and should not delay surgical intervention. Whilst sedation, hyperventilation and careful management of fluids and diuretics may help control intracranial pressure, if there is a significant haematoma contributing to and compromising cerebral perfusion, it requires evacuation.

The indication for surgery is intracranial hypertension in acute traumatic haematoma, and the presence of symptoms in chronic subdural haematoma.

Craniotomy

Acute haematomas exerting a mass effect and compromising cerebral perfusion require urgent evacuation by a craniotomy. Planning of the site of the burr holes is assisted by CT localization. Burr holes are created and the bone-flap is lifted. The haematoma is identified and evacuated using a soft suction tip catheter. An integral part of operating on an extradural haematoma is to stitch the dura up to the surrounding bone edge to obliterate the extradural space,

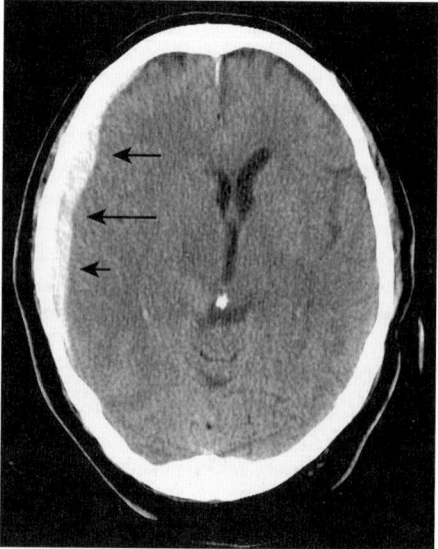

Fig. 9.23 CT of the head showing a right-sided subdural haematoma (arrows).

preventing re-collection. The bone-flap is then replaced, and the wound closed in layers.

With acute subdural haematomas, the underlying brain often swells, obliterating the space. As part of the craniotomy procedure, an intracranial pressure monitor is generally inserted to guide subsequent ITU management.

Chronic subdural haematomas have liquefied, formed clot no longer being present. Therefore they can generally be evacuated through burr holes. Indeed, in an elderly patient who is well with an acute or subacute haematoma, one may elect to wait, to allow it to liquefy and permit drainage via burr holes, and avoid submitting the patient to a craniotomy. Occasionally a chronic subdural haematoma can re-collect because the haematoma cavity contains membranes with friable new vessel formation. In these cases a craniotomy may be performed to remove the membranes.

Prognosis

It is notoriously hard to prognosticate in individual cases of acute head injury. Outcome depends not only on the head injury but on any other injuries that may have been sustained. In general, however, extradural haematomas have a better prognosis than acute subdural and intra-cerebral bleeds, and the outcome of an extradural haematoma depends critically on the patient's conscious level prior to surgery, which will reflect any underlying brain injury.

i FURTHER INFORMATION

Committee on Trauma of the American College of Surgeons. ATLS. Chicago: American College of Surgeons, 2002.

REFERENCES

(1) *Alderson P, Roberts I. Corticosteroids in acute traumatic brain injury: systematic review of randomised controlled trials. BMJ 1997; 314:1855–1859.*
(2) *Roberts I, Yates D, Sandercock P, et al. Effect of intravenous corticosteroids on death within 14 days in 10008 adults with clinically significant head injury (MRC CRASH trial): randomised placebo-controlled trial. Lancet 2004; 364: 1321–1328.*

Subarachnoid haemorrhage

Epidemiology

The incidence of spontaneous subarachnoid haemorrhage (SAH) has been estimated to be up to 16 per 100 000 per year. There is a degree of variation due to different diag-nostic criteria and the extent to which older patients with stroke-like illnesses are investigated.

Pathology

The causes of spontaneous subarachnoid haemorrhage vary with age. The most common cause (approximately 75%) is rupture of a saccular aneurysm (Fig. 9.24). These aneurysms typically form at the major branch points of arteries around the circle of Willis, causing high-pressure arterial bleeding.

Approximately 10% are due to rupture of an arteri-ovenous malformation (Fig. 9.25). These malformations are considered to be embryological defects, and patients with such defects present with subarachnoid haemorrhage at a younger age. As blood is shunted through the arteriovenous malformation into a relatively low-pressure venous system, the intracranial bleeding tends to be at a lower pressure.

In a proportion of cases, no vascular abnormality is iden-tified, and a number may be associated with atherosclerotic disease, hypertension or the use of anticoagulants.

Clinical features

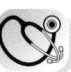

The classical presentation is a sudden-onset, unusual headache that is generally severe, typically associated with nausea and vomiting, and with symptoms and signs of

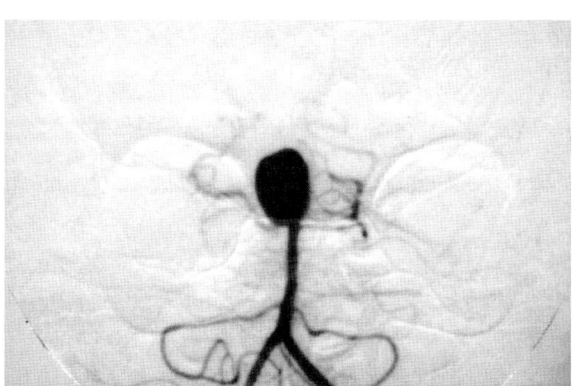

Fig. 9.24 Angiogram demonstrating a basilar artery tip aneurysm.

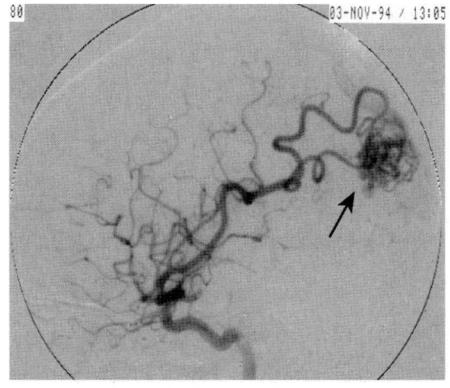

Fig. 9.25 Angiogram demonstrating a cerebral arteriovenous malformation (arrow).
Courtesy of Mr John Wattam, Royal Hallamshire Hospital, Sheffield, UK.

meningism. Many patients deteriorate in conscious state with the ictal event with a severity that can range from mild impairment to deeply comatose. It is estimated that 30% of patients never regain consciousness or suffer an apoplectic death as a result of the subarachnoid haemorrhage. In addition, particularly if there is bleeding into the brain substance, there may be focal neurological signs such as a hemiparesis.

Investigations
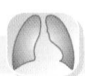

CT of the head
Approximately 90% of subarachnoid haemorrhages are detectable on a CT scan (Fig. 9.26) and the pattern of blood may give a clue to the pathogenesis of the bleed such as an arteriovenous malformation or an aneurysm.

Lumbar puncture
A minor or herald bleed from an aneurysm may be of small volume and undetectable on a CT scan. Therefore if the CT scan does not show any evidence of blood and the history is suggestive of subarachnoid haemorrhage, a lumbar puncture is performed to look for blood or its xanthochromic breakdown products.

Cerebral angiography
If blood is detected on lumbar puncture, cerebral angiography is required to screen for an aneurysm or arteriovenous malformation to prevent a subsequent catastrophic haemorrhage. The timing of angiography and indeed subsequent

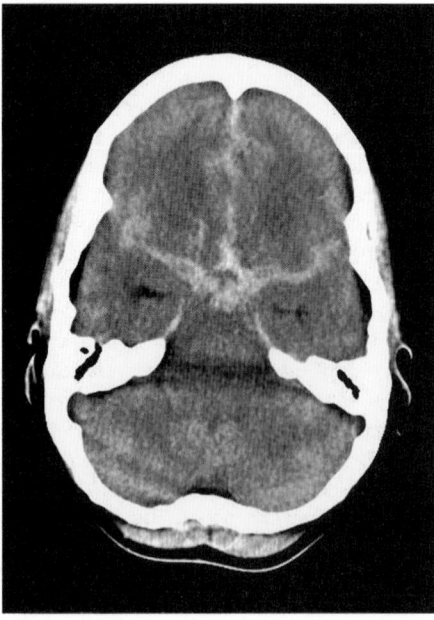

Fig. 9.26 CT scan of a subarachnoid haemorrhage due to rupture of an anterior communicating aneurysm.
Courtesy of Dr Stuart Coley, Royal Hallamshire Hospital, Sheffield, UK.

treatment will depend on a number of factors including the patient's general condition and age.

Management

Early consultation is required with supervising neurosurgical services. Patients may require prompt angiography to formally diagnose the cause and site of a haemorrhage.

Hydration
The initial management is medical to stabilize the patient. The patient should be kept well hydrated.

Nimodipine
Nimodipine should be given to the administration of nimodipine, a calcium channel blocker, which can help protect against delayed ischaemic neurological deficits.

Endovascular and surgical management of aneurysms
The timing of intervention after subarachnoid haemorrhage has been the subject of debate. With high-pressure bleeds, there is a significant incidence of further haemorrhage. In general, second haemorrhages are more catastrophic than the initial events and have worse outcomes. Therefore there has been a drive towards early angiography and treatment. However, patients in a poor clinical state may be better served by a late approach to allow for some recovery before therapeutic intervention. In addition, between the third and tenth day after a bleed, the major cerebral arteries may be constricted (vasospasm) and intervention in this period may carry additional risks.

The treatment of aneurysms has advanced significantly in recent years with the advent of endovascular techniques. Currently, coils are deployed to reinforce the aneurysm from within the blood vessel lumen. This has the advantage of a minimally invasive approach compared to traditional open cranial surgery and clipping (a clip is placed around the aneurysm neck to exclude it from the circulation). Not all aneurysms are equally suitable for either of these two treatments (depending on the shape and size of the aneurysm).

Management of arteriovenous malformations
The management of arteriovenous malformations is more elective as the bleeding risks are reduced in a low-pressure system (unless there is a large haematoma exerting a mass effect on the brain). Management options are more diverse and may include surgical resection, endovascular embolization and stereotactic radiosurgery to induce an obliteration of the malformation.

Prognosis

The most important factor in determining the prognosis is the patient's clinical state at presentation. Age is a significant contributory factor. As age increases, the morbidity and mortality are also increased.

Epilepsy

A seizure is an abnormal paroxysmal discharge of cerebral neurones that results in a clinical event, and epilepsy is a tendency to develop recurrent seizures.

Epidemiology

The incidence of epilepsy is 46 per 100 000 persons per year in the UK. It is more common in developing countries, in the very young and the elderly. It occurs equally in both sexes. The prevalence of epilepsy in the UK is 4% (4000 per 100 000),[1] and the lifetime cumulative incidence is approximately 3%.

Pathology

Epilepsy is a multifactorial disorder, and the risk factors associated with its development are listed in Table 9.31. The International League Against Epilepsy (ILAE) classification system devised a system to differentiate epilepsy syndromes according to clinical seizure type and EEG findings, dividing epileptic seizures into two broad categories: focal (epileptic activity confined to a local area of the brain) and generalized seizures (epileptic discharges involving both hemispheres widely and from the onset).[2]

Focal epilepsy (partial or localized epilepsy) may have an abnormal underlying focal abnormality such as cerebral tumour or congenital abnormality acting as a focus for abnormal and paroxysmal discharges. If the abnormal discharge spreads to both hemispheres it becomes generalized (secondary generalization). In addition, focal seizures are divided into those with preservation of consciousness (simple) and those with impairment of consciousness (complex).

Table 9.31	Risk factors for epilepsy
Congenital brain abnormalities	
Learning disability	
Head injury	
Cerebrovascular disease	
Dementia	
Meningitis/encephalitis	
Cerebral tumour	
Multiple sclerosis	
Alcohol excess	
Recreational drugs	
Family history	

Primary generalized epilepsy may be triggered by emotional stress, alcohol, fatigue, flashing lights or menstruation. Seizures of this type are generalized from onset and more commonly have a genetic basis, usually polygenic rather than a Mendelian trait.

Scope of disease

Epilepsy is associated with increased mortality, accidental injury and hospital admissions. The 2–3-fold increase in mortality may be due to drowning, accidental injury, status epilepticus or sudden unexplained death in epilepsy (SUDEP).

Status epilepticus is a medical emergency and is defined as prolonged seizure activity lasting longer than 30 minutes or repeated seizures with no recovery in between. The incidence of SUDEP is 1 in 1000 epileptic patients per year, possibly due to central apnoea or a cardiac arrhythmia. It is associated with all types of epilepsy, and the risk increases with disease severity.

Epilepsy also has social implications: driving is restricted, certain occupations are not permitted (heavy goods vehicle driver, airline pilot) and it may be associated with social stigma.

Clinical features

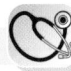

Focal seizures

The presentation of a focal seizure varies according to the part of the brain affected. Features include rhythmic jerking of an arm (frontal cortex), sensory disturbance (parietal lobe), abnormal sensation rising from the abdomen known as epigastric aura (temporal lobe), a feeling of déjà-vu (temporal lobe), a sensation of panic, abnormal taste, or visual disturbance (occipital lobe).

Focal seizures can become generalized, leading to tonic-clonic seizures. After the symptoms of the initial focal seizure (the 'aura'), the patient loses consciousness and develops the generalized tonic-clonic seizure. Initially the patient stiffens (tonic phase) and then all four limbs rhythmically jerk (clonic phase). During a generalized seizure, injuries may be sustained, the tongue may be bitten and urinary incontinence can occur. The generalized seizure usually lasts for 2–3 minutes followed by a period of post-ictal confusion, drowsiness or headache. Patients often feel a need to sleep and full recovery may take 1–2 hours. The rate of generalization of the abnormal discharge may be so fast that an aura is not experienced.

Complex partial seizures are focal seizures with an alteration in consciousness (loss of awareness) without tonic-clonic seizure. Automatisms such as lip smacking or plucking at clothes occur.

Generalized seizures

Idiopathic generalized seizures consist of absence seizures, myoclonic jerks, generalized tonic-clonic, tonic, clonic and atonic seizures. Paroxysmal discharges are generalized from onset and no aura is experienced.

Typical absence seizures (petit mal) are brief blank spells that last a few seconds. They usually begin in childhood and during attacks there is a 3 per second spike and wave pattern on the EEG. In many patients attacks cease in adolescence.

Generalized tonic-clonic seizures occur without an aura (warning) and are primary from the onset.

Myoclonic jerks are brief movements, usually of the limbs. They often occur in the morning and specific enquiry should be undertaken as not all patients may be aware that they are abnormal.

In clonic seizures, convulsive movements are experienced. In tonic seizures, only the rigidity of the body and limbs occurs. In atonic seizures there is sudden loss of tone, and the patient falls without warning, often leading to injury.

A combination of absence seizures, myoclonic jerks and generalized tonic-clonic seizures is seen in juvenile myoclonic epilepsy (JME).

The differential diagnosis of a seizure is listed in Table 9.32.

Initial investigations

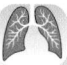

CT/MRI of the brain

CT or MRI is required to screen for a structural abnormality in patients over the age of 25 years and for patients with focal seizures.

Table 9.32	Differential diagnosis of a seizure
Syncope Vasovagal	There is often a trigger (having blood taken) and prodromal symptoms such as blurring of vision, light-headedness, or nausea. The patient is usually upright. Loss of consciousness is short-lived and recovery is quick. Urinary incontinence can occur if the bladder is full
Cardiac	This may be due to an arrhythmia (sick sinus syndrome) or a structural problem such as aortic stenosis. It can occur in any posture and convulsive movements can occur
Migraine	This may be mistaken for a simple partial seizure, especially when the migraine aura is not followed by a headache
Pseudo-seizure	These attacks are psychogenic in origin and misdiagnosis can lead to inappropriate treatments and admissions to intensive care
Transient ischaemic attack	These may be mistaken for partial seizures

Electrocardiogram (ECG)

This should be performed in all patients, particularly to exclude the prolonged QT syndrome.

Electroencephalography (EEG)

In between seizures (interictal) the EEG may be abnormal, for example a 3 Hz spike and wave pattern may be seen in idiopathic generalized epilepsy (Fig. 9.27). The interpretation of the EEG is operator dependent and the sensitivity (20–91%) and specificity (13–99%) vary widely.[3] In addition, the EEG may also identify the origin of focal seizures (Fig. 9.28).

Ambulatory EEG may be useful in patients who are having frequent episodes as an EEG may be recorded during one of the attacks, confirming or refuting the diagnosis of a seizure.

Initial management

Patient education

It is important to advise patients regarding safety around the home (avoid deep baths), safety in recreation (avoid

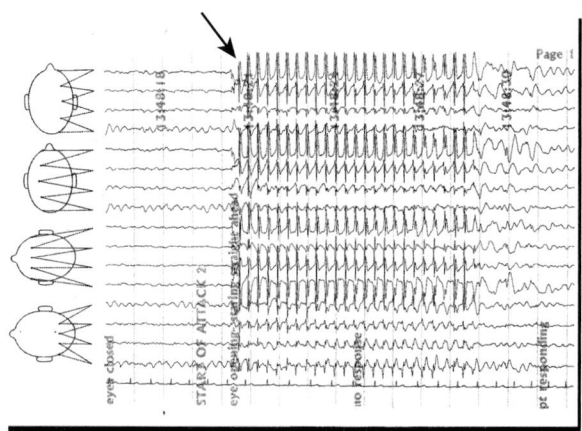

Fig. 9.27 EEG in a patient with primary generalized epilepsy. A run of 3 per second spike and wave is seen in all leads (arrow).

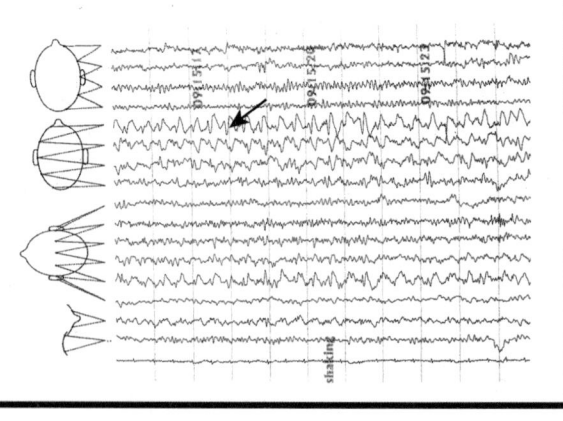

Fig 9.28 EEG in a patient during a focal seizure (complex partial) showing a left temporal focus. Large-amplitude sharp waves can be seen on the left (arrow).

swimming or fishing alone) and safety at work (avoid working at great height or with dangerous machinery). Driving regulations must be discussed. Patients must be fit-free for 1 year or have only nocturnal seizures for 3 years before they can regain their driving licence. Women of child-bearing age must be counselled regarding contraception as many of the antiepileptic medications interfere with the oral contraceptive pill. Also there are increased teratogenic risks with antiepileptic medications, particularly with sodium valproate.

Medical management

Anticonvulsant medication

The initial drug of choice for focal seizures is carbamazepine. Lamotrigine, sodium valproate, phenytoin, levetiracetam, topiramate and pregabalin are useful second-line or adjunctive agents.

The first-line treatment for idiopathic generalized epilepsies is sodium valproate. Lamotrigine, levetiracetam and topiramate are useful second-line drugs. Ethosuximide may control absences.

Ideally treatment should be simple (monotherapy) with minimal side effects. Medication should be increased to the maximum tolerated dose before switching to an alternative drug, and combination therapy should only be prescribed when at least two or more drugs have been tried as monotherapy without good control of seizure activity.

⚡ CLINICAL ALERT

Status epilepticus is a medical emergency. The airway and breathing should be assessed, and the pulse and blood pressure should be monitored. Oxygen should be administered. Initial treatment is with an intravenous benzodiazepine (lorazepam 4 mg or diazepam 10 mg), and this may be repeated after 2 minutes if seizures persist. Hypoglycaemia and other metabolic abnormalities should be corrected. Intravenous thiamine should be administered if there is a history of alcoholism.

If seizure activity remains, intravenous infusion of phenytoin (or fosphenytoin) should commence and continuous cardiac monitoring is required due to the risk of arrhythmia. If the seizures persist, admission to an intensive care unit for intubation and ventilation will be required.

Surgical management

Anteromesial temporal lobe and localized neocortical resections

Surgery should be considered for those patients refractory to medical treatment, particularly those with an identified structural abnormality such as an arteriovenous malformation or brain tumour. Patients with mesial temporal sclerosis, which gives rise to complex partial seizures (temporal lobe epilepsy), are good candidates for the consideration of surgery, particularly if they have a history of a prolonged febrile convulsions and localizing EEG and MRI abnormalities.

Surgery for epilepsy entails resection of a maximum of 6.5 cm of the anterior lateral non-dominant temporal lobe or 4.5 cm of the dominant temporal lobe. The mesial resection includes the amygdala and the anterior 3–4 cm of the hippocampus. Postoperatively 58% of patients are expected to be free from seizures impairing awareness at 1 year (compared to 8% receiving medical therapy) and randomized trials indicate better quality of life after surgery compared to medical therapy alone.[4] Surgery, however, is associated with the risk of memory impairment, language deficit (dominant hemisphere) and stroke.

Vagal nerve stimulation

Vagal nerve stimulation may be attempted in patients with poor seizure control on currently available medication who are not candidates for surgery. Approximately 18% become seizure free with intermittent vagal nerve stimulation.[5]

Prognosis

Remission with antiepileptic drugs can be achieved in approximately 75% of patients although this is dependent on the aetiology. Lower rates of remission are observed with epilepsy associated with learning disabilities.

Reduction in life expectancy can be up to 2 years for patients with epilepsy but can increase up to 10 years if the predisposing cause has been identified, e.g. stroke or congenital deficit.[6]

ℹ FURTHER INFORMATION

www.nice.org.uk National clinical guidelines for epilepsy: The diagnosis and management of the epilepsies in adults and children in primary and secondary care. October 2004.

www.sign.ac.uk SIGN 70: Diagnosis and management of epilepsy in adults. A national clinical guideline, 2003.

REFERENCES

(1) *MacDonald BK, Cockerell OC, Sander JW, Shorvon SD. The incidence and lifetime prevalence of neurological disorders in a prospective community-based study in the UK. Brain 2000; 123 (Pt 4): 665–676.*
(2) *Proposal for revised clinical and electroencephalographic classification of epileptic seizures. From the Commission on Classification and Terminology of the International League Against Epilepsy. Epilepsia 1981; 22: 489–501.*
(3) *Gilbert DL, Sethuraman G, Kotagal U, Buncher CR. Meta-analysis of EEG test performance shows wide variation among studies. Neurology 2003; 60: 564–570.*
(4) *Wiebe S, Blume WT, Girvin JP, et al. A randomized, controlled trial of surgery for temporal-lobe epilepsy. New England Journal of Medicine 2001; 345: 311–318.*
(5) *Murphy JV, Torkelson R, Dowler I, Simon S, Hudson S. Vagal nerve stimulation in refractory epilepsy: the first 100 patients receiving vagal nerve stimulation at a pediatric epilepsy center. Archives of Pediatric and Adolescent Medicine 2003; 157: 560–564.*
(6) *Gaitatzis A, Johnson AL, Chadwick DW, Shorvon SD, Sander JW. Life expectancy in people with newly diagnosed epilepsy. Brain 2004; 127: 2427–2432.*

Movement disorders

Movement disorders are characterized by involuntary movements or loss of accuracy and speed in the execution of movements. Normal voluntary movements are initiated by the motor cortex but are controlled and modified by the complex relationships between the cerebral cortex, cerebellum and basal ganglia.

Ataxia

Ataxia is a clinical feature that results from cerebellar dysfunction, characterized by loss of coordination and accuracy of the execution of movements.

Epidemiology

Ataxia is a common neurological complaint that affects both sexes equally.

Hereditary ataxias are divided into autosomal recessive (Friedreich's ataxia, ataxia telangiectasia, abetalipoproteinaemia, ataxia and oculomotor apraxia) and autosomal dominant (spinocerebellar ataxias or SCAs 1–28).

Pathology

The end result of most diseases associated with ataxia is the destruction of Purkinje cells, which are large cells located in the grey matter of the cerebellum. The Purkinje cells provide the sole output (which is inhibitory and mediated by GABA) through approximately 160 000 synapses. Other disease processes that can also result in ataxia include cerebellar white matter inflammation (multiple sclerosis) and demyelination or dysfunction of the vestibular system (viral labyrinthitis, benign positional vertigo). When ataxia is due to dysfunction of the vestibular system, it is usually associated with positional vertigo, hearing loss and dizziness. Vestibular dysfunction tends to produce transient or intermittent symptoms.

Severe loss of posterior column sensation may result in sensory ataxia, although in practice it can be difficult to distinguish between sensory and cerebellar ataxia.

Clinical features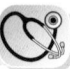

Ataxia can affect the limbs and gait. Patients usually complain of loss of balance that is exacerbated in the dark. The accuracy of limb movements is impaired, resulting in dropping of objects, inability to cope with fine movements and falls. Prominent nystagmus may result in oscillopsia (jumpy vision). Additional features such as postural dizziness and urinary frequency may imply autonomic involvement as seen in the cerebellar variant of multiple system atrophy. Stiffness and spasticity can also be a feature in some ataxias due to spinal cord involvement (spinocerebellar ataxia). A detailed family history is essential in identifying hereditary ataxias.

Prolonged and excessive alcohol intake is one of the most common causes of ataxia, and certain drugs (phenytoin, carbamazepine, lithium) are associated with ataxia.

Clinical examination usually reveals nystagmus (vertical or horizontal) during eye movements. There may be mild tremor of the head (titubation) and dysarthria (slow and segmented speech with variable intonation). Finger–nose testing reveals loss of accuracy of movement with intention tremor on reaching the target, and a similar finding is seen on heel–shin testing with both feet. Truncal ataxia results in inability to remain seated. The gait is broad based, and patients cannot stand on one leg at a time or walk on a straight line (tandem walk). Repetitive movements are clumsy and slow (dysdiadochokinesia).

Initial investigations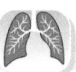

Initial investigations are directed by the mode of onset of ataxia and whether the ataxia is focal or global. Sudden onset of unilateral ataxia may be secondary to stroke, necessitating the relevant investigations. Progressive unilateral ataxia can be secondary to a tumour affecting one cerebellar hemisphere. The following investigations should be done in those patients presenting with gradual onset of generalized ataxia in the absence of a family history.

Full blood count
Macrocytosis may suggest excessive alcohol intake, hypothyroidism or B_{12} deficiency, all of which can cause ataxia. Anaemia may suggest gluten sensitivity.

Serum B_{12}
Subacute combined degeneration of the spinal cord as a result of B_{12} deficiency may be associated with a significant degree of ataxia.

Thyroid function tests
Hypothyroidism can manifest with ataxia.

Liver function tests
Elevated gamma glutamyltransferase can also suggest excessive alcohol intake.

Vitamin E levels
Deficiency can result in ataxia.

Anti-gliadin antibodies
Gluten sensitivity may account for up to 40% of patients with sporadic ataxia (p. 268). A gluten-free diet can be beneficial.

Thiamine levels
Thiamine deficiency is usually secondary to alcohol abuse and may cause Wernicke's encephalopathy with ataxia as a prominent feature.

CT or MRI of the brain
MRI is the preferred mode of imaging the posterior fossa, as it is able to assess the presence of cerebellar atrophy (Fig. 9.29), stroke, tumour or inflammatory causes such as multiple sclerosis.

Further investigations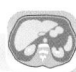

Genetic testing
Genetic testing for both recessive and dominant hereditary ataxias, even in the absence of a family history, may reveal abnormalities in up to 20% (sporadic ataxias).

Further investigations for malignancy
Rapidly progressive ataxia may be seen as a paraneoplastic syndrome (immune mediated), and further investigations looking for malignancy (particularly ovarian and lung) may be indicated

Varicella zoster, Epstein–Barr and human immunodeficiency virus serology
Post-infection cerebellitis can be seen after chickenpox and Epstein–Barr virus infections as well as after atypical

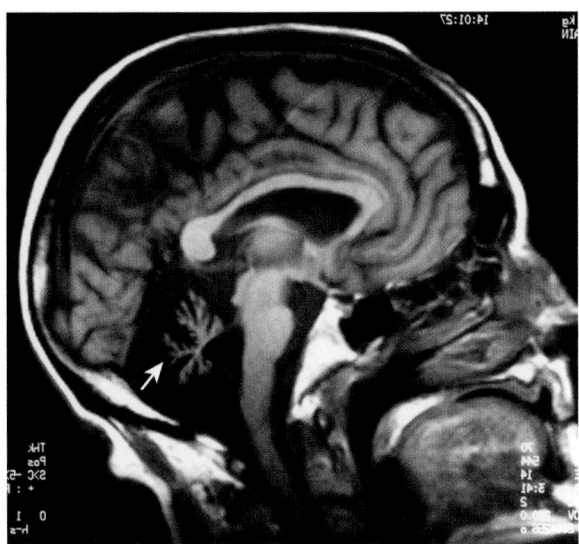

Fig. 9.29 A sagittal MRI scan showing cerebellar atrophy (arrow) in a patient presenting with ataxia.

pneumonias (usually self limiting). Serological testing for those infections may be useful. Ataxia can be seen in HIV infection.

Lumbar puncture
Prion diseases can present with ataxia but with additional features of rapidly progressive cognitive decline. The diagnosis can be aided by CSF examination.

Other metabolic investigations
Rare causes of ataxia include cerebrotendinous xanthomatosis (high cholestanol) and adult-onset Tay–Sachs disease (hexosaminidase deficiency on white cell enzyme testing). Most of these metabolic conditions tend to have an early onset (childhood).

Medical management

Treatment of the underlying cause
Management is directed to the underlying cause. Immune-mediated ataxias (paraneoplastic, gluten ataxia) are amenable to treatment that is instituted before permanent damage occurs. Treatment of the cancer may result in resolution or improvement of the ataxia. A gluten-free diet in patients with gluten ataxia can also result in improvement. Ataxia due to intoxication with drugs such as phenytoin and carbamazepine can improve on reduction of the dose or stopping the medication. Prolonged use of phenytoin may result in permanent cerebellar dysfunction. Acute cerebellar ataxia following alcohol intoxication may be seen in the context of Wernicke's encephalopathy and may respond to thiamine supplementation. Vitamin E supplementation may improve ataxia due to vitamin E deficiency.

Prognosis

Loss of Purkinje cells is permanent, and most ataxias that are degenerative (including familial ataxias) tend to progress and are irreversible.

Friedreich's ataxia

The most common inherited ataxia is Friedreich's ataxia, accounting for half of all inherited ataxias. It results from a genetic mutation (tri-nuclear (GAA) repeat expansion) on chromosome 9. Its estimated prevalence is 2 per 100 000 but the carrier frequency is as high as 1000 per 100 000. It is considered a multisystem disease because of involvement of other organs such as the pancreas (diabetes mellitus) and heart (cardiomyopathy). The mean age at onset is 15 years.

In addition to ataxia these patients have optic atrophy, peripheral neuropathy and skeletal abnormalities such as scoliosis. It is a disabling disease leading to physical dependence, so that by the age of 25 more than half of patients will be confined to a wheelchair.

Ataxia

Parkinsonism (akinetic rigid syndromes)

Tremor

Tics

Chorea

Dystonia

Myoclonus

Autosomal dominant spinocerebellar ataxias (SCA)

The autosomal dominant spinocerebellar ataxias are a heterogeneous group of diseases that result from different genetic defects. They usually present in adolescence or late adulthood, although some subtypes (SCA6) may not present until later on in life (40–50 years). The age of onset distinguishes them from the autosomal recessive ataxias, most of which are of early onset (before the age of 25). So far 24 different types have been described (SCA1–SCA24). The prevalence of dominant ataxias ranges from 0.9 to 1.3 per 100 000. The most common types in Europe are SCA1, SCA3 and SCA6 but with significant geographical differences. SCA6 presents with a pure ataxia, whilst others like SCA1 and SCA3 are associated with pyramidal and extrapyramidal symptoms and signs (dystonia, spasticity, rigidity, bradykinesia).

Parkinsonism (akinetic rigid syndromes)

There are many causes of Parkinsonism, including idiopathic Parkinson's disease, post-encephalitis (encephalitis lethargica) and diffuse damage to the white matter of the brain as in hydrocephalus or cerebrovascular disease. Some neurodegenerative disorders such as multiple system atrophy and progressive supranuclear palsy can produce Parkinsonism. Parkinsonian features are also seen in manganese poisoning and after repeated head injury in boxers.

Idiopathic Parkinson's disease

Epidemiology

The incidence of idiopathic Parkinson's disease is approximately 20 per 100 000 per year with a prevalence of 150 per 100 000. The prevalence increases with age. The disease usually presents between the ages of 50 and 70. Both men and women are equally affected.

Pathology

Idiopathic Parkinson's disease is associated with loss of pigmented neurones in the substantia nigra and locus caeruleus with degeneration of the dopaminergic pathway. There are also Lewy bodies (eosinophilic cytoplasmic inclusions) in other parts of the brain. It is probably the only disease that is less common in smokers but a pathological explanation for this is not yet available. Drugs that block dopaminergic receptors (antipsychotics, antiemetics) can cause a Parkinsonian syndrome.

Scope of disease

Impairment of mobility and loss of postural reflexes often lead to falls and injuries. The disease has a higher prevalence of dementia when compared to healthy control populations. The complications of treatment include postural hypotension, hallucinations and troublesome on/off phenomena including dyskinesias.

Clinical features

Patients complain of generalized slowness of movement (bradykinesia) during everyday activities and at work. In addition they may complain of stiffness (rigidity) and tremor, which is prominent at rest and may disappear with movement. The triad of bradykinesia, rigidity and tremor forms the main features of this disease. These features are usually asymmetrical but gradually progress to affect all four limbs. Additional symptoms include hypersalivation.

Drug enquiry (neuroleptic medication, antiemetics) is essential in excluding drug-induced Parkinsonism. Several risk factors for cerebrovascular disease may suggest a vascular aetiology.

On examination, patients usually have an expressionless face and soft monotonous speech. They adopt a flexed posture and have a slow and festinant gait. Initiation of walking may be difficult and there is absence of arm swinging. Examination of the limbs often reveals a resting tremor (frequency of 4–6 Hz), cogwheel rigidity on passive movement and slowness of repetitive movements.

Initial investigations

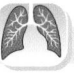

The diagnosis is clinical, and confirmation of the disease usually follows from evidence of response to treatment which distinguishes idiopathic Parkinson's disease from other Parkinsonian syndromes.

Further investigations

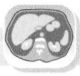

CT or MRI of the head

Imaging is required for patients with symptoms or signs of secondary disease. Other structural pathologies that can lead to symptoms of Parkinsonism include basal ganglia tumours, extensive ischaemic damage and hydrocephalus.

Copper studies

Wilson's disease can mimic Parkinsonism, and copper studies should be performed for young patients with Parkinsonian features.

Autonomic function tests

Autonomic function tests may help distinguish idiopathic Parkinson's disease from multiple system atrophy. The latter is characterized by additional evidence of autonomic dysfunction and symmetrical signs, often without tremor.

Apomorphine challenge

Apomorphine is the most powerful dopamine agonist but can only be administered intradermally. Its effects are almost immediate and thus it can be used as a diagnostic tool in demonstrating clinical responsiveness where idiopathic Parkinson's disease is suspected clinically. Some clinicians prefer a challenge with oral L-dopa preparations over a period of several weeks.

Medical management

Drug treatment does not alter the progression of the disease but can significantly alleviate the symptoms, particularly earlier on in the disease process.

L-DOPA and a dopa-decarboxylase inhibitor

L-dopa is a precursor of dopamine that is able to cross the blood–brain barrier. To avoid the peripheral dopaminergic adverse effects (nausea, vomiting, cardiac arrhythmias), L-dopa is administered in conjunction with a dopa-decarboxylase inhibitor (benserazide, carbidopa) that remains in the systemic circulation and does not cross the blood–brain barrier. L-dopa is the most powerful drug in the treatment of idiopathic Parkinson's disease.

Dopamine agonists

Dopamine agonists (bromocriptine, pergolide, ropinirole, pramipexole, cabergoline, apomorphine) can be used alone or in combination with L-dopa. They are less effective than L-dopa but can be used as the first line (particularly in young individuals) when treatment is clinically indicated or in combination with L-dopa in more advanced disease.

Monoamine oxidase inhibitors

Selegiline is a selective inhibitor of the enzyme monoamine oxidase B that results in an increase in cerebral dopamine. It is a useful agent in reducing dyskinesias.

Parenteral apomorphine

Parenteral apomorphine (a direct acting agonist) is useful in sparing the use of L-dopa and other dopamine agonists in dopa-induced psychosis and for advanced disease with severe fluctuations. It is intensely emetic and is therefore co-administered with an antiemetic which does not cross the blood–brain barrier (domperidone).

Anticholinergic agents

Anticholinergic drugs (trihexphenidyl) are less effective and limited by their extensive side effect profile (dry mouth, memory loss, etc.).

Surgical management

Stereotactic ablation and deep brain stimulation

Neurosurgical intervention is targeted at three sites: the thalamus, globus pallidus and subthalamic nucleus. Surgery involves either ablation or deep brain stimulation, with an aim to reduce or eliminate the abnormal output discharges from the basal ganglia to the cortex and brainstem. Therefore, surgery attempts to control the disease, and does not modify the underlying neurodegenerative process.

Surgery can be of benefit in severe disease when optimal medical therapy cannot provide acceptable disease control. Further studies are currently underway to evaluate the effects of surgical intervention.[1]

Prognosis

Patients with idiopathic Parkinson's disease have a reduced lifespan as a result of the disease. Patients eventually become bed bound and the cause of death is usually pneumonia.

REFERENCE

(1) Stowe RL, Wheatley K, Clarke CE, et al. Surgery for Parkinson's disease: lack of reliable clinical trial evidence. Journal of Neurology Neurosurgery and Psychiatry 2003; 74: 519–521.

Tremor

A tremor is an involuntary, oscillating and rhythmic movement of one or more parts of the body. It may be present at rest (e.g. Parkinson's disease) or during voluntary movement (intention tremor of cerebellar disease). It can be associated with neurodegenerative or systemic diseases or occur in isolation (e.g. benign essential tremor, physiological tremor). The most common causes of tremor are benign essential tremor, idiopathic Parkinson's disease, drugs (sodium valproate, lithium, amiodarone), thyrotoxicosis, sympathetic stimulants (salbutamol inhaler, caffeine), liver failure, CO_2 retention (seen in respiratory failure and chronic obstructive pulmonary disease) and hypoglycaemia.

Benign essential tremor is a coarse tremor (5–8 Hz) that becomes more prominent during sustained posture and worsens on action. It is common, with a prevalence of 300 per 100 000 and is often familial (autosomal dominant). It can improve with alcohol and worsen under observation or stress. Patients seek medical advice due to fear of the diagnosis of Parkinson's disease and social embarrassment (tremor is worse on holding a glass or a cup of drink). Reassurance as to the aetiology and the use of a beta-blocker and primidone may be beneficial.

Tics

Tics are abrupt, repetitive, stereotyped, coordinated but inappropriate jerk-like movements. They are easy to imitate and can be voluntarily suppressed for a time, usually at the expense of inner tension. Muscles around the eye, face, neck and shoulders are the most commonly affected. Males are three times more often affected than females. The onset is in childhood or adolescence. There is no pharmacological treatment. Reassurance, explanation and occasionally behavioural therapy can be useful.

Gilles de la Tourette syndrome is a rare familial disorder characterized by multiple tics which develop in childhood or adolescence. These are accompanied by explosive stereotyped verbal utterances (usually swear words) and sounds (grunts). The syndrome can be characterized by obsessive-compulsive behaviour (seen in 50% of cases).

Chorea

Chorea is a brief, highly organized, semi-purposeful movement of the whole or part of a limb that may be accompanied by facial dyskinesia. Choreic movements are probably due to lesions in the caudate nuclei. Causes of chorea are listed in Table 9.33.

Huntington's disease is an autosomal dominant neurodegenerative condition affecting males and females equally. The prevalence is about 6 per 100 000. Patients present with gradual onset of chorea often associated with behavioural, affective or psychotic disorders. In addition to chorea it is characterized by progressive dementia. Genetic testing is readily available and genetic counselling is essential for all family members of the affected individual. Tetrabenazine and sulpiride can be useful for the chorea but otherwise treatment is supportive.

Dystonia

Dystonia is characterized by sustained muscle contraction causing abnormalities of posture or movement. It can be divided into idiopathic or secondary (Table 9.34).

Table 9.33	Causes of chorea
Drugs	
L-dopa and dopamine agonists (treatment of idiopathic Parkinson's disease)	
Neuroleptics	
Anticonvulsants	
Oral contraceptive pill	
Sydenham's rheumatic chorea (St Vitus dance)	
Huntington's disease	
Systemic lupus erythematosus	
Antiphospholipid syndrome	
Wilson's disease	
Thyrotoxicosis	
Pregnancy	
Acanthocytosis	
Polycythemia rubra vera	

Table 9.34	Causes of dystonia
Idiopathic	
Idiopathic focal dystonia	
Spasmodic torticollis	
Writer's cramp	
Blepharospasm	
Idiopathic generalized dystonia	
Dystonia musculorum deformans	
Secondary	
Neurological diseases	
Juvenile Parkinsonism	
Hallervorden–Spatz disease	
Juvenile Huntington's disease	
Wilson's disease	
Drugs (antiemetics)	

Idiopathic focal dystonias include spasmodic torticollis, writer's cramp and blepharospasm, but they can affect almost any part of the body. Dystonia may be generalized (dystonia musculorum deformans). Idiopathic focal dystonia may run in families and certain types have been genetically characterized. It can be triggered by overuse, trauma or surgery to the affected part.

Marked variation in severity, early age of onset and familial tendency may suggest dopa-responsive disease. This form can be controlled with the use of L-dopa. Focal dystonias may be treated with botulinum toxin injections of the affected muscles. Such injections provide temporary relief and need to be repeated at regular intervals.

There is evidence that the motor processing in the medial pallidum is defective and this has led to the use of pallidal brain stimulation as a possible treatment option.

Myoclonus

Myoclonus is an involuntary, brief, sudden, shock-like contraction of muscles or a group of muscles which usually produces movement. The contractions can be isolated, repetitive and irregular or rhythmic. They are associated with a range of neurological diseases but can also be physiological (benign hypnagogic myoclonus occurs on falling asleep). Causes of myoclonus include juvenile myoclonic epilepsy, Creutzfeldt–Jakob disease, Alzheimer's disease, renal failure, hepatic encephalopathy and post-cerebral anoxia. Myoclonus can be seen in association with other movement disorders such as ataxia (myoclonic ataxia). It may respond to clonazepam or sodium valproate.

Multiple sclerosis

Multiple sclerosis (MS) is a chronic demyelinating disease that follows a fluctuating and unpredictable course. It is a major cause of disability in young adults.

Epidemiology

There is marked geographical variation in MS, characterized by increasing frequency with increasing latitude north or south from the Equator. Scotland has the highest incidence of MS in the world (12 per 100 000) compared to 6 per 100 000 in England.[1,2]

The age of onset is usually between 20 and 40 years though primary progressive MS tends to occur after the age of 40. The risk of developing MS is also increased if a first-degree relative (sibling or parent) is affected.

Pathology

The basic pathological change in MS is patchy degeneration of the myelin sheath resulting in 'plaques' of demyelination. As a consequence, nerve impulse transmission is delayed.

The exact aetiology of MS is unknown. It is thought to be an autoimmune disorder mediated by T cells associated with specific HLA antigen. Environmental factors also play a role: moving at a young age from an area of low risk to high risk can also increase the risk. A possible viral agent is therefore thought to play a role but no single agent has been conclusively identified.

Scope of disease

The frequency of complications that can result from MS increases with severity and duration of the disease (Table 9.35).

Clinical features

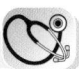

The clinical features of MS depend on the site of demyelination. Symptoms are often exacerbated by heat or exercise (Uhthoff's phenomenon).

Unilateral visual loss can occur due to demyelination of the optic nerve, the most common cause of optic neuritis. There is gradual loss of vision with red colour desaturation. Eye movements may be painful and examination of the eye can reveal an afferent pupillary defect with normal fundus. Eventually optic atrophy develops.

Motor involvement may cause a spastic paraparesis or unilateral weakness. Spasticity may be a marked problem. The clinical signs are of an upper motor neurone lesion,

Table 9.35	Complications of multiple sclerosis and treatment options
Complication	**Treatment**
Spasticity	Physiotherapy, antispasmodic agents (baclofen, tizanidine)
Fatigue	Fatigue management programmes, amantadine, modafinil
Bladder dysfunction—urgency, frequency, incontinence, nocturia	Oxybutynin, desmopressin (for nocturia), intermittent self-catheterization, suprapubic catheter
Paroxysmal (trigeminal neuralgia) or chronic pain	Neuropathic pain medications, e.g. amitriptyline, gabapentin, pregabalin
Depression	Counselling, antidepressants
Tremor	Severe tremor may require surgery (insertion of a thalamic stimulator)
Erectile dysfunction	Sildenafil
Constipation	Dietary modification, lactulose
Epilepsy	Anticonvulsants
Cognitive dysfunction	

that is increased tone, clonus, hyperreflexia and extensor plantar responses.

Sensory disturbance is common with sensory loss or, more often, non-specific paraesthesia. Neck flexion may cause lightning pains shooting down the body (Lhermitte's phenomenon).

Brainstem and cerebellar involvement can give rise to vertigo, vomiting, dysarthria, incoordination and ataxia. Eye movements may be abnormal with internuclear ophthalmoplegia or nystagmus.

Urinary symptoms are common, particularly frequency and urgency.

The diagnosis of MS depends on lesions being disseminated in time and space. After one clinical attack the diagnosis of MS cannot be made (this is referred to as a clinically isolated syndrome) unless an MRI scan also indicates lesions disseminated in time and space.

Disease subtypes

There are four types of MS. The majority of patients will start with the relapsing remitting type (80–90%). An attack (relapse) is followed by a remission during which disability does not progress. A relapse lasts for a minimum of 24 hours but usually lasts several weeks. Recovery from a relapse can be complete or partial and a second attack can cause the same or new symptoms.

Secondary progressive MS is characterized by slow deterioration with increasing disability (in addition there may still be relapses). Primary progressive MS is a form of MS with no history of relapses or remissions and a slow and insidious course; it occurs in approximately 10%. Benign MS does not tend to get worse over time or result in permanent disability.

Initial investigations

MRI of the brain and spinal cord
MRI of the brain (and spinal cord if there are symptoms suggestive of spinal involvement) is an excellent tool for evaluating a patient with suspected MS, as 95% with clinically definite MS will have an abnormal brain MRI scan.[3] New lesions can be identified by the use of gadolinium contrast (Fig. 9.30). MRI can also assist in the evaluation of the prognosis of the disease. After the first attack of demyelination, an abnormal MRI scan suggests a high risk of developing MS (83% risk at 10 years), but with a normal scan the risk is 11% at 10 years.[4]

Visual evoked potentials (VEPs)
A delay in the visual evoked potentials is indicative of demyelination, particularly if this is asymmetrical. VEPs can be abnormal even if there is no history of clinical involvement.

Lumbar puncture
Oligoclonal bands (unmatched in the serum) may be present in the cerebrospinal fluid. This is indicative of inflammation within the central nervous system and is not specific to demyelination although oligoclonal bands are present in 95% of clinically definite cases of MS. The lymphocyte count and protein level can be slightly raised.

Initial management

Multidisciplinary team management
Patient education, counselling and the support of a multidisciplinary team is crucial for patients with MS. Physiotherapy, occupational therapy and specialist MS nurses can all help with emotional and physical support.

Medical therapy
There is no cure for MS and treatment is aimed at relieving symptoms, preventing relapses and delaying disease progression.

Corticosteroids
A short course of high-dose methylprednisolone (oral or intravenous) is given to shorten the relapse time but corticosteroids have no effect on disease progression.

Disease-modifying agents
Interferon-beta
The most commonly given disease-modifying agent is interferon-beta, which both reduces relapse rate and delays disease progression.[5] The indications for treatment are relapsing remitting MS if the patient is able to walk independently (at least 100 metres without assistance) and has had at least 2 clinically significant relapses in the last 2 years. It is not currently recommended in the treatment of

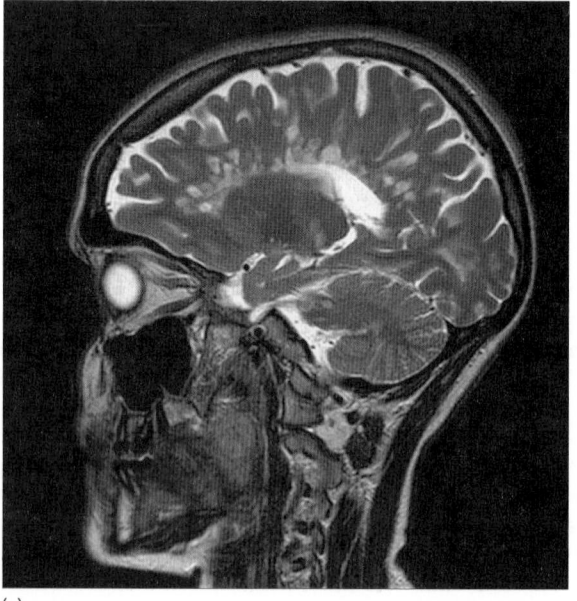
(a)

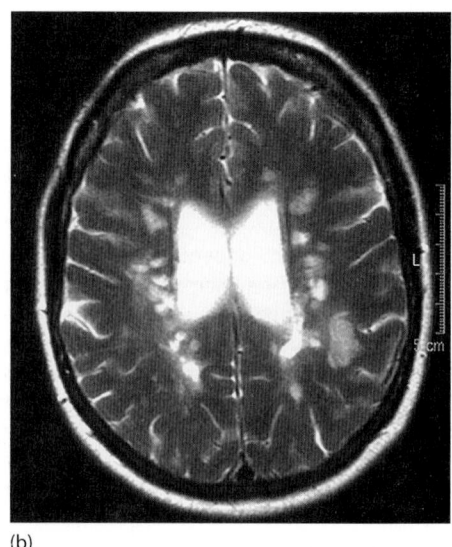
(b)

Fig. 9.30 MRI of multiple sclerosis. Numerous periventricular plaques of demyelination seen on (a) a T2 sagittal MRI scan, and (b) a T2 axial MRI scan. Courtesy of Dr Stuart Coley, Royal Hallamshire Hospital, Sheffield, UK.

clinically isolated MS or secondary progressive MS unless the patient has had at least 2 clinically significant relapses in the last 2 years, is able to walk 10 metres without assistance, and the disability from slow disease progression is minimal.[6]

Other disease-modifying agents

Other treatments include glatiramer acetate, azathioprine, mitoxantrone and plasma exchange.

Prognosis

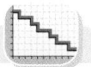

The overall life expectancy of patients with MS is shortened by 5–7 years; however, the disease process is very variable and ranges from no disability and few relapses to frequent relapses, rapid progression of disability and early death.

The main indicator of a poor prognosis is the onset of the progressive phase of disease. Other indicators include frequent relapses in the first 2 years, short intervals between attacks and female sex.

i FURTHER INFORMATION

Compston A, Ebers G, Lassman H, McDonald I, Matthews B, Wekerle H. McAlpine's Multiple sclerosis, 3rd edn. Edinburgh: Churchill Livingstone, 1998.

REFERENCES

(1) Rothwell PM, Charlton D. High incidence and prevalence of multiple sclerosis in south east Scotland: evidence of a genetic predisposition. Journal of Neurology Neurosurgery and Psychiatry 1998; 64: 730–735.
(2) Mumford CJ, Fraser MB, Wood NW, Compston DA. Multiple sclerosis in the Cambridge health district of East Anglia. Journal of Neurology Neurosurgery and Psychiatry 1992; 55: 877–882.
(3) Ormerod IE, Miller DH, McDonald WI, et al. The role of NMR imaging in the assessment of multiple sclerosis and isolated neurological lesions. A quantitative study. Brain 1987; 110 (Pt 6): 1579–1616.
(4) O'Riordan JI, Thompson AJ, Kingsley DP, et al. The prognostic value of brain MRI in clinically isolated syndromes of the CNS. A 10-year follow-up. Brain 1998; 121 (Pt 3): 495–503.
(5) Randomised double-blind placebo-controlled study of interferon beta-1a in relapsing/remitting multiple sclerosis. PRISMS (Prevention of Relapses and Disability by Interferon beta-1a Subcutaneously in Multiple Sclerosis) Study Group. Lancet 1998; 352: 1498–1504.
(6) Guidelines for the use of beta interferon in multiple sclerosis. Association of British Neurologists, 2001.

Infections of the central nervous system

Meningitis

Meningitis is the inflammation of the meninges, and can result from infection with bacteria, viruses, fungi, protozoa or parasites or infiltration with malignant cells.

Epidemiology

Haemophilus influenzae was the most common pathogen causing meningitis in the age group 3 months to 5 years. Since the introduction of the *Haemophilus influenzae* type b (Hib) vaccine the incidence of *Haemophilus influenzae* meningitis has dramatically declined.

Neisseria meningitidis (meningococcal meningitis) is most frequent in the 2–24-year-old age group. The UK recently introduced a programme to vaccinate children against meningococcal serogroup C strains, which has reduced the incidence of this capsular type. Serogroup B meningococcus, however, is currently the most common cause of bacterial meningitis.

Streptococcus pneumoniae (pneumococcal meningitis) commonly affects those under 5, adults over 45 years, those with head injury or recent ear infection or the immunocompromised.

Pathology

Viruses are the most common cause of meningitis. Bacterial pathogens include *Neisseria meningitidis, Streptococcus pneumoniae, Haemophilus influenzae* and *Listeria monocytogenes*. Group B streptococci, *E. coli* and Listeria are the most common pathogens that affect neonates.

Bacterial invasion of the meninges may result by extension from nearby infections (nasopharynx or ear), via the blood stream or by external communication with CSF (intracranial surgery, basal skull fracture, intracranial shunt). Immunocompromised patients are also at higher risk.

Common viral causes include enteroviruses, Epstein–Barr virus and mumps.

Chronic meningitis (symptoms over weeks to months) may result from infection with *Mycobacterium tuberculosis, Borrelia burgdorferi, Treponema pallidum, Leptospira* or brucella. In addition, fungal infection with *Cryptococcus neoformans* (now the second leading cause of death in

615

HIV-positive patients worldwide) or malignancy may result in subacute or chronic meningitis.

Scope of disease

Hydrocephalus and seizures may complicate the acute stages of bacterial meningitis. Long-term consequences include cranial nerve palsy, hearing loss (up to 40%), epilepsy and permanent brain damage with cortical blindness, sensory or motor impairment (from cerebral infarction) or learning difficulties.

Clinical features

Acute meningitis presents with fever, headache, photophobia and neck stiffness. Bacterial meningitis is a medical emergency causing rapid progression to altered consciousness and coma over a few hours. Viral meningitis is usually a less severe self-limiting illness.

On examination there may be painful neck stiffness. Kernig's sign may be elicited: with the patient in the supine position, the hip is flexed to 90° and the knee is flexed to 90° then extended. A positive Kernig's sign is when spasm in the hamstring muscles leads to inability to straighten the knee. Septic shock can occur, particularly with meningococcal septicaemia, where a purpuric rash may also be present.

Initial investigations

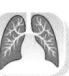

Full blood count
The white cell count may be elevated.

Erythrocyte sedimentation rate/C-reactive protein
The non-specific markers of inflammation may be elevated.

Urea and electrolytes
Renal impairment is suggested by a raised creatinine and may indicate impending shock. Acidaemia is unusual.

Blood cultures
These may be positive in patients with bacterial meningitis, especially with pneumococcal and meningococcal septicaemia.

Throat swabs
These may identify carriage of the responsible bacterial or viral organisms.

Meningococcal polymerase chain reaction (PCR)
A sample of whole blood is sent for PCR analysis to detect meningococcal DNA.

Lumbar puncture
A lumbar puncture should only be performed if there is no evidence of raised intracranial pressure. In bacterial meningitis the cerebrospinal fluid is usually turbid, with an elevated white cell count that is predominantly a neutrophilia. The cerebrospinal fluid protein level is also elevated and the glucose is low. Bacteria may be seen on a Gram stain or subsequent cultures (Table 9.36) or identified by latex agglutination. The causes of lymphocytic meningitis are listed in Table 9.37.

PCR on cerebrospinal fluid can aid in the diagnosis of meningitis (meningococcal, pneumococcal, enterovirus, herpes simplex and varicella). A sample should be sent for mycobacterial culture if tuberculous meningitis is suspected.

Further investigations

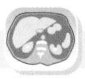

CT of the head
CT of the head is indicated when there is focal neurology or evidence of raised intracranial pressure prior to lumbar puncture.

Initial management

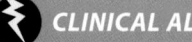 **CLINICAL ALERT**

Bacterial meningitis is a medical emergency. Treatment should be instigated as soon as the diagnosis is suspected, and not delayed by waiting for the results of a lumbar puncture.

Intravenous antibiotics
Empirical intravenous cefotaxime or ceftriaxone 2 g should be administered as soon as possible. Amoxicillin (2 g, 3 times daily) should be added in patients over 65 years or

Table 9.36	CSF findings in meningitis

	Bacterial	Viral	Tuberculous	Cryptococcal
White cells	Neutrophils*	Lymphocytes	Lymphocytes	Lymphocytes
Protein	Elevated	Normal/slightly elevated	Elevated	Elevated
Glucose	Reduced	Normal	Reduced	Reduced
Specific test	Gram stain and culture	PCR	Prolonged culture for tuberculosis	Indian ink stain/cryptococcal antigen

* A lymphocytic picture is seen if meningitis is due to *Listeria monocytogenes*.

Table 9.37	Causes of lymphocytic meningitis
Partially treated bacterial meningitis	
Viral meningitis	
Listeria meningitis	
Tuberculous meningitis	
Cryptococcal meningitis	
Malignant meningitis	
Syphilis	
Encephalitis	
Multiple sclerosis	
Sarcoidosis	

in the immunosuppressed to cover *Listeria*. Antibiotic regimens should be modified depending on the organism identified.

Immunomodulation

A moderate benefit has been demonstrated for all patients with bacterial meningitis treated with intravenous corticosteroid (dexamethasone 10 mg given 20 minutes prior to, or with, the first antibiotic dose and continued 6-hourly for the next 4 days).[1] Subgroup analysis revealed a significant benefit for pneumococcal meningitis, therefore current advice is to consider steroid treatment when pneumococcal meningitis is suspected and when confident that the correct antimicrobial agents are being used.[2]

Secondary prevention

Close contacts (household members, kissing contacts) should receive rifampicin or ciprofloxacin (depending on age) for secondary prevention of meningococcal meningitis. Vaccination can be considered in patients infected with group C meningococcus or if there is evidence of an outbreak.

Medical management

Tuberculous meningitis

Tuberculous meningitis should be treated with quadruple antituberculosis treatment for 2 months (isoniazid, rifampicin, pyrazinamide plus streptomycin/ethambutol/ethionamide) followed by continuation therapy with isoniazid and rifampicin for 10 months.[3] Corticosteroids are recommended for severe disease.

Anticonvulsants

Seizures should be treated with anticonvulsants (p. 607).

Intensive care

Transfer to a critical care unit should be considered if there is any evidence of raised intracranial pressure, shock or respiratory failure, as careful fluid volume, inotropic or ventilatory support may be required.

Surgical management

Surgical intervention may be required if hydrocephalus develops. This is more common with tuberculous meningitis.

Prognosis

Prognosis is dependent on the causative organism. Viral meningitis has an excellent prognosis with <1% mortality and little morbidity. Bacterial meningitis, however, has a mortality of 25% and can be associated with significant morbidity.[4]

Notification

Notification of cases of meningitis should be made to the consultants in communicable disease control (CDCC).

i FURTHER INFORMATION

www.britishinfectionsociety.org UK meningitis clinical guidelines.

REFERENCES

(1) *De Gans J, Van de Beek D. European Dexamethasone in Adulthood Bacterial Meningitis Study Investigators. Dexamethasone in adults with bacterial meningitis. New England Journal of Medicine 2002; 347: 1549–1556.*
(2) *British Infection Society. Early management of suspected bacterial meningitis and meningococcal septicaemia in adults. www.britishinfectionsociety.org/meningitis*
(3) *Joint Tuberculosis Committee of the British Thoracic Society. Chemotherapy and management of tuberculosis in the United Kingdom: recommendations 1998. Thorax 1998; 53: 536–548.*
(4) *Durand ML, Calderwood SB, Weber DJ, Miller SI, Southwick FS, Caviness VS Jr, Swartz MN. Acute bacterial meningitis in adults. A review of 493 episodes. New England Journal of Medicine 1993; 328: 21–28.*

Encephalitis

Encephalitis is an acute inflammatory process of the brain (encephalon).

Epidemiology

Encephalitis tends to affect children or young adults. The incidence is 0.1 per 100 000 per year.

Pathology

Encephalitis is usually due to a viral infection. The most commonly implicated virus is herpes simplex. Other causes include varicella zoster, influenza A, measles, mumps and enteroviruses. HIV can cause subacute encephalitis or increase the risk of encephalitis due to cytomegalovirus infection. Rarely, prion diseases (Creutzfeldt–Jakob disease) can also cause encephalitis.

Scope of disease

Seizures can occur as a complication of encephalitis.

Clinical features

The symptoms of encephalitis are non-specific, and include fever, headache, behavioural changes, seizures, focal neurological signs or altered conscious levels.

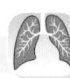

Initial investigations

Full blood count
The white cell count may be raised.

MRI of the brain
MRI is the imaging tool of choice and may reveal cerebral oedema, usually of the temporal lobe.

Lumbar puncture
A lumbar puncture should be performed unless contra-indicated due to evidence of raised intracranial pressure. The cerebrospinal fluid is abnormal with lymphocytosis and elevated protein levels. The cerebrospinal fluid glucose concentration is usually normal. Cerebrospinal fluid PCR for herpes simplex should be performed.

Electroencephalography
The EEG may reveal diffuse slowing or periodic complexes with encephalitis (Fig. 9.31).

Medical management

Aciclovir
Immediate treatment with intravenous aciclovir (an anti-viral agent) is crucial to prevent long-term sequelae. This is a specific treatment for herpes simplex encephali-tis. For CMV encephalitis intravenous ganciclovir can be used.

Anticonvulsants
Seizures should be treated with anticonvulsants (p. 607) and patients may need high-dependency unit care.

Prognosis

The mortality of herpes simplex encephalitis was 70% with severe morbidity in surviving patients (epilepsy, memory impairment, behavioural or personality change). Since the introduction of aciclovir the prognosis has been greatly improved, though mortality and severe morbidity rates remain high (30%).[1]

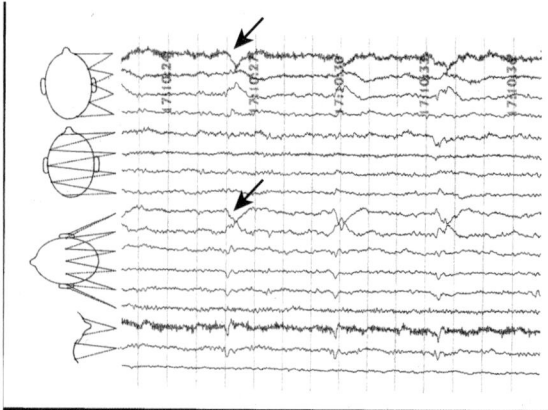

Fig. 9.31 EEG in a patient with herpes simplex encephalitis. Periodic complexes in the right temporal region can be seen (arrows).

REFERENCE

(1) McGrath N, Anderson NE, Croxson MC, Powell KF. Herpes simplex encephalitis treated with acyclovir: diagnosis and long term outcome. Journal of Neurology Neurosurgery and Psychiatry 1997; 63: 321–326.

Cerebral abscess and subdural empyema

Bacterial infections include cerebral abscesses and subdural empyemas. Whilst rare, they are frequently misdiagnosed because of the subtlety of radiological signs.

 CLINICAL ALERT

Bacterial infections resulting in intracranial pus are life-threatening emergencies requiring urgent diagnosis, frequently surgical drainage and appropriate antibiotic therapy.

Epidemiology

Cerebral abscess is rare. It can occur at any age, equally in both sexes. Subdural empyemas are more common in adolescent males.

Pathology

Infection can spread into the cranium and lead to a cerebral abscess or subdural empyema by three routes: direct (from adjacent structures), haematogenous (from a distant site) and via external penetrating trauma.

Direct spread can occur from infection of the paranasal or mastoid air sinuses or the middle ear. Haematogenous spread can lead to multiple cerebral abscesses, and is associated with chronic suppurative lung conditions, congenital cyanotic heart disease, pulmonary arteriovenous fistulae and bacterial endocarditis. Penetrating trauma introduces infection directly into the cranium (hence compound depressed skull fractures are debrided).

Direct infections from the air sinuses and haematogenous spread frequently involve streptococci and are often mixed infections with anaerobes. Infections from penetrating trauma often involve staphylococcal or *Enterobacter* organisms.

The greatest change in intracranial sepsis is probably opportunistic infection related to HIV. When there are multiple intracranial lesions, *Toxoplasma* is the most likely cause. Other infective organisms in this setting include *Nocardia*, tuberculosis, *Cryptococcus*, *Listeria* and fungi.

Scope of disease

A cerebral abscess can rupture into the ventricle, resulting in ventriculitis and hydrocephalus and leading to an increase in mortality (90%). Seizures and focal neurological deficits can also occur.

Clinical features

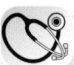

Patients with cerebral abscesses present with symptoms from sepsis, raised intracranial pressure and features of the source of infection. Symptoms include fever, malaise, headache, altered consciousness, seizures and focal neurological deficits.

Patients with subdural empyemas typically present with pyrexia and seizures, often with a background of paranasal air sinus infection.

A detailed clinical assessment also includes the identification of any potential source of the infection.

Initial investigations

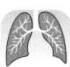

Full blood count
A raised white cell count is common.

Markers of inflammation
The ESR is usually elevated.

Blood cultures
Blood cultures are performed before antibiotics are commenced in an attempt to identify causative organisms.

CT of the head
The diagnosis is generally made with CT scanning (Fig. 9.32). When sepsis is suspected, both non-contrast and contrast scans should be performed. An abscess may start as a low-density region of cerebritis, but evolves with liquefaction

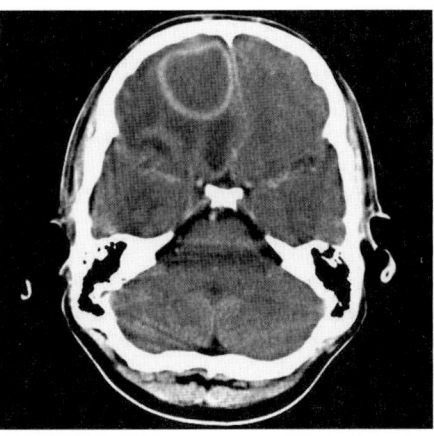

Fig. 9.32 Cerebral abscess on contrast enhanced CT scan. The abscess is seen as a right frontal low-density area with ring enhancement and surrounding oedema.
Courtesy of Mr D Bhattacharyya, Royal Hallamshire Hospital, Sheffield, UK.

necrosis to form a ring enhancing lesion which may be missed if contrast is not given.

The radiological changes of a subdural empyema can be very subtle and limited to an apparently small collection of fluid in the subdural space.

Further investigations

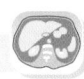

Direct pus cultures
As a rule, an organism should be identified in every case, and this may require the culture of pus obtained from surgical drainage.

Investigations of underlying disease
Further investigations are appropriate to identify any underlying source of infection such as a chest X-ray for patients with a history of suppurative lung disease.

Medical management

Antibiotics
Empirical therapy with a third-generation cephalosporin and metronidazole is indicated if the infection is diagnosed early in the cerebritic phase, when there is no formed pus or when the abscess is small (less than 2 cm in diameter). Antibiotics should be modified when culture results are available.

Anticonvulsants
Given the risk of seizures, anticonvulsant prophylaxis is recommended.

Steroids
The use of steroids to reduce oedema and any potential mass effect is controversial.

Surgical management

The indications for surgical drainage are diagnostic (to identify the pathogen) and therapeutic. The aim is to decompress the abscess, reduce its mass effect and drain the necrotic pus, especially if the abscess is situated adjacent to the ventricle (to prevent intraventricular rupture).

Needle aspiration

Deep abscesses and assessable lesions are preferentially drained by needle aspiration through a burr hole. Aspiration may decrease the duration of antibiotic therapy, but may require repeated aspirations due to reaccumulation of pus.

Excision of the abscess

Superficial abscesses in non-eloquent areas may be drained by an open procedure that involves a craniotomy and excision of the contents and wall of the abscess.

Open debridement

Open debridement is indicated to evacuate any foreign material when an abscess has formed from penetrating trauma.

Burr hole or craniotomy drainage

Treatment of a subdural empyema includes drainage either by burr holes or a craniotomy.

Treatment of the underlying condition

In addition to treating any abscess or empyema, drainage of any associated sinus infection should be considered.

Prognosis

With modern imaging and antibiotics, mortality is less than 10%. The long-term risk of seizures has been estimated to be as high as 50%.

SECTION 9.11 Intracranial tumours

Intracranial tumours can be primary or secondary. Primary intracranial neoplasms can vary from being benign to rapidly growing malignant tumours. Secondary tumours are much more common.

Epidemiology

The incidence of cerebral metastases may be as high as 64 per 100 000 per year, although many of these tumours arise in the context of disseminated metastatic spread and therefore may never be treated by neurological or neurosurgical services. The incidence of primary intracranial tumours is 10 per 100 000 per year.[1]

Pathology

Tumours that most commonly metastasize to the brain include breast carcinoma, lung carcinoma, colorectal carcinoma, testicular tumours, renal cell carcinoma and malignant melanoma.

The most common intrinsic primary brain tumours arise from neuroepithelial cells (gliomas) and may be subdivided according to the cell of origin if well differentiated, e.g. astrocytic tumours. Gliomas are graded from 1 (low grade) to 4 (high grade, e.g. glioblastoma multiforme) as listed in Table 9.38.

The most common extrinsic tumour is a meningioma, which arises from the arachnoid layer of the meninges. This tends to be a benign slow-growing tumour, although rarely it can have atypical or frankly malignant characteristics.

In addition, a number of other types of tumour may arise (Table 9.38).

Scope of disease

The features of an intracranial tumour can arise from destruction of normal brain parenchyma leading to neurological deficits, or abnormal electrical activity leading to seizures. In addition, the enlargement of the tumour may lead to raised intracranial pressure.

Clinical features

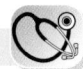

The most common symptom is raised intracranial pressure, and patients may complain of progressive headache that is worst in the morning (isolated headache is uncommon), nausea, vomiting or decreased consciousness. Intracranial tumours may present with progressive focal neurological signs specific to the tumour location. Patients with frontal lobe tumours may present with personality changes. Visual field defects or limb paralysis may occur. In addition, patients can also present with seizures.

Initial investigations

CT/MRI of the head

Contrast enhanced CT or MRI is required for a radiological diagnosis. The origin of the tumour, particularly whether it is from outside the brain pressing in (such as meningiomas,

Table 9.38	Primary intracranial tumours
Tumour type	**Example**
Neuroepithelial tumours (gliomas)	
Astrocytic tumours	Pilocytic (grade I)
	Astrocytoma (grade II)
	Anaplastic astrocytoma (grade III)
	Glioblastoma multiforme (grade IV)
Oligodendroglial tumours	Oligodendroglioma (grade II)
	Anaplastic oligodendroglioma (grade III)
Ependymal tumours	Ependymoma (grade II–IV)
Tumours of the choroid plexus	Choroid plexus papilloma
	Choroid plexus carcinoma
Primitive neuroectodermal tumours	Medulloblastoma (grade IV)
Tumours of the meninges	Meningioma
Cranial nerve tumours	Vestibular schwannoma (acoustic neuroma)
Tumours of the sellar region	Pituitary adenoma
	Craniopharyngioma
Haematological tumours	Primary central nervous system lymphoma

acoustic neuromas), or whether it is intrinsic arising from the brain substance itself, is an important discriminating feature. Patterns of enhancement may give an indication of tumour grade. The location of the tumour is also important in considering the likely cell type of origin. Multiple lesions generally suggest a metastatic process, although gliomas can have a multifocal appearance on occasion.

Care should be taken with radiological interpretation as ring enhancing lesions can be a necrotic tumour, cerebral abscess or rarely an area of cerebral infarction (stroke).

Further investigations

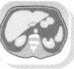

Brain biopsy

Once a space-occupying lesion is identified and if radiological diagnosis is not possible, brain biopsy is usually required to obtain a tissue diagnosis. This is usually done under imaging guidance.

Initial management

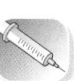

Management of cerebral oedema

Initial therapy may be required to reduce cerebral oedema. Surrounding cerebral oedema caused by rapidly growing tumours may contribute to the symptoms and physical signs. This can be reduced by steroid use (usually dexamethasone 8 mg, 2 times daily).

Intravenous mannitol is occasionally used to reduce increased intracranial pressure. This, however, is a temporary measure and is often used prior to emergency surgery.

Surgical management

Craniotomy and surgical excision

The aims of surgery are to obtain a tissue diagnosis, relieve intracranial pressure and debulk the tumour to facilitate adjuvant treatment. Depending on the tumour size, location and type, complete removal may be achieved (meningioma, vestibular schwannoma). More commonly debulking of the tumour without complete removal is achieved, which can provide symptomatic relief.

Medical management

Radiotherapy

This can extend survival for primary malignant brain tumours and occasionally offer cure for certain tumour types, e.g. medulloblastoma, a primitive neuroectodermal tumour found in the posterior fossa affecting children.

Chemotherapy

Chemotherapy generally has a palliative role in the treatment of intracranial tumours and is usually offered following surgery and radiotherapy for progressive symptoms. Exceptions to this include treatment of primary central nervous system lymphomas and oligodendrogliomas. Chemotherapy is also used as first-line treatment in paediatric gliomas to avoid the complications of radiotherapy.

Anticonvulsants

Antiepileptic drugs may also be required to control seizures.

Prognosis

Prognosis varies according to the type, tumour site, age of the patient and presenting symptoms. Meningiomas are slow-growing tumours that may be successfully treated by surgery and therefore have an excellent prognosis. Low-grade gliomas (astrocytoma WHO grade II) have a median survival of 8–10 years. High-grade gliomas (glioblastoma multiforme) have a median survival of 3 months, though this can be extended by radiotherapy to 12 months.

> **RECENT ADVANCES**
>
> *Extensive research is taking place on newer therapeutic options such as immunotherapy, anti-angiogenesis therapy, targeted toxins and gene therapy.*

REFERENCE

(1) *MacDonald BK, Cockerell OC, Sander JW, Shorvon SD. The incidence and lifetime prevalence of neurological disorders in a prospective community-based study in the UK. Brain 2000; 123 (Pt 4): 665–676.*

SECTION 9.12 Hydrocephalus

Hydrocephalus is an accumulation of cerebrospinal fluid that results in raised intracranial pressure and enlargement of the ventricular system. It arises from either a blockage to the normal cerebrospinal fluid circulation or inadequate cerebrospinal fluid reabsorption. It is rarely due to excess cerebrospinal fluid production.

Epidemiology

The prevalence of infantile hydrocephalus has been reported to be 53 per 100 000.[1]

Pathology

Non-communicating (or obstructive) hydrocephalus occurs due to a blockage of cerebrospinal fluid circulation so that the ventricles enlarge. Cerebrospinal fluid does not circulate over the surface of the brain and is not in continuity with the lumbar cistern. In such circumstances a lumbar puncture is dangerous as it will increase the differential in pressures, potentially resulting in brain shift and herniation. Conversely, with a communicating hydrocephalus there is free flow of cerebrospinal fluid from the ventricular system over the surface of the brain and down to the lumbar cistern. In this case a lumbar puncture may be a useful diagnostic and indeed therapeutic manoeuvre.

A range of tumours, particularly those located in the third and fourth ventricles, can cause obstructive hydrocephalus. In addition, congenital malformations such as Arnold–Chiari malformation may also give rise to obstructive hydrocephalus.

Communicating hydrocephalus may result from infection (most notably bacterial meningitis) or haemorrhage (either spontaneous or from head injury), which may cause blockage of the arachnoid villi and failure of CSF resorption.

Clinical features

The clinical features of hydrocephalus depend on the underlying cause, site and rate of development. In childhood the cranial sutures have not yet fused and so hydrocephalus can manifest as an increasing head circumference.

In the adult, rapid development of hydrocephalus manifests with headache and decreasing level of consciousness, the symptoms of acute raised intracranial pressure. If hydrocephalus arises more slowly, visual failure may also be part of the syndrome. The elderly have a predisposition to develop low-grade hydrocephalus, so-called 'normal pressure hydrocephalus', although this may be a physiological misnomer. It manifests with dementia with early gait apraxia and urinary incontinence. The importance of this condition is that it is potentially treatable but often difficult to distinguish from cerebral atrophy and other more common causes of dementia.

Investigations

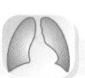

CT/MRI of the brain
Dilated ventricles may be seen on CT (Fig. 9.33), but MRI allows better visualization of the posterior fossa, which may be the site of obstruction.

Lumbar puncture
In suspected cases of normal pressure hydrocephalus, after a mass lesion has been excluded, a lumbar puncture with cerebrospinal fluid drainage may aid in diagnosis. Symptomatic improvement can be assessed objectively by a timed walk.

Management

Cerebrospinal fluid drainage
Consideration needs to be paid to the underlying cause of the hydrocephalus. If the patient is symptomatic from the hydrocephalus, then the management relies on diverting the cerebrospinal fluid. This may be by a shunt, which drains cerebrospinal fluid from the ventricular system into a body cavity, most commonly the peritoneum.

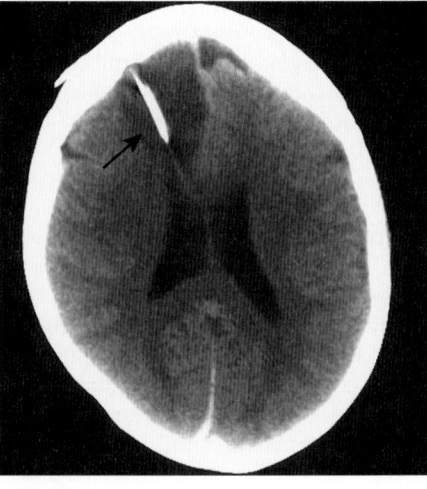

Fig. 9.33 CT scan of a patient with hydrocephalus treated with an external ventricular drain (arrow).

Where there is an obstruction at the level of the aqueduct or fourth ventricle, it may be possible to perform an internal diversion ventriculostomy, a window in the front end of the third ventricle to allow a bypass of the fluid.

Prognosis

This depends on the underlying cause of the problem. The shunt can be complicated by obstruction, infection and overdrainage, resulting in low-pressure headaches or subdural haematoma.

REFERENCE

(1) *Fernell E, Hagberg B, Hagberg G, von Wendt L. Epidemiology of infantile hydrocephalus in Sweden. I. Birth prevalence and general data. Acta Paediatrica Scandinavica 1986; 75: 975–981.*

SECTION 9.13   Diseases of the spinal cord

Syringomyelia

A syringomyelia is a cystic expansion (syrinx) of the central canal in the spinal cord (Fig. 9.34). It may result from abnormal CSF flow and therefore is associated with Arnold–Chiari malformations. Other associated pathologies include spinal tumours and arachnoiditis from previous injury. Most commonly, the cyst develops in the cervical spine and subsequent expansion may compromise the lateral spinothalamic tract giving a cape-like loss of pain and temperature sensation. There may be a lower motor neurone pattern of weakness affecting the arms/hands, with an upper motor neurone pattern of weakness below this. The syrinx can also extend cranially to affect the brainstem. Management is to address any associated hydrocephalus or a Chiari malformation or less commonly to shunt and drain the syrinx.

The spinal cord can be affected by inflammatory lesions (e.g. transverse myelitis, sarcoidosis), tumours or deficiency states such as low B12 (subacute combined degeneration of the cord). It can also be affected by degenerative conditions such as hereditary spastic paraparesis and Friedreich's ataxia.

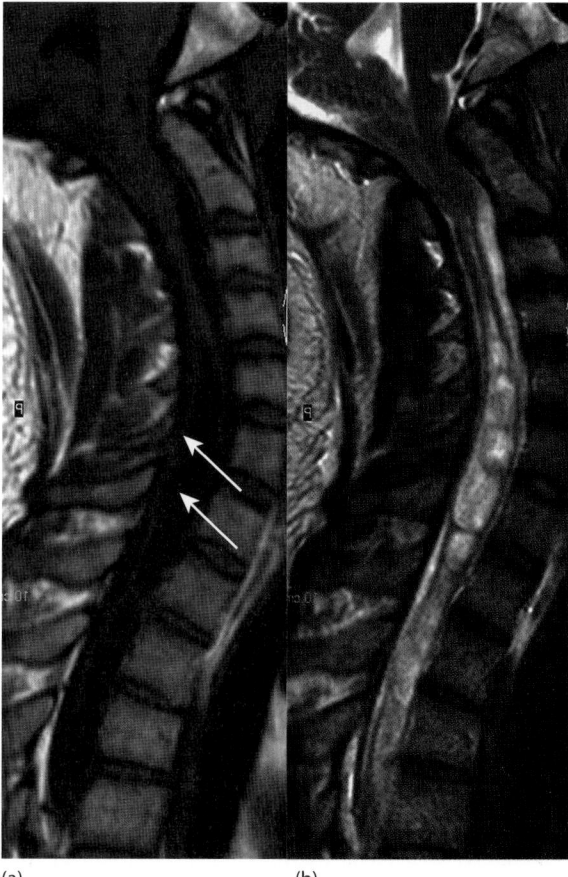

(a)   (b)

Fig. 9.34a, b MRI of a syrinx. (a) T1 and (b) T2 weighted MRI of the spine showing that fluid-filled cavities are present within the spinal cord (arrows).
Courtesy of Mr D Bhattacharyya, Royal Hallamshire Hospital, Sheffield, UK.

SECTION 9.14 # Diseases of the peripheral nerves

Peripheral neuropathies

Peripheral neuropathy can be idiopathic or secondary to an underlying disease process (60%) (Table 9.39). Therefore, identification and treatment of any underlying disease may result in improvement of the peripheral neuropathy.

Epidemiology

Peripheral neuropathy is common: the prevalence is 8% (8000 per 100 000) and it occurs equally in both sexes.[1] Only a small proportion of patients with peripheral neuropathy are referred to a neurology unit for detailed evaluation.

Pathology

The disease process resulting in peripheral neuropathy can affect the nerve fibres (axons) and/or their sheaths (myelin). It can affect both cranial and peripheral nerves and their spinal roots.

The dorsal (sensory) and ventral (motor) spinal roots of each segment of the spinal cord come close together in the intervertebral foramen to form the spinal nerve. Damage of spinal nerves at this level can result from osteophytic compression or disc prolapse, e.g. L5 nerve root compression from lumbar disc prolapse causing loss of sensation over the lateral aspect of the leg, absent ankle reflex and weakness of dorsiflexion.

The two roots fuse to form the spinal nerve, which may then join other spinal roots to form larger nerves. These form a plexus of nerves (e.g. brachial plexus) that subsequently divides into peripheral nerve trunks (e.g. median nerve) supplying both motor and sensory innervation to muscle and skin.

The peripheral nerve trunks contain many fascicles. Each fascicle contains nerve fibres consisting of axons, some of which have a myelin sheath acting as electrical insulation. Thus a total lesion of one fascicle results in only a minor deficit whereas damage to a large number of fascicles (e.g. nerve trunk transection due to a knife wound) will cause both motor and sensory loss in the distribution of that nerve.

Each fascicle is surrounded by perineurium, acting as an effective barrier, and each fascicle has its own connective tissue stroma, the endoneurium. The intraneural blood supply (vasa nervorum) is a rich plexus fed at intervals by nutrient arteries. Widespread disease of small blood vessels can produce nerve ischaemia resulting in nerve dysfunction (e.g. diabetes mellitus, vasculitis due to polyarteritis nodosa).

Damage to the axon causes an axonal neuropathy (e.g. neuropathy due to alcohol abuse). As a result the distal part of the axon degenerates first, the myelin sheath distally breaks down and the nerve cell body undergoes central chromatolysis. The muscles supplied by that nerve will eventually become atrophic, e.g. loss of the thenar eminence in chronic severe carpal tunnel syndrome.

Damage to myelin (demyelinating neuropathy) can be seen in some neuropathies such as Guillain–Barré syndrome

Table 9.39	Causes of peripheral neuropathies

Hereditary

Hereditary motor and sensory neuropathies (HMSN) I–VII

Hereditary liability to pressure palsies

Hereditary sensory and autonomic neuropathies

Familial amyloid polyneuropathies

Acquired

Metabolic
  Diabetes mellitus
  Hypothyroidism
  Porphyria

Vitamin deficiencies
  Vitamin B_{12}
  Thiamine
  Vitamin E

Neoplastic/paraneoplastic
  Associated with any cancer
  Paraproteinaemia/myeloma

Immune mediated
  Guillain–Barré syndrome
  Chronic inflammatory demyelinating polyradiculopathy
  Multifocal motor neuropathy with conduction block
  Vasculitic (in isolation or commonly associated with systemic vasculitis)
  Sarcoidosis
  Gluten sensitivity
  Associated with connective tissue diseases

Toxic
  Heavy metals (lead, arsenic, thallium)
  Alcohol
  Drugs

Infections
  Leprosy
  Lyme disease
  HIV
  Hepatitis C

Associated with organ failure
  Renal failure
  Hepatic failure
  Critical illness polyneuropathy

(acute demyelinating polyradiculopathy), where the myelin sheath is damaged but the axon usually remains intact or is only partially damaged. The recovery may be rapid, but residual deficits may ensue.

Some neuropathies can be mixed axonal and demyelinating (e.g. diabetic neuropathy).

In metabolic, degenerative and toxic neuropathies the largest and longest fibres are the most vulnerable. The nerve fibres 'die back' from the periphery giving the classic symptoms and signs of distal and symmetrical 'glove and stocking' sensory and motor dysfunction. Whilst this is the most common form of neuropathy, sometimes nerve involvement can be patchy and affect individual nerves resulting in single (e.g. ulnar nerve entrapment at the elbow) or multiple mononeuropathies (mononeuritis multiplex as seen, for example, in rheumatoid vasculitis).

Scope of disease

Distal motor weakness from peripheral neuropathy (e.g. foot drop) increases the risk of tripping and falling. Loss of pain sensation predisposes to repeated trauma and this can lead to neuropathic joint deformities (Charcot joint).

Clinical features

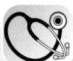

Clinical assessment consists of defining the duration, distribution and severity of peripheral nerve involvement (Figs 9.35 and 9.36) and determining the underlying aetiology.

Patients may complain of 'pins and needles' (paraesthesia), unpleasant sensations such as burning or hypersensitivity (dysaesthesia) or numbness as well as distal weakness (tripping, dropping things). Patients may also complain of the symptoms of other diseases that are the likely cause of their peripheral neuropathy such as diabetes, hypothyroidism (p. 411) and gluten sensitivity. The rapidity of onset and progression may alert to the possibility of a systemic illness (e.g. polyarteritis nodosa) or an underlying malignancy (paraneoplastic neuropathies).

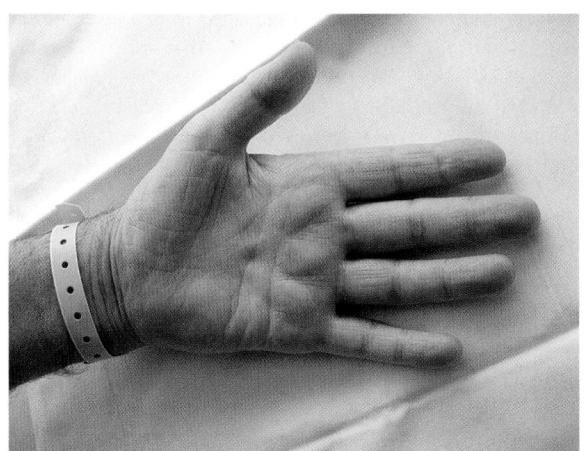

Fig. 9.35 Left median nerve lesion. Image of the palm showing wasting of the thenar eminence.

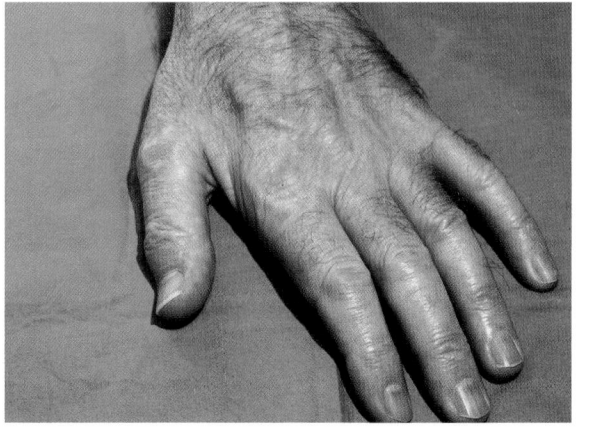

Fig. 9.36 Left ulnar nerve lesion. Image of the dorsum of the hand showing wasting of the first dorsal interosseous muscle.

A family history may suggest a hereditary motor and sensory neuropathy. A detailed drug history is required to exclude any offending medication (e.g. phenytoin, amiodarone) that has peripheral neuropathy as an adverse effect. Enquiry as to the level of alcohol intake is imperative as alcohol abuse is a common cause of peripheral neuropathy.

On examination, assessment of all sensory modalities may provide clues to the aetiology (e.g. loss of vibration and joint position sense in B_{12} deficiency). Global sensory loss in a glove and stocking distribution is most commonly seen in most metabolic or toxic neuropathies. Predominant or exclusive motor involvement with distal weakness and loss of reflexes may be seen in heavy metal poisoning (lead neuropathy). Asymmetry of nerve involvement may suggest multiple mononeuropathy (e.g. as seen in Wegener's granulomatosis) or an individual nerve root pathology (wrist drop due to trauma of the radial nerve).

Initial investigations

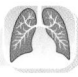

Full blood count
Macrocytosis may indicate vitamin B_{12} deficiency or excessive alcohol intake.

Markers of inflammation
Elevated ESR may suggest an ongoing inflammatory disease process (e.g. vasculitis).

Urea and electrolytes
Chronic renal failure can cause peripheral neuropathy, and systemic vasculitis causing peripheral neuropathy may be associated with renal failure.

Liver profile
Elevated gamma-glutamyltransferase may indicate alcohol abuse. Elevated transaminases may suggest hepatitis.

Random plasma glucose

This is used to screen for diabetes, which is probably the most common cause of peripheral neuropathy in developed countries.

Serum B$_{12}$ levels

Vitamin B$_{12}$ deficiency can cause peripheral neuropathy and subacute combined degeneration of the spinal cord.

Thyroid stimulating hormone

Serum TSH levels may reveal hypothyroidism (causing sensorimotor axonal neuropathy) or thyrotoxicosis (associated with predominantly motor neuropathy).

Serum paraprotein screen

Both monoclonal gammopathy of undetermined significance and myeloma are associated with peripheral neuropathy.

Autoimmune and vasculitic screen

This investigation aims to diagnose connective tissue diseases and vasculitides, important causes of a peripheral neuropathy which tends to be asymmetrical (mononeuropathy multiplex).

Anti-gliadin antibodies

Up to a quarter of patients with coeliac disease on a gluten-free diet have evidence of peripheral neuropathy, but gluten neuropathy may exist without an enteropathy (presence of anti-gliadin antibodies).

Chest X-ray

A peripheral 'coin' lesion may suggest lung cancer, and bilateral hilar lymphadenopathy may indicate sarcoidosis.

Nerve conduction studies and electromyography

This investigation should help confirm the clinical suspicion of a peripheral neuropathy as well as the pattern of nerve involvement (e.g. sensory vs motor or mixed). In addition it can distinguish between demyelinating (slow conduction) and axonal (reduced amplitude) neuropathies. Such distinction is important because of the therapeutic implications.

Further investigations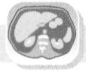

Thermal thresholds

This investigation is useful if a small fibre neuropathy is suspected, as seen in diabetes.

Lumbar puncture for cerebrospinal fluid examination

This should be done in patients with demyelinating neuropathies where an immune-mediated pathogenesis is suspected (e.g. Guillain–Barré syndrome). The cerebrospinal fluid protein level in such cases may be elevated. If there is clinical suspicion, CSF examination may reveal the presence of abnormal cells in an infiltrative process (sacral plexus infiltration from cancer) or the presence of infection (e.g. borreliosis).

Screening for malignancy

Paraneoplastic antibodies such as anti-Hu may have a role in the pathogenesis. Whole body imaging with CT and PET scanning may be necessary to detect occult cancer.

Rare vitamin deficiencies/excess

Less common causes include vitamin E deficiency, thiamine deficiency and pyridoxine (vitamin B$_6$) excess.

Infective causes

Peripheral neuropathy can be seen in the context of HIV infection, hepatitis C, leprosy and Lyme disease (infection with *Borrelia* following a tick bite).

Medical management

Treatment of underlying cause

Management depends on the underlying cause of the peripheral neuropathy (e.g. optimal glycaemic control in diabetic neuropathy results in improvement); this can be found in the appropriate section.

Supportive care

Supportive and symptomatic care are also important and include drugs for unpleasant dysaesthesiae, decompression of entrapment neuropathies, physiotherapy to optimize mobility and ensure safety, and the use of aids such as ankle splints to help foot drop.

Prognosis

The course of the disease depends very much on the underlying cause. In general, neuropathies with axonal loss (e.g. alcohol related) are said to be less likely to recover fully by comparison to demyelinating neuropathies (e.g. Guillain–Barré syndrome). There are notable exceptions; e.g. axonal neuropathy related to hypothyroidism may fully recover with thyroxine replacement.

When no underlying cause is found, patients should remain under regular review. Re-investigation may be indicated if the neuropathy progresses, e.g. to exclude the development of diabetes mellitus in a patient with subclinical glucose intolerance or the development of symptomatic malignancy in previously occult cancer. Spontaneous recovery is rare but stabilization is common if investigations remain normal.

REFERENCE

(1) Martyn CN, Hughes RA. *Epidemiology of peripheral neuropathy. Journal of Neurology Neurosurgery and Psychiatry* 1997; 62: 310–318.

Genetic neuropathies

The genetic neuropathies are a rapidly evolving field because of advances in chromosomal linkage and gene identification. Hereditary motor and sensory neuropathies (HMSN) are commonly referred to as Charcot–Marie–Tooth (CMT) disease. The nomenclature remains confusing as CMT type 1 is also known as HMSN type I. CMT type 2 (same as HMSN II) is an inherited axonal neuropathy, which is less common than CMT 1.

There are other inherited neuropathies (HMSN III–VII, hereditary autonomic neuropathies and familial amyloid polyneuropathies) but these are rare.

Epidemiology

HMSN type I is by far the most common inherited neuropathy with an estimated prevalence of 1:2500. It affects both sexes equally, and the onset of symptoms occurs in the first or second decade of life.

Pathology

HMSN type I is inherited as an autosomal dominant disorder that results from duplication in chromosome 17p11.2–12. Approximately 20% are due to spontaneous mutations (no family history). The neuropathy is demyelinating, resulting in reduced conduction velocities. In hereditary neuropathy with liability to pressure palsies, the underlying genetic abnormality is deletion rather than duplication of the same portion of chromosome 17 that causes CMT 1.

Clinical features
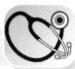

The chronicity and early onset of these neuropathies usually results in skeletal abnormalities such as pes cavus (Fig. 9.37) and hammer toes. Patients with hereditary neuropathies often seek medical advice because of foot

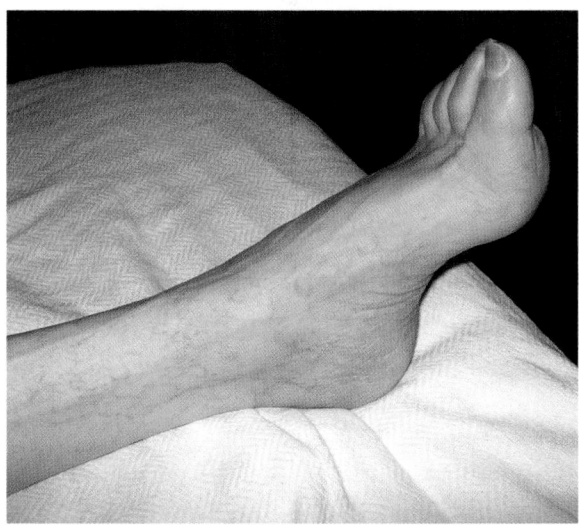

Fig. 9.37 Pes cavus.

deformities causing pressure changes and painful calluses. Distal muscle weakness and atrophy in the legs is very prominent ('inverted champagne bottle' appearance). Contrary to acquired neuropathies, these patients may not often complain of sensory symptoms even if the neurophysiological assessment shows severe disease. It is estimated that up to 25% of patients are asymptomatic.

Investigations
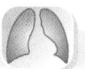

Neurophysiological studies
Neurophysiological studies may reveal peripheral nerve disorders.

Management

Supportive treatment
Treatment is supportive for all the inherited neuropathies.

Genetic counselling
Most genetic centres offer diagnostic genetic testing (chromosome 17p11.2–12 duplication in HMSN type I) as well as genetic counselling for the patient and his or her family.

Prognosis

The prognosis is that of slow progressive disease in the majority.

Chronic inflammatory demyelinating polyradiculopathy

Chronic inflammatory demyelinating polyradiculopathy (CIDP) is a disease of unknown aetiology that primarily affects myelinated nerves producing symptoms of weakness and sensory loss sometimes associated with arm tremor. With time, axonal loss may occur producing permanent disability. CIDP responds to treatment with corticosteroids, plasma exchange or intravenous immunoglobulins as well as other immunosuppressive agents.

Variants of CIDP include multifocal motor neuropathy with conduction block characterized by exclusively motor nerve involvement and conduction block (failure of conduction through a peripheral nerve as seen on neurophysiological assessment). Intravenous immunoglobulins are very effective in this condition, which is not responsive to corticosteroids

Guillain–Barré syndrome

Guillain–Barré syndrome is a rare immune-mediated neuropathy that can follow any infection, most commonly

Campylobacter jejuni enteritis. The infection usually resolves prior to the development of neurological symptoms, which are those of a rapidly ascending weakness with or without sensory loss and with loss of reflexes. Mildly affected patients may not require any specific treatment and can expect to recover fully within weeks or months. More severely affected patients may require supportive treatment for respiratory failure, cardiovascular disturbance and thromboembolism. Such patients may also make a full recovery but this tends to be over several months. Plasma exchange and intravenous immunoglobulins have proven beneficial in expediting recovery.[1,2] Up to 50% of patients may have evidence of residual damage of peripheral nerves on neurophysiological testing.

REFERENCES

(1) *Hughes RA, Raphael JC, Swan AV, Doorn PA. Intravenous immunoglobulin for Guillain-Barre syndrome. The Cochrane Database of Systematic Reviews 2004: CD002063.*
(2) *Raphaël JC, Chevret S, Hughes RAC, Annane D. Plasma exchange for Guillain-Barré syndrome. The Cochrane Database of Systematic Reviews 2002, Issue 2 Art no: 10.1002/14651858.CD0017982.*

SECTION 9.15 Diseases of muscle and the motor end plate

Weakness is the main presenting symptom of disease of muscle. The distribution and characteristics of the muscle weakness and its associated features (pain, absent reflexes) assist in formulating a diagnosis. This section covers genetically determined myopathies (muscular dystrophies and myotonia) as well as disorders of the neuromuscular junction (myasthenia gravis and Lambert–Eaton myasthenic syndrome). Many myopathies are acquired, and some of the conditions that can result in myopathy are discussed in the relevant chapters (Table 9.40).

Myasthenia gravis

Myasthenia gravis is a chronic autoimmune disease of the neuromuscular junction. It affects the skeletal (voluntary) muscles of the body and is characterized by fatigable muscle weakness.

Epidemiology

The incidence of myasthenia gravis is 1 per 100 000 per year, women being more frequently affected than men. It can present at any age, although in men it tends to occur in later life (>60 years old) and in women it has two peaks—between the ages of 16 and 35, and after 65 years of age.

Pathology

Neuromuscular transmission relies on the arrival of an action potential at the nerve terminal with the subsequent release of the excitatory neurotransmitter, acetylcholine, which crosses the neuromuscular junction. Acetylcholine binds to the acetylcholine receptors on the motor end plate; an action potential is then initiated leading to muscle contraction. Acetylcholine is broken down by acetylcholinesterase.

Table 9.40	Causes of myopathy

Inherited

Muscular dystrophy
Myotonic dystrophy
Inherited metabolic myopathy
   Glycogen storage disorders
   Lipid metabolism disorders
Ion flux disorders
   Hypokalaemic periodic paralysis
   Hyperkalaemic periodic paralysis
   Paramyotonic congenita

Acquired

Endocrine
   Diabetes
   Thyrotoxicosis
   Hypothyroidism
   Cushing's disease
   Addison's disease
   Vitamin D deficiency
Drugs and toxins
   Alcohol
   Steroids
   HMG-CoA reductase inhibitors (statins)
Inflammatory
   Polymyositis
   Dermatomyositis
   Inclusion body myositis
   Infections (e.g. HIV)

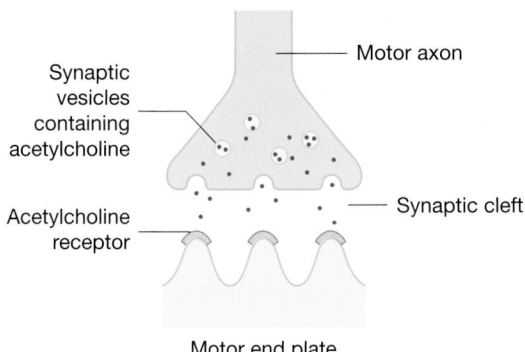

Fig. 9.38 The neuromuscular junction. Myasthenia gravis is an autoantibody-mediated post-synaptic disorder of the neuromuscular junction.

Myasthenia gravis is an autoantibody-mediated post-synaptic disorder of the neuromuscular junction (Fig. 9.38). IgG anti-acetylcholine receptor antibodies are detectable in 85% of patients and result in blockade and destruction of acetylcholine receptors. Seronegative myasthenia gravis is also antibody mediated but there are antibodies against muscle-specific kinase and other unknown antigens.

The thymus gland is frequently abnormal in patients with antibody-positive myasthenia gravis. Early onset disease (less than 40 years of age) is associated with thymic hyperplasia, and thymomas are present in 10% of cases.

Myasthenia gravis may be induced by treatment with penicillamine. It is also associated with rheumatoid arthritis, systemic lupus erythematosus, type 1 diabetes and thyrotoxicosis.

Scope of disease

The main complication of myasthenia gravis is the myasthenic crisis. This is characterized by respiratory difficulties, when ventilatory support may be required. Myasthenic crisis may be the presenting complaint of newly diagnosed myasthenia gravis. It may, however, be triggered by infection, pregnancy, emotional stress or the use of certain drugs such as aminoglycoside antibiotics (e.g. gentamicin) in patients with pre-existing myasthenia. In addition, there is a risk of aspiration pneumonia when there is bulbar weakness.

Clinical features

Myasthenia gravis may affect any voluntary muscle although the external ocular muscles, bulbar muscles, neck and shoulder girdle muscles are those most frequently affected.

The most common presenting complaint is diplopia and ptosis, and the eyes may be the only affected sites of the body (ocular myasthenia). Generalized myasthenia may result in facial weakness (myasthenic snarl), dysarthria (nasal speech), dysphagia, regurgitation of fluids through the nose (due to palatal weakness), neck weakness lead-ing to a forward head tilt, limb weakness and breathing difficulties.

Symptoms become worse with prolonged use. Dysphagia and difficulties in chewing increase through the course of a meal, ptosis is worse at the end of the day, and dysarthria worsens during a telephone conversation.

On examination, muscle wasting is rare and the reflexes are retained. There is no sensory loss and the classic feature is muscle fatigability. Testing of muscle strength therefore may initially be normal but weakness may become apparent after repeated exercise.

Initial investigations

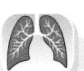

Acetylcholine receptor antibodies
The diagnosis of myasthenia gravis is definite if these antibodies are present; however, they are negative in 15% of generalized myasthenia and in 50% of ocular myasthenia cases.

Electromyography
In myasthenia gravis repetitive nerve stimulation results in a decrement of compound muscle action potential, however it is normal in ocular myasthenia.

Single fibre electromyography
This is more sensitive than EMG, and the orbicularis oculi can be tested. An increase in jitter is suggestive of myasthenia.

Edrophonium (Tensilon) test
Edrophonium is a short-acting anticholinesterase that can be used to test the reversibility of muscle weakness. It should be used with caution in those with asthma or bradycardia as its adverse effects include bronchoconstriction, increased bronchial secretions, bradycardia and asystole, abdominal cramps and excessive sweating (p. 395).

Pulmonary function tests
Forced vital capacity should be checked if there are any concerns regarding breathing. A low or rapidly falling FVC may indicate that ventilation is required.

Further investigations

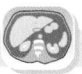

CT of the thorax
CT of the thorax is indicated in patients with positive acetylcholine receptor antibodies due to the association with thymoma (p. 173) and thymic hyperplasia.

Medical management

Anticholinesterase
Pyridostigmine is the anticholinesterase of choice. Symptomatic relief is often achieved. Gastrointestinal side effects

Myasthenia gravis

Lambert–Eaton myasthenic syndrome

Muscular dystrophy

629

such as abdominal cramps can be treated with an antimuscarinic agent such as propantheline.

Immunomodulation

If pyridostigmine is inadequate for symptomatic control then immunosuppression is required. This is achieved with prednisolone starting at a low dose and increasing gradually to 1.5 mg/kg on alternate days. Generalized myasthenia may worsen when steroids are introduced, and ideally patients should be admitted to hospital for initiation of prednisolone treatment. The target dose should be maintained until symptoms improve, and then the dose is slowly reduced. Ocular myasthenia does not usually require such a high dose of prednisolone.

Azathioprine (2.5 mg/kg) is often introduced as a steroid-sparing agent. It should be introduced early as its effects can take up to a year to appear.[1] Alternative immunosuppressants are ciclosporin and methotrexate.

> ### ⚡ CLINICAL ALERT
>
> *During a myasthenic crisis management of the airway is vital. Patients may require ventilatory support. Short-term relief of symptoms can be obtained by plasma exchange or with intravenous immunoglobulin therapy. Adjustments are then made to the pyridostigmine or immunosuppressive regimen.*

Surgical management

Thymectomy

Thymectomy is indicated for patients with an associated thymoma (p. 173). Patients without a thymoma may also obtain remission or symptom improvement following thymectomy, however randomized trials are awaited to evaluate the efficacy of surgery in this regard.[2]

Prognosis

The prognosis for ocular myasthenia is good: many develop complete remission or significant improvement on treatment. The overall remission rate is 21% at 10 years.[3] Mortality is still associated with generalized myasthenia though the prognosis has improved with immunosuppressive treatment. The overall survival probability at 5, 10 and 20 years is 81%, 69% and 63% respectively.[4]

i FURTHER INFORMATION

Hanna MG. Neuromuscular disease; muscle. Current Opinion in Neurology 2001; 14: 539–575.

REFERENCES

(1) *Palace J, Newsom-Davis J, Lecky B. A randomized double-blind trial of prednisolone alone or with azathioprine in myasthenia gravis. Myasthenia Gravis Study Group. Neurology 1998; 50: 1778–1783.*
(2) *Gronseth GS, Barohn RJ. Practice parameter: thymectomy for autoimmune myasthenia gravis (an evidence-based review): report of the Quality Standards Subcommittee of the American Academy of Neurology. Neurology 2000; 55: 7–15.*
(3) *Beghi E, Antozzi C, Batocchi AP, et al. Prognosis of myasthenia gravis: a multicenter follow-up study of 844 patients. Journal of Neurological Science 1991; 106: 213–220.*
(4) *Christensen PB, Jensen TS, Tsiropoulos I, et al. Mortality and survival in myasthenia gravis: a Danish population based study. Journal of Neurology Neurosurgery and Psychiatry 1998; 64: 78–83.*

Lambert–Eaton myasthenic syndrome

Lambert–Eaton myasthenic syndrome is a rare autoantibody-mediated pre-synaptic disorder of the neuromuscular junction. The autoantibody target is voltage-gated calcium channels, and the syndrome is associated with small cell carcinoma of the lung.

Lambert–Eaton myasthenic syndrome presents with difficulties walking due to proximal muscle weakness and is associated with autonomic dysfunction (constipation, impotence and dry mouth). Fatigue is not a feature, muscle strength can actually improve on testing, and reflexes are depressed or absent but can also reappear on testing of the muscle. EMG reveals increment of the initially reduced compound muscle action potential after maximum voluntary contraction and anti-voltage-gated calcium channel antibodies can be detected.

Muscular dystrophy

Compared to Duchenne's muscular dystrophy, Becker's (X-linked) is a less severe genetic disorder of dystrophin. The severity of the disease is variable and correlates with the reduction of dystrophin protein. The onset is between 5 and 25 years, and although most patients are unable to walk after the age of 25, many have a normal life expectancy. Clinical features include limb girdle weakness with pseudohypertrophy of the calf muscles.

The muscular dystrophies are a group of inherited disorders of muscle characterized by progressive weakness and degeneration of skeletal muscles. Duchenne's muscular dystrophy, an X-linked recessive disorder, is the most common form affecting children whereas myotonic dystrophy is the most common form affecting adults. Other varieties of X-linked, autosomal dominant and autosomal recessive muscular dystrophies are briefly described. In addition other forms of muscle disease can produce myotonia such as channelopathies (disorders of the ion channels).

Facio-scapulo-humeral dystrophy is an autosomal dominant disease that develops from childhood and progresses into adulthood. The abnormality is detected on chromosome 4. There is weakness of the facial muscles, shoulder and limb girdle muscles, often in an asymmetrical fashion. The progression is very slow and life expectancy is normal.

Limb girdle dystrophy is a heterogeneous group that is inherited as an autosomal recessive or dominant form. The onset of limb girdle weakness occurs between 10 and 20 years old and gradually becomes more severe over 20–25 years. It is associated with a reduced life expectancy.

Duchenne's muscular dystrophy

Epidemiology

The incidence of Duchenne's muscular dystrophy is approximately 29 per 100 000 live male births.

Pathology

Duchenne's muscular dystrophy is an X-linked recessive disorder of the dystrophin gene that results in a marked reduction of the dystrophin protein in muscle.

Scope of disease

With time, patients become increasingly disabled, develop contractures and scoliosis and are at an increased risk of respiratory infection and failure. The myocardium may be affected resulting in cardiomyopathy.

Clinical features

Initial presenting features include difficulties in walking, running and climbing stairs or frequent falls. This condition is usually apparent by the age of 4, and those affected may demonstrate Gowers' sign, climbing up their legs with their hands to rise from the floor. On examination a waddling gait may be evident (due to pelvic muscle weakness) and there may be pseudohypertrophy of the calf muscles and weakness of the shoulder girdle muscles.

Initial investigations
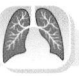

Creatine kinase
This is elevated by 100–200 times in Duchenne's muscular dystrophy (it is only slightly raised in limb girdle or facio-scapulo-humeral dystrophy).

Muscle biopsy
Dystrophic features—including variation in muscle fibre size, fibre necrosis and regeneration—may be demonstrated.

Electromyography
Myopathic changes are seen, characterized by small-amplitude and short-duration motor unit potentials.

Initial management
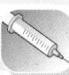

Supportive treatment
There is no curative treatment available and management remains supportive. Initially psychological support needs to be offered to the parents and family. Physical aids may be required to improve mobility and splints for muscle contractures.

Genetic counselling
Genetic screening and counselling is offered to establish the carrier status in female members of the family.

Medical management

Corticosteroids
Corticosteroid therapy improves muscle strength and function in the short-term and so aids in prolonging ambulation.[3]

Non-invasive ventilation
When respiratory function begins to decline, non-invasive ventilatory support such as nocturnal intermittent positive pressure ventilation has been shown to prove both quality and duration of life.[1]

Surgical management

Scoliosis surgery
Surgery to correct scoliosis improves respiratory function and quality of life in selected patients with severe spinal deformity.[2]

Prognosis

This disease is slowly progressive and by the age of 10 the patient will be severely disabled and require a wheelchair. By the age of 25 half of those affected will have died from respiratory infection or cardiac failure.[1]

REFERENCES

(1) Eagle M, Baudouin SV, Chandler C, Giddings DR, Bullock R, Bushby K. Survival in Duchenne muscular dystrophy: improvements in life expectancy since 1967 and the impact of home nocturnal ventilation. Neuromuscular Disorders 2002; 12: 926–929.
(2) Cervellati S, Bettini N, Moscato M, Gusella A, Dema E, Maresi R. Surgical treatment of spinal deformities in Duchenne muscular dystrophy: a long term follow-up study. European Spine Journal 2004; 13: 441–448.
(3) Glucocorticoid corticosteroids for Duchenne muscular dystrophy. Cochrane Database Syst Rev. 2004; (2):CD003725.

Myotonic dystrophy

Myotonic dystrophy (dystrophia myotonica) is characterized by muscular atrophy and myotonia (the continued contraction of muscle after voluntary effort has ceased, e.g. slowness in relaxing hand grip).

Epidemiology

The incidence of myotonic dystrophy is approximately 5 per 100 000 per year.

Pathology

Myotonic dystrophy is an autosomal dominant multisystem disorder (Fig. 9.39). It is caused by the expansion of a trinucleotide repeat in the myotrophin protein kinase gene on chromosome 19, resulting in an abnormal chloride channel function on the muscle membrane. Myotonic dystrophy is a genetic disorder that demonstrates anticipation: each successive generation develops the condition with increasing severity and at an earlier age.

Scope of disease

Associated features of myotonic dystrophy include frontal balding in men, ptosis, cataracts, sensorineural deafness, cognitive slowing, dysphagia and constipation (due to involvement of the smooth muscle of the oesophagus and colon), impaired pulmonary function, endocrine abnormalities (thyroid dysfunction and diabetes mellitus), gonadal atrophy, cardiomyopathy and conduction defects.

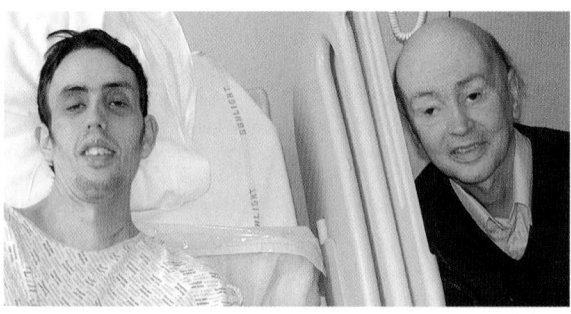

Fig. 9.39 Father and son with myotonic dystrophy. The disease is inherited as an autosomal dominant condition.

With progressive disease, myotonic dystrophy carries an increased risk of death from respiratory infection and cardiac failure.

Clinical features

This is a disease of variable severity. Patients tend to become symptomatic between the ages of 20 and 50 years. The presenting complaint is usually hand weakness or difficulty walking. There is slowly progressive muscle weakness and atrophy that is initially distal (Fig. 9.40). Patients may also present with one of the associated features, e.g. cataract.

On examination there is facial myopathy with wasting of the masseters, temporal and sternomastoid muscles (Fig. 9.41). Patients are areflexic, myotonia is present, and percussion myotonia may be demonstrated—tapping the thenar eminence gives rise to a long-lasting indentation.

Initial investigations
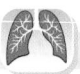

Creatine kinase
This is elevated by 2–10 times in dystrophia myotonica, unlike the other hereditary myotonias.

Electromyography
This is abnormal with high-frequency discharges and myopathic changes are seen in wasted muscles.

Muscle biopsy
Dystrophic changes are seen with splitting of muscle fibres with central nuclei.

Further investigations
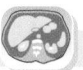

Electrocardiogram
A 12 lead ECG is performed to screen for the presence of conduction block.

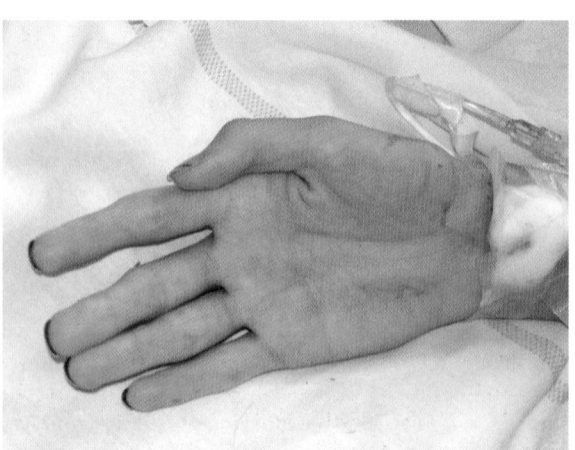

Fig. 9.40 Wasting of the small muscles of the hand.

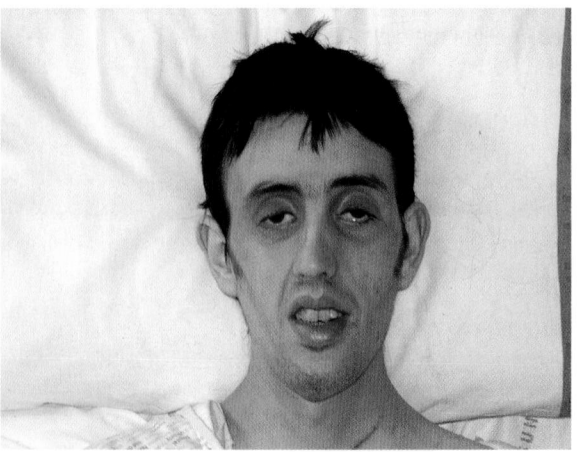

Fig. 9.41 A patient with myotonic dystrophy showing bilateral ptosis and facial myopathy.

Muscular dystrophy

Motor neurone disease

Hereditary spastic
paraparesis

Thyroid function tests

Thyroid function tests are performed to screen for hypo-thyroidism or hyperthyroidism.

Random blood glucose

A random blood glucose is performed to screen for the development of diabetes mellitus.

Initial management

Screening for complications

Annual review should be performed with review of the ECG, eyes and monitoring of thyroid function to screen for complications. The onset of conduction block may necessitate the insertion of a pacemaker.

Physical support

Occupational therapy and physiotherapy are required to optimize function and mobility.

Genetic screening

Currently preclinical and antenatal diagnosis is possible, therefore genetic analysis and counselling should be offered to family members.

Medical therapy

The mainstay of treatment is supportive measures.

Non-invasive ventilation

With progressive disease, non-invasive ventilatory support may be required.

Antimyotonic agents

Mexiletine, phenytoin or procainamide may help improve symptomatic myotonia (it is frequently asymptomatic).

Prognosis

The disease is slowly progressive and patients may be disabled 15–20 years after diagnosis. The 10-year survival probability is 80%, and the mean age at death is 53 years.[1]

REFERENCE

(1) *Mathieu J, Allard P, Potvin L, Prevost C, Begin P. A 10-year study of mortality in a cohort of patients with myotonic dystrophy. Neurology 1999; 52:1658–1662.*

SECTION 9.16 Neurodegenerative diseases

The neurodegenerative diseases are a group of diseases that begin insidiously, following normal neural function, and pursue a gradually progressive course that may continue for months to many years. It is usually impossible to determine the date of onset. The family of the patient may attribute the onset of the symptoms to a specific event (e.g. a surgical procedure, minor trauma) but on close questioning there are often subtle symptoms that predate the event. As a rule these diseases run a progressive course and with very few exceptions are not influenced by any medical or surgical intervention. Dementia (p. 593) can be seen as part of other neurological entities such as idiopathic Parkinson's disease, progressive supranuclear palsy, Huntington's disease, prion disease, and motor neurone disease.

Motor neurone disease

Motor neurone disease, also known as amyotrophic lateral sclerosis, is characterized by progressive degeneration of the upper and lower motor neurones. The majority of cases are sporadic but up to 5% have a familial history due to mutation of the superoxide dismutase gene.

Epidemiology

The prevalence is 10 per 100 000, and the disease presents in patients at an approximate age of 55. It is approximately twice as common in men.

Pathology

The aetiology remains obscure and may include environmental, infective, toxic and immunological causes. Glutamate excitotoxicity and free radical injury is a current focus of research.

Clinical features

The initial presenting feature is wasting and weakness of a hand or leg, leading to difficulties with turning a key in a lock or coping with buttons or a foot drop. The onset is insidious and the weakness is progressive and may be asymmetrical. Muscle fasciculations are prominent early in the disease process. Speech disturbance occurs when bulbar muscles are affected, and impairment of respiratory muscle strength results in hypoventilation and CO_2 retention. With time, swallowing is affected leading to weight loss and risk of aspiration, and progressive paralysis results in increasing difficulties with mobilization.

Clinical examination reveals a mixture of upper (weakness, increased tone, brisk reflex, extensor plantar response) and lower motor neurone dysfunction (weakness, wasting, absent reflexes, fasciculations) in the absence of any sensory involvement. Cognitive decline and dementia can be seen in the context of motor neurone disease, implying that the pathology is not exclusively confined to the motor neurones.

Investigations

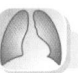

The diagnosis is usually clinical with support from neurophysiological assessment.

Electrodiagnostic studies
The principal features are chronic partial denervation and widespread fasciculation potentials with normal sensory potentials.

Management

The care of patients with motor neurone disease is challenging because of rapid progression, impending respiratory difficulty and severe loss of function with inability to communicate and feed. A multidisciplinary team approach (neurologist, nurse, dietitian, physiotherapist, speech therapist, respiratory physician) is essential.

Nutrition
Appropriate measures to prevent aspiration with progressive bulbar disease include insertion of a PEG feeding tube (p. 236). Adequate nutritional intake is essential and may prolong survival in addition to reducing the risk of aspiration.

Riluzole
Riluzole is an antiglutamate agent that slows the progression of motor neurone disease, and may improve survival.[1]

Non-invasive ventilation
Non-invasive ventilation is required for patients with respiratory failure. It improves the quality of life and prolongs survival.

Prognosis

The median time from diagnosis to death is 4 years, and the 5-year survival is 25%.

REFERENCE

(1) Bensimon G, Lacomblez L, Meininger V. *The ALS/Riluzole Study Group. A controlled trial of riluzole in amyotrophic lateral sclerosis. New England Journal of Medicine* 1994; 330: 585–591.

Hereditary spastic paraparesis

Hereditary spastic paraparesis has a prevalence of up to 10 per 100 000. The most common inheritance mode is autosomal dominant. Patients complain of lower limb spasticity, which impairs their walking ability. A large number will have evidence of distal wasting with pes cavus. The diagnosis is based on the clinical picture, the exclusion of spinal and brain pathology on imaging and the presence of other affected members of the family. There is considerable familial heterogeneity: some family members have only minimal signs (e.g. just pes cavus and brisk reflexes) whilst others are severely affected.

Diseases of the eye

10

Jodhbir S Mehta, Ben Burton

SECTION 10.1 ## Introduction

Applied basic sciences of the eye

Anatomy

The eye is an important organ for sight. The anatomy of the eye is divided into three sections: the external anatomy (Fig. 10.1), the internal anatomy (Fig. 10.2) and the anatomy of the fundus.

Physiology

Cornea

The cornea is transparent as a result of destructive interference patterns set up by regularly aligned and spaced collagen fibres. If this spacing and alignment is interrupted, the cornea will become cloudy (corneal oedema or trauma). To keep the cornea dehydrated and transparent, numerous endothelial cells pump water out of the cornea and into the anterior chamber. These may be damaged in disease or following surgical trauma and do not regenerate. The cornea is also transparent because it does not contain any blood vessels. This lack of a blood supply also means that it is an immunologically privileged site. Corneal allografts are relatively well tolerated without the need for HLA matching or immunomodulation.

Aqueous secretion and drainage

The ciliary body just behind the iris is constantly producing watery aqueous which circulates from behind the iris through the pupil and drains through the trabecular meshwork which is situated in the angle between the iris and the inner surface of the cornea. If this circulation through the pupil is obstructed (angle closure glaucoma or seclusio pupillae) then the pressure will increase dramatically from a normal range of 10–21 mmHg up to 60 or 70 mmHg with damage to the optic nerve (causing glaucoma, p. 669). Pressure may also increase if the trabecular meshwork is obstructed by blood or if it does not drain fluid effectively (primary open angle glaucoma or following steroid use). In certain circumstances the ciliary body may stop producing fluid, the pressure in the eye will drop to zero and the eye eventually becomes blind and shrunken (phthisis bulbi), a common end stage for many severe eye problems (trauma, endophthalmitis, retinal detachment).

Photoreceptor function

The retina has photoreceptors that detect light of different wavelengths and pass signals to the brain via the optic nerve. Rods are photoreceptors that only work in the dark and are very sparse in the fovea. Loss of photoreceptors (retinitis pigmentosa) causes night blindness and loss of the peripheral visual field.

Cones may be red sensitive, green sensitive or blue sensitive. They are more common at the fovea and macula and are essential for normal daylight vision and colour perception. Hereditary conditions may affect only the cone system, leaving patients with poor daylight vision but relatively good night vision. Some patients may be missing one type of cone or have abnormal cone function for one wavelength. This most commonly occurs as an X-linked

635

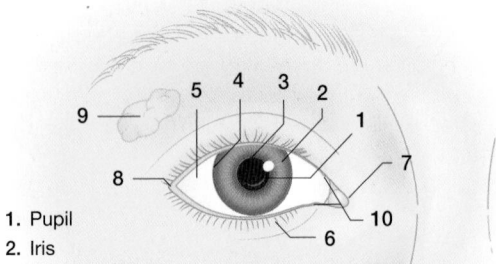

1. Pupil
2. Iris
3. Cornea (transparent tissue in front of the iris and pupil)
4. Limbus (where the clear cornea meets the white sclera)
5. Sclera (white with overlying episclera and conjunctiva)
6. Meibomian glands (in upper and lower eyelids with orifices at the lid margin)
7. Medial canthus
8. Lateral canthus
9. Site of lacrimal gland
10. Puncti (leading to canaliculi and then nasolacrimal duct)

Fig. 10.1 Important anatomical structures of the eye: 1, pupil; 2, iris; 3, cornea (transparent tissue in front of the iris and pupil); 4, limbus (where the clear cornea meets the white sclera); 5, sclera (white with overlying episclera and conjunctiva); 6, meibomian glands (in upper and lower eyelids with orifices at the lid margin); 7, medial canthus; 8, lateral canthus; 9, site of lacrimal gland; 10, puncti (leading to canaliculi and then nasolacrimal duct).

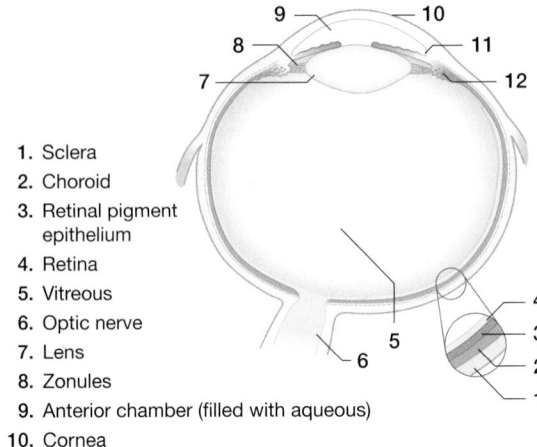

1. Sclera
2. Choroid
3. Retinal pigment epithelium
4. Retina
5. Vitreous
6. Optic nerve
7. Lens
8. Zonules
9. Anterior chamber (filled with aqueous)
10. Cornea
11. Trabecular meshwork, 'angle' between iris and cornea (Drains aqueous from the eye)
12. Ciliary body (secretes aqueous into the eye)

Fig. 10.2 Anatomy of the inner eye: 1, sclera; 2, choroid; 3, retinal pigment epithelium; 4, retina; 5, vitreous; 6, optic nerve; 7, lens; 8, zonules; 9, anterior chamber (filled with aqueous); 10, cornea; 11, trabecular meshwork—'angle' between iris and cornea (drains aqueous from the eye); 12, ciliary body (secretes aqueous into the eye).

condition in which males are unable to reliably distinguish red from green. It affects 1 in 8 men and can be tested for using Ishihara pseudoisochromatic plates.

Afferent pupillary defect

Normally, when a bright light is shone into one eye, both pupils constrict. There is a common pathway from the optic nerves to the midbrain, where the signal from both eyes is added and an identical neural signal is transmitted via parasympathetic fibres travelling with the IIIrd nerve to both irises causing pupillary constriction. If there is damage to the whole retina or the optic nerve then this constriction will not be induced by bright light to the same degree as normal (an afferent papillary defect). It is not caused by cataract, vitreous haemorrhage or occipital cortex lesions and therefore the afferent pupillary defect is useful in localizing the site of damage in an eye with poor vision. An afferent papillary defect is best examined using a very bright light in a dark room and swinging the light from one pupil to the other. In health, both pupils will remain small whichever eye the light is shone into. If one eye has optic nerve damage then both pupils will enlarge when the light is swung to shine in the affected eye, and both pupils will constrict when the light is swung to shine into the healthy eye.

Tears

Tears are constantly being secreted at a slow rate onto the surface of the eyes from the lacrimal gland. Tears contain oxygen, which is important for corneal health, and a tight-fitting contact lens which prevents the circulation of tears will result in an ischaemic corneal epithelium which is at increased risk of developing infection or inducing corneal vascularization. Tears also contain antibodies and other antibacterial components. An eye with no tears will quickly become painful and risks infection and permanent damage. Tears spread evenly over the surface of the cornea because of the oil secreted by the meibomian glands in the eyelids. In blepharitis these commonly become blocked or secrete abnormally thick oil which functions poorly, resulting in a patchy tear film and stinging eyes.

Symptoms of eye disease

The red eye

The red eye is a very common presenting feature and associated symptoms often reveal the diagnosis (Table 10.1). The associated symptoms include pain, visual loss, reduced vision, photophobia (diseases of the corneal epithelium or anterior uvea), stickiness or watering of the eye.

Enquiries of the duration will differentiate between acute and chronic conditions. A past medical history should be obtained for iritis, episcleritis, scleritis, herpes simplex, marginal ulcers and corneal erosions. Extraocular symptoms may indicate underlying disease such as nausea, vomiting (acute angle closure glaucoma), joint pains from rheumatoid arthritis (scleritis), ankylosing spondylitis (iritis) and sarcoidosis (iritis).

On examination, the pattern of redness is assessed (Table 10.2). The position of the lids is assessed for abnormalities such as ectropion or entropion, the position of the lashes

Applied basic sciences
of the eye

**Symptoms of
eye disease**

Examination of the eye

Table 10.1 Causes of a 'red eye'

Painful red eye	Causes
Associated with reduced or loss of vision	Severe inflammation Severe acute anterior uveitis Infective endophthalmitis Acute angle closure glaucoma Central corneal abscess Central corneal ulcers
Associated with minimal or no loss of vision	Peripheral corneal ulcer Early anterior uveitis (iritis) Anterior scleritis Keratitis or central abrasion Corneal erosions

Non-painful red eye	Causes
Associated with purulent discharge	Infective conjunctivitis Bacterial Viral Chlamydial
Associated with itching, stickiness and watering	Allergic conjunctivitis Hay fever Acute allergy
Associated with photophobia or lacrimation	Keratitis Herpes simplex Corneal abrasion Early iritis
Associated with general grittiness	Blepharitis Blepharoconjunctivitis Sicca syndrome
Associated with a sector of redness	Marginal ulcers Episcleritis Pterygium Pinguecula Subconjunctival haemorrhage Rosacea keratitis

Table 10.2 Clinical assessment of red eye

Site/nature of redness	Likely aetiology
Fornices	Conjunctivitis
Segmental redness near the limbus	Focal keratitis
Segmental redness	Episcleritis
Limbal or circumferential redness (ciliary)	Iritis or glaucoma
Brawny red appearance	Scleritis
Interpalpebral redness	Dry eyes
Confluent redness	Subconjunctival haemorrhage

angle closure glaucoma), keratic precipitates with iritis, flare and cells with iritis and for a fluid level suggestive of hypopyon in severe iritis, endophthalmitis or infected ulcers. The pupil is examined for its shape and reaction to light, which may be impaired with acute angle closure glaucoma and iritis. The fundus should be dilated and examined if loss of vision is not compatible with the amount of anterior segment disease.

Visual loss

Causes of severe visual loss are listed in Table 10.3. Most patients will not be able to distinguish between central loss of vision (Table 10.4) and blurring of vision (Table 10.5) hence diagnostic groups will overlap. It is important to establish if there is monocular or binocular visual loss, as it will indicate if the lesion is in front of (monocular) or behind the chiasma (binocular). If the visual loss is monocular, it is important to determine if there is loss of a visual field, segmental loss or central visual loss. If the visual loss is binocular, then further assessment should be undertaken to determine the pattern of field loss (bitemporal hemianopia or homonymous hemianopia).

In addition, it is important to determine if there is complete visual loss or blurred vision. Associated symptoms should be enquired about; for example, pain on eye movement is typical of optic neuritis. Younger patients may have a central serous retinopathy (CSR) and optic neuritis whilst older patients are more likely to have age-related macular degeneration and anterior ischaemic optic neuropathy. The speed of onset is important: sudden onset indicates a vascular cause such as occlusion or haemorrhage. Gradually

Table 10.3 Causes of severe visual loss

Vascular	Anterior ischaemic optic neuropathy Ischaemic central retinal vein occlusion Central retinal artery occlusion Vitreous haemorrhage
Inflammatory	Optic neuritis
Infiltrative, compressive, inherited, nutritional	Optic neuropathy
Ocular	Retinal detachment

Table 10.4 Causes of central loss of vision

Degenerative	Macular hole Age-related macular degeneration
Inflammatory	Optic neuritis
Ocular	Central serous retinopathy
Vascular	Ciilioretinal artery occlusion
Infiltrative, compressive, inherited, nutritional	Optic neuropathy

(trichiasis), contour of lid (blepharitis), conjunctiva (oedema with chemosis), papillae and follicles. The upper lid should be everted to look for foreign bodies and papillae. The cornea is examined, and appears dull with acute angle closure glaucoma (due to oedema). Epithelial defects can occur with abrasions, ulcers and herpes infection. The anterior segment is assessed for depth (it is shallow in acute

Table 10.5	Causes of blurred vision
Cornea	Surface disease (dry eyes) Corneal oedema/scarring Keratoconus
Lens	Cataract
Refractive error	
Anterior chamber	Iritis (protein/cells) Blood
Vitreous	Haemorrhage Intermediate uveitis (cells)
Retina	Retinitis/choroidoretinitis Vein/artery occlusions Diabetic retinopathy
Optic nerve	Optic neuritis/neuropathy

enlarging defects over days occur with retinal detachment, and progressive dimming of vision over hours to a few days is characteristic of optic neuritis and optic neuropathy.

Visual acuity should be assessed. Patients with hemianopic defects have normal or only mildly reduced acuity. Improvement in vision through a pinhole indicates that a refractive error is present. A relative afferent pupil defect indicates optic nerve disease or extensive retinal damage. Desaturation of colour vision indicates early optic nerve disease or late macular disease. Lesions of the macula will cause a positive scotoma (i.e. patients are aware of an obstruction/distortion) whereas optic nerve lesions will cause a negative scotoma (i.e. patients are not aware constantly of an obstruction and only notice if it is pointed out).

The eye should be inspected. Lens opacification would suggest a cataract, and the absence of a fundal view occurs with vitreous haemorrhage and very dense cataracts. Examination of the fundus may reveal multiple retinal haemorrhage with central retinal vein occlusion, retinal pallor and a cherry red spot with central retinal artery occlusion. An elevated mobile grey retina occurs with retinal detachment, and abnormal disc swelling with anterior ischaemic optic neuropathy, optic neuritis and neuropathy. Retinal pigment epithelial changes at the macula are indicative of age-related macular degeneration, and a central retinal hole indicates a hole in the macula. Diabetic retinopathy is suggested by microaneurysms, haemorrhages, exudates and oedema.

Homonymous hemianopia

Homonymous hemianopia (Table 10.6) commonly indicates damage to the occipital cortex or optic radiation and rarely that of the optic tract or lateral geniculate body. Temporal lobe lesions predominately cause an upper field loss, and parietal lobe lesions cause a lower field loss. Patients are unaware of objects coming from the side of the field defect, therefore patients would find reading difficult with right-sided field defects. Visual acuity is only slightly reduced as half the macular fibres are still intact, colour vision is unaffected and there should not be any relative afferent pupillary defect.

Table 10.6	Causes of homonymous hemianopia
Vascular	Thrombosis Haemorrhage Embolism
Inflammation	
Neoplasia	Primary Metastatic

Bitemporal hemianopia

Bitemporal field loss usually indicates disease of the optic chiasm or bilateral retinal disease (Table 10.7). The field loss is usually asymmetrical and can be predominantly superior or infero-temporal depending on the direction (anterior or posterior) of the chiasmal compression. Patients may have blurring in the temporal fields or reduced acuity or colour perception with a relative afferent pupillary defect. Examination may reveal bilateral temporal pallor. Large tumours will cause pituitary dysfunction and oculomotor nerve palsies.

Temporary visual loss

The causes of temporary visual loss (seconds to hours) are listed in Table 10.8. Typically there is abrupt onset of visual loss progressing over a few seconds to involve whole or part of the visual fields in one or both eyes. In the area the vision is dimmed or the lost sight returns in seconds or minutes, occasionally hours. The duration of attack may

Table 10.7	Causes of bitemporal hemianopia
Neoplasia	Pituitary adenoma Craniopharyngioma Meningioma
Vascular	Aneurysm

Table 10.8	Causes of transient visual loss
Vascular	Thromboembolism Carotid artery disease (amaurosis fugax) Heart valve disease Atrial fibrillation Vertebrobasilar stroke Vasculitis Giant cell arteritis Systemic lupus erythematosus
Neurological	Papilloedema Migraine
Haematological	Hyperviscosity Polycythaemia Thrombocythaemia Plasma cell myeloma Anaemia
Ocular	Intermittent angle closure

vary but typically embolic causes last seconds to minutes, migraine lasts for minutes, papilloedema lasts for seconds and is related to posture, acute angle closure glaucoma lasts minutes to hours. Precipitating factors may include posture (papilloedema), turning the head (carotid sinus disease) or red wine (migraine). Associated symptoms may include headache (papilloedema, giant cell arteritis), visual aura (migraine) and haloes around lights (angle closure glaucoma).

Flashes and floaters

Flashes and floaters are common symptoms. A sudden onset is characteristic of posterior vitreous detachment, retinal tears and retinal haemorrhage (Table 10.9). If floaters are seen after flashing lights, a retinal tear must be excluded since there is risk of progression to retinal detachment. Patients who are short sighted may have floaters for some time. Diseases such as diabetes and hypertension are associated with vitreous haemorrhage, and sarcoid is associated with vitreous inflammation. Detailed examination of the retina should be performed with slit-lamp biomicroscopy.

Ocular pain

Pain may come from an inherent problem within the eye or orbit or be referred from orbital structures (Table 10.10). Associated symptoms such as loss of vision usually indicate a severe inflammatory process such as scleritis, endophthalmitis, ischaemia or acute glaucoma. Associated photophobia may be due to ciliary spasm in bright lights (iritis, corneal lesions). Diplopia indicates involvement of ocular muscles, nerves or lesions of the orbital cavity (orbital cellulitis). A history of surgery to the eye may predispose to infections such as endophthalmitis and cellulitis.

Examination of the eye

Inspection

The lid may be ptotic (droopy) or swollen, or the eye protruding (proptosis) on inspection (best examined by standing behind the patient with the patient seated). Erythema of the lid may indicate localized lid infection or underlying orbital or intraocular infection or inflammation. Note any ocular deviation.

Visual acuity

Distance vision is assessed in the unaided eye, with glasses and through a pinhole (corrects any refractive error) by a

Table 10.9	Causes of flashes and floaters
Ocular	Posterior vitreous detachment Retinal tear/detachment
Vascular	Vitreous haemorrhage
Inflammation	Uveitis

Table 10.10	Causes of ocular pain
Symptoms	**Causes**
Severe aching ocular pain, patient unable to sleep	Endophthalmitis Anterior/posterior scleritis Cluster headache/ Raeder's syndrome Orbital cellulitis
Sharp ocular pain, photophobia, watering, and a foreign body sensation	Corneal abrasions Foreign bodies Viral/bacterial keratitis Contact lens problems
Throbbing pain and photophobia	Acute iritis Corneal ulcers Neovascular glaucoma

Associated diplopia and pain	Orbital myositis/cellulitis
	Superior orbital fissure
	   syndrome
	Acute thyroid
	   ophthalmopathy

Severe throbbing pain with nausea and vomiting	Acute glaucoma Migraine
Retrobulbar aching pain on moving the eye	Retrobulbar neuritis Cavernous sinus syndrome
Lancing pain around the eye and face	Trigeminal neuralgia Postherpetic neuralgia

Snellen chart (Fig. 10.3). The chart is designed to be read at a distance of 6 metres, and the top line is designated as 6/60 (which means that the top line can be read at 6 metres which a normal eye is able to read at 60 metres). If the patient is unable to read the top row, the chart can be brought to 3 metres and recorded as 3/60 (which means that the top line can be read at 3 metres which a normal eye is able to read at 60 metres).

For patients who are illiterate, a Snellen 'E' chart can be used in which rows of the letter E are oriented in four different directions; the patient is given a letter E and asked to orientate it as the examiner points to the chart. For children, a board with different letters is given to the child or parent; the examiner points to a letter on the chart and the child is asked to point to the corresponding letter on the board.

Increasing severity of vision loss is recorded as counting fingers, hand movements and light perception.

Near vision is assessed using a standard print test and defined as the smallest type that can be read comfortably in good light at 33 cm.

Colour vision

Colour vision is a function of retinal cones. Diseases affecting the macular area (high cone density) will reduce both colour vision and visual acuity, whereas lesions of the optic nerve will reduce colour vision with initial preservation of distance visual acuity. Colour vision is assessed by Ishihara pseudoisochromatic plates, recording the number of plates seen divided by number of plates shown.

Applied basic sciences of the eye

Symptoms of eye disease

Examination of the eye

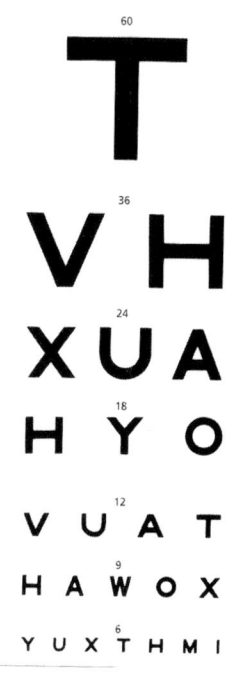

Fig. 10.3 A Snellen chart.

639

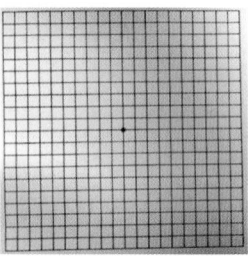

Fig. 10.4 An Amsler grid.

Visual fields

Visual fields are assessed clinically using the confrontation method. The patient is seated a metre away from the examiner with one eye occluded. The patient is asked to look directly at the examiner's eye. The examiner's finger is brought in from the periphery at all four quadrants, and the point where the finger is visible should be the same for the patient and examiner.

The extent of the blind spot should be mapped, and colour desaturation is assessed with a red pin in each hemifield for bitemporal defects and central or centrocaecal scotomas.

Macular function is assessed using an Amsler grid, a 20 × 20 grid of 5 mm squares with a central fixation dot (Fig. 10.4). Patients are asked to fixate on the dot with spectacles on one eye at a time and to comment on any distorted or missing lines.

Pupil reaction

The pupil size should be noted in bright and in dim light, noting any anisocoria (difference in pupil size). Anisocoria that is greater in darkness is due to failure of the smaller miotic pupil to dilate (sympathetic paresis, e.g. Horner's syndrome). Anisocoria that is greater in light is due to failure of the larger pupil to constrict (parasympathetic paresis). If the difference in pupil size is the same in both lighting conditions the diagnosis is usually essential anisocoria, which is of no neurological significance.

The relative afferent pupil response compares the afferent pathway of both eyes. The amplitude of the pupil response (light reflex) is normally the same whichever eye is illuminated. The relative afferent pupil response is not affected by media opacities or vitreous haemorrhage and if one pupil is damaged it is still possible to examine for a relative afferent pupil response by observing the unaffected pupil alone.

Slit-lamp biomicroscope

A slit lamp is a binocular microscope mounted horizontally with a light source which can provide diffuse light or slit beams of various heights and widths as well as various angles of incidence. There are filters that vary the wavelength of light. Examination starts by assessing the position of the eyelids and lid margin. Further detailed examination of the cornea and anterior chamber, e.g. for cells and flare (protein), is then performed. With additional lenses, the vitreous and fundus can also be examined. With the attachment of a Goldmann tonometer the pressure in the eye can also be checked.

Direct ophthalmoscopy

Direct ophthalmoscopy is a useful basic examination. The red reflex can be sought and examination of the optic disc, macula and lens can be made. However, the view is not stereoscopic so appreciation of retinal fluid is difficult, and detailed examination of the peripheral retina and the anterior segment is challenging.

Binocular indirect ophthalmoscopy

Binocular indirect ophthalmoscopy gives a stereoscopic view of the fundus and allows a more peripheral view. The pupil is dilated and with scleral indentation, a dynamic examination is performed.

SECTION 10.2 Investigations for eye disease

Ophthalmic investigations may be divided into the parts of the eye they examine, the orbit/globe or the visual pathways in the brain.

Anterior segment investigations

Conjunctival swabs

Swabs are taken for conjunctival disease, commonly to check for bacterial, viral or chlamydial infections.

Corneal scrapes

Corneal scrapes are performed on corneal ulcers. Samples are taken with a sterile needle and plated directly. A Gram stain sample is taken, placing the sample on a glass microscope slide. Plates used are blood agar (most ocular pathogens), chocolate agar (*Haemophilus*, *Neisseria*) and Sabouraud's medium (fungal).

Corneal topography

Corneal topography measures the curvature of the cornea to estimate the refractive power. It is essential in contact lens fitting, refractive surgery, and to calculate intraocular lens power for cataract surgery. Automated machines give quantitative assessment of the corneal power (Fig. 10.5).

Pachymetry

Pachymetry is the measurement of corneal thickness, an indication of the integrity of its function. The cornea is normally thinnest in the centre and increases in thickness towards the limbus.

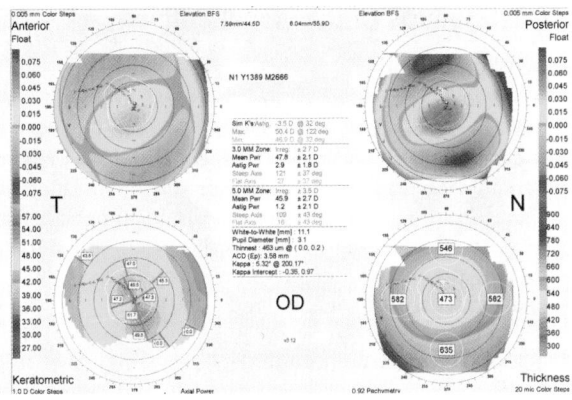

Fig. 10.5 Corneal topography results.

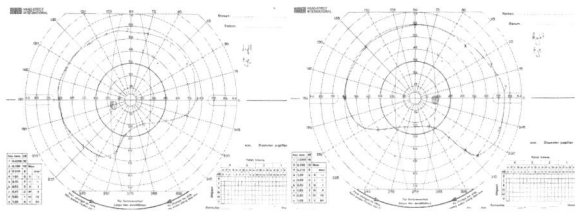

Fig. 10.6 Perimetry results.

Posterior segment investigations

Visual fields (perimetry)

The perimeter is a three-dimensional structure extending 60° nasally, 90° temporally, 50° superiorly and 70° inferiorly (Fig. 10.6). Assessment of visual fields for quantitative analysis determines the size, shape and depth of any field loss. Normal visual acuity is sharpest at the centre and declines progressively towards the periphery, with a blind spot located temporally between 10° and 20°. A scotoma is a defect in the visual field. An absolute scotoma is an area of total loss of vision, a relative scotoma one of reduced sensitivity in which some targets are seen.

Fundus fluorescein angiography

Fluorescein angiography is an invaluable test for retinal vascular disease, vein occlusions, macular disease, choroidal disease and ocular tumours. A fluorescent dye is injected intravenously; as it enters the retinal vasculature, a camera shines a blue light onto the retina which reacts with the molecules of dye to emit a light energy of longer wavelength. This is then captured by the camera and can be stored digitally. Sequential photographs show the dye entering and leaving the retinal vasculature, allowing the assessment of blood flow. The phases of blood flow are pre-arterial, arterial, arteriovenous (capillary) and venous (Fig. 10.7). Fluorescein is the dye most commonly used; indocyanine green has specific use for the choroidal circulation.

Investigations of the orbit and globe

Computed tomography (CT)

CT is the imaging modality of choice for the orbit, and is useful in the assessment of globe ruptures, intraocular foreign bodies, orbital wall fractures and space-occupying lesions. The use of contrast may help with vascular lesions.

Ultrasonography

B scan ultrasound allows imaging of the intraocular contents by placing a probe over a closed eyelid (Fig. 10.8). It is useful in globe trauma, in retinal assessment when no fundal views are available (due to dense cataract or vitreous haemorrhage) and in the assessment of intraocular masses (tumours, scleritis). Colour flow Doppler will aid in assessment of vascular lesions of the globe and orbit.

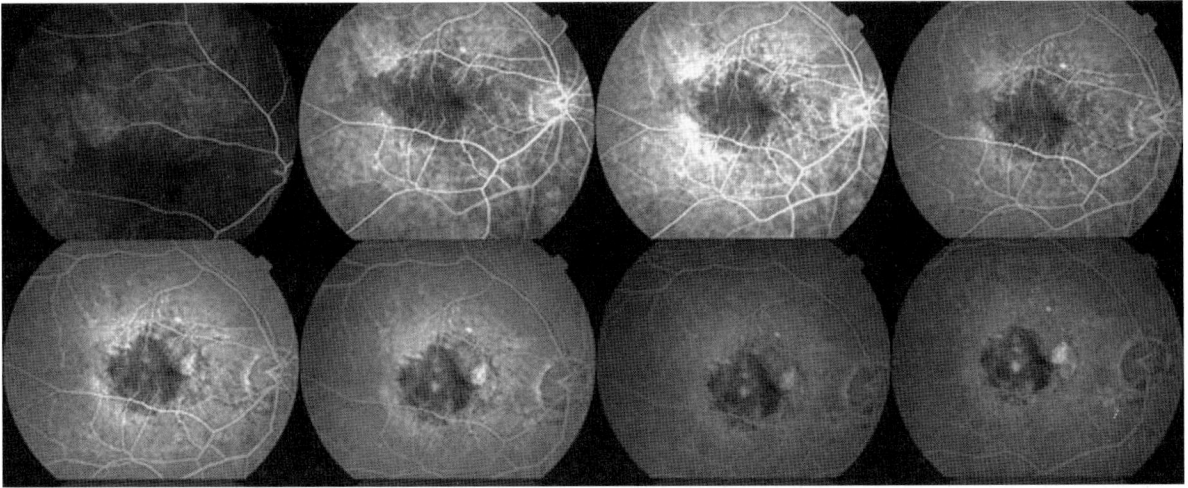

Fig. 10.7 Fundus fluorescein angiography.

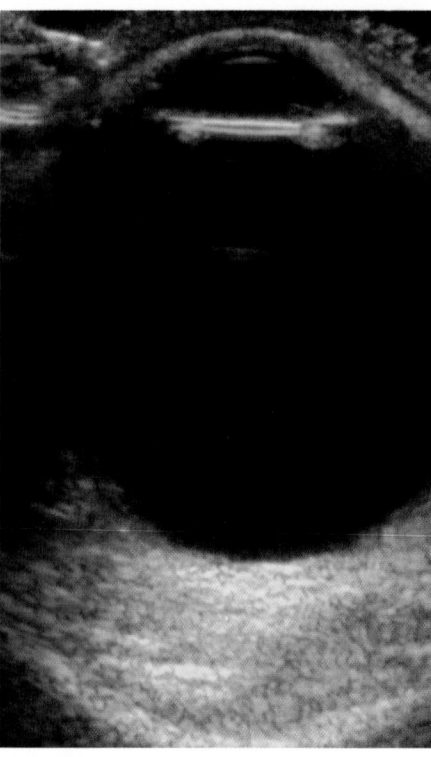

Fig. 10.8 Corneal ultrasound.

Investigations of the visual pathway

Electrophysiology

The nervous system generates electrical impulses and these can be detected by electrodes in preset positions along the visual pathway and recorded. The visual evoked potential measures the response of the entire afferent pathway from retina to cortex and is useful in optic nerve disease to assess for demyelination. The electroretinogram measures the function of the photoreceptor layer of the retina and is useful in inherited retinal diseases.

Magnetic resonance imaging

MRI is the imaging technique of choice for optic nerve and intracranial pathology causing ophthalmic signs, e.g. cavernous sinus disease, pituitary disease or demyelination.

SECTION 10.3 · Manifestations of eye disease

The dry eye

Epidemiology

Symptoms of a dry eye are very common.

Pathology

Symptoms of a dry eye and tear film insufficiency are commonly due to meibomian gland dysfunction. Other causes such as mucin deficiency and true aqueous deficiency are rare.

Meibomian oil glands in the eyelids usually produce enough thin oil to stabilize the tear film between blinks. Disorders of oil gland function usually arise from infection (staphylococcal blepharitis or meibomianitis), resulting in unstable tear films with very short break-up times and corneal drying between blinks. Reflex aqueous overproduction may then occur causing a seemingly paradoxical watering dry eye.

Reduced production of mucin (an important component of the tear film–corneal interface) can occur with vitamin A deficiency and conjunctival scarring, e.g. Stevens–Johnson syndrome. True tear aqueous deficiency may occur as part of Sjögren's syndrome or sarcoidosis.

Clinical features

Patients with dry eyes often complain of a burning, stinging or foreign body sensation in the eyes. On examination, the eye may be red and sometimes watery (paradoxical watering).

Schirmer's test measures the amount of tear absorbed by a piece of filter paper slipped inside the lower lid for 5 minutes. The normal wetting distance is over 10 mm. Rose Bengal drops can be used if there is suspicion of devitalized epithelial cells. However, Rose Bengal causes pain for several hours afterwards.

Investigations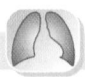

In general, investigations are required only to confirm the presence of associated diseases.

Management

Identify and treat underlying cause

Blepharitis, vitamin deficiencies and connective tissue diseases should be treated if present.

Lubricating eye drops

Hypromellose or other lubricating eye drops and ointments can be used 4–6 times per day. Severely affected patients may require lubricating drops every 10 minutes.

Punctal occlusion

Occlusion of the punctum can be achieved temporarily by silicone plugs and works by reducing the drainage of tears. Permanent occlusion is achieved by cautery.

Prognosis

Many patients are only symptomatic for brief periods (e.g. with recurrent blepharitis). A minority have permanently dry and painful eyes, and a few develop blindness from dry eyes (this is more common with vitamin A deficiency or measles in developing countries).

SECTION 10.4   Diseases of the eyelids

Disorders of the eyelids are common. They can arise from infection or inflammation, or occur as a part of ageing (Table 10.11). The miscellaneous causes are detailed below.

Sebaceous cysts (cysts of Moll/Zeis) are small fluid-filled cystic lesions found on the anterior lid margin. They present as a small well-defined nodule in the anterior eyelid. They are all benign and easily removed by surgical excision.

A chalazion is a chronic inflammatory lesion caused by blockage in the meibomian gland orifices and stagnation of sebaceous secretion. It is associated with acne rosacea and seborrhoeic dermatitis. A chalazion presents as a round firm lesion in the tarsal plate of the eyelid. With infection, the lid becomes swollen and tender due to abscess formation. Small lesions can be treated by hot compress and topical antibiotics, but large lesions require incision and curettage. Systemic antibiotics are required for recurrent lesions or associated cellulitis, and biopsies are usually performed to exclude malignancy in recurrent lesions.

A stye is a small abscess caused by acute staphylococcal infection of the eyelash follicle and its associated gland of Zeis or Moll. A stye presents as a tender inflamed swelling in the eyelid which points anteriorly. There may be associated preseptal cellulitis. Hot compresses and surgical excision of the infected follicle with systemic antibiotics may be required.

Xanthelasmata are yellowish subcutaneous plaques of cholesterol and lipid which typically occur on the medial aspect of the eyelids. They may indicate underlying hypercholesterolaemia and are removed surgically with laser or with trichloroacetic acid.

Blepharitis

Blepharitis is an eruption producing inflammation of eyelids and eyelashes. The lifetime prevalence is as high as 25%. Blepharitis is associated with staphylococcal infection and abnormal meibomian oil gland function. It is more common in patients with acne rosacea. Patients present with a gritty burning sensation in the eye with watering and crusting on the eyelids. Blepharitis is alleviated with regular lid cleaning using sodium bicarbonate solution, topical antibiotics (chloramphenicol), artificial tear drops (hypromellose) and topical steroids. Patients with associated acne rosacea should receive oral doxycycline. Blepharitis is usually a chronic and recurrent disease.

Trichiasis

Trichiasis is a posterior misdirection of previously normal lashes. Secondary trichiasis occurs with blepharitis, trachoma, following chemical burns or Stevens–Johnson syndrome. It causes a corneal epitheliopathy which may lead to corneal

Table 10.11	Diseases of the eyelids
Aetiology	**Condition**
Infection/inflammation	Chalazion, stye
Haemangiomas	Port wine stain, capillary haemangioma
Tumours	Squamous cell papilloma, basal cell carcinoma, squamous cell carcinoma, sebaceous gland carcinoma, Kaposi's sarcoma
Inflammation of the eyelashes	Trichiasis, blepharitis
Abnormal position of the eyelids	Entropion, ectropion, ptosis
Others	Xanthelasmata, cysts

643

ulceration and infectious keratitis. Treatment involves epilation or, more effectively, electrolysis or laser thermoablation.

Ectropion

Ectropion is the outward turning of the eyelid. It is associated with epiphora (watering of the eyes), chronic conjunctivitis and corneal exposure. An ectropion may be congenital, involutional, cicatricial or paralytic.

Senile ectropion is similar to senile entropion with excessive horizontal lid laxity but associated with medial or lateral canthal tendon laxity. Treatment is by eyelid shortening with or without conjunctivoplasty.

Cicatricial ectropion is caused by scarring or contracture of skin, pulling the eyelid away from the globe. The causes include tumours, trauma and burns. Surgical correction involves excision of scar tissue and transposition flaps or free skin grafting if a large defect is present.

Paralytic ectropion caused by facial nerve palsy may cause exposure keratopathy, incomplete lid closure (lagophthalmos), epiphora and retraction of the eyelids. Temporary reversible causes such as Bell's palsy are treated with artificial tears or temporary tarsorrhaphy. Permanent causes such as acoustic neuroma are treated by surgical correction reducing the horizontal and vertical palpebral apertures (using gold weight to lower the aspect of the upper eyelid, or by the use of an augmented lateral canthal sling).

Entropion

Entropion is inversion of the eyelid. An entropion may be congenital, involutional (senile), cicatricial (scarring) or spastic. Senile entropion is the most common type. It affects the lower lid, due to a combination of horizontal lid laxity, weakness of the lower lid retractors and overriding of the preseptal over the pretarsal portion of orbicularis muscle. Cicatricial entropion is due to scarring of the palpebral conjunctiva which pulls the eyelid towards the globe. It may be due to ocular cicatricial pemphigoid, Stevens–Johnson syndrome, trachoma or chemical injuries. Spastic entropion is caused by spasm of orbicularis oculi from ocular irritation, and is usually reversible when the irritation is corrected. Surgical correction of entropion is by the insertion of everting sutures on the eyelid, with or without horizontal shortening of the eyelid. The treatment of cicatricial entropion is usually more complex and may require mucous membrane grafting.

Ptosis

Ptosis is an abnormally low position of the upper lid in relation to the globe.

Epidemiology

Ptosis is a common clinical problem.

Pathology

The causes of ptosis are neurogenic, aponeurotic, mechanical and myogenic (Table 10.12).

Clinical features

A small ptosis is usually asymptomatic, but a large ptosis may interfere with vision. The duration of the ptosis will distinguish between congenital and acquired cases. It is important to enquire about associated symptoms of underlying disease; for example, diplopia or variability in the degree of ptosis is characteristic of myasthenia gravis (p. 628).

On examination, the palpebral aperture should be measured. The amount of upper lid movement and level of skin crease will enable differentiation of causes, i.e. aponeurotic ptosis will have a high skin crease while congenital may not have one at all; in myogenic, neurogenic and congenital ptosis the upper lid movement will be reduced while in aponeurotic it may well be normal.

Investigations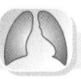

In general, investigations are only required to determine the underlying cause of suspected neurogenic or myogenic ptosis.

Management

Müllerectomy

A small ptosis (2 mm) may be repaired by Müllerectomy. Müller muscle is a smooth muscle with a sympathetic nerve supply causing the ptosis in Horner's syndrome. It may be resected by a transconjunctival approach.

Resection of the levator palpebrae muscle

A larger ptosis will require resection of the levator palpebrae muscle. In children with dystrophic levator function or adults with muscle dystrophy the eyelid may be raised by transferring the attachment of the tarsus to the frontalis muscle. This is achieved with a sling made from non-

Table 10.12	Causes of ptosis

Neurogenic
  IIIrd nerve palsy
  Horner's syndrome	

Aponeurotic Senile dehiscence of levator aponeurosis	
Mechanical Dermatochalasis (redundancy of upper lid skin)	

Myogenic
  Congenital dystrophy
  Myasthenia gravis
  Myotonic dystrophy
  Chronic progressive external ophthalmoplegia	

absorbable material such as Prolene or autologous fascia lata from the thigh.

Prognosis

The majority of causes of ptosis are irreversible. Good results, however, can be achieved with corrective surgery.

Haemangiomas of the eyelids

Port-wine stains are soft subcutaneous demarcated pink lesions that darken from red to purple. They are present at birth and are composed of large thin-walled vessels and capillaries. The overlying skin may be coarse. Lesions involving the first or second division of the trigeminal nerve are associated with glaucoma and 5% are associated with Sturge–Weber syndrome. Cosmetic treatment with argon laser can reduce the amount of discolouration in severe cases.

Strawberry naevus is a capillary haemangioma that may involve the eyelids and present at birth. It usually continues to grow until the child is 1 year of age before spontaneously involuting. Occasionally it may extend into the orbit, and if there is a threat to vision (obstruction of the visual axis, optic nerve compression or exposure keratopathy) then intralesional steroid injections may be given to promote faster regression.

Tumours of the eyelids

Epidemiology

Tumours of the eyelid are common. Approximately 5–10% of all skin cancers occur in the eyelid. Of the eyelid tumours, only 15% are malignant. Basal cell carcinomas (BCC) account for 90% and squamous cell carcinoma for 9%.

Pathology

The papilloma is the most common benign tumour of the eyelid. Of malignant tumours, basal cell and squamous cell carcinomas are the most common.

Approximately 90% of basal cell carcinomas are located in the head and neck region, and around the eyelid they are found in increasing frequency in the lower lid, medial canthus, and upper eyelid followed by the lateral canthus. BCC is a slow-growing and locally invasive tumour that does not metastasize.

The squamous cell carcinoma is much less common than BCC. It has a predilection for the lower lid, especially in elderly patients with a fair skin complexion and a history of chronic sun exposure. It may arise de novo or from precancerous dermatosis (e.g. actinic keratosis). It is a more aggressive tumour that metastasizes to regional lymph nodes.

Kaposi's sarcoma and sebaceous gland carcinomas are much rarer. Sebaceous gland carcinomas usually arise from meibomian glands and have a predilection for the upper eyelid, whereas Kaposi's sarcoma is a vascular tumour frequently associated with AIDS.

Clinical features

A papilloma usually presents as a slow-growing pedunculated skin lesion. Basal cell carcinoma can be nodular, ulcerative or sclerosing. The nodular lesion is a firm, raised, indurated nodule with hyperkeratosis and dilated blood vessels on its surface. The ulcerative lesion has a raised, rolled border with an ulcerated centre that may bleed with minor trauma. The sclerosing lesion is a diffuse spreading, flat indurated plaque with margins that are difficult to delineate.

Squamous cell carcinoma presents as a hard nodule or a scaly patch which develops crusting erosions and fissures. Shallow ulceration develops with a red base and an indurated elevated border. Regional lymph node examination is vital.

Sebaceous gland carcinoma presents similarly to a recurrent chalazion before assuming a nodular appearance. The nodule enlarges gradually or spreads by infiltrating into the dermis. The associated thickened and inflamed areas may be mistaken for chronic blepharitis (p. 643).

Kaposi's sarcoma usually presents as a small violet-brown lesion which may be mistaken for a naevus or haematoma.

Investigations

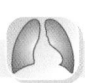

Photographs

Photographs taken prior to treatment are essential for documentation.

CT of the head

CT is required if there are any signs of orbital extension (restriction of orbital movement) and in patients with aggressive sebaceous gland carcinomas.

Biopsy

Incisional biopsy of any suspicious lesion is often undertaken prior to subsequent wide excision.

Management

Surgical excision

Surgical excision of the entire tumour is the treatment of choice. Mohs' micrographic surgery allows excision with serial horizontal sections from the undersurface of the tumour. Small residual defects can be closed directly, but larger defects require rotation flaps or even lid sharing procedures. Skin grafts may be required to reconstruct the anterior (e.g. auricular skin) and posterior lamellae (e.g. buccal membrane). Extensive infiltrating lesions will require exenteration (removal of globe and orbital contents).

Radiotherapy and chemotherapy

Radiotherapy and chemotherapy are reserved for patients who refuse surgery, with the exception of Kaposi's sarcoma where low-dose radiotherapy is an effective treatment modality.

Prognosis

Since the advent of Mohs' excision the recurrence rate of a basal cell carcinoma is 1% and a squamous cell carcinoma 2.9% at 5 years. Local metastatic spread is extremely rare in basal cell carcinomas. Regional lymph node metastasis is reported in up to 21% of patients with squamous cell carcinomas.

SECTION 10.5   Disorders of the lacrimal system

Disorders of the lacrimal system are listed in Table 10.13.

Epidemiology

Congenital obstruction of the lacrimal drainage system may be present in up to 50% of newborn infants. It may be bilateral in one third. Due to the variety of causes of acquired lacrimal system obstruction an exact epidemiological figure is not known. However, lid malposition is the most common cause of epiphora (watery eye).

Pathology

Diseases causing obstruction of the lacrimal system can occur at the level of the punctum, canaliculus or nasolacrimal duct.

Primary obstruction of the lacrimal system can arise from medial obstruction of the common canaliculus (chronic dacryocystitis) or lateral obstruction (idiopathic pericanalicular fibrosis) in which the entire common canaliculus can become obstructed. Obstruction of the individual canaliculus can also occur with trauma, drugs (fluorouracil) or infection (herpes simplex).

Secondary obstruction refers to a patent system where the drainage is affected from the abnormal position of the eyelid, such as punctal eversion from an involutional ectropion.

Nasolacrimal duct obstruction may be due to involutional stenosis, naso-orbital trauma and chronic sinus disease. Dacryocystitis is usually secondary to blockage of the nasolacrimal duct.

Table 10.13	Disorders of the lacrimal system
Epiphora	
Punctal obstruction	
Canalicular obstruction	
Nasolacrimal duct obstruction	
Infection	
Dacryocystitis	

Clinical features

Disorders of the lacrimal system usually present with excessive watering (epiphora).

It is important to assess if the watering occurs in a medial position (lacrimal system problem) or in a lateral position (lid problem, such as ectropion). Acute dacryocystitis presents as sudden onset of a painful tense swelling at the medial canthus associated with epiphora. Chronic dacryocystitis presents as recurrent unilateral conjunctivitis.

On examination, the eyelids are assessed for ectropion, trichiasis and lower lid laxity. Compression of the lacrimal sac may cause reflux of mucopurulent material, indicating the development of a mucocele.

The height of a tear strip may give an indication to outflow obstruction. Using a slit-lamp, the punctum is assessed for malposition, stenosis or obstruction. The fluorescein disappearance test is performed by placing drops of fluorescein into the conjunctival sac. Normally, very little or no dye remains after 2 minutes. The presence of dye indicates inadequate drainage. Direct assessment of lacrimal drainage is performed using a saline-filled syringe fitted with a lacrimal cannula. It is inserted into the lower canaliculus and passed to the medial wall of the lacrimal sac. If injected saline passes into the nose, no obstruction (or partial obstruction) is present. With total obstruction, the saline refluxes through the upper punctum and distension of the lacrimal sac occurs.

Investigations

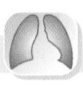

Dacryocystography

Contrast medium (Lipiodol ultra fluid) is injected into one of the canaliculi and posteroanterior and lateral radiographs are taken. Digital subtraction (bone-free) images are obtained that detail the lacrimal system, identifying any obstruction, diverticulum, fistula or lacrimal sac stones.

Lacrimal scintigraphy

Lacrimal scintigraphy is obtained by labelling tears with technetium-99m and using a gamma camera to monitor their progress through the drainage system.

Management

Antibiotics

An intravenous or oral combination of penicillin, flucloxacillin and metronidazole is required for initial management of acute dacryocystitis, often prior to dacryocystorhinostomy.

Punctal dilatation

Punctal stenosis can be dilated with a Nettleship dilator.

Ampullotomy

An ampullotomy should be considered with recurrent stenosis after two dilatations. Snip ampullotomy is performed with a single vertical snip in the posterior wall of the ampulla or a vertical and horizontal cut in the ampulla to widen the stenosis.

Dacryocystorhinostomy

Dacryocystorhinostomy is a procedure to address obstruction of the lacrimal sac that is distal to the internal opening of the common canaliculus. The lacrimal sac is incised and an opening is made between the lacrimal sac and the middle turbinate. Tubes are placed through the canaliculi and the new opening and left in the nose for 8 weeks. In adults the symptom-free success rate after external dacryocystorhinostomy is over 90%.

RECENT ADVANCES

Transnasal dacryocystorhinostomy is popular as it avoids an external incision. However, the 80% long-term patency rates are slightly lower than with conventional approaches.

Prognosis

The majority of congenital obstructions resolve by 4–6 weeks after birth. Approximately 90% of patients with obstructions at 1 year will be cured after one procedure (nasolacrimal system probing). Very few patients will require silicone intubation or external dacryocystorhinostomy.

SECTION 10.6 Diseases of the conjunctiva

Conjunctivitis

Epidemiology

Conjunctivitis is extremely common. Almost everyone will experience conjunctivitis during his or her lifetime.

Pathology

The vast majority of cases of conjunctivitis are due to a self-limiting viral infection. Rarely, after adenoviral conjunctivitis, tiny white spots develop on the cornea approximately 2 weeks after the initial infection causing blurred vision and a sensation of a foreign body. This usually resolves spontaneously over a few months but may clear faster with topical steroids. Other common causes are bacterial infection and allergies (Table 10.14).

In developing countries, recurrent chlamydial infection leads to trachoma, a major cause of preventable blindness worldwide. Chronic recurrent infections result in entropion and trichiasis. The in-turned eyelashes rub on the cornea causing corneal scarring and eventually blindness. Trachoma spreads in conditions of poor hygiene, and simple measures such as hand washing are effective at reducing reinfection rates.

Rare causes include Stevens–Johnson syndrome, pemphigoid, pediculosis pubis, molluscum contagiosum and as a presentation of graft versus host disease.

Clinical features

Patients with viral or bacterial conjunctivitis present with red eyes that feel gritty but are not usually painful. The eyelids are stuck together in the morning from sticky discharge produced by either one or both eyes. The vision is normal once the discharge is wiped away. There may be a history of an accompanying cold or sore throat. Bacterial conjunctivitis is usually difficult to differentiate from viral conjunctivitis. A feature that favours the diagnosis of bacterial conjunctivitis is a quick clinical response to antibiotic eye drops. Patients with allergic conjunctivitis present with itchy and watering eyes. There is often a clear history of allergen exposure (animals, pollen). On examination, chemosis (fluid under the conjunctiva) may be evident if the eyes have been rubbed a lot.

647

Table 10.14   Causes and management of acute conjunctivitis

Cause	Specific clinical features	Management
Viral (adenovirus)	Gets worse for 4–7 days then improves over 2–3 weeks	Topical lubricants (hypromellose) and topical steroids (severe disease)
Viral (herpes simplex)	Vesicles around the eye, unilateral, painful pre-auricular lymph node	Oral aciclovir for 10 days
Bacterial (staphylococcus or streptococcus)	Gets worse for 4–7 days then improves over 2–3 weeks	Topical chloramphenicol drops for 1 week
Bacterial (gonococcal)	Hyperacute onset, copious purulent discharge, corneal perforation may occur	Systemic antibiotics (ceftriaxone) and intensive topical treatment
Allergic conjunctivitis	Itchy discharge that is watery or stringy but not purulent	Topical sodium cromoglicate for a month, allergen avoidance

Table 10.15   Causes and management of chronic conjunctivitis

Cause	Specific clinical features	Management
Chlamydia	Non-specific follicular conjunctivitis. History of recent sexual contact or dysuria	Refer to STD clinic for systemic treatment (azithromycin) and genitourinary investigations
Trachoma (from recurrent chlamydial infection)	Scarring on the inside of the lids may lead to trichiasis (eyelashes rubbing on the cornea) risking corneal scarring and blindness. A leading cause of preventable world blindness, especially in underdeveloped countries	Azithromycin. Surgery on the eyelids may be required to prevent further damage to the cornea
Allergy to eye drops	Itchy sore red eyes. The skin below the eye is often indurated as the eye drop spills from the eye during administration	Use of preservative-free eye drops (allergy is usually to the preservatives in the eye drops)
Vernal keratoconjunctivitis	Chronic allergic conjunctivitis affecting children and young adults. Often worse in spring. Patients present with bilateral, large cobblestone papillae under lids	Long-term topical steroid drops for patients with severe disease

 CLINICAL ALERT

Features that suggest a more serious cause for conjunctivitis are vesicles around the eye (herpes simplex), accompanying urethral discharge (gonococcal or chlamydial infection) or conjunctivitis that lasts for more than a week (Table 10.15).

Investigations

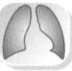

No investigations are required for patients with mild conjunctivitis.

Eye swab
Patients with severe or chronic conjunctivitis should have an eye swab to screen for bacterial infection (Gram stain and cultures). A specific swab should be taken for *Chlamydia* cultures.

Management

The management of conjunctivitis is according to best initial clinical assessment of the aetiology. Specific management is detailed in Tables 10.14 and 10.15.

Prognosis

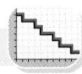

Untreated viral and staphylococcal or streptococcal conjunctivitis usually resolves within 7 days without complications, although it can occasionally last for up to 5 weeks. Allergic conjunctivitis recurs with repeat exposure to the allergen; in most cases this results in symptomatic disease only. In certain rare forms of chronic allergic conjunctivitis, permanent visual loss can occur. Conjunctivitis from chlamydial infection responds well to antibiotics, but patients need additional screening for other sexually transmitted diseases.

SECTION 10.7 Diseases of the sclera

Scleritis

Epidemiology

Scleritis is rare, and typically presents in patients aged about 50.

Pathology

Scleritis is a localized inflammation of the sclera. In 25% it is associated with underlying disease (Table 10.16); in the remainder, the cause is unknown. The vision can be normal but may be grossly reduced by glaucoma, cataract, associated uveitis, retinal oedema, choroidal folds and occasionally exudative retinal detachment. The sclera can become thin with anterior scleritis and predispose to perforation of the globe. Necrotizing scleritis without inflammation (associated with rheumatoid arthritis) can also result in perforation following minor trauma (scleromalacia perforans).

Scleritis should not be confused with the much more common episcleritis (inflammation of the layer immediately beneath the conjunctiva). Episcleritis is a self-limiting process that resolves quickly with topical steroid drops.

Table 10.16	Diseases associated with scleritis
Rheumatoid disease	
Wegener's granulomatosis	
Polyarteritis nodosa	
Systemic lupus erythematosus	
Syphilis	
Gout	
Ophthalmic surgery	
Ankylosing spondylitis	

Clinical features

In anterior scleritis the eye is red. In posterior scleritis, the eye may appear normal. In both conditions the pain can be severe enough to wake patients from sleep (a characteristic feature). It affects both eyes in 50%.

On examination, the eyeball is painful to touch and the vision is usually normal. Phenylephrine drops (10% concentration) applied to the eye will result in a white eye after 10 minutes in most cases of conjunctivitis, but with scleritis the deeper scleral vessels will not be affected and the eye remains red.

Investigations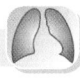

B-scan ultrasound

A B-scan ultrasound is useful to detect thickening of the sclera in posterior scleritis.

Further investigations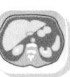

A history will guide further investigations of any underlying disorders (Table 10.16).

Management

Non-steroidal anti-inflammatory drug

Flurbiprofen 100 mg tds is prescribed for most patients.

Immunomodulation

Systemic steroids are required for patients with thinning of the cornea or those who fail to improve with NSAIDs. Cyclophosphamide may be useful in patients with Wegener's granulomatosis.

Prognosis

Visual loss may occur in up to 40%, and 35% develop recurrent disease.

Diseases of the cornea

The cornea is a transparent avascular structure. It is kept relatively dehydrated by endothelial cells which pump water out of the cornea, allowing the collagen fibres to maintain their regular structure for corneal transparency. Visual impairment can result as a complication of the healing process from corneal injury or due to the deposition of calcium. The corneal epithelium does not regenerate after damage (e.g. during cataract surgery), and the cornea becomes oedematous and hazy. Eventually blisters form on its surface and can rupture, leaving painful epithelial defects (bullous keratopathy). Moreover the normal healing response involves ingrowth of blood vessels and deposition of opaque fibrotic scar tissue that can also impair vision. Calcium deposition (band keratopathy) is a rare cause of blurred vision (e.g. chronic uveitis, hypercalcaemia) and sometimes a painful eye.

An advantage of corneal avascularity is that corneal transplants carry a much lower risk of rejection compared to internal organ transplantation.

Herpes simplex infection

Epidemiology

Ocular infection with herpes simplex tends to affect young adults.

Pathology

Corneal infection with herpes simplex virus causes a dendritic ulcer. The sensory nerves to the cornea are also damaged by the infection. A single episode of infection results in a dendritic ulcer which heals to leave a small superficial scar that does not usually affect the vision. Recurrent attacks may lead to corneal vascularization. Significant scarring of the cornea can lead to loss of vision and neurotrophic epithelial defects which may not heal.

Clinical features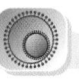

Patients present with a unilateral foreign body sensation in one eye. There is usually a history of cold sores on the face. Subsequent attacks may be less painful as the corneal nerves are progressively damaged with each episode.

On examination, the eye is red and a dendritic ulcer may be present, which can be seen on fluorescein staining (Fig. 10.9). Loss of corneal sensation is a useful sign in equivocal cases. Rose Bengal drops will light up the borders of a dendritic ulcer much more than a normal epithelial defect. Unfortunately Rose Bengal drops cause severe eye ache for several hours and should not be used routinely.

> **⚡ CLINICAL ALERT**
>
> *Dendritic ulcers that are misdiagnosed and treated with topical steroids will enlarge massively to become geographic ulcers.*

Investigations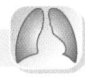

Microbiology

The diagnosis is clinical but may be confirmed by sending a swab for virology in difficult cases.

Management

Aciclovir

Oral aciclovir for 10 days is all that is required for most cases. Long-term oral aciclovir prophylaxis may reduce the risk of further attacks in patients with recurring disease.

Immunomodulation

Topical steroids (prednisolone 0.5%) are prescribed for patients with lesions on the visual axis to reduce scarring and visual loss. Steroid treatment must be covered by antiviral treatment, and it may take weeks to wean the patient off this treatment.

Corneal grafting

Loss of vision due to corneal scarring can be corrected by a corneal graft. In the setting of chronic herpes simplex

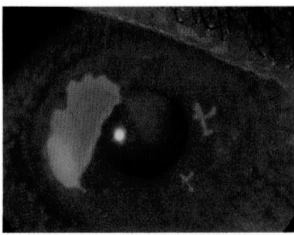

Fig. 10.9 Herpes simplex ulceration. Right eye photograph after fluorescein staining and examination with a blue light showing a large geographic ulcer and multiple dendritic ulcers due to herpes simplex virus.

infection, graft rejection is more likely due to the presence of corneal revascularization. Moreover, recurrent herpes keratitis in the graft can lead to further scarring.

Prognosis

Patients with less than two attacks have an excellent prognosis. Others with multiple recurrent attacks often suffer with a degree of permanent visual loss in the affected eye.

Herpes zoster ophthalmicus

Epidemiology

Herpes zoster ophthalmicus is uncommon; the incidence increases with age.

Pathology

Herpes zoster ophthalmicus results from the reactivation of dormant herpes zoster virus in the first division of the trigeminal nerve following previous chicken pox infection. The result can be simple conjunctivitis, corneal microdendrites, anterior uveitis, neurotrophic keratitis, glaucoma, scleritis or rarely acute retinal necrosis.

Clinical features

Patients present with a painful unilateral vesicular rash (shingles) over the forehead and upper eyelid. The eye is not always involved. If the side of the nose has vesicles on it (Hutchinson's sign) the risk of eye involvement is greater. Features of eye involvement range from a red eye (conjunctivitis) to an acute painful eye (keratitis) or visual loss (retinal necrosis).

Investigations
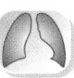

Microbiology
The diagnosis is clinical, but can be confirmed by sending vesicular fluid for virology.

Management

Aciclovir
If the rash has been present for less than 4 days, oral aciclovir (800 mg 5 times per day for 10 days) should be prescribed.

Prognosis

The ocular problems usually resolve completely but can recur years after the initial infection.

Corneal ulceration

Corneal ulceration is also known as microbial keratitis (inflammation of the cornea).

Epidemiology

Corneal ulceration usually occurs in young adults who wear contact lenses (developed countries) or following minor trauma in agricultural workers (developing countries).

Pathology
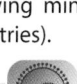

The majority (95%) of patients who develop corneal ulceration wear contact lenses. The contact lens limits the amount of oxygen from the air reaching the front of the avascular cornea, a problem that is compounded if lenses are worn during sleep (less oxygen is available to diffuse from the blood vessels on the inside of the closed eyelids).

In a normal eye the bacteria that build up on the inside of inadequately cleaned lenses are washed away by tears. With tight-fitting contact lenses, this process is impaired, and bacteria can accumulate. Moreover, the normal protective function of hypoxic corneal epithelial cells is impaired, predisposing the individual to corneal infection from relatively benign bacteria.

Pseudomonas can lead to aggressive infection with ulceration that can perforate if inadequately treated. *Acanthamoeba* is a rare but particularly virulent contact lens-related corneal infection that can lead to blurred vision, severe scleritis and diffuse keratitis. Dormant cyst formation in the cornea is impervious to current medical therapy, and late diagnosis may result in enucleation for pain relief.

Clinical features

Patients usually present with severe pain, lacrimation and sometimes blurred vision in one eye. There is usually a history of contact lens use, often overnight wearing, improper cleaning or inappropriate use of disposable lenses (wearing them for several days instead of one day only). On inspection, the eye is usually red, and it is important to perform a thorough examination of the cornea by lifting the upper lid to examine the superior cornea. Close inspection may reveal a fluffy white circle (the ulcer) on the cornea (Fig. 10.10), and accumulation of pus can manifest as a hypopyon (Fig. 10.11). The ulcer stains with fluorescein dye and becomes prominent on ultraviolet light examination.

Investigations
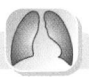

Microbiology
After instillation of topical anaesthesia, a corneal scrape should be sent urgently for Gram stain, culture and

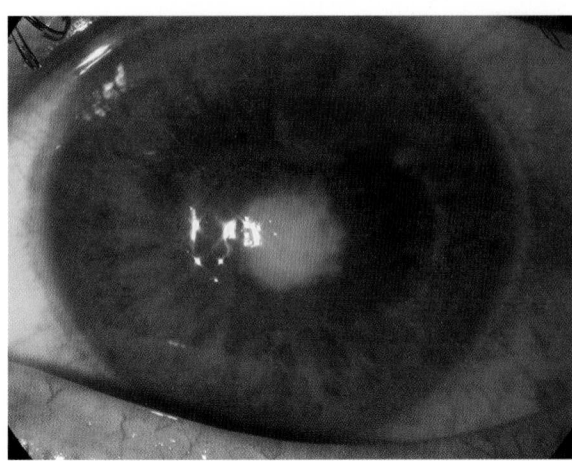
Fig. 10.10 A patient with a central corneal ulcer from contact lens wear.

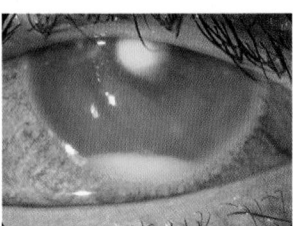
Fig. 10.11 Collection of inflammatory white blood cells in the anterior chamber (hypopyon) due to a central corneal ulcer.

sensitivity, especially if *Pseudomonas* is suspected. Fungal keratitis should be considered in immunocompromised patients or following agricultural injuries. The corneal scrape may also have a therapeutic role in reducing the bacterial load in the cornea.

Management

Patient education
Patients should be advised not to wear contact lenses, or change to rigid gas-permeable lenses which have a better safety record than the more comfortable soft lenses.

Antibiotics
Hourly topical ofloxacin is required for 48 hours (even through the night). The patient should be reviewed within 48 hours if *Pseudomonas* is suspected. Approximately 95% will improve by 48 hours, after which the frequency of the drops can be reduced. Lack of compliance with the topical regimen carries a poor response to treatment, and admission to hospital (for intensive drop regimens) may be required. *Acanthamoeba* infection requires prolonged treatment with topical chlorhexidine.

Prognosis

Most patients make an excellent recovery. Lesions on the visual axis can result in permanent loss of vision from scarring.

Recurrent corneal erosion syndrome

Epidemiology

Recurrent corneal erosion syndrome usually occurs in adults.

Pathology

Recurrent corneal erosion syndrome is a recurrent painful epithelial defect that occurs as a complication of a single episode of trauma to the cornea. The initiating cause is usually a scratch that damages and takes off the surface layer of epithelium from the cornea. Although the cornea quickly regenerates, the new epithelium is irregular and not fully adherent to the surface of the cornea. The loose epithelium may stick to the inside of the eyelid during sleep and, when the eye is opened, tears off a further corneal layer resulting in another painful epithelial defect.

Clinical features

Patients may complain of a sharp pain from the front of the eye, lacrimation and a red eye, usually occurring on waking and often improving by lunchtime (as the defect re-epithelializes). The defect may be seen with the help of fluorescein dye and ultraviolet light.

Investigations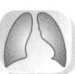

No investigations are required.

Management

Antibiotics
Topical chloramphenicol to the affected eye (for 5 days) is prescribed when the eye becomes painful.

Lubricating eye ointment
Lubricating eye ointment (e.g. simple eye ointment) every night for 3 months is first-line treatment, often with topical hypromellose to lubricate the eye during the day.

Bandage contact lenses
Cases that recur despite medical treatment may benefit from the use of bandage contact lenses.

Excimer laser resurfacing
Excimer laser resurfacing of the cornea can be used to ablate the irregular epithelial area leaving a smoother, more adhesive surface for the new epithelium to regenerate. Approximately 75% resolve with laser treatment.

Prognosis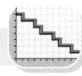

Most patients improve with non-surgical measures.

Pterygium

A pterygium is a wing of fibrovascular tissue that grows across the cornea.

Epidemiology

Pterygium is increasingly common with age and exposure to hot dry sunny environments.

Pathology

Sunlight and constant irritation cause elastotic degeneration of conjunctiva. The result is a wing of fibrovascular tissue that grows slowly across the cornea.

A pinguecula is a small yellow lump under the conjunctiva which may occasionally become inflamed and be confused with a pterygium. It does not migrate onto the cornea and rarely requires anything but reassurance.

Clinical features

The patient usually notices a triangular wing of tissue on the eye (Fig. 10.12). It is often simply a cosmetic problem, but can cause blurred vision. Occasionally the eye may be red and inflamed.

Investigations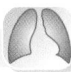

No investigations are required.

Management

Patient education

Patients with asymptomatic pterygium require no treatment other than reassurance.

Ocular lubricants

Ocular lubricants such as topical hypromellose (qds) or topical steroids (prednisolone 0.5% qds) may make the eye more comfortable.

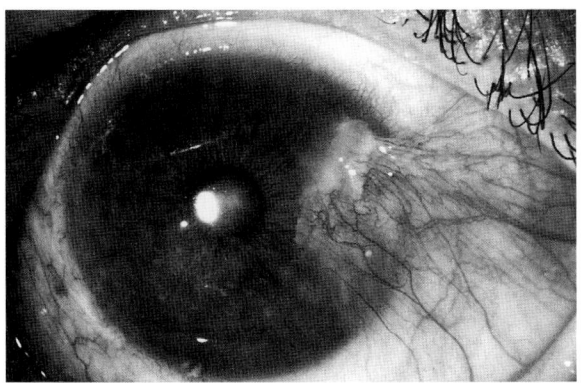

Fig. 10.12 Right eye showing a large nasal pterygium.

Surgical excision

Surgical excision is relatively straightforward and indicated when the visual axis is threatened by the pterygium or if there is a cosmetic defect. Recurrence following surgery is common, but can be reduced by transplanting normal autologous conjunctiva into the site from which the pterygium was removed.

Prognosis

For most patients, the pterygium is simply a cosmetic defect and surgery is not required. Permanent visual loss is rare.

Corneal graft

Indications

The corneal transplant is often the end-stage treatment for numerous corneal diseases. Historically, the most common indication was bullous keratopathy following cataract surgery. Currently keratoconus is the most common indication.

Patient preparation

Patients are admitted to hospital; informed consent is required. There are two main types of graft, full thickness and deep lamellar keratoplasty. The full thickness graft obtained from a cadaveric donor is most commonly used.

Procedure

A central circle of the recipient cornea is cut away and replaced with the donor cornea (Fig. 10.13). This is sutured in place and the sutures are left for at least a year before removal. If the patient has healthy endothelial cells (e.g. keratoconus) then a deep lamellar keratoplasty may be performed. The vision may not be quite as sharp as with a full thickness procedure but there is less graft rejection and endothelial cell failure.

Complications

The main risks are infection, corneal graft rejection (decrease in sight, eye pain and a red eye), recurrence of the original pathology (e.g. herpes simplex in the graft), secondary glaucoma, microbial keratitis of the graft and endothelial cell failure. Large amounts of astigmatism are common and several operations may be needed to correct this.

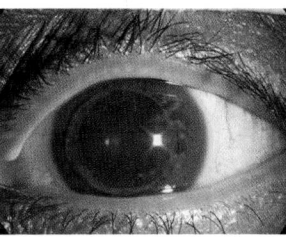

Fig. 10.13 Left eye photograph showing a clear functioning corneal graft.

Post procedure care

No immunosuppression is required as the corneal is an immunoprivileged site. A protective plastic eye shield is given to the patient to wear when sleeping for about 2 weeks. Patients may be sensitive to light and a pair of plain dark glasses is recommended.

Prognosis

In general good results are achieved with corneal grafting. Rejection is uncommon and usually occurs in the first year after the operation, following a change of treatment, after removal of stitches, or as a result of eye infection or injury.

SECTION 10.9 | Diseases of the uvea

Uveitis is inflammation of the uvea, the pigmented part of the eye which is made up of the iris, ciliary body and choroid. When any of these structures is inflamed it is usually possible to see inflammatory cells in the vitreous or anterior chamber. Approximately 75% of all uveitis is anterior uveitis, which predominantly affects the iris and ciliary body; this is also known as iritis or iridocyclitis (Fig. 10.14). The remaining 25% is made up of a number of more serious conditions such as intermediate uveitis, posterior uveitis or panuveitis. Most conditions that cause posterior uveal inflammation can also cause some signs of anterior uveitis, hence anterior uveitis can only be diagnosed after the back of the eye has been examined to exclude more serious pathology. Infection inside the eye often presents as a uveitis, typically a panuveitis, but is normally referred to as an endophthalmitis.

Epidemiology

Anterior uveitis has an annual incidence rate of 8 per 100 000 per year and typically affects young adults.

Pathology

The aetiology of anterior uveitis is thought to be idiopathic or autoimmune in 50%. The systemic and ocular associations of anterior uveitis are presented in Table 10.17. HLA-B27 associated anterior uveitis represents the largest group, and ankylosing spondylitis is the most commonly associated disease in the UK.

If posterior synechiae are allowed to develop they may become continuous (360°) around the pupil margin, preventing the normal circulation of aqueous from the ciliary bodies into the anterior chamber. The iris is pushed

Anterior uveitis

Anterior uveitis is the inflammation of the iris and ciliary body. It is also known as iritis or iridocyclitis.

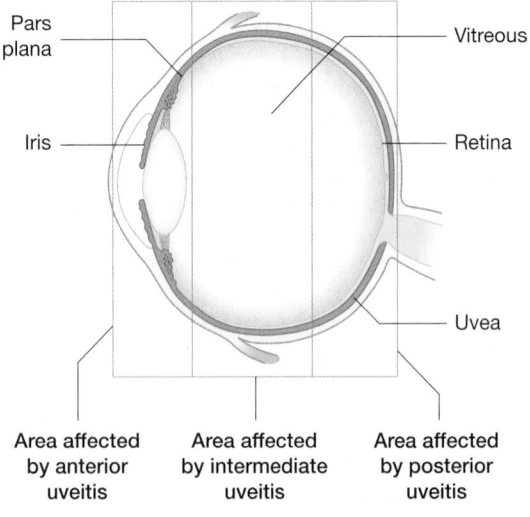

Fig. 10.14 Anatomical divisions of uveitis.

Table 10.17	Associations of anterior uveitis
Systemic associations	
HLA-B27	
Ankylosing spondylitis	
Reiter's syndrome	
Inflammatory bowel disease	
Psoriatic arthritis	
Juvenile idiopathic arthritis	
Herpes simplex/zoster infection	
Ocular ischaemia	
Sarcoidosis	
Syphilis	
Tuberculosis	
Leprosy	
Non-systemic associations	
Fuchs' heterochromic cyclitis	
Posner–Schlossman syndrome	
Cidofovir treatment	
Traumatic uveitis	
Hypermature cataract	
Post eye surgery (cataract surgery)	

forwards, closing off the drainage angle, and intraocular pressure rises causing an acute glaucoma.

Keratic precipitates may develop; these are clumps of inflammatory cells settling on the inside of the cornea. They are usually inferiorly placed and white in colour. In granulomatous conditions (e.g. sarcoidosis) they take on a distinctive 'mutton fat' appearance. In severe attacks, a hypopyon may form as a result of inflammatory cells settling in vast numbers (Fig. 10.11).

Clinical features

Anterior uveitis usually presents with photophobia, eye pain, blurred vision and a red eye. The acute episode typically worsens over a few days, but may follow a chronic grumbling course. Some patients, particularly those with juvenile idiopathic arthritis, may be asymptomatic (therefore screening is required). Patients with uveitis should not have sticky discharge from their eye although lacrimation is common.

Features suggestive of underlying associated disease include rash, joint problems, erythema nodosum (sarcoidosis), back pain and stiffness (ankylosing spondylitis), bloody diarrhoea (inflammatory bowel disease), shortness of breath (sarcoidosis), herpetic vesicles around the eyelids, mouth or genital ulcers (syphilis, Behçet's disease) and urethritis (Reiter's syndrome).

On examination, there is usually nothing to see at the bedside except a red eye. Occasionally (with a bright light), keratic precipitates and posterior synechiae (Fig. 10.15) may be present (an irregular shaped pupil due to the iris being stuck down to the lens). There will be no corneal staining with fluorescein unless there is infection with herpes virus. However, slit-lamp examination may reveal flare (protein leak into the anterior chamber) and anterior chamber activity (cells floating in the anterior chamber).

Investigations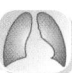

An otherwise well patient with anterior uveitis needs no investigations.

Management

Topical steroid eye drops
Anterior uveitis is treated with topical steroid drops (e.g. dexamethasone 0.1%), initially one drop every hour but reducing slowly in frequency over 6 weeks. The uveitis should respond within a few days.

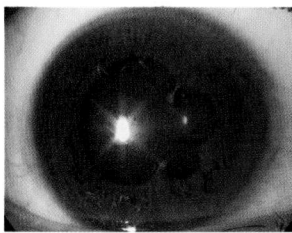

Fig. 10.15 Photograph showing posterior synechiae.

Subconjunctival steroid injections
More severe cases may require subconjunctival steroid injection (betamethasone 4 mg).

Dilating drops
Dilating drops (cyclopentolate 1% tds) are used for the first week to prevent or break posterior synechiae. The dilating drops cause a temporary paralysis of accommodation leading to blurred near vision in most patients.

Prognosis

Anterior uveitis usually has a benign course if treated appropriately. Full visual recovery is the rule but recurrent attacks are common. The exception to this is patients with juvenile idiopathic arthritis where the course is chronic. Cataract surgery has a particularly poor prognosis in this group and significant long-term visual impairment is common.

Intermediate uveitis

Intermediate uveitis is used to describe the location of inflammation between the anterior and posterior aspects of the uveal tract (Fig. 10.14).

Epidemiology

Intermediate uveitis is rare.

Pathology

Diseases associated with intermediate uveitis are sarcoidosis, multiple sclerosis, inflammatory bowel disease and Lyme disease. Visual loss is mainly due to cystoid macular oedema (fluid in the retina) and vitreous opacities.

Clinical features

Patients with intermediate uveitis present with floaters and gradual onset of blurred vision. Pain is not a major feature and the eye is usually white. At the bedside, examination is essentially normal but in severe cases the view of the retina will be blurred with a direct ophthalmoscope. The inflammation is centred on the uvea just posterior to the iris, and inflammatory cells and debris can be seen in the vitreous jelly with a slit lamp. Clumps of vitreous cells floating in the vitreous are called 'snow balls'. Sheets of white exudative material ('snowbanks') can sometimes be seen in the far periphery of the retina and over the pars plana (pars planitis).

Investigations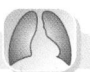

Investigations are directed to identifying any associated or underlying cause, of which sarcoidosis is the most common (p. 140).

Management

Immunomodulation

Oral prednisolone is usually prescribed only when vision has dropped to below 6/12; this is usually due to the development of cystoid macular oedema. A reducing course of prednisolone starting at 40 mg per day is often prescribed.

Patients with unilateral disease may be managed with orbital floor depot steroid injections (triamcinolone) or by intraocular steroid injections.

Prognosis

The majority (66%) of patients with intermediate uveitis maintain vision that is better than 6/12 with appropriate treatment.

Posterior uveitis

Posterior uveitis encompasses inflammation of the retina and choroid.

Epidemiology

Posterior uveitis is rare.

Pathology

There are many causes of posterior uveitis, listed in Table 10.18. The common pathology is inflammation of the fundus. Retinal detachment or vitreous haemorrhage may also occur. All forms of uveitis can cause cataract and glaucoma.

Infections that can lead to posterior uveitis include toxoplasmosis, tuberculosis, syphilis and AIDS. In addition, patients with AIDS are also predisposed to cytomegalovirus retinitis, toxoplasmosis and *Pneumocystis carinii* retinitis. Endophthalmitis is detailed on page 657.

Sympathetic ophthalmia occurs from exposure of disrupted uveal tissue to antigen-presenting cells following trauma. This autoimmune phenomenon usually presents a few months after serious eye trauma (e.g. ruptured globe) but can occur years after the initial event.

Clinical features

Posterior uveitis typically presents like an intermediate uveitis but often the visual loss is more severe and the onset is faster. Direct ophthalmoscopy may reveal a hazy view with retinal vessel sheathing, choroidal infiltrates, disc swelling, retinal haemorrhages and exudates. Slit-lamp examination will also show cells in the vitreous. Panuveitis is posterior uveitis with a significant anterior component.

With toxoplasmosis retinochoroiditis there is often an old chorioretinal scar from previous subclinical attack. A

Table 10.18	Management of the different causes of posterior uveitis and panuveitis
Cause	**Management**
Toxoplasmosis	Systemic steroids and antimicrobial therapy (pyrimethamine, folinic acid and sulfadiazine)
Sarcoidosis	Systemic steroids
Behçet's disease	Systemic steroids, and other immunomodulating agents
Sympathetic ophthalmia	Systemic steroids
Tuberculosis	Antituberculous treatment, and systemic steroids
Cytomegalovirus	Systemic ganciclovir and foscarnet
Herpes simplex virus	Aciclovir
Herpes zoster virus	Aciclovir
Syphilis	Penicillin, systemic steroids
Idiopathic retinal vasculitis	
Candida endophthalmitis	Intravitreal amphotericin, followed by systemic antifungal treatment
Bacterial endophthalmitis	Intravitreal antibiotics

focal area of white retinal infiltrate (retinitis) is seen with a brisk vitreitis (cells in the vitreous). Behçet's disease is characterized by optic disc swelling with an occlusive retinitis. Approximately 33% have a hypopyon despite having a white eye. In miliary tuberculosis, choroidal tubercles can be seen on fundoscopy but anterior uveitis is more common. Sympathetic ophthalmia presents with bilateral granulomatous anterior uveitis but pale subretinal lesions can be seen on fundoscopy.

Investigations

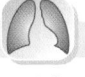

Investigations are directed to the underlying aetiology (Table 10.18).

Management

Immunomodulation

Treatment of posterior uveitis will depend on the cause (Table 10.18). Often high-dose steroids (prednisolone 80 mg per day) or other immunomodulating agents (azathioprine 50 mg tds) may be needed.

Prognosis

The prognosis of posterior uveitis and panuveitis depends upon the aetiology.

Endophthalmitis

Endophthalmitis is infection of the inside of the eye, leading to panuveitis.

Epidemiology

Bacterial and candidal endophthalmitis are uncommon.

Pathology

Bacterial endophthalmitis can occur from septic emboli from an infected heart valve, as a complication of intraocular surgery (especially previous glaucoma filtration surgery). Intravenous drug users who dilute their heroin with lemon juice (which is usually contaminated with candida) are at particular risk of developing a candidal endophthalmitis. Critically ill patients in the ITU are also at risk of candidal endophthalmitis.

Clinical features

Patients with endophthalmitis present with eye pain, photophobia, loss of vision and a red eye often with a small hypopyon. Intraocular infection with *Propionibacter acnes* occurs during cataract surgery and follows a chronic course, often presenting as a mild postoperative uveitis weeks after surgery which responds initially to topical steroids. Candidal endophthalmitis develops slowly, with floaters and mild blurring of vision being the first symptoms (some patients can be asymptomatic). It will usually turn into a panuveitis if untreated.

Investigations

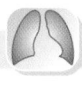

Vitreous sample

A vitreous sample is taken for microbiology.

Management

Identify and correct underlying cause

Any underlying disease that is predisposing to sepsis should be treated. If the offending agent is an intraocular lens, the implanted lens usually has to be removed to prevent recurrence of infection.

Intravitreal antibiotics

Intravitreal antibiotics are injected, and intravitreal amphotericin is followed by systemic antifungal treatment for candidal endophthalmitis.

Prognosis

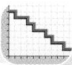

The prognosis depends on the organism involved but is often very poor.

SECTION 10.10 # Diseases of the lens

Cataract

A cataract is defined as any opacity in the crystalline lens. It is the most common cause of treatable blindness in the world.

Epidemiology

Cataract is very common and the prevalence increases with age from 4000 per 100 000 at the age of 52–64 years to 45 000 per 100 000 at the age of 65–74 years.[1]

Pathology

Over 90% of cataracts are age related (senile cataract) and no underlying cause can be identified. Cataracts are only rarely congenital but more often occur as a result of ocular or systemic disease (Table 10.19). They may be described by anatomical location of the opacity (Fig. 10.16) and stage of maturation.

Clinical features

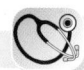

Cataracts cause painless visual loss which typically occurs over a period of years but may develop within a few weeks, particularly after trauma. Visual acuity will usually be reduced and may worsen in conditions of bright light as a result of glare from the cataract. Younger patients with posterior subcapsular cataracts may complain of glare from oncoming headlights at night as a presenting symptom. This can prevent night driving before visual acuity is reduced. Patients with early cataract formation may notice that they need to change their glasses more frequently. A previous history of any eye disorder, drugs history and systems review may identify underlying disease associated with cataract formation.

On examination, the cataract may be visible as an opacity in the lens but cataract alone does not cause an abnormal pupillary response to light or accommodation. Hence the presence of a cataract does not explain a relative afferent pupillary defect and other causes must be

Table 10.19	Causes of cataract
Senile cataract (most common)	

Congenital cataract (rare)
   Genetic
   Maternal infection (rubella or toxoplasmosis)	

Ocular causes	
Chronic or recurrent uveitis	
Acute angle closure glaucoma	
Retinal detachment	
Ocular trauma (including intraocular surgery)	
Radiotherapy	
Systemic causes	
Diabetes (most common systemic cause)	
Drugs (corticosteroids—eye drops or tablets)	
Down's syndrome	
Galactosaemia	
Wilson's disease	
Fabry's disease	
Myotonic dystrophy	

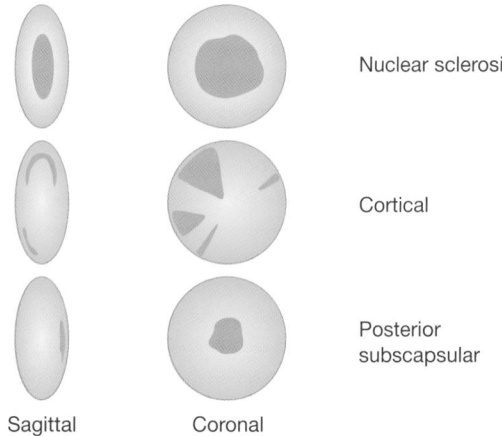

Fig. 10.16 Anatomical location of a cataract.

Nuclear sclerosis

Cortical

Posterior subscapsular

Sagittal   Coronal

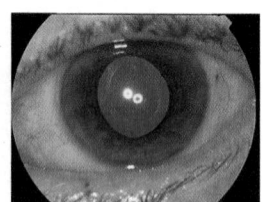

Fig. 10.17 An intraocular lens.

B-scan ultrasound

If the retina cannot be adequately visualized on dilated fundoscopy, an ultrasound scan of the eye is required if surgery is to be considered as a screening measure for retinal detachment or vitreous haemorrhage.

Initial management

Not all patient with cataracts require surgery, and surgery should not be performed simply because an optometrist has seen some lens opacity. An explanation of the slowly progressive nature of the condition and its treatment is required. It is no longer necessary to wait for a cataract to become ripe as surgical techniques have improved and, in normal circumstances, the final outcome will be the same even if surgery is delayed. If the patient is not keen on surgery then new glasses may help in early cases.

Surgical management

Symptomatic visual impairment is the main indication for surgery. However, the decision to operate is not based on the severity of visual loss alone, but on the impact of visual impairment on the desired activities of the patient. Other indications are rare but include the treatment of phacomorphic glaucoma, ruptured lens capsule, dislocated lens and to allow visualization and treatment of retinal pathology such as diabetic retinopathy.

Cataract surgery is increasingly performed as a day case procedure with local anaesthesia or just anaesthetic eye drops. Sutureless phacoemulsification has largely replaced extracapsular cataract extraction in developed countries. Cataract removal is followed by intraocular lens implantation to replace the extracted native lens with a synthetic lens.

Phacoemulsification

This is currently the preferred technique. A high-frequency ultrasound probe is used to emulsify and aspirate the lens. A small incision is made in the cornea, the probe is introduced into the anterior chamber of the eye and the lens is gradually cored out. When the core of the lens has been removed the lens capsule is cleaned and a flexible intraocular lens is implanted.

The power of the intraocular lens is calculated preoperatively based on ultrasound measurements of the length of the eye and the curvature of the cornea. When implanted, it unfolds within the eye and is positioned inside the old lens capsule. As the initial incision is small, sutures are not normally required to secure the wound.

Extracapsular cataract extraction

This procedure requires a more extended incision into the cornea, as the cataract is removed in one piece, followed by implantation of a rigid intraocular lens in its place (Fig. 10.17). The wound is sutured and this usually causes some astigmatism which improves when the sutures are removed 3 months later.

Patients are usually given chloramphenicol and dexamethasone drops for 4 weeks to prevent infection or exces-

determined. On direct ophthalmoscopy, the cataract appears as black flecks against the red reflex. It is best seen from about 1 metre away from the patient in a darkened room. Slit-lamp examination may reveal further clues to the aetiology of the cataract and allows anatomical localization of the opacity within the lens.

Initial investigations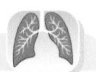

Routine investigations are not usually required unless there is suspicion of underlying disease.

sive inflammation. Four weeks after phacoemulsification surgery, patients are advised to see an optometrist as the majority will require glasses for reading, distance vision or both. Unlike the native lens, the implanted intraocular lens is unable to accommodate.

Postoperatively, 95% recover full visual acuity. The chance of cataract surgery leading to worse vision is 1%, and 5% of patients may require more than one operation to achieve a satisfactory result.

Complications are the same for both procedures. Major complications that potentially lead to blindness are endophthalmitis (1 in 3000), retinal detachment (1 in 3000) and choroidal haemorrhage (1 in 3000). Postoperative anterior uveitis occurs commonly causing photophobia, blurred vision and a red eye. This usually resolves with a longer course of steroid eye drops but endophthalmitis must first be excluded.

Posterior capsular opacification is a late complication that develops several years later in approximately 20%. The original lens capsule (holding the synthetic lens) loses its clarity as a result of epithelial migration across the posterior capsule surface. Significant visual deterioration can result and is treated by creating a small hole in the opaque capsule with a YAG laser.

RECENT ADVANCES

Multifocal lenses and accommodating intraocular lenses are not yet of proven benefit and risk sacrificing optimal vision in an attempt to avoid the need for reading glasses.

Prognosis

The natural history of a developing cataract is very variable and many patients are quite happy to tolerate mild blurring for more than 10 years whilst others will insist on immediate surgery despite minimal opacity. Cataract surgery is one of the most effective surgical procedures ever developed but despite this it still carries a small risk of blindness and all patients should be adequately counselled prior to agreeing to have surgery.

REFERENCE

(1) *Kahn HA, Leibowitz HM, Ganley JP, Kini MM, Colton T, Nickerson RS, Dawber TR. The Framingham eye study II. American Journal of Epidemiology 1997; 106: 33–41.*

SECTION 10.11 Diseases of the retina

Diabetic retinopathy

Epidemiology

Diabetic retinopathy is the most common cause of blind registration in the working population (20–65) in the UK. Diabetic retinopathy affects approximately 40% of type 1 diabetics and 20% of type 2 diabetics.

Pathology

Risk factors for developing diabetic retinopathy are increased duration of diabetes, poor glycaemic control, high blood pressure and hyperlipidaemia. There is no single explanation for the toxicity of glucose to retinal vasculature but there is an alteration in the retinal capillary pericyte to endothelial cell ratio, capillary cell death and microvascular occlusion. The resultant ischaemia stimulates release of vasoactive growth factors such as vascular endothelial growth factor, making the blood vessels become increasingly permeable, leaking fluid into the retina (macular oedema). New vessels may grow along the retinal surface or into the vitreous (proliferative retinopathy).

Scope of disease

Macular oedema results in blurred vision. New vessels bleed, causing a vitreous haemorrhage and loss of vision or tractional retinal detachment as they mature and fibrose, pulling the retina off. Diabetic retinopathy may become much worse during pregnancy or just after glycaemic control is improved (e.g. after switching to insulin).

Clinical features

Patients with type 2 diabetes typically develop predominantly macular oedema whilst patients with type 1 diabetes tend to develop proliferative retinopathy. Retinopathy has traditionally been graded as background, pre-proliferative and proliferative (when new vessels are present).

Many patients develop background diabetic retinopathy without sight-threatening complications and are detected during screening examinations for diabetic eye disease. Typical changes of background (non-proliferative) diabetic retinopathy are dot and blot haemorrhages, microaneurysms, hard exudates (Fig. 10.18), venous beading, cotton wool spots (Fig. 10.19) and intraretinal microvascular abnormalities.

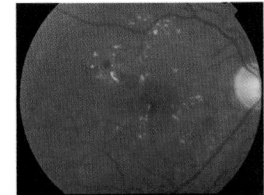

Fig. 10.18 Right eye fundus photograph showing moderate non-proliferating diabetic retinopathy: hard exudates are visible as yellow spots with haemorrhage and microaneurysms.

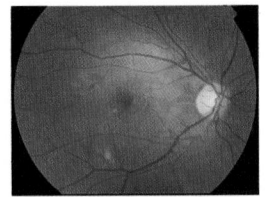

Fig. 10.19 Right eye fundus photograph showing cotton wool spots with venous beading.

659

Dot haemorrhages and microaneurysms appear identical on direct ophthalmoscopy but may be differentiated by fluorescein angiography. Hard exudates are lipid deposits which occur in the presence of macular oedema. Cotton wool spots represent microinfarcts and disappear after a few weeks. Veins develop a beaded appearance when they cross areas of ischaemic retina (capillary closure) and are a particular risk factor for developing new vessels (Fig. 10.20). Intraretinal microvascular abnormalities are dilated capillaries within the retina and are a precursor of retinal new vessels.

Diabetic maculopathy may be ischaemic or non-ischaemic with oedema, microaneurysms and hard exudates near the macula. Some patients have both oedema and ischaemia. Retinal thickening is visible with a slit-lamp biomicroscope. Changes nearer to the fovea will have a greater effect on vision.

New vessels appear either at the optic disc or growing off the larger retinal veins. New vessels may also develop on the iris, giving rise to rubeotic glaucoma.

If there is haemorrhage in the vitreous or subhyaloid haemorrhage then there are almost certainly new vessels growing somewhere which need treatment.

Initial investigations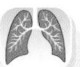

Random blood glucose
Patients may present with advanced diabetic retinopathy without ever having been diagnosed, so random blood glucose estimation should be performed.

Further investigations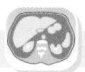

Fluorescein angiography
Fluorescein angiography may be useful in patients with visual loss from maculopathy as it will differentiate untreatable ischaemic maculopathy from treatable non-ischaemic maculopathy. New vessels are much easier to identify with fluorescein angiography.

Initial management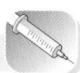

Modification of risk factors
Optimal glycaemic, blood pressure, lipid and obesity management should be the initial aim.

Surgical management

Laser therapy
Laser treatment is indicated for patients with oedematous non-ischaemic macula. It may prevent further visual loss and improves vision in 15%. It is thought to work by stimulating retinal pigment epithelium cells to pump excess fluid out of the retina more efficiently. Grid laser treatment for macular oedema reduces the risk of further visual loss by 50%.[1]

Panretinal photocoagulation
Panretinal photocoagulation to the peripheral retina is used to treat neovascularization (proliferative retinopathy). This destroys most of the peripheral retina but spares the macula and optic disc (Fig. 10.21). Once the retina is destroyed by the laser it ceases to produce growth factors and the new vessels regress. Patients are left with a constricted visual field, and if both eyes are treated they may lose their entitlement to drive. Panretinal photocoagulation reduces the risk of severe visual loss by 50%.[2]

> **RECENT ADVANCES**
>
> *Intraocular steroid injections are currently being evaluated for macular oedema to determine if they reduce vascular permeability[3] and help retain vision long term.*

Vitrectomy
Vitrectomy is required to clear persistent vitreous haemorrhage and to remove fibrotic membranes causing or threatening to cause tractional retinal detachment.

Prognosis

The prognosis is related to the disease subtype and treatment received, as detailed above.

Screening
Patients develop asymptomatic retinal changes long before they develop visual loss, and early treatment is essential. All patients should have dilated fundoscopy annually, by their general practitioner, qualified optometrist, diabetic physician or eye clinic. Type 1 diabetics are not normally screened for the first 5 years after developing diabetes but type 2 diabetics should be screened immediately upon the diagnosis of diabetes.

REFERENCES

(1) *Treatment techniques and clinical guidelines for photocoagulation of diabetic macular edema. Early Treatment Diabetic Retinopathy Study Report Number 2. Early Treatment Diabetic Retinopathy Study Research Group. Ophthalmology 1987; 94: 761–774.*
(2) *Photocoagulation treatment of proliferative diabetic retinopathy. Clinical application of Diabetic Retinopathy Study (DRS) findings, DRS Report Number 8. The Diabetic Retinopathy Study Research Group. Ophthalmology 1981; 88: 583–600.*
(3) *Massin P, Audren F, Haouchine B, et al. Intravitreal triamcinolone acetonide for diabetic diffuse macular edema: preliminary results of a prospective controlled trial. Ophthalmology 2004; 111: 218–224; discussion 224–225.*

Hypertensive retinopathy

Epidemiology

Approximately 20% of adults have chronic hypertension, and associated hypertensive retinopathy is common.

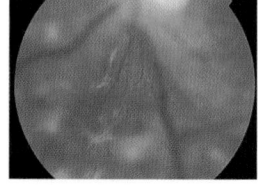

Fig. 10.20 Photograph of the left optic disc. New vessels are forming at the disc.

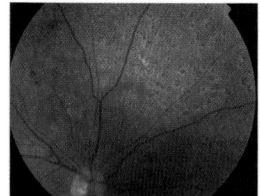

Fig. 10.21 Right eye fundus photograph showing laser scars after panretinal photocoagulation.

Pathology

Chronic hypertension results in arteriosclerotic changes of the retinal arterioles; the changes are graded 1–4 (Table 10.20). Grades 1 and 2 are common and occur in chronic hypertension whilst grades 3 and 4 are rare and occur in acute severe sustained hypertension (e.g. malignant hypertension due to bilateral renal artery stenosis).

The retinal arteries and vein share a common adventitial sheath. As the artery becomes harder it compresses the more pliable vein which develops arteriovenous nipping that may progress to branch retinal vein occlusion. Retinal emboli also occur as a result of carotid atherosclerosis. Other ocular complications of systemic hypertension are listed in Table 10.21.

Clinical features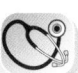

Patients with grade 1 or 2 hypertensive retinopathy are asymptomatic, and patients with grade 3 or 4 disease may present with blurred vision.

Patients may have an elevated blood pressure. On fundoscopy there is narrowing of the arteries with silver wiring. This is an increased, almost shiny, reflectance from the surface of the larger retinal arteries. Arteriovenous nipping occurs and in severe cases retinal haemorrhages, dot or flame shaped, may occur. Macular exudates in a star shape and disc oedema are much less common and are only seen with very high blood pressure.

An important aspect of detecting early hypertensive retinal changes is that it confirms long-standing hypertension that requires treatment (p. 68), differentiating it from white coat hypertension.

Table 10.20	Grading of hypertensive retinopathy
Grade 1	Silver wiring and narrowing of arteries
Grade 2	Arteriovenous nipping
Grade 3	Retinal haemorrhages, macula star of hard exudates, cotton wool spots
Grade 4	As grade 3, but with optic disc swelling

Table 10.21	Ocular complications related to systemic hypertension
Branch retinal vein occlusion	
Central retinal vein occlusion	
Branch retinal artery occlusion	
Central retinal artery occlusion	
Retinal artery macroaneurysm	
Anterior ischaemic optic neuropathy	
Serous retinal detachment (very high blood pressure only)	
Ocular ischaemic syndrome	

Investigations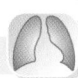

Hypertensive retinopathy is a clinical diagnosis, and no further investigations are required for the ocular disease. The investigations for hypertension are listed on page 69.

Management

Blood pressure control

The mainstay of management is blood pressure control (p. 69). No specific ophthalmic treatment is required. Very rapid control of blood pressure should be avoided in patients with very high blood pressure as optic nerve or cerebral infarction may result due to altered autoregulation of blood flow.

Prognosis

The prognosis for vision is good for grade 1 and 2 disease. Even for patients with grade 3 or 4 retinopathy, some visual recovery can be expected as long as the blood pressure is not dropped too precipitously.

> ***i*** **FURTHER INFORMATION**
>
> *Luo BP, Brown GC. Update on the ocular manifestations of systemic arterial hypertension. Current Opinion in Ophthalmology 2004; 15: 203–210.*

Retinal artery occlusion

Branch and central retinal occlusions occur as a result of emboli (Table 10.22). The risk factors are atherosclerosis, cardiac valve disease and atrial fibrillation. Branch retinal artery occlusions are often asymptomatic but may cause a peripheral field defect. Fundoscopy may reveal an embolus, usually lodged at the bifurcation of a vessel. No specific ophthalmic treatment is needed.

Central retinal artery occlusion has similar risk factors to branch retinal artery occlusion, with giant cell arteritis as a rare cause. Patients present with sudden loss of vision.

Table 10.22	Types of retinal emboli
Cholesterol	Bright glistening yellow fragments—from aorta or carotid, rarely cause vascular occlusion
Platelet–fibrin	Dull grey, fragmented, elongated—from heart valves or arteries, also seen in coagulopathies
Calcific	Large, chalky-white often seen at optic disc—cardiac valves, occasionally from carotid or aorta

Often they will have 'count fingers' vision or worse. There is often an afferent pupillary defect. Some patients have sparing of their cilioretinal artery which supplies a tiny area of the central macula; although these patients may have perfect 6/6 central vision, the field of vision is so small that it is useless. Fundoscopy will show narrow retinal arteries, a cherry red spot at the macula and a subtle whitening of the retina which disappears with the cherry red spot after about 6 weeks. It is easy to mistake the appearance of central retinal artery occlusion for a normal retina. There is no haemorrhage. Immediate treatment attempts to dislodge the embolus by massage of the globe, rebreathing from a paper bag (to increase blood carbon dioxide to induce retinal artery dilatation) and intravenous acetazolamide (to lower the intraocular pressure) but none has been shown to be effective. Occasionally the emboli clear themselves and vision improves within 24 hours, otherwise the visual loss is usually permanent. Further treatment is aimed at preventing occlusion in the other eye and is similar to the prevention of embolic strokes (p. 599).

Retinal vein occlusion

Epidemiology

Retinal vein occlusion is a common cause of visual loss. The prevalence of retinal vein occlusion is 700 per 100 000 between the ages of 49 and 60 years and 4600 per 100 000 at 80 years.[1] It occurs equally in both sexes, with branch retinal vein occlusion 3 times more common than central retinal vein occlusion.

Pathology

Retinal vein occlusion occurs due to obstruction of the central or branch retinal vein by a thrombus. The main risk factors are hypertension, hyperlipidaemia, diabetes, increasing age, raised intraocular pressure, hyperviscosity syndromes (rare) and periphlebitis (sarcoid and Behçet's—rare).

Clinical features

Patients present with sudden loss of vision (central retinal vein occlusion) with a visual acuity of 6/24 to 6/60, or loss of part of their field of vision (branch retinal vein occlusion). Branch retinal vein occlusion can be asymptomatic in the elderly, but may cause macular oedema.

Fundoscopy reveals numerous flame-shaped haemorrhages (Fig. 10.22) often with cotton wool spots. In branch retinal vein occlusion these changes only affect one quadrant of the retina or occasionally just the macula. In central retinal vein occlusion the whole retina will be affected and disc swelling may occur.

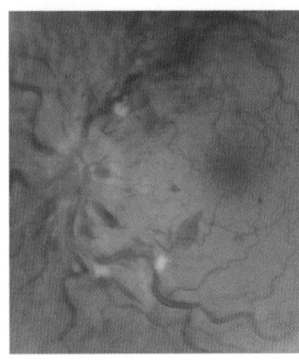

Fig. 10.22 Left eye colour fundus photograph showing central retinal vein occlusion with multiple flame haemorrhages and venous tortuosity.

Investigations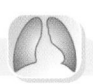

The main aim of investigation is to determine the source or risk factors associated with thrombus formation.

Full blood count/markers of inflammation
A high haemoglobin level may be due to polycythaemia (hyperviscosity). The ESR is a non-specific marker of inflammation.

Urea and electrolytes
Abnormal renal function may detect dehydration causing hyperviscosity or end organ damage from hypertension or diabetes.

Random blood glucose
Diabetes is a known risk factor for retinal vein occlusion.

Serum lipid profile
Hyperlipidaemia is a known risk factor for retinal vein occlusion.

Further investigations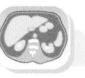

Patients less than 50 years should also have a thrombophilia screen, and if necessary screening for systemic lupus erythematosus (p. 492) and sarcoid (p. 725).

Management

Identify and correct underlying disorder
An important aspect in the management is to identify and correct any underlying disorder or risk factor associated with retinal vein occlusion.

Panretinal photocoagulation
In patients with branch retinal vein occlusion, macular grid laser treatment is indicated if there is no spontaneous improvement within 3 months. New retinal vessels can be treated with sector panretinal photocoagulation.

In patients with central retinal vein occlusion, spontaneous improvement can occur in young patients but vision usually remains at 6/60 or worse in older patients. Patients are at high risk of new vessel growth and rubeotic glaucoma, therefore panretinal photocoagulation should be performed as soon as new vessels appear.

FURTHER INFORMATION

Retinal Vein Occlusion Guidelines. The Royal College Of Ophthalmologists. March 2004. www.rcophth.ac.uk

REFERENCE

(1) *Mitchell P, Smith W, Chang A. Prevalence and associations of retinal vein occlusion in Australia. The Blue Mountains Eye Study. Archives of Ophthalmology 1996; 114: 1243–1247.*

Retinitis pigmentosa

Epidemiology

The prevalence of retinitis pigmentosa is approximately 25 per 100 000. The age of onset is usually in early adulthood but it can be quite variable.

Pathology

Retinitis pigmentosa is a common phenotype to many different genetic abnormalities of rod photoreceptor function. The inheritance can be autosomal dominant, autosomal recessive, X-linked, mitochondrial or genetically more complex. It is associated with Usher's syndrome in 12%, Bardet–Biedl syndrome in 4% and learning difficulties in 11%[1]; further associations are listed in Table 10.23.

Clinical features

Patients present with progressive bilateral night blindness and constriction of the peripheral visual field. The disease slowly progresses over decades to blurred vision and eventually blindness in a proportion.

Fundoscopy reveals a pale optic disc, attenuated retinal vessels and a 'bone spicule' appearance from clumps of retinal pigment epithelium cells in the peripheral retina (Fig. 10.23). Cataract and macular oedema may occur.

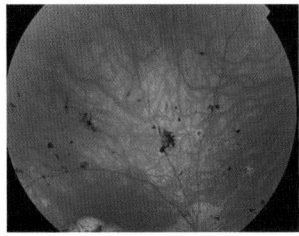

Fig. 10.23 Retinitis pigmentosa.

Table 10.23	Diseases associated with retinitis pigmentosa
Syndrome	**Features**
Usher's syndrome	Sensorineural deafness
Refsum's disease	Phytanic acid storage disease. Deafness, ataxia, peripheral neuropathy, ichthyosis
Abetalipoproteinaemia	Acanthocytes, ataxia, restricted eye movements, fat malabsorption
Kearns–Sayre syndrome	Limitation of eye movements, ptosis, heart block
Laurence–Moon–Bardet–Biedl syndrome	Polydactyly, mental retardation, obesity, hypogonadism

Investigations

Electrophysiological testing
This will show a reduced a-wave on electroretinogram reflecting abnormal rod photoreceptor function. Some patients have predominantly cone abnormalities, called 'cone dystrophies' or 'cone–rod dystrophies'.

Management

No treatment is effective at preventing disease progression.

Acetazolamide
Oral acetazolamide may reduce macular oedema in affected patients.

Cataract surgery
Surgery is beneficial in patients with established cataracts.

Prognosis

The prognosis depends on the gene defect. Some patients maintain some useful vision into old age whilst others are registered blind in their twenties.

REFERENCE

(1) *Haim M. Epidemiology of retinitis pigmentosa in Denmark. Acta Ophthalmologica Scandinavica Suppl 2002; 233: 1–34.*

Retinal tears

Epidemiology

The incidence of retinal detachment is approximately 5 per 100 000 per year in the general population. The incidence increases with age, and peaks at 55 years. It is slightly more common in men, and males are more likely to suffer with traumatic detachments.[1]

Pathology

A hole or tear in the retina usually occurs because of traction from the vitreous jelly. The vitreous jelly is attached to the peripheral retina a few millimetres posterior to the iris and at the optic disc head. Retinal tears are more common in late middle age when the vitreous shrinks and separates away from its attachment at the optic disc head (posterior vitreous detachment). In most cases the hole remains flat on the retina but in some patients fluid from within the eyeball seeps through the hole and lifts the retina.

A small retinal detachment usually progresses over a few days to total retinal detachment. As the photoreceptors are no longer in contact with their supporting retinal pigment epithelium cells or choroidal blood supply they no longer function normally.

Rarely a macular hole develops, particularly in post-menopausal women. Although retinal detachment from this is rare, the fovea is involved and consequently vision is often reduced to 6/60.

Patients at increased risk of retinal detachments include those with severe myopia, Marfan's, Stickler's and Ehlers–Danlos syndrome. Retinal detachment can also occur as a complication of cataract surgery and eye trauma.

Clinical features

Symptoms of posterior vitreous detachment include flashing lights and floaters. If retinal detachment occurs, the patient usually complains of a net curtain effect which obscures part of the vision in one eye.

Examination by dilated fundoscopy should be performed by an ophthalmologist within 24 hours as early treatment improves the possibility of visual recovery. On examination, single or multiple, well-circumscribed round or oval lesions may be seen within the posterior fundus. The lesions are typically dome-shaped elevations with a yellow to orange colour. A reddish 'halo' is often seen around the base of the detachment with overlying pigment defects such as clumping or mottling.

Investigations

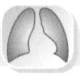

Most patients with retinal detachments require no investigations.

Ultrasound of the orbit

This is a useful investigation when the retina cannot be seen because of dense cataract or blood in the vitreous.

Ultrasound may (occasionally) be helpful to exclude underlying choroidal melanoma, particularly in patients with long-standing retinal detachment.

Surgical management

Laser therapy

If a small hole or tear is detected, laser can be applied around the retinal break. This stimulates fibrous adhesions between the retina, retinal pigment epithelium and Bruch's membrane, preventing the spread of fluid and consequent retinal detachment.

Scleral buckling

Scleral buckling is a technique to address retinal detachment. Usually, a silicon band is sutured to the outside of the eye to press the peripheral sclera towards the detached retina, fluid is drained from beneath the retina, and laser is applied to stop further fluid leaking under the retina.

Vitrectomy

Alternatively the vitreous can be removed and the retina floated back into position using a gas bubble or silicon oil. The retinal hole is then sealed by laser or cryotherapy. The gas bubble may take 6 weeks to dissolve and during this time patients should not fly (the bubble expands at high altitude). If patients with gas in their eye need another general anaesthetic the anaesthetist should be warned not to use nitrous oxide as this may also cause the gas bubble to expand.

Vitrectomy and intraocular gas can also close a macular hole to improve vision to about 6/12. Patients are required to posture face down constantly for 10 days to keep the bubble in the correct position to tamponade the hole.

Prognosis

The prognosis depends on how much retina has detached at the time of surgery. If the macula has been detached for more than 24 hours, the chance of full visual recovery is small even with anatomically successful surgery. A vision of 6/60 is typical in these cases. If the detachment is repaired before the macula detaches, then vision of 6/12 or better can be expected.

REFERENCE

(1) *Mowatt L, Shun-Shin G, Price N. Ethnic differences in the demand incidence of retinal detachments in two districts in the West Midlands. Eye 2003; 17: 63–70.*

Diseases of the macula

Age-related macular degeneration

Epidemiology

Age-related macular degeneration is the most common cause of severe loss of vision in developed countries. The prevalence increases with age and the condition tends to occur in patients over the age of 50. Approximately 30% of adults over the age of 75 have a degree of age-related macular degeneration.

Pathology

The two forms of age-related macular degeneration are 'dry', which is more common (90%) and less serious, and 'wet'. In both types, abnormal yellow to grey deposits (drusen) accumulate on Bruch's membrane which separates the highly vascular choroid from the retina. This prevents adequate nutrition of the retina from the choroid vasculature and the removal of harmful waste products of phototransduction.

The pathogenesis is not yet adequately understood, and no clear risk factors have been identified except for increasing age and smoking. In dry age-related macular degeneration (geographic atrophy) the retinal pigment epithelial cells atrophy and the overlying photoreceptors cease to work without pigment epithelial cell support. In wet age-related macular degeneration a choroidal neovascular membrane grows from the choroid through Bruch's membrane into the subretinal space. These vessels may bleed, causing a large fibrotic scar at the macula which results in devastating loss of central vision.

Clinical features

Patients with dry age-related macular degeneration present with gradual mild to moderate central visual loss. The central scotoma increases in size very slowly over a period of years. Fundoscopy will usually reveal drusen near the macula and a pale well-circumscribed area of retinal pigment epithelial cell atrophy. It is usually bilateral.

Patients with wet age-related macular degeneration usually have asymptomatic drusen for some years before a choroidal new vessel develops. The first symptom is of visual distortion in that straight lines look kinked or bent. This is due to fluid leaking from the new vessels lifting the retina a little. Over weeks or months the new vessels bleed under the retina and the resulting macular scar destroys all central vision. Wet age-related macular degeneration usually presents unilaterally but second eye involvement is common. Fundoscopy may show a green to grey macular lesion, often with a small area of retinal haemorrhage in the early stages. A white fibrovascular scar is seen in end-stage disease (Fig. 10.24).

Investigations

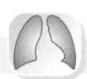

Dry age-related macular degeneration is a clinical diagnosis and needs no further investigations.

Fluorescein angiography

The presence of wet age-related macular degeneration can be confirmed by fluorescein angiography. This demonstrates leakage of dye from the abnormal subretinal blood vessels which are usually not visible on fundoscopy (Fig. 10.25).

Management

Vision aids

Patients with age-related macular degeneration may benefit from low-vision aids, as there is no proven therapy for established dry age-related macular degeneration.

Nutritional supplementation

High-dose vitamins C and E, beta carotene and zinc supplements may reduce the risk of visual loss in non-smoking patients with certain high-risk retinal features.[1] There may be an increased risk of cancer with vitamin supplementation in smokers.

Direct argon laser therapy

Patients with wet age-related macular degeneration can be treated with laser if the new vessels are detected before extensive bleeding and scar formation has occurred. Direct

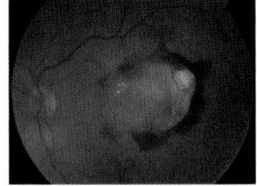

Fig. 10.24 A fibrovascular scar of age-related macular degeneration is seen on the right of the subretinal haemorrhage.

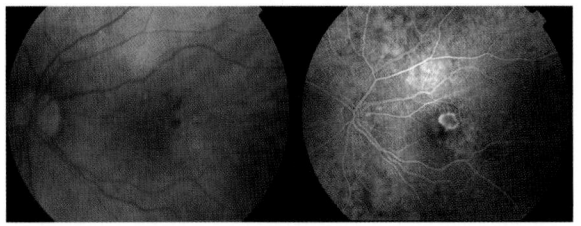

Fig. 10.25 Fluorescein angiography. On the left posterior pole colour photograph, a subretinal haemorrhage is barely visible but is clearly delineated on the fluorescein angiogram on the right.

argon laser destroys the new vessels and the overlying retina but there is a high recurrence rate.

Photodynamic therapy

Photodynamic therapy is useful for a small subgroup of patients with wet age-related macular degeneration with well-defined 'classic' choroidal neovascularization. It involves injection of verteporforin, a light-sensitive dye, which accumulates in the new vessels. When a less intense laser is directed at the new vessels, the dye is activated to release free radicals which close off the new vessels without damaging the overlying retina.

Retinal translocation

Retinal translocation works by rotating the whole retina by 30°, so that the fovea is no longer over the new vessels. This works well in some patients, but carries the risk of total loss of vision in a significant number.

Prognosis

Although central vision is permanently lost, peripheral vision which is useful for navigation and maintaining independence is almost always preserved in both wet and dry age-related macular degeneration.

REFERENCE

(1) *Age-Related Eye Disease Study Research Group. A randomized, placebo-controlled, clinical trial of high-dose supplementation with vitamins C and E, beta carotene, and zinc for age-related macular degeneration and vision loss: AREDS report no. 8. Archives of Ophthalmology 2001; 119: 1417–1436.*

SECTION 10.13 # Diseases of the orbit

Idiopathic orbital inflammation

Idiopathic orbital inflammation is a non-specific inflammatory process that involves the soft tissue components of the orbit. Bilateral involvement may be associated with polyarteritis nodosa, Wegener's granulomatosis, sarcoidosis, tuberculosis and Sjögren's syndrome. Clinical features are similar to orbital cellulitis, however patients are usually well with little pain and the eye is not warm to touch. Oral steroids lead to symptom resolution in up to 75%. Radiotherapy and chemotherapy may be used as an adjunct to steroids in patients with severe disease. The course is variable with spontaneous remission, intermittent episodes of activity or severe prolonged inflammation.

Preseptal and orbital cellulitis

Preseptal cellulitis is infection of the anterior orbit that does not penetrate the orbital septum whilst orbital cellulitis is an infection of the soft tissues behind the orbital septum.

> **⚡ CLINICAL ALERT**
>
> *Orbital cellulitis is a medical emergency requiring hospital admission. There is potential for blindness and intracranial infection.*

Epidemiology

Preseptal cellulitis is common. In adults it usually arises from a superficial source such as an infected chalazion or traumatic inoculation. Orbital cellulitis is much more rare: 90% of cases are associated with sinus disease in both adults and children.

Pathology

Preseptal cellulitis usually occurs as a complication of eyelid infection (e.g. chalazion) and is commonly associated with sinus disease, infection from adjacent structures (dacryocystitis, dental infection) or after trauma (surgery).

Preseptal cellulitis can spread deeper to cause orbital cellulitis. The most common causative organisms are *Streptococcus*, *Staphylococcus* and *Haemophilus* species (in children). Complications from orbital cellulitis include intracranial infection (meningitis, brain abscess, cavernous sinus thrombosis), subperiosteal abscess formation (Fig. 10.26), and ocular complications such as retinal vascular occlusion, exposure keratopathy and optic nerve inflammation.

Clinical features

Patients with preseptal cellulitis may have a history of initial eyelid infection or infection of an adjacent structure that has spread to the eye. On examination, there may be periorbital swelling without proptosis, with normal ocular motility, visual acuity and pupil reaction (Fig. 10.27).

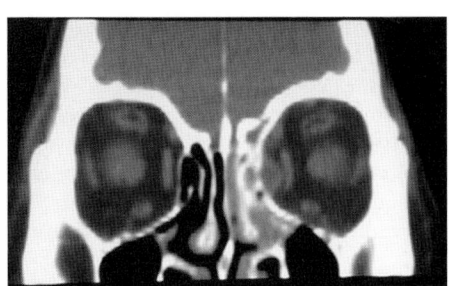

Fig. 10.26 CT of a periosteal abscess.

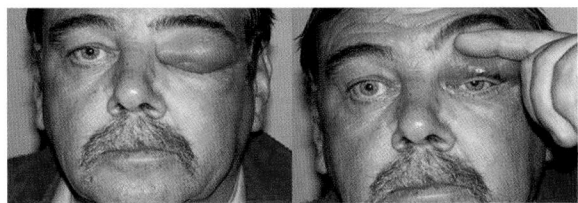

Fig. 10.27 Preseptal cellulitis.

With orbital cellulitis, the patient is usually unwell and pyrexial. On examination the eyelids are swollen, erythematous, warm and tender to palpation. Ocular movements are restricted and painful. As the disease progresses, visual acuity may be diminished, accompanied by a relative afferent pupillary defect.

Investigations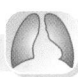

Full blood count
The white cell count is usually elevated with the infection.

Blood cultures
Blood cultures are performed in an attempt to isolate the offending bacteria.

CT of the head
A CT scan of the orbit, sinuses and brain can identify the site and extent of disease, as well as allow for the planning of any surgical intervention.

Management

ENT liaison is vital in the management of patients with orbital cellulitis.

Antibiotics
Oral treatment suffices for preseptal infection but orbital cellulitis requires admission and intravenous ampicillin (children) or a cephalosporin and metronidazole (adults).

Surgical drainage
Surgical drainage is required for abscess and patients with decreasing vision who do not respond to antibiotics. Concomitant drainage of the sinus may also be required.

Prognosis

Most patients respond well to appropriate medical and surgical treatment. Surgical drainage, if indicated, with appropriate medical management leads to dramatic clinical improvement within 24 hours.

Thyroid eye disease

Epidemiology

Thyroid eye disease is the most common cause of proptosis.

Pathology

Proptosis is the result of Graves' disease, due to the production of eye-specific autoantibodies. There is enlargement of extraocular muscles, proliferation of orbital fat and cellular infiltration of interstitial tissues by macrophages and lymphocytes (congestive stage) followed by degeneration of muscle fibres (fibrotic phase). There are two stages in the disease: the active stage when the eyes are red and painful (usually remits within 3 years), and a quiescent stage when the eyes are not red but a painless motility defect of variable severity may be present.

Clinical features

Proptosis is usually asymptomatic and noticed by the patient or by friends and relatives. On examination there may be eyelid retraction of both upper and lower lids, soft tissue involvement with conjunctival injection over the extraocular muscles, chemosis (conjunctival oedema), swollen eyelids, an axial proptosis that can lead to exposure keratopathy, optic neuropathy and restrictive myopathy (30% of patients have restricted eye motility due to oedema in the active phase and fibrosis in the quiescent phase).

Investigations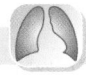

Thyroid function tests and thyroid antibodies
Approximately 80% of patients with proptosis have clinical or biochemical evidence of thyroid dysfunction due to Graves' disease.

Management

Management of underlying disorder
The management of Graves' disease is detailed on page 412.

Topical lubricants
Topical lubricants may help to prevent exposure keratopathy in mild cases of proptosis.

Immunomodulation

Oral or intravenous steroids are used when acute proptosis is sight threatening. Adjunctive ciclosporin may also be necessary.

Radiotherapy

Radiotherapy to the orbit may be used in patients who do not respond to oral steroids.

Orbital decompression

Orbital decompression surgery was formerly indicated only for patients with sight-threatening optic neuropathy. However, improvement in surgical technique with a reduction in major complications has now made this the treatment of choice for patients with stable advanced proptosis. It may be followed by squint surgery and eyelid surgery since orbital decompression surgery will affect the musculature and eyelids. Orbital decompression involves removal of 2–3 parts of the orbital wall. Squint surgery is performed on patients with stable deviations for 6 months and no active disease.

Prognosis

The correction of thyroid function abnormalities is vital in the care of the patient. Smoking has been shown to be an exacerbating factor in thyroid patients with respect to their eye signs and must be stopped. Ophthalmopathy may progress despite achieving a euthyroid state. In the majority of patients the disease stabilizes over weeks to months but there may be an ongoing chronic irritation due to surface problems. In a long-term follow-up study, 50% of patients perceived that their eyes looked abnormal and 38% were dissatisfied with their appearance.

Optic nerve tumours

The most common optic nerve tumours are gliomas and meningiomas. Gliomas are associated with neurofibromatosis type 1. Meningiomas tend to splint the optic nerve, restricting the motility of the eye, and progress to intra-orbital disease. Patients present with gradual progressive visual loss, and examination may reveal disc oedema which may progress to disc pallor and proptosis. CT will demonstrate the lesion, and MRI can delineate any extension through to the optic chiasm. Patients are kept under close observation to monitor tumour growth. If there is no evidence of tumour growth, no treatment is required. Radiotherapy is indicated for meningiomas that are progressive, and surgical excision is recommended for growing tumours associated with poor vision. The prognosis is variable; most gliomas remain indolent.

Tumours of the orbit

Tumours of the orbit can be benign cystic lesions (dermoid, mucocele), benign tumours (adenoma, haemangioma) or malignant (rhabdomyosarcoma) (Table 10.24).

A dermoid is a benign cystic lesion caused by embryonic displacement of the epidermis to a subcutaneous location along embryonic lines of closure. Dermoids are lined by stratified squamous epithelium, have a fibrous wall and contain dermal appendages (e.g. sweat glands).

A mucocele is a slowly expanding cystic accumulation of mucoid secretions and epithelial debris which erodes the wall of the sinuses. They cause symptoms by encroaching on surrounding tissues.

Adenomas are the most common benign lacrimal tumours. Although malignant tumours are rare, they have a similar presentation. A distinguishing feature for malignancy is usually the onset of pain. The rhabdomyosarcoma is the most common primary malignant orbital tumour in children.

Metastatic tumours to the orbit

Metastatic tumours to the orbit are commonly from neuroblastoma and acute myeloid leukaemia in children, breast, bronchus, prostate, skin melanoma, gastrointestinal tract and kidney in adults. Patients usually present with an orbital mass with ocular displacement and cranial nerve palsies. CT scanning and biopsies will help confirm the diagnosis. The main aim of treatment is preservation of vision and pain control. Radiotherapy and chemotherapy may be required. The prognosis is poor and the 1-year mortality is high.

Table 10.24	Features and management of orbital tumours	
Type	**Clinical features**	**Management**
Dermoid	Painless enlarging mass Progressive proptosis	Surgical excision
Mucocele	Proptosis, diplopia, epiphora and globe displacement	Surgical evacuation and drainage/obliteration of affected sinus
Adenoma	Painless, smooth, firm, non-tender, slowly progressive swelling in the upper outer quadrant	Surgical excision
Rhabdomyosarcoma	Rapidly progressive proptosis within the first decade of life. There is a mass in the upper part of the orbit	Radiotherapy and chemotherapy
Retinoblastoma		Surgical excision
Melanona		Radiotherapy

Glaucoma

Glaucoma is an optic neuropathy with characteristic morphological changes at the optic nerve head that may be associated with loss of visual function and raised intraocular pressure.

> **⚡ CLINICAL ALERT**
>
> *Acute angle closure glaucoma is a medical emergency that can lead to irreversible visual loss if untreated. The history is of an acute painful eye and blurred vision. On examination the eye is tense with a dull corneal reflex. It requires immediate ophthalmic referral.*

Epidemiology

Primary open angle glaucoma is the most common form in North America and Europe with a prevalence of 10% in the eighth decade. The incidence is increased in Afro-Caribbeans, diabetics, myopes and those with a family history. Primary angle closure glaucoma is more common in the Chinese population.

Pathogenesis

The primary abnormality associated with glaucoma is damage to the optic disc leading to visual field loss and eventual blindness. The cause of the damage varies with different glaucoma subtypes. Primary open angle glaucoma (POAG) results from microscopic damage and impaired aqueous humour outflow. The optic disc may be damaged due to raised intraocular pressure affecting the microcirculation (indirect ischaemic theory) or direct damage from the raised intraocular pressure as the nerve fibres pass through the optic nerve head (direct mechanical theory).

In primary angle closure glaucoma, the obstruction of aqueous outflow results from closure of the drainage angle by the peripheral iris. The pathogenesis of normal tension glaucoma is not fully understood but is believed to be a reduction in vascular perfusion to the optic nerve head that results in glaucomatous atrophy despite 'normal' intraocular pressure.

Secondary glaucoma (Table 10.25) is due to the build-up of material such as pigments, pseudoexfoliative debris, white blood cells, protein (inflammatory) or vessels (neo-vascular) in the trabecular meshwork.

Clinical features

Primary open angle glaucoma
This is a chronic, slowly progressive, usually bilateral disease with insidious onset. A significant proportion of patients will be asymptomatic until significant and irreversible field loss occurs. Occasionally patients may have eye ache from high intraocular pressure.

Normal tension glaucoma
The presentation of normal tension glaucoma is similar to that of primary open angle glaucoma but patients may have a history of hypotension (acute blood loss or myocardial infarction). Patients are often asymptomatic and tend to be referred late as the intraocular pressure is in the normal range.

Table 10.25	Classification of glaucoma		
Congenital		**Acquired**	
	Open angle	*Narrow angle*	
Primary	**Primary**	**Primary**	
Primary congenital glaucoma (PCG)	Primary open angle glaucoma (POAG)	Intermittent angle closure glaucoma (IACG)	
Secondary	Juvenile onset POAG	Acute angle closure glaucoma (AACG)	
Neurofibromatosis	Normal tension glaucoma (NTG)	Chronic angle closure glaucoma (CACG)	
Sturge–Weber syndrome	**Secondary** Pseudoexfoliative glaucoma (PXF) Pigmentary glaucoma (PDS) Neovascular glaucoma (NVG) Inflammatory glaucoma	**Secondary** Neovascular glaucoma (NVG) Inflammatory glaucoma	

Acute angle closure glaucoma

Acute angle closure glaucoma is characterized by peri-ocular pain associated with rapidly progressive visual impairment. There may be associated nausea and vomiting and patients occasionally present with abdominal pain. Some patients present with blurred vision as the only symptom. Typically the intraocular pressure is over 50 mmHg with corneal oedema and a fixed mid-dilated pupil due to iris ischaemia.

On examination, visual acuity often remains normal until primary open angle glaucoma is advanced, when it is markedly reduced. The intraocular pressure is normal in normal tension glaucoma, mildly elevated in primary open angle glaucoma and chronic angle closure glaucoma (22–40 mmHg), and markedly elevated in acute angle closure glaucoma (40+ mmHg).

Optic disc assessment is performed by slit-lamp bio-microscopy. Glaucoma causes a progressive loss of retinal nerve fibres, increasing the size of the optic cup to disc ratio (vertical and horizontal).

Gonioscopy is the clinical examination of the drainage angle performed with a special lens. The angle can be graded to evaluate functional status and degree of closure and assess the risk of future closure.

Initial investigations

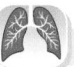

Refraction

Patients who are long sighted are at risk from acute angle closure glaucoma.

Perimetry (visual fields)

Computerized perimetry is the method of choice. Early defects include scotoma within the central 30° field in areas continuous with an upward or downward extension of the blind spot or nasal defects/paracentral scotomas. Later the scotomas coalesce to form arcuate defects which arc from the blind spot around the macula. Commonly a ring or double arcuate scotoma is present and field loss spreads to involve the periphery so that only a central island remains (hence maintaining reasonable visual acuity but with a severely restricted field). Further progression results in loss of the entire field.

Further investigations

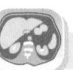

Phasing

Although intraocular pressure normally fluctuates (intra-ocular pressure is higher in the morning), the fluctuation is more pronounced in glaucoma patients, and phasing is a useful method to quantify the fluctuation in pressure. It is also useful in distinguishing between primary open angle and normal tension glaucoma.

Optic nerve head imaging

Confocal scanning laser ophthalmoscopy and optical coherence tomography allows the reconstruction of the surface shape of the optic nerve head, enabling quantitative analysis of the area of the neuroretinal rim, optic cup volume, disc area and retinal nerve fibre layer thickness.

Medical management (Table 10.26)

Beta-blockers

Beta-blockers such as timolol, betaxolol and levobunolol act by decreasing aqueous secretion. They are used as first-line treatment for all types of glaucoma.

Prostaglandin analogues

Prostaglandin analogues such as latanoprost, bimatoprost and travoprost act by increasing uveoscleral outflow. They are suitable for all types of glaucoma. Side effects include increased iris pigmentation (should be used with care in patients with blue iris), increase in eyelash growth and periocular pigmentation.

Carbonic anhydrase inhibitors

Carbonic anhydrase inhibitors such as acetazolamide act by reducing aqueous secretion. Acetazolamide is typically used when acute lowering of pressure is required (e.g. acute angle closure glaucoma), and may also be used orally as an interim measure to acquire target intraocular pressure before definite treatment. Dorzolamide is a topical formulation, not as effective as acetazolamide, and is used as second-line treatment.

Parasympathomimetic agents

Pilocarpine opens the angle by mechanical contraction of the pupil, pulling the peripheral iris away from the trabecula.

Table 10.26	Glaucoma—management summary
Initial management	
At-risk patients, e.g. those with family history, should be screened at optometrists regularly (yearly)	
Medical therapy	
1. Beta-blockers or prostaglandin analogues—for first-line therapy	
2. Pilocarpine—for patients with narrow angles	
3. Topical carbonic anhydrase inhibitors/alpha-2-agonists—for adjunct treatment to obtain further lowering of intraocular pressure	
4. Hyperosmotic agents—for emergency lowering of intraocular pressure	
Non-medical therapy	
1. Nd:Yag iridotomy—for patients with angle closure glaucoma	
2. Argon laser trabeculoplasty—for patients not controlled on medication but unfit for surgery	
3. Trabeculectomy—primary procedure for optimal intraocular pressure control	
4. Cyclodiode laser/tube surgery—for patients with 1 or more failed trabeculectomy procedures	

It is mainly reserved for patients with narrow angles (acute angle closure glaucoma).

Alpha-2-agonists

Alpha-2-agonists such as apraclonidine and brimonidine act by reducing aqueous production. They can be used in all types of glaucoma, usually as an adjunctive agent. Apraclonidine has a high incidence of ocular toxicity with follicular conjunctivitis and periocular dermatitis, and tachyphylaxis rapidly occurs. Brimonidine may cause systemic effects such as dry mouth, fatigue, drowsiness and hypotension.

Hyperosmotic agents

Hyperosmotic agents such as glycerol, isosorbide mononitrate and mannitol lower intraocular pressure by increasing serum osmolality to draw water from the vitreous. They are usually used to lower the intraocular pressure acutely before definitive treatment.

Surgical management

Argon laser trabeculoplasty

Direct argon laser treatment of the trabecular meshwork is usually reserved for patients with uncontrolled intraocular pressure despite maximal tolerated medical treatment who are unfit for surgery. The recurrence rate is approximately 50% by 5 years.

Nd:YAG iridotomy

Laser is used to make peripheral iridectomies in patients with acute angle closure glaucoma, both in the affected and contralateral eye, as it is a bilateral disease.

Cyclodiode laser

Trans-scleral cyclodiode laser can be used to ablate the ciliary body in patients with end-stage glaucoma, poor visual prognosis or failed multiple filtering/tube surgery.

> **RECENT ADVANCES**
>
> *Treatment of the ciliary processes by an endoscopic diode laser allows direct visualization of the treated areas and a more graded treatment. Longer follow-up data on safety and efficacy are needed.*

Goniotomy

Goniotomy is performed by making an incision in the angle to create a communication between the anterior chamber and Schlemm's canal. It is used for the treatment of primary congenital glaucoma.

Trabeculectomy

Trabeculectomy is the creation of a new channel (fistula) for aqueous outflow between the anterior chamber and the sub-Tenon's space. It is the primary procedure of choice for patients with uncontrolled progressive glaucoma.

The use of the antimetabolites 5-fluorouracil (5-FU) and mitomycin C has improved the success rates of trabeculectomy by altering the effects of wound healing in causing premature failure of trabeculectomy blebs by fibrotic scarring.[1]

Tube surgery

Tubes (Molteno, Ahmed, Baerveldt) are plastic devices that create a communication between the anterior chamber and the sub-Tenon's space. The fluid drains down the tube into a plate from which it is absorbed. Tube surgery is mainly used for complicated secondary glaucoma or in patients with multiple failed filtering procedures (trabeculectomy). Complication rates are higher than conventional filtering procedures.

Prognosis

Glaucoma is a progressive disease, and poorly controlled intraocular pressure causes progressive visual loss.[2] It is assumed that lowering the intraocular pressure may modify the rate of change. Primary open angle glaucoma is associated with a poor prognosis, especially in Afro-Caribbean patients who tend to present at a younger age. Primary congenital glaucoma is associated with a good prognosis in 60%. In the remaining patients, visual loss occurs due to optic nerve damage, anisometropic amblyopia and corneal scarring.

ℹ FURTHER INFORMATION

Hitchings RH. Glaucoma. London: BMJ Publications, 2000.

REFERENCES

(1) *Kitazawa Y, Kawase K, Matsushita H, Minobe M. Trabeculectomy with MMC: A comparative study with 5FU. Archives of Ophthalmology 1991; 109: 1693–1698.*
(2) *Katz J, Gilbert D, Quigley HA, Sommer A. Estimating progression of visual field loss in glaucoma. Ophthalmology 1997; 104: 1017–1025.*

SECTION 10.15 Ocular trauma

Epidemiology

Ocular trauma is often seen in children, and occurs more often in men compared to women.

Pathology (Table 10.27)

Blunt trauma is probably the most common cause. The degree of tissue damage is related to the energy of the injury. Anteroposterior compression of the globe with objects smaller than the orbital rim (e.g. golf balls) can cause severe injuries. Blunt injuries to the ocular surface will cause abrasions or subconjunctival haemorrhage due to damage to the superficial vessels. Surface injuries include subtarsal foreign bodies, conjunctival lacerations and corneal foreign bodies. Blow-out fractures of the orbit commonly affect the floor or the medial wall. Penetrating eye injuries are the most severe and may or may not be associated with an intraocular foreign body.

Chemical injuries are common; the severity will depend on the nature of the chemical involved and how rapidly treatment is started. Acids tend to cause less severe injuries than alkalis since they react with protein and hence are impeded from further penetration into the eye. Superglue injuries are usually due to accidental instillation and should be referred to an ophthalmologist. Arc eye from ultraviolet exposure from welding arcs or sunbeds causes a delayed loss of corneal epithelial cells.

Clinical features

A usual trauma history must be taken including any previous ocular history, pre-morbid vision, whether any protective eyewear was worn. Examination may need to be performed after topical anaesthesia and any abrasion demarcated with fluorescein drops and examination with a blue light.

The upper lid is everted for examination for foreign bodies. Examination of the anterior chamber may show cells and flare (iritis) or hyphaema (blood in the anterior chamber). Blood will cause a rise in intraocular pressure. Damage to the pupil (traumatic mydriasis) and lens dislocation/cataract may also be found. Fundal examination may show vitreous haemorrhage, retinal oedema (commotio), choroidal rupture, retinal tears or optic nerve contusion. Visual loss can occur with severe injuries.

Orbital injuries cause pain in the direction of action of the bruised or entrapped muscle. With orbital floor fractures (Fig. 10.28), there may be numbness over the lower lid and gum area, diplopia, limitation of ocular movement and enophthalmos (sunken globe).

Chemical injuries mainly cause damage to the anterior segment with lid erythema, swelling, conjunctival chemosis, epithelial loss, limbal ischaemia, corneal epithelial loss, sclera ischaemia and anterior chamber inflammation.

Arc eye causes severe ocular pain, photophobia and watering. There is usually lid oedema, erythema, conjunctival chemosis, injection and corneal epithelial loss.

Increasing pain or a reduction in vision after a few days may indicate underlying infection and patients must be referred.

Investigations
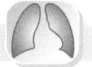

X-ray of the head
Plain films are performed if there is any suggestion of retained foreign bodies.

Ultrasound of the eye
An ultrasound may detect non-metallic foreign bodies.

CT of the head
If the posterior border of a subconjunctival haemorrhage cannot be seen, CT of the head is required to screen for a base of skull fracture. Orbital fractures will need further assessment by CT.

Table 10.27	Types of ocular trauma
Non-penetrating injuries	Blunt trauma (contusion) Surface injuries Blow-out fractures
Penetrating injuries	Intraocular foreign body
Burns	Chemical Thermal Radiation—arc eye Glue injuries

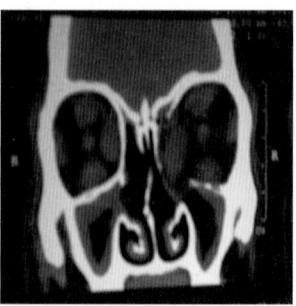

Fig. 10.28 CT of a left orbital floor fracture.

Management

Simple abrasions

Simple abrasions will heal within a few days. Patients should be given cyclopentolate drops to help relieve pain caused by ciliary spasm with oral analgesia and an antibiotic ointment, e.g. chloramphenicol, for prophylaxis and lubrication. Temporary padding may aid healing. Arc eye is treated in the same way as a corneal abrasion and there will be complete recovery within 24 hours.

Conjunctival laceration

Small lacerations will heal spontaneously but larger defects (5 mm or more) may need suturing, especially if they are vertical in orientation. All cases must be referred to an ophthalmologist to exclude underlying scleral perforation.

Corneal foreign bodies

A corneal foreign body should be removed under direct visualization with a slit-lamp after topical anaesthesia (e.g. tetracaine).

Penetrating eye injuries

Corneal lacerations, hyphaemas and penetrating eye injuries require specialist review and initial surgery to restore the structural integrity of the globe. The risk of sympathetic ophthalmitis (a bilateral inflammation that may follow an injury to one eye if it is not removed early) is very small and responsive to modern high-dose immunosuppression.

Eyelid lacerations

Eyelid lacerations need to be cleaned with normal saline and all foreign bodies removed to examine the extent of the injury. Broad-spectrum oral antibiotics are needed prophylactically, especially in bite injuries. Surgery can be deferred for up to 48 hours if the wound is covered by a moist dressing. Referrals to an ophthalmologist should be made for full thickness lacerations, lacerations involving the lid margin, and those with damage to the nasolacrimal system.

Chemical injuries

Chemical injuries should be irrigated immediately with at least 2 litres of physiological saline for at least 30 minutes. The pH should be tested with litmus paper before and after irrigation. Topical anaesthesia and an eyelid speculum are required to ensure that the lids are doubly everted. Any retained materials must be removed. All patients must be referred to an ophthalmologist.

Superglue injuries

Superglue does not penetrate deeply, and tears often prevent adhesion. The eyelids are often stuck together. The glue is brittle when dry and the lids are separated carefully with forceps by direct visualization on the slit-lamp. Any associated abrasion is treated as above.

Prognosis

The prognosis of severely damaged eyes can be difficult at initial presentation and patients should understand that visual rehabilitation may require many operations over months or years. Most trauma patients require specialist review by an ophthalmologist.

SECTION 10.16   Neuro-ophthalmology

Pupil abnormalities

Argyll Robertson pupil

The Argyll Robertson pupil is a complication of neurosyphilis. It is now a rare disease characterized by bilateral small and irregular pupils with an absent light reflex and normal accommodation. The pupils are difficult to dilate. Management is directed to the underlying syphilis infection.

Holmes–Adie pupil

The Holmes–Adie pupil is due to denervation of the postganglionic supply to the sphincter pupillae and ciliary muscle. It is unilateral in 80% and typically affects healthy young adults. It may occur as a complication of viral infection. Vision is normal, but the affected pupil is large and regular and the light reflex is absent. Pharmacological testing with dilute 0.1% pilocarpine in both eyes will cause constriction in only the affected pupil (denervation hypersensitivity). No treatment is required.

Horner's syndrome

Horner's syndrome results from the disruption of the sympathetic pathway to the eye (Table 10.28). The clinical features are unilateral mild ptosis (denervation of Müller's muscle in the upper lid) and miosis (constricted pupil on the affected side) with a normal pupil light reaction. There is reduced ipsilateral sweating (for lesions proximal to the superior cervical ganglion). The lesion can be confirmed with topical cocaine; cocaine prevents reuptake at the noradrenergic terminal, hence a normal pupil will dilate

Table 10.28	Causes of Horner's syndrome by anatomical location
Central nervous system Brainstem demyelination Brainstem stroke Syringomyelia	
Level of T1 Pancoast tumour (of the lung apex)	
Superior cervical ganglion Compression from cervical lymphadenopathy Surgery (carotid endarterectomy) Trauma	
Carotid sympathetic plexus Carotid aneurysm	

whereas the Horner's pupil will not. Topical hydroxyamphetamine differentiates a first/second order neurone lesion from a third order neurone lesion. Hydroxyamphetamine causes the release of transmitters from the adrenergic terminal endings; a third order lesion pupil will hence not dilate but a first/second order one will. Topical adrenaline assesses denervation supersensitivity. A dilute solution of adrenaline will cause dilatation in a third order lesion patient but minimal effect in a first/second order lesion.

Optic neuropathy

Diseases of the optic nerve usually manifest as reduced visual acuity, visual field defects (central/centrocaecal scotoma) and impaired colour vision. Patients tend to develop a relative afferent pupil defect. The causes are listed in Table 10.29.

Optic neuritis

Optic neuritis is the inflammation of the optic nerve.

Epidemiology

Optic neuritis is a common cause of visual loss in the young.

Pathology

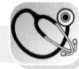

The most common cause of optic neuritis is demyelinating disease such as multiple sclerosis. Approximately 74% of women and 34% of men with optic neuritis develop multiple sclerosis after 15 years.

Clinical features

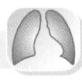

In early disease, patients may notice that colours do not appear as bright (colour desaturation); as the disease progresses, vision is affected. With mild disease, impairment to vision is maximal after 1–2 weeks, and may be reduced to counting fingers. The classic presentation of severe disease is acute monocular visual loss, associated with periocular discomfort that is worse on moving the eye. Ophthalmoscopy may be normal or papillitis may be seen (blurred optic disc margins).

Investigations

MRI of the head
Up to 70% of patients with optic neuritis have abnormal MRI with evidence of demyelination.

Management

Observation
When presenting visual acuity loss is mild, no treatment is needed as visual recovery occurs within 6 weeks.

Immunomodulation
With poor visual acuity, bilateral involvement or incomplete improvement from previous attacks, intravenous steroids are administered to hasten the speed of recovery. The long-term prognosis, however, is not altered by steroids.

Prognosis

In general, the prognosis is good: 75% of patients recover visual acuity up to 6/9 or better. Colour vision may remain abnormal, and mild optic atrophy may develop with time.

Table 10.29	Classification and causes of optic neuropathy	
Type of optic neuropathy		**Cause**
Optic neuritis Retrobulbar neuritis (normal optic nerve head) Papillitis (disc swelling) Neuroretinitis (optic papillitis and macular star)		Inflammation, demyelination, infection (measles, mumps, chicken pox)
Ischaemic optic neuropathy (microvascular occlusion of the blood vessels supplying the optic nerve head)		Arteritis, autoimmune
Toxic optic neuropathy		Malnutrition or drug induced

Arteritic anterior ischaemic optic neuropathy

Arteritic anterior ischaemic optic neuropathy is due to giant cell arteritis. The general features are detailed on page 517. Ophthalmic features are caused by arteritis of the blood vessels that supply the optic nerve. Optic neuropathy usually occurs within the first few weeks of onset of giant cell arteritis, and 65% of untreated patients become blind in both eyes within a few weeks. The optic head becomes oedematous, and within 2 months the swelling resolves and the disc becomes atrophic. Patients with giant cell arteritis may present with amaurosis fugax, central retinal artery occlusion, cortical blindness or extraocular nerve palsies. Ophthalmoscopy reveals a pale and swollen optic nerve head which may be surrounded by splinter haemorrhages. Treatment with steroids is aimed to prevent blindness to the fellow eye. Current regimens are intravenous methylprednisolone (1 g for 3 days) followed by oral steroids (80 mg) on a reducing dose to maintenance at 10 mg for 12 months. The duration of treatment is longer if there are symptoms of residual disease or a persistently elevated ESR.

Non-arteritic anterior ischaemic optic neuropathy

The causes of non-arteritic anterior ischaemic optic neuropathy (optic nerve ischaemia not due to giant cell arteritis) are either autoimmune or unknown (idiopathic). Approximately 1% of patients with systemic lupus erythematosus present with an optic neuropathy, and the disease process can be progressive. Patients present with painless loss of vision, and the typical field defects are altitudinal hemianopia. One third of patients will have normal or reduced visual acuity; the rest will have moderate to severe visual impairment. Colour vision is reduced in proportion to the level of reduction of visual acuity. On ophthalmoscopy, there is a diffuse or sectorial swelling of the optic disc. With time, the swelling may resolve leaving the involved portion of the disc pale. Treatment is of the underlying disease and the prognosis is better than arteritic ischaemic optic neuropathy as there is no further visual loss in most patients.

Toxic optic neuropathy

Toxic optic neuropathy can be caused by deficiency of vitamins (commonly B_{12}/B_1) and folate in alcoholics or induced by drugs (ethambutol, isoniazid, chloroquine). Patients present with slowly progressive bilateral visual and colour impairment. On ophthalmoscopy, mild disc oedema with a centrocaecal scotoma may be present. The management is directed to the underlying cause, hydroxycobalamin and multivitamin replacement in patients who are undernourished, and stopping any offending drug associated with optic neuropathy. The prognosis is good for patients with early disease, with complete resolution of visual impairment. Advanced disease with optic atrophy is usually unresponsive to treatment.

Disorder of the control of eye movement

Conjugate movements are binocular movements in which the two eyes move synchronously and symmetrically in the same direction. Saccadic (scanning) eye movements occur when the objects are placed on the fovea rapidly (when the eye moves from one object to another); control is achieved from the premotor cortex of frontal motor area to the horizontal gaze centre (in the pontine paramedian reticular formation). Pursuit (tracking) eye movements maintain fixation on the target once it has been located by the saccade; movement is slow. The control is from the occipital cortex to the horizontal gaze centre. The vestibular-ocular reflex maintains eye position with respect to any changes of the head and body; the control is from labyrinth and proprioceptors in the neck to the horizontal gaze centre.

Gaze palsies caused by supranuclear disturbances do not result in diplopia. Horizontal movements are generated by the horizontal gaze centre, and the output is to the ipsilateral VIth nucleus and via the medial longitudinal fasciculus to the contralateral IIIrd nerve nucleus. Lesions of the medial longitudinal fasciculus will cause an internuclear ophthalmoplegia (reduced adduction on the ipsilateral side and ataxic nystagmus on the contralateral side). Unilateral lesions are usually vascular, and bilateral lesions are due to demyelination. Vertical movements are mediated from the vertical gaze centre in the midbrain. Up-gaze palsies can be caused by lesions of the dorsal midbrain (e.g. pinealomas) and down-gaze palsies can occur from bilateral midbrain damage (e.g. Steele–Richardson syndrome, stroke).

Nystagmus

Nystagmus is the repetitive involuntary oscillation of the eyes (Table 10.30).

Optic chiasmal disease

Diseases of the optic chiasm may be due to direct compression or demyelination. The causes are listed in Table 10.31. Patients with optic chiasmal disease tend to present with desaturation of colour vision and bitemporal hemianopia. Other features are specific to the underlying disease, such as endocrine abnormalities associated with pituitary adenomas or proptosis with meningiomas. MRI of the head is usually required as the main mode of investigation, together with endocrine tests for patients with suspected

Table 10.30 | Causes of nystagmus

Type of nystagmus	Features	Causes
Pendular	Velocity is equal in each direction	Impairment of vision in early life (e.g. congenital cataracts, albinism)
Jerk	Slow drift and a corrective fast phase	Physiological (extremes of gaze)
Optokinetic	A jerk nystagmus induced by moving, repetitive stimuli across the visual field	Motor imbalance of the rectus muscles, e.g. vestibular dysfunction
Ataxic nystagmus	Horizontal jerk nystagmus which occurs in the abducting eye of a patient with an internuclear ophthalmoplegia	E.g. Alcohol intoxication, CNS disorders, e.g. multiple sclerosis
Downbeat	The fast phase beats downwards	Lesions at the cranio-cervical junction (e.g. Arnold–Chiari malformation)
Upbeat	Fast phase beating upward	Drugs (phenytoin), posterior fossa lesions
Gaze-control	Nystagmus not present when the individual looks straight but appears as the eyes look to the side	Gaze-evoked (e.g. cerebellar) or gaze-paretic (e.g. brainstem damage)

endocrine disorders (p. 397). The management is of the underlying cause.

Retro-chiasmal diseases

Retro-chiasmal diseases refer to diseases of the cerebral cortex that affect the optic tract and optic radiation. The optic tracts arise from the posterior aspect of the chiasm and extend around the cerebral peduncles to terminate in the lateral geniculate body. The optic radiations arise from the lateral geniculate body to the occipital lobe. Lesions of the optic tracts may involve the ipsilateral cerebral peduncle and are associated with contralateral pyramidal signs (weakness, paralysis, upgoing plantar reflexes). The visual field defect is an incongruous (asymmetrical) homonymous hemianopia. As the optic radiations lie progressively closer, the hemianopic defects become more congruous (symmetrical). The inferior fibres of the optic radiations (superior field) pass through the temporal lobe to the occipital lobe. Therefore, lesions at this location tend to produce quadrantanopia (a quarter visual field defect). Temporal lobe space-occupying lesions can lead to seizures, receptive dysphasia and upper quadrantanopia.

As the superior fibres pass through the parietal lobe to the occipital lobe, space-occupying lesions of the parietal lobe can lead to agnosia, acalculia, right–left confusion and lower quadrantanopia. The occipital lobe representation is of peripheral visual field anteriorly (supplied by the posterior cerebral artery) and macular vision posteriorly (the middle and posterior cerebral arteries). Strokes in this location can cause a congruous homonymous hemianopia with macular sparing.

Table 10.31 | Disorders affecting the optic chiasm

Compression

Tumours
   Pituitary adenoma
   Meningioma
   Craniopharyngioma
   Metastatic tumour

Aneurysms

Sphenoidal sinus mucocele

Demyelination

Refractive error

In a normal eye the curved surface of the cornea and the lens sharply focus images on the retina, allowing clear vision. Most eyes when relaxed are in focus for distance, and accommodation is required to focus on closer objects. Accommodation involves constricting the ciliary muscles (posterior to the insertion of the iris) which relax tension on the zonules that support the lens. As a result, the lens becomes fatter and rounder (innate elasticity) increasing the focusing power.

Most dilating eye drops (e.g. tropicamide) paralyze not only the iris constrictor muscles but also the ciliary muscles (cycloplegia) causing blurred vision for close objects for a few hours.

Myopia

Epidemiology

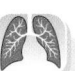

Myopia, also known as short-sightedness, is very common. Approximately 26% of the population suffers with myopia.[1]

Pathology

In a myopic eye, the image is focused in front of the retina either because the focusing power of the lens or cornea is too great or the length of the eye is too long. The severity of the myopia stops progressing in most patients by the mid twenties.

In a small proportion, pathological myopia occurs, and the disease severity continues to progress after the mid twenties. High myopia is associated with both retinal detachment and myopic retinal degeneration, where large non-functioning atrophic patches develop in the thinned retina around the optic disc and macula.

Scope of disease

Patients with myopia usually have eyes that are larger than normal, increasing the risk of retinal detachment and open angle glaucoma. Patients with myopic degeneration may slowly progress to very poor vision for which there is no treatment. High myopia is also associated with loss of vision from the development of choroidal neovascular membranes.

Clinical features

Myopic patients can focus on near objects but cannot see clearly in the distance.

On examination the eyeball may appear abnormally large. Fundoscopy often reveals peripapillary atrophy (which is benign), and a few patients may have myopic degeneration (Fig. 10.29).

Initial investigations

No investigations are required unless there are features of rare associated conditions such as Marfan's syndrome, homocystinuria or Ehlers–Danlos syndrome.

Initial management

Glasses and contact lenses

In most patients myopia is correctable with glasses with negative power corrective lenses. Very high myopia is best corrected with contact lenses as they cause less optical aberration. Difficulty in handling contact lenses limits their use in the elderly.

Complications associated with contact lenses include sight-threatening infective corneal ulceration (especially with *Pseudomonas* or *Acanthamoeba* infections) and contact lens intolerance.

Surgical management

Laser refractive surgery

Laser surgery works by removing a very thin layer of the cornea to alter its curvature and subsequently the refractive power. This can be done by lifting a thin flap before applying the laser and then reapplying the flap or by scraping off the epithelium and applying the laser directly onto the corneal surface. Although most patients are delighted with the results, a few will suffer from glare and difficulty with driving at night. None of these techniques prevents presbyopia (p. 678).

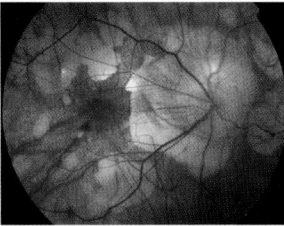

Fig. 10.29 Right eye colour fundus photograph showing myopic retinal degeneration.

Prognosis

Unless pathological myopia occurs, the disease severity stops progressing in the majority by the mid twenties.

Hypermetropia

Epidemiology

Hypermetropia, also known as long-sightedness, is common. Children are usually born a little hypermetropic but become emmetropic (normal) within the first few years of life. Approximately 10% of the adult population are hypermetropic.[1]

Pathology

In a hypermetropic eye the image is focused behind the retina. This is because the focusing power of the lens or cornea is too little or the length of the eye is too short.

Scope of disease

Patients with hypermetropia usually have eyes that are smaller than normal and are at increased risk of acute angle closure glaucoma. Care should be taken when using dilating drops in older long-sighted patients as it is possible to induce an attack of angle closure glaucoma in predisposed individuals.

Clinical features

Patients with hypermetropia see clearly in the distance (by accommodating) but are unable to focus on near objects. Symptoms of intermittent headaches, seeing haloes, blurred vision or eye pain may be due to intermittent angle closure glaucoma, often brought on by low light levels when the iris dilates.

On examination the eye may appear abnormally small and the optic disc may appear crowded. Occasionally, these findings may be mistaken for optic disc swelling (pseudopapilloedema).

Investigations

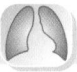

Investigations are not routinely required.

Initial management

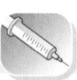

Glasses and contact lenses

In most patients, hypermetropia is correctable with glasses with positive power corrective lenses. Young patients with hypermetropia may be able to see clearly by accommodation but frontal headache after reading is an early sign that glasses are required. Contact lenses may also be used, with the same complications as listed on page 651.

Surgical management

Laser refractive surgery

Laser refractive surgery is described on page 671, although only fairly low levels of hypermetropia (3 dioptres) can be corrected using photorefractive techniques.

Clear lens extraction

Hypermetropia can be treated surgically by clear lens extraction and insertion of a synthetic intraocular lens but this is rarely done as patients are still likely to need reading glasses after surgery and the operation is not without risk (see cataract surgery, p. 658).

Prognosis

Most patients maintain good vision throughout their life but they are likely to require reading glasses from a relatively early age (e.g. 35 years); this is called premature presbyopia.

REFERENCE

(1) *Kempen JH, Mitchell P, Lee KE, et al; Eye Diseases Prevalence Research Group. The prevalence of refractive errors among adults in the United States, Western Europe, and Australia. Archives of Ophthalmology* 2004; 122: 495–505.

Presbyopia

With age, the lens in the eye loses its ability to change focus, and patients cannot focus on near objects. Reading glasses (positive lens) are required by the age of 40–50 years and earlier in patients with hypermetropia. Patients with a pre-existing refractive error require bifocals, which are glasses with a lens for distance vision in the upper part of the glasses and a relatively more positive-powered lens in the lower part of the glasses for focusing on near objects, i.e. reading.

Astigmatism

Astigmatism occurs with abnormalities in the shape of the cornea which result in asymmetric focus, for example a greater focal power in the vertical plane than the horizontal plane. Patients may present with blurred vision or frontal headache and the vision may be only partially corrected by glasses. Contact lenses can correct a much greater degree of astigmatism than glasses. Laser refractive surgery can usually improve astigmatism but should be avoided in patients with keratoconus.

Keratoconus

Keratoconus is a rare condition in which the cornea is abnormally thin and stretches slowly over many years. The end result is a cornea that resembles one end of a rugby ball in shape. The image focused by this cornea is blurred from a high degree of astigmatism. Hard contact lenses may be adequate in the early stage of the disease but some patients will require a corneal graft operation to maintain adequate vision.

Amblyopia

Epidemiology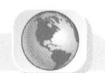

Amblyopia is also known by the lay term 'lazy eye' and is a common, usually unilateral, condition.

Pathology

In childhood, when brain development occurs, each eye needs a focused image on the retina in order for the brain to learn to use the information from the eye properly. Amblyopia occurs if an image is impaired in one eye by refractive error, congenital cataract, ptosis or suppression due to squint. The brain ignores the blurred image from the affected eye and amblyopia develops. This is usually irreversible after 8 years of age.

Clinical features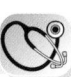

The eye appears structurally and physiologically normal but the patient is unable to see normally from it, despite using the correct glasses, as the brain ignores the visual information transmitted down the optic nerve.

If the patient has a squint, the eyes will not be looking at the same target as each other and the brain will not be able to fuse the two images. This will result in double vision unless the image from one eye is ignored (suppressed). Suppression from a squint can lead to amblyopia, although poor vision from amblyopia can also result in a squint.

Investigations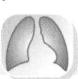

No investigations are required to diagnose amblyopia.

Management

Glasses and address any underlying cause
If amblyopia is detected early, treatment involves glasses if necessary and removing any possible visual obstruction such as cataract or ptosis.

Eye patch
If no improvement occurs, and the patient is under the age of 8, then an eye patch can be worn over the good eye to force the brain to use the amblyopic eye. This should be done carefully and under supervision as there is a risk of inducing amblyopia in the good eye.

Prognosis

Amblyopia is correctable if detected and treated early by addressing the underlying cause. There is not much point wearing an eye patch after the age of 8 years as vision is very unlikely to improve.

Squints

A squint (strabismus) is an abnormal deviation of the eye.

Epidemiology

Approximately 2% of the population suffer with varying degrees of a squint.

Pathology

A squint may be concomitant or incomitant, depending on the deviation of the eye with the position of the gaze. In a concomitant squint the deviation is constant regardless of the position of gaze. This is a typical squint of childhood and patients do not have double vision because the image of one eye is suppressed. In an incomitant squint, the deviation varies according to the direction of gaze, usually due to a paretic muscle or muscle underaction.

Clinical features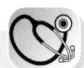

It is important to distinguish monocular diplopia from binocular, and whether the diplopia is horizontal or vertical. Sudden onset of diplopia may be associated with ischaemia, and intermittent diplopia may be associated with tiredness (phoria). Diplopia can also be associated with fatigue (myasthenia) and may be progressive (compressive lesion) or stationary (thyroid eye disease). Pain associated with a squint may be due to idiopathic orbital inflammation or aneurysm of the posterior communicating artery (causing IIIrd nerve palsy). Associated neurological symptoms such as abnormalities of gait, balance, urinary problems and headache may be due to multiple sclerosis (internuclear ophthalmoplegia), or raised intracranial pressure (VIth nerve palsy).

Examination may reveal an abnormal head posture (left head turn for a left lateral rectus weakness), abnormal eye

679

alignment (globe displacement with orbital tumour and thyroid eye disease), proptosis (thyroid eye disease or tumour), enophthalmos (orbital fracture), ptosis (IIIrd nerve palsy, myasthenia) or eyelid retraction (thyroid eye disease). Globe injection and chemosis are associated with thyroid eye disease and idiopathic orbital inflammation.

Ocular motility examination will establish the weak or restricted muscle. The cover–uncover test is performed with the patient fixating on a near or distance target. The patient's eye is covered and uncovered; if the uncovered eye moves to take up fixation there is a manifest squint. If there is not a manifest squint, the alternate cover test is used to reveal a phoria (tendency for eyes to deviate into a squinting position normally prevented when both eyes are open). Each eye is occluded alternately several times. In a latent squint the occluded eye drifts under the occluder and has to move to regain fixation.

Investigations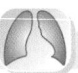

Hess chart
A Hess chart test is performed by dissociating the two eyes by red and green filters. A target is presented in one colour (e.g. red) and the patient is then asked to position a pointer of another colour (e.g. green) in the same position as the initial target. Once the target is presented in all position of gaze, the colour of the pointer and target is reversed and the other eye examined.

Refraction
If the phoria is intermittent it is important to refract the patient as an outward squint may be found in uncorrected myopia and an inward squint with uncorrected hypermetropia.

Management

Glasses
Patients with refraction errors are managed by appropriate glasses, prisms and exercises to aid near focusing.

Address underlying cause
It is important to treat or address any underlying cause of a squint, e.g. myasthenia, as this may correct the symptoms without any further treatment.

Squint surgery
Surgery is contemplated if the deviation is stable for 6 months. The principles of squint surgery are to weaken muscles (recession, myomectomy), to strengthen them (resection) or to alter their mode of action (transposition).

Prognosis

The recovery of a squint depends on the underlying cause (Table 10.32). Squints associated with refraction errors are easily corrected. Occasionally, addressing the underlying cause (myasthenia, multiple sclerosis) may improve the squint. Some causes of a squint are refractory to treatment (tumours).

Table 10.32	Causes of diplopia
Nerve palsies	
IIIrd, IVth, VIth nerve palsies	
Ischaemia	
Compressive lesions	
Arteritis	
Raised intracranial pressure	
Congenital	
Demyelination	
Cavernous sinus disease (meningioma, aneurysm, pituitary tumour)	
Neoplasms	
Consecutive	
Old muscle imbalance	
Breakdown of phoria	
Previous squint surgery	
Tethering of muscle	
Trauma (orbital fractures)	
Thyroid eye disease	
Myositis/orbital disease	
Idiopathic orbital inflammation	
Orbital tumours	
Orbital cellulitis	
Neuromuscular junction	
Myasthenia gravis	

Diseases of the kidney and urinary system

11

Sampi Mehta, Fiona Dallas, Derek Rosario, Albert Ong

SECTION 11.1 **Introduction**

Applied basic sciences of the renal and urinary system

The kidneys

The kidneys are lobulated organs approximately 11 cm (length) by 6 cm (width) by 3 cm (thickness). They weigh approximately 150 g in the adult and lie on the posterior abdominal wall. The hila of the kidneys lie on L1 (the transpyloric plane). The collecting ducts of the renal parenchyma drain into the medulla, which in turn forms the minor calyces, which in turn form the major calyces. Urine drains into the pelvis of the kidney and into the ureters. The blood supply comes from the renal arteries, which arise directly from the aorta and give off branches to the adrenals and ureter before dividing into the lobar arteries of the kidney (Fig. 11.1). The left renal vein crosses in front of the aorta and drains into the inferior vena cava and receives the gonadal, lumbar and adrenal veins. The right renal vein drains directly into the vena cava.

The kidneys receive one quarter of the cardiac output. Approximately 180 litres of water are filtered daily, necessitating accurate concentration. Failure of this concentration would rapidly result in dehydration and death. The kidneys usually produce 1–3 litres of urine daily, with the correct amount of electrolytes to maintain homeostasis. The glomerular filtration rate depends on the pressures within the kidney. This pressure remains stable despite alterations in systemic blood pressure.

$$\begin{array}{ccccc} \text{Glomerular} & = & \text{glomerular} & - & (\text{oncotic} & + & \text{Bowman's} \\ \text{filtration} & & \text{capillary} & & \text{pressure} & & \text{space} \\ \text{pressure} & & \text{pressure} & & 25 \text{ mmHg} & & \text{pressure}) \\ & & 45 \text{ mmHg} & & & & 10 \text{ mmHg} \end{array}$$

The final volume of urine passed is affected by antidiuretic hormone (ADH) and aldosterone levels. ADH is released when an increase in plasma osmolality is detected in the hypothalamus. This may be in response to dehydration or reduced cardiac output, or due to other factors such as nausea, nicotine or antidepressants. ADH is released from storage in the posterior pituitary. It acts on the collecting duct cells via cAMP, increasing water re-absorption.

Reduced perfusion pressure in the kidney results in the secretion of renin in the juxtaglomerular apparatus. Renin acts on angiotensinogen, releasing angiotensin I. The angiotensin I is converted to angiotensin II, which is a powerful vasoconstrictor. The adrenal zona glomerulosa then produces more aldosterone. Aldosterone activates the Na^+/K^+ exchange, increasing sodium retention, and thus fluid retention. The physiological functions of the individual nephron sites are listed in Table 11.1.

Erythropoietin

Erythropoietin is a hormone produced by the peritubular fibroblasts in response to hypoxia. It stimulates erythropoiesis. Both acute and chronic renal failure can lead to inappropriately low erythropoietin production.

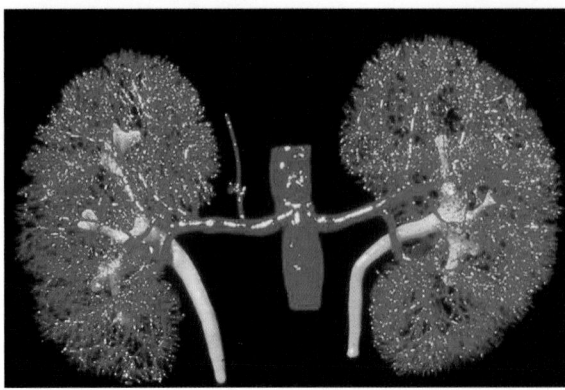

Fig. 11.1 A cast model illustrating the vascular supply of the kidneys.

Vitamin D

Vitamin D is produced in the skin as vitamin D_3 (cholecalciferol). After conversion in the liver to 25-hydroxy-D_3, it is only made active within the kidney. The tubules convert it into 1,25-dihydroxy-D_3. This conversion is regulated by parathyroid hormone, serum phosphate and a feedback mechanism. Vitamin D metabolism is abnormal in chronic renal failure, leading to renal osteodystrophy.

Prostaglandin PGE_2 is a vasodilator produced in the kidney. It is thought to regulate intrarenal blood flow and may affect sodium and water homeostasis. Kallikrein is also produced by the kidney and is thought to affect salt and water homeostasis.

The collecting system

The collecting system consists of three groups of calyces draining the upper, middle and lower poles of the kidney. These come together to form the renal pelvis. The pelvis drains via the pelvi-ureteric junction into the ureter. The ureters course anteromedially initially and follow the tips of the transverse processes of the lower four lumbar vertebrae to the ipsilateral sacro-iliac joint at the pelvic brim. Here the ureter crosses the bifurcation of the common iliac arteries

and courses laterally as it enters the pelvis. On the left, the ureter runs in the root of the mesentery of the sigmoid colon. In the female, the ureter passes under the uterine artery and turns medially, running 1.5 cm anterior to the uterine cervix, entering the bladder approximately 2.5 cm from the midline. The proximity of the ureters to pelvic structures makes the ureter susceptible to injury during procedures such as excision of the rectum or gynaecological surgery. Knowledge of the course of the ureters is important in the interpretation of calcifications on plain abdominal films when screening for urinary calculi. There are three areas of narrowing of the ureter where calculi may lodge: the pelvi-ureteric junction (PUJ), the point of crossing the iliac vessels and the vesico-ureteric junction.

In contrast with the high pressures encountered in the nephron, the pressure in the renal pelvicalyceal system is low, typically around 14 cmH_2O. Because of this, drainage of the collecting system may be impaired if the pressure in the bladder is consistently high during filling, leading to obstructive renal failure. The vesico-ureteric junction has a muscular valve-like function that prevents retrograde reflux of urine during bladder contraction (voiding) thus protecting the collecting system from the relatively high pressures generated during voiding.

The lower urinary tract

The lower urinary tract is defined as the bladder, distal sphincter mechanism (DSM) and urethra. The bladder neck mechanism and prostate gland in the male are intimately related and are often considered to be a single functional unit, which is sometimes referred to as the pre-prostatic sphincter. The lower urinary tract in the male includes the bladder neck and prostate gland. There are a number of smaller glands draining into the urethra in both males and females. These may develop infection or inflammation leading to abscess formation, diverticula, fistulae or strictures.

The bladder

The bladder is a muscular organ (detrusor muscle) consisting of a body and a base. The body is the muscular part (fundus or dome), which is readily distensible and responsible for storage, as well as providing the contractile force for expulsion of urine. The detrusor muscle of the bladder is a functional syncytium of smooth muscle with multiple interwoven bundles. The trigone is a triangular area at the base of the bladder bounded by the twin ureteric orifices above and the internal urethral meatus below. The superficial trigonal muscle consists of specialized muscle cells, distinct from the detrusor. The function of this area is contraction during micturition, thereby occluding the ureteric orifices and preventing vesico-ureteric reflux.

The wall of the urinary bladder consists of three layers: the outer serosa, an adventitial layer of connective tissue; the muscularis propria, which is smooth muscle termed the detrusor muscle; and the innermost mucosa consisting of the subepithelial lamina propria and the transitional cell epithelium.

Table 11.1	Physiological function at individual nephron sites
Site	**Physiological function**
Glomerulus	Formation of filtrate
Proximal tubule	Absorption of water (60–80%), glucose, amino acids, HCO_3, PO_4, Na^+, K^+, Ca, urea Excretion of H^+
Loop of Henle	Countercurrent system to adjust fluid balance
Distal tubule	Absorption of $Na^+/Cl^-/Ca/Mg$/water
Collecting duct	Fine tuning of $K^+/H^+/HCO_3$/water Excretion of drugs, metabolites, urea and amino acids

The mucosa of the bladder and urethra consists of transitional epithelium (urothelium) and an underlying lamina propria of loose connective tissue. The urothelium is up to six cells in thickness; the exact thickness depends on the degree of filling of the bladder. The urothelium was initially thought to be completely impermeable and inert. More recent evidence indicates that ionic and drug transport takes place across the urothelium.

The bladder does not possess a rigid serosal layer. It is surrounded by several well-defined fascial layers that, on the one hand, separate the bladder from adjacent organs and, on the other, hold it in position. The retropubic aspect of the bladder is covered by a layer termed the superior hypogastric wing, which extends laterally as far as the vascular pedicles of the bladder and posteriorly as far as the dome of the bladder. The dome and posterior aspect of the bladder are covered by the inferior hypogastric wing, which roofs over the lateral pedicles and extends posteriorly to the presacral fascia. The fascia under these coverings is loose and tenuous, allowing expansion of the urinary bladder as it fills. It follows that any pathological condition that results in thickening of these fasciae, e.g. radiotherapy, could lead to a reduction in bladder capacity. The nerves from the pelvic plexus run forward within the presacral fascia to reach the lateral pedicles of the bladder. The base of the bladder and prostate gland are relatively fixed and held in place anteriorly by the more rigid endopelvic fascia and posteriorly by Denonvilliers' fascia.

In order to provide a low-pressure reservoir, the bladder must be compliant enough to accommodate a high volume of urine with only minimal rises in intravesical pressure. During storage, contributory factors for compliance are the visco-elastic properties of the tissues, the intrinsic ability of smooth muscle to maintain a constant tension over a wide range of stretch, and neural control of muscle tone via afferents passing from free nerve endings within the walls of the bladder.

The bladder neck

The most distal portion of the bladder base is referred to as the bladder neck. Muscle fibres from the bladder neck penetrate the base of the prostate and intermingle with its musculature. The bladder neck and proximal prostatic smooth muscle in the male are impossible to separate histologically. Functionally this constitutes a single unit of clinical significance, the pre-prostatic sphincter. The primary role of the pre-prostatic sphincter is to prevent retrograde ejaculation. It will serve as a urinary sphincter and maintain continence following ablation of the distal sphincter mechanism, as occurs with a post pelvic fracture urethral distraction defect. Resection of the bladder neck at transurethral resection of the prostate will result in retrograde ejaculation in around 90% of men. There is no well-defined bladder neck in the female, supporting the theory that the bladder neck is a genital sphincter enabling ejaculation rather than having a primary role in continence.

The prostate gland

The prostate gland is made up of glandular elements, responsible for secretory function, and stromal elements which include smooth muscle and connective tissue. The smooth muscle of the stroma comprises approximately 40% of the mass of the prostate gland. The innervation of this smooth muscle is primarily noradrenergic (sympathetic) in common with the innervation of the bladder neck. The normal prostate in the post-pubescent male has a volume of approximately 20 mL. It is composed of three zones (see Fig. 11.27). The peripheral zone accounts for 70% of the volume of the young adult prostate, and is the site of origin of 60–70% of all carcinomas of the prostate. The central zone consists of around 25% of the gland volume. The central zone surrounds the ejaculatory ducts from the base of the prostate to their opening on the verumontanum, a prominence clearly visible on the posterior urethral wall at cystoscopy. The transitional zone is a small area adjacent to the urethra. Benign prostatic hyperplasia originates as nodular hyperplasia of the transitional zone. These nodules enlarge to form the main mass of tissue and the diffuse enlargement of the transitional zone accounts for the increase in size of the prostate gland with age. As the transitional zone enlarges, the peripheral zone is compressed posteriorly as can be seen on transrectal ultrasound (see Fig. 11.28). Thus, in the elderly male, the peripheral zone may account for 30% or less of the prostate volume, as the volume of hyperplastic tissue rises. On cystoscopy, the prostatic urethra extends between the bladder neck proximally and the verumontanum distally. The verumontanum, which is a prominence at the level of the opening of the ejaculatory ducts, is an important anatomical landmark during transurethral surgery of the prostate. The distal sphincter mechanism lies immediately distal to the verumontanum and cutting past this point at the time of endoscopic prostatic resection runs the risk of incontinence due to sphincter damage. In a man with benign prostatic hyperplasia, the hyperplastic tissue protrudes into the urethral lumen in a characteristic manner. On either side one can see a cushion of tissue, which surgeons refer to as the lateral 'lobes' of the prostate. Posteriorly, there is often a prominence arising from the floor of the prostatic urethra which may protrude through the bladder neck. This is often referred to as the 'median lobe' of the prostate. These descriptive terms are useful in describing the surgical approach to transurethral manipulations of the prostate but have no true anatomical significance.

The distal sphincter mechanism

The distal sphincter mechanism or urethral sphincter proper (rhabdosphincter) is similar in both males and females. It is approximately 2.5 cm long and is integral to the wall of the urethra. It is discrete from the levator ani muscles of the pelvic floor. It is placed rather eccentrically, being relatively deficient dorsally. The distal sphincter mechanism is approximately 2.5 cm long and receives its somatic innervation via the pudendal nerves, as well as sympathetic and parasympathetic innervation arising from the pelvic plexus.

Autonomic innervation

The lower urinary tract receives a dense autonomic innervation via the sacral parasympathetic outflow (sacral micturition centre (SMC) situated at spinal levels S2–4) and the splanchnic sympathetic nerves (T10–L2). The nerves intermingle in the hypogastric plexus before joining the individual branches to the end organ. Damage to this plexus during surgical dissection in the pelvis results in lower urinary tract dysfunction. The motor supply to the detrusor muscle is predominantly parasympathetic (cholinergic) and is responsible for detrusor contraction during micturition. The motor supply to the bladder neck mechanism and prostatic smooth muscle is predominantly sympathetic (noradrenergic). The somatic nucleus innervating the distal sphincter mechanism (Onuf's nucleus) is situated in the sacral anterior motor horn adjacent to the nucleus innervating the muscles of the pelvic floor. There is a third population of nerves, the non-adrenergic non-cholinergic (NANC) nerves, which appear to play an important role in neuromodulation. Several peptide transmitters have been described within this population of nerves but their exact role in lower urinary tract function has yet to be delineated.

Symptoms of renal and urological disease

Loin pain

Lateralizing abdominal or flank pain is classically associated with renal and ureteric disease but can also be caused by a wide variety of gastrointestinal conditions.

Ureteric colic may result from passage of a stone, blood clot or tissue. It is characterized by pain of relatively rapid onset (minutes to hours) and is usually described as the worst pain ever experienced. The term 'colic' is a misnomer as it is usually constant with frequent exacerbation rather than intermittent (true colic). The pain most often radiates from the loin anteriorly to the lower abdomen and into the labium in the woman and testicle in the man. Radiation of pain to the testicle is said to be characteristic of ureteric pain, but testicular pain (e.g. from a torsion) can also cause flank pain. Similarly, in women, diseases of the ovaries can result in pain that is indistinguishable from ureteric colic. The site and severity of the pain is not related to site or severity of obstruction nor to the size of the stone being passed. Associated features such as pallor, tachycardia and nausea are usually present, but hypotension may suggest a ruptured aortic aneurysm as the differential diagnosis. Other conditions that may present with similar pain include biliary colic, pancreatitis, mesenteric infarction and ruptured aortic aneurysm.

'Renal pain' is more difficult to characterize and is often referred to as a dull aching in the loin. Other conditions including musculoskeletal disease can present with similar symptoms and differentiation between the two can be difficult.

Macroscopic (frank) haematuria

Frank haematuria is the visible presence of blood in the urine. Approximately 20% of patients with frank haematuria have a urological malignancy. The timing of the bleeding in relationship to the urinary stream may indicate the location of the bleeding point. Urethral bleeding (e.g. benign prostatic hyperplasia) precedes the main stream or is heaviest at initiation of the urinary stream. Bleeding that is uniformly mixed in with the stream is usually of renal or bladder origin. Terminal haematuria is an unusual problem associated with a bleeding lesion at or near the bladder neck, triggered by contact with the contracting bladder. Haematuria in conjunction with loin pain points usually points to a renal or ureteric origin, most likely due to a renal cell carcinoma or ureteric calculi. The classic triad of haematuria, loin pain and a loin mass is now an uncommon presentation of renal cancer.

Microscopic haematuria

Microscopic haematuria is not a symptom, but the presence of red blood cells in the urine that is detected on microscopy. The point prevalence of microscopic haematuria in men aged 18–33 years is around 1%, and the prevalence in men aged 50 and over is around 20%. Currently, microscopic haematuria is a term used synonymously with 'dipstick' positive haematuria, and the significance of this finding usually relates to the history and age of the individual in whom it is detected. The chance of finding significant pathology in the younger age group is less than 1%, compared with the older age group where urological malignancy can be found in approximately 8% and other significant pathology (nephropathy, urolithiasis, urinary tract infection) in approximately 25%.

Haemoejaculate

The presence of blood within a man's ejaculate is alarming but rarely of any significance. This symptom is often seen described erroneously as haemospermia. The origin of blood is rarely apparent on clinical examination but in a younger man one should be particularly vigilant as to the possibility of testicular malignancy. In the older man, prostate cancer should be considered. Reassurance is often the only treatment that is required.

Lower urinary tract symptoms

Lower urinary tract symptoms were previously described as irritative and obstructive. Although there were some advantages with this approach, the terms implied some underlying knowledge of the pathophysiology involved. This implication is not justified, as the symptoms of lower urinary tract disease are not specific to any particular condition. Symptoms are best considered according to the phase of the micturition cycle in which they occur. Pain related to the lower urinary tract may be experienced during any phase of micturition.

Storage symptoms

These include urgency, frequency, nocturnal frequency (nocturia), incontinence and suprapubic pain. The degree of urgency should be evaluated empirically as well as the pattern of any incontinence. Pain related to bladder filling is characteristic of sensory abnormalities of the bladder but may point to other diseases such as transitional cell carcinoma of the bladder or endometriosis.

Pre-void symptoms

Pre-void symptoms include suprapubic pain and hesitancy. Sensory conditions of the bladder are most often associated with pelvic pain that is most marked either just preceding or immediately following voiding. Hesitancy is the inability to initiate voiding on demand causing a delay in initiation of the urinary stream. This symptom is very typical of benign prostatic obstruction and increasing hesitancy may indicate impending acute retention of urine.

Voiding symptoms

Voiding symptoms include straining to void, a poor urinary stream, intermittency of stream, dysuria, strangury and terminal dribbling. Straining to void is of doubtful significance in men. Dysuria is defined as a burning sensation felt urethrally during voiding. Strangury is a much more unpleasant sensation of painful micturition associated with a mass lesion in the bladder such as a stone, tumour, clot or foreign body. The most common cause of strangury is the presence of the balloon of an indwelling urethral catheter.

Post-void symptoms

Post-void symptoms include pain and post-micturition dribbling. Post-void pain felt suprapubically or urethrally may be caused by inflammatory bladder conditions or mass lesions within the bladder. Post-micturition dribbling of urine is characterized by the leakage of a small volume of urine, classically after walking away from the toilet. It probably reflects loss of tone in the periurethral musculature and responds to behavioural therapy.

Examination of the renal system

Inspection

Advanced acute renal failure may be associated with a reduced consciousness, whilst end-stage uraemia can produce hiccups and uraemic encephalopathy (flapping tremor and twitching). Uraemic frost is extremely rare. Patients with chronic renal impairment develop anaemia with pallor and a 'dirty' uraemic tinge to their skin, occasionally mistaken for sun-tanned skin. Anorexia is a common problem and patients are often malnourished, having had to adhere to a restrictive diet.

Vasculitic rashes associated with disease that can cause glomerulonephritis are purpuric and tend to be on the lower limb. There may be splinter haemorrhages, visible in the nails, with either vasculitis or subacute bacterial endocarditis. A typical butterfly facial rash occurs with systemic lupus erythematosus (SLE), which is associated with renal disease. Patients with renal impairment on long-term steroids can have fragile skin with purpura and ecchymoses. Jaundice from liver disease may be part of hepatorenal syndrome. Livedo reticularis is associated with cholesterol embolization and occurs most frequently over the legs. Tertiary hyperparathyroidism with phosphate retention causes pruritus leading to multiple scratch marks.

Patients on haemodialysis have an arterio-venous (AV) fistula, usually in the forearm or antecubital fossa. A constant thrill may be present and a bruit auscultated over the fistula. New fistulae may be audible before the thrill has had time to develop. There may be scars from previous failed fistulae. Long-standing fistulae can become grossly enlarged with massive blood flows through them, leaving the hand cold and underperfused. Synthetic grafts are also used for haemodialysis access: a semi-rigid Teflon graft may be palpable either in the forearm or upper thigh with an audible bruit. Tenckhoff catheters for peritoneal dialysis are inserted in the suprapubic midline region, and the insertion of each catheter results in an additional small scar in the upper abdomen.

If kidneys have been removed, there is usually a large nephrectomy scar either in the loin or across the anterior abdominal wall; laparoscopic techniques produce smaller multiple incisions. Ascites may be part of generalized fluid overload associated with nephrotic syndrome.

 CLINICAL ALERT

Arterio-venous fistulae are 'lifelines' and care should be taken not to place tourniquets around the limb in case the blood supply drops and they fail. Likewise, phlebotomy and blood pressure measurement should be avoided in the fistula arm.

Palpation

Normal kidneys lie posteriorly on either side of the vertebral column between T12 and L3. The right kidney is marginally lower than the left, and both kidneys are not normally palpable except in thin individuals. Palpable kidneys are usually enlarged, obstructed or transplanted. The most common cause of enlarged kidneys is autosomal dominant polycystic kidney disease, in which the kidneys can take up much of the intra-abdominal space. Occasionally, they may be mistaken for hepatomegaly or splenomegaly. The kidney can be tender if obstructed (hydronephrosis) or infected (pyelonephritis/pyonephrosis). Abdominal aortic aneurysms are associated with retroperitoneal fibrosis and vascular disease. Transplanted kidneys are anastomosed in the pelvis to the iliac vessels. They are superficial and their outline can be clearly palpated in the iliac fossa. The infected or rejecting transplanted kidney is usually tender and enlarged. Failed transplants may be left in situ so a patient may have several palpable pelvic masses.

The presence of a palpable bladder in a comfortable patient without a desire to void is diagnostic of chronic retention of urine. The distended bladder is palpable as a non-compressible, non-pulsatile smooth ovoid midline mass arising out of the pelvis. The full bladder is dull to percussion. Structures that are commonly mistaken for the bladder include a gravid or fibroid uterus, a large ovarian cyst and an aortic aneurysm. It is important to re-examine the patient following insertion of a urethral catheter. Failure of the mass to disappear should always raise doubt as to whether the original mass was indeed the bladder. A 'bimanual' examination is performed under anaesthesia with one hand on the abdomen, the other in the vagina (female) or rectum (male).

In the uncircumcised, the prepuce is retracted to inspect the glans for tumour or infection. A phimosis may prevent this, although it is normal for the prepuce to be unretractable in children younger than 4 years (see p. 761). Lesions secondary to sexually transmitted infections may be present (e.g. warts). The position of the urethral meatus is noted excluding hypo- or epispadias. The penile shaft is palpated for Peyronie's plaques or dense urethral strictures. Priapism is clinically obvious, as is a fractured penis.

The scrotum and contents should be examined in conjunction with penile and groin examination. The scrotal skin may be affected by sebaceous cysts, and the groin creases are liable to fungal infections. The testes are gently bimanually palpated, confirming presence of normal size and anatomy and also any abnormal swellings. Details of specific scrotal pathology can be found on page 765. In the standing position the spermatic cord is inspected for a varicocele, which typically feels like a 'bag of worms'.

Digital rectal examination is an essential part of the assessment of the lower urinary tract. Explanation of the procedure is essential prior to examination. Examination is carried out with the patient in the left lateral position or resting on a couch (crouch position). Inspection of the perineum for soiling, skin excoriation and pressure sores gives valuable clues as to the individual's general social functioning (e.g. elderly person living alone). Loss of sensation of the perianal skin, loss of anal tone and an absent voluntary squeeze may indicate neurological disease contributing to the symptoms. Following careful inspection, the pulp of the gloved, lubricated index finger is gently pressed against the anus. The patient is instructed to strain downwards as if passing a stool and the finger is then gently inserted per anum. A systematic sequence of examination should always be followed including palpation superiorly and laterally for pelvic masses, of the rectal mucosa in all directions and finally focusing anteriorly on the prostate gland in male patients. The normal prostate gland is about the size of a chestnut and has a consistency similar to a well-done fillet steak. Enlargement of the gland causes it to push backwards against the anterior rectal wall, from which it is separated by Denonvilliers' fascia. The most important features on palpation are the surface, firmness and regularity of the gland. The size of the gland is misleading and is usually of little diagnostic significance. Approximately 50% of localized palpable abnormalities (nodules) turn out to be cancers. An irregularly enlarged prostate gland, particularly with an ill-defined margin, is suspicious for locally advanced prostate cancer (see p. 758). A tender boggy prostate suggests prostatitis.

Female pelvic examination should always be performed with a chaperone present, in a relaxed environment. The patient's knees are flexed and abducted, as though undergoing a smear. The external genitalia and introitus are inspected for ulcers, warts, discharge and atrophic changes. The urethral meatus is inspected for caruncles, cysts and mucosal prolapse. Pelvic floor descent (i.e. cystocele and rectocele) is assessed during a gentle Valsalva manoeuvre. On coughing, urinary leak of stress incontinence may be apparent. A bimanual examination is performed with one hand on the abdomen. The clinician assesses for mobility and abnormal masses. The uterus, ovaries and cervix are also assessed.

Other systems

The cardiovascular system

Examination of the cardiovascular system provides important information about a patient's fluid status and the presence of cardiac failure from fluid overload. When fluid overloaded, peripheral oedema may be present, the jugular venous pressure (JVP) is elevated, and there is crepitation in the lung fields from pulmonary oedema. On auscultation of the heart, there may be a gallop rhythm and a fourth heart sound with tachycardia. The blood pressure is usually elevated unless there is left ventricular failure. Dehydration can result in low blood pressure, tachycardia and low volume pulse pressure. Pericarditis can occur with advanced uraemia and cause a pericardial rub.

The respiratory system

Fluid overload is confirmed with pulmonary oedema and pleural effusions. Rarely, peritoneal dialysate may leak through the diaphragm to cause marked pleural effusion. This can be differentiated from other causes of pleural effusion by testing for glucose (peritoneal dialysis fluid has supraphysiological concentrations of glucose). Acute renal failure with pulmonary haemorrhage, such as with Wegener's granulomatosis, is often accompanied by epistaxis and haemoptysis.

The rheumatological system

Rheumatoid arthritis may cause renal failure through both the disease process and the medication used. Gouty tophi suggest hyperuricaemia. Chronic renal replacement therapy is associated with calcium phosphate deposits, which may erode through the skin.

The nervous system

Chronic renal failure is associated with peripheral sensory neuropathy. There may also be a glove and stocking distribution with diabetes. Fundoscopy may confirm changes of hypertension or diabetes, and cholesterol emboli may (rarely) be seen.

Investigations for renal and urinary tract disease

Assessment of renal function

Serum creatinine

Estimation of urea and electrolytes is the most commonly used screening investigation for renal impairment. Measurement of plasma creatinine is the simplest way to assess renal function. The normal serum creatinine ranges from 60 to 120 μmol/L and the function of approximately 60% of glomeruli must be lost before any appreciable rises in serum creatinine occur.

Glomerular filtration rate

Often, more accurate assessment of renal function such as an estimate of glomerular filtration rate is required. The normal glomerular filtration rate (GFR) is remarkably constant from day to day. It is, however, affected by age, gender and build. It is normally corrected (indexed) to body surface area (GFR/1.73 m^2). The glomerular filtration rate naturally declines with age from a peak of 130 mL/min in young adults. Pregnancy is accompanied by a temporary 50% increase in glomerular filtration rate due to increased cardiac output and glomerular hyperfiltration.

Creatinine clearance

It is difficult to perform a direct measure of the glomerular filtration rate. Since creatinine, produced by skeletal muscle cells, is readily filtered from the kidneys with minimal reabsorption, creatinine clearance is often used as an indirect measure of glomerular filtration rate. Creatinine clearance is calculated from a 24-hour urine collection and serum creatinine result. The creatinine clearance (Ccr) is calculated as:

$$Ccr = Ucr/Pcr \times V$$

where Pcr is the plasma concentration of creatinine, Ucr is the urine creatinine concentration and V is the urine flow rate. In clinical practice the accuracy is often limited by the completeness of the urine collection.

The creatinine clearance can also be approximated from the serum creatinine taking into account sex, age and weight using the Cockroft–Gault formula. This precludes the need for a 24-hour urine collection, but is less accurate in obese individuals, children and patients on low-protein diets. The formula for men is provided below; in women, the constant of 1.04 is used instead of 1.23.

$$Ccr = \frac{1.23 \times (140\text{-age}) \times (\text{weight in kg})}{Pcr\ (\mu mol/dL)}$$

^{51}Cr-EDTA estimation of glomerular filtration rate

If a 24-hour urine collection is not possible (e.g. in patients with ileal conduits after cystectomy), the glomerular filtration rate may be calculated using ^{51}Cr-EDTA.

Reciprocal plots for monitoring renal function

Reciprocal plots are often used to monitor renal function over time. Due to the reciprocal relationship between serum creatinine and glomerular filtration rate, initial decline in glomerular filtration leads to minimal increases in serum creatinine until the glomerular filtration is 60% of normal, when serum creatinine suddenly climbs. To overcome this problem, the reciprocal of the serum creatinine ($1/P_{cr}$) is plotted to obtain a linear relationship with decreasing glomerular filtration rate. Reciprocal plots may be used to estimate an approximate date when renal function deteriorates sufficiently for the initiation of dialysis. Deviations from the expected rate of decline can occur with reversible causes of acute deterioration (e.g. urinary tract infection or obstruction).

 FURTHER INFORMATION

Walser M. Assessing renal function from creatinine measurements in adults with chronic renal failure. American Journal of Kidney Diseases 1998; 32: 23–31.

Blood tests

Urea and electrolytes (U&Es)

The standard urea and electrolytes profile measures sodium, potassium, chloride, urea and creatinine. Urea is the nitrogenous waste derived mainly from dietary protein and tissue breakdown. Elevated levels may correspond with renal impairment, but as many conditions can lead to a rise in urea, it is not always a good indicator of renal function. Serum creatinine has been discussed above.

Serology

Screening for causes of glomerulonephritis and nephrotic syndrome requires a multitude of serological tests. The more common tests are listed in Table 11.2.

Table 11.2	Serological tests for glomerulonephritis	
Investigation	**Result**	**Possible aetiology**
Anti-streptolysin O (ASO) titres	Elevated	Post-streptococcal glomerulonephritis
Anti-neutrophil cytoplasmic antibodies (ANCA)	Elevated cytoplasmic cANCA (positive for proteinase 3), and peripheral pANCA (positive for myeloperoxidase)	Wegener's granulomatosis, bacterial endocarditis, cystic fibrosis, inflammatory bowel disease, anti-GBM disease
Anti-glomerular basement membrane (GBM) antibodies	Present	Goodpasture's disease
Autoantibodies	Elevated double-stranded DNA antibodies	Systemic lupus erythematosus
Serum complement	Low	Systemic lupus erythematosus, subacute bacterial endocarditis, membranoproliferative glomerulonephritis type II, cryoglobulinaemia, post-streptococcal glomerulonephritis
Rheumatoid factor	Present	Rheumatoid disease and other inflammatory conditions

Urine tests

Inspection

The first part of urinalysis is direct visual observation. Normal, fresh urine is pale to dark yellow or amber in colour and clear. A red or red-brown (abnormal) colour could be due to blood, food dyes, eating fresh beetroot (beeturia), a drug (e.g. rifampicin) or the presence of either haemoglobin or myoglobin. Turbidity or cloudiness may be caused by excessive cellular material or protein in the urine or may develop from crystallization or precipitation of salts upon standing at room temperature or in the refrigerator.

Urinalysis

Currently, dipstick urine testing is the most commonly used initial screening urine test. The sticks are impregnated with reagents that react with a known or suspected constituent within the urine, allowing qualitative and semi-quantitative analysis.

pH

The glomerular filtrate of blood plasma is usually acidified by renal tubules and collecting ducts from a pH of 7.4 to about 6 in the final urine. However, depending on the acid–base status, urinary pH may range from as low as 4.5 to as high as 8.0.

Specific gravity

Specific gravity (which is a measure of solute concentration) measures the ability of the kidney to concentrate or dilute the urine. Specific gravity between 1.002 and 1.035 on a random sample should be considered normal. Low values are characteristic of diabetes insipidus, and high values indicate relative dehydration if kidney function is normal. In end-stage renal disease, specific gravity tends towards 1.007 to 1.010, i.e. that of plasma.

Protein

Normally, only small plasma proteins filtered at the glomerulus are reabsorbed by the renal tubule. However, a small amount of filtered plasma proteins and protein secreted by the nephron (Tamm–Horsfall protein) can be found in normal urine. Normal total protein excretion is quantified by 24-hour collection and does not usually exceed 150 mg/24 hours.

Glucose

Less than 0.1% of glucose normally filtered by the glomerulus appears in urine (<130 mg/24 h). Glycosuria (excess sugar in urine) most commonly indicates diabetes mellitus but may reflect a low renal threshold for glucose.

Ketones

Ketones (acetone, acetoacetic acid, β-hydroxybutyric acid) resulting from either diabetic ketosis or some other form of calorie deprivation (starvation) are easily detected.

Nitrite

Urine normally contains nitrates. Certain microorganisms (e.g. *E. coli*) possess enzymes that convert nitrates to nitrites. A positive **nitrite** test therefore indicates that bacteria may be present in significant numbers in urine. Compared with microscopy and culture, the **nitrite** test has a specificity of over 90% for detecting bacteriuria, but a sensitivity of 85%.

Leukocyte esterase

Leukocyte esterase is an enzyme produced by neutrophils. A positive leukocyte esterase test results from the presence of white blood cells either as whole cells or as lysed cells, i.e. it signifies pyuria. It is possible to have significant urinary tract infection without significant pyuria, hence a negative leukocyte esterase test on its own does not reliably rule out infection. In combination with nitrites, it has a sensitivity of over 90% in detecting urinary tract infection.

Urine microscopy and culture

A clean-catch, midstream urine specimen (MSU) is the recommended form of collection to identify urinary tract infection. The first half of the voided urine is discarded and the collection vessel is introduced into the urinary stream to catch a midstream specimen.

Red blood cells

Haematuria is the presence of red cells in urine. Usually, some red cells will find their way into the urine of healthy individuals. However, when detected, the presence of red cells should be considered abnormal unless contamination can be ruled out. The abnormal red cells may appear dysmorphic (oddly shaped) if their origin is glomerular rather than from the collecting system.

White blood cells

Abnormal numbers of leukocytes may appear with infection in either the upper or lower urinary tract or with acute glomerulonephritis. White cells from the vagina, especially in the presence of vaginal and cervical infections, or the external urethral meatus in men and women may contaminate the urine. If two or more leukocytes per high-power field appear in non-contaminated urine, the specimen is probably abnormal. The presence of sterile pyuria is commonly due to a partially treated urinary tract infection (antibiotic effect); however, if persistent it should alert the clinician to the possibility of a bladder stone, bladder tumour or fastidious organism requiring specialized culture techniques (e.g. tuberculosis, *Neisseria*).

Epithelial cells

Renal tubular epithelial cells, usually larger than granulocytes, contain a large round or oval nucleus and normally slough into the urine in small numbers. However, with nephrotic syndrome and in conditions leading to tubular degeneration, the number appearing in urine is increased. Transitional epithelial cells from the renal pelvis, ureter or bladder have more regular cell borders, larger nuclei and smaller overall size than squamous epithelium. Abnormal transitional cells are found in the urine particularly with high-grade transitional cell carcinoma or carcinoma in situ.

Casts

Urinary casts are formed only in the distal convoluted tubule or the collecting duct (distal nephron). Hyaline casts are composed primarily of a mucoprotein (Tamm–Horsfall protein) secreted by tubule cells and are found in healthy individuals. Disease states that predispose to cast formation include low renal flow, high salt concentration and low pH. Protein casts with long, thin tails formed at the junction of Henle's loop and the distal convoluted tubule are called cylindroids. Red blood cells may stick together and form red blood cell casts with glomerulonephritis, leakage of red cells from glomeruli or severe tubular damage. White blood cell casts are typical for acute pyelonephritis but may also be present with glomerulonephritis. Their presence indicates inflammation of the kidney.

Bacteria

Urine culture is the gold standard in the definition of bacterial urinary tract infection. Significant bacteriuria is defined by the presence of more than 10^5 organisms per mL in pure culture. Pyuria is diagnostic of urinary tract infection. Multiple organisms usually reflect contamination.

Diagnostic imaging

Ultrasound

Ultrasound is often the first imaging technique of choice for the investigation of patients with renal disease as it is non-invasive, quick and avoids radiation and nephrotoxic contrast media. It is limited by patient cooperation and patient size and the results are operator dependent.

The renal outlines should be smooth and 9–12 cm long in adults. Asymmetry of renal size is associated with unilateral renal artery stenosis or congenital hypoplasia. Small, shrunken, scarred kidneys occur with chronic disease such as long-term hypertension, chronic pyelonephritis or reflux. Ultrasound can differentiate between cystic and solid masses and qualify the nature of the cysts. Enlarged kidneys are frequently due to polycystic kidney disease, but the presence of one or more simple cysts can occur normally with age. The calyces and ureters are not clearly identified unless there is obstruction. Increased brightness of the cortex may indicate glomerulonephritis. Colour Doppler allows the assessment of renal vascular flow and identification of renal artery stenosis.

Plain abdominal film

A plain abdominal film is often used as a baseline investigation for patients presenting with symptoms suggestive of ureteric calculi. Approximately 90% of ureteric calculi are radio-opaque as they contain calcium, but it can be difficult to distinguish them from abdominal calcification or phleboliths. In general, ureteric calculi appear as calcification that occurs along the anatomical lie of the ureters.

Computed tomography (CT)

CT of the abdomen and pelvis is used to evaluate cysts, solid masses, calculi, renal vasculature and in renal trauma. A non-contrast CT scan can be used to detect ureteric stones. Secondary signs such as ureteral dilatation and perinephric stranding may indicate the presence of ureteric calculi that are not directly visible. Stones in the pelvis can reliably be distinguished from phleboliths by the presence of an oedematous cuff surrounding the calculus (the 'rim' sign). In contrast, phleboliths exhibit a tail of high attenuation (the 'comet' sign). Unlike plain radiography, uric acid stones are readily visible.

Contrast enhanced CT (Fig. 11.2) is the imaging technique of choice in evaluating complex renal cysts for malignancy (p. 706). Helical CT allows an arterial phase prior to standard imaging. Sequenced scans can be obtained, detailing the renal parenchyma, cortico-medullary junction, and the renal venous phase. Enhancement of a mass lesion of greater than 10 Hounsfield units is usually indicative of malignancy. Other features suspicious of renal malignancy are coarse calcification and thick-walled, ill-defined margins. 'Hyperdense' renal cysts that contain high quantities of

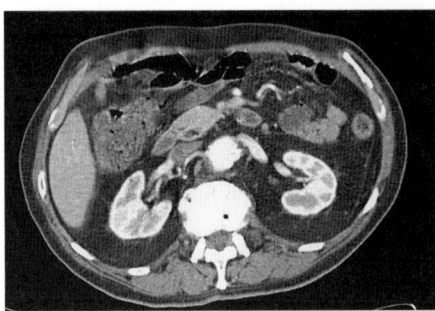

Fig. 11.2 Contrast enhanced CT of the kidneys.

blood and protein may be confused with renal cell carcinoma, however (unlike carcinoma) they do not enhance with contrast.

Non-enhancing wedge-shaped sections with substance loss indicate infarction. The perinephric and para-aortic region is readily seen on CT, which may help to identify lymphadenopathy or congenital abnormalities.

CT is also the imaging modality of choice in surveillance of the retroperitoneum for nodal metastases associated with testicular cancer and to identify alternative diagnoses for patients with suspected ureteric colic or upper tract obstruction with no evidence of stone (e.g. aortic aneurysm, retroperitoneal fibrosis or appendicitis).

Magnetic resonance imaging (MRI)

MRI may be used for the assessment of renal masses, staging of renal carcinoma, evaluation of the renal vasculature and urography. In staging renal cancers, MRI is considered to be equivalent to CT scanning, and superior for the diagnosis of angiomyolipoma and assessment of the renal vein or vena cava for tumour.

MRI is now the imaging modality of choice for staging bladder cancer. It can accurately assess spread beyond the detrusor muscle, defining T2 and T3 disease. Images typically show extension of tumour into the perivesical fat with T3 disease. MRI is also used to stage prostate cancer, but may not detect or may underestimate extracapsular extension. Both CT and MRI are unable to differentiate changes associated with microscopic capsular invasion from non-malignant inflammatory reaction.

MRI has also been used in conjunction with cystoscopy and urethrography to evaluate urethral diverticula in women, and can provide three-dimensional reconstruction of complex circumferential urethral lesions. MRI can also be used to identify undescended intra-abdominal testes, and used as an adjunct to ultrasound in differentiating a scrotal mass from haematoma.

Magnetic resonance angiography (MRA), using T1-weighted images with gadolinium contrast, will outline renal vessels allowing the diagnosis of renal artery stenosis. Excellent views of the renal vasculature are possible. Gadolinium is safer than iodinated contrast with impaired renal function.

Intravenous urogram (IVU)

Also known as an intravenous pyelogram, the IVU is a well-established method of imaging the urological tract. Contrast is injected intravenously and excreted by the kidneys, outlining the renal pelvis, ureters and bladder. A plain X-ray is taken prior to contrast as a control image, as the excreted contrast will obscure any renal tract calcification. Modern contrast agents are of low osmolarity and take less than a minute to reach the kidney. The second film is the nephrogram, which represents renal uptake. After 5 minutes a further film is obtained showing renal excretion and the ureteric filling. At this point ureteric compression may be applied by inflating a belt worn around the waist to impede contrast drainage and distend the pelvicalyceal system and proximal ureters for better imaging. When the compression is released, the system drains and further films are obtained. The bladder fills after about 30 minutes, and a bladder film may reveal filling defects. A post-void or 'post-micturition' film allows visualization of the lower ureters.

Pyelography

Pyelography is indicated after an inconclusive IVU where doubt remains as to a suspicious filling defect in the pelvis or to better determine the lower extent of an obstructive lesion. It involves direct injection of contrast into the urinary tract, either via a fine catheter inserted into the ureter at cystoscopy (retrograde) or via renal puncture or nephrostomy (antegrade). Fluoroscopy allows detailed imaging of the urinary tract independent of renal function. Patients lie on a tilt table and gravity aids contrast movement.

Cystourethrography

A formal cystogram requires direct retrograde instillation of contrast into the bladder via a catheter. It may be used to identify traumatic rupture or post-surgical leakage, or as a part of pressure flow urodynamics to determine the presence of ureteric reflux, nature of urinary incontinence or bladder outflow obstruction. A micturating cystourethrogram (MCUG) may be performed in the paediatric patient to identify urethral valves or vesicoureteric reflux. The urethra may be imaged at the end of a cystogram on voiding as a micturating cystourethrogram (MCUG). An ascending urethrogram may be performed by inserting a 12 F Foley catheter into the penile fossa navicularis and the balloon inflated slightly to occlude the urethral meatus. When contrast is instilled, the urethra is outlined, identifying traumatic or obstructive lesions (e.g. strictures or tumour), diverticula or fistulae. In the female, this is anatomically not possible and complex double balloon catheters have been developed to trap contrast in the urethra under pressure, which may open a collapsed urethral diverticulum (positive pressure urethrography). It is often used in conjunction with urethrocystoscopy.

Angiography

Due to the increasing availability of MRA and CT angiography, 'conventional' angiography for the diagnosis of urological tract disease is becoming rare. Transfemoral renal vein cannulation is still performed for renin sampling in renovascular hypertension. Indications for conventional angiography are for embolization of large renal tumours, embolization of uncontrollable bleeding and the investigation of renal artery stenosis, renal artery aneurysm, arteriovenous fistulae and renal trauma.

Renal isotope studies

Isotope renography relies on the kidney's ability to filter or secrete a radionucleotide. It is therefore a study of uptake, transit and elimination. The study itself provides information on either static (DMSA) or dynamic (MAG3 or DTPA) function (Table 11.3). The kidneys and bladder are imaged using a gamma camera. Currently ^{99m}Tc-MAG3 is the most commonly used agent.

A normal renogram is characterized by rapid uptake followed by slower 'renal handling', after which the kidney drains and activity declines. The drainage phase marks the beginning of bladder activity, which continues to rise inversely to renal activity. An obstructed system may not affect uptake, but handling and drainage will be impaired. If the uptake is reduced to background activity, the kidney is deemed to be 'non-functioning'. Misleading obstructive traces may occur, where no true obstruction is present.

A type I (normal) trace is when rapid uptake is followed by transit and then prompt and complete washout. A type II (obstructed) trace with rapid uptake is followed by a slow and steady rise that continues despite administration of diuretic.

Physiological investigations

Urodynamics

Urodynamics is the study of the physiological and pathological factors involved in the transport, storage and evacuation of urine. Simple tests are non-invasive investigations, which can be carried out with a minimum of equipment and are sufficient evaluation for the vast majority of patients with symptoms of lower urinary tract dysfunction. Complex tests are invasive or require highly specialized equipment and are reserved for the more complicated cases.

Simple urodynamic tests
Frequency–volume charts
A frequency–volume chart is a micturition diary, which records the time and volume of each void together with

relevant symptoms and events such as urgency, incontinence episodes and pad usage. It allows the patient to focus on his or her symptoms and provides the clinician with an objective record of the patient's symptoms. A time period of a minimum of 2 days is recommended but a period of between 3 and 7 days is preferable. From the diary the average functional bladder capacity (i.e. the typical volume voided), voiding frequency and, if the patient's time in bed is recorded, day and night urine production and nocturia can be determined. Self-reported volumes have been found to agree well with measured voided volumes.

Post-void residual urine
Under normal circumstances, the bladder empties completely at the end of micturition. The presence of residual urine at the end of voiding is a non-specific indicator of inefficient detrusor action. Residual urine is most conveniently measured using a portable ultrasound machine. These are readily available and can provide automated calculation of residual urine based on the dimensions of the bladder visualized post voiding. Causes of increased residual urine are interrupted voiding, non-physiological testing (over-filling the bladder or insufficient privacy), detrusor hypo-contractility, outflow obstruction and dyssynergic voiding.

Uroflowmetry
Uroflowmetry is a non-invasive test and represents the minimum urodynamic assessment in the patient with suspected bladder outflow obstruction. It is a measure of the final result of micturition and therefore is influenced by several factors, i.e. detrusor contractility, presence of obstruction and completeness of sphincter relaxation. The most reliable uroflow results are obtained on voided volumes of between 150 and 400 mL. The peak flow rate (Qmax) is the single most valuable measurement; however, in assessing this, the flow rate pattern and the volume voided must be taken into account. Examples of normal and typical abnormal uroflowgrams are shown in Table 11.4. In clinical practice, uroflowmetry is used as a screening test in the detection of outflow obstruction. In men with lower urinary tract symptoms, the presence of a peak flow rate of less than 10 mL/s is highly predictive of bladder outflow obstruction.

Complex urodynamic tests
Pressure flow investigations
As uroflowmetry may be influenced by impaired detrusor contractility, only a pressure-flow study will determine if

Table 11.3	Radionucleotides for renal isotope imaging	
Nucleotide	**Renal handling**	**Information**
DMSA	Secreted by tubules	Split renal function and structure (e.g. scarring)
DTPA	Filtered by glomerulus	Diagnosis of obstruction or renovascular hypertension
MAG3	Filtered and secreted	Split renal function, diagnosis of obstruction or renal artery stenosis

DMSA, dimercaptosuccinic acid; DTPA, diethylenetriamine pentaacetic acid; MAG3, mercaptoacyl triglycine.

Table 11.4	Predicted percentage obstruction by maximum urinary flow (Qmax)		
Qmax on uroflowmetry	<10 mL/s	10–15 mL/s	>15 mL/s
% Obstructed on pressure-flow analysis	88	54	24
% Unobstructed on pressure-flow analysis	12	46	76

detrusor functioning is adequate or if the low flow recorded was due to obstruction. Approximately 25% of symptomatic men will have a reduced flow rate secondary to impaired detrusor activity and approximately 5–10% will be obstructed despite having a peak flow rate of between 15 and 20 mL/s recorded on uroflowmetry.

Pressure-flow studies are by their nature invasive and involve the insertion into the bladder of a filling and measuring line (dual-lumen catheters are often used). The detrusor pressure is a measure of the pressure exerted by the detrusor muscle itself and is calculated as the difference between the pressure exerted by the abdominal musculature and the pressure recorded by the bladder line. A fine transducer is inserted, usually into the rectum, to determine abdominal pressure. Whilst this is only an approximation of true intra-abdominal pressure it is of sufficient value in clinical practice. In all pressure-flow studies the reference point is the level of the superior border of the symphysis pubis. The single most important parameter for the diagnosis of obstruction is the subtracted detrusor pressure recorded at the time of peak flow. This may be plotted against peak flow in a pressure-flow plot.

Videocystometrography

The addition of X-ray screening facilities and filling the bladder with contrast allows the visualization of the urinary tract during filling and provocative tests such as coughing and voiding. In women with incontinence, cystography allows visualization of the bladder neck and base, which facilitates planning of the appropriate surgical procedure. In men, the advantages of video pressure-flow studies are that one can visualize the site of obstruction and therefore distinguish between anatomical strictures and functional obstruction due to bladder neck or detrusor sphincter dyssynergia. Bladder neck dyssynergia is revealed on a video study by performing a 'stop test' during which the patient interrupts voiding by contraction of the distal sphincter. In the normal patient, 'milk back' of urine occurs into the bladder prior to shutting of the bladder neck. With bladder neck dyssynergia there is trapping of urine in the prostatic urethra. True detrusor sphincter dyssynergia results from incoordinated detrusor and sphincter function and is seen in patients with neurological disease. The upper tracts can be visualized in cases of vesico-ureteric reflux.

SECTION 11.3 Diagnostic procedures

Renal biopsy

Indications

The definitive diagnosis of many renal conditions is only possible with a renal biopsy. The indications are listed in Table 11.5. For proteinuria, biopsy is usually indicated for patients with more severe disease with 1.5–3.5 g proteinuria per day. Diabetic patients rarely require biopsy unless diabetic retinopathy is absent or if there are other features suggesting an alternative diagnosis. Systemic disorders with active urinary sediments (e.g. vasculitis) may require biopsies to monitor disease progression. Isolated haematuria due to glomerulonephritis is usually associated with benign conditions such as IgA nephropathy or thin membrane disease, and biopsy is indicated only if patients develop hypertension, declining glomerular filtration rate or significant proteinuria. If two small kidneys are seen on ultrasound, these are rarely biopsied as the disease process is too advanced to be treatable.

Patient preparation

Ultrasound should be used to confirm the presence of two kidneys. Very rarely a single kidney may be biopsied if renal function is declining with no apparent cause. Systolic blood pressure should be controlled, and blood should be sent for clotting screen and group and save. Uraemic patients may have a prolonged bleeding time, and temporary improvement can be achieved by infusing desmopressin (DDAVP) 20 μg immediately prior to biopsy.

Procedure

The patient lies prone with a pillow under the abdomen, and the left kidney is localized using real-time ultrasound. Local anaesthetic is infiltrated down to the capsule along the needle track and the patient holds their breath whilst the biopsy is taken. The biopsy gun is aimed at the lower pole, checking the position using ultrasound real-time scanning, and several cores are taken from the same area of the kidney.

Table 11.5	Indications and contraindications for renal biopsy

Indications

Unexplained acute renal failure

Acute renal failure not responding to treatment

Adult with nephrotic syndrome

Renal disease as part of a systemic disorder

Transplant dysfunction

Contraindications

Uncontrolled bleeding disorder

Uncontrolled hypertension

Uncooperative patient

Morbid obesity

Single kidney

The cores should contain cortex rather than medulla. This may be confirmed at the time of sampling using light microscopy to ensure adequate specimens with sufficient glomeruli for diagnosis. Samples are sent for histology, immunological staining and electron microscopy. Preliminary diagnoses may be available within 24 hours.

Complications

The overall complication rate is 5%. Serious complications include death (1 in 10 000) and significant bleeding requiring nephrectomy (0.05%). Macroscopic haematuria occurs in up to 4%, significant haematoma in 2%, bleeding requiring blood transfusion in 1% and intrarenal arteriovenous fistula formation in 1%.[1]

Post-procedure care

Patients are kept on bed rest for between 6 and 24 hours. Ideally, the patient is kept well hydrated to reduce the chance of clots. Retroperitoneal bleeding causes pain and hypotension but no overt blood. If this is suspected, urgent CT abdomen is indicated as ultrasound will not always show the haematoma. If an AV fistula is formed at the biopsy site, a bleeding source can be seen on angiography and the site can be embolized.

REFERENCE

(1) *Hergesell O, Felten H, Andrassy K, et al. Safety of ultrasound-guided percutaneous renal biopsy - retrospective analysis of 1090 consecutive cases. Nephrology Dialysis Transplantation 1998; 13: 975–977.*

Cystourethroscopy

Indications

Flexible cystoscopy is performed for investigation of lower urinary tract symptoms (e.g. new-onset frequency/nocturia) and anatomy (e.g. urethral stricture). All patients with haematuria require cystoscopy to exclude lower urinary tract malignancy.

Patient preparation

Patients are admitted as a day case procedure for flexible cystoscopy (Fig. 11.3) under intraurethral local anaesthetic (gel). Rigid cystoscopy requires general or regional anaesthesia. It may be performed as a day surgical procedure although intervention (e.g. resection of bladder tumour) may necessitate admission. Informed consent is required for rigid cystoscopy.

Procedure

Visualization of the bladder and urethra may be performed using a flexible (16 F) or rigid (22–26 F) cystoscope. The urethra is pre-lubricated with lidocaine gel and the flexible scope is advanced via the urethral meatus. Irrigation fluid flows through the scope to dilate the urethra and distend the bladder to make visualization possible. Once in the bladder, a detailed inspection is performed; the scope may be advanced in a J fashion against the dome of the bladder to view the bladder neck. Any suspicious or abnormal findings are documented. A small working channel allows limited intervention, such as diathermy ablation or biopsy.

Rigid cystoscopy provides superior images to flexible scopes, owing to its rod-lens construction. It is larger than a flexible scope and cystoscopy is usually performed under anaesthesia. Irrigation with 1.5% glycine allows good visualization and, being non-ionic, permits current to pass during electrosurgical procedures. The scope sheath is wide enough to accept one of many different specialized components which allow specific interventions. Biopsies can be taken, tumours and prostates resected, calculi crushed and ureters accessed for upper tract endoscopy or radiology.

Complications

Complications with flexible cystoscopy are rare, although patients are warned about the risk of urinary tract infection. Rigid cystoscopy runs the risk of bleeding, infection and bladder perforation.

Post-procedure care

Following diagnostic flexible cystoscopy, patients are allowed home once voiding. After a rigid cystoscopy, patients are discharged once roused from anaesthetic although if a significant resection has been performed the bladder will require catheterization and irrigation with saline.

Ureteroscopy

Ureteroscopy is endoscopic examination of the ureter and renal pelvis. It may be performed with a flexible or 'semi-rigid' endoscope.

Indications

Ureteroscopy is performed to visibly diagnose lesions in the upper urinary tract, to obtain tissue biopsy for histological diagnosis or for fragmentation and removal of an impacted

Renal biopsy

Cystourethroscopy

Ureteroscopy

Percutaneous nephrostomy

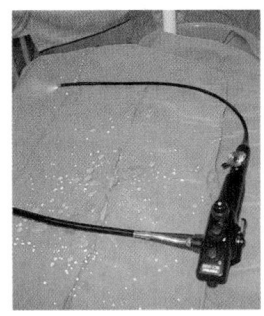

Fig. 11.3 A flexible cystoscope.

ureteric calculus. A stent may be inserted to facilitate renal drainage.

Patient preparation

Ureteroscopy can be performed under general, regional or local anaesthesia. The patient is placed in the lithotomy position, prepared with Betadine and draped. Antibiotics are given on induction (e.g. gentamicin 120 mg i.v.). Radiological screening is required to ensure correct passage of wires and scope.

Procedure

Visualization of the ureters is usually performed via the bladder but may be performed via a percutaneous nephroscope. A cystoscopy is performed prior to ureteroscopy and a 'safety' wire may be passed to the renal pelvis. The ureteroscope is passed transurethrally, into the bladder. A guidewire can be passed through the scope into the ureteric orifice to assist scope passage; the scope is advanced following the wire. High-pressure irrigation distends the ureter to accept the 7 F scope. The rigid scope can reach the renal pelvis but is generally not considered appropriate for major intrarenal procedures.

Flexible ureteroscopes are much smaller and can reach all parts of the renal pelvis. A working channel allows wires or laser fibres to be used. Ureteroscopes may be used for diagnostic procedures to investigate filling defects or stenosis. Lasers are now commonly used to fragment stones or ablate small tumours. A host of baskets exist to allow stone extraction. A ureteric stent may be left in situ to facilitate renal drainage (Fig. 11.4).

Complications

Dysuria is common following ureteroscopy. Patients are warned about the risk of ureteric perforation and the need for a ureteric stent or rarely nephrostomy.

Post-procedure care

For purely diagnostic ureteroscopy, patients are usually allowed home once recovered. If an intervention has been performed, a stent may be left in the ureter and will require removal using a flexible cystoscope at a later date.

Percutaneous nephrostomy

Percutaneous nephrostomy is the insertion of a drainage tube into the collecting system of the kidney, via cutaneous puncture.

Indications

The procedure may be carried out electively to provide access to the collecting system for the treatment of stones (percutaneous nephrolithotomy) or as a diagnostic procedure where it is combined with pressure measurement of the renal pelvis (Whitaker test). More commonly in urology, percutaneous nephrostomy may be performed as an emergency to relieve obstructive renal failure (particularly in the setting of pelvic malignancy) or to drain a pyonephrosis (an obstructed infected renal pelvis).

Patient preparation

Patients require admission to hospital, and informed consent. A clotting screen is performed to exclude a bleeding diathesis. Prophylactic antibiotics are required (e.g. cefuroxime 1.5 g i.v.) prior to nephrostomy.

Procedure

The patient is placed in the prone or prone oblique position on the fluoroscopy table with the arms above the head. A small pillow or foam pad is placed under the flank to be punctured to open the renal angle. The soft tissue space between the 12th rib and the iliac crest is palpated. Using ultrasound, a point for skin puncture is identified from where a lower or mid pole calyx is identified for puncture. Care is taken to ensure that adjacent organs (liver, spleen and colon) are not injured. Under sterile conditions, the skin and deep subcutaneous tissues are infiltrated with local anaesthetic. A 19 G needle is guided into the target calyx using ultrasound. Following successful puncture, a small volume of contrast is injected to outline the collecting system and a guidewire is advanced into the ureter. The sheath of the puncturing needle is then secured within the collecting system. The needle track is dilated and an 8 F pigtail nephrostomy catheter is inserted. A closed drainage system is attached (Fig. 11.5).

Complications

Serious complications are uncommon and include puncture of adjacent organs. A small amount of bleeding is common but usually insignificant. Occasionally, rigors and other manifestations of Gram-negative sepsis occur during manipulation despite prophylactic antibiotics and are presumably due to dissemination of organisms. Late complications include small renal artery aneurysms and arterio-venous fistulae.

Post-procedure care

Hourly blood pressure and heart rate measurement is performed for 4 hours after the procedure to ensure the patient remains haemodynamically stable. Objective improvement of renal function is required (lowered serum creatinine). If external urinary drainage is permanent, patients are required to 'manage' drainage bags. If antegrade stents are planned, this is performed as a staged procedure.

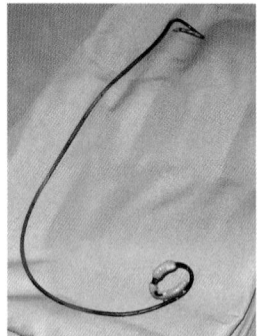

Fig. 11.4 An encrusted ureteric stent.

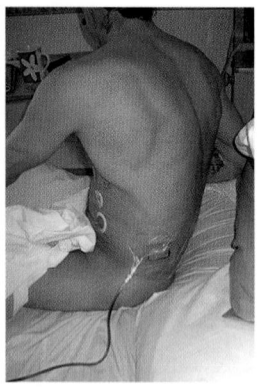

Fig. 11.5 Percutaneous nephrostomy in situ.

Therapeutic procedures

Urethral catheter drainage

Indications
The indications for insertion of a urinary catheter include acute urinary retention and elective monitoring of urine output (renal failure, shock, surgery). Relative contraindications include known urethral strictures and urethral trauma.

Patient preparation
Urethral catheterization is usually performed using topical (lidocaine gel) anaesthesia, and an explanation of the procedure may help relieve any associated anxiety.

Procedure
Sterile precautions are required to minimize the risk of introducing infection. Male patients are positioned supine, and a sterile drape with a small hole to allow the penis through is placed on the groin. The foreskin is retracted and the glans is cleaned with saline. Topical lidocaine gel is instilled directly into the urethra, providing anaesthesia and lubrication. Female patients are positioned in a lithotomy position, and a sterile drape is placed across the genitalia. The labia are gently retracted and the external urethral meatus identified and cleaned with saline.

A 14 G Foley catheter is then removed from its plastic sterile sheeting and introduced into the urethra. The catheter is advanced into the bladder, and (only) when urine is seen to drain, the balloon side arm is filled with 10 mL of saline. The catheter is gently retracted until resistance is felt when the balloon is in contact with the bladder wall, and the drainage lumen attached to a urine collecting bag. Smaller (8–12 F) and larger (28 F) two- and three-way catheters may be required in differing clinical situations.

Complications
Complications are uncommon and include the introduction of urinary infection, haematuria from trauma to the urethra or prostate, and the creation of false passages.

Post-procedure care
It is important to ensure that urine flows freely from the catheter and that any associated haematuria is mild and transient.

 CLINICAL ALERT

If no urine drains, this suggests that the catheter may be blocked, the catheter tip is outside the bladder or there is no urine in the bladder (patient is anuric).

Suprapubic catheter drainage

Suprapubic catheter (SPC) insertion is the insertion of a drainage tube into the bladder via cutaneous puncture over a distended bladder in the lower abdomen.

Indications
The procedure may be carried out electively to defunction the lower urinary tract or as a diagnostic procedure for imaging and pressure studies of the bladder or urethra (antegrade micturating cystourethrography). More commonly, suprapubic catheterization is carried out as an emergency to relieve acute retention of urine where urethral catheterization is unsuccessful or undesirable.

Suprapubic catheterization should not be carried out if urine cannot be aspirated on preliminary puncture with a seeker needle. In the presence of unexplained haematuria or a previous history of bladder cancer, suprapubic catheterization is CONTRAINDICATED!

Patient preparation
The procedure is performed under local anaesthesia using aseptic precautions.

Procedure
The patient is placed supine and the bed tilted head down to bring the lower abdomen horizontal. The bladder is palpated above the pubis, and a mark is made in the midline 2 cm above the pubic symphysis. It is important to remain in the midline to avoid vascular injury. Using an 18 G needle directed vertically, a trial puncture is carried out. If urine is aspirated, the procedure can proceed. Under no circumstances should suprapubic catheterization proceed in the face of inability to aspirate urine at this stage without further assessment. If required, ultrasound may be used to direct the needle towards the bladder.

Under aseptic conditions, the skin and subcutaneous tissues are infiltrated with local anaesthetic. In overweight patients it may be necessary to hold back the 'apron of fat' from the lower abdomen with the flat of the left hand to facilitate the whole procedure. A small stab incision (1 cm) is made through the skin, subcutaneous fat and linea alba. Using an introducer, the bladder is punctured with a trocar directed vertically in the midline (Fig. 11.6). A catheter attached to a drainage bag is advanced through the sheath into the bladder once the trocar has been removed and the retaining balloon is inflated. The catheter is secured with a silk stitch, which may be changed after 10 days (Fig. 11.7).

695

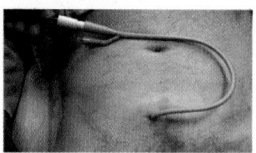

Fig. 11.7 Suprapubic catheter in situ.

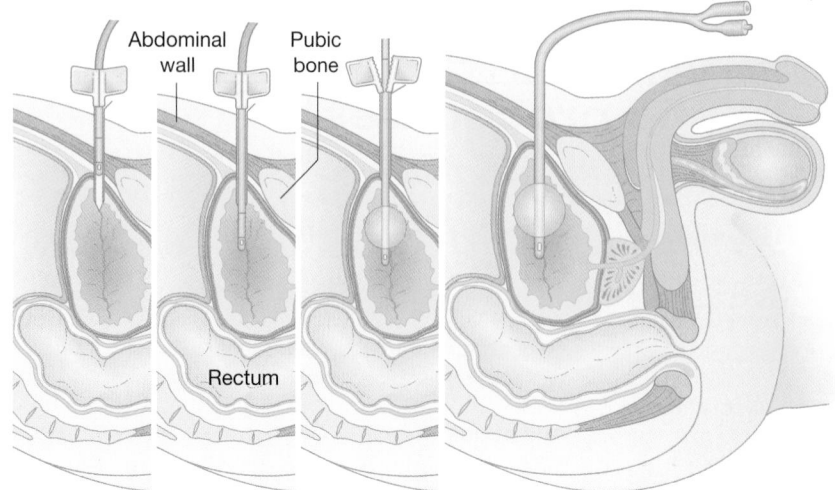

Abdominal wall

Pubic bone

Rectum

Fig. 11.6 Suprapubic catheter insertion.

Complications

Serious complications following suprapubic catheterization are rare. Perforation of a viscus (small bowel, sigmoid colon) and vascular injury (aortic puncture) may occur.

Post-procedure care

After insertion of a suprapubic catheter, patients are kept under observation to ensure good urine drainage and that no bleeding or symptoms of peritonitis (abdominal pain, rigidity) develop.

SECTION 11.5 Manifestations of renal and urinary tract disease

Nephrotic syndrome

Nephrotic syndrome is a manifestation of glomerular disease, defined by proteinuria (>3.5 g per day), hypoalbuminaemia (<30 g/L), generalized oedema and hyperlipidaemia. It is also associated with hypercoagulability, although this is not formally part of the syndrome.

Epidemiology

The incidence of nephrotic syndrome varies depending on the individual underlying pathology (Table 11.6).

Pathology

In the majority of children with nephrotic syndrome, the underlying cause is glomerulonephritis due to minimal change disease. A minority of adults develop nephrotic syndrome as a complication of systemic disease such as diabetes or systemic lupus erythematosus (SLE).

Urinary protein losses lead to hypoalbuminaemia, resulting in lowered plasma oncotic pressure and extravasa-

tion of fluid into the interstitial space. Clinically this is apparent as pitting oedema or anasarca (total body oedema). The liver increases albumin synthesis, but it is often insufficient to compensate for the large urinary protein losses. There are associated increases in plasma clotting factors, fibrinogen and plasma viscosity predisposing to thrombosis. Hyperlipidaemia (most prominently hypercholesterolaemia) results from loss of high-density lipoprotein (HDL) in the urine and increased production of low-density lipoprotein (LDL) and very low-density lipoprotein (VLDL).

Scope of disease

The degree of renal impairment varies according to the underlying disease giving rise to the nephritic syndrome. Acute renal failure is uncommon but can occur as a result of hypovolaemia (especially with rapidly progressive glomerulonephritis). Intravascular thrombosis can occur leading to renal, deep vein, peripheral venous and arterial thromboses. Infection is a common complication, usually presenting as pneumonia or cellulitis. Over time, protein–calorie malnutrition can develop.

Table 11.6	Causes of nephrotic syndrome

Primary glomerular disease
  Minimal change disease (most common cause in children)
  Membranous glomerulonephritis
  Focal segmental glomerulosclerosis

Systemic disease
  Diabetes (most common cause in adults)
  Systemic lupus erythematosus
  Amyloid disease

Drugs
  NSAIDs
  Penicillamine
  Gold (2% of patients receiving gold therapy)

Neoplasm
  Any solid organ tumour
  Leukaemia
  Lymphoma

Infection
  Malaria
  Streptococcal
  Hepatitis B and C
  HIV

Vascular
  Malignant hypertension

Clinical features

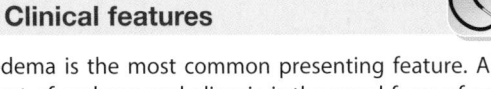

Oedema is the most common presenting feature. Abrupt onset of oedema and oliguria is the usual form of presentation in children, whereas in adults an insidious onset is more common. Patients may notice frothy urine due to proteinuria.

When assessing patients with nephrotic syndrome, it is important to identify the underlying cause. A careful history should screen for offending drugs and associated systemic disease, infection or malignancy. In addition, a careful history should screen for symptoms of potential complications such as infection and deep vein thrombosis.

On examination, the distribution of the oedema may be dependent (localized in the legs and genitalia) or generalized (face and eyelids). Fluid in the abdominal cavity results in ascites.

Initial investigations

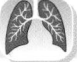

Urinalysis
A dipstick test will be strongly positive for protein. Granular and hyaline casts with occasional erythrocytes are seen on microscopy. A 24-hour collection should then be sent to estimate the creatinine clearance and quantify the 24-hour protein loss.

Serum albumin
The serum albumin levels will be low.

Serum lipid profile
Serum lipids will be elevated, especially cholesterol levels.

Serology
Serological markers are required to screen for the underlying aetiology: ASO titre, autoantibodies, complement, rheumatoid factor, ANCA and anti-GBM antibodies (see p. 146).

Renal ultrasound
Ultrasound is required to confirm that both kidneys are of normal size such that a renal biopsy can be performed.

Further investigations

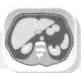

Renal biopsy
Renal biopsy (p. 692) is recommended in adults for histological diagnosis and assessment of prognosis. In children, minimal change disease is assumed and biopsy is not generally performed unless a trial of steroid therapy is unsuccessful.

Initial management

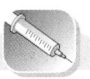

Identify and treat underlying cause
It is important to identify and manage the underlying cause, for example blood sugar control in diabetics.

Nutrition
A low-salt, high-calorie diet is recommended. Low-protein diets are not indicated.

Monitoring
Daily weights and U&Es are performed to monitor fluid losses (aim for 1 kg per day) and to assess changes in serum electrolytes.

Medical management

Diuretics
Oral or intravenous diuretics are administered for symptomatic relief.

Immunomodulation
The treatment of nephrotic syndrome is directed to the underlying cause. Once histological diagnosis has been achieved, oral corticosteroids are usually the first-line therapy for steroid-responsive causes, e.g. minimal change disease. The dose of steroid can be titrated down according to clinical response. Response is measured by reduction in proteinuria and an improvement in serum albumin.

In steroid-resistant causes (e.g. membranous nephropathy), immunosuppression with other agents such as chlorambucil or ciclosporin may be required.

Protective agents such as proton pump inhibitors are administered to patients receiving high doses of steroids as prophylaxis against gastric and duodenal ulceration.

Nephrotic syndrome

Nephritic syndrome

Acute renal failure

Chronic renal failure

697

Anticoagulation

Anticoagulation is indicated whilst the serum albumin is less than 20 g/dL, if the patient is immobile and for all patients with membranous nephropathy. Low molecular weight heparin or warfarin is administered to patients until remission of the disease is achieved.

Prevention of infection

Patients should receive pneumococcal vaccination. In addition, prophylactic penicillin is given to children with relapsing nephrotic syndrome.

Hyperlipidaemia

Patients should receive a statin (HMG CoA reductase inhibitors) while they have features of nephrotic syndrome.

Prognosis

The prognosis is variable and depends on the underlying disease. Even within a disease process such as membranous nephropathy, prognosis can be affected by the degree of proteinuria, HLA type and serum creatinine at presentation.[1] Approximately 15% of patients with membranous glomerulonephritis require dialysis within 5 years. Patients with minimal change disease often experience complete resolution of the disease. Membranoproliferative glomerulonephritis and focal segmental glomerulosclerosis carry a poor prognosis, with up to 50% progressing to renal failure within 10 years.[2] Heavy proteinuria is predictive for the progression to chronic renal failure and dialysis.

REFERENCES

(1) Schieppati A, Mosconi L, Perna A, et al. Prognosis of untreated patients with idiopathic membranous nephropathy. New England Journal of Medicine 1993; 329: 85–89.
(2) Tune BM, Mendoza SA. Treatment of the idiopathic nephrotic syndrome: regimens and outcomes in children and adults. Journal of the American Society of Nephrology 1997; 8: 824–832.

Nephritic syndrome

Nephritic syndrome is characterized by acute onset fluid overload, proteinuria and haematuria.

Epidemiology

Acute nephritic syndrome associated with post-streptococcal glomerulonephritis is most commonly seen in childhood. Acute nephritic syndrome was the presenting complaint of 29.2% of elderly patients with glomerulonephritis in a recent study.[1]

Pathology

The individual pathology depends on the underlying process (see Table 11.7). Some nephritides can cause both nephritic and nephrotic syndrome, e.g. IgA.

Table 11.7	Causes of nephritic syndrome
Common causes	
Post-streptococcal glomerulonephritis	
IgA nephropathy	
Less common causes	
Membranoproliferative glomerulonephritis	
Lupus nephritis	
Crescentic glomerulonephritis	

Clinical features

The proteinuria is not in the nephrotic range but still leads to hypertension and peripheral oedema. Examination demonstrates signs of fluid overload including raised JVP. Haematuria is more likely than with nephrotic syndrome, with the urine appearing brown rather than red.

Initial investigations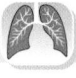

Urinalysis
An active sediment is found, with red blood cells, protein and possibly red cell casts.

Urea and electrolytes
These may be normal or elevated depending on the degree of inflammation.

Serum albumin
The serum albumin level is normal.

Renal ultrasound
Renal ultrasound should show two normal-sized kidneys. In cases of glomerulonephritis, the kidneys may show increased echogenicity.

Serology
A full glomerulonephritis screen should be sent (p. 712).

Further investigations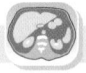

Biopsy
Biopsy may not be indicated if the history gives a clear cause such as post-streptococcal glomerulonephritis. Impaired renal function, failure to resolve or other systemic features are indications for a renal biopsy.

Management

Management of underlying disease
Management is for the underlying disease process. Patients with post-streptococcal disease settle with just supportive treatment. Dialysis is rarely needed.

Prognosis

Prognosis depends on the underlying process. Children with post-streptococcal disease do well whereas patients with crescentic glomerulonephritis are more likely to need ongoing renal support or renal replacement.

REFERENCE

(1) *Prakash J, Singh AK, Saxena RK, Usha. Glomerular diseases in the elderly in India. International Urology and Nephrology 2003; 35: 283–288.*

Acute renal failure

Although there is no exact definition of acute renal failure, it is often regarded as the rapid (hours to days) loss of glomerular function and inability (of the kidney) to excrete nitrogenous waste or maintain fluid electrolyte homeostasis. An almost universal feature is an acute rise in serum urea and creatinine (nitrogenous waste) from baseline, and other definitions have included a 50% drop in premorbid glomerular filtration rate, serum creatinine more than 500 µmol/L and the need for dialysis.

Epidemiology

Due to a lack of standardization of the definition of acute renal failure, it is difficult to determine the epidemiology. Moreover, patients with acute renal failure may exist in the community without referral to a renal unit or hospital.

The overall hospital incidence of acute renal failure has been reported as 21 per 100 000 per year[1]; the incidence increases with age and is equal in both sexes. Acute renal failure accounts for 5% of acute hospital admissions, and develops in up to 10% of patients hospitalized for other conditions.

Pathology

The aetiology of acute renal failure is often divided into pre-renal, renal and post-renal causes (Table 11.8). Intrinsic renal failure is less common than pre-renal or post-renal causes.

Pre-renal acute renal failure develops in a setting of reduced effective extracellular fluid volume, and the most common cause is hypovolaemia due to fluid loss. Once the mean arterial pressure drops below 80 mmHg, there is a corresponding drop in renal blood flow. At this point, autoregulation cannot be sustained and the glomerular filtration rate falls.

Renal or intrinsic renal causes of acute renal failure are due to disease processes affecting the kidney. The most common is acute tubular necrosis from nephrotoxic drugs. Once the onset of acute tubular necrosis has occurred, no current treatment has been shown to reduce the duration of renal failure.

Table 11.8	Causes of acute renal failure
Pre-renal	
Hypovolaemia	
Sepsis	
Cardiogenic	
Haemorrhage	
ACE inhibitors	
Hepatorenal syndrome	
Renal	
Acute tubular necrosis	
Rapidly progressive glomerulonephritis	
Vasculitis	
Nephrotoxic medication	
Radiocontrast	
Multiple other rarer causes	
Post-renal	
Obstruction	
Ureter	
Bladder	
Urethra	

Post-renal acute renal failure is due to obstruction of the flow of urine. The most common cause is back pressure from benign prostatic hypertrophy. Diseases such as urinary calculi may cause more proximal obstruction (of a single ureter), and affect the function of only one kidney.

In practice, the aetiology of acute renal failure is often multifactorial; for example, patients with renovascular disease are at particular risk of loss of perfusion pressure when NSAIDs are administered (Fig. 11.8).

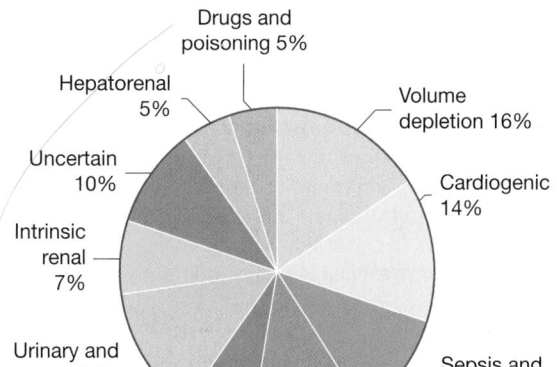

Fig. 11.8 Causes of acute renal failure.

Scope of disease

Life-threatening complications of acute renal failure include hyperkalaemia leading to ventricular arrhythmia and gross fluid overload leading to pulmonary oedema. If the pre-renal acute renal failure is not treated promptly, patients may progress to intrinsic renal failure (acute tubular necrosis).

Clinical features

Many patients are asymptomatic or minimally symptomatic (thirst, frothy urine) and acute renal failure is diagnosed from elevated serum urea and creatinine. In hospital, oliguria (defined as an hourly urine output less than 0.5 mL per kg of body weight) is often the earliest presenting feature of acute renal failure (in patients who are catheterized).

When assessing a patient with acute renal failure, it is important to establish the underlying cause. Dehydration and bleeding as pre-renal causes may be evident from the history. Not all patients respond to dehydration by increased thirst and this mechanism can be lost with age or decreased consciousness. Evaluation of the possibility of periods of prolonged hypotension is important as it predisposes patients to acute tubular necrosis. A history of potential 'third space' fluid losses (bowel obstruction, ileus after gastrointestinal surgery) should also be considered.

A drug history (renal causes) should include the use of NSAIDs (either short- or long-term), known nephrotoxic agents such as contrast medium and over-the-counter preparations and traditional herbal remedies. There may be symptoms of underlying systemic disorders (rash or joint problems) that are associated with renal disease. Past medical history should include any recent procedures or surgery, foreign travel (considering malaria or other infective causes) and any previous renal problems.

In men, symptoms of bladder outflow obstruction (p. 755) may indicate prostatic hypertrophy as an underlying cause. A family history of pelvi-ureteral junction obstruction is relevant.

Examination findings may also give clues to the aetiology of acute renal failure. Estimating the risk of pre-renal causes of acute renal failure is best undertaken by assessment of the patient's fluid status. Patients, especially younger ones, may not develop any signs of fluid loss until about 10% of their circulating volume has been lost, with postural hypotension as the only sign of hypovolaemia. Increasing severity of hypovolaemia is suggested by tachycardia, low JVP, low blood pressure, reduced skin turgor and dry mucous membranes.

Alternatively, a patient with fluid overload may have features such as peripheral oedema, a gallop rhythm, fine crackles in the chest and a history of orthopnoea. Skin changes suggestive of underlying diseases include rash with SLE or livedo reticularis with cholesterol emboli. Vasculitis produces purpuric and nail fold infarcts.

A palpable bladder suggests the presence of at least 500 mL of urine and may account for a post-renal cause for the acute renal failure (p. 701). Obstruction may also be due to pelvic pathology such as ovarian or prostatic carcinoma so a pelvic and rectal examination should also be performed.

Inpatient fluid charts should be scrutinized, noting blood pressure, presence of postural hypotension and urine output. Caution is needed as the charts may not be accurate, and the patient may not be able to give a clear history. If possible, previous serum biochemistry should be found for comparison. The patient may have had blood tests previously either via his or her general practitioner or other hospitals.

Initial investigations

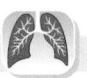

Urea and electrolytes

Both urea and creatinine rise with acute renal failure. Typically the creatinine will rise by 100 μmol per day in patients who are anuric, and this is often accompanied by hyperkalaemia, raised uric acid and hyperphosphataemia.

Biochemical differential diagnoses include gastrointestinal bleeding, corticosteroid use with concomitant systemic infection or volume depletion. However, in these circumstances there is a relatively higher increase in blood urea compared with creatinine. Rhabdomyolysis is a condition that generates creatine so serum creatinine is disproportionately high. Malnourished patients may not generate as much urea due to reduced muscle mass, so their relative rise in urea is less than the creatinine rise in acute renal failure.

Full blood count and blood film

Thrombocytopenia and red cell fragments on the blood film accompany haemolytic uraemic syndrome and thrombotic thrombocytopenic purpura (p. 723). Anaemia is more common with chronic rather than acute renal failure.

Serology

If glomerulonephritis is suspected, a nephritic screen should be sent (p. 712).

Urinalysis

A urine dipstick tests positive for blood in rhabdomyolysis due to the presence of myoglobin. Urinary sediment with minimal levels of blood and protein suggests a pre-renal or post-renal cause. Blood and protein are associated with infection but also glomerular disease, interstitial nephritis or malignancy. Red cell casts accompany glomerular bleeding. Hyaline casts may be benign but can be associated with acute tubular necrosis and most pre- and post-renal causes. Eosinophils in urine occur with acute interstitial nephritis.

Electrocardiogram

Changes associated with hyperkalaemia include tented T waves, widening QRS complexes, and a sine wave pattern. Absence of these findings, however, does not indicate that the serum potassium level is safe.

Chest X-ray

The chest X-ray is a useful screening investigation for pulmonary oedema, infection or malignancy. Acute renal failure can occur in the context of septicaemia, and the presence of metastases may mean that haemodialysis would not be appropriate.

Plain abdominal film

A plain abdominal film (kidneys, ureter and bladder) may reveal an obstructive cause such as radio-opaque renal stones (p. 743).

Renal ultrasound

An ultrasound scan is a highly sensitive test to screen for a post-renal cause. Hydronephrosis is seen clearly with ultrasound, although the exact site of potential obstruction may be unclear. Measurement of renal size can help evaluate the duration of the condition, with small kidneys suggesting a more chronic problem. Increased renal size occurs with glomerulonephritis, amyloid and diabetic kidney disease.

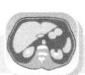

Further investigations

CT scan

CT can be used to identify the exact site of obstruction, or to identify abdominal or retroperitoneal pathology that is not seen on ultrasound (e.g. retroperitoneal fibrosis). Contrast should be avoided if possible.

Renal biopsy

Patients with suspected intrinsic renal disease should undergo a renal biopsy once their condition has been stabilized. Biopsy is only performed in patients with suspected pre-renal or post-renal cause when there is a delayed recovery and an alternate diagnosis needs to be considered.

Initial management

Urinary catheterization

Urinary catheterization immediately resolves obstruction due to benign prostatic hyperplasia and is essential for monitoring of urine output. The residual bladder volume should be noted, and any subsequent input and output documented at hourly intervals. If a catheterized patient develops anuria, the catheter must be flushed to ensure it is not blocked.

Fluid resuscitation

Intravenous fluids are needed to resuscitate patients with hypovolaemia. Colloid or intravenous saline is infused until the normal circulating volume is restored. Ongoing losses are measured, and replacement should include the total daily output plus approximately 1 litre. Adequate fluid resuscitation should ensure a urine output more than 0.5 mL/kg/h and a systolic blood pressure more than 100 mmHg.

Resuscitation should improve urine output and serum biochemistry within a few hours. If improvement is delayed, the patient may need their treatment plan altering.

Later in the disease patients can become polyuric, e.g. when obstruction is relieved. Fluid losses must also be fully replaced as volume depletion at this point could delay renal recovery.

Central venous pressure (CVP) monitoring

Monitoring of central venous pressures with a CVP line allows more accurate assessment of fluid status, especially in patients who lose large volumes into a 'third space' such as the bowel, or in patients with diarrhoea where volume cannot be accurately measured. A CVP of 10–12 mmHg indicates sufficient circulating volume.

Identify and address underlying cause

Where possible, it is important to identify and correct any underlying cause. Any proven nephrotoxic drugs should be stopped. Many other drugs can cause interstitial nephritis so the need for any other medication should be reviewed.

Medical management

Management of fluid status

Patients who are fluid overloaded require restriction of fluid intake (<1 litre/day) and diuretic therapy. The fluid restriction includes all water intake and may seem over-restrictive to the patient. A daily weight loss of 1 kg is ideal.

Intravenous furosemide is administered as extensive oedema may interfere with the absorption of oral diuretics. As the glomerular filtration rate declines, the doses required may be much higher (e.g. 250–500 mg furosemide over 3 hours). Thiazide diuretics such as metolazone or bendrofluazide may improve the diuresis in conjunction with furosemide. Over-diuresis may result in postural hypotension and consequent reduction in renal perfusion.

Management of hyperkalaemia

Patients with hyperkalaemia should receive 10 mL of 10% calcium gluconate intravenously to stabilize the cardiac membranes to reduce the risk of arrhythmias. The effect is short-lived (but can be repeated) and does not affect the serum potassium level.

Hyperkalaemia can be addressed initially with intravenous insulin and dextrose (10 units of Actrapid in 50 mL of 50% glucose). The insulin promotes potassium and glucose influx into cells, whilst the dextrose prevents the development of hypoglycaemia. The effect lasts a few hours, and care must be taken to monitor blood sugars to avoid hypoglycaemia.

A loop diuretic leads to increased potassium excretion, and nebulized salbutamol can also be used to reduce serum potassium levels by promoting entry into the intracellular space. A cation exchange resin such as calcium resonium decreases absorption of potassium from the gastrointestinal tract. It takes 24 hours or more to act, and can be given rectally if oral administration is not possible.

All potassium-retaining drugs and supplements should be discontinued, a low-potassium diet should be instigated and the serum potassium should be checked frequently to ensure the level is improving.

Management of acidaemia

Acidaemia can be corrected initially with intravenous 1.4% of sodium bicarbonate as part of the fluid resuscitation. Sodium bicarbonate lowers serum potassium by driving the potassium into the cells but it should be avoided in fluid overloaded patients as the sodium promotes fluid retention. Lesser acidosis can be corrected with oral bicarbonate, typically 500–600 mg sodium bicarbonate 3 times daily. Haemodialysis corrects the acidosis most effectively but is also more invasive.

Management of hypocalcaemia and hyperphosphataemia

Hyperphosphataemia is treated with phosphate-binding agents (p. 727) and a low-phosphate diet. All drug doses should be altered according to the calculated glomerular filtration rate.

Dopamine

Dopamine was thought to have beneficial effects when infused at a low dose (1–3 µg/min/kg) since it is a renal vasodilator. Whilst dopamine increases urine output in acute renal failure, it does not alter the requirement for dialysis or influence survival.[2] Dopamine is now rarely used in acute renal failure.

Renal replacement therapy

The indications for renal replacement therapy are listed in Table 11.9. Note that the value of the serum creatinine itself is not an indication for renal replacement. The usual mode of renal replacement in the emergency setting is haemodialysis, which can be achieved in a matter of minutes after placing of a femoral dialysis catheter.

If the patient is not haemodynamically stable (low systolic blood pressure) or has multiple problems, he or she may be more appropriately managed on HDU or ICU with continuous venovenous haemofiltration (CVVH) or continuous venovenous haemodialysis (CVVHD). These modes of therapy are less likely to induce cardiac arrhythmias or cardiovascular collapse.

Table 11.9	Indications for dialysis in acute renal failure
Hyperkalaemia not responding to medical treatment	
Fluid overload not responding to medical treatment	
Deteriorating renal function despite active medical management	
Anuria	

Prognosis

The prognosis for recovery from acute renal failure depends on patient age and the cause and degree of renal failure. Survival at 2 years may be as low as 19% in high-risk patients (elderly patients with comorbidity), and is still only 80% in low-risk patients. Creatinine does not always return to baseline in those who recover, and there can be chronic deterioration.

i FURTHER INFORMATION

Thadhani R, Pascual M, Bonventre JV. Acute renal failure. New England Journal of Medicine 1996; 334: 1448–1460.

REFERENCES

(1) *Liano F, Pascual J. Epidemiology of acute renal failure: a prospective, multicenter, community-based study. Madrid Acute Renal Failure Study Group. Kidney International 1996; 50: 811–818.*
(2) *Friedrich JO, Adhikari N, Herridge MS, Beyene J. Meta-analysis: Low-dose dopamine increases urine output but does not prevent renal dysfunction or death. Annals of Internal Medicine 2005; 142: 510–524.*

Chronic renal failure

Chronic renal failure is a persistent and irreversible reduction in overall renal function. It is now divided into five stages, stage 5 being end-stage renal failure (ESRF) and the requirement for renal replacement therapy (Table 11.10).

Epidemiology

Chronic renal failure is becoming more prevalent, and the incidence increases with age. With advances in medical care, more patients now survive serious illnesses such as myocardial infarction or major surgery. These patients now survive with comorbidities, which include chronic renal failure. This has immense implications for future planning of renal services.

Pathology

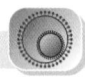

Many conditions causing acute renal failure (Table 11.11) can be controlled but not cured, leaving patients with a steady reduction in glomerular filtration rate despite medical intervention. Chronic renal failure is a multisystem disorder and the effects are summarized in Table 11.12.

Scope of disease

Reduced renal function leads to reduced production of 1,25-dihydroxy-D_3, leading to reduced absorption of calcium from the diet, and stimulating parathyroid hormone (PTH) release. The excessive PTH causes calcium

Table 11.10	Stages of renal failure	
Stage 1	Normal GFR with other evidence of kidney damage	GFR 90 mL/min/1.73m^2
Stage 2	Slight decrease in GFR with other evidence of kidney damage	GFR 60–90 mL/min/1.73m^2
Stage 3	Moderate decrease in GFR with or without evidence of kidney damage	GFR 30–60 mL/min/1.73m^2
Stage 4	Severe decrease in GFR with or without other evidence of kidney damage	GFR 15–30 mL/min/1.73m^2
Stage 5	Established end-stage renal failure	GFR <15mL/min/1.73m^2

Table 11.11	Causes of chronic renal failure
Diabetes	
Hypertension	
Glomerulonephritis	
Pyelonephritis	
Polycystic kidney disease	

Rare causes
  Vasculitis
  Metabolic disorders
  Malignancy
  Hereditary	

and phosphate release from the skeleton and the renal tubules continue to lose calcium into the urine. This leads to a vicious cycle where hypocalcaemia and hyperphosphataemia lead to further overstimulation of the parathyroid glands.

As the glomerular filtration rate drops, the kidney does not produce sufficient erythropoietin, resulting in anaemia, and with disease progression the kidney is unable to maintain acid–base homeostasis.

Malnutrition is common and cardiovascular risk is much higher in patients with chronic renal failure. Approximately 50% will die from a cardiovascular event. Reduced excretion of uric acid and high doses of diuretics predispose to the development of gout.

Women with chronic renal failure ovulate erratically and many stop menstruating. The conception rate is low, with poor pregnancy outcomes and high rates of fetal loss. Young women with mild renal impairment may have to decide to have their children earlier than anticipated (before further decline in glomerular filtration rate) or wait until they have had a renal transplant.

Psychological problems are common in patients with chronic renal failure. They are often tired and may be unable to continue their normal level of activity. Employment levels are low and financial difficulties are common.

Clinical features

As patients experience a decline in their renal function, they develop a wide range of symptoms (Table 11.12). The common presenting features are problems with fluid balance and non-specific symptoms such as tiredness or poor appetite. Renal failure may be found incidentally such

Table 11.12	Clinical features of chronic renal failure	
Location	**Effect of disease**	**Clinical features**
Blood	Reduction in erythropoietin	Anaemia
	Impaired platelet function	Bruising
Cardiovascular	Fluid overload	Pulmonary oedema
	Deposition of urate in the pericardium	Uraemic pericarditis
	Calcium deposition in blood vessels	Accelerated atherosclerosis
Bones	Hyperparathyroidism	Renal osteodystrophy, subperiosteal bone resorption, bone cysts
Nervous	Unknown	Restless legs
	Unknown	Peripheral neuropathy (sensory)
	Accelerated atherosclerosis	Erectile dysfunction
Muscle	Electrolyte imbalance	Cramps
Nails	Unknown	Half white and half brown nails
Skin	Phosphate accumulation	Pruritus
	Pseudoporphyria/bullous drug reactions	High-dose diuretic
	Unknown	Dry skin

703

as when investigating patients for hypertension or anaemia.

Initial investigations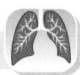

Urea and electrolytes

Serial U&Es allow the physicians to track any decline in renal function. 24-hour urine collections for protein and creatinine clearance also help with monitoring disease progression.

Renal ultrasound

Renal ultrasound will identify the number and size of the kidneys. If patients present with two small kidneys there is rarely any benefit from a kidney biopsy as the disease process will not be reversible.

Initial management

Multidisciplinary management

Addressing the problems associated with chronic renal failure necessitates a multidisciplinary approach. Patients may present at any stage of chronic renal failure. Early referral to a renal unit is preferable, as patients who are referred late tend to have a poorer prognosis.

Patient education

There is quite a lot of information that needs to be imparted to patients with chronic renal failure: the natural history of the disease and information with regards to renal replacement therapy. Compliance with medication is a common problem as patients may be taking 30 or more tablets per day.

Fluid balance

Not all patients have fluid overload, but many have reduced excretory capacity and require fluid restriction to 1.5 litres per day. This restriction includes water in any form. In some patients, a 2–3 kg increase over their 'dry' weight is sufficient to cause dyspnoea, particularly if there is anaemia or cardio-respiratory comorbidity.

Renal diet

Chronic renal failure patients need to follow a limiting diet to control serum phosphate or potassium. Phosphate is present in milk, cheese, yoghurt, bony fish and shellfish. Potassium is high in fresh fruit (especially bananas and strawberries), nuts, chocolate, red wine, crisps and chips, and vegetables. Avoidance of all of the above can make it difficult to have an adequate intake of calories. Chronic renal failure is associated with changes in taste perception, exacerbated by the acidosis. The role of dietitians is vital in chronic renal failure, both for education and the avoidance of malnutrition.

Medical management

Patients with stage 1 or 2 renal failure rarely progress to need renal replacement, but will need measures to prevent or slow any decline in GFR. Treatment of hypertension and anaemia can delay the need for renal replacement therapies.

Management of renal bone disease

Treatment of renal bone disease (Fig. 11.9) starts with low-phosphate diets and phosphate binders, taken before meals to reduce dietary phosphate absorption. Calcium and aluminium based phosphate binders are associated with hypercalcaemia and dementia respectively. Newer phosphate binders (e.g. Renagel) are effective and have a better side effect profile but are expensive. In general, phosphate control is often difficult because of poor compliance due to the side effects (gastrointestinal upset) and the chronicity of treatment.

Alfacalcidol, a synthetic vitamin D, is administered to suppress parathyroid hormone production. This is taken daily or at 'pulsed' weekly intervals. As alfacalcidol increases both phosphate and calcium, good phosphate control should precede its use. Parathyroidectomy may be necessary if hyperparathyroid bone disease cannot be controlled medically.

Management of renal anaemia

As oral iron is not well absorbed, intravenous iron is the initial treatment of choice for patients with renal anaemia. Multiple sequential doses of 100–200 mg are administered until iron stores are replete. If patients remain anaemic, erythropoietin is started.

Erythropoietin (EPO), now available as a recombinant protein, has dramatically cut the number of blood transfusions used in patients with chronic renal failure. Erythropoietin is given intravenously or subcutaneously, 1–3 times weekly (newer preparations with longer half-lives are given every 2–4 weeks). Erythropoietin is costly and side effects include hypertension. Resistance can develop and is more common in patients with hyperparathyroidism, poor dialysis adequacy, aluminium toxicity, infection and with drugs causing marrow suppression.

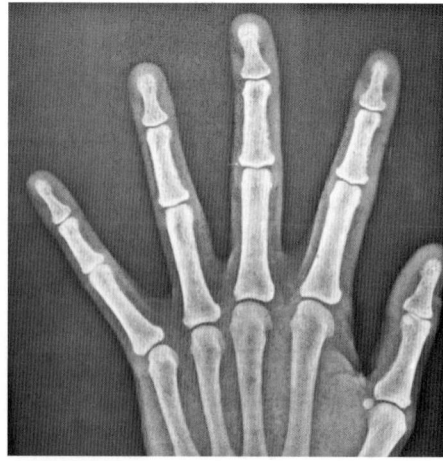

Fig. 11.9 Renal osteodystrophy. The translucent appearance of the bone is due to bone resorption with renal failure.

Recently pure red cell aplasia (PRCA)[2] has been identified as an unfortunate response to subcutaneous EPO, resulting in severe resistance to EPO and hence profound anaemia. The use of intravenous EPO is associated with a lower risk of PRCA. PRCA is very rare—only a few cases worldwide—but has implications for future anaemia treatment.

Management of cardiovascular disease

Hypertension is primarily related to chronic fluid overload, and patients often require multiple antihypertensive agents. Good hypertension control is associated with a slower decline in glomerular filtration rate[3] and ACE inhibitors are a safe option (except in patients with renal artery stenosis) provided that serum creatinine is monitored.

Statins (HMG CoA reductase inhibitors) are recommended to lower the risk of coronary disease, although it is controversial whether the development of atherosclerosis is modifiable by statin therapy, as atherosclerosis associated with renal impairment is partly related to the calcium deposition.

Management of acidosis

Correction of the acidosis improves nutritional status and reduces bone loss. Oral sodium bicarbonate (500–600 mg tds) is often administered for this purpose in patients who do not require dialysis. Concomitant diuretics are often required as the sodium load from sodium bicarbonate can exacerbate fluid retention and worsen hypertension. Once dialysis has started sodium bicarbonate should no longer be required.

Management of gout

Allopurinol 100–300 mg daily (depending on glomerular filtration rate) is used as prophylaxis for gout. NSAIDs should be avoided in treating acute episodes of gout as they could worsen renal failure.

Management of cramps

Chronic renal failure, an elderly population and high doses of diuretics make cramps a frequent problem. Quinine sulphate (300 mg) and reducing the dose of diuretics (if possible) may help.

Management of restless legs

Patients with chronic renal failure may experience 'restless legs' where the lower limbs are twitchy and restless, making sleep difficult. Clonazepam (0.5–1 mg) at night can help. Clonazepam addiction is uncommon but tolerance may develop.

Prognosis

The prognosis depends on the stage of the renal failure and the underlying condition. Many elderly patients with stage 2 or 3 renal failure never progress to needing renal replacement due to other comorbidities causing their demise. Sometimes, despite good control of hypertension and anaemia, patients progress rapidly through to stage 5 and need to start on renal replacement therapies. An increasing amount of nephrology practice consists of the outpatient care of patients with chronic renal failure and multiple other medical problems.

REFERENCES

(1) *Ansell D, Feest T, Byrne C (eds). Renal Registry Report 2002. Bristol: UK Renal Registry, 2002.*
(2) *Casadevall N, Nataf J, Viron B, et al. Pure red-cell aplasia and antierythropoetin antibodies in patients treated with recombinant erythropoetin. New England Journal of Medicine 2002; 346: 469–475.*
(3) *Collins AJ. Cardiovascular mortality in end-stage renal disease. American Journal of Medical Science 2003; 325: 163–167.*

SECTION 11.6

Congenital and genetic abnormalities of the kidney

Autosomal dominant polycystic kidney disease

The most common hereditary cause of chronic renal failure is autosomal dominant polycystic renal disease (Fig. 11.10).

Epidemiology

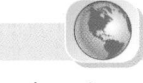

The prevalence of autosomal dominant polycystic renal disease is 100 per 100 000 and accounts for 8.9% of patients under 65 starting on renal replacement therapy.[1]

Pathology

Autosomal dominant polycystic renal disease has 100% penetrance but variable expression. It does not skip generations. Currently, two genes have been identified: the *PKD1* gene is located on chromosome 16 and accounts for up to 90% of cases; the *PKD2* gene is located on chromosome 4, accounting for 10–15%. The genes encode for the polycystin 1 and 2 proteins that are present in many tissues other than the kidney. Cysts arise in any part of the kidney, in contrast to the autosomal recessive version (p. 707) where cysts only arise from the distal tubule and collecting ducts.

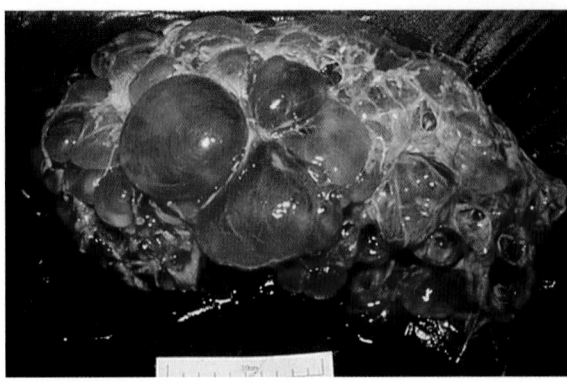

Fig. 11.10 Polycystic kidney disease.

Scope of disease

There is no increased risk of neoplasia within polycystic kidneys, but there is a higher incidence of berry aneurysms with 10% of families having a positive history for subarachnoid haemorrhage. Patients with autosomal dominant polycystic kidney disease are more likely to develop mitral valve prolapse, inguinal hernias, and aneurysms in their vertebral and coronary vessels.

Clinical features

As genetic methods are used to diagnose the disease, it is now known that many people remain disease free despite having the gene. Symptomatic patients with polycystic renal disease may present with hypertension, loin pain, recurrent urinary infections or haematuria. Pain or gross haematuria can occur from bleeding into a cyst. Infections can be recurrent and resistant to standard antibiotics. Initially the kidneys are normal in size but can grow up to 5 kg or more. The enlargement of the kidneys is also associated with flank pain, a feeling of 'fullness' and chronic abdominal discomfort. Hypertension usually accompanies the cystic changes and becomes more common as the renal size increases. On examination, the polycystic kidneys may be palpable in the flanks.

Initial investigations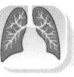

Urea and electrolytes

The urea and creatinine is normal early in the disease and rises as the disease progresses and more renal parenchyma is lost.

Full blood count

Haemoglobin levels may be normal as erythropoietin production is relatively spared compared with other patients with similarly impaired renal function.

Ultrasound of the abdomen

Ultrasound will confirm cystic lesions in the kidney. Strict age-related diagnostic criteria regarding the number of

cysts are used as benign simple cysts can develop in the normal population. The cysts are bilateral and distributed throughout the structures of the kidney. Over time, cyst expansion and the onset of interstitial fibrosis lead to massive kidney enlargement. Liver cysts may also be present but these do not usually lead to liver dysfunction. Pancreatic cysts are present in 10%.

CT of the abdomen

Occasionally, CT of the abdomen may be required to diagnose polycystic kidney disease (Fig. 11.11) or screen for other concomitant pathology.

Further investigations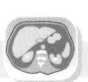

Cerebral angiography

If there is clinical suspicion of an expanding aneurysm, angiography should be performed. Patients with a strong family history of aneurysm rupture are associated with particular genetic mutations and are at higher risk of subarachnoid haemorrhage. Routine screening for berry aneurysms in asymptomatic patients is not required.

Genetic testing

Genetic testing by linkage or mutational analysis confirms the diagnosis, especially where the radiological features are equivocal.

Family screening

Once a patient is identified as having autosomal dominant polycystic renal disease, ultrasound screening should be offered to other family members, along with genetic counselling. Antenatal testing is not usually performed in view of the late onset of symptomatic disease.

Initial management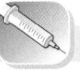

At present, there is no specific treatment for the gene defect or for slowing disease progression. Treatment is directed to that of associated complications.

Analgesia

Chronic pain in the flanks is hard to treat and can lead to dependence on opiate analgesia.

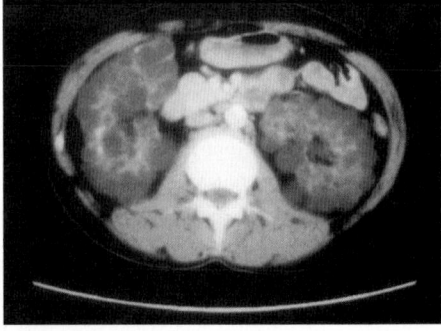

Fig. 11.11 CT of polycystic kidney disease.

Urinary tract infection

Prolonged courses of antibiotics may be required to treat urinary tract infection as the antibiotics may have difficulty penetrating the cyst wall.

Medical management

Aspiration of cysts

Individual cysts are rarely punctured as therapy, although very large painful cysts can be drained under ultrasound guidance.

Renal replacement therapy

Renal failure progresses more quickly in males, patients with PKD1 and those presenting before the age of 30 years. PKD2 patients develop end-stage renal failure about 15 years later than PKD1 patients. Overall, patients cope well with dialysis.

Surgical management

Renal transplantation

Patients with end-stage renal disease are suitable candidates for transplantation. Occasionally the native kidneys are removed prior to the patient being accepted on a transplant waiting list to make sufficient room for the subsequent transplant.

Prognosis

Poor hypertension control is associated with a faster decline in renal function (glomerular filtration rate). Renal impairment usually develops in adulthood and up to 50% of patients will need renal replacement therapy by the age of 70.

REFERENCE

(1) Ansell D, Feest T, Byrne C. *The Renal Registry Fifth Annual Report 2002.* Bristol: UK Renal Registry, 2002.

Autosomal recessive polycystic kidney disease

The incidence of autosomal recessive polycystic kidney disease is estimated to be 1 in 20 000 live births. The disease is due to a gene located on chromosome 6. In its most extreme form, cystic disease is associated with pulmonary hypoplasia and the infant soon dies from respiratory problems. Less severe forms are compatible with life, but these children develop hypertension and renal failure. Renal replacement may not be required until adolescence. Autosomal recessive polycystic kidney disease may present in later childhood, often with portal hypertension and

hepatomegaly. The outlook for neonates is poor, with perinatal mortality of up to 50%. Once the infant has survived the first few months, the prognosis is better and patients cope well with renal replacement or renal transplantation. Children found to have autosomal recessive polycystic kidney disease are treated for both renal and liver dysfunction, and may benefit from combined renal and hepatic transplantation.

Alport syndrome

Epidemiology

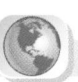

Alport syndrome is a rare inherited disorder of type IV collagen.

Pathology

The inheritance can be either X-linked or autosomal recessive, with over 200 identified genetic mutations on chromosome 2. Abnormalities of type IV collagen result in the formation of thickened layers of glomerular basement membrane, usually associated with progressive renal disease. X-linked Alport is the more common mode of inheritance and renal replacement is eventually required for affected men; women are usually mildly affected and may develop symptoms at a later age. Deafness is always accompanied by renal disease and develops in 50%. Hearing is usually normal in childhood. Other potential abnormalities include anterior lenticonus and leiomyomatosis in the oesophagus and genitals.

Clinical features

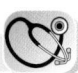

Patients usually present with macroscopic or microscopic haematuria. The glomerular damage is progressive, with associated hypertension and proteinuria and declining renal function.

Investigations

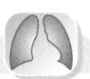

The clinical picture, renal biopsy and genetic testing make the diagnosis.

Renal biopsy

Renal biopsy may be used to confirm the diagnosis, but with a positive family history renal biopsy is not necessarily indicated.

Genetic testing

DNA analysis can be used for carrier detection and prenatal diagnosis.

Ultrasound of the kidneys

The presence of haematuria necessitates ultrasound screening of the renal tract to exclude other structural lesions.

Management

Blood pressure control

Treatment in general is supportive, with control of blood pressure to minimize disease progression.

Renal replacement therapy

Patients with established renal failure will require dialysis.

Renal transplantation

Patients with end-stage renal disease due to Alport syndrome can be considered for transplantation. Anti-GBM nephritis (p. 711) due to an immunological response to the type IV collagen can occur in the transplanted kidney, but this is rare (less than 5%).

Prognosis

Of the patients with X-linked Alport's syndrome, evidence of glomerular disease will exist in 98%, and 99% have haematuria. End-stage renal failure develops in 76%, and 54% eventually require transplantation.[1]

i FURTHER INFORMATION

Pescucci C, Longo I, Bruttini M, et al. Type-IV collagen related diseases. Journal of Nephrology 2003; 16: 314–316.

REFERENCE

(1) *Jais JP, Knebelmann B, Giatras I, et al. X-linked Alport syndrome: natural history in 195 families and genotype-phenotype correlations in males. Journal of the American Society of Nephrology 2000; 11: 649–657.*

Tuberous sclerosis

Epidemiology

Tuberous sclerosis is an autosomal dominant condition, with a prevalence of 10 per 100 000.

Pathology

Tuberous sclerosis is associated with renal tumours, skin disease, epilepsy, learning difficulties, cardiac and brain tumours, and results from a *TSC1* or *TSC2* gene mutation. The *TSC1* gene (hamartin gene) is located on chromosome 9, and the *TSC2* gene (tuberin gene) is located on chromosome 16. Spontaneous mutations account for over half of cases, so a positive family history is not essential.

Renal angiomyolipomas are benign tumours of the kidney, invading only local structures, without distant metastases. They are not exclusive to tuberous sclerosis, but multiple angiomyolipomas strongly suggest the diagnosis. They can cause haemorrhage, and lead to hypertension and renal impairment by distortion of the renal architecture. Renal carcinomas are more frequent with tuberous sclerosis. They can be bilateral and present early (under the age of 30) with a poor prognosis due to early metastases. Cystic disease leading to renal failure is rare unless associated with contiguous deletion of *PKD1* in TSC2 patients.

Clinical features

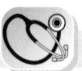

Patients present with skin (white skin patches, facial fibroangiomatous rash, skin fibromatous plaques) and neurological problems (seizures), but most also have renal involvement.

Investigations

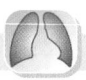

Ultrasound of the abdomen

Renal cysts are commonly seen on ultrasound or CT scanning. Without the other features of tuberous sclerosis, the condition may be mistaken for autosomal dominant polycystic kidney disease.

Management

Patient education

Patients need to be informed about the diagnosis and complications associated with tuberous sclerosis. Management of this condition is largely supportive.

Regular surveillance

Annual ultrasound or CT scanning is usually performed as surveillance for renal tumours. Pregnancy is associated with rapid growth of the angiomyolipomas and close supervision is needed.

Nephrectomy

Surgery is only indicated for renal carcinoma or in cases of uncontrollable bleeding.

Prognosis

Most people with tuberous sclerosis have a normal life expectancy. Regular surveillance is required for brain and kidney tumours.

i FURTHER INFORMATION

Sampson JR, Maheshwar MM, Aspinwall R, et al. Renal cystic disease in tuberous sclerosis: role of the polycystic kidney disease 1 gene. American Journal of Human Genetics 1997; 61: 843–851.

Nail–patella syndrome

Nail–patella syndrome is a rare autosomal dominant disease due to a gene on chromosome 9 that encodes a transcription factor LMX1B. The clinical features include abnormalities of the nails (absent, hypoplastic, dystrophic, ridged, pitted, discoloured or separated), patellae (small, irregularly shaped or absent), other bones (elbow abnormalities, talipes, and iliac horns on X-ray) and kidneys (haematuria to progressive glomerulopathy and end-stage renal disease), and glaucoma. The diagnosis can be confirmed with electron microscopy of the renal biopsy showing specific changes in the glomerular basement membrane. Treatment is supportive and the condition does not recur in renal transplants.

 FURTHER INFORMATION

Sweeney E, Fryer A, Mountford R, Green A, McIntosh I. Nail patella syndrome: a review of the phenotype aided by developmental biology. Journal of Medical Genetics 2003; 40: 153–162.

Von Hippel–Lindau disease

Von Hippel–Lindau disease is an autosomal dominant disorder associated with retinal haemangiomas, cerebellar haemangioblastoma, renal carcinoma, and cysts of the kidney, liver, pancreas and epididymis. The prevalence is 2–3 per 100 000 and spontaneous mutations are rare. Patients commonly have renal cysts but these seldom lead to renal failure. Incidental multiple bilateral renal clear cell carcinomas may be detected on screening, rather than with the usual symptoms of haematuria or pain. These tumours tend to occur in patients under the age of 40. Renal preservation surgery is often advocated.

Membranous glomerulonephritis

Focal segmental glomerulosclerosis

IgA nephropathy

Membranoproliferative glomerulonephritis

Minimal change disease

Post-streptococcal glomerulonephritis

Rapidly progressive glomerulonephritis

SECTION 11.7   Glomerular diseases

Glomerulonephritis is inflammation of the glomeruli. Disorders of glomerular structure and function occur with many systemic diseases, and are termed secondary glomerulonephritis. When the renal glomerulus is the sole or predominant cause, the disease process is termed primary glomerulonephritis.

Due to lack of international acceptance, the classification of glomerular diseases is not standardized. Clinical classifications concentrate on the presentation of the disease (nephrotic or nephritic syndrome) and response to treatment (steroid responsive, non-steroid responsive), whilst pathological classifications concentrate on a combination of aetiology (post-streptococcal) and histological findings on renal biopsy (minimal change disease, membranous glomerulonephritis).

Histological findings are important for the classification for glomerular disease, as it is often predictive of the clinical course, response to treatment and prognosis. Based on microscopy, the disease process can be focal (affecting some glomeruli), diffuse (affecting all glomeruli) or segmental (affecting only part of the glomerulus). In addition, cellular proliferation, basement membrane changes and the presence of sclerosis are useful features to classify the appearance of glomerular diseases (Table 11.13).

An immune pathogenesis is common to many of the glomerular diseases. Glomerular damage results from antibody-mediated damage (IgA nephropathy), cell-mediated injury and complement.

 FURTHER INFORMATION

Couser WG. Glomerulonephritis. Lancet 1999; 353: 1509–1515.

Table 11.13	Aetiology of glomerulonephritis
Primary glomerulonephritis	
Minimal change glomerulonephritis	
Focal segmental glomerulosclerosis	
Membranous nephropathy	
IgA nephropathy	

Rapidly progressive glomerulonephritis
    Anti-glomerular basement membrane disease
    Pauci-immune glomerulonephritis	

Post-streptococcal	
Membranoproliferative	
Secondary glomerulonephritis	
Lupus nephritis	

709

Membranous glomerulonephritis

Membranous glomerulonephritis is synonymous with epi-membranous and extra-membranous glomerulonephritis.

Epidemiology

Approximately 25% of glomerulonephritis in adults is due to membranous glomerulopathy. It is uncommon before the age of 30 years.

Pathology

Approximately 80% of membranous glomerulonephritis is idiopathic. The rest is caused by systemic disease, drugs, infection and malignancy (Table 11.14). The characteristic feature of membranous glomerulonephritis is diffuse thickening of the walls of the capillary loop due to electron-dense deposits. Characteristic spikes of basement membrane are seen on light and electron microscopy.

Clinical features

The majority of patients present with nephrotic syndrome or the associated complications of nephrotic syndrome such as infection and thrombosis (p. 696). Less commonly patients may also present with asymptomatic proteinuria (frothy urine) or haematuria. On examination, hypertension may be evident. In elderly patients, it is important to screen for clinical features of malignancy.

Investigations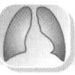

Urea and electrolytes
Serum creatinine may be elevated.

Table 11.14	Causes of membranous glomerulonephritis

Malignancy
  Lung
  Colon
  Breast
  Stomach
  Prostate
  Ovarian
  Lymphoproliferative disorders	

Infection
  Malaria
  Hepatitis B	

Drugs
  Gold
  NSAIDs
  Captopril
  Penicillamine	

Systemic disease
  Diabetes mellitus
  Systemic lupus erythematosus
  Sarcoid	

Urinalysis
Dipstick testing may be positive for blood and protein. A 24-hour urine collection is required to quantify the severity of proteinuria.

Renal biopsy
A renal biopsy is usually performed to establish the diagnosis.

Screening for malignancy
Screening for underlying malignancy is important in elderly patients and includes a chest film, gastroscopy and blood film. Clinical features of malignancy may not present for up to 2 years after the onset of membranous nephropathy.

Management

Identify and address any precipitating cause
Correcting any underlying cause (such as infection or cancer) may lead to resolution of the glomerulonephritis.

Anticoagulation
Anticoagulation with warfarin or heparin is required until remission occurs as patients are at a high risk of venous thrombosis.

Immunomodulation
Membranous nephropathy may respond to prolonged high doses of steroids. Other immunosuppressants such as ciclosporin, chlorambucil or cyclophosphamide might help to induce remission.

Prognosis

Up to 25% of patients develop a spontaneous remission. At 10 years, about 25% of patients with idiopathic membranous glomerulonephritis will have progressed to end-stage renal failure, and 25% will either be receiving dialysis or will have died.[1]

REFERENCE

(1) Honkanen E, Tornroth T, Gronhagen-Riska C, Sankila R. Long-term survival in idiopathic membranous glomerulonephritis: can the course be clinically predicted? Clinical Nephrology 1994; 41: 127–134.

Focal segmental glomerulosclerosis

Focal segmental glomerulosclerosis is synonymous with focal sclerosing glomerulonephropathy.

Epidemiology

Focal segmental glomerulosclerosis (FSGS) is an increasing cause of nephrotic syndrome in adults and accounts for about 3.3% of patients starting on renal replacement in the USA.[1]

Pathology

The causes of focal segmental glomerulosclerosis are primary or secondary (Table 11.15). The histological appearance is capillary collapse and replacement with collagen and mesangial matrix (sclerosis) that occurs in segments (segmental) of some glomeruli (focal).

Clinical features

Patients with glomerulonephritis due to FSGS tend to present with nephrotic syndrome (p. 697). Patients may have haematuria and hypertension.

Investigations

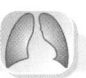

Serology
A serological screen is obtained to identify any underlying condition.

Renal ultrasound
The kidneys are usually normal in size.

Renal biopsy
The diagnosis can be confirmed by renal biopsy, but there is a risk of false negative biopsy results due to the focal nature of the disease.

Management

There is no specific treatment for focal segmental glomerulosclerosis; immunomodulation is the main approach. The management of nephrotic syndrome is detailed on page 697–698.

Immunomodulation
Approximately 30% of patients respond to steroids, and 25% achieve remission whilst taking ciclosporin (relapse is common as soon as it is discontinued) or alkylating agents. Ciclosporin is nephrotoxic and requires careful monitoring of levels, especially with chronic use.

Prognosis

Focal segmental glomerulosclerosis tends to be progressive, with approximately half of patients reaching end-stage renal failure by 10 years. Focal and segmental glomerulosclerosis can quickly recur in patients receiving renal transplants.

REFERENCE

(1) Kitiyakara C, Kopp JB, Eggers P. *Trends in the epidemiology of focal segmental glomerulosclerosis. Seminars in Nephrology* 2003; 23: 172–182.

IgA nephropathy

IgA nephropathy is synonymous with Berger's disease.

Epidemiology

IgA nephropathy is a common cause of glomerulonephritis, found in up to 40% of renal biopsies. It is usually sporadic but can be familial.

Pathology

The pathogenesis is abnormal circulating IgA that is deposited in renal mesangium, but the aetiology is unknown. The renal tissue itself is normal, but granular IgA deposition leads to diffuse mesangial cell proliferation. Other known conditions that can lead to mesangial deposition include Henoch–Schönlein purpura and alcoholic liver disease. IgA nephropathy is associated with immune-mediated disorders such as rheumatoid arthritis, coeliac disease and inflammatory bowel disease.

Clinical features

Patients often present with macroscopic or microscopic haematuria. Increasing urine screening in the general population is revealing more cases of suspected IgA nephropathy. Patients with isolated haematuria without proteinuria should be investigated for other causes (p. 684). Later presentation is with proteinuria, hypertension and impaired renal function.

Investigations

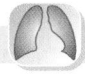

Urinalysis
Urine dipstick testing is positive for blood and protein. A 24-hour collection is required to quantify the amount of proteinuria. Proteinuria of nephrotic syndrome severity is rare (less than 10%).

Serology
Serology is performed to screen for other underlying causes for the glomerulonephritis, and includes ASO titre, ANCA, anti-GBM antibodies, autoantibodies, rheumatoid factor and complement levels.

Table 11.15	Causes of focal segmental glomerulosclerosis
Primary	
Secondary	
Reflux nephropathy	
Analgesic nephropathy	
HIV	
Heroin use	
Obesity	
Sickle cell disease	

Renal ultrasound

Renal ultrasound screens for the presence of two kidneys, is able to estimate the size (assessment of chronicity associated with small kidneys), and is able to exclude causes for haematuria such as tumours.

Renal biopsy

A renal biopsy is indicated for patients with an elevated serum creatinine and/or proteinuria >1 g/24 hours.

Management

Supportive management and monitoring

There are no proven strategies for reducing the production of the abnormal IgA, and no treatment has been shown to alter the progression of chronic IgA nephropathy. Management is largely supportive with good blood pressure control. Mild cases may be monitored as outpatients with clinical assessment, U&Es and 24-hour urine collections. A renal biopsy should be performed if the serum creatinine rises, or if there is more than 1–2 g of proteinuria in 24 hours.

Control of hypertension

Good control of hypertension may slow the progression of renal disease; the drug of choice is an ACE inhibitor.

Immunomodulation

On the rare occasions when IgA is associated with a crescentic glomerulonephritis and rapid decline in renal function, immunosuppression may be attempted to preserve renal function. Plasma exchange, prednisolone (30–60 mg/day), ciclosporin, azathioprine and cyclophosphamide have each been used without any conclusive evidence of benefit.[1]

Prognosis

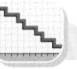

The majority of patients have a good prognosis, but disease progression is very variable ranging from a mild benign disorder to aggressive glomerulonephritis and requirement for dialysis within months.

REFERENCE

(1) *Goumenos DS, Davlouros P, El Nahas AM, Ahuja M, Shortland JR, Vlachojannis JG, Brown CB. Prednisolone and azathioprine in IgA nephropathy—a ten-year follow-up study. Nephron Clinical Practice 2003; 93: C58–68.*

Membranoproliferative glomerulonephritis

Membranoproliferative glomerulonephritis (MPGN) is synonymous with mesangiocapillary glomerulonephritis (MCGN).

Epidemiology

Membranoproliferative glomerulonephritis is increasingly uncommon in the West. It can present in childhood, or later as part of a chronic immune complex disorder.

Pathology

There are two types of membranoproliferative glomerulonephritis. The histological appearance of type I disease is characterized by splitting of the basement membrane, and the causes are classified as primary or secondary (Table 11.16). Type II disease seems to be a distinct entity with long segments of staining deposits (dense deposit disease). Although the cause of type II disease is unknown (idiopathic), it is associated with low plasma C_3, circulating C_3 nephritic factor and partial lipodystrophy.

Clinical features

Patients may present with nephrotic syndrome (with haematuria, hypertension and renal impairment), nephritic syndrome or acute renal failure.

Investigations

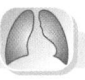

Urinalysis

Protein and blood is usually detected on dipstick testing of the urine. A 24-hour urine collection is required to estimate proteinuria and calculate the glomerular filtration rate.

Serology

Complement levels are low, and C_3 nephritic factor is present.

Renal biopsy

Renal biopsy will confirm the diagnosis.

Management

Supportive treatment

Patients with mild proteinuria and normal renal function do not require treatment apart from control of blood pressure.

Table 11.16	Causes of membranoproliferative glomerulonephritis
Idiopathic (primary)	
Secondary	Cryoglobulins
	Systemic lupus erythematosus
	Hepatitis B and C
	Sickle cell disease
	Chronic lymphocytic leukaemia
	Malignancy

Immunomodulation

Patients with nephrotic syndrome or impaired glomerular filtration rate receive prednisolone and antiplatelet agents although there is limited evidence for these.

Prognosis

In general, the prognosis is poor. Approximately 50% are in end-stage renal failure requiring dialysis or dead by 5 years. Membranoproliferative glomerulonephritis may recur in patients receiving renal transplant.

Minimal change disease

Minimal change disease is synonymous with lipoid nephrosis.

Epidemiology

Minimal change disease is the most common cause of glomerulonephritis in children, and accounts for up to one third of adult cases.

Pathology

The cause of minimal change disease is unknown. It is thought to be caused by antibody-mediated injury in genetically susceptible individuals in view of the association with atopy, HLA DR3 in Europe and DR8 in Japan. Light microscopy and immunological investigations are normal. The only significant change on electron microscopy is fusion (effacement) of the foot processes (podocytes).

Clinical features

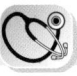

Patients almost always present with nephrotic syndrome (p. 697); there is no hypertension and renal function is usually normal. Patients may also present with complications of nephrotic syndrome such as infection and thrombosis.

Investigations

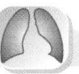

Full blood count

The haemoglobin concentration may be elevated due to haemoconcentration.

Urea and electrolytes

Serum urea and creatinine are usually normal unless severe hypovolaemia and pre-renal renal failure occurs.

Urinalysis

Dipstick urine testing is positive for protein, and 24-hour collection reveals heavy proteinuria of usually more than 3.5 g per day.

Renal biopsy

A renal biopsy is usually performed in adults to screen for other causes of glomerulonephritis.

Management

Immunomodulation

Prednisolone (30–60 mg daily) is given orally and the dose is tailed off once recovery begins. Steroid-resistant cases (5% of the total) may need agents such as cyclophosphamide, ciclosporin or mycophenolate mofetil to induce remission.

Prognosis

The prognosis is good and disease remission usually occurs within 1–3 weeks. Approximately 90% of adults will achieve remission within 5 months. Often patients have frequent relapses, but renal failure is unusual.

Post-streptococcal glomerulonephritis

Post-streptococcal glomerulonephritis is synonymous with diffuse exudative proliferative glomerulonephritis and post-infectious glomerulonephritis.

Epidemiology

Post-streptococcal glomerulonephritis is rare in the West. It is more common in males and tends to occur in children.

Pathology

Post-streptococcal glomerulonephritis is an immune complex mediated glomerulonephritis that develops 10–14 days after a throat or skin infection with certain (nephritogenic) strains of β-haemolytic streptococci. The histological appearance is diffuse proliferative glomerulonephritis and prominent polymorphic infiltration.

Clinical features

Patients tend to present with acute nephritic syndrome with haematuria, peripheral oedema and hypertension. This usually resolves, but can rarely progress to cardiac failure, hypertensive encephalopathy or acute renal failure.

Investigations

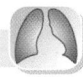

Anti-streptolysin O titre

ASO titres are usually elevated.

Plasma complement levels

Plasma C_3 and C_4 are low.

Renal biopsy

The history, presence of positive ASO titre and low C_4, and presentation are typical so biopsy is reserved for very severe cases to exclude alternative diagnoses.

Management

Supportive care is required. Management of nephritic syndrome is detailed on page 698.

Penicillin

Penicillin is administered for acute streptococcal infection.

Prognosis

This is usually a self-limiting condition and the glomerulonephritis usually settles spontaneously within 1 or 2 weeks. Less than 5% of patients need temporary renal support, but 20% of adult patients are left with mild proteinuria or microscopic haematuria.

Rapidly progressive glomerulonephritis

Rapidly progressive glomerulonephritis (RPGN) is also known as diffuse crescentic glomerulonephritis.

Epidemiology

Rapidly progressive glomerulonephritis is uncommon.

Pathology

Rapidly progressive glomerulonephritis can be primary (idiopathic) or secondary to systemic disease (Table 11.17). The classic histological appearance is the presence of 'crescents' and necrosis in the glomeruli (Fig. 11.12). The 'crescents' are cells, fibrin and collagen in the Bowman's space; eventually this leads to irreversible obliteration of the glomerular capillary tuft.

Clinical features

Patients usually present with haematuria and proteinuria with rapid deterioration of renal function to oliguric or anuric renal failure within days.

> ### ⚡ CLINICAL ALERT
>
> *Rapidly progressive glomerulonephritis must be treated as an emergency to preserve the remaining nephrons as there is brisk loss of renal tissue and function.*

Investigations

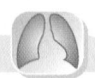

Urinalysis

Blood and protein may be found on dipstick testing of the urine.

Table 11.17	Causes of rapidly progressive glomerulonephritis
Primary (idiopathic)	
Secondary	
Goodpasture's disease	
Wegener's granulomatosis	
Systemic lupus erythematosus	
Henoch–Schönlein purpura	
IgA nephropathy	
Post-streptococcal glomerulonephritis	

Urea and electrolytes

The serum urea and creatinine may be normal in the early stages of the disease, but quickly rise.

Serology

A serology screen (p. 710) is sent to screen for any underlying cause.

Renal biopsy

Renal biopsy is performed urgently, and histology confirms the diagnosis.

Management

Plasma exchange

Repeated plasma exchange is performed in conjunction with immunomodulation.

Immunomodulation

Methylprednisolone (500 mg i.v. daily for 3 days) is administered in pulsed doses.

Prognosis

In general the prognosis is poor with many patients developing end-stage renal failure.

i FURTHER INFORMATION

Bolton WK. Rapidly progressive glomerulonephritis. Seminars in Nephrology 1996; 16: 517–526.

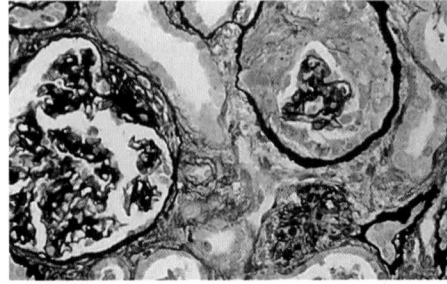

Fig. 11.12 A renal biopsy of crescentic glomerulonephritis.

SECTION 11.8 Acute tubular necrosis

Acute tubular necrosis is an important cause of acute renal failure and results from ischaemia or injury (usually drug induced) of the renal tubular cells (Table 11.18).

Epidemiology

Acute tubular necrosis is one of the most common causes of acute renal failure.

Pathology

Although the medulla receives less blood flow than the cortex and is relatively hypoxic, the oxygen levels are sufficient to maintain tubular metabolism. A slight decrease in renal medullary blood flow (and accompanying hypoxia) or increased metabolic activity (and oxygen consumption) can be sufficient to compromise tubular function, the pars recta being the most vulnerable region because it is normally exposed to the lowest normal oxygen tension. Tubular ischaemia results in structural damage to the cells, with desquamation and apoptosis.

Decreased medullary blood flow can cause pre-renal failure; if this is allowed to progress, the medullary metabolism is affected and acute tubular necrosis develops. The injury to the epithelial cells is established and addressing the renal insult does not reverse the damage.

Acute tubular necrosis can also be caused by direct nephrotoxic injury to the tubular cells, usually by drugs such as aminoglycosides or endogenous nephrotoxins such as uric acid (acute urate nephropathy).

Although acute tubular necrosis may develop in the presence of a single renal insult, it is more common for

there to be a combination of insults such as sepsis, dehydration, increased catabolism, hypotension, nephrotoxic agents and typically as part of a multi-organ failure.

Clinical features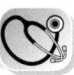

Acute oliguric renal failure (p. 700) is the usual presentation of patients with acute tubular necrosis.

Initial investigations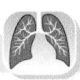

Urea and electrolytes
Serum urea and creatinine are usually increased. Daily electrolyte and fluid balance charts are used to monitor progress. High serum potassium indicates the need for renal replacement therapy.

Arterial blood gases
Acidaemia is an indication for renal replacement therapy.

Ultrasound scan
An ultrasound scan is useful to exclude obstruction as a cause of acute tubular necrosis.

Initial management

Identify and address any precipitating cause
Patients with pre-renal acute renal failure should have the circulating volume replaced and cardiac output, oxygenation and blood pressure should be optimized. If possible, all nephrotoxic drugs should be stopped.

Medical management

Furosemide
Although furosemide can increase water excretion, the solute clearance is not improved and it does not hasten recovery. Patients may not respond to the usual doses and if furosemide is prescribed, higher doses may be required.

Dopamine
Dopamine increases urine output in acute renal failure, but does not alter the recovery period, reduce the requirement for dialysis or influence survival.[1]

Renal replacement therapy
During haemodialysis the blood pressure often drops and tubular oxygenation may worsen. Therefore haemodial-

Table 11.18	Causes of acute tubular necrosis
Ischaemia	
Haemorrhage	
Septic shock	
Cardiogenic shock	
Severe dehydration	
Nephrotoxins	
Drugs	
Aminoglycosides	
Contrast media	
Ciclosporin	
Endogenous nephrotoxins	
Haemoglobinuria	
Myoglobinuria	
Urate nephropathy	

715

ysis is only used for defined indications (uncontrollably high serum potassium, severe acidaemia), as unnecessary haemodialysis may delay recovery of acute tubular necrosis. If haemodialysis is required, the use of biocompatible haemodialysis membranes is associated with improved survival.[2]

Prognosis

Complete recovery of the tubular function can take between 6 and 12 weeks and occurs in a significant proportion of patients. Correcting the precipitating cause alone may not influence the recovery if there has been prolonged ischaemia and tubular necrosis. The necrotic debris must be cleared and the tubules regenerate. Patients

may be supported with dialysis in the interim. In a small proportion, native renal function does not recover and, in many, renal function does not return to baseline. In patients with severe disease who are ventilator and renal replacement therapy dependent, the mortality can be as high as 80%, usually due to bleeding, infection and other comorbidities.

FURTHER INFORMATION

Firth JD. Medical treatment of acute tubular necrosis. Quarterly Journal of Medicine 1998; 91: 321–323.

REFERENCES

(1) *Friedrich JO, Adhikari N, Herridge MS, Beyene J. Meta-analysis: Low-dose dopamine increases urine output but does not prevent renal dysfunction or death. Annals of Internal Medicine 2005; 142: 510–524.*
(2) *Subramanian S, Venkataraman R, Kellum JA. Influence of dialysis membranes on outcomes in acute renal failure: a meta-analysis. Kidney International 2002; 62: 1819–1823.*

SECTION 11.9 Acute interstitial nephritis

Acute interstitial nephritis, also known as tubulointerstitial nephritis, is a group of diseases in which the predominant renal lesion detected on renal biopsy is inflammation of the tubules and interstitium.

Epidemiology

Acute interstitial nephritis is uncommon, accounting for less than 2% of acute renal failure cases, and approximately 6% of all renal biopsies. It is slightly more common in men and in the elderly.[1] It is rare in childhood, possibly a reflection of lesser numbers of medications.

Pathology

Acute interstitial nephritis can be primary (idiopathic) or more commonly secondary to drugs (Table 11.19). Less commonly, it is precipitated by infection or systemic disease (SLE, sarcoid).

Clinical features

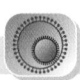

Classically, patients present with acute renal failure with features of hypersensitivity (eosinophilia, rash and aching joints). The majority have haematuria. Acute and chronic

renal failure are common at presentation (up to 45%); nephrotic and nephritic syndrome are less common (less than 12%).[1]

A careful drug history may identify the offending agent that has commenced within the previous few weeks. A systems enquiry is also important to screen for any underlying infection or associated disease.

Table 11.19	Drug causes of acute interstitial nephritis

Antibiotics
  Cephalosporins
  Penicillins
  Sulphonamides
  Vancomycin	

NSAIDs	

Anticonvulsants
  Phenytoin
  Carbamazepine	

Diuretics
  Furosemide
  Thiazides	

Allopurinol	
Azathioprine	

Investigations

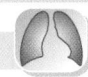

Urinalysis
Urine dipstick testing shows red blood cells. Urine microscopy may demonstrate eosinophils.

Ultrasound of the kidneys
The kidneys are usually normal in size, but may show increased echogenicity.

Renal biopsy
Renal biopsy is usually reserved for patients with a protracted recovery period to confirm the diagnosis and exclude other pathology.

Management

Identify and address precipitating cause
Renal function usually recovers once the offending drug is withdrawn although creatinine does not necessarily return to baseline. However, identification of the agent responsible can be difficult in patients with polypharmacy.

Immunomodulation
The use of corticosteroids is controversial as patients often improve without the need for immunomodulation. In some patients, renal function may continue to decline despite corticosteroids.

Prognosis

In general, early identification and withdrawal of the offending drug often leads to rapid improvement of renal function with or without corticosteroids.

> **REFERENCE**
>
> **(1)** Davison A, Jones C. *Acute interstitial nephritis in the elderly: a report from the UK MRC glomerulonephritis register and a review of the literature. Nephrology Dialysis Transplantation* 1998; 13 Supplement 7: 12–16.

Renal tubular acidosis

Fanconi's syndrome

Bartter's syndrome

Liddle's syndrome

Gitelman's syndrome

Salt-wasting nephropathy

SECTION 11.10   Tubular disorders

Renal tubular acidosis

The renal tubular acidoses (RTA) are a group of disorders characterized by a defect in urinary acidification.

Epidemiology

The renal tubular acidoses are rare and often present in childhood as 'failure to thrive'. Later presentations in adulthood can be as metabolic acidosis with a normal anion gap.

Pathology

The kidney usually buffers the body's acid–base balance using bicarbonate and can normally acidify urine to a pH of below 5.5.

In distal (type 1) RTA, there is an inability to secrete H^+ ions in the distal tubule due to primary or secondary diseases such as analgesic nephropathy.

In proximal (type 2) RTA, there is a defect in the proximal tubule leading to reduction in both hydrogen excretion and bicarbonate reabsorption.

In type 4 RTA, the distal tubule is unable to cope with H^+ or K^+ exchange and serum aldosterone is usually low. Drugs, including NSAIDs and ACE inhibitors, are common causes of type 4 RTA.

Type 3 is rare and not discussed further.

Clinical features

In type 1 disease, systemic acidosis leads to leaching of the skeletal calcium. The combination of calciuria, alkaline urine and low urinary citrate levels leads to the development of renal stones (calcium phosphate) and nephrocalcinosis. The hypokalaemia leads to episodes of weakness or collapse. Patients with type 4 RTA are less acidotic than patients with type 1, and usually have some degree of renal impairment.

Investigations

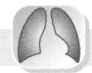

Urea and electrolytes
Serum potassium may be low or elevated depending on the subtype of RTA (Table 11.20). Low chloride levels are part of the characteristic chronic hypochloraemic metabolic acidosis.

Arterial blood gas
An acidaemia with a normal anion gap is the characteristic finding.

Random urine pH
Renal tubular acidosis is suggested by a high random urine pH; a normal result, however, does not exclude the diagnosis.

717

Table 11.20	Types of renal tubular acidoses		
Type	**Name**	**Serum potassium**	**Causes**
1	Distal	Low	Primary Drugs (amphotericin) Systemic disorder (Sjögren's syndrome, systemic lupus erythematosus)
2	Proximal	Low	Fanconi's syndrome Amyloidosis Vitamin D deficiency
3	A subset of type 1	Low	
4	Hyporeninaemic hypoaldosteronism	High	Diabetes mellitus Chronic renal impairment Drugs (ciclosporin)

Urine acidification test

Confirmation of suspected renal tubular acidosis (any type) is by formal urinary acidification testing or administration of ammonium sulphate.

Management

Identify and address any underlying cause

The acidosis and hypokalaemia may not warrant drug treatment; dietary advice may suffice. The drugs responsible may need to be withdrawn.

Bicarbonate

Oral bicarbonate is administered for patients with moderate to severe acidosis.

Potassium supplementation

Oral potassium supplementation is given to patients with hypokalaemia.

Prognosis

Type 4 is the most benign, not necessarily needing treatment other than dietary modifications. Type 1 is intermediate and the acidosis can be corrected with bicarbonate. Type 2 is much more resistant to correction, leading to long-term acidosis and a worse prognosis.

Fanconi's syndrome

Fanconi's syndrome may be congenital or acquired. The congenital causes are all rare, metabolic, and tend to present in early childhood. Acquired cases are frequently due to drugs such as chemotherapy agents, heavy metals and herbal medicine. Proximal tubular dysfunction results in leakage into the urine of amino acids, phosphate, glucose and bicarbonate. In children, chronic loss of these electrolytes results in failure to thrive, rickets, osteomalacia and acidosis. Adults tend to present with bone pain, polyuria and polydipsia. Correction of the underlying disorder will often lead to an improvement in the tubular disorder.

Bartter's syndrome

Bartter's syndrome is a rare autosomal recessive disease characterized by a transport defect in cells of the thick ascending limb of the loop of Henle. Patients tend to present in infancy or early childhood with profuse vomiting, dehydration, failure to thrive and short stature. Serum chloride and potassium are low, and an alkalosis is present. Treatment is with correction of electrolyte disorders, a loop diuretic and ibuprofen.

Liddle's syndrome

Liddle's syndrome is a rare autosomal dominant disorder of the distal tubule that leads to pseudohyperaldosteronism. Patients develop polyuria and hypertension; children can present with failure to thrive. Serum renin and aldosterone levels are low and there is hypokalaemia and metabolic alkalosis. Treatment is life-long, with salt restriction and amiloride.

Gitelman's syndrome

Gitelman's syndrome is a rare autosomal recessive defect in the distal convoluted tubule leading the kidney to lose magnesium, sodium, potassium and chloride. It is not associated with renal impairment. Patients present in adolescence with hypokalaemia, hypochloraemia and alkalosis. Treatment is with thiazides and supplementation with magnesium.

Salt-wasting nephropathy

Pseudohypoaldosteronism type I is rare and presents in the neonate with failure to thrive. Patients are extremely ill with severe salt wasting, hyperkalaemia, hypotension and metabolic acidosis. Renin and aldosterone levels rise, with no response to exogenous mineralocorticoids. Sodium supplements are required for treatment.

Drug-induced kidney disease

Patients with previously normal baseline renal function may develop renal impairment following administration of a wide variety of drugs. The reaction may be anticipated, as certain drugs are recognized as nephrotoxic, or it may be idiosyncratic.

Aminoglycosides

Aminoglycosides can cause acute tubular necrosis, especially in combination with diuretics. Close supervision is needed when prescribing aminoglycosides with any degree of impaired excretory function.

Non-steroidal anti-inflammatory agents

NSAIDs can cause acute or chronic renal failure. In vulnerable patients with comorbidities, the addition of NSAIDs is sometimes sufficient to precipitate acute tubular necrosis and acute renal failure. Chronic usage can lead to glomerulonephritis or papillary necrosis.

Lithium

Acute lithium toxicity can be precipitated by the addition of many other drugs, including diuretics and NSAIDs. Severe toxic levels and deliberate overdoses can be treated by haemodialysis. Haemodialysis clears the drug and should reverse toxicity.

Chronic usage can also affect the tubules causing nephrogenic diabetes insipidus or chronic tubulointerstitial nephropathy.

The kidney and systemic disease

Pauci-immune vasculitis

The kidney can be affected by several vasculitides (diseases associated with vasculitis) causing rapidly progressive glomerulonephritis. The term 'pauci-immune vasculitis' refers to the fact that immunoglobulin and immune deposits are not found in the glomeruli (in contrast to Goodpasture's disease).

Epidemiology

Pauci-immune vasculitis is more common than Goodpasture's disease but remains rare with an incidence of 0.8 per 100 000 per year.[1] Patients are usually more than 50 years old and more commonly male.

Pathology

Diseases that result in pauci-immune vasculitis include polyarteritis nodosa, microscopic polyangiitis, Wegener's granulomatosis and Churg–Strauss syndrome. The predominant sites for the vasculitis are small vessels (small arteries to capillaries) including the glomerular capillaries. Extra-renal sites often involve the skin (vasculitic rash) and lungs (alveolar haemorrhage). The exact mediator of tissue injury has not been identified, and on renal biopsy, crescents and segmental necrosis occur (rapidly progressive glomerulonephritis).

Clinical features

Patients can present with acute glomerulonephritis ranging from haematuria to rapidly progressive glomerulonephritis and the signs and symptoms of end-stage renal failure. Patients may complain of malaise, lethargy and flu-like symptoms. On examination, purpura may be evident, often on the legs, with ulceration.

Sometimes vasculitis is more insidious, and the main features are of upper or lower respiratory tract disease. Respiratory involvement may present as sinusitis, epistaxis or haemoptysis (Wegener's granulomatosis). Vasculitis in the gastrointestinal tract causes abdominal pain, blood loss and symptoms of ischaemia.

Investigations

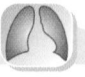

Full blood count
Churg–Strauss syndrome can present with asthma and eosinophilia (more than 1.5×10^9/L).

Urea and electrolytes
Urea and creatinine are elevated, and need to be requested daily as deterioration can occur rapidly.

Urinalysis
Blood and protein are found on urine dipstick testing. There may be erythrocyte casts on microscopy.

Serology
ANCA is not specific to an individual vasculitis, so an overall picture of the patient's clinical condition, serology and histology is needed to make a diagnosis. If both anti-GBM and ANCA are positive, it is safer to assume anti-GBM disease (Goodpasture's disease) and to treat accordingly. With Wegener's granulomatosis, serology shows predominantly cANCA antibodies specific for proteinase PR3. Both pANCA and cANCA may be present with microscopic polyangiitis. With Churg–Strauss syndrome pANCA is more likely to be positive than cANCA.

Renal ultrasound
Renal ultrasound is performed as a screening investigation to confirm the presence of two normal sized kidneys prior to biopsy.

Renal biopsy
Rapidly progressive glomerulonephritis is characterized by crescents and necrosis.

Management

Immunomodulation
Steroids may be used in isolation or with another agent such as cyclophosphamide. As with all such regimens, infection must be excluded before immunosuppression is started. Steroids and cyclophosphamide are given either orally or intravenously and treatment needs to be tailored to the disease activity seen on renal biopsy. Cyclophosphamide is discontinued after a few months and may be replaced with less toxic drugs such as azathioprine.

Inflammatory markers such as C-reactive protein (CRP) and ANCA titres are used to monitor remission and disease activity respectively. Once remission is achieved, the doses of immunosuppression are gradually reduced and monitoring continues using ANCA, CRP and levels of protein and blood in the urine.

If remission is not achieved, immunosuppression is withdrawn fairly quickly as its risks will then outweigh the benefits.

Plasma exchange
Plasma exchange (and intravenous immunoglobulin) has less of a clearly identified role and is sometimes used in patients with aggressive glomerulonephritis.

Prevention of relapse
Acute infection can induce relapse, and infection should be treated aggressively. Eradication of nasal staphylococcus reduces the risk of relapse of Wegener's granulomatosis 7-fold.[2]

Management of relapse
A rise in ANCA titre is a positive predictor for a relapse, and up to half of patients will relapse at some point. If this is detected early by routine monitoring, smaller doses of immunosuppression may be prescribed.

Renal transplantation
Renal transplantation is a suitable option for patients with vasculitis but carries a higher risk of graft failure due to recurrence of disease in up to 5% of transplants.

Prognosis

The overall 2-year survival of patients with pauci-immune vasculitis is 75% but many require dialysis.[3] Prompt treatment of Wegener's granulomatosis will achieve remission in up to 90%. In general, long-term frequent relapses are associated with poorer prognosis.

REFERENCES

(1) Pettersson EE, Sundelin B, Heigl Z. Incidence and outcome of pauci-immune necrotizing and crescentic glomerulonephritis in adults. Clinical Nephrology 1995; 43: 141–149.
(2) Stegeman CA, Tervaert JW, Sluiter WJ, Manson WL, de Jong PE, Kallenberg CG. Association of chronic nasal carriage of Staphylococcus aureus and higher relapse rates in Wegener granulomatosis. Annals of Internal Medicine 1994; 120: 12–17.
(3) Falk RJ, Hogan S, Carey TS, Jennette JC. Clinical course of anti-neutrophil cytoplasmic autoantibody-associated glomerulonephritis and systemic vasculitis. The Glomerular Disease Collaborative Network. Annals of Internal Medicine 1990; 113: 656–663.

Goodpasture's disease

Goodpasture's disease results from anti-glomerular basement membrane (GBM) antibodies, whereas Goodpasture's syndrome is the combination of nephritis and pulmonary haemorrhage.

Epidemiology

Goodpasture's disease is rare with an incidence of less than 0.1 per 100 000 per year. It affects men more than women, and usually presents over the age of 50.

Pathology

Patients with Goodpasture's disease develop auto-antibodies to their glomerular basement membrane. The aetiology for the development of anti-GBM antibodies is unknown, but is associated with genetic (HLA-DR2) and environmental (occupational exposure to hydrocarbons) factors.

Anti-glomerular basement membrane (GBM) antibodies with immunoglobulin are deposited along the glomerular basement membrane leading to rapidly progressive glomerulonephritis (p. 714). They are also found in the circulation and other tissues. Lung haemorrhage can be fulminant with profound hypoxia, and the disease occasionally affects the cochlea, eyes and brain.

Clinical features

Patients present with rapidly declining renal function or end-stage renal failure with anuria, and this may be accompanied by pulmonary symptoms such as cough or dyspnoea. Smokers are more likely to develop haemoptysis and pulmonary haemorrhage.

Investigations

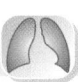

Full blood count
Pulmonary haemorrhage may be sufficient to cause anaemia.

Urea and electrolytes
Urea and creatinine are elevated and need to be requested daily as deterioration can occur rapidly.

Serology
Anti-GBM antibodies are found in the serum. False positive results can occur from vasculitis due to other causes. ANCA may be positive. Titres of anti-GBM antibodies are also used to monitor disease activity during treatment.

Urinalysis
Blood and protein are found on urine dipstick testing. There may be erythrocyte casts on microscopy.

Chest X-ray
Alveolar haemorrhage presents as diffuse shadowing on a plain chest film.

Lung function tests
A diffusion factor (K_{CO}) less than 30% predicted usually indicates lung haemorrhage.

Renal ultrasound
Renal ultrasound is performed as a screening investigation to confirm the presence of two normal sized kidneys prior to biopsy.

Renal biopsy
Biopsy is vital, and a rapidly progressive glomerulonephritis is characterized by crescents and necrosis. A high proportion of crescents correlates with poorer prognosis.

Management

Since the disease is known to be due to anti-GBM antibodies, the treatment involves removing these antibodies then trying to suppress their formation.

Management of fluid status
Control of both hypertension and fluid status is vital.

Plasma exchange
Plasma exchange is performed daily to remove the anti-GBM antibodies for up to 3 weeks.

Immunomodulation
Immunosuppression is started as soon as possible. High-dose pulsed methylprednisolone (500 mg intravenously on 3 consecutive days) is used prior to converting to oral prednisolone (up to 60 mg daily). Oral cyclophosphamide may also be used.

As immunomodulating regimens leave the patient vulnerable to infection, the neutrophil count needs to be closely monitored; some recommend prophylactic anti-fungal agents with co-trimoxazole to prevent *Pneumocystis carinii* pneumonia. Prophylactic proton pump inhibitors reduce the risk of gastrointestinal bleeding due to the steroids, and patients can become overtly diabetic.

Renal replacement therapy
Patients may require haemodialysis for elevated serum potassium, acidaemia or fluid overload.

Renal transplantation
Patients with anti-GBM antibodies may be considered for transplantation, but only if their anti-GBM titres become negligible to minimize the risk of recurrence in the transplanted kidney.

Prognosis

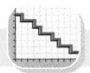

Anuric patients are unlikely to recover their native kidney function. Plasma exchange and immunosuppression may improve lung haemorrhage but have little effect on the kidneys. Recovery of renal function is more likely with early treatment, serum creatinine less than 200 µmol/L on presentation and only few crescents on renal biopsy.[1]

REFERENCE

(1) *Merkel F, Pullig O, Marx M, Netzer KO, Weber M. Course and prognosis of anti-basement membrane antibody (anti-BM-Ab)-mediated disease: report of 35 cases. Nephrology Dialysis Transplantation 1994; 9: 372–376.*

Systemic lupus erythematosus

Epidemiology

Approximately 50% of patients with systemic lupus erythematosus (SLE) eventually develop renal disease.

Pathology

A wide variety of renal diseases are associated with SLE, including glomerulonephritis, interstitial nephritis, renal vein thrombosis and renal artery stenosis. The classification of lupus glomerulonephritis is provided in Table 11.21. Immune complexes and complement (C_3, C_4 and C_{1q}) are found on immunological staining and electron microscopy.

Clinical features

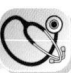

The clinical picture does not necessarily reflect the level of renal damage or inflammation. Lupus nephritis is only an occasional presenting feature of SLE. More commonly patients may have mild incidental proteinuria, therefore testing for SLE is an important aspect in the investigation of glomerulonephritis (p. 492). Less commonly patients can present in acute renal failure.

Investigations

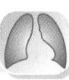

Urea and electrolytes
Serum creatinine is usually normal in the early stages of the disease.

Urinalysis
Urinary dipstick testing may reveal blood or protein. A 24-hour urine collection is required to quantify the severity of the proteinuria.

Renal biopsy
Renal biopsy is a key investigation to confirm the diagnosis and to classify the type of lupus nephropathy. Lupus glomerulonephritis may alter in time from one class of nephritis to another. Therefore patients may need a series of biopsies to monitor their disease.

Table 11.21	Classification of lupus glomerulonephritis
Class I (minimal change)	
Class II (mesangial disease)	
Class III (focal proliferative)	
Class IV (diffuse proliferative)	
Class V (membranous)	

Management

Class I and II disease
Classes I and II have a mild course and may not require treatment, but the severity of proteinuria and inflammatory markers needs to be monitored.

Class III and IV disease
Classes III and IV are more aggressive forms of the disease with a worse prognosis. There is a limited evidence base so treatment is empirical with immunomodulation. Patients should receive steroids and an additional immunomodulating agent such as ciclosporin or azathioprine. Cyclophosphamide may be given orally or intravenously (in pulses).

The progress is monitored by inflammatory markers, dsDNA, complement levels, proteinuria and creatinine. Once proteinuria improves, the immunosuppression is reduced but steroids and azathioprine may be required at lower maintenance doses.

Renal transplantation
Patients maintained on dialysis are often suitable for transplantation. Lupus rarely recurs in renal transplants and the immunosuppression regimen may be adapted for the treatment of SLE in addition to reducing the risk of transplant rejection.

Prognosis

Renal failure usually develops within the first 10 years of lupus nephropathy. Approximately 10% of patients will need dialysis eventually. After 10 years, renal disease severe enough to require dialysis is rare. The 5- and 10-year survival rates of patients with lupus nephritis are 84% and 72% respectively.[1] Deaths are predominantly from cardiovascular disease.

REFERENCE

(1) Bono L, Cameron JS, Hicks JA. The very long-term prognosis and complications of lupus nephritis and its treatment. *Quarterly Journal of Medicine* 1999; 92: 211–218.

Hyperuricaemia and gout

Hyperuricaemia can lead to acute renal failure by precipitation of uric acid crystals and chronic renal failure from tubulointerstitial nephritis, and is associated with the formation of uric acid stones. In addition, renal failure causes hyperuricaemia and secondary gout.

Epidemiology

Gout is extremely common in chronic renal failure, whereas chronic urate nephropathy is much less common and is a rare cause of chronic renal failure.

Pathology

Acute urate nephropathy

Any condition that causes uric acid release can cause acute urate nephropathy. A common example is acute urate nephropathy due to tumour lysis syndrome after chemotherapy. Although uric acid is normally freely filtered by the kidneys, destruction of tumour cells leads to the release of a high uric acid load that can overwhelm the reabsorption mechanisms in the distal tubule. When this occurs, uric acid is deposited as crystals leading to acute renal failure.

Chronic urate nephropathy

Patients with gout have long-standing elevations of serum uric acid. As urate crystals are irritants, they provoke a fibrotic inflammatory reaction when deposited within renal parenchyma. This occasionally leads to interstitial nephritis and renal impairment. Filtration of urate decreases proportionally with the decline in glomerular filtration rate, and high doses of diuretics further increase serum uric acid levels.

Rarely, familial hyperuricaemia can lead to interstitial fibrosis, medullary cystic kidney disease and progressive renal failure. This autosomal dominant condition results from mutations in a gene on chromosome 16 which encodes for the protein uromodulin.

Clinical features

Patients may have asymptomatic hyperuricaemia or symptoms of gout (p. 506). In acute urate nephropathy, patients may have clinical features of the underlying condition. When hyperuricaemia and chronic renal failure coexist at presentation, it becomes difficult to differentiate between gout with secondary renal impairment and chronic renal failure with secondary gout.

Investigations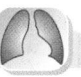

Urea and electrolytes

Serum urea and creatinine are normal in the early stages of the disease, and rise with the onset of acute or chronic renal failure.

Serum uric acid

Serum uric aid is elevated.

Management

Acute urate nephropathy

Prevention is preferable by commencing allopurinol before chemotherapy. Patients should be well hydrated prior to chemotherapy to minimize the uric acid concentrations and to ensure a good diuresis. Treatment of established disease is with aggressive rehydration, and dialysis may be required to clear the uric acid load.

Chronic urate nephropathy

Chronic urate nephropathy is usually secondary to gout, and the management of patients without renal impairment is detailed on page 507. As NSAIDs are contraindicated in patients with impaired renal function, colchicine or prednisolone may be used for acute gout instead.

Prognosis

Patients with acute urate nephropathy usually recover their renal function, although this depends on their baseline creatinine and whether other nephrotoxic agents have been used. Patients with chronic urate nephropathy may progress to end-stage renal failure but this is unusual. The exception to this is hereditary hyperuricaemia, which can progress to end-stage renal failure in early adulthood.

Haemolytic uraemic syndrome and thrombotic thrombocytopenic purpura

Haemolytic uraemic syndrome (HUS, p. 821) is a rare condition resulting in acute renal failure. It shares features with thrombocytopenic thrombotic purpura (TTP), with the same pathophysiology.

Epidemiology

The most common age for HUS is childhood, with reducing incidence as age increases. HUS is associated with *E. coli 0157* (D+ HUS) and its incidence varies with the seasons.

Pathology

Platelet thrombi form and settle throughout the body, but especially in the kidney with HUS and in the brain with TTP. These microvascular thromboses are triggered by endotoxins, causing cytokine release.

Clinical features

HUS is a triad of microangiopathic haemolytic anaemia, low platelets and renal failure; in addition TTP also includes fever and neurological symptoms. The likelihood of developing acute renal failure correlates with a raised white cell count on presentation.

Investigations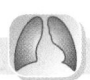

Investigations for the diagnosis of HUS and TTP are presented on page 821.

Urea and electrolytes

Urea and creatinine are elevated.

Management

Supportive management

The management of HUS and TTP is supportive. In general, typical D+ HUS is a self-limiting disease with an excellent prognosis and usually full recovery of renal function.

Patients with significant fragments detected on blood film or impaired renal function will usually require a series of plasma exchanges or supportive haemodialysis.

Prognosis

Patients with typical childhood D+ HUS are expected to recover fully. Only half of patients with atypical D− HUS will recover their renal function. TTP has a mortality of 10–28% despite plasma exchange, and the overall prognosis depends on the underlying cause.

Plasma cell myeloma

Plasma cell myeloma and related disorders cause acute and chronic renal failure. In some patients it is reversible, but a high proportion of patients remain on dialysis.

Epidemiology

Approximately 50% of patients with plasma cell myeloma (p. 809) already have a degree of renal impairment when they present with the malignancy.

Pathology

Patients with plasma cell myeloma have many predisposing features to renal failure such as dehydration and hypercalcaemia and are at increased risk of renal impairment secondary to contrast and nephrotoxic drugs (e.g. NSAIDs). The associated high tumour load and any infection further interfere with renal function.

Urinary light chains aggregate in the distal tubule and, at a critical concentration, casts precipitate (cast nephropathy) in the renal tubules. Dehydration and diuretic usage accelerate cast formation and increasing proteinuria correlates with the risk of renal failure. Proportionally more patients with light chain myeloma develop renal failure.

Clinical features

Patients often present with renal failure and a myriad of non-specific symptoms. They are often frail, hypercatabolic and prone to infections. Cast nephropathy presents as acute renal failure often needing immediate supportive therapy.

Initial investigations

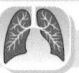

Urea and electrolytes

Baseline U&Es are raised, often with hyperkalaemia and hypercalcaemia.

Urinalysis

Dipstick testing will not detect light chains in the urine so urine is also tested for Bence Jones protein, which is present in more than 50%.

Protein electrophoresis

Protein electrophoresis of serum will identify an intact paraprotein and identify the immunoglobulin as usually IgG or IgA.

Skeletal X-rays

Plain X-rays are the best way of identifying lytic lesions. A 'skeletal survey' consists of images of the skull, chest, pelvis and proximal long bones.

Ultrasound of the kidneys

The kidneys are usually normal in size at presentation.

 CLINICAL ALERT

The diagnosis of plasma cell myeloma related renal disease should be suspected in any patient over 40 with unexplained renal failure, negative dipstick testing and normal-sized kidneys.

Further investigations

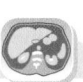

Bone marrow aspirate

The bone marrow aspirate can be diagnostic and shows patchy and variable levels of infiltration by plasma cells.

Renal biopsy

Renal biopsy is usually indicated in most patients with myeloma and renal failure, although in some patients the risks may outweigh the potential benefits (due to possible infection and bleeding) when the diagnosis has already been made. Renal biopsy may reveal the presence of casts and be able to quantify the extent of the disease and prognosis. In addition, other concomitant diseases can be excluded.

Initial management

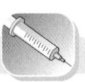

Rehydration

Rehydration is the initial treatment for patients with renal impairment to avoid further cast formation.

Identify and address any precipitating cause

Any nephrotoxic drugs should be stopped. If radiological contrast use is unavoidable, the patient should be well hydrated before the procedure.

Medical management

Chemotherapy

Dexamethasone (40 mg/day for 5 days) has an immediate effect on the plasma cells.

Further chemotherapy, such as melphalan or vincristine, adriamycin and dexamethasone (VAD) may be planned but takes longer to have an effect.

Bisphosphonates

Bisphosphonates are administered to lower the serum calcium levels in patients with hypercalcaemia.

Renal replacement therapy

Renal replacement therapy (haemodialysis) may be required acutely for patients with elevated serum potassium, acidaemia or pulmonary oedema. Some frail patients are unable to tolerate haemodialysis and chronic ambulatory peritoneal dialysis (CAPD) should be considered.

Plasma exchange

Plasma exchange may be used to treat the acute renal injury but the evidence is equivocal (p. 736).

Surgical management

Renal transplantation

Most patients are unsuitable for renal transplantation. In general, only young patients with disease remission are suitable for consideration for renal transplantation.

Prognosis

Once the patient is oliguric and dialysis dependent, the chance of recovery of renal function is small. The median survival with end-stage renal failure is 9 months. Approximately one third of patients die within 3 months of referral and one third live longer than 1 year. Low serum albumin and thrombocytopenia at presentation is associated with poor prognosis.

 FURTHER INFORMATION

Irish AB, Winearls CG, Littlewood T. Presentation and survival of patients with severe renal failure and myeloma. Quarterly Journal of Medicine 1997; 90: 773–780.

Sarcoid

Renal disease associated with sarcoid (p. 418) is mainly due to hypercalcaemia. Hypercalciuria promotes the formation of renal stones, and calcium is also deposited within the interstitial tissues (nephrocalcinosis). Granulomas can also produce an interstitial nephritis (p. 717). Sarcoid renal disease usually presents with pain from renal stones or with acute renal failure. The finding of nephrocalcinosis

may be incidental. Supportive treatment of acute renal failure (p. 699) and specific therapy for the hypercalcaemia is required. Prednisolone (up to 60 mg daily) is used to correct the hypercalcaemia, and the withdrawal of steroids may take several months.

Sickle cell disease

Epidemiology

Sickle cell nephropathy affects over 50% of patients with sickle cell disease, and 4.2% develop end-stage renal failure.[1]

Pathology

Nephropathy caused by sickle cell disease is multifactorial and can be caused by sickling within the medulla, release of myoglobin with rhabdomyolysis, and papillary necrosis in response to ischaemia (50%). Sickling within the glomerular capillaries leads to focal segmental glomerulosclerosis (FSGS).

Clinical features

Patients present with haematuria from the sickling. Haemoglobin and myoglobin are released into the urine. Sickle cell patients are also prone to dehydration due to polyuria, and can present with acute renal failure. A third form of presentation is with nephrotic syndrome (p. 697) due to focal segmental glomerulosclerosis.

Investigations
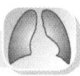

Urea and electrolytes
Serum urea and creatinine are usually raised.

Urinalysis
Urinary dipstick testing can detect haemoglobin and myoglobin. Urine microscopy may show haemoglobin casts, and urine should be cultured to screen for infection.

Ultrasound of the kidneys
Ultrasound is a safe investigation to detect papillary necrosis but is not as sensitive as an intravenous urogram.

Intravenous urogram
An intravenous urogram may show papillary necrosis, but the addition of contrast carries the risk of worsening renal failure. Patients should be well hydrated prior to the investigation.

Management

The standard regimen for treatment of acute renal failure (p. 699) is followed.

Rehydration

Haematuria usually settles spontaneously, but patients should also be adequately hydrated.

Immunomodulation

Focal segmental glomerulosclerosis sometimes responds to steroids and ACE inhibitors, but recovery is unlikely.

Renal replacement therapy

Some patients with rhabdomyolysis need temporary dialysis. Most patients needing renal replacement do so long term.

Renal transplantation

Transplantation is possible, with long-term graft survival similar to that of patients without sickle cell disorders. However, the risk of vascular problems remains high after renal transplantation.

Prognosis

Approximately 5% of patients with sickle cell disease develop end-stage renal failure.[2] The prognosis of patients on dialysis is poor due to vascular problems and multi-system disorders, with a 3-year survival of approximately 59%.

i FURTHER INFORMATION

Scheinman JL. Sickle cell disease and the kidney. Seminars in Nephrology 2003; 23: 66–76.

REFERENCES

(1) *Sklar AH, Campbell H, Caruana RJ, Lightfoot BO, Gaier JG, Milner P. A population study of renal function in sickle cell anemia. International Journal of Artificial Organs 1990; 13: 231–236.*
(2) *Powars DR, Elliott-Mills DD, Chan L, Niland J, Hiti AL, Opas LM, Johnson C. Chronic renal failure in sickle cell disease: risk factors, clinical course, and mortality. Annals of Internal Medicine 1991; 115: 614–620.*

Rhabdomyolysis

Rhabdomyolysis occurs from damage to skeletal muscle and is an important and treatable cause of acute renal failure.

Epidemiology

Rhabdomyolysis is the underlying cause of up to 3% of acute renal failure in hospital.[1]

Pathology

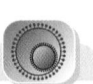

The causes of rhabdomyolysis are listed in Table 11.22, but the common primary insult is the breakdown of skeletal

Table 11.22	Causes of rhabdomyolysis
Crush injuries	
Trauma	
Prolonged immobilization/coma	
Compartment syndrome	
Prolonged seizures	

Drugs
  Heroin
  Ecstasy	

Environmental
  Snakebites
  Hyperthermia	

Genetic
  McArdle's syndrome
  Carnitine palmityl transferase deficiency	

muscle with release of myoglobin into the circulation. The myoglobin is filtered by the kidney and obstructs the renal tubules causing acute tubular necrosis (see p. 715). Higher myoglobin loads correlate with the severity of the decline in creatinine clearance, a situation that is often made worse by associated conditions such as dehydration and acidosis.

Clinical features

Patients may have been found collapsed or immobile on the floor, or there may be a history of trauma, alcohol excess, crush injury or either overdose of recreational drugs or para-suicide. On examination, evidence of trauma may be obvious. A history of injury or ischaemia with a swollen tight calf may be due to compartment syndrome. Urine becomes dark brown due to the presence of myoglobin, but a proportion of patients are anuric.

Initial investigations

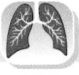

Urea and electrolytes and serum calcium

Urea and electrolytes are raised, and the serum creatinine is disproportionately high due to its release from dead myocytes. The muscle damage causes hyperkalaemia, hyperphosphataemia and hypocalcaemia. The serum potassium must be checked daily.

Creatinine kinase

Creatinine kinase is markedly elevated. Significant rhabdomyolysis is associated with levels in excess of 15 000 u/mL.

Urinalysis

Urine dipstick testing may be false positive for blood due to the presence of myoglobin. In the laboratory, myoglobin is detected in the urine samples and no red blood cells are seen on microscopy.

Initial management

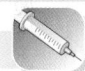

Intravenous fluids and mannitol

Intravenous fluids to maintain good hydration encourage the excretion of the myoglobin. Mannitol and alkalinization of the urine may reduce the need for renal replacement therapy.

Identify and address any precipitating cause

Fasciotomy or surgical release of compartment syndrome may be required. In rhabdomyolysis due to opiate overdose, the circulating opiate is not excreted in the urine due to acute renal failure. Respiration must be monitored, and naloxone infusion may be required to reverse the effects of opiate overdose.

Medical management

Correction of electrolyte abnormalities

Phosphate binders, a low-potassium diet and oral calcium/alfacalcidol are used to manage hyperphosphataemia, hyperkalaemia and hypocalcaemia respectively. During the recovery phase, patients become hypercalcaemic due to the remobilization of the calcium from the muscle, so at this stage calcium supplements are withdrawn.

Renal replacement therapy

If the myoglobin concentration is too high, or when treatment is delayed, the cumulative damage becomes more pronounced. Daily haemodialysis may be required to clear the high solute load.

Prognosis

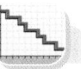

Patients with anuric rhabdomyolysis nearly always recover their renal function. Approximately 3 weeks after the onset of anuria, the patient's tubules recover from the acute tubular necrosis and urine is passed. Patients may become polyuric, and adequate hydration during recovery is essential.

i FURTHER INFORMATION

Zager RA. Rhabdomyolysis and myohemoglobinuric acute renal failure. Kidney International 1996; 49: 314–326.

REFERENCE

(1) *Woodrow G, Brownjohn AM, Turney JH. The clinical and biochemical features of acute renal failure due to rhabdomyolysis. Renal Failure 1995; 17: 467–474.*

Amyloidosis

Renal amyloid deposition is found in light chain (AL) and secondary (AA) amyloidoses, and occurs in up to 50% of patients with amyloidosis (p. 467). Glomerulosclerosis results from the deposition of AL amyloid in the mesangium and glomerular basement membrane of the kidney. Apart from symptoms of the underlying disease, the renal manifestations include proteinuria and nephrotic syndrome (p. 696). Elderly patients may present with severe oedema. Investigations are similar to those for suspected myeloma (p. 810). Renal biopsy is usually required to confirm the diagnosis and carries an increased risk of bleeding at the biopsy site. Management is supportive rather than curative. The underlying disease should be identified and addressed. Most patients are supported with renal replacement therapy and rarely receive renal transplantation. Orthostatic hypotension and low-output cardiac failure can make haemodialysis precarious. Chronic ambulatory peritoneal dialysis may be more acceptable but survival is not improved. The prognosis of patients with AL amyloid is poor; the median survival is approximately 12 months.

Malignancy-associated renal disease

Renal disease may arise primarily due to the neoplasia or secondary to the drugs (cisplatin, ifosfamide) used in the treatment. Glomerulonephritis can also be associated with cancer. Up to 20% of patients with membranous disease have an underlying malignancy such as breast, gastrointestinal and lung cancers. Curing the cancer may induce remission of the nephritis but prognosis is more closely related to the underlying cancer.

In addition, tumours such as pelvic cancers can obstruct the urinary tract, leading to post-renal renal failure. Malignancy can cause renal failure by tumour infiltration of the kidneys. Unless the primary tumour is amenable to treatment, patients are not usually suitable for dialysis because of the poor prognosis and concurrent comorbidities (the exceptions are those with amyloid or myeloma). In exceptional circumstances, patients who present at end-stage renal failure with newly diagnosed but terminal cancer may be dialyzed as a humanitarian measure whilst they adjust to their diagnosis.

Infection

Systemic infection is a recognized cause of both acute and chronic renal failure. Moreover, the treatment of renal disease often involves immunomodulation, exposing the patient to increased risk of infection.

Malaria

Plasmodium malariae infection is associated with membranoproliferative glomerulonephritis or membranous nephropathy. Despite treatment of the parasite, the nephropathy is progressive and up to half of these patients

727

reach end-stage renal failure within the following 5 years. *Plasmodium falciparum* has a more acute effect, causing haemolysis, myoglobin release and 'black water fever', resulting in acute tubular necrosis (p. 715). It can cause a temporary glomerulonephritis that responds well to antimalarial therapy.

Hepatitis

Hepatitis B produces a variety of forms of glomerulonephritis including membranoproliferative, IgA and membranous glomerulonephritis. Treatment with interferon-alfa may induce remission. Both immunosuppression and renal transplantation are contraindicated, and the prognosis depends on the histology seen on renal biopsy. Immunization against hepatitis B is encouraged in renal patients before they reach end-stage renal failure. Response to the vaccine is better before renal failure becomes severe. Hepatitis C is associated with cryoglobulinaemia and membranoproliferative glomerulonephritis. Interferon may help but a proportion of patients invariably progress to end-stage renal failure and are not candidates for transplantation.

Endocarditis

Bacterial endocarditis is associated with immune complex-related proliferative glomerulonephritis. This can be complicated by the use of high doses of antibiotics such as gentamicin, which can also cause acute interstitial nephritis. Eradication of the infection should lead to resolution of the renal failure, but sometimes this will not improve until the valve is replaced surgically.

Human immunodeficiency virus (HIV)

Infection with HIV can cause various glomerulonephritides, a more aggressive variation known as human immuno-deficiency virus nephropathy (HIVAN) and rarely IgA or membranoproliferative glomerulonephritis. Glomerulonephritis may be the first presentation of patients with HIV. Patients with human immunodeficiency virus nephropathy are more often young African or Afro-Caribbean men, and account for 1% of patients starting dialysis in the USA. The pathology of glomerulonephritis in HIV is usually due to focal segmental glomerulosclerosis and patients may present with nephrotic syndrome. The cause of human immunodeficiency virus nephropathy is not clear; it may be due to direct damage from the HIV or cytokine release. Patients present with very heavy proteinuria, rapid decline in renal function and progression to dialysis within 6 months. The management is largely with antiretroviral therapy. Patients are not currently suitable for transplantation due to the risks associated with further immunosuppression. Advances in retroviral therapy mean that transplantation may be considered in the future.

SECTION 11.13 Renal and urothelial tumours

This section focuses on benign and primary malignant tumours of the kidney, renal pelvis and ureters (urothelial tumours). Urothelial tumours of the bladder are presented on page 733. Tumours of the kidney are often classified into benign, malignant, inflammatory and vascular (Table 11.23).

Benign renal tumours

Epidemiology

Autopsy studies estimate the incidence of small benign cortical adenomas to be 7–23%; the incidence increases with age with a male predominance. Oncocytomas are rare tumours whose incidence is estimated to be 1 in 1000. Simple renal cysts represent 70% of all benign renal masses.

Pathology

Common benign tumours of the kidneys are simple cysts, oncocytomas and angiomyolipomas. Cysts in the renal parenchyma are the most common benign renal mass lesions. They may be single or multiple and are usually of little concern. An oncocytoma is a well-differentiated, eosinophilic, granular cell renal tumour that arises from the collecting tubules of the nephron. Angiomyolipomas are yellow to grey tumours consisting of unusual blood vessels, adipose tissue and smooth muscle that are associated with tuberous sclerosis.

Less common benign tumours are adenomas (well-circumscribed tumours of clear cells), fibromas (tumours consisting of small cortical capsular nodules) and haemangiopericytomas that may secrete renin and cause hypertension.

Table 11.23	Tumours of the kidney

Benign tumours

Simple cyst (70%)

Adenoma

Angiomyolipoma

Oncocytoma

Fibroma

Pseudotumour (rare)

Reninoma (rare)

Juxtaglomerular tumour (rare)

Malignant tumours

Renal cell carcinoma

Renal urothelial cell carcinoma

Wilms' tumour

Lymphoma

Haemangiopericytoma

Metastatic (lung cancer)

Inflammatory/infective

Bacterial abscess

Tuberculosis

Xanthogranulomatous pyelonephritis

Vascular

Renal artery aneurysm

Arterio-venous malformation

Haemangioma

Haemangiopericytoma

Table 11.24	Radiological appearances and risk of malignancy*	
I	Benign	Simple cyst
II	Probably benign	Septated; minimal calcification; non-enhancing high density or obviously infected
III	Suspicious	Multiloculated haemorrhagic; coarse or pleomorphic calcification; non-enhancing or solid component
IV	Probably malignant	Marginal irregularity and enhancing solid component (renal cell carcinoma)

* From Bosniak MA. The use of the Bosniak classification system for renal cysts and cystic tumors. Journal of Urology 1997; 157: 1852.

Benign renal tumours

Renal cell carcinoma

Urothelial carcinoma of the upper urinary tract

Urethral tumours

Clinical features

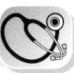

Most benign renal tumours are asymptomatic and detected incidentally. Occasionally hormone-secreting tumours such as renin-secreting juxtaglomerular tumour may present with hypertension, typically in young patients.

Investigations

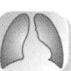

Imaging is the mainstay in diagnosing and differentiating benign from malignant renal tumours. Surgery is indicated for large tumours. A tissue diagnosis may be sought in patients who are infirm or those with poor renal reserve, but carries a risk of tumour seeding along the biopsy port and the possibility of coexisting renal cell carcinoma within the same kidney.

Ultrasound of the kidney

Ultrasound is effective at distinguishing cystic from solid masses. Benign simple cysts appear as smooth well-defined round or oval-shaped masses, with no internal echoes.

CT of the abdomen

CT allows accurate distinction of benign and malignant renal cysts according to Bosniak's classification (Table 11.24).

Management

Conservative management

Simple cysts and small (<4 cm) angiomyolipomas are benign and do not require further treatment. They may be observed radiologically and symptomatically; intervention is indicated if tumours grow or become symptomatic.

Surgical excision

Surgical excision is indicated for symptomatic masses, suspected renal adenomas larger than 3 cm and suspicious oncocytomas. 'Nephron-sparing' surgery (e.g. partial nephrectomy or wedge resection) is preferred for benign tumours. Symptomatic simple renal cysts can be treated by aspiration and sclerotherapy. Occasionally renal embolization may be required to stem bleeding from a large haemorrhagic angiomyolipoma.

Prognosis

Most benign renal tumours run an indolent course. Observation for symptoms and growth is all that is required. Prognosis is favourable unless the tumour undergoes malignant transformation. A large (>3 cm) solid renal cortical adenoma requires excision as it may have foci of renal cell carcinoma with metastatic potential.

Renal cell carcinoma

Epidemiology

Renal cell carcinoma accounts for 3% of all adult malignancies. The highest rate is found in North America and Scandinavia where the incidence is approximately 5–10 per 100 000 per year.[1] It is one and a half times more common in men and the peak age of presentation is 50–60 years.

Pathology

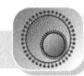

Renal cell carcinomas most commonly arise from the proximal convoluted tubule (85%). The solid–cystic round tumours are typically unilateral, as bilateral lesions occur in less than 2%. The pathological subtypes are listed in Table 11.25.

The risk factors for the development of renal cell carcinoma are smoking, obesity and acquired cystic disease. In addition, genetic predisposition (3p26 deletion) and familial forms (von Hippel–Lindau, hereditary papillary renal cell carcinoma) exist.

Scope of disease

Local

Increase in the size of the primary tumour can result in an abdominal mass. Infiltration into the blood vessels can cause haematuria, and the large size can also cause abdominal pain. Local infiltration can occur up the inferior vena cava leading to vena cava obstruction and also into the left renal vein, obstructing the flow of the testicular vein and resulting in the formation of a varicocele.

Metastatic

Metastases occur in up to 40% of patients at presentation and are classically to the lungs (causing dyspnoea), bone (pathological fractures) and brain (focal neurological symptoms).

Paraneoplastic

Associated paraneoplastic syndromes include polycythaemia (erythropoietin production), hypercalcaemia and Cushing's syndrome (Table 11.26). Hepatic necrosis may occur in the absence of metastases (Stauffer's syndrome), which usually improves following nephrectomy. Persistent fever may also be the initial presenting complaint.

Clinical features

Approximately 60% of organ-confined renal cancers are asymptomatic and discovered incidentally. The classic triad of pain, haematuria and an abdominal mass occurs in less than 10% and usually indicates advanced disease. Pyrexia and malaise are common symptoms.

Table 11.25	Pathological subtypes of renal cell carcinoma
Clear cell (80%)	
Papillary (14%)	
Sarcomatoid (most aggressive)	
Chromophobe (4%)	
Oncocytic (2%)	
Collecting duct (<1%)	

Table 11.26	Paraneoplastic manifestations of renal cell carcinoma
Secreted hormone	**Clinical feature**
Prolactin	Gynaecomastia
Adrenocorticotrophic hormone	Cushing's syndrome
Parathyroid hormone	Hypercalcaemia
Erythropoietin	Polycythaemia
Renin	Hypertension

The frequencies of the presenting clinical features are haematuria (50%), pain (40%), abdominal mass (30%), hypertension (22%), a paraneoplastic syndrome (10%) and an acute varicocele (2%).

On examination an abdominal mass may be palpable in the flanks and, rarely, a varicocele may be present. Signs of advanced disease include caput medusae and bilateral lower limb oedema from inferior vena cava obstruction.

Initial investigations

Full blood count

Anaemia is a common finding, and polycythaemia is a rare paraneoplastic feature of renal cell carcinoma.

Markers of inflammation

The erythrocyte sedimentation rate (ESR) is usually raised in advanced disease.

Urea and electrolytes

The renal function is usually preserved with normal urea and creatinine.

Liver profile

Mild abnormalities in the liver profile are common.

Urinalysis

Dipstick testing of the urine may reveal blood.

Intravenous urogram

An IVU may reveal a distortion in the outline of the kidney or calyceal pattern.

Abdominal ultrasound

An ultrasound scan can distinguish between a solid and a cystic lesion (Fig. 11.13). Solid lesions are more likely to be associated with malignancy, and an ultrasound scan is also able to assess for renal vein and inferior vena cava involvement.

Further investigations

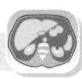

Chest X-ray

A plain chest film is a useful screening investigation for pulmonary metastases but CT is more sensitive.

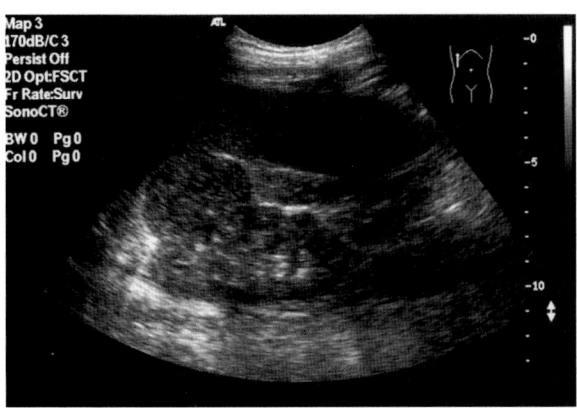

Fig. 11.13 Renal cell carcinoma. A lobulated lesion is seen on the ultrasound scan

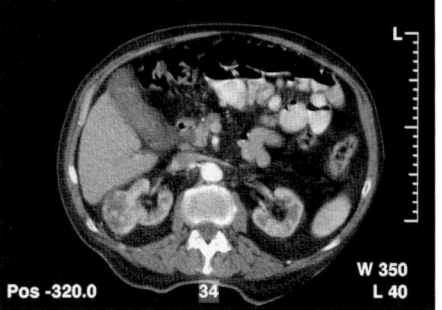

Fig. 11.14 CT of renal cell carcinoma. The lobulated lesion is visible in the right kidney

CT of the abdomen and thorax

CT of the abdomen can evaluate lesions that are equivocal on initial investigation. The malignant risk of renal cyst can be assessed with Bosniak's classification (p. 729). CT is also the investigation of choice to stage a renal cell carcinoma (Fig. 11.14). Preoperative needle biopsy is not recommended, due to the theoretical risk of tumour seeding along the needle tract and possibility of false negative biopsy due to sampling error.

TNM staging of renal cell carcinoma

T—Primary tumour

Tx	Primary tumour cannot be assessed
T0	No evidence of primary tumour
T1	limited to the kidney; <7 cm
T2	limited to the kidney; >7 cm
T3	Confined to Gerota's fascia, invades into adrenal or perinephric tissue, extends into renal vein or inferior vena cava
T4	Beyond Gerota's fascia

N—Nodal involvement

N1	Single regional lymph node involvement
N2	More than one regional node involvement

M—Metastasis

M0	No distant metastases
M1	Distant metastases

MRI of the abdomen

MRI is superior to CT for assessing renal vein and inferior vena cava involvement in lesions greater than 3 cm.

Surgical management

Nephrectomy

Surgical excision (Fig. 11.15) is the only curative option for organ-confined renal cell carcinoma and is offered to all patients who are fit enough for surgery. Radical (curative) surgery removes the mass, the perinephric fat and Gerota's fascia. Partial nephrectomy ('nephron-sparing' surgery) may be feasible in selected cases (e.g. polar tumours, solitary kidney).

The transperitoneal anterior approach is commonly used to facilitate early ligation of the artery and vein in large hypervascular tumours. The patient is positioned supine and the kidney approached by a transverse abdominal incision. The artery and vein are ligated and the kidney or part of the kidney is excised (partial nephrectomy).

Supradiaphragmatic caval extension requires cardiopulmonary bypass for complete excision, and adrenalectomy is indicated for upper pole tumours or if there is involvement of the adrenal glands.

RECENT ADVANCES

Intraoperative ultrasound may identify multifocal tumour warranting a radical nephrectomy. Laparoscopic nephrectomy has become the operation of choice.

Medical management

In general, radiotherapy, chemotherapy and immune therapy are offered to patients with metastatic disease. In selected cases pulmonary metastases have regressed following excision of the primary tumour.

Radiotherapy

In patients with metastatic disease, radiotherapy may reduce local tumour size and delay local recurrence. It is effective for palliation of skeletal metastases, but no survival benefit has been shown.

Chemotherapy

Although renal cell carcinoma is considered chemoresistant, the use of α-interferon, 5-fluorouracil and interleukin-2 has been reported.[9]

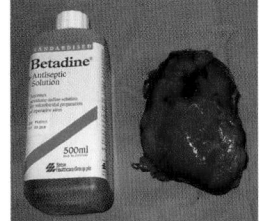

Fig. 11.15 Excised specimen of renal cell carcinoma.

731

Immune therapy

Immune therapy relies upon host immune factors modifying the cancer. Interferon-alfa, interleukin-2 and lymphocyte activated killer cells (LAK) have all produced promising results in a clinical trial setting.[2]

Prognosis

The main prognostic factors in renal cell carcinoma are stage, size, nuclear grade, cell type, vena caval or renal vein involvement, renal pelvic invasion and whether the mass is symptomatic. In patients with metastatic disease, a solitary isolated pulmonary metastasis in fit patients can carry a 5-year survival of almost 70% after complete resection, whilst for those with disseminated metastatic disease a 20% 5-year survival can be expected.

Following radical nephrectomy, overall survival is approximately 60%. Five-year survival is approximately 85% for stage 1 disease, 80% for stage 2, 35% for stage 3 and 10% for stage 4 disease.

REFERENCES

(1) *Landis SH, Murray T, Bolden S, Wingo PA. Cancer statistics: 1999. CA Cancer Journal for Clinicians 1999; 49: 8–31.*
(2) *Yang JC, Rosenberg SA. An ongoing prospective randomized comparison of interleukin-2 regimens for the treatment of metastatic renal cell cancer. Cancer Journal from Scientific American 1997; 3(suppl): 579–584.*

Urothelial carcinoma of the upper urinary tract

Tumours of the urothelium can occur anywhere from the renal pelvis to the urethra. This section deals with urothelial tumours in the renal pelvis and ureters.

Epidemiology

Renal pelvic and ureteric urothelial cancers account for 5% of all upper urinary tract malignancies. Urothelial carcinoma is 3 times more common in men with a peak age of presentation between 60 and 70 years.

Pathology

The majority of ureteral cancers arise in the distal one third and up to 50% are associated with synchronous bladder cancer. The risk factors for upper tract urothelial tumours are the same as for bladder cancer (p. 749), with the addition of Balkan nephropathy. The histological subtypes are transitional cell (>90%), squamous (5–10%) and primary adenocarcinoma (<1%).

Clinical features

The most common symptom is frank haematuria (80%) or flank pain (30%). Less common symptoms include dysuria

and bladder outflow obstruction. On examination, a palpable mass invariably indicates advanced disease.

Investigations
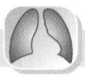

The key investigations of urothelial tumours are urinalysis, cystoscopy and IVU.

Urinalysis

Urine analysis for microscopy and cytology is important, as microscopic haematuria may be present. Malignant cells may be seen on cytology. In addition, concomitant urinary tract infections are common.

Intravenous urogram

An IVU is the investigation of choice. A filling defect or obstruction (20%) is readily visible, and rarely more than one filling defect is seen (synchronous and metachronous tumours).

Cystoscopy, ureteroscopy and retrograde pyelography

Cystoscopy and retrograde pyelography evaluates the bladder, images the lower ureter and allows samples to be retrieved (brush biopsy) for histology. In addition, ureteroscopy provides direct visualization and formal biopsy of equivocal lesions.

Abdominal CT/MRI

Abdominal CT provides the necessary information for staging, and MRI provides better resolution for soft tissue changes in tumours close to the bony pelvis. More recently CT has established a place in primary diagnosis as well as local staging.

Management

Radical nephro-ureterectomy

Radical nephro-ureterectomy is the treatment of choice in view of the multifocal nature of this disease and difficulties associated with follow-up of segmental resection. The surgical approach may require two incisions, in the loin and in the iliac fossa; however, the nephrectomy may be performed laparoscopically for renal pelvic tumours, the ureteric orifice can be resected cystoscopically, to detach the ureter from the bladder. During nephrectomy the distal ureter is 'plucked' from the perivesical tissue.

Segmental resection

Segmental resection or distal ureteral resection and a Boari flap (a fold of bladder is used to create a tube to act as a substitute for the distal ureter) or psoas hitch may be an option for a patient with a solitary kidney. This more conservative approach may also be adopted in high-risk patients with low-grade tumours.

Laser or diathermy ablation

This is a minimally invasive option in selected patients. Minimally invasive treatment (e.g. endoscopic ablation) may be preferred in patients who are a poor anaesthetic risk or in those with poor renal reserve (e.g. solitary kidney). Regular uretero-renoscopy and laser (Nd:YAG) or diathermy ablation can delay progression and relieve symptoms but may cause ureteric stricturing.

Systemic chemotherapy
A palliative option for advanced disease is a systemic chemotherapeutic regimen such as M-VAC (Adriamycin, cisplatin, methotrexate and vinblastine).

Topical chemotherapy
A further palliative option is topically chemotherapeutic agents. Mitomycin can be directly instilled into the collecting system, either percutaneously or via a retrograde catheter.

Radiotherapy
A further palliative option is radiotherapy. This may reduce local recurrence rates and palliate symptoms, but it has little effect on overall survival.

Prognosis
The overall 5-year survival is 100% for T1, 80% for T2 and 30% for T3 disease. Despite systemic chemotherapy only 5% of patients with metastatic disease survive 5 years. High-grade tumours carry a worse prognosis.

Urethral tumours
Primary urethral malignancies are rare. Most are squamous carcinomas arising secondary to squamous metaplasia associated with long-standing stricture disease. Transitional cell tumours of the urethra usually arise in association with direct invasion or tumour seeding from bladder cancer. The most common symptom is bleeding per urethra, which may discolour urine or semen. Advanced disease may cause urethral obstruction and urinary retention. Treatment involves a combination of surgical excision, radiotherapy and chemotherapy. However, many of these tumours are locally invasive or have metastasized at the time of presentation, and the prognosis is often poor.

SECTION 11.14 Renovascular disease

Atheromatous renovascular disease
Renal vessel disease occurs as part of generalized atherosclerosis (Fig. 11.16), and is an increasingly recognized cause of chronic renal impairment in the elderly.

Epidemiology
Renovascular disease usually affects people over the age of 50. It accounts for up to 30% of end-stage renal failure in patients over 60 years old, but may be silent or clinically insignificant.[1] It is often found incidentally when patients undergo angiography for extra-renal reasons such as iliac vessel imaging.

Pathology
The risk factors for atheromatous renovascular disease are those of atherosclerosis; the disease is more common in smokers, diabetics and patients with hyperlipidaemia. Patients often have coexistent hypertension, ischaemic heart disease and peripheral vascular disease.

The site of stenosis is often the proximal renal artery, within 1 cm of the junction with the aorta (the ostium). Once blood flow to the kidney is reduced below the limit of auto-regulation, the kidneys start to atrophy. Chronic progression results in a shrunken small kidney with scarring and fibrosis. Once there is 60% narrowing of the internal diameter of the renal artery, the rate of renal artery occlusion is 5% per year.

Scope of disease
'Flash' pulmonary oedema is a dramatic presentation with dyspnoea and hypotension developing overnight, possibly due to a surge of renin and angiotensin. Renal artery stenosis is also a secondary cause of hypertension.

Clinical features
The majority of patients have asymptomatic disease. As the disease progresses, declining renal function and mild proteinuria are common. Presentation with flash pulmonary oedema is rare.

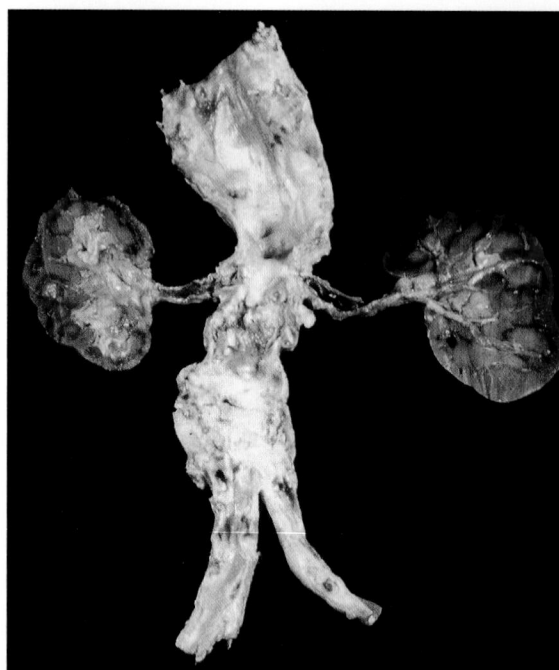

Fig. 11.16 Pathology specimen of renal artery stenosis. The diffuse involvement of the aorta and branches are visible as part of a generalized atherosclerotic process.

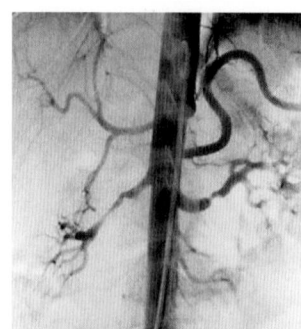

Fig. 11.17 Angiogram showing bilateral renal artery stenosis.

Examination may reveal evidence of widespread vascular disease such as abdominal bruits or loss of pulses. Hypertension may be evident.

 CLINICAL ALERT

Initiation of ACE inhibitor therapy is detrimental in renal artery stenosis. ACE inhibitors cause vasodilatation of the afferent vessels. As patients rely on the internal renal gradient to perfuse their kidneys, starting ACE inhibitors abolishes this gradient, dropping perfusion pressure profoundly.

Initial investigations

Urinalysis
Urine dipstick testing may reveal non-specific mild proteinuria.

Urea and electrolytes
Serum urea and creatinine are often elevated.

Ultrasound of the kidneys
The kidneys may be asymmetrical in size if one is affected more than the other. Alternatively, both may be small.

Further investigations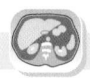

MRI
MR angiography is the screening investigation of choice for renovascular disease. It is safe and avoids the use of potentially nephrotoxic contrast.

Renal artery angiogram
A renal artery angiogram (Fig. 11.17) is usually performed as part of an intervention (angioplasty or stenting).

Medical management

Address underlying risk factors
Hypertension and hyperlipidaemia should be controlled.

Angioplasty or stenting
The aims of angioplasty or stenting are to halt the decline in renal function, cure the refractory hypertension and prevent the need for dialysis. Angioplasty of a single functioning kidney with proximal renal artery stenosis is a very high-risk procedure, but may be indicated in the presence of rapid decline in glomerular filtration rate, flash pulmonary oedema or severe hypertension.

Despite angioplasty, only 25% will improve their serum creatinine and it is rare for patients to improve sufficiently to stop requiring renal replacement therapy. Complications include cholesterol emboli and dissection of the renal artery. Re-stenosis occurs in up to 30% of patients by 2 years.

Surgical management

Revascularization
Surgical revascularization of renal vessels is associated with a high complication rate, and improvement in renal function occurs in only 25% of the patients.[2]

Prognosis

The prognosis of patients with renal artery stenosis is worse than that of the 'normal' dialysis population, with a 5-year survival of 18%. This is likely to be due to widespread atheroma resulting in increased cardiac deaths.

REFERENCES

(1) *van Ampting JM, Penne EL, Beek FJ, Koomans HA, Boer WH, Beutler JJ. Prevalence of atherosclerotic renal artery stenosis in patients starting dialysis. Nephrology Dialysis Transplantation 2003; 18: 1147–1151.*
(2) *Dejani H, Eisen TD, Finkelstein FO. Revascularization of renal artery stenosis in patients with renal insufficiency. American Journal of Kidney Diseases 2000; 36: 752–758.*

Fibromuscular dysplasia

Fibromuscular dysplasia is a rare form of renal vascular disease (about 1% of all cases). It occurs in young patients and is 7 times more common in women. Patients present with severe hypertension. Angiography demonstrates 'beading' of the renal artery and angioplasty is very successful in controlling hypertension.

Cholesterol emboli

Arterial interventions (e.g. angiography and vascular surgery) can dislodge atherosclerotic plaques leading to a shower of microemboli that settle in small vessels, including the renal vessels, resulting in a reduced glomerular filtration rate. Patients with systemic cholesterol emboli may present with acute renal failure and livedo reticularis. Extra-renal features include abdominal pain, amaurosis fugax, transient ischaemic attacks, skin ulceration and nodules. The diagnosis is suggested by the history, eosinophilia and eosinophiluria, and is confirmed by the cholesterol emboli in renal, muscle or skin biopsies. Treatment is that of the underlying cause. The renal failure may be insidious and irreversible.

Haemodialysis

Peritoneal dialysis

| SECTION 11.15 | **Renal replacement therapy** |

Indications for renal replacement therapy

Patients with renal failure can cope very well with a gradual drop in the glomerular filtration rate, but once it falls below 25 mL/min, renal replacement should be planned, and when it becomes less than 10 mL/min, dialysis is necessary. Renal replacement may need to be started earlier if fluid overload or hyperkalaemia cannot be managed medically, or if uraemic symptoms are unbearable. In general, patients with diabetes tend to need to start renal replacement earlier due to nausea and fluid overload. The underlying disease of patients commencing renal replacement therapy is summarized in Figure 11.18.

Contraindications for renal replacement therapy

Not every patient with end-stage renal failure is a candidate for dialysis. Frail elderly patients with significant comorbid conditions may not be fit enough for dialysis, and some patients may decline the offer of dialysis. Coexisting cognitive impairment due to dementia or psychiatric conditions may make compliance with strict dialysis regimens very difficult. Severe peripheral vascular disease or heart failure may make the actual process of dialysis difficult to perform or tolerate. The level of support also influences the decision for dialysis for elderly patients. Without a good overall social support network, dialysis may not be practicable. Patients in whom dialysis may be inappropriate should still receive therapy to improve their symptoms and quality of life.

Types of renal replacement therapy

The three modalities of renal replacement are haemodialysis, peritoneal dialysis and renal transplantation. An integrated approach is taken, as most patients use more than one modality. Transplantation is discussed on page 738.

Withdrawal of renal replacement

At some point, withdrawal of dialysis may be appropriate in some patients, but it is best managed using a multidisciplinary approach and involving the patient and family

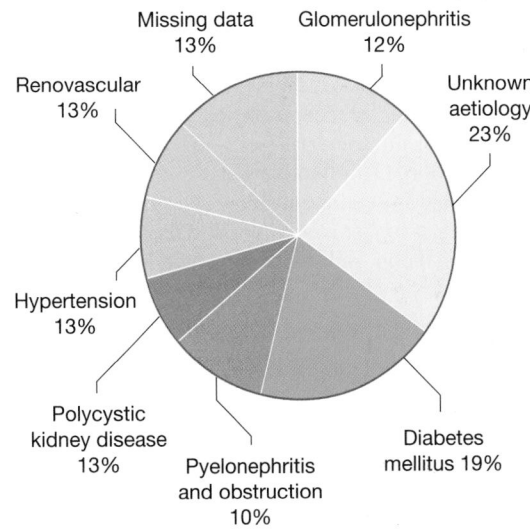

Fig. 11.18 Underlying causes for starting renal replacement therapy in the UK.

or care-givers. Withdrawal of dialysis accounts for up to 20% of dialysis patient deaths in the USA. Palliative care should be provided, with the involvement of hospice staff if possible, to achieve good symptom control.

Prognosis

The prognosis of patients on renal replacement therapy depends on comorbidities and age.

Haemodialysis

Haemodialysis treats nearly 15 000 people in the UK: i.e. 400 per million of population. The median age of patients on dialysis is 64 years. Haemodialysis is the most commonly used dialysis technique in an emergency.

Haemodialysis works by pumping the patient's blood through a dialyser, removing solute and excess fluid. The dialyser has a surface area of 0.8–2.1 m^2, allowing diffusion of molecules. Small molecules such as urea are easier to clear than large ones like β_2-microglobulin. In a standard dialysis regimen, the patient dialyses for 3–4 hours, 3 times every week. Ultrafiltration removes fluid over this time, at a rate of about 1 litre per hour. Removal of volumes greater than 3 litres per session can result in hypotension and collapse. The acidosis is corrected by bicarbonate in the dialysate; pre-set sodium and potassium levels are programmed to correct the patient's electrolyte abnormalities.

Most haemodialysis is done in a hospital setting (Fig. 11.19). Home haemodialysis is possible with the training of motivated patients. Solute clearance is better with more frequent dialysis, even if the sessions are shorter. The role of daily dialysis is being reviewed since there is evidence that it is associated with improved prognosis. However, this frequency is only possible with home haemodialysis, and it is more expensive due to the costs of the materials used. Longer (>6 hours) dialysis sessions are thought to improve hypertension and fluid control, but implementation may be constrained by available resources.

The patients require 'access' to connect them to the dialysis machine. In an emergency setting, a large-bore dual lumen central line is used, usually via the jugular or femoral vein. Long-term, an arterio-venous fistula (Fig. 11.20), formed as a minor operation, allows for better quality dialysis (due to higher blood flow, and thus larger volumes of processed blood) and avoids implanted foreign materials.

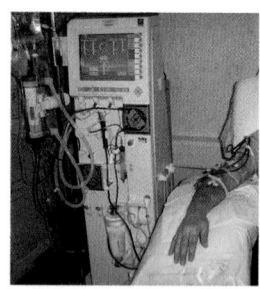

Fig. 11.19 Patient receiving haemodialysis.

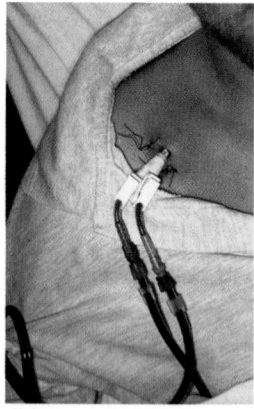

Fig. 11.21 A tunnelled haemodialysis line.

If there is no suitable site for an arterio-venous fistula, a polytetrafluoroethylene (PTFE) graft can be used as a bridge. Patients with very poor blood vessels may need to have tunnelled dialysis lines (Fig. 11.21) inserted (like Hickman lines) but they have a higher incidence of infection and poorer blood flows.

The complications of haemodialysis are listed in Table 11.27.

Continuous venovenous haemofiltration

Continuous venovenous haemofiltration (CVVH) is a continuous form of dialysis often employed in the ITU. This relies on convection rather than diffusion and is a gentler process. Haemodialysis requires a systolic blood pressure of >80–100 mmHg whereas CVVH can be performed whilst the patient is hypotensive or receiving inotropes.

Haemodiafiltration

A combination of convection and diffusion is used in haemodiafiltration. This can be carried out on a standard renal unit, not just in the ITU, and is invaluable in haemodynamically unstable patients.

Plasma exchange

Plasma exchange uses dialysis machines but does not clear solute. Instead, the circulating plasma is removed and replaced with fresh frozen plasma or similar colloid. This is in an effort to remove large molecules responsible for disease states such as thrombotic thrombocytopenic purpura, Goodpasture's disease, cryoglobulinaemia and Guillain–Barré syndrome.

Peritoneal dialysis

In the UK, approximately 5500 patients are currently receiving continuous ambulatory peritoneal dialysis (CAPD) or automated peritoneal dialysis (APD); their median age is 58 years.

Peritoneal dialysis uses the peritoneal membrane to clear solute and fluid by diffusion and convection. Ultrafiltration is manipulated by varying the concentrations of glucose in the dialysis fluid. A catheter (Tenckhoff catheter) is inserted into the peritoneal space to allow fluid to run in and out of the peritoneum in a sterile manner, and can be used 1–2 weeks after insertion. Earlier usage can be associated with leakage at the insertion site.

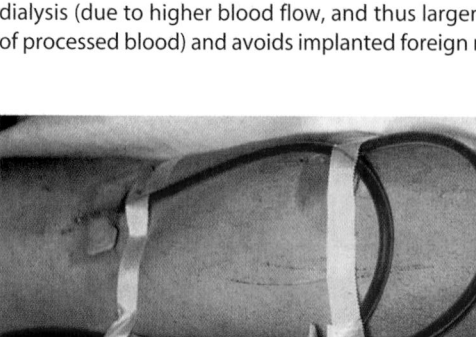

Fig. 11.20 Vascular access for haemodialysis is achieved via the arterio-venous fistula in the forearm.

Table 11.27	Complications of haemodialysis
Air embolism	
Bleeding	

Adverse effects of haemodialysis
   Muscle cramps
   Headaches
   Restless legs	

Vascular access
   Non-functioning fistulae
   Stenoses of fistulae
   Fistulae or PTFE graft infection
   No further suitable sites for vascular access	

Infection
   Systemic infection (*S. aureus* septicaemia)
   Endocarditis	

Social/psychological Difficulties with employment	

Patients with poor vision can perform peritoneal dialysis, but manual dexterity and a clean environment are necessary to perform the exchanges. Intra-abdominal sepsis is a contraindication for peritoneal dialysis due to the infection risk.

Continuous ambulatory peritoneal dialysis (CAPD)

CAPD involves 3–5 exchanges of peritoneal dialysis fluid daily by the patient (Fig. 11.22). The dialysate is left in the peritoneal cavity for several hours, then drained and replaced by fresh peritoneal dialysis fluid, so that dialysate is continuously present in the peritoneum. The exchange volumes used are between 1.5 and 3 litres each time, usually 2 litres.

Automated peritoneal dialysis (APD)

In APD, a machine is used to perform the exchanges automatically overnight. These exchanges are more rapid, each lasting 1–3 hours. Patients may require an additional exchange in situ during the day for extra solute clearance.

Complications of peritoneal dialysis

Peritoneal dialysis predisposes patients to peritonitis. The usual organism is coagulase-negative *Staphylococcus aureus* from skin contamination or exit site infection. This is treated by adding antibiotics directly to the dialysis fluid (intraperitoneal delivery). More severe infections occur with *Staphylococcus aureus* and Gram-negative organisms. Peritoneal dialysis may need to be temporarily stopped whilst a patient is infected, switching to haemodialysis. Repeated infections are associated with loss of diffusion capacity, and patients may need to change over to haemodialysis long term. Pseudomonal and fungal infections are very difficult to clear and invariably require removal of the catheter. Infection at the Tenckhoff exit site predisposes patients to peritonitis and can also be very resistant to treatment.

Native urine production contributes to solute and fluid clearance. Residual renal function tends to decrease over time so it can be difficult to ensure adequate dialysis with peritoneal dialysis if the patient has a large muscle mass and little urine output.

If peritoneal dialysis fluid is draining poorly, it is most often due to constipation. If drainage is still inadequate after laxatives, an abdominal film is required to screen for the position of the catheter tip, as it may move to an inappropriate site such as resting under the diaphragm, occluding the lumen. Surgery may be necessary to correct the position.

In patients with inguinal hernias, dialysate fluid may drain into the scrotum, which becomes grossly enlarged. Surgical correction is usually required. More rarely, fluid may track upwards into the pleural space. The high glucose concentration distinguishes this from other causes of pleural effusions.

Peritoneal dialysis has been thought to be a 'temporary' form of dialysis due to the limited lifespan of the peritoneal membrane. Some patients remain on peritoneal dialysis longer than 10 years, but the overall technique survival is less than 50% at 5 years. Approximately 38% stop dialysis due to infection, and 20% because of the inability to cope.

RECENT ADVANCES

New peritoneal dialysates are now available. The presence of glucose macromolecules (icodextrin) helps to achieve ultrafiltration. Amino acids in peritoneal dialysis fluid have a role in nutrition, and bicarbonate/lactate-buffered fluids may help patients with severe pain perform peritoneal dialysis exchanges.

Haemodialysis

Peritoneal dialysis

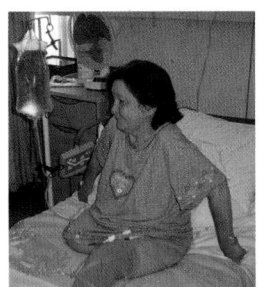

Fig. 11.22 A patient receiving peritoneal dialysis.

Renal transplantation

Indications

Patients reaching end-stage renal failure and needing renal replacement will usually be considered for a renal transplant. Screening for contraindications means that only a minority of patients on renal replacement are considered suitable recipients. Current contraindications include active malignancy, chronic sepsis and current infection (hepatitis B, hepatitis C, HIV).

Patient preparation

Patients must be suitable for a general anaesthetic and may need invasive cardiological tests prior to going onto the transplant list. A proportion of patients require angioplasty or coronary artery bypass surgery. End-stage renal failure patients have accelerated atherosclerosis and, since the transplant is anastomosed to the iliac vessels, Doppler scans or angiography of pelvic vessels may be needed to ensure that this is feasible.

Malignancy must be excluded: patients usually have to wait at least 3 years after curative cancer treatment to be considered for transplantation, since the immunosuppressive drugs promote neoplasia.

Patients should be counselled about the potential risks associated with transplantation and understand that a transplant is not a 'cure' but another form of renal replacement. Ideally this should be explained at this stage, rather than when a potential transplant has been identified, as patients may not think clearly due to the excitement of the situation.

Because of the national shortage of cadaveric transplants, live-related donation is encouraged. Family members (usually siblings and parents) may donate a kidney. There is extensive workup of the donor beforehand to check both the suitability of the kidney and the donor's health. Donation is a major operation and donors are monitored long term in case of potential future morbidity associated with a single kidney.

Procedure

Once a compatible organ is found, the recipient is brought to hospital urgently. There is an acceptable 'cold ischaemia' time, i.e. time from removal of the organ to connection to the recipient, of up to 30 hours but it is preferable that this time is as short as possible as it has a significant impact on long-term graft function.

The operation takes $2\frac{1}{2}$ or more hours, usually under general anaesthetic. The organ is transported in preservative solution at 4°C to prolong its viability. Before theatre, suitability of the renal vessels for anastomosis is checked. Multiple renal vessels make the operation technically more difficult and may lead to postoperative complications.

The renal vein and artery are anastomosed to the iliac artery and vein, and the ureter is anastomosed to the bladder, often with a J stent to prevent ureteric obstruction. This stent is removed postoperatively via cystoscopy once graft function is established.

Post-procedure care

The bladder is catheterized, and antibiotics are given along with the first immunosuppression, usually intravenous methylprednisolone. Prophylactic antivirals and antibiotics such as ganciclovir and co-trimoxazole are administered to prevent opportunistic infections

Patients do not necessarily need to be in the HDU or ITU unless there are complications. However, electrolytes (daily) and fluid status (hourly urine measurements) are monitored closely. CVP readings allow accurate estimation of fluid, with care being taken to avoid dehydration. Hyperkalaemia postoperatively is due to the muscle damage incurred with surgery releasing potassium; steroids also cause hyperkalaemia. Patients may need haemodialysis immediately postoperatively. The peritoneal cavity is not routinely opened during transplantation so it may still be possible to perform peritoneal dialysis as required.

The function of the native kidneys may cease following surgery because of the anaesthetic and peroperative hypotension. Delayed function is common, especially if there is prolonged cold ischaemia, and the patient may remain oliguric or anuric for days or even weeks.

Complications

Up to 50% have an episode of acute rejection, presenting as a decline in renal function, tenderness over the graft or a decrease in urine output. The treatment is high-dose methylprednisolone (0.5 g i.v. daily for 3 consecutive days) and an increase in the usual immunosuppression. Patients are more susceptible to opportunistic infection such as cytomegalovirus and *Pneumocystis carinii*, but more commonly have standard infections such as urinary tract infections (especially until the stent is removed) or pneumonias.

High-dose steroids may render a patient diabetic, and insulin is usually required rather than oral hypoglycaemic agents. Most patients are hypertensive post transplantation. Blood pressure control is essential for maintaining graft function. Patients who develop hyperlipidaemia will require statin therapy and dietary advice. Even when there is a favourable tissue cross-match, graft function may still decline over time. This has been attributed to the process termed 'chronic rejection' or ciclosporin nephrotoxicity. Some primary renal diseases may recur in the transplant with variable outcome. IgA recurs but rarely interferes with the long-term graft function, whereas focal segmental glomerulosclerosis can return within days leading to graft failure despite immunosuppression.

Immunosuppression is required for life, and involves a combination of prednisolone, ciclosporin and azathioprine. Newer agents such as mycophenolate mofetil (MMF), tacrolimus and sirolimus have expanded the scope of immunosuppression available. With time, the doses of agents can be reduced, and some units are keen to stop steroids altogether or cut the regimen to two drugs rather than three.

Prognosis

There is still a reduction in long-term survival despite normal graft function. One-year graft survival has improved to 85%, but death with a functioning graft (54% of all renal transplants lost) is a significant problem, mostly from cardiovascular disease rather than from the renal failure itself.

SECTION 11.17   Urinary tract infection

Bacteria may enter the urinary tract either by ascending via the urethra or descending via the kidney or through a fistulous tract to another hollow viscus (e.g. colo-vesical fistula). Urine flow and the protective nature of the urothelium act as a barrier to infecting organisms. As a result, in the normal patient, the proximal urethra and stored urine is sterile. The pathogens responsible for ascending bacterial infections possess adherin and digestive enzymes, which allow adhesion to the urothelium. This is the basis of bacterial virulence.

Bacterial cystitis

Although a urinary tract infection can occur anywhere from the renal pelvis, ureters, bladder to urethra, the term 'urinary tract infection' is often loosely used to refer to bacterial cystitis.

Epidemiology

The incidence of urinary tract infection increases with age, and is approximately 5 times more common in women than in men. Half of the female population will experience a urinary tract infection in their lifetime. The incidence in men is less than 1% per year until the age of 50 when benign prostatic hyperplasia develops.

Pathology

Simple bacterial urinary tract infection is usually the result of bacteria ascending through the urethra from the perineum. Women are more commonly affected due to the shorter female urethra, which is more readily contaminated by perineal flora. Other risk factors are structural abnormalities of the urinary tract (neuropathic bladder), urinary retention (benign prostatic hyperplasia) and instrumentation of the urethra.

The most common infecting organisms are bacteria such as *E. coli, S. saprophyticus, Proteus* species and *Klebsiella*. Rare causes include tuberculosis, anaerobes and *Neisseria gonorrhoeae*.

Scope of disease

Complications of bacterial cystitis include systemic sepsis and ascending infection to the kidneys (pyelonephritis).

Clinical features

Classic symptoms are frequency, urgency and dysuria. There may be suprapubic pain and occasional haematuria. With severe infection, patients may be unwell with fever and rigors. Clinical examination is often unremarkable and a detailed clinical assessment should attempt to identify any underlying cause.

Initial investigations

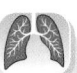

Urinalysis
Urine produced is 'dipped' for urinalysis (p. 688). A positive result for blood, protein, white cells and nitrites is strongly suggestive of active infection.

Midstream specimen of urine
A formal MSU should be sent for microscopy culture and sensitivity (MC&S). This allows bacteria to be cultured and antibacterial sensitivities obtained. The clinician should be aware that a negative urine culture does not exclude a urinary tract infection, and a partially treated infection may not always produce a positive culture.

Further investigations

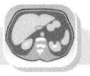

Further investigations are usually required for men who present with urinary tract infection (atypical population) to screen for structural abnormalities and for patients with severe infection to screen for complications.

Full blood count

Infection is often associated with a leukocytosis and neutrophilia.

Urea and electrolytes

Serum urea and creatinine allows an estimation of global renal function, which may become impaired with pyonephrosis.

Plain abdominal film

An abdominal kidneys, ureters and bladder (KUB) film is performed if urinary calculi are suspected. Struvite calculi are classically associated with urinary tract infections.

Abdominal ultrasound

Ultrasound is a non-invasive test that is used to identify structural anatomical abnormalities predisposing to urinary tract infection. Renal ultrasound identifies the presence of hydronephrosis and renal cortical thickness. Hydroureter can also be seen and often the ureter can be traced to the level of obstruction. Scanning the bladder can identify some bladder tumours (see urothelial tumours, p. 732) and can accurately estimate post-micturition residual urine.

Flexible cystoscopy

Flexible cytoscopy is indicated for urinary tract infections in men and recurrent infections in women. Those associated with haematuria require cystoscopic evaluation to rule out an underlying urothelial malignancy or fistula.

Initial management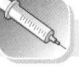

Patient education

Patients should be advised to increase fluid intake to promote hydrostatic clearance of the bladder. Alkalinizing the urine with bicarbonate of soda or intake of cranberry juice may be effective in preventing bacterial adherence.

Medical management

Empirical antibiotics

A short course of antibiotics (3–5 days) may be started without awaiting the results of MSU. Amoxicillin is a useful initial antibiotic that can be modified according to culture results. Trimethoprim is another antibiotic that may be prescribed in areas with a high frequency of penicillin-resistant organisms. Ideally, the MSU should be repeated following treatment to confirm eradication of the infection.

Maintenance antibiotics

Patients with recurrent or persistent urinary tract infection of no discernible anatomical cause may require long-term low-dose antibiotics (e.g. trimethoprim 100 mg od for 3 months) to reduce the bacterial load and prevent clinical infections.

Prognosis

The majority of patients respond to a short course of antibiotics. Approximately 25% will develop recurrent infection.

Acute pyelonephritis

Epidemiology

The incidence of pyelonephritis is 117 per 100 000 women and 24 per 100 000 men per year.[1] It is approximately 5 times more common in women, and the epidemiology reflects that of bacterial cystitis.

Pathology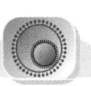

Infecting organisms colonizing the bladder may ascend the urinary tract to infect the renal pelvis, calyces and parenchyma, causing pyelonephritis. Many cases of pyelonephritis therefore are associated with a preceding history of cystitis. *E. coli* is the bacterium most commonly isolated. Complications from pyelonephritis include development of renal abscesses. Perinephric and renal abscesses may also develop from haematogenous spread.

Clinical features

Patients complain of high fever and loin pain in association with urinary frequency, dysuria and urgency. Loin pain is insidious and constant and does not (usually) radiate to the groins. It may be bilateral, often with one side worse than the other. Patients with renal abscesses are usually systemically unwell and, along with loin pain and fever, the abscess may point into the lumbar triangle or present as a psoas abscess.

Investigations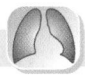

Urinalysis

Urinalysis indicates the presence of protein, nitrate and blood.

Midstream urine

An MSU is sent for culture to identify any infecting organism and provide antibiotic sensitivities for treatment.

Blood cultures

In septicaemic patients, blood cultures may confirm the organism.

Ultrasound of the kidneys

In cases where urinary obstruction or abscess is suspected an urgent ultrasound should be performed to exclude hydronephrosis or a drainable collection.

Plain abdominal film

An abdominal KUB film may identify radio-opaque calculi, which may be the source of infection.

Management

Intravenous fluids

Intravenous hydration is necessary in those who are vomiting or to resuscitate ill patients.

Antibiotics

High-dose intravenous antibiotics (gentamicin or ciprofloxacin) are often required to allow adequate tissue concentrations. Two weeks of oral antibiotics are usually commenced when patients improve.

Percutaneous drainage

Patients with a small renal abscess (pyonephrosis) require percutaneous drainage to prevent irreversible renal damage.

Surgical drainage

A large abscess may require surgical drainage.

Prognosis

The in-hospital mortality from pyelonephritis is 1.7% in men and 0.7% in women.[1] Most patients however, make an uneventful recovery.

REFERENCE

(1) *Foxman B, Klemstine KL, Brown PD. Acute pyelonephritis in US hospitals in 1997: hospitalization and in-hospital mortality. Annals of Epidemiology 2003; 13: 144–150.*

Xanthogranulomatous pyelonephritis

Xanthogranulomatous pyelonephritis results from a combination of renal calculi and chronic urinary infection. The chronic pyelonephritis that develops occurs from an intense granulomatous reaction that eventually replaces the kidney. A central focus of abscess and necrosis coalesce forming a complex mass, often radiologically similar to a renal carcinoma. Presentation is with unresolving loin pain and fever, usually in diabetic patients with a history of bacterial pyelonephritis. Patients are often unwell with septicaemia. A tender mass may be palpable in the loin and the abscess may point through the lumbar triangle. A plain abdominal KUB film may identify radio-opaque calculi and an irregular renal outline. Diagnosis is confirmed on CT visualization of the complex infiltrating mass and stone. Treatment is with intravenous antibiotics, diabetic control and nephrectomy, which is often difficult due to the intense inflammatory response.

Urinary calculi

Epidemiology

The prevalence of urinary calculi is approximately 3% of the general population. Calculi are 3 times more common in men and have a peak presentation between 40 and 50 years. The incidence is high in Europe, North America and Northern India.

Pathology

Many calculi (90%) form from a metabolic, infectious or structural abnormality. In most however, no cause is identified (idiopathic stone formation).

Metabolic abnormalities

Urine is a complex solution of inorganic ions and organic proteins. Crystallization, nucleation (the adherence of crystals) and subsequent aggregation of inorganic ions lead to stone formation. Calcium oxalate is present in 85% of stones and is the predominant constituent in 60% of calculi (Table 11.28). Calcium oxalate may crystallize when supersaturated (hypercalciuria, hyperoxaluria or low urine volumes) or in the presence of cell injury or infection. Any cause of hypercalcaemia, hyperuricaemia (gout), hypercalciuria or hyperoxaluria also predisposes to urinary tract calculi. The organic proteins (and inorganic compounds such as citrate) are natural inhibitors of stone formation that may be deficient in recurrent stone formers.

Inherited metabolic conditions such as cystinuria and hyperoxaluria also predispose to stone formation. Cystinuria is the underlying cause in approximately 3% of the stone-forming adult population.

Urinary tract infection

Urease-forming organisms alkalize the urine by converting urea into ammonium ions. Under these conditions, crystals of ammonium triple phosphate (ammonium, calcium and magnesium) may precipitate to form soft, large stones

741

Table 11.28	Composition and properties of common stones		
Crystal type	**Frequency**	**Radiodensity**	**Fragility (ESWL)**
Oxalates	65%		
Calcium oxalate monohydrate		Opaque	Intermediate
Calcium oxalate dihydrate		Opaque	Very fragile
Phosphates	10%		Intermediate
Calcium hydroxyphosphate		Very opaque	
Calcium hydrogen phosphate dehydrate		Very opaque	
Infective	20%		
Mg ammonium PO_4 hexahydrate		Slightly opaque	Intermediate
Urate	5%	Lucent	Fragile
Cystine	4%		
		Slightly opaque	Poor fragmentation
		Slightly opaque	Intermediate
Xanthine	<1%	Lucent	

NB The percentages add up to more than 100% as some stones are a mixture of crystal type

that occasionally fill the entire collecting system. Stones filling all the calyces resemble stag's antlers on X-ray (stag-horn calculi).

Structural abnormalities

Urinary stasis predisposes to nucleation and crystal aggregation with consequent stone formation. Medullary sponge kidney, pelvi-ureteral junction obstruction and vesico-ureteric reflux are structural abnormalities that predispose to stone formation.

Scope of disease

Calculi can obstruct the ureteric tract causing ureteric colic or haematuria. In addition, coexistent infection can lead to systemic sepsis.

Clinical features

Ureteric colic is characterized by severe pain (over minutes to hours) that originates in the loin and radiates to the lower abdomen (anteriorly) and into the scrotum, tip of penis or testis (men) or labium (women). Associated features such as pallor, tachycardia and nausea are usually present.

Microscopic or dipstick haematuria is present in approximately 95% during the acute phase. Frank haematuria is uncommon and may indicate 'clot colic' from a bleeding tumour proximal to the site of obstruction.

Coexistent infection may occur in a minority and, in addition to loin pain, patients may complain of fever, malaise and rigors. The most reliable clinical sign in this setting is that of severe renal tenderness on palpation of the flank.

When assessing a patient with ureteric colic, it is important to ascertain the presence of infection and any other underlying cause that predisposes to stone formation.

> ### ⚡ CLINICAL ALERT
>
> *In the presence of infection, an obstructed kidney will start to lose function irreversibly within 6 hours and may lose function completely within 48 hours. Treatment with antibiotics alone is not always effective as the infection occurs within an enclosed space. Therefore the combination of sepsis and obstruction (pyonephrosis) is of grave importance requiring urgent investigation and drainage via percutaneous nephrostomy.*

Initial investigations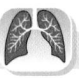

Urine dipstick testing

Although haematuria is often detected, its absence does not exclude the diagnosis of ureteric calculi.

Urine microscopy

Microscopy may reveal organisms that cause or coexist with the urinary calculi.

Full blood count

An elevated white cell count may indicate the presence of coexistent infection.

Urea and electrolytes

Urea and creatinine may be elevated in the presence of renal impairment secondary to severe sepsis or obstructive uropathy.

Spiral CT of the abdomen

Where available, spiral 'non-contrast' CT of the abdomen is the investigation of choice for suspected ureteric colic (Fig. 11.23). It can detect up to 99% of stones, even those lucent on plain film. Even if the original stone has passed, CT can detect secondary features such as fluid in the

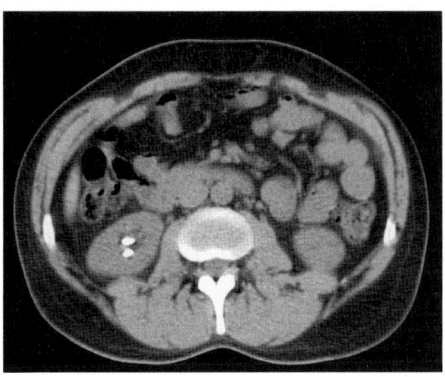

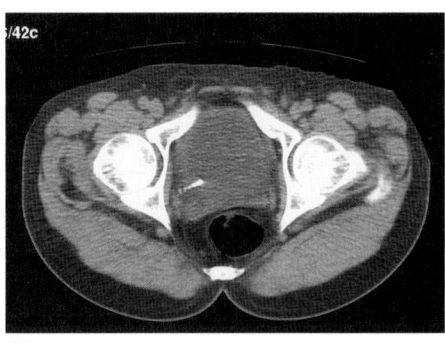

(b)

(a)

perinephric fat and residual dilatation of the collecting system from a passed stone. In approximately 30%, an alternative diagnosis for 'ureteric colic' will be identified on CT scanning.

Plain abdominal film

A KUB X-ray is simply a plain abdominal film that includes the entire pelvis. It is commonly stated that 90% of urinary calculi are visible on plain film; however, although 90% of calculi contain calcium, at best only 50% are diagnosed on plain film due to overlying bony shadows, the size of the stone and obscuring bowel shadows.

Further investigations

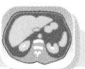

Ultrasound KUB

Although renal calcification produces classic acoustic shadowing, the ureters are shielded through most of their course by the vertebral processes and the bony pelvis except distally where they pass into the bladder (and urine jets can be visualized). Therefore, ultrasound is only preferred as the investigation of choice when radiation is contraindicated (pregnancy) or in the presence of pyonephrosis. Pyonephrosis is detected as echogenic debris within a dilated renal pelvis, suggesting pus rather than clear urine.

Intravenous urography

IVU is a useful investigation for demonstrating calyceal and ureteric anatomy such as a horseshoe or duplex system. It should be used to supplement spiral CT when planning surgical intervention. It is contraindicated in the presence of sepsis as the infected kidney does not effectively concentrate contrast. Moreover, the combination of intravenous contrast and sepsis increases the risk of acute tubular necrosis.

24-hour urine collection

Urinary calcium and phosphate concentrations should be performed for patients with recurrent urinary calculi; the normal level of calcium is 7–9 mmol and that of phosphate is 50 mmol. Urine should also be assayed for urate, cysteine (cystinuria) and oxalate (hyperoxaluria). A spot sample

nitroprusside test for urinary cysteine should be performed in recurrent stone formers or children.

Serum calcium

Serum calcium should be performed in all patients to exclude hypercalcaemia.

Uric acid levels

Serum urate should be performed in all patients to exclude hyperuricaemia.

Initial management

Analgesia

Effective pain control is an important aspect in the management of patients with acute ureteric colic. NSAIDs (e.g. diclofenac) or opiates (e.g. pethidine) are usually first-line treatment. Antispasmodics (e.g. hyoscine butylbromide) may be a useful adjunct.

Expectant management

Analgesia and observation is appropriate for patients with small stones without any evidence of coexistent infection or underlying structural abnormalities. Approximately 90% of stones less than 5 mm in size within 5 cm of the vesicoureteric junction will pass spontaneously. Only 10% of similar sized stones at the pelvi-ureteric junction will pass unaided. For uncomplicated stones, intervention is required for those with persistent pain or evidence of obstruction. An asymptomatic stone can be followed indefinitely, although most urologists would prefer treatment for stone clearance within 4–6 weeks.

Percutaneous nephrostomy

In a minority of patients with pyonephrosis, the indication for emergency drainage is a clinical picture of severe loin pain with fever, malaise and rigors in the presence of urinary infection with proven ureteric obstruction. Drainage is performed radiologically. Using an aseptic technique and local anaesthetic, the dilated renal pelvis is punctured using a needle. The Seldinger method is used, passing a guide-wire initially, then railroading a short pigtail stent into the renal pelvis. The wire is removed and the stent secured to the skin allowing external renal drainage. The nephrostomy allows renal drainage and can also be used as access to perform a 'nephrostogram' and insert an antegrade stent.

Surgical management

Upper urinary tract calculi

Extracorporeal shock wave lithotripsy (ESWL)

ESWL in many centres is the first-line treatment of patients with small to medium-sized renal simple stones (<2 cm) or simple upper ureteral stones. Contraindications to ESWL include pregnancy, morbid obesity, uncorrected coagulopathies, sepsis and upper urinary tract obstruction.

Lithotripsy is a procedure that involves focusing shock wave energy from a spark generator, piezo-electric dish or an electromagnetic plate so that it passes through the soft tissues of the body and is absorbed by the incompressible stone, causing it to fragment.

A small water-filled cushion with a silicone membrane provides air-free contact between the spark and the patient's skin.

ESWL is performed as an outpatient procedure. Stone visualization can be with fluoroscopy or ultrasound. Patients are positioned on a lucent X-ray screening table; once they are aligned, the water-filled balloon and shock focus is brought into contact with the skin. Repetitive shock waves cause discomfort and patients may require diclofenac suppositories or, rarely, intravenous sedation. Modern lithotriptors (e.g. Dornier HM3) can deliver high pressures over a wide area ensuring long-term stone-free rates of up to 90%.

Steinstrasse ('stone street') is the presence of multiple stone fragments in the ureter causing pain and obstruction. In the presence of sepsis, prompt renal drainage is required. Pre-ESWL stenting for a large stone burden (>2.5cm) can reduce the rate of subsequent complications. Stents should also be used in those with solitary kidneys. Further possible complications of ESWL include infection, bleeding and renal haematoma (25%), adjacent organ injury (e.g. pancreas, spleen and liver) and arrhythmias.

If unsuccessful, repeat ESWL should be considered for the simple stone. Up to 40% of residual stone fragments are cleared in this way. When ESWL has been ineffective, ureteroscopy or percutaneous nephrolithotomy should be considered for ureteric and renal stones respectively.

Percutaneous nephrolithotomy (PCNL)

Patients with renal stones greater than 2 cm are best served by PCNL, which carries stone clearance rates of between 70% and 100%. PCNL is also suited for patients with renal stones who have contraindications to ESWL, lower calyx stones or complex stones, e.g. 'staghorn' calculi, horseshoe kidney or stones within calyceal diverticula.

PCNL requires a general anaesthetic. The patient is positioned prone and with fluoroscopic guidance a needle tract is used to establish a nephrostomy tract (Fig. 11.24a).

The passage is widened to 30 F using either a balloon or graduated dilators (Fig. 11.24b). A sheath is inserted into the renal pelvis. The nephroscope (Fig. 11.24c) can then be passed into the renal pelvis and the stone extracted. Small stones can be retrieved intact; larger stones (>1 cm) require in situ fragmentation either by laser or lithotripsy. Once the stone is cleared, a flexible nephroscope can be used to inspect each calyx in turn. At the end of the procedure a nephrostomy tube is left in place to ensure renal drainage (Fig. 11.24d).

Complications of PCNL include bleeding from renal venules or arterioles that occasionally necessitates transfusion or arterial embolization, adjacent organ damage and local extravasation of irrigation fluid.

Open surgery

Open surgical excision is rarely performed these days (<1%). It should be considered in persistent complex calculi refractory to all endourological techniques or in situations where the site of the stone is exposed for other reasons. Exact techniques of open stone extraction are beyond the scope of this text, although where indicated, laparoscopic ('retroperitoneoscopic') techniques should be considered.

Ureteric calculi

Extracorporeal shock wave lithotripsy

Stones in the upper third of the ureter can be treated by ESWL with the patient supine, as described above. Distal third ureteric calculi may be treated by ESWL but the technique is less effective as patients have to be laid prone to avoid the shield of the sacrum; the shock wave traverses the pelvis to reach the ureter, thereby losing energy.

Endoscopic removal

Impacted ureteric calculi are best managed by ureteroscopic extraction, especially in the distal ureter. Ureteroscopy can be flexible or rigid and can be performed in the day case setting under general or regional anaesthesia. A safety guidewire should be passed in all but the simplest cases. Once visualized, the stone can be grasped in a basket (e.g. Segura, Dormia), as illustrated in Figure 11.25 and fragmented with in situ lithotripsy or laser tripsy. Use of a stent post procedure has little effect on stone passage rates. For mid and distal ureteral stones, ureteroscopic stone extraction is almost 100%.

Ureteroscopy can also be used to wash large ureteral stones back into the renal pelvis in anticipation for either PCNL or ESWL (the 'push bang').

Bladder calculi

Endoscopic removal

In the UK, stones in the bladder arise either from the upper tracts as ureteral calculi or secondary to foreign bodies (e.g. catheters). Small stones are easily crushed and washed out via a cystoscope (Fig. 11.26).

Most medium-sized bladder calculi (<3–4 cm) can be fragmented using a lithotrite or 'stone punch' (cystolitho-

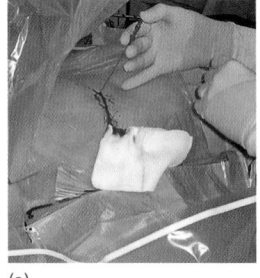

(a)

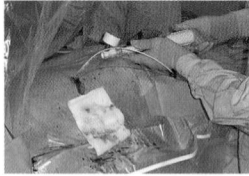

(b)

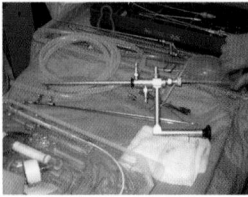

(c)

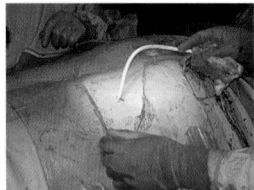

(d)

Fig. 11.24 Extraction of a renal stone by percutaneous nephrolithotomy.

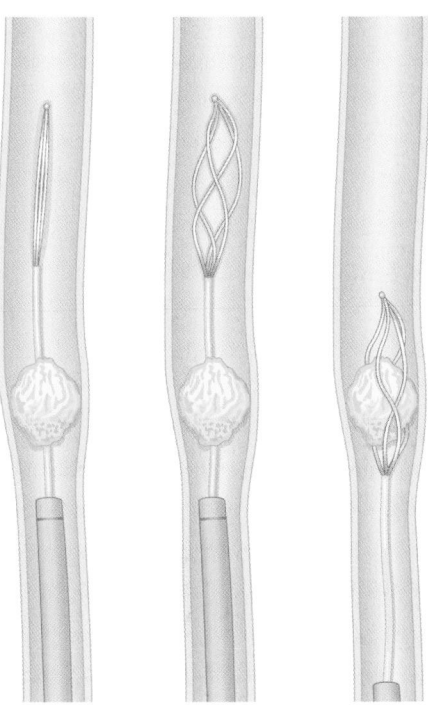

Fig. 11.25 Stone extraction using a basket.

lapaxy). The stone fragments may be removed cystoscopically with an Ellik's evacuator. Larger stones (>3–4 cm) do not allow sufficient purchase to fragment with the lithotrite. These stones are removed via a small suprapubic cystotomy. The calculus is extracted intact and the bladder sutured.

Urethral calculi

This rare entity can be managed cystourethroscopically. Calculi in the prostatic urethra are pushed back into the bladder and managed as for bladder calculi.

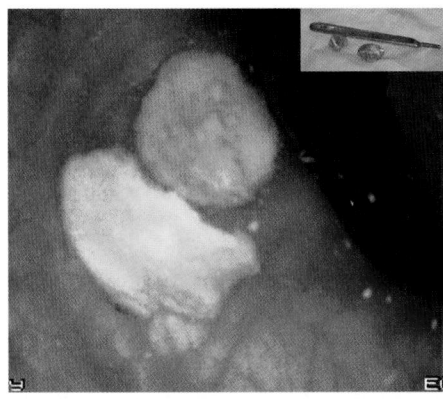

Fig. 11.26 Cystoscopic extraction of bladder calculi.

Medical management

The aims of medical therapy are to treat any underlying condition that predisposes to stone disease and also to prevent recurrence.

Increased fluid intake

Patients should be advised to increase their fluid intake to 3 L/day to maintain an output of at least 2 litres of urine volume a day.

Salt reduction

A high salt intake may increase urinary calcium considerably. Restriction to 150 mEq/day greatly lowers calcium excretion, thereby reducing stone formation. Foods containing 'hidden' sodium include canned soups, processed meats and fast food.

Calcium restriction

Hypercalciuria is present in up to 60% of those with calcium oxalate stones. However, in the normocalcaemic patient restriction of dietary calcium is of little benefit. Hypercalcaemia requires investigation and treatment. Minor changes in dietary calcium may not affect these levels substantially. Thiazide diuretics are effective in treating absorptive hypercalciuria because of their hypocalciuric action. Foods high in calcium include all dairy products, rhubarb and chocolate.

Hyperuricosuria

Allopurinol is a xanthine oxidase inhibitor that reduces endogenous uric acid production and therefore serum and urinary uric acid levels. The standard dose of 300 mg per day should be reduced in the presence of renal impairment. Restriction of animal proteins and therefore purines (e.g. red meat, fish or poultry) should be encouraged but is sometimes impractical.

Hypocitraturia

Citrate is required to inhibit crystallization of calcium salts and lower urinary saturation. Potassium citrate is able to restore normal urinary citrate levels in those with hypocitraturic calcium oxalate stones either secondary to renal tubular acidosis or secondary to thiazide use.

Hyperoxaluria

Primary hyperoxaluria is rare and treated with pyridoxine (B_6). In the more common 'enteric' form, urinary oxalate levels may be decreased by binding enteric oxalate with high doses of oral calcium or magnesium. The subsequent rise in urinary calcium should be managed by adequate oral fluid replacement as outlined above. The idiopathic form requires reduction of oral intake along with the above measures. Foods rich in oxalate include rhubarb, spinach, beetroot, chocolate and tea.

Prognosis

Following an acute episode, all patients are given advice on prevention of recurrence although studies have shown that at best only 20% of patients follow this information 2 years after receiving it. Patients with an identified underlying cause should be treated appropriately.

Of patients who pass a stone, 50% should expect to form more stones within the next 5 years. In patients with mild to moderate stone loads medical and surgical interventions can achieve over 90% remission from stone formation. However, despite this, the overall rate of recurrence of calcium oxalate stones is approximately 10% at 1 year, 35% at 5 years and 50% at 10 years.

SECTION 11.19 Diseases of the bladder

Neuropathic bladder disorders

The neuropathic or neurogenic bladder arises from disease processes that affect higher cortical, spinal or pelvic innervation to the bladder.

Epidemiology

As a neuropathic bladder may arise as a part of many clinical entities, the epidemiology is reflected by the underlying disorder. Specialist urological expertise is most commonly required in patients with spinal cord injury, of which there are approximately 800 new cases per year in the UK, affecting males 4 times more commonly than females with a peak incidence in the third decade.

Pathology

The process of voiding is controlled centrally in the cerebrum. It influences the pontine micturition centre (PMC), which in turn controls the sacral micturition centre (SMC).

Normally the bladder relaxes as it fills with urine and sphincter tone increases to prevent leakage. As a consequence, pressures in the bladder remain low until voiding commences. Bladder distension is associated with sensation and desire to void. Urgency can be suppressed by higher centres until it is socially convenient. During voiding the bladder actively contracts, pressures rise and the urethral sphincter relaxes. This relationship between the bladder and sphincter ensures an unobstructed flow with low bladder pressures.

In the neurogenic bladder, relaxation, sensation, contractility and sphincteric control are altered. The coordinated void may be lost causing dangerous pressure rises in the bladder predisposing to upper urinary tract dilatation, urinary tract infection, vesico-ureteric reflux, calculus formation and autonomic dysreflexia.

Clinical features

Neuropathic disorders of the bladder can arise entirely or as part of the underlying disorder (e.g. spinal stenosis or Parkinson's disease). A detailed clinical assessment is required to locate the site of any structural lesion, as voiding symptoms vary according to the location of the lesion (Table 11.29) and range from disrupted social awareness of voiding to a completely atonic bladder and incompetent sphincter.

Investigations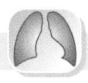

Urea and electrolytes

Elevated urea or creatinine suggests the development of renal impairment.

Urinalysis

Urine culture should be obtained as patients with neuropathic bladders are predisposed to infection. A 24-hour urinary creatinine clearance should be obtained to estimate glomerular filtration rate if the serum creatinine is elevated.

Abdominal ultrasound

Renal and bladder ultrasound is performed to exclude hydronephrosis secondary to obstructive uropathy or reflux. The bladder is assessed for trabeculation, diverticula and stone formation, which indicate features of dysfunctional voiding.

Pressure flow urodynamics

Formal urodynamic assessment of the lower urinary tract can detect detrusor sphincter dyssynergia (DSD), vesico-ureteric reflux, the 'fir tree' appearance of bladder trabeculation and incomplete bladder emptying.

Management

The main aims of treating the neuropathic bladder are to prevent the consequences of DSD (renal failure, urinary sepsis and calculus formation). This is done by lowering bladder resting pressures and ensuring efficient urinary emptying.

Permanent indwelling catheter

The use of indwelling catheters (either suprapubic or urethral) can be very effective in some patients, keeping their bladder pressure at zero. Suprapubic catheters are preferred to indwelling urethral catheters in women as the latter may erode the urethra rendering the patient incontinent. Complications of long-term catheterization include

Location	Site of lesion	Causes	Clinical features
Table 11.29	**Summary of neuropathic bladder disorders**		
Cerebrum	Above the pontine micturition centre	Cerebrovascular accident Dementia Parkinson's disease	Disrupted social awareness of micturition
Spinal cord	Above the sacral micturition centre	Spinal cord trauma Meningomyelocele Multiple sclerosis	Initially detrusor hyperreflexia then detrusor sphincter dyssynergia
Spinal cord	At or below the sacral micturition centre		Areflexic, incompetent bladder
Peripheral nerves	Distal to the spinal cord	Diabetes Prolapsed intervertebral disc	Areflexic bladder with or without competence

recurrent urinary tract infection, blockages which may precipitate autonomic dysreflexia, stone formation and a theoretical increased risk of bladder cancer.

Intermittent self-catheterization

Patients who have good hand function (i.e. most paraplegics) are usually able to perform intermittent self-catheterization to ensure good bladder drainage whilst maintaining continence. Pressure flow urodynamics should be performed to assess resting bladder pressure and bladder capacity.

Intermittent self-catheterization alone may not be sufficient to ensure adequate bladder emptying. In some, anticholinergic medication (e.g. oxybutynin/tolterodine) may be used to increase effective bladder capacity and reduce resting pressures. Patients should be warned as to side effects, in particular dry mouth, blurred vision and constipation.

A patient with a persistently high resting pressure and low capacity bladder despite maximal medical therapy may require an indwelling catheter or bladder augmentation surgery.

Transurethral sphincterotomy

DSD can be overcome by surgically incising or bypassing the urethral sphincter. The cut sphincter still contracts during the voiding phase but is unable to obstruct the bladder sufficiently to cause a rise in bladder pressure. Preserving the bladder and reducing bladder outflow obstruction comes at the cost of incontinence, and patients manage their urinary drainage by 'convene drainage' where the bladder contracts in a reflex manner emptying into the convene attached to a leg bag. This form of treatment is ideal for those with tetraplegia who are unable to perform intermittent self-catheterization.

Bladder augmentation

Augmentation surgery involves bivalving the bladder and using a patch of bowel to cover the defect (see Fig. 11.31, p. 753). This is performed to preserve the patient's continence, or to help patients already using intermittent self-catheterization with high resting bladder pressure. The pressure is reduced in the bladder at the cost of incomplete emptying; the patient is required to perform intermittent self-catheterization 5 times a day for life. As part of a continence-preserving procedure in patients with low cord lesions, additional procedures (e.g. colposuspension or artificial urinary sphincter) may be required to ensure continence due to poor sphincter tone.

Prognosis

Patients with an untreated neuropathic bladder secondary to spinal cord injury most commonly succumb either to obstructive renal failure or pneumonia. With regular follow-up and timely intervention a near normal life expectancy can be expected. Patients who undergo cystoplasty require lifelong bladder surveillance for detection of new tumours at the anastomosis line. Catheter appliances are generally well accepted but patients should be aware of the risks of urinary infection and calculus formation.

Urinary incontinence

Urinary incontinence is the involuntary loss of urine.

Epidemiology

The incidence of urinary incontinence increases with age; it affects up to 30% of the elderly in the community and 50% of those institutionalized.

Pathology

In a continent patient, the bladder relaxes to allow filling, storing urine at low pressures. The sensation to void can be suppressed until socially convenient. Voiding begins with relaxation of the urethral sphincter mechanism followed by an active and sustained bladder contraction. After the bladder empties, the sphincter contracts and urethral pressure rises, allowing continent bladder filling. If this cycle is deficient, urinary leakage may occur. Incontinence may occur in several pathophysiological circumstances leading to stress, urgency, continuous or overflow incontinence. Often the picture is mixed with different processes contributing to leakage.

Stress incontinence

Stress incontinence is the involuntary loss of urine associated with raised intra-abdominal pressure such as coughing, sneezing and laughing. It suggests weakness in the pelvic floor musculature or sphincter weakness. In women this may follow childbirth; in men sphincter weakness may be of neurological origin or follow prostatic or urethral surgery.

Urgency incontinence

Urgency incontinence is the involuntary loss of urine associated with extreme urgency. This is often associated with an overactive bladder (detrusor overactivity), although this may be a presenting feature for neurological disease.

Continuous incontinence

Continuous incontinence is the involuntary loss of urine regardless of urgency or raised intra-abdominal pressure. Continuous leakage may suggest complete sphincter deficiency (e.g. conus lesion in spina bifida) or a fistulous tract from the bladder to the vagina (vesico-vaginal fistula).

'Overflow' incontinence

'Overflow' incontinence can occur in men with chronic urinary retention. The bladder remains full and continence is maintained by virtue of the urethral resting pressure exceeding the bladder pressure. When the bladder is over-stretched an unstable contraction may occur, overcoming the urethral pressure, and the patient leaks. The leakage may occur at day or night (nocturnal enuresis) and a painless full bladder may be palpable.

Clinical features

The presenting symptom may be clearly obvious to the patient. However, in some cases it may be necessary to prove the presence of leakage and to determine the quantity of urine loss by the use of a pad test.

A detailed history should be obtained to determine the nature of leakage. Severe storage symptoms such as urgency, frequency and nocturia usually indicate urgency incontinence.

General examination usually reveals a well patient although those with obstructive renal failure may be uraemic or in congestive cardiac failure. Examination should include a full neurological assessment to exclude a central or peripheral nerve lesion. Abdominal examination is usually unremarkable but may reveal a painless distended bladder. Assessment of the external genitalia in the female should be directed at identifying the site of urinary loss and overall condition of the introitus and pelvic floor. Internal (per rectal and vaginal) examination is essential to exclude a pelvic mass, severe constipation or an abnormal prostate and to assess pelvic floor descent.

Initial investigations

The goal of investigating incontinence is to accurately determine the origin of the leakage by first identifying the presence of leakage and then to assess anatomy and function.

Urinalysis

Dipstick urine testing is performed to determine the presence of urinary blood, white cells, nitrates or glucose. A midstream urine should be sent for microscopy culture and sensitivity if urinalysis is abnormal.

Frequency volume chart

The patient monitors the quantity of urine produced and the frequency of micturition over a few days. Episodes of severe urgency or incontinence are also recorded. The chart provides documented evidence of the micturition pattern and allows a baseline to which therapeutic measures can be compared.

Pad test

A pad placed in the underwear is weighed before and after exercise. A sizeable increase in weight corresponds to urinary leakage.

Further investigations

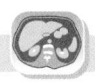

Ultrasound

A formal ultrasound should be performed to exclude anatomical abnormalities and assess the state of the upper tracts for hydronephrosis. A post void residual scan can be performed to screen for large volumes of residual urine associated with 'overflow' incontinence.

Intravenous urogram

An IVU may be performed to define normal anatomy and identify an ectopic ureteric opening or fistula.

Cystoscopy

In patients with a short history of irritative storage symptoms such as frequency and nocturia, flexible cystoscopy should be performed to exclude an intravesical cause such as a bladder tumour. Careful urethroscopy may identify the opening of a urethral diverticulum.

Videocystometrogram (VCMG)

A VCMG provides clear objective evidence of stress leakage. Rises in detrusor pressure associated with urgency may identify the overactive bladder. Instillation of contrast into the bladder during VCMG provides anatomical information relating to pelvic floor descent or the presence of fistula (e.g. vesico-vaginal fistula).

Management

Once the diagnosis has been made, treatment should be directed to the underlying anatomical abnormality. For example, continuous incontinence due to a fistula may require fistula repair with reconstructive surgery, ectopic ureters require reimplantation into the bladder, and patients with bladder outflow obstruction may require transurethral resection of the prostate.

Stress incontinence

Many cases of stress incontinence are related to a pelvic floor weakened through childbirth. Conservative methods such as weight reduction and pelvic floor exercises can be effective in up to 50% of mild cases. New medical pharmacotherapy is emerging with the advent of serotonin noradrenaline reuptake inhibitors (e.g. duloxetine).

Surgery is reserved for those with severe symptoms in whom conservative measures have failed. In the majority, the weakened pelvic floor causes bladder descent. Surgery is aimed either at elevating the bladder to its intraabdominal location by suspending the bladder neck, e.g. colposuspension, or providing urethral support e.g. tension-free tape procedure.

In those with intrinsic sphincter weakness, the urethra may be supported with urethral bulking agents (e.g. Macroplastique). If the urethral sphincter is deficient, an artificial sphincter may be required.

Urge incontinence

Bladder retraining regimens are often effective in mild cases of urge incontinence due to detrusor overactivity. Patients are instructed to resist the urge to void and, by increasing the intervals between voiding, increase their functional bladder capacity. 'Voiding by the clock' instructs the patient to void at set intervals, e.g. every 3 hours from 9 am. This gives patients a target time to hold their urine.

Anticholinergic medication (e.g. oxybutynin) is often used to 'desensitize' the bladder, allowing bladder retraining to be more effective. Patients should be warned as to side effects of dry mouth, blurred vision and constipation. Medication can be very effective, but many patients find these side effects intolerable. Anticholinergic medication is contraindicated in closed angle glaucoma.

Surgery is reserved for patients with severe symptoms in whom medical therapy has failed. Cystoscopically distending the bladder under anaesthetic (cysto-distension) may provide limited benefit. It also allows a formal cystoscopy to be performed and biopsies taken if required. Poor bladder capacity and compliance may be overcome by bladder augmentation surgery, e.g. clam cystoplasty or detrusor myomectomy. Results can be excellent but patients should be warned of complications of major surgery, the presence of mucus in the urine and the possible need for lifelong intermittent self-catheterization.

In cases refractory to all forms of treatment, urinary diversion via an ileal loop may be appropriate. However, in those unsuitable for or reluctant to undergo surgery, an indwelling urinary catheter may be appropriate. The great advantage of urinary catheters is their simplicity of use and effectiveness at keeping the bladder empty.

The main disadvantages of catheters are their need for regular change, problems with blockage or infections and urethral erosion. The catheter balloon may erode the urethra such that the patulous urethra becomes unable to retain the catheter. In such cases a suprapubic catheter may be required. Long-term catheterization has also been linked to formation of bladder calculi and squamous carcinoma of the bladder.

Prognosis

For mild stress urinary incontinence pelvic floor exercises using vaginal cones can achieve success rates of approximately 50%. Periurethral injectables have a short-term cure rate of up to 90%, although further 'booster' injections may be required. The success from Burch colposuspension surgery at 5 years approaches 90%. Artificial sphincters can be very effective although this has to be weighed against technically difficult surgery and the risk of infection, erosion and potential mechanical failure.

Bladder cancer

Epidemiology

The incidence of bladder cancer is rising; current estimated incidence in the UK is 20 per 100 000 per year. It is 4 times more common in men, and increases with age, classically affecting 'white collar' Caucasians of 60–70 years of age. Areas with high risk are linked to aetiological associations with smoking (Europe and North America) and schistosomiasis (North Africa).[1]

Pathology

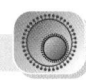

The latent period from exposure to development of cancer is approximately 25 years, and the risk factors are detailed in Table 11.30. Cigarette smoke contains known urothelial carcinogens, and regular exposure at least doubles the risk of cancer. Occupational exposure to beta-naphthylamine through the chemical, rubber and dye industries remains a common cause of cancer. Once absorbed, aromatic amines (β-naphthylamine and benzidine) are metabolized by the liver and activated in the urine. Schistosomiasis is responsible for many cases of squamous carcinoma in the Nile delta, and chronic irritation is thought to predispose to malignant change. Other causes of chronic irritation include infection, prolonged catheterization and calculi.

Table 11.30	Risk factors for bladder cancer

Increasing age (above 40 years)
Smoking
Occupation Chemical manufacture Dye industries Rubber manufacture
Drugs Cyclophosphamide Phenacetin
Chronic irritation of the bladder Chronic infection Prolonged catheterization Calculi
Schistosomiasis

The majority of bladder cancers are urothelial cell carcinomas. Urothelial tumours can originate anywhere from the renal pelvis, ureters to the urinary bladder and urethra. Squamous carcinoma (associated with schistosomiasis) accounts for approximately 5% and primary adenocarcinoma, 1–2%. Bladder cancers tend to be superficial papillary tumours (75%); infiltrative and invasive tumours are less common. The degree of histological differentiation is graded from G1 to G3 (well, moderately and poorly differentiated) and corresponds to increasing malignant potential. Carcinoma in situ may arise from the urothelium. In combination with high-grade (G3) tumours, it represents a more aggressive disease.

Scope of disease

Local

As tumours grow they may bleed, causing haematuria, or irritate the bladder and present with symptoms suggestive of a urinary tract infection. Local invasion may cause pain, infiltration into the ureters may present with obstructive renal failure, and invasion of the urethral orifice may cause bladder outflow obstruction.

Metastatic

Metastases from bladder tumours tend to be to the liver and lungs.

Paraneoplastic

Paraneoplastic symptoms such as persistent pyrexia are uncommon.

Clinical features

The most common presentation (85%) is intermittent, painless, frank haematuria. Symptoms of bladder irritation from the tumour can lead to urinary frequency, urgency, nocturia, dysuria or pain. Patients may present with dipstick-detected microscopic haematuria at a routine medical screening.

Initial investigations

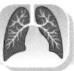

The combination of clinical assessment, KUB X-ray, renal ultrasound and flexible cystoscopy forms the basis of any haematuria clinic evaluation.

Full blood count

Haematuria sufficient to cause anaemia is uncommon. A leukocytosis may occur in the presence of urinary tract infection.

Urea and electrolytes

Elevated serum creatinine from renal impairment may suggest obstructive renal failure from tumour infiltration.

Urinalysis

Urine should be sent for microscopy, culture, sensitivity and cytology. A urinary tract infection is present in a third of patients with bladder cancers, and does not change the need for subsequent investigations.

Plain abdominal film

As part of basic investigations for haematuria, all patients require a KUB X-ray to exclude renal calculi.

Renal tract ultrasound

Renal tract ultrasound is used to exclude solid renal tumours.

Flexible cystoscopy

Flexible cystoscopy should be performed for all patients with suspected bladder cancer. It allows visual confirmation of the diagnosis. It is performed using local anaesthetic gel (Instillagel) as a day case procedure.

Further investigations

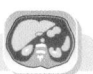

Further imaging is required for staging. Pertinent information includes the depth of the local invasion, involvement of the upper urinary tracts (3% have concomitant upper tract cancers) and identification of metastases.

⏵⏵⏵ Simplified staging of bladder cancer	
T—Primary tumour	
Tx	Primary tumour cannot be assessed
T0	No evidence of primary tumour
Ta	Non-invasive papillary carcinoma
Tis	Carcinoma in situ: 'flat tumour'
T1	Tumour invades subepithelial connective tissue
T2	Tumour invades (detrusor) muscle
T3	Tumour invades perivesical tissue
T4	Tumour invades any of the following: prostate, uterus, vagina, pelvic wall, abdominal wall
N—Regional lymph nodes	
N0	No regional node metastases
N1	Metastases in a single lymph node 2 cm or less
N2	Metastases in a single lymph node between 2 cm and 5 cm, or multiple lymph nodes each less than 5 cm
N3	Metastases in a single lymph node 5 cm or more
M—Distant metastases	
M0	No distant metastases
M1	Distant metastases

Chest X-ray

A plain chest film is required to exclude pulmonary metastases.

Intravenous urogram

Prior to transurethral resection an IVU is performed to exclude an upper tract urothelial tumour and to screen for filling defects from a bladder tumour (Fig. 11.27). If for

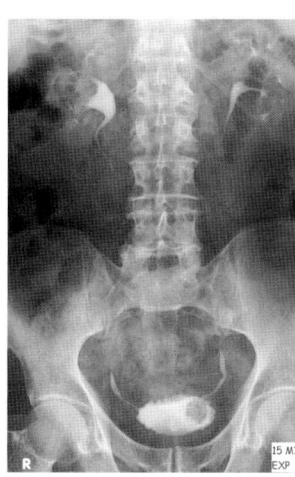

Fig. 11.27 The filling defect of a bladder tumour can be seen on the intravenous urogram.

any reason the IVU is suboptimal, a retrograde pyelogram may be performed at the time of transurethral resection.

MRI/CT of the pelvis

MRI is investigation of choice — CT is an alternative where MRI unavailable. Indication is solid tumour on cystoscopic or histologically proven invasive tumour. Image either before TURT or leave 2/5 after TURT to minimize surgical artefact.

Liver ultrasound

Liver ultrasound is performed to screen for liver metastases.

Initial management

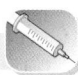

Transurethral resection of bladder tumour

Transurethral resection of bladder tumour (TURT) is both diagnostic and therapeutic. It is performed under general or regional anaesthesia and provides tissue for histology. Tissue samples need to include bladder muscle for staging. This carries the risk of bleeding and bladder perforation (intraperitoneal bladder perforation invariably requires exploratory laparotomy to exclude bowel injury).

Bimanual examination should be performed before and after resection to assess the size, position and mobility of the tumour mass. A repeat resection may be required a few weeks later to ensure adequate tissue for accurate staging.

Surgical management

Superficial bladder cancer

Superficial bladder cancer relates to pathological stages Ta and T1, with the exception of high-grade T1 disease (G3 pT1), which is considered invasive, especially in the presence of carcinoma in situ.

Endoscopic resection and adjuvant intravesical therapy

Endoscopic resection is the treatment of choice for superficial bladder cancer (Figs 11.28). Without adjuvant treatment, approximately 60% develop recurrence. Therefore a single administration of adjuvant intravesical mitomycin-C chemotherapy is given to all patients immediately post resection.

Patients should be followed up with regular flexible cystoscopy and any recurrences should be resected or fulgurated (Fig. 11.29). Radical cystectomy is usually considered if tumours continue to recur despite intravesical treatment or if new tumours show changes to muscle invasive disease.

Adjuvant intravesical chemotherapy

Currently, mitomycin-C or epirubicin is offered as a single instillation after endoscopic tumour resection to reduce the risk of recurrence, or as several weekly instillations as an extended treatment course. Although it may prolong the disease-free survival, it does not reduce disease progression.

Adjuvant intravesical BCG

Immunotherapy is used as adjuvant treatment after endoscopic resection; it is the primary treatment of choice for 'high risk' disease (e.g. G3 disease with carcinoma in situ) without evidence of invasion. Immunotherapy is performed using a live attenuated strain of bacillus Calmette–Guérin (BCG) instilled into the bladder weekly for 8 weeks. It produces an intense immunogenic response in the bladder wall. BCG instillation carries the risk of systemic absorption, rarely leading to tuberculosis. Tumour recurrence is reduced with intravesical BCG compared to mitomycin-C in patients at high risk of tumour recurrence.

Invasive bladder cancer

Muscle invasive bladder cancer relates to pT2 and above, and includes high-grade T1 tumours (G3 pT1). By definition, the tumour has invaded the detrusor muscle. One in four patients have muscle invasive disease, of which half will harbour micrometastases.

Cystectomy – treatment of choice

Radical cystectomy (includes excision of the bladder and all of the anterior pelvic organs, including hysterectomy in

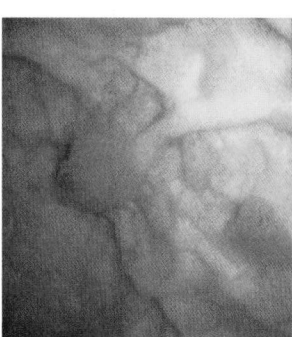

Fig. 11.28 Endoscopic view of a transitional cell tumour of the bladder.

Neuropathic bladder disorders

Urinary incontinence

Bladder cancer

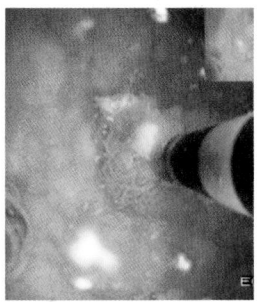

Fig. 11.29 Endoscopic ablation of a bladder tumour.

751

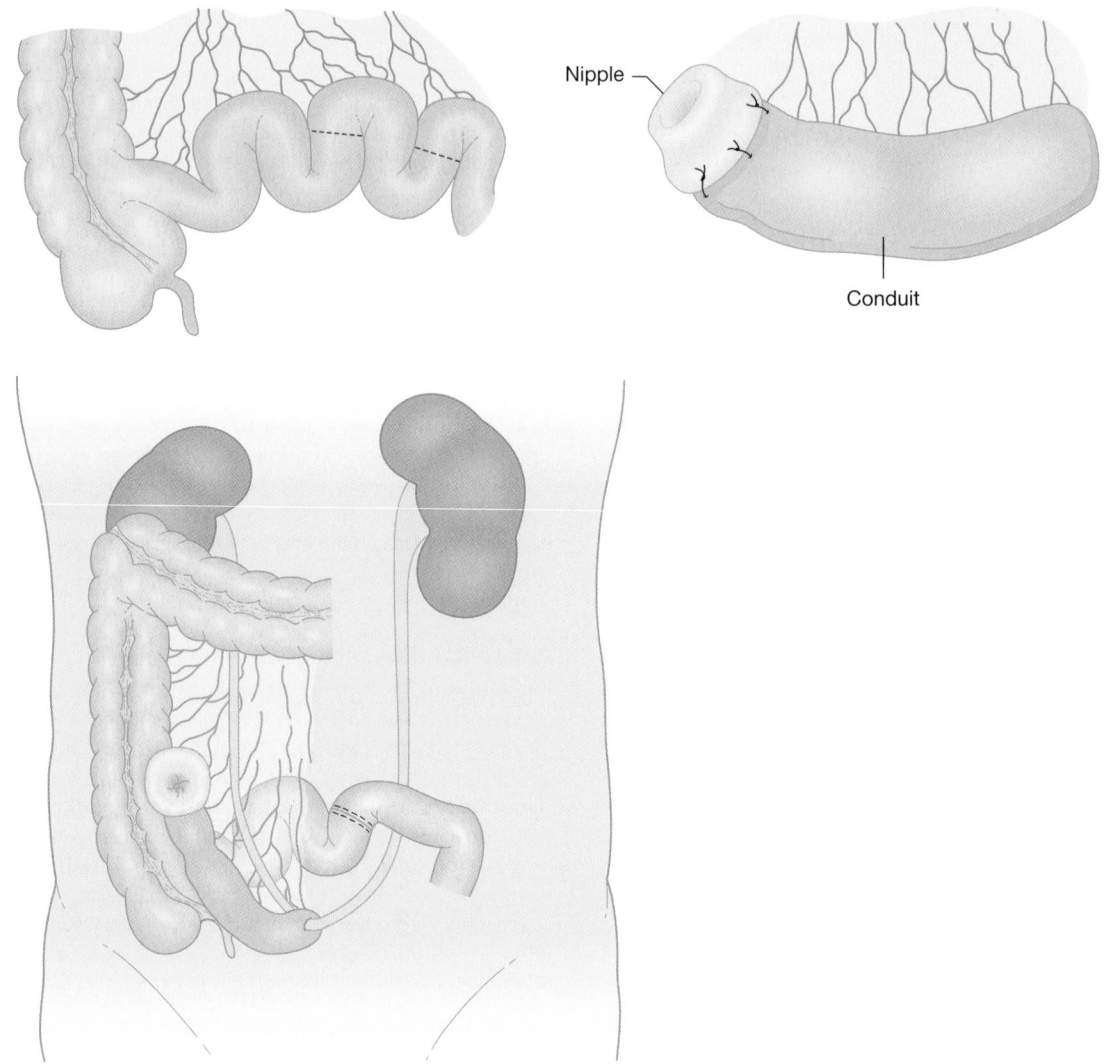

Nipple

Conduit

Fig. 11.30 Ileal conduit for urinary diversion.

females) is the treatment of choice for muscle invasive bladder cancer. There is a 90% 10-year recurrence-free survival for organ-confined disease. Regional lymph nodes (obturator, hypogastric and external iliac) are excised at the time of surgery. Urinary diversion is achieved either through an ileal conduit (Fig. 11.30), a continent reservoir for catheterization or orthotopic bladder reconstruction (using bowel, Fig. 11.31).

Partial cystectomy is reserved for specific tumours such as adenocarcinoma arising within a machal remnant or for isolated high grade superficial tumour in a diverticulum.

Systemic chemotherapy

Systemic chemotherapy may be used prior to (neoadjuvant) or following cystectomy (adjuvant). Neoadjuvant chemotherapy administered before surgery increases the overall 5-year survival probability after surgery by a further 5%.[3] Adjuvant chemotherapy using M-VAC (methotrexate, vinblastine, epirubicin and cisplatin) or Gem-Cis (gemcitabine and cisplatin) also improves survival.

Radiotherapy

Modern conformal radiotherapy offers the potential for cure for transitional cell carcinoma whilst preserving bladder function and causing reduced toxicity to surrounding tissues. Adenocarcinoma and squamous cancers are generally considered to be radioresistant. In selected cases primary radiotherapy may be equivalent to surgery although, overall, 5-year survival for T2–4 disease is about 30%. Surgery is associated with better overall survival rates, as recurrence with radiotherapy is common (60%).[4]

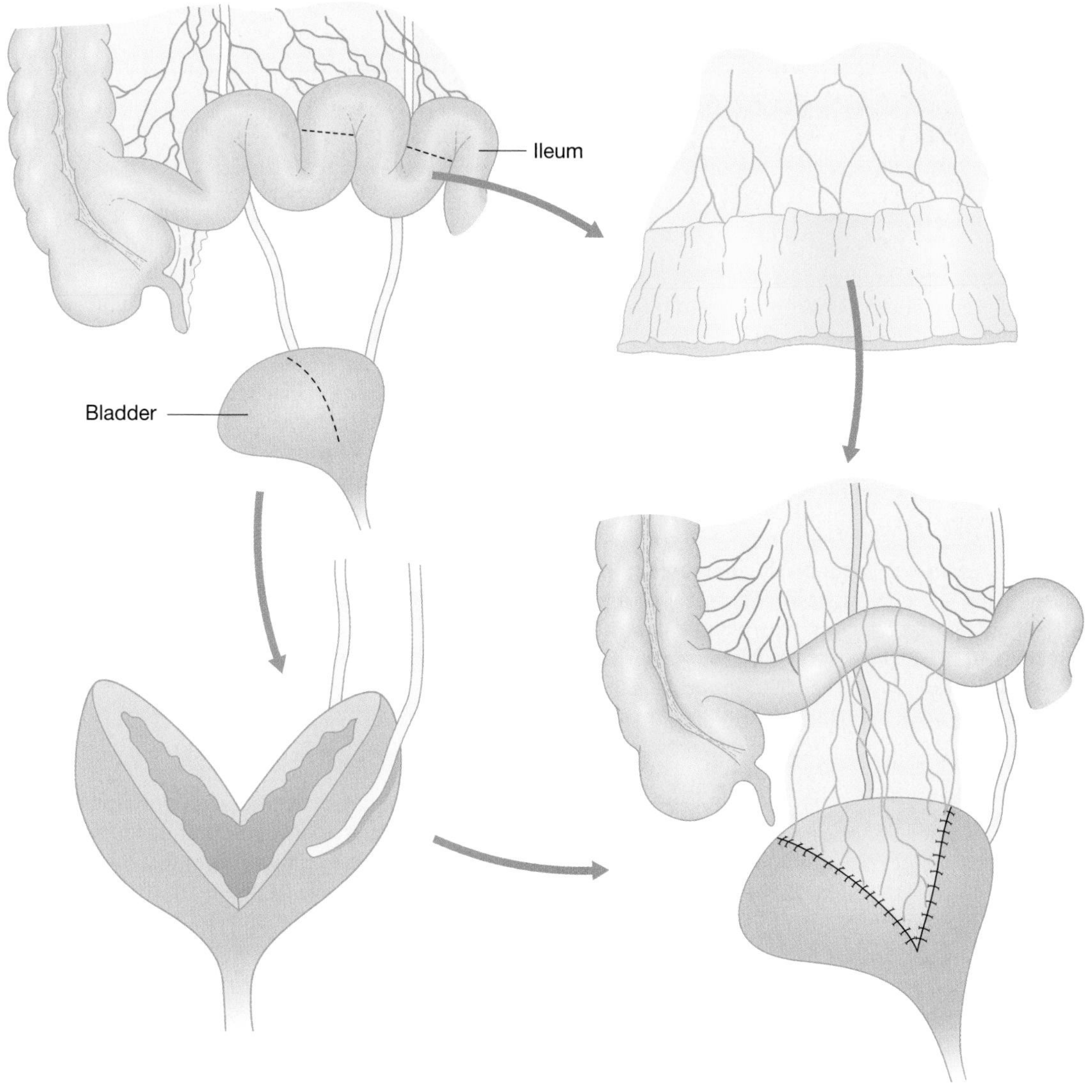

Bladder ——

Ileum ——

Fig. 11.31 Clam cystoplasty for bladder reconstruction.

Close cystoscopic follow-up is required to identify residual disease or recurrence, and if this is confirmed histologically, a 'fit' patient should be counselled towards 'salvage' cystectomy. Early results of the concurrent use of chemotherapy (chemo-sensitization) have shown improved response rates.

Prognosis

For adequately treated superficial (pTa, G1 or G2 pT1) bladder cancers in the absence of carcinoma in situ, the 5-year survival probability is approximately 95%. However, muscle invasion (pT2 and beyond) carries a much worse prognosis, with 50% and 20% 5-year survival for organ-confined and extravesical disease respectively.

REFERENCES

(1) *Parkin DM, Pisani P, Ferlay J. Global cancer statistics. CA Cancer Journal for Clinicians 1999; 49: 33–64.*
(2) *Shelley MD, Court JB, Kynaston H, Wilt TJ, Coles B, Mason M. Intravesical bacillus Calmette-Guerin versus mitomycin C for Ta and T1 bladder cancer. The Cochrane Database of Systematic Reviews 2003: CD003231.*
(3) *Neoadjuvant chemotherapy in invasive bladder cancer: a systematic review and meta-analysis. Lancet 2003; 361: 1927–1934.*
(4) *Shelley MD, Barber J, Wilt T, Mason MD. Surgery versus radiotherapy for muscle invasive bladder cancer. The Cochrane Database of Systematic Reviews 2001.*

Diseases of the prostate

Benign prostatic hyperplasia

Benign prostatic hyperplasia (BPH) is a histological entity characterized by an increase in both the stromal and glandular elements of the prostate gland, leading to an overall increase in its size. Benign prostatic enlargement is a clinical finding on rectal examination and is not necessarily associated with benign prostatic obstruction of urine flow, as defined by urodynamic studies.

Epidemiology

Benign prostatic hyperplasia is the most common benign tumour in men and the risk of its development increases with age. It is found in 70% of men aged 70 and the prevalence approaches 100% by 80 years of age. It is more common in Western societies than in the Far East; in the USA it is more common in the black population than the white.

Pathology

Benign prostatic hyperplasia arises as nodular growth in the periurethral glands of the transitional zone of the prostate (Figs 11.32, 11.33). Histological evidence can be found as early as the fourth decade of life. Development of benign prostatic hyperplasia probably results from an imbalance of growth factors (fibroblast growth factors and transforming growth factor β), oestrogen and increasing sensitivity of the ageing prostate to circulating androgens. Circulating testosterone is converted by the prostatic intracellular enzyme 5α-reductase to dihydrotestosterone (DHT), the major intracellular androgenic metabolite, and is the main stimulant for growth.

Although the symptoms associated with benign prostatic hyperplasia are often attributed to outflow obstruction, the association is not entirely accurate. Relief of symptoms does not always follow after prostatectomy and yet treatments that do not necessarily relieve outflow obstruction can result in improvement of symptoms (Fig. 11.34). It is likely that there are other mechanisms involved. Therefore objective evidence of obstruction is usually acquired prior to surgical treatment.

Scope of disease

The majority of patients with benign prostatic hyperplasia are asymptomatic. A smaller proportion of patients present with symptoms arising directly from urinary flow obstruction (voiding symptoms) or secondary to changes within the detrusor muscle of the bladder as a result of outflow obstruction (storage symptoms). Patients can also develop

Fig. 11.32 Cross-section of the prostate.

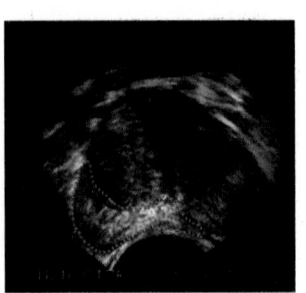

Fig. 11.33 Transrectal ultrasound of the prostate.

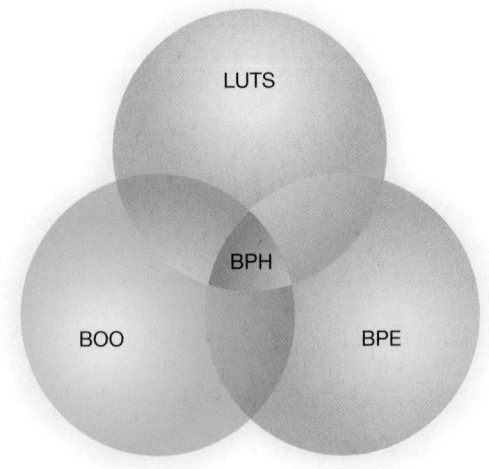

Fig. 11.34 There is considerable overlap in the clinical presentation of patients with benign prostatic enlargement (BPE), bladder outflow obstruction (BOO) and the development of lower urinary tract symptoms (LUTS); all three culminate in the syndrome of clinical benign prostatic hyperplasia (BPH).

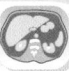

haematuria, stone formation, acute and chronic retention of urine and secondary renal impairment.

Clinical features

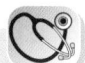

The most common form of presentation is with lower urinary tract symptoms (LUTS). Voiding symptoms include hesitancy (longer time to initiate the urinary flow), poor or intermittent stream of urine, straining, terminal dribbling, haematuria and dysuria. Storage symptoms include frequency of urine, urgency, nocturnal enuresis and incontinence. It is important to note that lower urinary tract symptoms are not specific to benign prostatic hyperplasia and can be caused by urethral strictures, urinary tract infections, bladder cancer, prostate cancer, or detrusor changes associated with aging.

Acute urinary retention is more common in the elderly and characterized by a painful total inability to void. Most patients have minimal urinary symptoms prior to the development of acute retention and on catheterization have a large amount of residual urine (600–1000 mL). Patients with chronic urinary retention may present with storage symptoms and may have a painless, palpable bladder on examination that may be associated with renal impairment.

On examination, the bladder may be palpable. The external genitalia are examined for phimosis, meatal stenosis or urethral induration as alternative causes for obstruction. A rectal examination is performed to assess the consistency and regularity of the prostate gland and to identify nodules suggestive of prostate cancer. The normal prostate feels rubbery, with a palpable median sulcus and discernible lateral margins. Although there is little correlation between the size of the prostate on rectal examination and the degree of obstruction, an enlarged prostate gland on clinical examination is an independent predictor of outcome following treatment.

Initial investigations

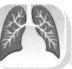

Urinalysis
A midstream specimen of urine should be taken for dipstick analysis, microscopy and culture to exclude infection or haematuria. The presence of haematuria should alert the clinician as to the possible presence of a bladder tumour or stones.

Urea and electrolytes
An elevated serum creatinine level implies renal impairment that can arise from obstruction to urinary flow (obstructive uropathy).

Prostate-specific antigen (PSA)
PSA estimation should be performed if there is a clinical suspicion of prostate cancer, but not routinely as an investigation for the evaluation of lower urinary tract symptoms. An elevated PSA in the range of 3–10 ng/mL is more commonly associated with benign prostatic hyperplasia (60–70%) than with prostate cancer (25–30%).

Further investigations

Urodynamic evaluation
Urodynamics refers to the objective documentation of urinary tract function and provides a rational basis for therapy. Urodynamic assessment for male lower urinary tract symptoms includes an assessment of urine flow rate by non-invasive uroflowmetry (Fig. 11.35), ultrasound assessment of residual urine and inspection of a detailed frequency–volume micturition diary.

The predictive value of uroflowmetry for the presence of obstruction on pressure-flow studies is indicated in Table 11.4 (p. 692). The outcome of bladder outlet surgery is better in men with a low flow rate than in those with flow rates greater than 15 mL/s. Full pressure-flow evaluation may be required in patients with failed previous surgery or concomitant pathology.

Abdominal film
A plain abdominal KUB film is performed if there is a suspicion of bladder calculi.

Abdominal ultrasound
Abdominal ultrasound is performed to identify hydronephrosis in patients with impaired renal function or a palpable bladder and to detect tumours in patients with haematuria.

Flexible cystoscopy
Flexible cystoscopy is indicated in selected patients with recent onset of storage symptoms or haematuria to exclude a lower urinary tract cancer.

Initial management

Urinary retention
A urinary catheter should be inserted to decompress the bladder and usually results in immediate relief of both acute and chronic retention. A trial without catheter alone is often unrewarding in acute retention, and surgery in the

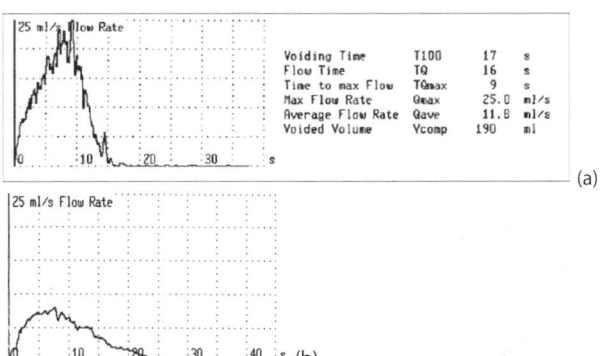

Fig. 11.35a, b (a) The normal male uroflow trace has rapid up and down strokes and a peak (Qmax) of greater than 20 mL/s. (b) In BPH and outflow obstruction, the uroflow trace has a low Qmax and prolonged 'tail'.

form of transurethral resection is usually indicated for relief of obstruction.

With chronic retention, the residual volume on catheterization may be in excess of 3 L, and a brisk diuresis may follow decompression. In this setting (5% of patients) fluid replacement with intravenous normal saline may be required.

Expectant management
Patients with mild symptoms may not require treatment. Over 5 years, 30% of patients with benign prostatic hyperplasia will experience progression of their symptoms, whilst 50% will remain static, and 20% will improve. Approximately 10% will experience an episode of acute retention. Patients need to be kept under follow-up to identify those with progressive disease.

Medical management

Drugs are aimed at reducing prostatic and bladder neck smooth muscle tone (α-adrenergic antagonists) or prostatic gland volume (5α-reductase inhibitors).

α-Adrenergic antagonists
Bladder outflow obstruction due to benign prostatic hyperplasia is partly due to the dynamic effect of the tone of the prostate smooth muscle mediated via α-adrenoreceptors. α-Adrenergic antagonists (e.g. alfuzosin, tamsulosin) lead to objective and subjective improvement in approximately 80%.

5α-Reductase inhibitors
5α-Reductase inhibitors (e.g. finasteride) block the conversion of testosterone to dihydrotestosterone and reduce prostate size with minimal effect on potency and libido. The use of finasteride is associated with symptomatic improvement (which may take from 6–9 months), with fewer patients undergoing surgery (10% to 5%) and developing acute urinary retention (7% to 3%) at 4 years.[1] The main clinical use is in the reduction of the risk of acute retention of urine in elderly unfit men and in those with a markedly enlarged prostate.

Combination therapy
It has recently been reported that the use of both doxazosin and finasteride results in significantly greater improvement in symptoms than either agent alone.[2]

Surgical management

Indications for surgical treatment include acute urinary retention, renal failure associated with hydronephrosis, recurrent urinary tract infection, recurrent haematuria and persistent symptoms.

Transurethral incision of prostate
Transurethral incision (bladder neck incision) is performed if there is bladder outflow obstruction due to benign prostatic hyperplasia with a resectable prostatic weight of less than 30 g. The bladder neck is divided with a single or double incision at the 7 or 5 o' clock position as far distally as the verumontanum. The results are comparable to transurethral resection.

Transurethral resection of the prostate
Transurethral resection of the prostate (TURP) is the standard surgical treatment for benign prostatic obstruction. It involves resection of the hyperplastic prostatic tissue from the bladder neck as far distally as the verumontanum. The prepared patient is anaesthetized with general or spinal anaesthetic and placed in stirrups. A resectoscope is inserted with diathermy attached. A formal cystoscopy is performed to exclude bladder lesions. The prostate is 'shaved' away in strips using the resecting loop, and haemostasis is performed. Resected 'chips' are evacuated from the bladder using an Ellik's evacuator. The specimen is sent for histology to exclude cancer. After sufficient tissue has been removed, a large (24 F) three-way catheter is carefully inserted and bladder irrigation attached. The catheter may be removed after a few days, when the haematuria has settled.

The success rate for symptomatic relief is 85%. Generally this procedure is safe, although it has an overall mortality of around 1% and morbidity due to transurethral resection syndrome (see below), haemorrhage, sepsis, clot retention, stricture formation (3%), urinary incontinence (1%), erectile dysfunction (15%), and retrograde ejaculation (90%).[3]

> ### ⚡ CLINICAL ALERT
> *Transurethral resection syndrome is due to absorption and breakdown of glycine (used as an irrigant) resulting in hypervolaemia and dilutional hyponatraemia. Clinically patients develop restlessness and confusion followed by convulsions, cardiac arrhythmia and pulmonary oedema. Mortality associated with transurethral resection syndrome is 50%. Measures to reduce the risk of transurethral resection syndrome include limiting the resection time to less than 1 hour, abandoning the procedure if there is excessive bleeding, and reducing the pressure of the irrigant in the bladder by lowering the level of the irrigation fluid. If the development of transurethral resection syndrome is suspected, resection should be discontinued, haemostasis obtained rapidly, the irrigant switched off and the patient transferred to a high-dependency unit for invasive monitoring together with cardiopulmonary support and the cautious use of diuretics or fluid restriction.*

Open retropubic prostatectomy
Open surgery via a lower midline or Pfannenstiel incision should be considered for patients with very large prostates (estimated resectable prostatic size greater than 80 g). This approach is preferred to TURP for large prostates because it is quicker and has a reduced risk of transurethral resection syndrome, as there is no need for irrigation with glycine.

Minimally invasive therapies

Due to the morbidity of TURP there has been considerable interest recently in the development of alternative, less invasive therapies. These include transurethral microwave thermal therapy (TUMT), transurethral needle (radio-frequency) ablation of the prostate (TUNA), high-intensity focused ultrasound (HIFU) and the insertion of self-retaining intraurethral stents (for patients with poor life expectancy or those who are unfit for surgery).

Prognosis

Drug treatment is associated with symptomatic improvements in the majority. Approximately 10% of patients will eventually require surgery.

REFERENCES

(1) *McConnell JD, Bruskewitz R, Walsh P, et al, The Finasteride Long-Term Efficacy and Safety Study Group. The effect of finasteride on the risk of acute urinary retention and the need for surgical treatment among men with benign prostatic hyperplasia. New England Journal of Medicine 1998; 338: 557–563.*
(2) *McConnell JD, Roehrborn CG, Bautista OM, et al, the Medical Therapy of Prostatic Symptoms (MTOPS) Research Group. The long-term effect of doxazosin, finasteride, and combination therapy on the clinical progression of benign prostatic hyperplasia. New England Journal of Medicine 2003; 349: 2387–2398.*
(3) *National Prostatectomy Audit. BJU 1995 Mar; 75 (3): 301–316.*

Prostate cancer

Epidemiology

Prostate cancer is a leading cause of cancer death in men. The peak age at presentation is 60–80 years. Patients rarely present before the age of 50 unless detected via case finding or screening. Regions with a high incidence include North America, Sweden, Australia and France (up to 137 per 100 000 per year). The incidence in Europe is up to 31 per 100 000 per year. Asian countries have the lowest incidence—up to 9.8 per 100 000 per year.[1]

The prevalence of asymptomatic (possibly latent) cancers is much higher: autopsy studies reveal small prostatic carcinomas in up to 29% of men between 30 and 40 years and 64% of men aged between 60 and 70 years.[2] The relationship between histologically detectable prostatic cancer and clinically detectable progressive disease is not clear, accounting for the uncertainty in optimum management of patients with early disease.

Pathology

Although no cause has been identified, prostatic cancer is associated with diet, genes and inflammation of the prostate.[2] The majority of prostate cancers are adenocarcinomas that arise in the peripheral part of the gland. Malignant potential is assessed by the Gleason grade (1–5), which is based on the histological appearance of well to poorly differentiated cancers. The Gleason score is the sum of the two most predominant Gleason grades in the biopsy sample (2–10).

Less frequently, transitional cell carcinoma of the prostatic urethra or bladder base invades locally to involve the prostate. Secondary deposits of lymphoma and melanoma have also been described.

Scope of disease

Local

Local extension of foci of prostatic cancer can lead to erectile dysfunction (pelvic autonomic plexus), intestinal obstruction (rectal encirclement), obstructive renal failure from ureteric obstruction and haemospermia. It is more common for prostate cancer to be detected incidentally as part of the diagnosis and treatment of benign prostatic hyperplasia rather than to directly cause symptoms of bladder outflow obstruction. Acute or chronic retention usually occurs in late disease due to the peripheral location of the tumour.

Metastatic

Spread to the bones can lead to pathological fractures, spinal cord compression (vertebral fractures from seeding via the venous plexus to the lumbar veins) or neurological symptoms (cerebral metastases). Liver or lung metastases and lymphangitis carcinomatosa of the lung can rarely occur.

Paraneoplastic

Hypercalcaemia can occur in patients with metastatic prostate cancer.

Clinical features

Currently, the most common form of presentation is incidentally or with PSA-detected asymptomatic disease. Prostate cancer may be detected on prostate biopsy or tissue samples sent from transurethral resection of the prostate for the treatment of benign prostatic hyperplasia.

Patients with locally advanced disease may present with perineal pain, intestinal obstruction or haemospermia. Systemic disease may be suggested by weight loss, fatigue, back pain or leg swelling from iliac vein or pelvic lymphatic occlusion.

Examination is usually normal in patients with early prostate-confined disease. Advanced disease is suggested by anaemia, lymphadenopathy (inguinal, supraclavicular), hepatomegaly, renal hydronephrosis and neurological signs.

Rectal examination is an important aspect of clinical staging. A malignant gland is usually asymmetrical, hard and nodular with obliteration of the medial sulcus. T1 cancers are impalpable, T2 tumours are confined to the capsule of the prostate, T3 tumours extend beyond the capsule, and T4 tumours are fixed to neighbouring structures. The sensitivity (ability to rule out) and specificity (ability to rule in) in the diagnosis of prostate cancer on rectal examination are 53% and 84% respectively.[3]

Benign prostatic hyperplasia

Prostate cancer

757

Modified TNM staging of prostate cancer

Clinical T category*

Tx	Primary tumour cannot be assessed
T0	No evidence of primary tumour
T1	Clinically inapparent tumour (not palpable or radiologically visible)
T2	Tumour confined within prostate
T3	Tumour extends through prostate capsule
T4	Tumour is fixed or invades adjacent structures other than the seminal vesicles

N category

N0	No regional lymph node metastases
N1	Regional lymph node metastases

M category

M0	No distant metastases
M1	Distant metastases

The clinical T category is presented as headings without division into subcategories.

Table 11.31	Upper limits of normal PSA levels according to age

Age (years)	PSA (ng/mL)
<50	2.5
50–59	3.5
60–69	4.5
70–79	5.5

Prostate biopsy

In all but the very frail with obvious advanced disease, it is important to obtain confirmatory tissue diagnosis prior to treatment. A digitally guided prostate biopsy can be performed in patients with advanced disease. Otherwise, biopsy is performed under transrectal ultrasound guidance. The internal gland anatomy is visualized and biopsies can be directed to the peripheral zone. Local anaesthetic is used prior to biopsy and patients should be warned about the risks of bleeding, infection and urinary retention.

Initial investigations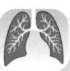

Serum prostate-specific antigen

PSA is a 34 kDa glycoprotein protease secreted from the epithelial cells that line the acini of the prostate, and is responsible for liquefying semen. PSA levels normally increase with age (Table 11.31), with benign prostatic hyperplasia, with urinary tract infection, with prostatic calculi and after ejaculation. Therefore an isolated elevated result does not necessarily indicate prostate cancer.

The risk of prostate cancer increases with rising PSA levels. The cut-off of 4 ng/mL has a sensitivity and specificity of 72% and 93% respectively for detecting prostate cancer.[3] In addition, the risk of extraprostatic disease increases with rising PSA levels. Extraprostatic disease occurs in 17% with PSA levels of less than 4 ng/mL,[3] increasing to 90% with PSA levels greater than 50 ng/mL.

RECENT ADVANCES

Efforts to increase the clinical utility for PSA estimation include expressing PSA in relation to the volume of the prostate (PSA gland density), change in PSA over time (PSA velocity), in relation to age (age-specific PSA) and the ratio between the free and total PSA.

Urinalysis

Midstream urine is sent for microscopy and culture and sensitivity to identify a urinary tract infection as a cause for an elevated PSA.

Further investigations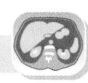

Transrectal ultrasound

Transrectal ultrasound can be used to stage prostate cancers to determine suitability for surgery. Most cancers appear hypoechoic, and extracapsular disease appears as glandular asymmetry with defects in the periprostatic fat layer.

MRI

MRI is emerging as a useful tool for preoperative local staging and provides valuable information on nodal status.

Bone scan

Radionuclide bone scanning is reserved for men with a PSA over 20 ng/mL or those with bone pain. False positive results can occur with osteoarthritis, Paget's disease and healing fractures.

RECENT ADVANCES

Three-dimensional and contrast enhanced transrectal ultrasound is currently being investigated as a tool for staging and diagnosis of prostate cancer.

Initial management

Expectant management

Not all patients with prostate cancer require treatment. 'Watchful waiting' is a suitable option for elderly patients with low-volume, low-grade cancer where life expectancy is unlikely to be affected. Regular monitoring of serum PSA is performed and hormone ablation treatment is offered if the serum PSA climbs or symptoms arise. This differs from 'active monitoring' where patients with biopsy-proven early prostate cancer who prefer to avoid the significant side effects of radical treatment opt to undergo close PSA surveillance. A rising PSA is an indication for radical treatment with curative intent.

Surgical management

Radical prostatectomy

Radical prostatectomy is the surgical removal of the whole prostate gland and seminal vesicles. It is surgery performed with a curative intent and is considered for patients with disease confined to the prostate (T1 or T2).

Open surgery is performed via either a retropubic or perineal approach. Laparoscopic techniques are emerging as minimally invasive means of prostatectomy. If the baseline PSA is over 10 ng/mL, laparoscopic lymph node sampling may be performed prior to radical prostatectomy to detect microscopic nodal involvement (in 10%).

Radical prostatectomy reduces mortality by 5% at 10 years. Although as yet the absolute reduction in the risk of death at 10 years is small, radical prostatectomy is associated with substantial reductions in the risks of metastasis and local tumour progression.[4]

RECENT ADVANCES

Laparoscopic and robotic approaches are currently being used for radical prostatectomy.

Medical management

Radiotherapy

Radical radiotherapy (in combination with androgen ablation) is a suitable option for patients who are high-risk candidates for open surgery, and may be a curative option for men with T3 disease. External beam radiotherapy is performed with CT-assisted planning. A three-field approach is commonly used (anterior and two opposed lateral portals) to irradiate the prostate and seminal vesicles, whilst attempts are made to shield the bladder, rectum and small bowel. As conventional external beam radiotherapy alone is associated with high recurrence, combination therapy is now preferred.[5]

Androgen ablation

Androgen ablation can be used in combination with radiotherapy as part of curative treatment or, more commonly, as a treatment option for patients with advanced symptomatic disease. 80% of prostate cancers are androgen

Benign prostatic hyperplasia

Prostate cancer

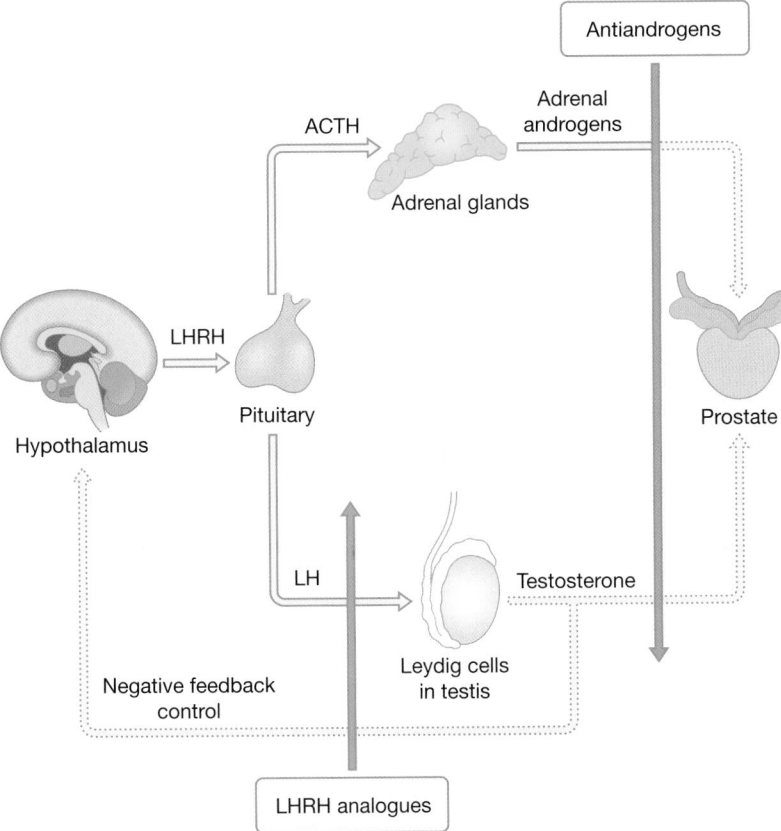

Fig. 11.36 Methods of androgen ablation. ACTH, adrenocorticotrophic hormone; LH, luteinizing hormone; LHRH, luteinizing hormone releasing hormone.

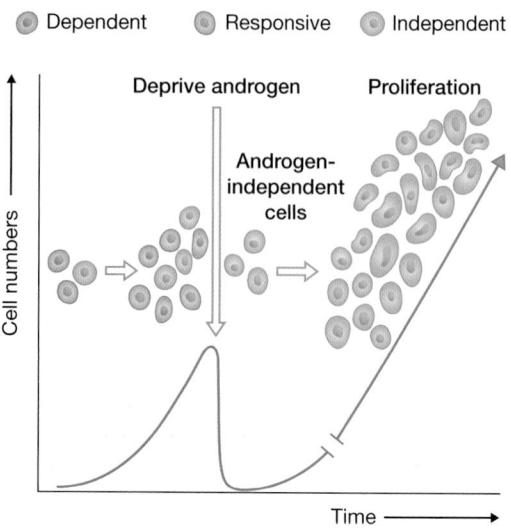

Fig. 11.37 Hormone escape disease.

sensitive, and androgen ablation can be achieved by bilateral orchidectomy or luteinizing hormone releasing hormone (LHRH) analogues (e.g. goserelin). In addition, antiandrogens (e.g. bicalutamide) can be administered to prevent the action of existing androgens (Fig. 11.36). Eventually, the cancer will become hormone refractory (hormone escape, Fig. 11.37).

Bilateral orchidectomy

Bilateral orchidectomy is performed via a midline scrotal incision. The testicles are either removed in toto or in a subcapsular fashion leaving only the tunica albuginea. Apart from the complications of surgery, patients may suffer considerable psychological morbidity as well as side effects of hormone deprivation (loss of libido, erectile dysfunction, hot flushes and lethargy).

LHRH analogues

LHRH analogues (e.g. goserelin, leuprolide) interfere with the negative feedback mechanism of the hypothalamic–anterior pituitary–gonadal axis. Initially there is a surge in luteinizing hormone (LH) secretion, which is rapidly followed by a downregulation and fall in LH and testosterone secretion to castrate levels. This transient surge can cause a tumour 'flare' which can accelerate disease progression, particularly of metastases. This is avoided by simultaneous use of an antiandrogen (e.g. cyproterone acetate) for 2 weeks.

Antiandrogens

Antiandrogens have a similar configuration to testosterone and act by blocking testosterone receptors. As well as side effects common to all forms of androgen suppression therapy, antiandrogens are also associated with gynaecomastia in 50%.

Maximum androgen blockade

Maximum androgen blockade is the suppression of both gonadal and adrenal androgens (which contribute up to 20% of circulating androgen). It is achieved by orchidectomy or administration of an LHRH analogue in conjunction with an antiandrogen. The addition of an antiandrogen has minimal impact on the overall 5-year survival.[6]

Combination radiotherapy and androgen ablation

The combination of radiotherapy and androgen ablation is associated with improvement in 5-year survival from 78% to 88% in patients with localized disease.[7] Clinical trials are underway to evaluate the use of combination therapy in patients with advanced and high-grade disease.

Chemotherapy

Bisphosphonate therapy has been shown to reduce the incidence of metastatic fractures. New chemotherapeutic agents (e.g. docetaxel) provide a further option for hormone-refractory prostate cancer, albeit with limited outlook.

Palliative care

Palliative radiotherapy is effective for pain of isolated bony metastasis, pathological fractures and spinal cord compression. Ureteric obstruction can be treated with high-dose dexamethasone or stenting, and colostomy may be required as a palliative measure for bowel obstruction.

Prognosis

If prostate cancer is detected and treated early with curative intent, a normal life expectancy can be expected in patients less than 65 years. Recurrence is common in patients with advanced cancer treated with hormone ablation, due to the proliferation of androgen-independent cells and the development of resistance to hormone treatment. The life expectancy of men with established hormone refractory disease is of the order of 12–18 months.

REFERENCES

(1) Hsing AW, Tsao L, Devesa SS. International trends and patterns of prostate cancer incidence and mortality. International Journal of Cancer 2000; 85: 60–67.
(2) Nelson WG, De Marzo AM, Isaacs WB. Prostate cancer. New England Journal of Medicine 2003; 349: 366–381.
(3) Mistry K, Cable G. Meta-analysis of prostate-specific antigen and digital rectal examination as screening tests for prostate carcinoma. Journal of the American Board of Family Practice 2003; 16: 95–101.
(4) Bill-Axelson A, Holmberg L, Ruutu M, et al, the Scandinavian Prostate Cancer Group Study No. 4. Radical prostatectomy versus watchful waiting in early prostate cancer. New England Journal of Medicine 2005; 352: 1977–1984.
(5) Mangar SA, Huddart RA, Parker CC, Dearnaley DP, Khoo VS, Horwich A. Technological advances in radiotherapy for the treatment of localised prostate cancer. European Journal of Cancer 2005; 41: 908–921.
(6) Maximum androgen blockade in advanced prostate cancer: an overview of the randomised trials. Prostate Cancer Trialists' Collaborative Group. Lancet 2000; 355: 1491–1498.
(7) D'Amico AV, Manola J, Loffredo M, Renshaw AA, DellaCroce A, Kantoff PW. 6-month androgen suppression plus radiation therapy vs radiation therapy alone for patients with clinically localized prostate cancer: a randomized controlled trial. JAMA 2004; 292: 821–827.

Disorders of the penis

Phimosis and paraphimosis

Phimosis is 'tightening' of the foreskin such that retraction behind the corona of the glans penis becomes difficult or impossible. A paraphimosis occurs when the tight foreskin is forcibly retracted behind the glans and reduction becomes difficult or impossible.

Epidemiology

Phimosis is relatively common in children, whereas a paraphimosis is less common and tends to occur in adults.

Pathology

The foreskin of an infant may normally be adherent to the glans of the penis until the age of 6 years. Phimosis causes balanitis or ballooning of the foreskin with micturition. The foreskin may appear atrophic and pale and eventually fibrose due to the development of balanitis xerotica obliterans.

In adults, a paraphimosis results from pulling a tight foreskin over the glans of the penis. The resulting constriction by the foreskin causes the glans to swell, compounding the difficulty of reducing the foreskin. With time, a band of skin may form behind the corona preventing the foreskin from being replaced.

Clinical features

Children with phimosis may complain of ballooning of the foreskin whilst micturating. Rarely, the condition can be so severe as to cause acute retention of urine. In adults, paraphimosis can occur after intercourse or masturbation or be iatrogenically caused during instrumentation of the urethra (e.g. after insertion of a catheter).

Investigations

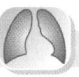

No investigations are required.

Management

Reduction of a paraphimosis
Initially the penis is covered in ice packs that are wrapped in towels (to prevent frost bite) and the glans is squeezed to reduce the oedema. Then the penis is grasped at the level of the constricting band. Gentle retraction of the band and pressure on the glans is applied, allowing the oedema to subside and reduction of the foreskin. A penile block with lidocaine may be effective, as may fenestrating the distal prepuce (multiple punctures of the oedematous tissue with a fine needle) to release the oedema.

Circumcision
Circumcision is surgical excision of the foreskin. It is the treatment of choice for children with urinary retention or balanitis xerotica obliterans from a phimosis, and usually offered as a treatment option for ballooning of the foreskin during micturition.

In adults, circumcision may be offered for a tight phimosis. Several techniques have been described. Surgical excision involves a circumferential incision just distal to the corona of the glans. The prepuce is retracted and a similar incision made approximately 1 cm proximal to the coronal sulcus. The intervening tissue is excised and the edges approximated with Vicryl Rapide. Immaculate haemostasis is essential, particularly at the frenulum, and care is taken not to excise too much tissue as a chordee can result.

> ⚡ **CLINICAL ALERT**
>
> *Circumcision should not be performed in patients with hypospadias as the prepuce may be required for urethral reconstruction.*

Prognosis

An untreated phimosis will usually progress and may completely obstruct urinary flow. Impairment of urinary flow predisposes to recurrent infection, stone formation and urinary retention. Surgery is invariably successful at removing the offending tissue. Complications include bleeding, infection and, rarely, meatal stenosis.

Peyronie's disease

Peyronie's disease is a benign fibromatous disorder characterized by inflammatory plaques affecting the tunica albuginea of the corpora cavernosa of the penis. This rare condition presents with pain or deformity on erection. Whilst flaccid, a lump may be palpable on the penis. In most, reassurance is all that is required as very few have deformities that preclude intercourse. Medical therapies such as colchicine or tamoxifen may relieve pain but are of limited value. Surgery is reserved for patients with stable disease and consists of plication (Nesbit), plaque excision and graft reconstruction or a penile prosthesis. Most patients have mild limiting symptoms, and only a few have disease of sufficient severity to require surgery

Penile cancer

Epidemiology

Penile cancer is rare, and accounts for 1% of all male cancers. It usually occurs after the age of 40 years.

Pathology

Squamous carcinoma is the most common type of penile cancer. Poor penile hygiene is the most established risk factor, and circumcision is well known to be protective. There are associations with HPV 16 infection, leukoplakia, erythroplasia of Queyrat and the Buschke–Löwenstein tumour.

Clinical features

Patients usually present with an ulcerative lesion in the coronal sulcus that bleeds and discharges. Fear or embarrassment may delay the presentation. Occasionally, patients may present due to an associated phimosis. On examination, advanced disease is suggested by the tumour invading the corpora or fungating through the skin, or the presence of inguinal lymphadenopathy.

Investigations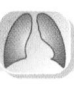

Biopsy
Biopsy (preferably excision biopsy) should be performed for all suspicious lesions.

Management

Circumcision
Circumcision alone may remove superficial disease that is confined to the foreskin.

Topical chemotherapy
Patients with carcinoma in situ may be successfully treated with topical 5-fluorouracil.

Superficial excision
In cases of minimally invasive disease, penile preserving techniques with superficial excision may be possible.

Radiotherapy
Radiotherapy may be used as radical or palliative treatment.

Penile amputation
In more advanced cases, partial or total penile amputation is necessary for local control. Penile reconstruction may be offered in the younger patient.

Systemic chemotherapy
Combination or single agent chemotherapy may be effective in metastatic disease but there is no universal agreement as to the agent of choice. Approximately 50% of patients with node-positive disease will respond to chemotherapy. Failure of lymph node response is an indication for surgical lymphadenectomy or radiotherapy.

Prognosis

The 5-year disease-free survival probability for organ-confined node-negative disease approaches 95%, falling to 30% in node-positive disease and less than 10% in patients with distant metastatic disease.

Erectile dysfunction

Erectile dysfunction or impotence is the inability to initiate or sustain a penile erection sufficient for sexual intercourse.

Epidemiology

The incidence of impotence increases with age: approximately 33% of men suffer with erectile dysfunction by 65 years, and 80% by 80 years of age.

Pathology

The origin of erectile dysfunction may be psychogenic or physical (neurogenic, endocrine, hormonal, arterial, cavernosal or drug induced). Mechanical defects such as trauma or Peyronie's disease occur only in the minority. Most men with erectile dysfunction have a combination of functional and physical causes.

Physical causes
Atherosclerosis can affect the internal pudendal artery and reduce penile arterial perfusion, leading to reduced rigidity and an increased time to erection. Perineal trauma and long-distance cycling may also affect perfusion to the penis. Erectile dysfunction can occur because large veins drain the corpora faster than they can be filled, and may also occur secondary to Peyronie's disease, diabetes, ageing or trauma (Fig. 11.38).

Psychogenic causes
Sexual activity is controlled by higher centres. These relay to spinal centres to either stimulate or inhibit erection. Excessive stimulation of sympathetic nerves is thought to contribute to erectile failure.

Clinical features

The medical history should focus on identifying an underlying cause such as atherosclerosis, diabetes or previous pelvic surgery. A medical and psychosexual history should be taken in conjunction with the patient and his partner.

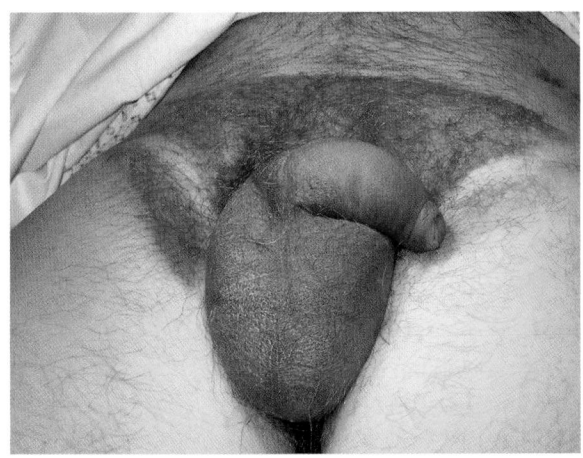

Fig. 11.38 Large perineal haematoma from a penile fracture.

General examination may indicate features of underlying disorders such as diabetes or peripheral vascular disease. Gynaecomastia or absence of secondary sexual characteristics may indicate an underlying endocrine disorder. Genital examination is required to ensure normal anatomy, and the bulbocavernosi reflex is tested to exclude a neurological disorder. A rectal examination should be performed to exclude prostate cancer in the older patient.

Investigations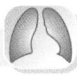

Random blood glucose
Elevated blood glucose may be due to diabetes.

Random serum testosterone
Serum testosterone, LH and prolactin focus on disorders of the hypothalamic–pituitary–gonadal axis. If a random serum testosterone is abnormal, a morning serum LH and testosterone estimation should be taken. A low testosterone and high LH indicate primary hypogonadism, and a low LH may indicate secondary hypogonadism (e.g. pituitary disorders). Patients with hyperprolactinaemia may present with erectile dysfunction and this may be secondary to a pituitary adenoma (0.3%) or drug therapy (e.g. metoclopramide and phenothiazine).

Colour Duplex ultrasound
Ultrasound can be performed to estimate blood flow in penile arteries before and after intracavernosal injection of a vasoactive agent.

Cavernosometry and cavernosography
A butterfly needle is inserted into the corpora and a vasoactive agent is injected followed by a saline infusion. Pressure and flow measurements are taken. When contrast is instilled a venous leak may be identified.

Arteriography
Under local anaesthetic, the iliac vessels are imaged following intracavernosal injection. Internal pudendal arteriog-

raphy can identify an occlusion, fistula or arterio-venous malformation.

Nocturnal penile tumescence studies
Various methods have been described to assess nocturnal tumescence, but the most popular is the 'Rigiscan' where two rings are placed on the penile shaft, one at the base, the other in the coronal sulcus, to measure changes in girth and rigidity in order to distinguish between physical and psychogenic erectile dysfunction.

Management

Psychosexual counselling
Psychosexual assessment and counselling may identify predisposing factors (e.g. traumatic sexual experience), precipitating factors (e.g. organic disease, ageing, depression) and maintaining factors (e.g. performance anxiety). Various behavioural therapies exist; these can be used in conjunction with cognitive and psychoanalytical techniques.

Testosterone replacement
Testosterone replacement therapy may be effective in those with low serum testosterone.

Vasodilator agents
Intraurethral administration of alprostadil pellets can cause cavernosal relaxation and arteriolar dilatation facilitating erection. Oral therapies also exist such as the centrally acting dopaminergic agents (e.g. apomorphine) and peripherally acting phosphodiesterase inhibitors (e.g. sildenafil). Response rates to sildenafil vary from 40% to 80% depending on the underlying aetiology.

Intracavernosal therapy
Alprostadil (Caverject) is the most commonly used agent for intracavernosal treatment. The solution is injected directly into the lateral aspect of the penile shaft, avoiding all vessels and nerves. Approximately 80% are able to achieve erections capable of intercourse but side effects can include prolonged erection (priapism), penile pain, bruising and corporal fibrosis.

Mechanical devices
Vacuum devices are effective for all aetiologies and have no contraindications. A clear plastic cylinder is placed over the penis with an air-tight seal at the base. A pump mechanism creates a vacuum in the chamber to expand the penis. A constriction ring is rolled down the chamber onto the base of the penis to ensure the erection is maintained. Vacuum devices are usually effective in over 75%, although the drop-out rate of this therapy is considerable. It does require a certain expertise, bruising may occur and the constriction band may obstruct ejaculation.

Surgery
Few patients require surgery. Semi-rigid or inflatable penile prostheses may be inserted into the body of the corpora.

Inflatable prostheses are less likely to erode; however, they are more expensive and technically more difficult to insert. Surgery results in all patients being able to produce an erection, but has no effect on libido. Penile arterial insufficiency can be overcome by anastomosing the inferior epigastric artery to vessels at the root of the penis.

Prognosis

The key to successful management is identifying the underlying aetiology. Approximately 60% will respond to psychotherapy alone, and vasodilator agents are effective in approximately 45%.

Priapism

Recurrent priapism often occurs in patients with sickle cell trait or disease.

Epidemiology

With the advent of oral agents for erectile dysfunction, priapism is now uncommon.

Pathology

Priapism is classified as ischaemic 'low flow' or post-traumatic 'high flow'. Low-flow priapism occurs due to impaired venous drainage from the corpora. High-flow priapism is not painful and is caused by the traumatic formation of an arterio-cavernosal fistula.

Clinical features

At presentation the diagnosis is usually obvious. The history may indicate recent use of intracavernous pharmacotherapy, sickle cell disease or leukaemia. In low-flow ischaemic priapism, the erection becomes increasingly painful after about 3 hours. Examination reveals a dusky painful erection with a soft glans.

> **CLINICAL ALERT**
>
> *Low-flow priapism is a urological emergency and requires immediate attention as corporal fibrosis occurs after 6 hours*

Investigations

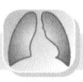

Corporal blood gas estimation
If there is any doubt as to the flow status of the priapism, blood should be aspirated from the corpora and sent for blood gas estimation. Dark deoxygenated blood is associated with low-flow priapism, whereas bright red oxygenated blood is associated with high-flow priapism.

Ultrasound of the corpora
Duplex scanning of the corpora pelvic arteriography confirms the flow status.

Management

Low-flow priapism
Exercise and ice packs
Exercise may divert blood to the gluteal muscles, and the patient is asked to exercise (run up and down the stairs a few times). The same effect may be achieved by placing ice packs around the penis.

Corporal aspiration
If exercise fails, corporal aspiration can be performed using a wide-bore needle. Dark blood indicates the low-flow state whilst bright red blood signifies high-flow priapism. If repeated aspirations are unsuccessful in resolving the erection, a tourniquet is applied to the penile base and after further aspiration, vasoconstrictors (phenylephrine 250 μg) injected directly into the corpora.

Surgical shunt
Failure of conservative measures requires a surgical shunt to connect the corpora to the glans. Corporo-spongiosal shunts may be performed by inserting a Tru-Cut needle through the glans into the body of the corpora or more formally by degloving the penis and creating a window between the two systems. Patients should be warned as to the risk of subsequent erectile failure.

High-flow priapism
Arteriography and selective embolization
In high-flow priapism, management is directed at identifying the site of the fistula by arteriography and selective embolization.

Prognosis

Untreated low-flow priapism causes corporeal fibrosis and impotence. The overall impotence rate in the low-flow state is up to 50% (20% in high flow). Almost all will regain potency if treated within 12 hours. After 36 hours, no patient will respond to α-adrenergics and all have some degree of fibrosis.

Most benign disorders of the scrotum present with either scrotal swelling (Table 11.32) or pain (Table 11.33). The examination of the scrotum will yield important information on the nature of a scrotal disorder. It should always be possible to define the superior aspect of a scrotal swelling; if one 'cannot get above it', it is likely that the swelling is inguinal in origin, as an indirect inguinal hernial sac is the remains of the processus vaginalis as it accompanies the testis in its descent. Large hernias of this type may extend into the scrotum, sometimes completely encasing the testis (p. 294). It should be possible to determine if the testicle is palpable separate from the swelling (epididymal cysts) or if it is not (hydrocele or tumour). The next is to determine if the swelling is painful, and if it transilluminates (hydrocele).

Table 11.32	Causes of scrotal swelling
True scrotal swellings	
Testicular tumour Hydrocele Epididymal cyst Haematocele Varicocele	
Direct inguinal hernia	

Table 11.33	Causes of scrotal pain
Testicular torsion	
Epididymitis	
Orchitis	
Torsion of a testicular appendage	
Testicular tumour	

Hydrocele

A hydrocele is an excessive amount of fluid that accumulates in the tunica vaginalis of the testes.

Epidemiology

A hydrocele is a common disorder with a peak age at presentation between 40 and 50 years.

Pathology

The causes of a hydrocele may be primary or secondary (Table 11.34). There are four main types of primary hydro-

celes. Congenital hydroceles (Fig. 11.39a) occur with a patent processus vaginalis that can fill intermittently with fluid (synonymous with an early inguinal hernia). In an infantile hydrocele (Fig. 11.39b), the processus vaginalis is obliterated at the deep ring causing a collection of fluid that surrounds the cord and testis. The vaginal hydrocele (Fig. 11.39c) is the most common with fluid within the tunica vaginalis that surrounds the testis without extending into the cord. Hydroceles of the cord (Fig. 11.39d) occur when a segment of the processus remains patent and adjacent obliteration causes an isolated fluid collection along the cord.

Clinical features

Presentation is that of a painless scrotal swelling that gradually increases in size. Patients seek advice when the swelling becomes uncomfortable or unsightly.

It is important to perform a detailed clinical assessment to screen for secondary causes of a hydrocele. On examination, it is possible to feel above the swelling, the testis is not palpable separately and the scrotum transilluminates.

Investigations

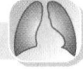

Scrotal ultrasound

If the testis is not palpable due to the size of the hydrocele, a scrotal ultrasound should be performed to exclude an underlying testicular malignancy.

Management

Many hydroceles do not require treatment. Intervention is required only for symptomatic relief.

Table 11.34	Classification of the causes of a hydrocele
Primary	
Patent processus vaginalis	
Secondary	
Systemic Heart failure	

Local
   Testicular tumour
   Infection
   Trauma	

765

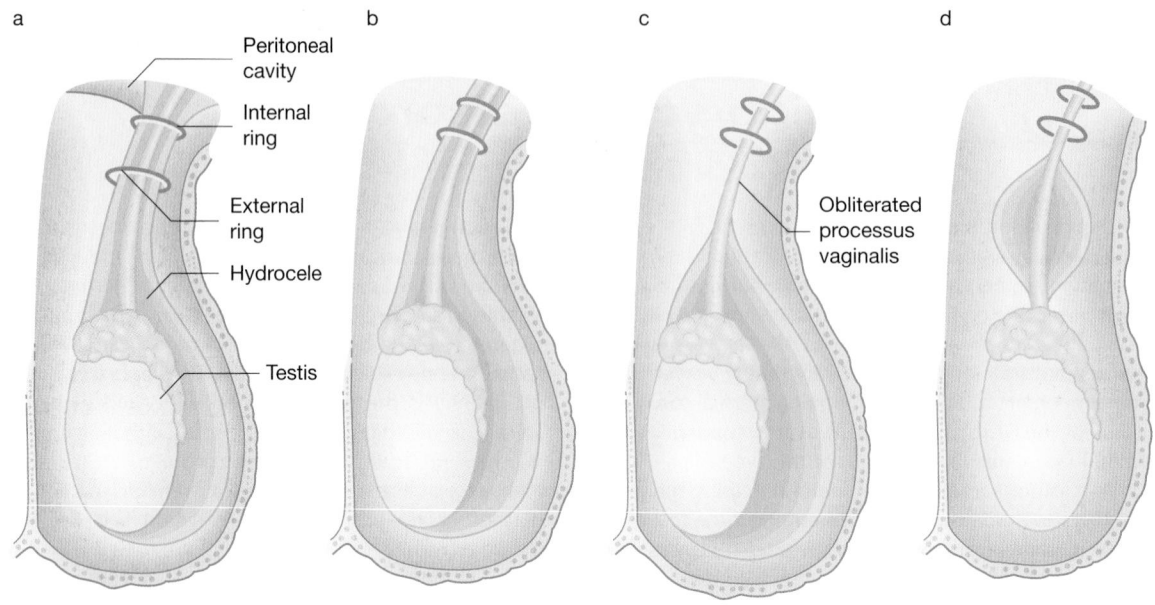

a   b   c   d

Peritoneal cavity

Internal ring

External ring

Hydrocele

Testis

Obliterated processus vaginalis

Fig. 11.39 Types of primary hydroceles: (a) congenital; (b) infantile; (c) vaginal; (d) hydrocele of the cord.

Needle aspiration

Needle aspiration of the hydrocele is the simplest treatment. Recurrent fluid re-accumulation is common, however, and repeated aspirations carry the risk of infection and bleeding. Needle aspiration is contraindicated when testicular malignancy is suspected.

Surgical excision

Surgery to obliterate or excise the sac is reserved for patients in whom the hydrocele is large enough to interfere with daily activity. For Jaboulay's repair a midline raphe (for bilateral) or transverse scrotal incision is made, the testis and sac are delivered, the sac is opened, trimmed, everted and secured with absorbable sutures to itself behind the cord. Recurrence after surgery usually suggests an alternative diagnosis (e.g. epididymal cyst). Complications include haematoma formation and wound infection.

Prognosis

Whilst many untreated patients have a persistent hydrocele, only a small proportion develop troublesome symptoms. In the few that develop significant symptoms and undergo surgery, the risk of recurrence is low.

Haematocele

A haematocele is blood within the tunica vaginalis of the testes. It occurs following trauma or intervention to the genital or inguinal area. In the post-traumatic haematocele the tunica albuginea may be often torn and blood fills the tunica vaginalis. On examination, the scrotum is dramatically swollen, with corresponding ecchymosis and tenderness. Haematoceles do not transilluminate. If pain and swelling preclude a physical examination, ultrasound or surgical scrotal exploration is required to confirm the integrity of the testis and evacuate the clot.

Varicocele

A varicocele is a dilatation of the pampiniform plexus of veins draining the testis.

Epidemiology

Varicoceles are common with a prevalence of 8000 per 100 000 and tend to occur in young adults.

Pathology

The majority of varicoceles are left sided (98%), possibly due to the vertical angle of the left gonadal vein as it enters the left renal vein or absent left terminal venous valve. A varicocele of recent onset raises the suspicion of proximal venous obstruction from a renal or retroperitoneal malignancy. It is widely believed that a possible rise in testicular temperature associated with varicocele may reduce spermatogenesis and cause infertility.

Clinical features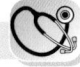

Most varicoceles produce no symptoms; a 'dull ache' is often the only complaint. When supine, the swelling may be absent or soft, but on standing it expands to feel like a 'bag of worms', and patients may notice it when standing to urinate.

Investigations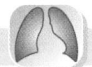

Scrotal ultrasound
Scrotal ultrasound is performed to confirm the diagnosis and identify a normal testis. An abdominal ultrasound scan is often performed in conjunction with the scrotal scan to exclude a renal mass.

Management

In general, no treatment is required for patients with asymptomatic varicoceles.

Gonadal vein embolization or ligation
Surgery is reserved for patients with troublesome symptoms. Varicocele ligation improves sperm counts but no significant differences in conception rates have been shown. Gonadal vein ligation can be performed with an open surgical or laparoscopic approach.

Radiologically controlled transfemoral gonadal vein embolization can be performed as a day case under local anaesthetic; it is usually attempted before surgery.

Prognosis

Most patients with varicoceles are asymptomatic or minimally symptomatic. Recurrences after surgery are rare but may arise due to patent collateral vessels.

Epididymal cysts and spermatoceles

Epididymal cysts arise as diverticula or retention cysts of the vasa efferentia and epididymal tubules, usually from the head of the epididymis (Fig. 11.40). Normally epididymal cysts are asymptomatic, or patients may notice a scrotal swelling. On examination, the cyst is a discrete firm swelling that is palpable separately posterior to the testis. It is possible to feel the top of the cyst (true scrotal swelling) and, if large, the cyst transilluminates. Epididymal cysts are often multiple and bilateral. If necessary, the clinical diagnosis can easily be confirmed by scrotal ultrasound. Excision of the cyst is reserved for patients with cysts that become large or painful. Cyst excision may result in impaired sperm transfer and should be avoided in men who wish to father children. Recurrence due to new cyst formation may occur occasionally necessitating epididymectomy.

Spermatoceles arise as epididymal cysts and contain spermatozoa. Consequently they transilluminate poorly and their aspirate is a 'lemon barley' colour. They are managed similarly to epididymal cysts.

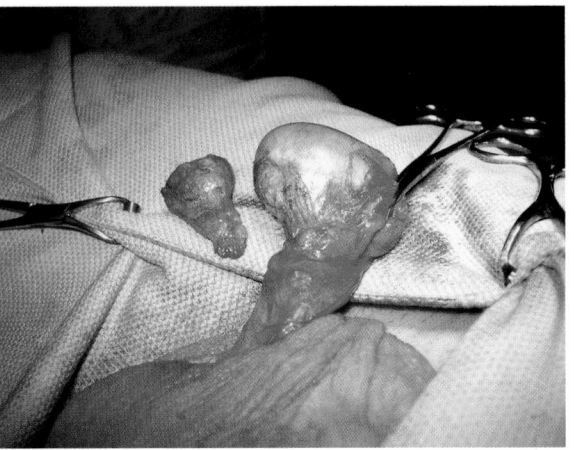
Fig. 11.40 Excised epididymal cyst.

Epididymo-orchitis

Epididymitis is usually caused by an acute infection of the epididymis, and orchitis (inflammation of the testis) may arise as an extension of epididymitis. Orchitis alone may arise from viral infections e.g. mumps.

Epidemiology

Epididymitis is uncommon before puberty, whilst orchitis can occur at any age.

Pathology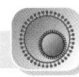

Infection of the epididymis may be bacterial, viral (varicella zoster in children) or chlamydial in origin. Infection gains access via the blood stream or genitourinary tract and into the vas deferens. The age of the patient invariably determines the infecting organism. In children bacterial causes are common and may indicate underlying structural urinary tract abnormalities. In the adult, sexually transmitted disease with organisms such as *Chlamydia* is the most common cause, and in the elderly, bacterial infection due to underlying bladder outflow obstruction or instrumentation.

Bacterial orchitis usually arises as an extension of bacterial epididymitis. Viral orchitis can be caused by mumps and coxsackie viruses. Mumps orchitis is usually bilateral and occurs after puberty. The resulting testicular oedema can cause patchy infarction of the seminiferous tubules and lead to sterility.

Clinical features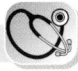

The patient complains of gradually worsening, constant throbbing pain over the scrotum (orchitis) that may later localize to the epididymis (epididymitis). There may be associated urinary frequency, urgency, dysuria, urethral discharge and pyrexia. Mumps orchitis may be associated with parotid swelling.

On examination, the scrotum is erythematous and the testicle is grossly enlarged and globally tender with orchitis, or there is localized tenderness with epididymitis. Occasionally it can be difficult to distinguish between orchitis and testicular torsion, and in these cases patients should be managed as for torsion with prompt evaluation (see below) in view of the risk of testicular infarction.

Investigations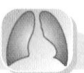

Urinalysis

A midstream urine specimen is sent for microscopy and culture to identify any offending organisms.

Urine for chlamydial RTPCR must be taken.

Management

Analgesia

Simple analgesia is usually required, and bed rest may be necessary for severe pain.

Antibiotics

Quinolone antibiotics (e.g. floxacin) are administered as empirical treatment if a bacterial cause is suspected. Tetracyclines (e.g. doxycycline) are usually prescribed to young adults for presumed chlamydial infection. Patients with suspected viral orchitis do not require antibiotic treatment but the public health authorities should be alerted if mumps is suspected.

Epididymectomy

Rarely, chronic epididymitis may occur following tuberculosis. Bilateral epididymectomy is reserved for when antituberculous therapy fails to resolve chronic infection.

Prognosis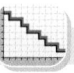

In the majority, epididymo-orchitis is a self-limiting disease that responds well to antibiotics. Mumps orchitis is associated with sterility in the minority.

Torsion of the testis and testicular appendages

Torsion is twisting of the testis along its mesorchium (mesentery).

Epidemiology

Testicular torsion can occur at any age, but the peak incidence is during the second decade.

Pathology

Torsion of the testis can occur within the tunica vaginalis (intravaginal) due to a high investment of the tunica leaving the spermatic cord unaffected, or on the spermatic cord (extravaginal) itself in neonates. A 'true torsion' of the testis alone, where the epididymis remains unaffected, is rare (5%). Torsion of the testis results in impairment of venous drainage, testicular oedema, haemorrhage, arterial occlusion and eventually irreversible infarction of the testis, usually within 7 hours.

Other testicular appendages such as the appendix testis (sessile hydatid of Morgagni), which is of mullerian duct origin, may also undergo torsion and present in an identical manner.

Clinical features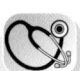

Patients present with sudden onset of spontaneous severe testicular pain associated with nausea and vomiting. There may have been preceding episodes, and an episode may occasionally follow local trauma, sports or coitus. On examination, the overlying scrotum has a bluish tinge; the testis lies high and horizontally in the scrotum. It is often impossible to palpate the testis due to pain or due to a reactive hydrocele.

Investigations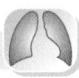

Ultrasound of the scrotum

Doppler ultrasound can be used to detect blood flow in the testicle. If torsion is suspected clinically, surgical exploration must be carried out without delay where there is clinical uncertainty.

Management

Analgesia

Opiate analgesics are usually required for severe pain.

Exploration of the testis

Emergency exploration is required for all suspected cases. A midline raphe incision allows access to both sides of the scrotum. The testis is examined, untwisted and fixed (three-point fixation with a non-absorbable suture). An orchidectomy is performed if the testis is frankly gangrenous. If torsion is present, the other testicle should also be fixed as 10% of cases will suffer the same consequence.

Prognosis

The prognosis relates directly to the time taken for surgical exploration. If surgery is performed within 12 hours after the onset of pain, the majority of testes are likely to retain some function. After 24 hours, testicular salvage is unlikely.

Testicular tumours

Scrotal tumours

Testicular tumours

Epidemiology

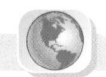

Testicular tumour is the most common cancer in men under the age of 35. It is more common in Caucasians, and the age-standardized incidence is increasing in Europe to 4900 per 100 000 per year.[1] The peak age at presentation is between 25 and 45 years. Testicular cancer is uncommon in men of Afro-Caribbean descent.

Pathology

The majority of testicular tumours are malignant, and the classification is provided in Table 11.35. Germ cell tumours are the most common type (90%). Both seminoma and non-seminomatous germ cell tumours originate from carcinoma in situ.

An undescended testis (cryptorchidism) is the most established risk factor for testicular cancer. It is present in approximately 10%, and increases the risk of testicular cancer 48 fold. A further 10% of those diagnosed with testicular cancer develop a malignancy in the contralateral testicle.

Table 11.35	WHO classification of testicular tumours*
Germ cell tumours	

Seminoma (40%)
    Classic
    Anaplastic
    Spermatocytic	

Nonseminomatous germ cell tumours (teratomas)
    Mature teratoma (teratoma differentiated, TD)
    Embryonal carcinoma with teratoma (malignant teratoma intermediate, MTI)
    Embryonal carcinoma (malignant teratoma undifferentiated, MTU)	

Choriocarcinoma (malignant teratoma trophoblastic, MTT)	
Mixed seminoma/teratoma	
Non germ cell tumours	
Leydig cell tumours (3%)	
Sertoli cell tumours (1%)	

* The classification system is based on the WHO classification; the terms used by the British Testicular Tumour Panel and registry classification are provided in brackets.

Scope of disease

Local

Direct extension of the testicular tumour is rare due to the enveloping tunica vaginalis. A secondary hydrocele may develop.

Metastatic

Lymphatic spread is predominantly to the retroperitoneal para-aortic nodes. Some lymphatic invasion can occur to the internal iliac nodes via lymph vessels associated with the testicular arteries. Inguinal nodes are not normally involved as they do not drain the testes.

Haematogenous spread can occur to the lungs (haemoptysis) and liver (jaundice), bone (back pain), brain and skin.

Paraneoplastic

Rarely, β-human chorionic gonadotrophin (β-hCG) secreting tumours cause gynaecomastia.

Clinical features

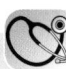

The most common presentation is a painless scrotal lump that arises from the body of the testis. Occasionally there may be an unrelated history of trauma that draws the patient's attention to the lump. Presentation is often delayed through embarrassment of the patient or an erroneous diagnosis of epididymitis. Patients may present with symptoms of advanced disease such as jaundice, abdominal swelling and haemoptysis.

On examination, a mass inseparable from the testis is easily palpable, unless obscured by a reactive hydrocele. The presence of hepatomegaly or supraclavicular lymphadenopathy implies advanced disease.

Initial investigations

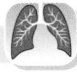

Serum tumour markers

The standard tumour marker profile for testicular cancers is α-fetoprotein and β-hCG; either one of these is raised in 90% of patients with testicular cancer (Table 11.36). Some seminomas produce placental alkaline phosphatase, although levels are not reliable in smokers. Lactate dehydrogenase may be used as a general marker of tumour bulk in patients with advanced disease.

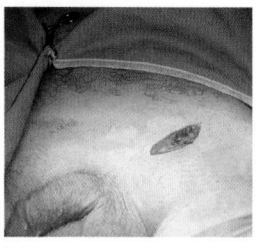

(a)

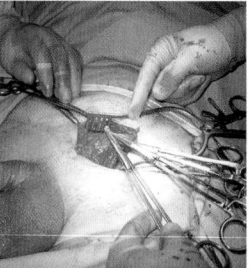

(b)

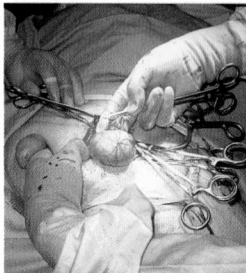

(c)

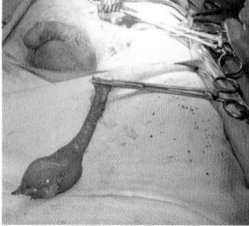

(d)

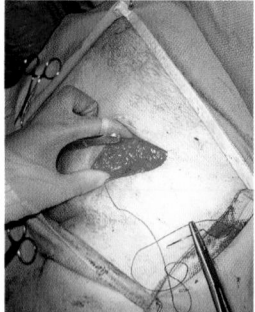

(e)

Fig. 11.41a–e Radical orchidectomy.

Scrotal ultrasound scan

Ultrasound of the scrotum will identify tumours as small as 2 mm. Assessment of tunica albuginea invasion is less accurate and better imaged on MRI.

Further investigations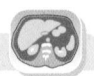

After the diagnosis is established, further investigations are performed to assess the anatomical extent for staging.

▶▶▶ Clinical staging of testicular tumours

T—Primary tumour

Tx	Primary tumour cannot be assessed
T0	No evidence of primary tumour
Tis	Intratubular germ cell neoplasia (carcinoma in situ)
T1	Tumour limited to the testis and epididymis without vascular invasion
T2	Tumour limited to the testis and epididymis with vascular/lymphatic invasion or tumour involving the tunica vaginalis
T3	Tumour invades the spermatic cord with or without vascular invasion
T4	Tumour invades the scrotum with or without vascular invasion

N—Regional lymph nodes

N0	No regional lymph node metastasis
N1	Metastasis with a lymph node mass 2 cm or less, and less than or equal to 5 positive nodes, none of which are greater than 2 cm
N2	Metastasis with a lymph node mass 2–5 cm, or more than 5 positive nodes, none of which are greater than 5 cm or evidence of extranodal extension of tumour
N3	Metastasis with a lymph node mass greater than 5 cm

M—Distant metastases

M0	No distant metastases
M1	Non-regional lymph node or pulmonary metastasis or visceral metastasis

S—Serum tumour marker

S0	Marker study levels are within normal limits
S1–3	Raised marker study levels (1–3 based on degree of elevation of AFP, HCG and LDH)

Stage grouping (simplified)

Stage I	T 1–4	N0	M0	S0
Stage IS	T 1–4	N0	M0	S1–3
Stage II	Any T	N1–3	M0	S0–1
Stage III	Any T	Any N	M1	Any S

Chest film

A plain chest film is a simple measure to identify pulmonary metastases.

CT/MRI of the chest, abdomen and pelvis

Screening CT (or MRI if available) of the chest, abdomen and pelvis is performed to identify any lymphadenopathy suggestive of retroperitoneal lymph node metastases.

Bone scan

A bone scan should be performed in patients with elevated levels of alkaline phosphatase or in those with bone pain.

Initial management

Radical inguinal orchidectomy

As a rule, an orchidectomy is performed prior to any further treatment for all types of testicular cancer to provide a confirmatory diagnosis, histological subtype and local stage. Through an inguinal incision (Fig. 11.41a) the spermatic cord is identified and isolated. It is clamped and doubly transfixed and divided at the level of the deep inguinal ring (Fig. 11.41b). This prevents tumour cell dissemination through testicular manipulation. The testis is delivered into the wound (Fig. 11.41c) and excised from the surrounding fascia and gubernaculum (Fig. 11.41d). The external oblique is repaired (Fig. 11.41e) and the skin is closed. Approximately 80% of patients with seminoma are cured by orchidectomy alone.

Medical management

Seminoma (stage I)

After orchidectomy, approximately 20% of patients with stage I seminoma will experience a relapse with surveillance alone. There is no consensus with regard to the ideal management as survival is equally good with all forms of adjuvant treatment. Adjuvant chemotherapy (carboplatin), irradiation of the retroperitoneal lymph nodes or retroperitoneal lymph node dissection reduces recurrence rates to less than 5%.

Seminoma (advanced disease)

After orchidectomy, radiotherapy may be offered to patients with stage II disease due to the radiosensitivity of the tumours. This also results in overall survival close to 100%, with disease-free survival probability of 95% and 89% at 1 and 6 years respectively.[2]

After orchidectomy, chemotherapy with bleomycin, etoposide and cisplatin (BEP) is the current treatment of choice for patients with metastatic disease.

Non-seminomatous germ cell tumours (stage I)

After orchidectomy, approximately 30% of patients will experience relapse with surveillance alone, usually in the retroperitoneum or lung. Further staging based on tumour marker levels and metastases can identify patients at low, intermediate and high risk.[3] Surveillance may be offered as

Table 11.36	Tumour markers of testicular cancers	
Marker	**Origin**	**Tumour**
α-fetoprotein (AFP)	Yolk sac elements	Teratoma (25%)
β-hCG (HCG)	Syncytiotrophoblasts	Choriocarcinoma (99%) Seminoma (10%)
Lactate dehydrogenase (LDH)		Seminoma
Placental alkaline phosphatase (PLAP)	Seminomatous gonadocytes	Seminoma (90%)

an option to low-risk patients and chemotherapy (BEP) or retroperitoneal lymph node dissection offered to patients at intermediate or high risk.

Non-seminomatous germ cell tumours (advanced disease)

After orchidectomy, patients with stage II disease may be offered surveillance or retroperitoneal lymph node dissection.

After orchidectomy, chemotherapy with BEP is the treatment of choice for patients with metastatic disease.

Surgical management

Retroperitoneal lymph node dissection

Retroperitoneal lymph node dissection is used both for staging and treatment. In early disease retroperitoneal lymph node dissection reduces recurrence rates, and in advanced disease it may improve survival. It is also used as adjuvant treatment for patients with Leydig and Sertoli cell tumours.

Retroperitoneal lymph node dissection is the surgical excision of the lymph nodes bounded by the renal arteries superiorly, the ureters laterally and the division of the iliac arteries inferiorly. Ipsilateral dissections are more limited. Patients should be warned about the risks of retrograde ejaculation due to damage to the sympathetic nerves.

Metastasectomy

There is a general consensus that surgical resection should be offered to patients with post-chemotherapy residual disease in the lung, mediastinum or neck. Pulmonary metastasectomy is associated with improved survival.[4]

Prognosis

The overall life expectancy of patients with stage I disease is normal. Recurrence occurs in approximately 20% and can be reduced to 5% or less with adjuvant treatment. The overall survival of patients with advanced disease is good with approximate 5-year disease-free survival probability of 80% with chemotherapy.[5]

Approximately 25% develop defective spermatogenesis, and 50% will be at least temporarily subfertile following orchidectomy. Adjuvant therapies further impair fertility with 25% becoming azoospermic after chemotherapy. Cryopreservation of sperm is possible before chemotherapy

and patients may be offered intracytoplasmic sperm injection to aid paternity.

FURTHER INFORMATION

Schmoll HJ, Souchon R, Krege S, et al. European consensus on diagnosis and treatment of germ cell cancer: a report of the European Germ Cell Cancer Consensus Group (EGCCCG). Annals of Oncology 2004; 15: 1377–1399.

REFERENCES

(1) Richiardi L, Bellocco R, Adami HO, et al. Testicular cancer incidence in eight northern European countries: secular and recent trends. Cancer Epidemiology Biomarkers and Prevention 2004; 13: 2157–2166.

(2) Classen J, Schmidberger H, Meisner C, et al. Radiotherapy for stages IIA/B testicular seminoma: final report of a prospective multicenter clinical trial. Journal of Clinical Oncology 2003; 21: 1101–1106.

(3) International Germ Cell Consensus Classification: a prognostic factor-based staging system for metastatic germ cell cancers. International Germ Cell Cancer Collaborative Group. Journal of Clinical Oncology 1997; 15: 594–603.

(4) Pastorino U, Buyse M, Friedel G, et al. Long-term results of lung metastasectomy: Prognostic analyses based on 5206 cases. Journal of Thoracic and Cardiovascular Surgery 1997; 113: 37–49.

(5) Williams SD, Birch R, Einhorn LH, Irwin L, Greco FA, Loehrer PJ. Treatment of disseminated germ-cell tumors with cisplatin, bleomycin, and either vinblastine or etoposide. New England Journal of Medicine 1987; 316: 1435–1440.

Scrotal tumours

Squamous carcinoma of the scrotum is rare and usually occurs from exposure to carcinogens. The first described association was with tar exposure in chimney sweeps and currently mineral oils have been implicated. The most common presentation is that of a locally invasive scrotal ulcer, which can metastasize to inguinal lymph nodes. Treatment is with wide surgical excision and ipsilateral inguinal lymphadenopathy. Adjuvant combination chemotherapy and radiotherapy (after surgery) is offered to patients with advanced stage disease. Survival is related to tumour stage and 70% of patients who undergo complete excision with early disease can expect a normal life expectancy.

Diseases of the haematological system

12

Mike Greaves, Dominic Culligan

SECTION 12.1   # Introduction

It is important to have an understanding of the changes in blood and bone marrow in disease, as many systemic disorders can influence the blood and bone marrow. In this chapter, the physiology and pathology of blood and bone marrow are discussed, and the symptoms and signs of haematological disease, relevant investigations and their management are reviewed.

Applied basic science of the haematological system

As an organ, blood is unique as it is in contact with almost all the tissue in the body. The non-nucleated cells of the blood, erythrocytes and platelets, and the nucleated cells, are produced principally in the bone marrow (leukocytes) and in the lymphoreticular system (lymphocytes).

Erythrocytes

The red cells are the most abundant cell type in the blood. The principal content of the red cell is haemoglobin. The deformable, non-nucleated, biconcave discs have features that render them ideal for oxygen carriage and delivery. The shape of the cell is maintained by structural proteins, such as spectrin, which form a cytoskeleton, and enzyme systems protect the haemoglobin from irreversible oxidation.

Haemoglobin is the oxygen-carrying pigment, and the haem component of haemoglobin is responsible for oxygen carriage. Haem is composed of a protoporphyrin ring structure with an iron atom. The molecular structure of haemoglobin evolves through fetal life and early infancy as the requirements for oxygen transfer from placenta differ from those from the lung. After 1 month of age, red cell precursors synthesize predominantly haemoglobin A. Haemoglobin is composed of four haem groups each with its own polypeptide chain.

Haemoglobin A is the predominant haemoglobin in adults with the structure $\alpha_2\beta_2$. Up to 2.5% of the haemoglobin in adults is composed of haemoglobin A2, with 2 δ chains ($\alpha_2\delta_2$), and 1% of the haemoglobin is composed of haemoglobin F with 2 γ chains ($\alpha_2\gamma_2$).

Erythrocytes are the progeny of marrow normoblasts. Their normal lifespan in the circulation is 120 days. Senescent red cells are removed by the reticuloendothelial system, and haem is metabolized to bilirubin, iron and amino acids. The iron of haem is re-utilized in haem synthesis, and globin is degraded to its constituent amino acids.

Immature erythrocytes are identifiable in a stained blood film as red cells with a purplish tinge due to residual RNA from the normoblast stage. They are referred to as reticulocytes when stained with a supravital stain (such as methylene blue). Reticulocytes are polychromatic cells that are more easily identified by the presence of characteristic inclusions. These young cells become indistinguishable from mature red cells after 48 hours. When bone marrow production of erythrocytes is increased, the proportion of polychromatic cells, or reticulocytes, in the peripheral blood becomes greater than 1% or 100×10^9/L. This usually occurs after acute haemorrhage or increased red cell destruction (haemolytic anaemia). When released from bone marrow, the immature red cell also contains a remnant of nuclear material that has the appearance of a single deeply stained inclusion known as a Howell–Jolly body. Because these nuclear remnants are removed by the reticuloendothelial cells on first passage through the spleen, Howell–Jolly bodies are not normally apparent on the blood film. However, they are prominent in hyposplenism, for example after splenectomy.

Leukocytes

Leukocytes are the nucleated cells of the peripheral blood. Neutrophil leukocytes are the most abundant ($2.0–7.5 \times 10^9$/L) except in infancy when lymphocytes predominate. In adults the normal lymphocyte count is $1.0–3.0 \times 10^9$/L. Monocytes ($0.15–0.6 \times 10^9$/L) are also prominent cellular blood components in health whereas eosinophil and basophil leukocytes make up only a small proportion of nucleated blood cells.

The primary role of leukocytes is protection against infection or infestations through the phagocytic capacity of neutrophil granulocytes, monocytes and the immune competence of B and T lymphocytes.

Neutrophil precursors and neutrophils spend 14 days in the bone marrow, but have a half-life of 6–9 hours in the blood. Therefore less than 10% of the total body neutrophils are in the circulation during health, but can be rapidly recruited from the bone marrow in response to cytokines. Lymphocytes have the longest survival of the blood cells, being measured in years.

Platelets

Platelets are non-nucleated and are the smallest blood cells, approximately one fifth the diameter of an erythrocyte. They circulate at a concentration of $150–400 \times 10^9$/L, and respond to agonists such as collagen, thrombin or adenosine diphosphate (ADP) by changing their shape to spiny spheres, adhering to the subendothelium and aggregating with fellow platelets (the primary haemostatic response to vascular injury).

Platelets are rich in intracellular granules that contain clotting factors and cytokines that promote the tissue repair process through stimulation of fibroblasts and vascular smooth muscle cells. Excessive or inappropriate platelet activation is controlled by mediators released by the vascular endothelium such as nitric oxide and prostaglandin I_2. The average lifespan of the platelet in the circulation is 10 days.

The bone marrow and haemopoiesis

In the infant and young child, practically all of the bones contain haemopoietically active marrow. In the adult, haemopoiesis is restricted to the bones of the axial skeleton (vertebrae, ribs, sternum, skull, sacrum, pelvis and proximal femora), however the mainly fatty marrow of other bones is capable of haemopoiesis when requirements for blood cells are increased.

Within the bone marrow, erythrocytes, leukocytes and platelets are derived from a common, self-replicating pluripotential stem cell. By a series of cell divisions, cells committed to each line are produced and further divisions result in the mature cells of the erythrocytes, granular leukocytes, megakaryocytes, T and B lymphocytes. Pluripotential stem cells possess the ability to renew and differentiate into all cellular components of blood.

The committed haemopoietic cell lines are erythropoietic, via normoblasts, thrombopoietic, via megakaryocytes, and leukopoietic, sequentially via myeloblasts, promyelocytes, myelocytes and metamyelocytes in the case of neutrophil leukopoiesis.

Peripheral blood cell counts are maintained within close limits in health, but the bone marrow is highly responsive to increased requirements (erythrocytes after acute haemorrhage and leukocytes in infection). Haemopoiesis is controlled by an orchestra of cytokines and hormones such as the interleukin family, the colony stimulating factors (GM-CSF) which increase stem cell commitment to granulocyte and monocyte production, thrombopoietin which stimulates platelet production and erythropoietin (a glycoprotein hormone produced by the kidney). The production of erythropoietin is increased in response to a reduced oxygen tension (anaemia or hypoxia) in the blood that reaches the kidney, and the result is an increase in the number of cells committed to the erythroid line, reduced maturation time and early release of erythrocytes from the bone marrow.

RECENT ADVANCES

It is now believed that stem cells exhibit plasticity—the ability to differentiate into non-haemopoietic cells such as muscle, liver and vascular cells. Attempts are being made to utilize this property in tissue repair (such as the treatment of heart failure) and novel approaches to treatment of disease (regeneration of nerve tissue for nerve injuries and islet cells for diabetes).

Plasma and coagulation

In a sample of peripheral blood which is centrifuged or allowed to sediment, the red cells comprise around 35–45% of the total volume (the haematocrit), the platelets and white cells 2–5% (the buffy coat), and the remaining 50% or more is plasma. Major components of plasma include the proteins of the coagulation and fibrinolytic systems.

As blood must be fluid, losses of blood through breaches of the vascular system must be minimized. Primary haemostasis (the rapid plugging of defects in small vessels) is the function of platelets. In order to secure haemostasis the platelet plug must be consolidated by the generation of insoluble fibrillar fibrin from fibrinogen, its soluble plasma protein precursor. In order to facilitate haemostasis whilst minimizing the risk of unwanted clot formation, a complex system of activators and inhibitors in plasma has evolved.

In the generation of fibrin, the coagulation proteins interact in a biological amplification system and several of the reactions are catalyzed by negatively charged phospholipid surfaces such as activated platelets. Clotting inhibitors such as antithrombin and protein C act at various stages of the coagulation reaction to damp down the process and control thrombin formation. The ability of antithrombin to inhibit thrombin and other coagulation factors is enhanced by glycosaminoglycans (heparan) that are present on endothelium.

Thrombin is a key enzyme in coagulation because it acts in a feedback loop to activate several of the other coagulation factors and is therefore pivotal in the amplification process and also activates protein C resulting in the inhibition of further thrombin formation.

In the face of a potent stimulus to coagulation the inhibitory mechanisms are overwhelmed and thrombin generation proceeds, leading to digestion of fibrinogen and fibrin clot formation. The final step in consolidation of the clot is the cross-linking of fibrin by the action of factor XIII. Coagulation activation in vivo is initiated principally through tissue factor, an integral cell membrane protein which is not normally expressed by vascular endothelial cells but is expressed by subendothelial cells and smooth muscle as well as most other cells.

As soon as blood leaks from a vessel it is exposed to tissue factor that in turn activates factor VII. This pathway is the principal route to thrombin formation in vivo. The much slower pathway for fibrin generation through activation of factors XII or XI on contact with subendothelial components is of relatively minor importance.

A further check on unwanted thrombus and thrombus extension is provided by the fibrinolytic mechanism, and the key enzyme is plasmin. Its precursor plasminogen, as well as the principal physiological fibrinolytic activator t-PA (tissue plasminogen activator), is bound to fibrin during clot formation, thus localizing fibrinolysis and minimizing any systemic effect. Plasmin digests cross-linked fibrin into peptides of variable molecular weight; one such fibrin degradation product is the D-dimer.

Symptoms of haematological disease

In medical practice in general the presence of disease in a system or organ and the likely diagnosis can frequently be determined from a thorough assessment of the clinical history and a full physical examination. Diseases of the blood and bone marrow are not exceptions to this general rule and investigations are often confirmatory only, or used to assist in subclassification. Investigations should be focused and determined by the results of the clinical assessment. The symptoms of haematological disease are varied, and grouped according to the predominant disease process.

Anaemia

The principal symptom of anaemia is tiredness, but it is not specific as a significant proportion of apparently healthy individuals will admit to lethargy in response to direct questioning. Moreover, severe anaemia can be well tolerated or asymptomatic if it develops over a long period of time. Due to reduced oxygen carriage, anaemia can precipitate symptoms of underlying disease such as angina, peripheral claudication and heart failure, especially in older patients.

In haemolytic anaemia the patient may have jaundice or the passage of unusually dark urine due to increased urobilinogen. Rarely, red urine is passed due to haemoglobinuria in intravascular haemolysis.

Symptoms in other systems may indicate the likely haematological diagnosis and its cause, for example altered bowel habit and blood-stained faeces due to carcinoma of the colon as the underlying cause for iron deficiency anaemia.

Haematological malignancy

Many neoplasms of the haematopoietic and lymphoid tissue, diseases of marrow infiltration and hypoplastic anaemias typically present with symptoms of bone marrow failure. Symptoms of anaemia may be due to failure of erythropoiesis. Recurrent or resistant infections can result from neutropenia and bleeding from thrombocytopenia.

Other common symptoms of haematological malignancy may be more specific, such as drenching night sweats of a severity to disrupt sleep and require a change of bed linen and night attire, a frequent feature of lymphoproliferative disorders. However, even such dramatic symptoms are not entirely specific for haematological disease as they occur in some other diseases such as AIDS and tuberculosis.

Lymphadenopathy may be part of an acute self-limiting illness such as infectious mononucleosis. Persistent and progressive lymphadenopathy, often accompanied by systemic symptoms such as weight loss, may indicate a more sinister diagnosis such as lymphoma. It should be noted, however, that lymph nodes may be palpable in the anterior triangle of the neck and inguinal regions in thin, healthy subjects. Splenomegaly is a feature of many haematological diseases, both benign and malignant.

Disorders of haemostasis and coagulation

Predictably, diseases of the coagulation and fibrinolytic mechanisms present with symptoms of bleeding or thrombosis. Directed questions are a much more reliable guide to the presence of a bleeding disorder than coagulation screening tests.

Easy bruising is a common manifestation in disorders of primary haemostasis and blood coagulation. However, easy bruising is a common but non-specific complaint that is also noted in healthy individuals, and a feature of conditions with no identifiable coagulopathy or defect of primary haemostasis due to abnormalities of the blood vessels or their supporting tissues (such as corticosteroid associated bruising). Features of bruising which are suggestive of significant haematological disease include bruises that are unusually large (for example more than 5 cm in diameter) especially when they occur on the trunk, without recognized trauma, and when bruising is accompanied by unexplained bleeding from other sites such as menorrhagia or recurrent epistaxis.

Epistaxis and gingival bleeding are common features in patients with bleeding disorders. However, occasional nosebleeds are also common in healthy children, and gingival bleeding after tooth brushing is also common in healthy individuals. Symptoms of greater diagnostic significance are when epistaxis is spontaneous and chronic, and when oral bleeding occurs in the presence of good dental hygiene with no evidence of gingival disease.

Although menorrhagia is a common and problematic manifestation of bleeding disorders, it is in fact most often due to endometrial, uterine or hormonal causes rather than a coagulopathy. Furthermore menstrual bleeding is difficult to quantify. When menstruation continues for more than 7 days or when heavy losses occur for more than 3 days, bleeding may be pathological. Excessive post partum blood loss may be a presenting feature of disorders of primary haemostasis or coagulation also, although obstetric causes of bleeding are more common.

Spontaneous bleeding into major joints (haemarthrosis) and spontaneous muscle haematomas are characteristic of severe haemophilia, and rarely occur in other bleeding disorders.

Haematuria, haemoptysis, haematemesis, melaena and rectal bleeding are relatively uncommon manifestations of bleeding disorders and almost never the presenting feature. They are usually caused by local pathology such as peptic ulceration in haematemesis and melaena.

The occurrence of unexpected bleeding after trauma, especially surgical trauma, may give important clues to the presence of an abnormal predisposition to bleeding. Conversely, normal haemostasis after surgery or accidental trauma provides evidence that haemostatic mechanisms were intact at that time. Dental extractions and tonsillectomy are commonly performed procedures and the clinical history should therefore include direct questions regarding bleeding complications after these operations. If there was no unusual bleeding after these procedures, it is unlikely that a significant bleeding disorder was present.

In addition to determining the likely presence of a bleeding disorder from the clinical history, it is often possible to determine whether the condition is an abnormality of primary haemostasis, fibrin formation or its premature dissolution. Spontaneous skin petechiae are a feature of severe thrombocytopenia (platelets $<20 \times 10^9$/L), whereas spontaneous haemarthrosis almost always indicates the presence of a severe bleeding disorder due to coagulation factor deficiency. In general, defects of primary haemostasis result in predominantly mucosal bleeding and skin bruising (although such bleeding also occurs in severe coagulation factor deficiency, muscle and joint bleeds generally dominate the clinical picture).

Family history and social history

A number of haematological conditions are hereditary, such as von Willebrand's disease (autosomal dominant), antithrombin deficiency and thalassaemia.

Occupational exposure to benzene and related chemicals is an occasional cause of bone marrow failure.

Examination in haematological disorders

Inspection

Anaemia may cause skin pallor; however, due to natural variations in skin colour it is not a reliable physical sign. A better indication may be given by examination of the oral mucous membranes and the conjunctiva of the lower eyelid, but even experienced clinicians may fail to diagnose significant anaemia from the physical examination. In haemolytic anaemias there may be clinical jaundice, best seen by examination of the sclerae. In polycythaemia there may be obvious facial plethora.

Examination of the mouth may also reveal smooth tongue (atrophic glossitis, Fig. 12.1) and cracking at the corners of the mouth (angular stomatitis, Fig. 12.1) in chronic iron deficiency anaemia, and inflamed buccal mucosa in megaloblastic anaemia.

Chronic iron deficiency anaemia occasionally causes koilonychia, a curious nail deformity with a concave or spoon-shaped configuration.

Close attention should be paid to the lymph node areas (neck, axillae and inguinal regions) as lymphadenopathy is an important physical sign, for example in lymphoma.

Examination of skin and joints may reveal evidence of a bleeding disorder, including purpuric or petechial rash in severe thrombocytopenia and/or abnormal bruising. Acute haemarthrosis and chronic joint damage with deformity can result from recurrent joint bleeding in severe haemophilia. Skin infiltration is an occasional finding in haematological malignancies, especially lymphomas.

Splenomegaly is a common feature of several benign and malignant disorders of the blood and bone marrow (Table 12.1). Massive splenomegaly is defined as a grossly enlarged spleen that reaches the pelvic brim. Intraabdominal lymphadenopathy may be palpable as abdominal masses in lymphoma, and other masses such as

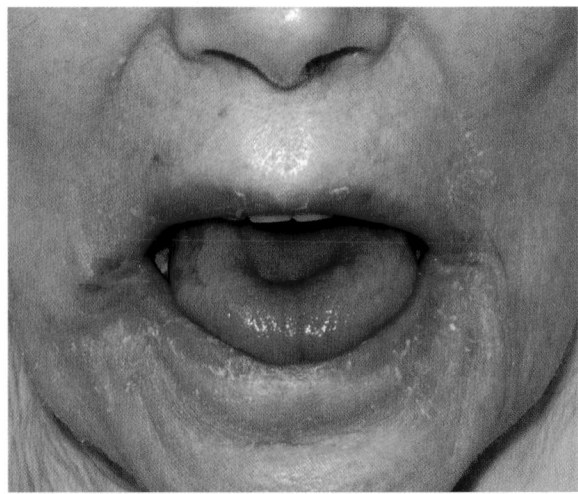

Fig. 12.1 Angular cheilitis and atrophic glossitis.

Table 12.1	Some causes of splenomegaly in haematological disease

Massive splenomegaly*

Myelofibrosis

Chronic myeloid leukaemia

Lymphoma

Chronic malaria

Splenomegaly

Haemolytic anaemia

Haemoglobinopathies

Haematological malignancies

Infection

* Any cause of massive splenomegaly will initially present with mild enlargement of the spleen.

advanced colorectal cancer or uterine fibroids may indicate the cause of iron deficiency anaemia.

In the cardiovascular system, severe anaemia causes a resting tachycardia or a systolic murmur due to hyper-dynamic circulation and there may be evidence of congestive cardiac failure.

In the respiratory system there may be evidence of chronic or recurrent infection due to leukopenia from haematological malignancy or bone marrow failure. Careful assessment may also provide an explanation for abnormal blood count findings such as secondary polycythaemia due to chronic hypoxia from obstructive pulmonary disease.

Peripheral neuropathy may be present in deficiency of vitamin B_{12}, most commonly due to pernicious anaemia. Less commonly there may be optic atrophy, features of subacute combined degeneration of the cord (abnormal gait and balance due to degeneration in the posterior and lateral columns of the spinal cord) and even dementia.

In many cases the physical examination may reveal the cause of an abnormal blood count which is due to systemic disease and not due to primary disease of the blood and bone marrow. Examples are rheumatoid arthritis causing anaemia of chronic disease, liver disease causing macrocytosis and bacterial sepsis causing neutrophil leukocytosis.

Blood tests

Diagnostic imaging

Investigation of haematological diseases

Blood tests

The full blood count

As many diseases can influence the blood, the full blood count is among the most commonly requested laboratory investigations in clinical practice. In modern laboratories, the full blood count is routinely performed by automated cell-counting equipment.

The concentrations of haemoglobin, erythrocytes, leukocytes and platelets are measured, and the size of erythrocytes and proportion of red cells to plasma (the haematocrit) determined. The proportion of leukocytes of each category (differential white cell count) is measured from cell size and granule content. Abnormal cells such as nucleated red cells and leukaemic blast cells are detected. Some machines can also measure the concentration of reticulocytes.

Examination of a stained blood film by light microscopy may provide additional diagnostic information, for example abnormally shaped red cells in sickle cell disease, the characteristic atypical mononuclear cells in infectious mononucleosis and abnormal leukocytes for the subclassification of leukaemias.

The data generated by automated cell counters have a high degree of accuracy and precision. The normal ranges are established by calculation of the mean and two standard deviations from the mean in a large cohort of healthy subjects. By definition, 2.5% of haematologically normal individuals will be slightly above and 2.5% will be slightly below the normal reference range. Therefore, minor abnormalities in the full blood count are not necessarily indicative of disease, and the results of laboratory investigations should always be interpreted in the clinical context. The range of normal values also differs between laboratories, with gender (e.g. lower haemoglobin concentration, red cell count and haematocrit in adult females) and at different stages of life (e.g. higher haemoglobin concentration, red cell count and haematocrit in neonates).

The full blood count includes numerical values which indicate the average size and haemoglobin content of erythrocytes. These parameters are very valuable in determining the likely causes of common anaemias (p. 779) and are calculated automatically from the haemoglobin concentration, red cell concentration and haematocrit of the whole blood sample as follows:

Mean corpuscular volume (MCV) in femtolitre (fL) = Haematocrit (l/l) / Red cell concentration (per litre)

Mean corpuscular haemoglobin (MCH) in picograms (pg) = Haemoglobin concentration (g/l) / Red cell concentration (per litre)

Mean corpuscular haemoglobin concentration (MCHC) in grams per ilitre (g/l) = Haemoglobin concentration (g/l) / Haematocrit (l/l)

Erythrocyte sedimentation rate

The erythrocyte sedimentation rate (ESR) is generally performed in the haematology laboratory. It is the rate at which red cells sediment by gravity in plasma in 1 hour.

Increased aggregation and sedimentation occur in the presence of high concentrations of immunoglobulin and fibrinogen (an acute phase reactant). The ESR is increased in a wide variety of inflammatory and neoplastic conditions, but is entirely non-specific. A normal value can never be used to exclude the presence of significant disease. Direct measurement of plasma viscosity provides equally useful data and has replaced ESR measurement in some diagnostic laboratories.

Dietary haematinics

These are the essential dietary components for haemoglobin synthesis and haemopoiesis. The most important clinically are iron, vitamin B_{12} and folates. Their concentrations can be measured in serum. Body iron stores can also be assessed by the measurement of the concentration of storage iron, ferritin, in serum.

Tests for haemolysis

Red cell destruction (haemolysis) results in an increased unconjugated bilirubin concentration in serum and increased urinary urobilinogen. Lactate dehydrogenase (LDH) is released from the red cells and its concentration in serum is increased. The concentration of haptoglobin (a haemoglobin-binding protein which scavenges extracellular haemoglobin) is reduced. Because erythropoiesis is increased in response to the anaemia there is a reticulocytosis.

In chronic intravascular haemolysis, iron from released haemoglobin passing through the renal tubules may be detected in cellular debris within a sample of urine by staining of the sediment for iron (haemosiderinuria).

Direct antiglobulin test

The direct antiglobulin test (DAT or Coombs' test) utilizes antibody raised against human immunoglobulin or complement to detect immunoglobulin deposited on the surface of red cells. In the presence of cell surface immunoglobulin, addition of anti-human immunoglobulin causes clumping of the red cells. The test is used to distinguish haemolytic anaemias with an immune pathogenesis from those in which other mechanisms are involved. For example, the test is positive in autoimmune haemolytic anaemia but not in haemolysis caused by physical damage to red cells passing through a faulty cardiac valve prosthesis.

Haemoglobin electrophoresis

Haemoglobin electrophoresis is employed in the diagnosis of haemoglobinopathies (thalassaemias, sickle disorders). For example in sickle cell disease, the principal haemoglobin is Hb S, and the single amino acid difference from Hb A results in altered electrophoretic mobility.

Serum immunoglobulins

Lymphoproliferative disorders are clonal diseases and frequently accompanied by the presence of a monoclonal immunoglobulin (paraprotein). This is a typical finding in plasma cell myeloma. In some cases of myeloma the monoclonal immunoglobulin consists only of light chains (Bence Jones protein) and can be detected in urine.

Immunological phenotyping

Immunological phenotyping is the classification of leukocytes in blood, bone marrow and other tissue by their antigenic profile. It is performed using a flow cytometer. A range of monoclonal antibodies is employed. It is of great value in the diagnosis and classification of haematological malignancies.

Clotting times

The function of the components of the coagulation system can be assessed by measuring the time required for clotting of re-calcified plasma prepared from a blood sample anticoagulated with sodium citrate. The citrate binds calcium ions which are required at several points in the mechanism, and the addition of calcium allows fibrin formation to take place.

The two principal screening tests are the activated partial thromboplastin time (APTT) and the prothrombin time (PT). To estimate the APTT, the intrinsic pathway is activated by surface contact, for example by the addition of kaolin (chalk powder providing a massive surface area for contact), and phospholipid is added to substitute for the role of platelets in coagulation; the time taken for the plasma to clot is measured. Clotting through the intrinsic and common pathways in the APTT involves all clotting factors other than factor VII and factor XIII.

To estimate the PT, tissue factor and phospholipid are added to the plasma sample. Clotting occurs through the extrinsic and common pathways. The test assesses factors VII, V, X, II and fibrinogen only.

In some circumstances it is necessary to assay the concentration of individual clotting factors to reach a precise diagnosis, for example factor VIII in haemophilia.

Skin bleeding time

Primary haemostasis (platelet function) is assessed in vivo by measuring the duration of bleeding from a standardized skin incision. Normal is less than around 8 minutes.

Fibrin degradation products

The quantitation of fibrin degradation products (FDP) forms part of the laboratory assessment in suspected disseminated intravascular coagulation. Also, the plasma concentration of a product of digestion of cross-linked fibrin, D-dimer, is used as part of the evaluation of possible deep vein thrombosis or pulmonary embolism. Although lacking specificity, the test is sensitive and a negative result indicates that venous clot is very unlikely to be present.

Bone marrow aspiration

Bone marrow aspiration is detailed on page 779.

Diagnostic imaging

Radiological imaging is an essential tool in the assessment of many haematological malignancies. The plain X-ray of the axial skeleton is useful diagnostically in plasma cell myeloma, as the typical lytic bone lesions are often easily visible. Imaging by CT or MRI or PET is employed to stage haematological malignancies.

SECTION 12.3   Diagnostic procedures

Bone marrow aspiration and trephine biopsy

Indication

Examination of bone marrow is indicated as part of the diagnostic work-up of haematological malignancies with suspected marrow involvement, the investigation of some anaemias and pancytopenia and the diagnosis of diseases such as chronic idiopathic myelofibrosis.

Patient preparation

The procedure requires informed consent. General anaesthesia is required for infants and children; in adults the procedure can be carried out with local anaesthetic.

Procedure

Patients are positioned supine on one side and the field is prepared with antiseptic solution and draped. The marrow can be aspirated into a syringe through a needle inserted into a marrow cavity (usually sternum or pelvis, or the tibia in infants and small children), smeared on a slide and stained by a method similar to that for peripheral blood.

A trephine biopsy acquires a core of tissue from the posterior superior iliac spine using a wide-bore cutting needle. Further information, particularly on the structure and cellularity of the marrow, can be obtained by preparation of sections of a marrow trephine biopsy.

Complications

There is often a degree of discomfort caused by the pressure exerted to penetrate the bone cortex and from the negative pressure induced within the marrow cavity during aspiration. Complications other than residual soreness and some bruising are uncommon.

Post procedure care

The procedure can be performed as a day case, and children may be allowed home when they have recovered from the general anaesthesia.

SECTION 12.4   Anaemias

Anaemia may be defined as a haemoglobin concentration less than 13.0 g/dL in an adult male and 11.5 g/dL in an adult female, although there are slight variations in normal ranges between laboratories. The lower limits of normal haemoglobin concentration are higher in neonates and lower in young children.

A low haemoglobin concentration usually reflects a reduction in the body red cell mass except in pregnancy, when both red cell mass and plasma volume increase (the latter to a greater degree resulting in haemodilution). Although the haemoglobin concentration is lower than in the non-pregnant state in the physiological 'anaemia' of pregnancy, red cell mass and overall oxygen-carrying capacity is increased to support the increased metabolic requirement of the mother and fetus.

In some causes of anaemia, the production of leukocytes and platelets may also be reduced, resulting in pancytopenia. An example is megaloblastic anaemia, where the defect in nucleic acid synthesis affects all cell lines causing pancytopenia, in contrast to iron deficiency and thalassaemias, where the only limitation is in haemoglobin synthesis.

Clinical features

The consequence of anaemia is tissue hypoxia. The severity of the anaemia alone is not the most important determinant of symptoms, but rather the rate of development of the anaemia and the presence of any coexistent disease.

Rapid-onset anaemia produces more symptoms, as the body does not have time to compensate for the reduction in oxygen-carrying capacity. Dyspnoea is the main symptom, and anaemia can precipitate symptoms of occult coexistent disease such as angina and claudication. Other symptoms include weakness, lethargy and pallor.

On examination, there may be pallor of the mucous membranes, but this sign has a low sensitivity (difficult to rule in anaemia). A hyperdynamic circulation may be in evidence with a bounding pulse, cardiomegaly and a systolic flow murmur. Some features are specific to the type of anaemia, such as the jaundice of haemolytic anaemias, nail changes of iron deficiency and the neurological manifestations of B_{12} deficiency.

Investigations

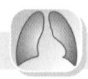

Full blood count, red cell indices and blood film

The mainstay of investigation is the full blood count to confirm the diagnosis. The red cell indices can be utilized to subclassify the anaemias and to focus on the more likely causes (Table 12.2). Using the mean cell volume (MCV), anaemias are classified into microcytic, normocytic or macrocytic.

The white cell count and platelet counts discriminate isolated anaemia from pancytopenia. There may be increased neutrophil and platelet counts, for example in blood loss anaemia or anaemia of chronic disease due to an inflammatory process.

The blood film may give additional important clues to the underlying aetiology. Specifically, variations in red cell shape (poikilocytosis) provide diagnostic clues, for example fragmented red cells (schistocytes) in some types of non-immune haemolytic anaemia, spherical red cells (spherocytes) in immune haemolytic anaemia and hereditary spherocytosis and sickle or crescent shaped cells in sickle cell disease. Another important feature is polychromasia, a purple tinge typical of newly formed red cells due to their content of residual RNA. Increased polychromasia indicates a relative excess of young erythrocytes due to increased haemopoiesis, usually as a response to blood loss or haemolysis.

Bone marrow aspiration

Examination of a sample of bone marrow by microscopy provides additional information and is useful when the blood count and film do not provide adequate diagnostic information. For example it is of value when the anaemia may be due to bone marrow infiltration by malignancy or fibrosis, or due to marrow failure.

Microcytic anaemias

Iron deficiency anaemia

Epidemiology

Iron deficiency is the most common cause of anaemia worldwide, especially in underdeveloped countries (due to low dietary intake). It is more common in women due to iron loss from menstrual bleeding.

Pathology

Iron is an essential nutritional requirement. The body stores are regulated mainly by absorption (duodenum and upper jejunum), as no active excretion occurs. There are small daily losses in the urine, faeces and sweat.

The daily requirements of iron are 1 mg for the adult male, 2 mg for menstruating adult females and 3 mg in pregnancy. Although a typical Western diet contains 10–20 mg of iron per day, less than one third is absorbed. The haem iron in meat is readily absorbed, but the inorganic iron in vegetables and cereals is complexed to amino and organic acids. It requires release

Table 12.2	Classification of anaemia		
Microcytic anaemias	**Macrocytic anaemias/macrocytosis**		**Normocytic anaemias**
MCV <80 fL	MCV >95 fL		MCV 80–95 fL
Iron deficiency	Megaloblastic anaemia B_{12} deficiency Folate deficiency		Acute blood loss
Sideroblastic anaemia	Macrocytosis[a] Alcohol Liver disease Cytotoxic drugs		Anaemia of chronic disorders[b]
Thalassaemia			Haemolytic anaemias
Anaemia of chronic disorders[b]			Hypoplastic anaemia
			Bone marrow infiltration: Leukaemias Myeloproliferative states Non-haematological malignancies

[a] Macrocytosis may occur without anaemia in these situations.

[b] Anaemia of chronic disorders is a common anaemia. It occurs in chronic inflammatory diseases, such as rheumatoid arthritis, chronic infections and malignancy. The haemoglobin is rarely <8.0 g/dL and the MCV is low normal or generally only slightly subnormal, unlike in iron deficiency.

and reduction from the trivalent (Fe^{3+}) to the divalent state (Fe^{2+}) for absorption, a process that is promoted by stomach (hydrochloric) acid and ascorbic acid in food.

In developed countries, poor iron intake may be contributory but is rarely the sole cause for iron deficiency. Chronic blood loss is a more important cause. As 1 mL of blood contains 0.5 mg iron, daily losses of 10 mL may be sufficient to cause a negative iron balance and depletion of iron stores.

The initial depletion of iron stores is an asymptomatic process (latent iron deficiency), and anaemia develops only when the reticuloendothelial stores (haemosiderin and ferritin) are completely depleted. The symptoms of anaemia only manifest after haemoglobin levels start to fall.

Scope of disease

Iron deficiency is common in many menstruating women, and iron deficiency anaemia is a common presentation of chronic occult gastrointestinal bleeding. Rarely, iron deficiency causes a post-cricoid mucosal web in the oesophagus causing dysphagia (Paterson–Brown-Kelly syndrome).

Clinical features

The symptoms of anaemia depend on the speed of onset and the presence of coexisting disease (p. 779). A dietary history is essential to estimate the daily iron intake, and a systems review should focus on any cause of chronic blood loss (Table 12.3).

On examination, features of iron deficiency include angular cheilitis (painful cracking at the corners of the mouth), atrophic glossitis (smooth tongue) and koilonychia (spoon-shaped deformity of the nails). An abdominal and rectal examination is required in view of the possible presence of a gastrointestinal cause for blood loss.

Table 12.3	Major causes of iron deficiency
Chronic blood loss	
Gastrointestinal	
Peptic ulcer	
Angiodysplasia of colon	
Stomach cancer	
Colorectal cancer	
Uterine	
Menorrhagia	
Increased requirements	
Childhood	
Pregnancy	
Malabsorption	
Gastrectomy	
Coeliac disease	
Malnutrition	

Initial investigations

Full blood count, blood film and red cell indices

Anaemia occurs only after all the body iron stores are depleted. Iron deficiency results in a microcytic hypochromic picture on the blood film. Iron deficient haemopoiesis, with a fall in the MCV, MCH and MCHC, may antedate the development of anaemia.

The platelet count may be elevated, especially in the presence of continuing blood loss.

Serum ferritin

Where there is doubt, tissue iron depletion can be confirmed by measurement of serum ferritin, a protein–iron complex. A small amount derived from the storage pool of body iron is detectable in plasma and is an accurate indicator of body iron stores.

Iron deficiency anaemia

Anaemia of chronic disorders

Megaloblastic anaemia

Red cell enzymopathies

Autoimmune haemolytic anaemia

Microangiopathic haemolytic anaemias

Hereditary spherocytosis

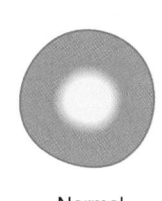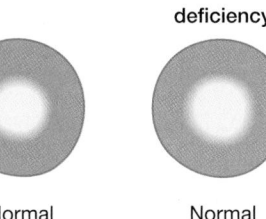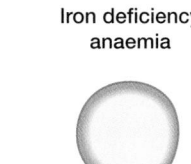

Red cell iron (peripheral film and indices)

Normal	Latent iron deficiency	Iron deficiency anaemia
Normal	Normal	Hypochromic, microcytic MCV↓, MCH↓, MCHC↓

Fig. 12.2 Development of iron deficiency anaemia.

Iron stores (bone marrow macrophage iron)

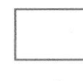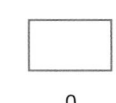

| ++ | 0 | 0 |

Low serum ferritin concentration confirms iron deficiency. However, as ferritin is also an acute phase response protein, serum ferritin levels may be normal or high despite tissue iron depletion in the presence of infection, inflammation and neoplasia.

Serum iron and total iron-binding capacity

In the presence of iron deficiency, serum iron is low and the total iron-binding capacity is high (a useful investigation to differentiate iron deficiency from anaemia of chronic disease).

Further investigations

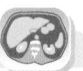

Bone marrow aspiration

Bone marrow examination is not required, other than in complicated cases where a multifactorial pathogenesis of anaemia is suspected. Under these circumstances, bone marrow examination with staining for iron is helpful. In iron deficiency no iron is present in bone marrow.

Investigation for the underlying cause

In males and post-menopausal females in whom the diet is adequate, gastrointestinal bleeding must be excluded. Testing for occult blood in samples of faeces is inadequate and upper and lower gastrointestinal imaging or endoscopy are usually indicated.

Initial management

Treatment of the underlying cause

The underlying cause should be identified and treated, for example by dietary correction, treatment for menorrhagia or peptic ulcer disease, or surgery when appropriate for gastrointestinal malignancy.

Medical management

Oral iron supplementation

Ferrous sulphate 200 mg 3 times daily is effective in most cases. Each 200 mg tablet contains 67 mg of iron. The side effects include nausea, abdominal pain, diarrhoea or constipation. Also, oral iron stains the faeces a black colour. Where there is intolerance, alternative formulations such as ferrous fumarate or slow-release preparations can be tried.

The response to treatment is limited by the haemopoietic capacity of bone marrow. Haemoglobin increases typically at 1 g/dL per week, and oral iron should be continued for 3 months after the normal haemoglobin level has been restored, in order to replace iron stores. Continuing iron supplementation may be required if blood loss is ongoing. Failure of the haemoglobin level to increase most commonly indicates poor compliance or a wrong diagnosis (usually anaemia of chronic disease).

Intravenous iron

Parenteral iron replacement is necessary only in exceptional circumstances such as when there is intolerance of oral iron or severe malabsorption. All preparations for intravenous use carry a risk of anaphylactic reaction, and the response to treatment is no faster than with oral iron therapy.

Packed cell transfusion

With significant ongoing blood loss or severely symptomatic disease, blood transfusion may be required. In general, however, transfusion of blood products is a last resort.

Prognosis

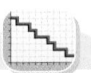

Adequate iron replacement and correction of the underlying cause will lead to the resolution of anaemia. The prognosis is determined by the nature of the underlying disease and its extent, for example carcinoma of the colon.

Anaemia of chronic disorders

Epidemiology

Anaemia of chronic disorders is a common cause of anaemia.

Pathology

The underlying pathogenesis is cytokine-induced failure of transfer of iron from reticuloendothelial cells to normoblasts. This may occur secondary to chronic inflammatory diseases such as connective tissue disorders, chronic infections and malignancies (Table 12.4).

Table 12.4	Some causes of anaemia of chronic disorders
Chronic infection	
Tuberculosis	
Osteomyelitis	
Endocarditis	
Lung abscess	
Chronic inflammation	
Systemic lupus erythematosus	
Rheumatoid disease	
Sarcoid	
Inflammatory bowel disease	
Malignancy	
Lymphomas	
Sarcomas	
Most carcinomas	

Clinical features

Although the degree of anaemia is rarely severe, patients are often symptomatic with lethargy and reduced exercise tolerance. A past medical history may immediately identify any potential underlying causes, or these may be evident on a detailed systems review.

Investigations

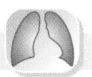

Full blood count, blood film and red cell indices

The full blood count typically reveals a mild to moderate normocytic anaemia with a haemoglobin rarely less than 8 g/dL. There may be a degree of microcytosis and hypochromia, but rarely as prominent as in iron deficiency anaemia.

Reactive neutrophil leukocytosis (elevated neutrophil count) and thrombocytosis (elevated platelet count) can occur due to inflammation.

Erythrocyte sedimentation rate/C-reactive protein

The non-specific markers of inflammation are usually raised.

Serum B_{12} and red cell folate

Serum B_{12} and red cell folate levels are normal (unless coexistent deficiency occurs).

Serum ferritin

With chronic inflammation, serum ferritin may not accurately reflect the iron stores. Because it is an acute phase reactant protein, it can be elevated, despite reduced tissue iron stores.

Serum iron and total iron-binding capacity

Both serum iron and total iron-binding capacity may be reduced (in contrast to iron deficiency, in which the serum iron is reduced but the total iron-binding capacity is increased).

Determining the underlying disease

If the anaemia is detected as an incidental finding with no clinical feature indicating the likely cause, further investigation should be directed towards identifying the occult inflammatory, infective or malignant disease that is likely to be present.

Management

Identify and treat any underlying disease

Successful treatment of the underlying disorder leads to improvement in the haemoglobin concentration.

Recombinant erythropoietin administration

In patients with severe chronic renal failure, a comparable but often more severe normocytic anaemia results from failure of erythropoietin secretion. The anaemia in this subset of patients often responds to regular subcutaneous recombinant erythropoietin administration. Moreover, the quality of life also improves, especially of those on dialysis.

Packed cells transfusion

Exceptionally, regular blood transfusion may be required for relief of severe symptoms of anaemia. Relief is temporary and repeated transfusions are required with their attendant risks, including iron overload.

> **RECENT ADVANCES**
>
> *There is interest in the possibility that the use of erythropoietin may be effective in some cases of intractable anaemia of chronic disease.*

Prognosis

The prognosis is related to the underlying cause. Anaemia usually resolves if the underlying cause is identified and successfully treated.

Macrocytic anaemias

Megaloblastic anaemia

The megaloblastic anaemias are characterized by the presence of megaloblasts (abnormally large and morphologically abnormal haemopoietic cells) in the bone marrow due to defective DNA synthesis secondary to vitamin B_{12} or folate deficiency.

Epidemiology

Megaloblastic anaemia is the second most common cause of anaemia. Pernicious anaemia accounts for most cases of megaloblastic anaemia with a prevalence of 1.9% (1900 per 100 000) in the general population aged 60 years and above; it is approximately twice as common in women.[1]

Pathology

Rapidly dividing cells, such as haemopoietic cells, are especially vulnerable to defective DNA synthesis, a process that requires vitamin B_{12} and folate. Vitamin B_{12} is a coenzyme involved in the methylation of homocysteine to methionine and the conversion of methylmalonyl CoA to succinyl CoA (Fig. 12.3). During the former reaction, methylcobalamin loses its methyl group and this is replaced from methyltetrahydrofolic acid, the principal form of folic acid in plasma.

Vitamin B_{12}

Vitamin B_{12} consists of a group of compounds called the cobalamins that are synthesized by microorganisms. B_{12} is present only in animal produce, and peptic digestion in the

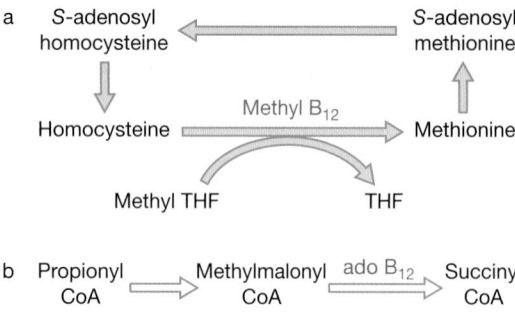

Fig. 12.3 Biochemical reactions of vitamin B$_{12}$.

stomach assists its release from food. Subsequently it becomes bound to intrinsic factor, a glycoprotein produced by gastric parietal cells. The cobalamin and intrinsic factor complex binds to receptors on the mucosal cells of the terminal ileum where B$_{12}$ is absorbed.

The causes of B$_{12}$ deficiency are listed in Table 12.5. Nutritional deficiency of vitamin B$_{12}$ sufficient to cause megaloblastic anaemia is rare and confined to fastidious vegans. Body stores of vitamin B$_{12}$ far exceed requirements and deficiency takes years to develop. The most common cause is Addisonian pernicious anaemia, an autoimmune disease associated with a combination of parietal cell antibodies (causing parietal cell destruction with failure of intrinsic factor production), antibodies that inhibit the binding of intrinsic factor to B$_{12}$ and antibodies that inhibit the binding of the intrinsic factor–B$_{12}$ complex to the terminal ileum. The end result is failure of B$_{12}$ absorption.

Folate

Most foods contain folate, but vegetables and fruits are especially rich sources. Dietary folates are very sensitive to heat, and cooking markedly depletes the folate content of food. Absorption occurs in the proximal small bowel, and body stores are relatively modest. As a result, deficiency can develop within weeks, in contrast to the years that are required before B$_{12}$ deficiency develops.

The causes of folate deficiency are listed in Table 12.6. The principal cause is poor intake, especially with excessively processed and intensively cooked diets deficient in fresh produce.

Table 12.5	Main causes of B$_{12}$ deficiency
Malabsorption	
Pernicious anaemia	
Gastrectomy	
Crohn's disease (with terminal ileitis)	
Ileal resection	
Poor intake	
Vegans (rare)	

Table 12.6	Main causes of folate deficiency
Poor intake	
Elderly	
Special diets	
Malabsorption	
Coeliac disease	
Increased requirement	
Pregnancy	
Malignancies	
Haemolytic anaemias	
Inflammatory disease	
Increased losses	
Liver disease	

Scope of disease

The white cell and platelet counts may be moderately reduced in patients with megaloblastic anaemia. B$_{12}$ deficiency can lead to a symmetrical peripheral neuropathy, subacute combined degeneration of the cord, optic atrophy and dementia. The neurological manifestations occasionally occur despite minimal abnormalities in the blood count.

Clinical features

Symptoms are principally of anaemia (p. 779). The degree of thrombocytopenia and leukopenia is rarely sufficient to cause bleeding or infection. A sore mouth with generalized erythema of the glossal (tongue) and buccal mucosa can occur.

In vitamin B$_{12}$ deficiency paraesthesia and peripheral neuropathy may be present. Less commonly spasticity, unsteadiness and altered gait occur due to subacute combined degeneration of the spinal cord (damage of the posterior and lateral columns). Visual disturbances (due to optic atrophy), dementia and weight loss (due to the effects of the vitamin deficiency on intestinal mucosal cells) can also occur.

Initial investigations

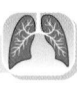

Full blood count, blood film and red cell indices

In megaloblastic anaemia, the haematological picture is identical for B$_{12}$ or folate deficiency. The full blood count reveals anaemia with raised MCV, and pancytopenia may be evident with reduced platelet and leukocyte counts. Oval macrocytes and hypersegmented neutrophils (exaggerated lobulation of the nucleus) are visible on the blood film.

Macrocytosis is not specific to megaloblastic anaemia; other common causes are alcohol abuse, liver disease and hypothyroidism.

Serum B$_{12}$

A low serum concentration of vitamin B$_{12}$ confirms deficiency.

Red cell folate

Folate can be measured in serum or the red cells. As serum folate can rapidly recover after a folate-rich meal, assay of red cell folate is a better indicator of body folate status.

Liver profile

Unconjugated hyperbilirubinaemia and increased lactate dehydrogenase may be observed with megaloblastic anaemia.

Further investigations

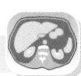

Bone marrow aspiration

Most cases of uncomplicated megaloblastic anaemia can be diagnosed from the blood count and haematinic assays. Marrow examination is rarely essential.

Aspirated bone marrow is hypercellular; the red cells are larger than normal at each stage of development with primitive chromatin patterns of the nuclei. There are also abnormal maturation and accompanying morphological changes in the white cell series and megakaryocytes due to megaloblastic haemopoiesis.

Schilling test

A Schilling test is a useful investigation of B$_{12}$ absorption when no obvious cause (gastrectomy, ileal resection) is identifiable.

Initially, an intramuscular injection of B$_{12}$ is administered to replace the body stores, followed by an oral dose of radiolabelled vitamin B$_{12}$ (first stage). A 24-hour urine collection is performed and the radioactivity of the urine is measured. If the urine excretion of radioactive B$_{12}$ is less than normal, the test is repeated with an oral dose of radiolabelled vitamin B$_{12}$ together with intrinsic factor (second stage).

The presence of normal quantities of radioactive B$_{12}$ in the urine indicates normal B$_{12}$ absorption, and the test can be stopped after the first stage. In pernicious anaemia, the urine excretion of radiolabelled B$_{12}$ is reduced in the first stage, and returns to normal in the second stage when the test is repeated with oral intrinsic factor. Disorders of the terminal ileum are associated with a reduction of urine excretion of radiolabelled B$_{12}$ in both stages as intrinsic factor cannot compensate for impaired intestinal absorption.

Gastrointestinal endoscopy

Further gastrointestinal investigations are required to determine the cause of folate deficiency or B$_{12}$ deficiency in the absence of any other identifiable cause. Coeliac disease is the most common underlying gastrointestinal diagnosis (p. 269).

Initial management

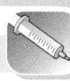

Identify and treat any underlying cause

It is important to determine any underlying pathology that can lead to B$_{12}$ or folate deficiency. Dietary advice should be given to patients with poor intake of folate or increased requirements.

> **⚡ CLINICAL ALERT**
>
> *In severe megaloblastic anaemia cardiomyopathy can occur. Fluid volume loads are poorly tolerated and may precipitate severe cardiac failure. In general, red cell transfusion should be avoided. If essential, transfusion should be undertaken cautiously (small volume and slow infusion).*

Medical management

B$_{12}$ replacement

Megaloblastic anaemia due to B$_{12}$ deficiency is treated by replacement with intramuscular injections of 1 mg of hydroxocobalamin. Initially, this is performed 3 times a week for 2 weeks. The maintenance dose is 1 mg every 3 months continued for life.

Folate replacement

Megaloblastic anaemia due to folate deficiency may be treated by 5 mg of oral folic acid once daily.

> **⚡ CLINICAL ALERT**
>
> *In vitamin B$_{12}$ deficiency folic acid should not be administered without vitamin B$_{12}$ as it can precipitate the onset of neurological complications associated with B$_{12}$ deficiency.*

Prognosis

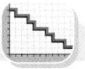

Haematological abnormalities are completely reversed by appropriate folate or vitamin B$_{12}$ replacement. A marked increase in the reticulocyte count occurs 2–3 days after treatment is instituted and the response is maximal at 7 days, with a rise that is proportional to the severity of the anaemia. Haemoglobin concentration increases at about 1 g/dL each week, with gradual resolution of the macrocytosis. The white cell and platelet counts recover within days. However, the neurological features of vitamin B$_{12}$ deficiency may only be partly corrected.

There is a life-long slightly increased risk of stomach cancer in patients with pernicious anaemia.

REFERENCE

(1) *Carmel R. Prevalence of undiagnosed pernicious anemia in the elderly. Archives of Internal Medicine 1996; 156: 1097–1100.*

Haemolytic anaemias

The haemolytic anaemias are those in which there is a reduction in red cell lifespan. They can be conveniently classified into those in which there is an intrinsic red cell defect and those where red cells are normal but damaged by an outside influence (Table 12.7). Almost all intrinsic red cell defects are hereditary (except paroxysmal nocturnal haemoglobinuria) and all haemolytic anaemias due to mechanisms outside the red cell are acquired.

The immune haemolytic anaemias are acquired disorders in which premature red cell destruction is due to an antibody to a red cell antigen. Included are autoimmune haemolytic anaemia, neonatal alloimmune haemolytic anaemia, and haemolysis due to mismatched blood transfusion. The last two are alloimmune disorders where antibodies are formed against antigens that are foreign to the individual. The presence of antibody or complement on the red cell surface is confirmed by the direct antiglobulin or Coombs' test (p. 778).

Clinical features

Common to this group of diseases are anaemia, jaundice and splenomegaly. There is bile in the urine, which may turn brown on standing due to urobilinogen.

Pigment gallstones are a complication of chronically increased red cell destruction, and folate deficiency may arise due to increased requirements for haemopoiesis.

Investigations

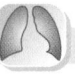

Full blood count, blood film

The anaemia is typically normocytic. Increased haemopoiesis in compensation for the anaemia results in red cell polychromasia. The reticulocyte count is increased. There may be red cell appearances typical of a particular kind of anaemia, for example microspherocytes in immune haemolysis and hereditary spherocytosis and fragmented red cells (also called schistocytes) in microangiopathic haemolysis.

Serum haptoglobin

Haptoglobin is a plasma protein that binds free haemoglobin. The haptoglobin–haemoglobin complex is removed by reticuloendothelial cells. In haemolysis haptoglobin is consumed and serum haptoglobin is reduced or absent

Liver profile

Serum (unconjugated) bilirubin is elevated as it is a breakdown product of protoporphyrin (from haem).

Faecal stercobilinogen

Faecal stercobilinogen is elevated due to excess bilirubin excretion, although it is not routinely measured.

Table 12.7	A classification of haemolytic anaemias
Haemolysis due to red cell abnormality	
Haemoglobin defects	
Thalassaemias	
Sickle cell disorders	
Enzyme defects	
G6PD deficiency	
Pyruvate kinase deficiency	
Membrane defects	
Hereditary spherocytosis	
Paroxysmal nocturnal haemoglobinuria	
Haemolysis due to abnormality outside the red cell	
Immune haemolytic anaemias	
Autoimmune haemolytic anaemia	
Neonatal alloimmune haemolytic anaemia	
Haemolysis due to mismatched blood transfusion	
Microangiopathic haemolysis	
Drugs, toxins and chemicals	
Snake bites	
Parasitic infection	
Malaria	

Urinalysis

Urine urobilinogen is elevated as the excreted bilirubin in the bile is partially reabsorbed and excreted in the urine as urobilinogen. In intravascular haemolysis, for example in microangiopathic haemolytic anaemia, haemoglobinuria may be present. In chronic intravascular haemolysis, iron from haemoglobin is present as haemosiderin in the urinary sediment. This is detected by staining of the sediment for iron (haemosiderinuria).

Bone marrow aspiration

There is erythroid hyperplasia which is an increase in the proportion of red cell precursors.

Red cell enzymopathies

Defects of red cell enzymes render erythrocytes susceptible to haemolysis due to damage by oxidant compounds. Although many red cell enzyme deficiencies have been recorded, the more common are glucose-6-phosphate dehydrogenase (G6PD) and pyruvate kinase (PK) deficiency.

Glucose-6-phosphate dehydrogenase (G6PD) deficiency

Epidemiology

G6PD deficiency is among the most common human enzyme disorders with the highest prevalence in African,

Mediterranean and Chinese populations. The marked geographical variation in prevalence is thought to be due to a relative protection from falciparum malaria in carriers. It is inherited as an X-linked disorder and female heterozygotes are usually asymptomatic.

Pathology

Deficiency of or defective G6PD results in the impaired reduction of glutathione, a peptide that protects the red cell membrane from oxidative damage. There are over 400 variants of this enzyme with reduced activity, and the severity of the disease varies between genotypes.

The common isoenzyme is designated type B (Western), and is functionally normal. Africans (as well as black Americans) have a high prevalence of type A. The two isoenzymes differ by a single amino acid. A further variant is found in Mediterranean populations and is associated with a tendency to acute haemolysis after ingestion of fava (broad) beans.

Scope of disease

Acute self-limiting haemolysis is the most common clinical feature. Neonatal jaundice and chronic haemolysis are less common features.

Clinical features
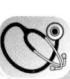

The main clinical features are anaemia and jaundice due to acute haemolysis. Acute haemolysis may be precipitated by the ingestion of oxidant drugs (for example antimalarials, sulphonamides), surgery and infection. Because the bone marrow response to anaemia is normal and reticulocytes contain a higher concentration of G6PD, episodes of haemolysis are usually self-limiting.

Initial investigations
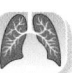

Full blood count and blood film
The blood picture is normal between haemolytic episodes. During a haemolytic crisis, there is red cell polychromasia and poikilocytosis is increased. Bite cells (erythrocytes with bite-shaped defects) and blister cells (erythrocytes with surface blebs) result from membrane damage due to the formation of oxidized, denatured haemoglobin. When an appropriate stain is used, denatured haemoglobin is visible within erythrocytes as inclusions attached to the cell membrane. These inclusions are called Heinz bodies. Biochemical features of haemolysis are also present (p. 778).

Further investigations
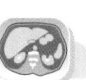

G6PD measurements
Diagnosis of G6PD deficiency is confirmed by measurement of the G6PD content of red cells. This should not be performed during an acute haemolytic episode as the G6PD content of reticulocytes may be normal, leading to a misleading result.

Initial management

Identify and correct precipitating cause
Management of G6PD deficiency centres on avoidance of precipitating causes through education of patients and doctors. Patients with the Mediterranean variant learn to avoid fava beans. During an acute haemolytic crisis, the offending agent should be identified and stopped. A high urine output should be maintained.

Packed cells transfusion
Red cell transfusion is rarely required.

Prognosis

Health is generally good between haemolytic episodes and survival is normal in the majority of cases.

Pyruvate kinase deficiency

Epidemiology

Pyruvate kinase deficiency affects many races but is less common than G6PD deficiency. The inheritance is autosomal recessive and heterozygote carriers are asymptomatic.

Pathology

Pyruvate kinase deficiency causes impaired glycolysis and red cell energy production resulting in chronic haemolysis. A product of the metabolic impairment is increased erythrocyte 2,3-DPG. This results in reduced oxygen affinity of haemoglobin, a right shift of the oxygen-haemoglobin dissociation curve, and increased oxygen delivery to the tissues. Therefore the anaemia is less symptomatic than would be expected from the severity of the reduced haemoglobin level.

Clinical features

The main clinical features are chronic haemolytic anaemia with jaundice and pigment gallstones.

Investigations
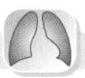

Full blood count and blood film
There is anaemia and red cell poikilocytosis (contracted cells) and polychromasia on the blood film. There are also biochemical abnormalities due to haemolysis.

Enzyme assay
Pyruvate kinase deficiency is confirmed by direct measurement of the enzyme.

Management

Folate supplementation is administered to avoid mega-loblastic anaemia as a complication of high red cell turn-over and increased folate requirements. Splenectomy may be indicated in patients requiring repeated transfusions. Although it is not curative, splenectomy usually results in a sustained increase in haemoglobin concentration.

Prognosis

In general, the prognosis is good with a normal life expectancy.

Autoimmune haemolytic anaemia

Autoimmune haemolytic anaemia results from red cell haemolysis due to the formation of anti-red cell antibodies.

Epidemiology

Autoimmune haemolytic anaemia is a fairly common autoimmune disease, with an epidemiology that varies with the underlying cause (Table 12.8).

Pathology

In the majority, there is no identifiable cause for the formation of red cell antibodies and the term 'idiopathic autoimmune haemolytic anaemia' is used. In these cases, a personal or family history of autoimmune disease such as rheumatoid arthritis, systemic lupus erythematosus or autoimmune thyroid disease often exists. Occasionally, autoimmune haemolytic anaemia may be precipitated by drugs or arise as a complication of lymphoproliferative disorders such as chronic lymphocytic leukaemia.

Warm antibody immune disorder

The most common form of autoimmune haemolysis results from warm antibody autoimmune disorder, due to IgG

Table 12.8	Causes of autoimmune haemolytic disorders
Warm antibody immune disorder	
Idiopathic	
Secondary	
Autoimmune disease (systemic lupus erythematosus, rheumatoid disease)	
Drugs (penicillin, quinine, methyldopa)	
Lymphoproliferative disorders (chronic lymphocytic leukaemia, lymphoma)	
Cold antibody immune disorder	
Idiopathic	
Secondary	
Infection (infectious mononucleosis, mycoplasma pneumonia)	
Lymphoma	

autoantibodies reactive at 37°C. The antibody-coated cells bind to macrophages of the reticuloendothelial system because they have receptors for the Fc portion of immunoglobulin. Phagocytosis results in loss of part of the erythrocyte membrane. As the surface area of the cell reduces, it assumes a spherical shape to maintain cellular integrity. These microspherocytes are less deformable, become trapped in the spleen, and are removed completely by phagocytosis.

Warm IgG antibodies may also develop as a result of drug treatment by three different mechanisms: the drug binding directly to the erythrocyte and acting as a hapten (e.g. penicillin), the drug promoting the formation of an immune complex with IgG which binds non-specifically to the red cell (quinine), or the drug inducing an autoantibody which recognizes a normal red cell antigen, usually a protein of the rhesus blood group system (methyldopa).

Cold antibody immune disorders

Cold antibody immune disorders are due to red cell IgM antibodies (usually directed at the 'I' antigen of the red cell surface) that are most active at 4°C. Although they are less active at higher temperatures, they are still able to bind to complement and agglutinate red cells at 30°C, the temperature of the peripheral tissues. Red cell agglutination (usually in cooler parts of the body) results in sluggish blood flow and reduced oxygen saturation. On re-entering the warmer central circulation, the IgM antibody may detach from the red cell, but if complement has bound to the red cell, the complement cascade proceeds to damage the cell membrane, leading to chronic haemolysis. Acute cold antibody haemolysis may occur as a complication of infection, especially with *Mycoplasma pneumoniae* and Epstein–Barr virus (EBV).

Scope of disease

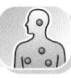

Jaundice can occur as a result of red cell degradation, and pigment gallstones can occur.

Clinical features

The clinical features of warm and cold antibody disease differ.

Patients with warm antibody disease usually present with pallor, jaundice and splenomegaly. The severity of the anaemia (rate of haemolysis) is variable ranging from subclinical disease to life-threatening anaemia. A detailed drug history, family history and systems enquiry and examination are required to ascertain the presence of precipitating factors and coexistent autoimmune or lymphoproliferative disease (lymphadenopathy).

Patients with cold antibody disease may also be anaemic and have blue extremities (fingers, toes, nose and ears), especially in cold temperatures. The severity of the disease is determined by the temperature at which the antibody remains active. In extreme cases, ischaemia and ulceration of the extremities can occur.

Initial investigations

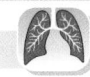

Full blood count, blood film

In warm antibody disease, the blood picture is of a normochromic, normocytic chronic anaemia, with microspherocytes and increased polychromasia. The reticulocyte count is raised and there is biochemical evidence of haemolysis (p. 778).

In cold antibody disease the features are a normochromic, normocytic anaemia, with marked agglutination of red cells on the blood film. Agglutination is no longer evident when the blood film is prepared at 37°C (the term 'cold haemagglutinin disease' is commonly applied).

Direct antiglobulin test

The direct antiglobulin test is performed by incubating red cells with Coombs' reagent, a mixture of monoclonal antibodies directed against IgG and C_3. In the presence of IgG or C_3, the monoclonal antibodies induce haemagglutination which can be visualized under light microscopy (positive test). The direct antiglobulin test is positive with IgG and C_3 (in approximately one third) in warm antibody disease and positive for C_3 alone in cold antibody disease. Haemolysis associated with a negative direct antiglobulin test usually indicates a non-autoimmune cause such as haemoglobinopathy, malfunctioning heart valve prosthesis and severe burns.

Initial management

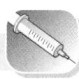

Identify and treat underlying cause

When autoimmune haemolytic anaemia is caused by an offending drug, withdrawal generally results in resolution of the anaemia over a period of weeks. When autoimmune haemolytic anaemia occurs as a complication of lymphoproliferative disease, treatment of the underlying malignancy may improve the haemoglobin concentration. Patients with cold antibody disease should avoid exposing their extremities to the cold.

Medical management

Immunomodulation

In symptomatic patients corticosteroids are the main treatment in warm antibody cases. Prednisolone is initiated at 1 mg per kg body weight and the dose is gradually reduced when remission has been achieved.

If relapse occurs despite corticosteroid therapy, long-term immunomodulatory treatment with a steroid-sparing immunosuppressive such as azathioprine may be considered to minimize the side effects of chronic steroid therapy.

Surgical management

In patients with warm autoimmune haemolytic anaemia that does not improve with immunomodulation therapy, splenectomy is recommended to reduce the rate of haemolysis. Splenectomy is not effective for patients with cold antibody disease as the complement-sensitized cells are destroyed in the liver and many other sites.

Prognosis

The prognosis of the disease is related to the underlying cause. Patients with a single episode caused by an identified offending agent have a good prognosis with avoidance of the precipitating agent. The clinical course of patients with idiopathic autoimmune haemolytic anaemia is variable. Most have long survival.

Microangiopathic haemolytic anaemias

Microangiopathic haemolytic anaemias are characterized by red cell damage due to trauma as they traverse the microvasculature. Comparable damage to red cells may result from malfunctioning mechanical heart valve prostheses.

Epidemiology

Anaemia of this type is uncommon.

Pathology

Trauma to erythrocytes may occur as they circulate through damaged small blood vessels, for example in the kidney in haemolytic uraemic syndrome (p. 821), and more diffusely in the systemic circulation in thrombotic thrombocytopenic purpura (p. 822), malignant hypertension and systemic vasculitis. In disseminated intravascular coagulation (p. 821) fibrin strands are deposited within the lumen of blood vessels and erythrocytes are damaged during passage through the fibrin mesh. Platelets are also consumed, resulting in thrombocytopenia.

March haemoglobinuria refers to intravascular haemolysis due to erythrocyte damage in the vessels of the feet during long-distance running or marching. In conditions with localized red cell trauma there is no thrombocytopenia. Other examples are listed in Table 12.9.

Table 12.9	Causes of microangiopathic haemolysis
Diffuse disorders of the microcirculation	
Thrombotic thrombocytopenic purpura	
Disseminated intravascular coagulation	
Malignant hypertension	
Systemic vasculitis	
Localized disorders of the circulation	
Haemolytic uraemic syndrome	
Mechanical heart valves	
Vascular prostheses	
March haemoglobinuria (repetitive tissue trauma)	

Clinical features

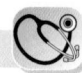

Anaemia and jaundice are common but the principal clinical features depend upon the cause, for example organ failure, including manifestations of cerebral ischaemia in thrombotic thrombocytopenic purpura and renal failure in haemolytic uraemic syndrome.

Investigations

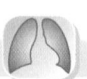

Full blood count, blood film

There is a normocytic anaemia. Numerous schistocytes (damaged red cells, with a ragged edge) are visible on the blood film. There is polychromasia and usually thrombocytopenia.

Direct antiglobulin test

The direct antiglobulin test (p. 789) is negative.

Biochemistry

The biochemical features of haemolysis are present. Serum lactate dehydrogenase is markedly increased.

Management

Identify and treat precipitating cause

The management depends on the underlying or precipitating cause. In haemolytic uraemic syndrome management is supportive with red cell transfusion and renal support, and complete recovery is possible. In thrombotic thrombocytopenic purpura intensive plasma exchange therapy is employed.

When severe haemolysis occurs due to a mechanical heart valve prosthesis, repeat valve replacement surgery may be necessary.

Prognosis

The prognosis depends on the underlying cause. In most cases, removal of the offending cause leads to recovery of anaemia.

Hereditary spherocytosis

Epidemiology

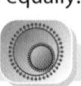

Spherocytosis is the most common hereditary haemolytic anaemia among Caucasians, affecting both sexes equally.

Pathology

Hereditary spherocytosis is characterized by spherical red cells with a short lifespan. It can be caused by a number of genetic defects in the structural proteins of the red cell membrane, the most common being a defect in spectrin.

The inheritance is autosomal dominant with variable penetration.

In some variants the erythrocytes are elliptical (hereditary elliptocytosis). Both spherocytes and elliptocytes are less deformable than normal red cells, impeding their passage through the splenic microcirculation. As a result, the abnormal cells are retained in the spleen and prematurely phagocytosed.

Clinical features

The main clinical features are anaemia and jaundice. The severity of the anaemia varies according to the genetic defect, ranging from subclinical disease to severe anaemia. Pigment gallstones can result from chronic haemolysis. In general the symptoms of patients with elliptocytosis are milder. On examination, splenomegaly is usually present.

Investigations

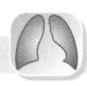

Full blood count, blood film

The full blood count reveals a normocytic anaemia. Polychromasia is evident on the blood film due to increased erythrocyte production. A high proportion of the red cells appear spherical and denser than biconcave erythrocytes, with loss of central pallor. The reticulocyte count is increased.

Direct antiglobulin test

Spherocytes are not specific to hereditary spherocytosis, and may also occur in immune haemolytic anaemias. In hereditary spherocytosis, the direct antiglobulin test is negative, however.

Osmotic fragility test

The osmotic fragility test is useful where there is doubt about the presence of spherocytes. Red cells are exposed to a range of solutions with different osmolarity and lysis is recorded. Spherocytes are more sensitive than normal to lysis under osmotic stress.

Management

Folate supplementation

In most cases of spherocytosis no treatment is required. Folate supplementation is advisable as the compensatory erythroid hyperplasia leads to increased folate requirements.

Splenectomy

Splenectomy is reserved for patients with severe symptoms, and is avoided in infants and young children. Removal of the spleen usually results in resolution of anaemia. However there is a life-long risk of morbidity and mortality from infection with encapsulated microorganisms and malaria. Immunization against pneumococcus, meningococcus and *Haemophilus influenzae* is undertaken routinely, and low-dose prophylactic penicillin or erythromycin is administered for life.

Prognosis

In general the prognosis is good after splenectomy with a normal life expectancy.

Paroxysmal nocturnal haemoglobinuria

Paroxysmal nocturnal haemoglobinuria is an acquired intrinsic red cell abnormality that leads to haemolytic anaemia. The principal features of paroxysmal nocturnal haemoglobinuria are red cell haemolysis, bone marrow hypoplasia and thrombosis.

Epidemiology

Paroxysmal nocturnal haemoglobinuria is a rare condition that usually presents in adults (equally in both sexes), with an incidence that increases with age.

Pathology

Paroxysmal nocturnal haemoglobinuria occurs as a result of an acquired mutation of the 'PIG-A' gene within a stem cell clone. The progeny lack α-1,6-N-acetylglucosaminyltransferase, an enzyme required for the synthesis of a phosphatidyl inositol which anchors several proteins to the red cell membrane, including some that are responsible for complement degradation. The end result is red cells that are abnormally sensitive to lysis by complement.

Platelets are affected also, and patients with paroxysmal nocturnal haemoglobinuria are prone to thrombosis. The bone marrow is often hypoplastic.

Clinical features

Despite its name, acute nocturnal haemolysis is rarely obvious. Typical features are chronic anaemia due to haemolysis and pancytopenia due to bone marrow hypoplasia. Portal, hepatic or cerebral venous thrombosis also occurs.

Investigations

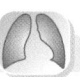

Full blood count, blood film

A normochromic normocytic anaemia is present, with features of chronic haemolysis on the blood film (p. 778). The reticulocyte response may be suppressed due to accompanying bone marrow failure. Biochemical markers of haemolysis may be present (p. 778)

Urinalysis

Haemosiderinuria is typically present, as with other causes of chronic intravascular haemolysis.

Acid lysis (Ham's test)

Erythrocytes tend to lyse at low pH (which activates complement): a positive Ham's test.

Direct assay of phosphatidyl inositol-linked antigens

Deficiency of phosphatidyl inositol-linked antigens on blood cells can be confirmed by flow cytometry analysis. For example CD59.

Management

Paroxysmal nocturnal haemoglobinuria is a chronic condition and in many cases treatment is supportive.

Iron and folate supplementation

Urinary iron losses are increased, as haemosiderin, and should be replaced by oral supplementation. Folate requirements are increased due to the high red cell turnover, and oral folic acid is administered.

Anticoagulation

Venous thrombosis is treated in the usual way with heparin and warfarin. Long-term anticoagulation, maintaining an international normalized ratio (INR) of 2–3, is often indicated due to a high rate of recurrent thrombosis.

Bone marrow transplantation

In the most severe cases allogeneic bone marrow transplantation can be considered.

Eculizumab

Eculizumab is a monoclonal antibody directed against C5. It reduces complement mediated haemolysis and improves anaemia.

Prognosis

The prognosis is variable but paroxysmal nocturnal haemoglobinuria is generally a life-shortening disease. Death from thrombotic complications is common.

Haemolytic disease of the newborn

Haemolytic disease of the newborn results from the passage of maternal IgG antibody against fetal red cell antigens across the placenta. Binding of antibody to target antigens, in the ABO or rhesus blood group systems, results in lysis of the fetal red cells.

Epidemiology

Haemolytic disease of the newborn was a common cause of fetal and neonatal haemolytic anaemia. With improved detection, and treatment with anti-D therapy in rhesus-negative women, the overall incidence of haemolytic disease of the newborn has reduced considerably.

Currently, immune antibodies against the ABO blood group system (anti-A or -B) are more common but fortunately haemolysis is less severe than with antibodies to rhesus D.

Pathology

Haemolytic disease of the newborn originates from the inheritance by the fetus from the father of a red cell antigen which is not present on the maternal red cells, leading to antibody development in the mother when fetal erythrocytes enter the maternal circulation, for example during parturition.

The most important antigen in this context is rhesus D, and approximately 15% of women are negative for the rhesus D antigen. Passage of fetal red cells into the maternal circulation occurs normally at delivery or as a result of miscarriage or operative intervention during pregnancy. Although sensitization to the 'foreign' (paternal) antigen may occur, there is usually no clinical consequence in the first pregnancy. Antibody production is stimulated during subsequent pregnancies with a rhesus D-positive fetus, and IgG antibodies can traverse the placenta from mother to fetus causing immune destruction of fetal red cells in utero.

Haemolytic disease of the newborn caused by ABO incompatibility can affect the first pregnancy, and the effect on subsequent pregnancies is variable. The disease is generally milder as the A and B antigens in the fetus are not fully developed at birth, and there is partial neutralization of the IgG antibodies by non-erythroid cells.

Clinical features

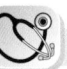

The main clinical feature is a haemolytic anaemia of variable severity occurring in utero. The most severe cases associated with a high titre of anti-D result in 'hydrops fetalis' and death in utero. The severe anaemia leads to cardiac failure, and hepatosplenomegaly occurs due to extramedullary haemopoiesis in liver and spleen.

In less severe cases of rhesus haemolytic disease and in ABO haemolytic disease of the newborn, anaemia is less severe and the neonate is jaundiced at birth. If untreated, the excess unconjugated bilirubin is deposited in the central nervous system (especially the basal ganglia) and causes kernicterus (spasticity and mental retardation).

Investigations

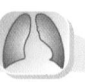

Neonate full blood count, blood film
Anaemia is evident, and the blood film has features of haemolysis with polychromasia and increased reticulocytes. Often nucleated red cells are prominent in the peripheral blood also, due to increased erythropoiesis in an attempt to keep pace with the markedly shortened red cell survival.

Neonate direct antiglobulin test
The direct antiglobulin test (p. 778) on the neonatal red cells is positive.

Maternal blood grouping and Rh-D antibody assay
Early detection of any pregnancy affected by rhesus haemolytic disease of the newborn is essential so that intrauterine treatment can be considered, to prevent hydrops fetalis. The maternal rhesus D status is determined routinely and the serum screened for anti-D in D-negative mothers.

If there is a rising titre of anti-D antibodies during pregnancy, fetal ultrasound and fetal blood sampling is performed to provide an assessment of the severity of haemolysis and the need for intrauterine transfusion to prevent fetal hydrops.

Management

Anti-D antibodies
Passive administration of IgG anti-D antibodies by intramuscular injection leads to the rapid removal of any fetal cells from the maternal circulation, before sensitization can occur. It is administered prophylactically during at-risk pregnancies or alternatively at the times of highest risk of feto-maternal bleeding, for example delivery.

Exchange transfusions
Treatment of the severely affected fetus is provision of unsensitized red cells by intrauterine transfusion and removal of bilirubin by exchange blood transfusion in the postnatal period.

Phototherapy
Mildly affected neonates with jaundice are treated by phototherapy. Exposure to light of an appropriate wavelength (425–475 nm) converts bilirubin to a water-soluble form that can be excreted in the bile and urine.

Prognosis

Prevention of the disease is possible with successful screening and treatment. Mildly affected neonates can be successfully treated by phototherapy. The outcome is generally good in the severely affected, provided intrauterine diagnosis is made early and appropriate antenatal therapy is instituted.

Haemoglobinopathies

The haemoglobinopathies arise from defective or variant haemoglobin synthesis (Table 12.10). This group of diseases includes the thalassaemias and sickle cell disorders. Thalassaemia results from a reduced rate of synthesis of structurally normal α- or β-globin chains, and sickle cell disease results from synthesis of variant haemoglobin due to a single point mutation in the genetic code resulting in an amino acid substitution.

In thalassaemia, anaemia is the principal manifestation. In sickle cell disease (Hb SS) haemoglobin becomes crystalline at low oxygen tension causing haemolysis and

Table 12.10	Haemoglobinopathies
Disease	**Abnormality**
Thalassaemia	Defective α or β chain production
Sickle cell anaemia	Hb SS
Hb C, Hb D, Hb E disease	Other point mutations causing synthesis of abnormal haemoglobin
Familial polycythaemia	Haemoglobin of increased oxygen affinity
Methaemoglobinaemia	Failure of reduction of haemoglobin

microvascular occlusion. Some point mutations result in unstable haemoglobin leading to chronic haemolysis with Heinz bodies, or haemoglobin of increased oxygen affinity causing familial polycythaemia due to reduced oxygen delivery, and in others haemoglobin which tends to the oxidized state (methaemoglobin) causing cyanosis; these are uncommon. Thalassaemias and sickle cell disease are very common disorders globally.

Thalassaemias

Thalassaemias are genetic disorders characterized by reduced rate of synthesis of the alpha or beta globin chains.

Epidemiology

Although thalassaemic genes are found in every racial group, they are particularly common in the Mediterranean region, Africa, the Middle East, the Indian subcontinent and South East Asia.

Pathology

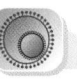

Thalassaemias arise from genetic defects that impair the regulation of globin structural gene expression. Haemoglobin production is also defective, resulting in microcytic hypochromic red cells. Moreover, the accumulation of excessive unaffected globin chains can lead to the haemolysis of erythrocytes.

Alpha-thalassaemia results from impaired α-globin chain synthesis, most commonly due to gene deletions. Each cell has four genes coding for α-globin (a pair on each chromosome 16), and the severity of disease corresponds to the number of genes deleted. Deletion of all four genes is incompatible with life (hydrops fetalis: lethal anaemia and severe congestive heart failure in utero) and deletion of three genes results in moderately severe anaemia and splenomegaly (haemoglobin H disease—haemoglobin H is tetramers of free β chain). Deletion of one or two genes results in alpha-thalassaemia trait, which is clinically silent with no or mild anaemia.

There are over 100 genetic defects responsible for beta-thalassaemia major. Only homozygotes for β-globin gene defects develop beta-thalassaemia; heterozygotes develop the thalassaemia trait.

Scope of disease

In beta-thalassaemia major the haemoglobin concentration may fall to around 3 g/dL by 3–6 months of age, when β-chain production normally takes over from the γ-chain haemoglobin of late fetal development.

In response to the defective haemoglobin synthesis and haemolysis, the red bone marrow is expanded, cortical bone is thinned and new bone is laid down on the outer aspect, especially in the skull vault, maxilla and frontal facial bones, resulting in bony deformities. Frontal bossing of the skull is most prominent, and fractures may develop in the long bones, vertebrae and ribs. Haemosiderosis occurs due to the ineffective erythropoiesis and iron accumulation from repeated red cell transfusions, resulting in failure of sexual development (iron deposition in endocrine organs and gonads), diabetes mellitus, liver and heart failure.

Clinical features

Homozygotes with beta-thalassaemia major have severe anaemia and develop complications such as growth failure or pathological fractures. Later in the course of the disease, complications from repeated red cell transfusions can lead to symptoms of diabetes, liver or heart failure.

On examination there may be characteristic facies with prominent frontal bossing of the skull and features of growth failure. Splenomegaly is usually prominent.

Thalassaemia intermedia is a genetically heterogeneous group with mild to moderate anaemia that usually does not require repeated red cell transfusions. Hepatosplenomegaly and iron overload may be present.

Patients with the alpha (one or two gene deletions) or beta (heterozygotes) thalassaemia trait have thalassaemia minor, no clinical disease, with normal or slightly reduced haemoglobin concentrations.

Investigations

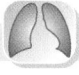

Full blood count, blood film and red cell indices
The characteristic feature of thalassaemia is a microcytic hypochromic blood picture. In beta-thalassaemia trait, there may be mild to no anaemia but marked microcytosis. The differentiation from iron deficiency is by demonstration of normal or increased iron stores as reflected by the serum ferritin.

In alpha-thalassaemia trait the red cell changes are subtle, often with only slightly reduced MCV. The free β chains in haemoglobin H disease form inclusion bodies that may be seen in a small proportion of red cells on the blood film using brilliant cresyl blue staining.

Haemoglobin electrophoresis
Haemoglobin electrophoresis is a technique that separates the subtypes of haemoglobin according to molecular

weight. The results are a profile of the haemoglobins usually expressed as percentages.

In beta-thalassaemia major, there is absent or very reduced haemoglobin A, with haemoglobin F as the main form of circulating haemoglobin. The haemoglobin A_2 levels are usually normal. Beta-thalassaemia trait is suggested by elevated (>2.5%) levels of haemoglobin A_2.

Haemoglobin H can be detected on electrophoresis (β_4), but patients with alpha-thalassaemia trait (1–2 deletions) have normal haemoglobin electrophoresis profiles. Alpha-thalassaemia trait is detected by a more complex assay which detects a reduced α/β synthesis ratio.

Initial management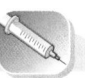

Education and genetic counselling

It is important to educate patients with thalassaemia with regard to the course and natural history of the disease. No treatment is required in thalassaemia trait but a formal diagnosis is important for genetic counselling. If both parents have beta-thalassaemia trait, there is a 25% change of each offspring developing thalassaemia major (homozygote).

Hepatitis B vaccination

In view of the need for repeated transfusions, vaccination for hepatitis B is recommended for all patients with thalassaemia major.

Medical management

Repeated red cell transfusion

In thalassaemia major treatment is supportive, with regular transfusion of red cells.

Minimizing iron accumulation

Iron chelation therapy with subcutaneous desferrioxamine is required to minimize the risk of organ damage from excess iron accumulation due to repeated red cell transfusions. The target is to keep the serum ferritin less than 1500 µg/L.

> **RECENT ADVANCES**
>
> *Orally administered iron chelators are currently being evaluated. They are much needed in less developed countries, where parenteral chelation therapy may not be available.*

Treatment of complications

Patients with end-organ damage may require insulin (diabetes), calcium or vitamin D supplementation (hypoparathyroidism).

> **RECENT ADVANCES**
>
> *Bone marrow or stem cell transplantation is potentially curative treatment but is often not an available option, especially in less developed countries.*

Surgical management

Splenectomy

Splenectomy is reserved for selected patients in an attempt to reduce the transfusion requirements.

Prognosis

Thalassaemia minor has a good prognosis compatible with normal life expectancy. The prognosis of patients with thalassaemia major, however, is poor, and death often occurs in childhood or early adult life despite transfusion support.

Sickle cell and related disorders

Sickle cell disease is a genetic disorder characterized by an abnormal haemoglobin (Hb S) that crystallizes at low oxygen tension.

Epidemiology

The sickle cell gene is common in Africa (west and central), the Mediterranean, the Middle East and parts of the Indian subcontinent. The gene is carried by 8% of black Americans and 30% of black Africans; the high prevalence in Africans is thought to be due to provision of a degree of protection against falciparum malaria.

Other point mutations of the β-chain gene give rise to haemoglobins C, D and E, commonly found in West Africa, India and South East Asia respectively. The gene for Hb C is often inherited with that for Hb S because of similar geographical location.

Pathology

Hb S (Hb $\alpha_2 \beta^s_2$) arises from the substitution of valine for glutamic acid in position 6 in the β chain of globin; the result is an unstable form of haemoglobin that aggregates and polymerizes at low oxygen levels. Carriers (heterozygotes: sickle cell trait) have less than 40% Hb S, but in the homozygote, the majority of the haemoglobin content of the erythrocytes is Hb S.

Deoxygenated sickle haemoglobin aggregates and distorts the red cell membrane causing the cell to adopt a sickle shape. These abnormal cells have a shortened lifespan. Moreover, due to their increased rigidity, sickle cells can occlude microvessels causing ischaemic injury.

Scope of disease

Painful crises occur due to bouts of increased sickling with microvascular occlusion. This can result in infarction of the bones, lungs, spleen or brain (leading to stroke). In one form, called acute chest syndrome, life-threatening hypoxia occurs due to microvascular occlusion in the pulmonary circulation. In sequestration crisis, sickled erythrocytes are retained in the spleen and/or liver with sudden worsening of anaemia.

Chronic haemolysis predisposes to pigment gallstones, and recurrent infarction leads to impairment of the function of the liver, spleen (auto-splenectomy) and kidneys.

Clinical features

Carriers of the sickle cell trait (heterozygotes) are asymptomatic, although haematuria due to renal papillary necrosis may occasionally occur. Sickle cells form only under conditions of extreme hypoxia in heterozygotes, for example distal to a lower limb tourniquet applied to achieve a bloodless field in orthopaedic surgery.

Patients with sickle cell disease (homozygotes) suffer with painful crises from an early age and may develop sequestration crises. Cholecystitis can occur due to pigment gallstones. On examination, anaemia and jaundice are usually present from infancy. Chronic ulceration of the lower leg is a frequent feature. Splenomegaly is present in children but by adult life acquired hyposplenism occurs due to recurrent infarction. There is a typical retinopathy which is usually asymptomatic.

Painful crises

Painful crises may occur spontaneously but are often provoked by hypoxia (altitude, surgery), infection, dehydration, acidosis or exposure to a cold environment. Exacerbation of anaemia and painful crises are also more frequent in pregnancy.

Severe pain in the long bones, abdomen or chest is the characteristic presentation, and ischaemic stroke or spinal cord infarction can also occur. The frequency of episodes varies greatly between individuals.

Acute chest syndrome is most often precipitated by pneumonia and clinical features are severe chest pain, hypoxia and pulmonary infiltrates on a plain chest radiograph.

Sequestration crises

When sequestration occurs in the blood vessels of the liver or (in children) spleen, patients present with upper abdominal pain with acute exacerbation of anaemia.

Haemoglobin C, D and E diseases

Homozygotes with haemoglobin C, D or E have chronic haemolysis and splenomegaly but no painful crises. Hb S-C disease behaves as a mild sickle disease with a particular tendency to venous thrombosis.

Investigations

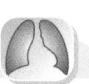

Full blood count and blood film

The full blood count and film is normal in heterozygotes. There is life-long anaemia in homozygotes, with haemoglobin levels ranging between 7 and 9 g/dL. Sickle cells are present and become more prominent during an acute

crisis. In the adult, features of hyposplenism (including Howell–Jolly bodies) are also evident on the blood film.

Sickle haemoglobin solubility test

A sickle haemoglobin solubility test is used as a rapid screen for sickle cell trait. Although sickle crisis is exceptionally rare in heterozygotes it is generally considered to be advisable to identify sickle cell trait prior to general anaesthesia in subjects of relevant ethnic origin.

Haemoglobin electrophoresis

Confirmatory diagnosis is obtained from haemoglobin electrophoresis. A single band of Hb S occurs in sickle cell disease, whilst two main bands (Hb S and Hb A) occur in patients with sickle cell trait.

Initial management

Prevention of sickle crises

Measures should be taken to avoid the factors known to precipitate sickle crises such as dehydration, infection and exposure to the cold. Special care is taken during surgery, hypoxia is avoided by adequate oxygenation, and distal limb tourniquets are contraindicated due to the possibility of precipitating an acute crisis on release of the tourniquet.

Folate supplementation

Folate supplementation is prescribed in view of the increased requirements in chronic haemolysis.

Medical management

Hydroxyurea

Long-term oral hydroxyurea, an antineoplastic drug, reduces the frequency of sickling episodes by increasing red cell Hb F concentration (which inhibits sickle cell formation) and its use is associated with a 40% reduction in mortality.[1]

Management of the acute painful crisis

Management of acute painful crisis is usually supportive. Oxygen is administered and adequate pain relief is essential, usually with opiate analgesics. Fluid replacement is important, as are antibiotics to treat any precipitating infections.

Exchange transfusions

In life-threatening situations, such as acute chest syndrome, exchange transfusion to reduce the proportion of sickle cells is required.

Bone marrow transplantation

Bone marrow transplantation is a potential cure for sickle cell disease, eliminating the clinical manifestations of the disease as well as disease-associated haemolytic anaemia. The overall and event-free survival at 11 years after bone

Paroxysmal nocturnal haemoglobinuria

Haemolytic disease of the newborn

Thalassaemias

Sickle cell and related disorders

marrow transplantation is 93% and 82% respectively.[2] Complications include graft-versus-host disease, haematological malignancy and gonadal dysfunction.

Prognosis

For patients who are homozygotes for sickle cell disease, the median age of death was 42 years for men and 48 years for women; the most common causes are organ failure, painful crises and acute chest syndrome.[3]

REFERENCES

(1) *Steinberg MH, Barton F, Castro O, et al. Effect of hydroxyurea on mortality and morbidity in adult sickle cell anemia: risks and benefits up to 9 years of treatment. JAMA 2003; 289: 1645–1651.*
(2) *Vermylen C, Cornu G, Ferster A, et al. Haematopoietic stem cell transplantation for sickle cell anaemia: the first 50 patients transplanted in Belgium. Bone Marrow Transplantation 1998; 22: 1–6.*
(3) *Platt OS, Brambilla DJ, Rosse WF, Milner PF, Castro O, Steinberg MH, Klug PP. Mortality in sickle cell disease—life expectancy and risk factors for early death. New England Journal of Medicine 1994; 330: 1639–1644.*

Hypoplastic anaemia

Primary hypoplastic or aplastic anaemia is characterized by anaemia, leukopenia and thrombocytopenia (pancytopenia) due to bone marrow failure associated with marrow hypocellularity.

Epidemiology

Hypoplastic anaemia is rare. It can affect any age group and both sexes.

Pathology

Hypoplastic anaemia results from failure or suppression of pluripotent stem cells resulting in pancytopenia. Pure red cell aplasia occurs when the defect is confined to cells committed to the erythroid series.

Bone marrow hypoplasia may be congenital or acquired. Acquired hypoplastic anaemia may be primary or secondary to some other disease or exposure. In the primary or idiopathic form of hypoplastic anaemia, T lymphocytes are involved in the suppression of stem cell development. Secondary causes are more common, as a result of known or idiosyncratic responses to drugs, ionizing radiation and chemicals or certain viral infections (Table 12.11).

Scope of disease

Depletion of all three cell lines can lead to anaemia, recurrent infections (low white cell count), and abnormal bruising and bleeding (low platelet count).

Table 12.11	Causes of bone marrow hypoplasia
Primary	
Congenital	
Idiopathic acquired	
Secondary	

Drugs
  e.g. Chemotherapy
  Chloramphenicol
  Phenylbutazone
  Gold	

Infection
  Parvovirus
  Hepatitis	

Irradiation Radiotherapy	
Chemicals Benzene	

Clinical features

Presenting features are typically anaemia (which may be severe), abnormal bleeding and severe, recurrent bacterial infections affecting the mouth and throat. A detailed drug, occupational and medical history is required to determine any underlying cause.

On examination, skin bruising, purpura and mucosal bleeding including epistaxis may be evident if thrombocytopenia is severe (platelet count less than 10×10^9/L). Splenomegaly is not a feature.

Initial investigations

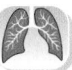

Full blood count, blood film
The full blood count reveals pancytopenia with normocytic red cells. Typical morphological changes of megaloblastic anaemia are absent. The reticulocyte count is low despite severe anaemia, indicating a failure of haemopoietic response.

Further investigations

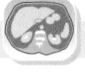

Bone marrow biopsy
A 'dry tap' may be obtained (an aspirate containing very little marrow). If marrow particles are present they appear hypocellular. Bone marrow trephine biopsy is essential to confirm the diagnosis. The marrow is markedly hypocellular and fat spaces predominate without any abnormal infiltrate.

Initial management

Identify and treat underlying cause
Possible causes should be sought, with special attention to recent use of medications. Occasionally, removal of the offending agent leads to recovery of the clinical condition.

Red cell and platelet transfusion

Symptomatic anaemia is treated with red cell transfusion. Bleeding associated with thrombocytopenia is treated with platelet transfusion.

Antibiotic therapy

Broad-spectrum antibiotics, antivirals or antifungals may be required to treat infections.

Medical management

Haemopoietic growth factors

Granulocyte colony stimulating factor (G-CSF) and granulocyte–macrophage colony stimulating factor (GM-CSF) can be used to increase the neutrophil count. They are usually ineffective in the most severe cases, which are, unfortunately, those with greatest need for treatment.

Immunomodulation

In idiopathic aplastic anaemia, treatment with antilymphocyte (ALG) and antithymocyte globulins (ATG) with methylprednisolone and ciclosporin produces a clinical improvement in 39%. The relapse rate is 38% after 11 years and malignant disease develops in 25% of the patients.[1]

Bone marrow or stem cell transplantation

In young patients with severe aplastic anaemia, bone marrow or stem cell transplantation from a matched donor (allogeneic bone marrow transplantation) is a potentially curative treatment option. Post-transplant patients have normal haematopoietic parameters, and the survival is 89% for patients without and 69% for patients with chronic graft-versus-host disease.[2] Complications include development of solid tumour malignancy in approximately 12%.

Prognosis

The prognosis is variable and usually related to the underlying cause. Successful identification and withdrawal or treatment of the underlying cause leads to recovery of the cell lines. In severe cases survival is short despite supportive therapy and spontaneous remission unlikely.

REFERENCES

(1) *Frickhofen N, Heimpel H, Kaltwasser JP, Schrezenmeier H. Antithymocyte globulin with or without cyclosporin A: 11-year follow-up of a randomized trial comparing treatments of aplastic anemia. Blood 2003; 101: 1236–1242.*
(2) *Deeg HJ, Leisenring W, Storb R, et al. Long-term outcome after marrow transplantation for severe aplastic anemia. Blood 1998; 91: 3637–3645.*
(3) *Fruchtman SM, Hurlet A, Dracker R, Isola L, Goldman B, Schneider BL, Emre S. The successful treatment of severe aplastic anemia with autologous cord blood transplantation. Biology of Blood and Marrow Transplantation 2004; 10: 741–742.*

Leukocytosis

Leukopenia

Disorders of white cell count

Leukocytosis

The numerical leukocyte count and differential count often provide a useful diagnostic guide in systemic disease. Some important causes of leukocytosis are listed in Table 12.12. Transient extreme levels of reactive leukocytosis, usually lymphocytosis, tend to occur in response to infection in childhood. Children and young adults develop a characteristic lymphocytosis with morphological peculiarities in infectious mononucleosis (p. 962). Marked reactive lymphocytosis is otherwise unusual in adults.

The response to bacterial sepsis in all age groups is the release of immature leukocytes; myelocytes and metamyelocytes in particular may appear in the peripheral blood. This is referred to as a 'left shift' in the myeloid series or a 'leukaemoid reaction' because of the similarity of the blood picture to chronic myeloid leukaemia.

In acute leukaemia, the leukocytosis is distinguished by the predominance of very primitive or immature leukocytes (blast cells), which are morphologically distinct from any normal component of peripheral blood.

Leukopenia

The normal neutrophil count varies according to population and is slightly lower in individuals of African ancestry. In neutropenia due to disease (Table 12.13) there is a risk of severe bacterial sepsis when the neutrophil count falls below 0.5×10^9/L. A mild degree of lymphopenia is

Table 12.12 Important causes of leukocytosis

Neutrophilia	Monocytosis	Eosinophilia	Lymphocytosis
Bacterial sepsis	Acute bacterial sepsis	Allergy	Viral infection
Tissue trauma	Chronic infection	Parasitic infection	Chronic bacterial infection
Tissue or organ infarction	Malignancy	Malignancy	Lymphoproliferative disease
Chronic inflammatory disease		Polyarteritis	
Acute haemorrhage		Hypereosinophilic syndromes	
Corticosteroid therapy			
Myeloproliferative disease			

common in sick individuals, and more severe lymphopenia occurs in collagen vascular disease, lymphomas and as a side effect of drugs such as immunosuppressants or cytotoxic agents. Marked lymphopenia is an important feature of infection with HIV.

Table 12.13 Important causes of leukopenia

Isolated neutropenia

Overwhelming sepsis
    Bacterial septicaemia

Autoimmune
    Rheumatoid disease (Felty's syndrome)

Drug induced
    Carbimazole (idiosyncratic reaction)

Cyclical
    Recurrent neutropenia in predictable cycles of
    approximately 4 weeks

As part of a pancytopenia

Bone marrow failure
    Acute leukaemia
    Marrow aplasia
    Chemotherapy

Megaloblastic anaemia
    Vitamin B_{12} or folate deficiency

Hypersplenism
    Systemic lupus erythematosus
    Portal hypertension

SECTION 12.6 Tumours of the haemopoietic and lymphoid tissues

Haematological malignancies are classified according to presentation (acute or chronic, with or without leukaemia) and their tissue of origin (myeloid or lymphoid). Recently the World Health Organization has refined the classification of tumours of the haemopoietic and lymphoid tissues to offer pathologists, haematologists, oncologists and geneticists a system based on their histopathological, immunological and genetic features.[1]

Table 12.14 outlines the main structure of the 2001 WHO system that classifies haematological malignancies by tissue of origin. In addition, common haematological malignancies are indicated in brackets.

In this section, the leukaemias are presented as a group of diseases subdivided into acute and chronic. To facilitate the presentation of the clinical management, the remaining haematopoietic and lymphoid tumours are presented according to tissue of origin in accordance with current WHO classification.

REFERENCE

(1) *Jaffe ES, Harris NL, Stein H, Vardiman JW. World Health Organization Classification of tumours of haematopoietic and lymphoid tissues. Lyon: IARC Press, 2001.*

Table 12.14	WHO headings for tumours of haematopoietic and lymphoid tissues*

Myeloid neoplasms

Acute myeloid leukaemia (AML)

Myelodysplastic syndromes

Myelodysplastic/myeloproliferative diseases

Chronic myeloproliferative diseases (including CML)

Lymphoid neoplasms

B-cell neoplasms

Precursor B-lymphoblastic leukaemia/lymphoma (B-ALL)

Mature B-cell neoplasms
  B-non Hodgkin lymphoma
  Plasma cell neoplasms

B-cell proliferations of uncertain malignant potential

T-cell and NK-cell neoplasms

Precursor T-lymphoblastic leukaemia/lymphoma (T-ALL)

Mature T-cell and NK-cell neoplasms
  T-non Hodgkin lymphoma

T-cell proliferations of uncertain malignant potential

Hodgkin lymphoma

Nodular lymphocyte predominant Hodgkin lymphoma
Classical Hodgkin lymphoma

Histiocytic and dendritic cell neoplasms

Langerhans cell histiocytosis

Mastocytosis

* Adapted from Jaffe ES, Harris NL, Stein H, Vardiman JW. World Health Organization Classification of tumours of haematopoietic and lymphoid tissues. Lyon: IARC Press, 2001.

Table 12.15	Risk factors for developing acute leukaemia

Hereditary
Down's syndrome (30-fold increased risk)

Fanconi's anaemia

Ataxia telangiectasia

Klinefelter's syndrome

Other haematological disease
Myelodysplastic syndrome

Myeloproliferative disease

Drugs and chemicals
Benzene

Alkylating agents

Radiation
Atom bomb survivors

Nuclear accidents

Therapeutic extended field irradiation (for lymphoma)

Acute leukaemias

Chronic leukaemias

Chronic myeloproliferative diseases

Plasma cell neoplasms

Myelodysplastic syndromes

Hodgkin lymphoma

Non-Hodgkin lymphomas

Leukaemia

Acute leukaemias

Acute leukaemias are a group of diseases arising from the malignant transformation of haemopoietic progenitor cells. Based on lineage, degree of maturation and the presence of known molecular abnormalities, they are divided into acute lymphoblastic leukaemia (ALL) and acute myeloblastic leukaemia (AML).

Epidemiology

Although both types can occur at any age, the incidence of ALL peaks in childhood (between 2 and 7 years) at 7 cases per 100 000 per year, whereas the incidence of AML increases with age, from 3 per 100 000 per year rising to 20 per 100 000 per year in those over 70 years of age.

Pathology

The leukaemic cell population arises from malignant transformation of either an undifferentiated bone marrow stem cell or an early progenitor cell committed to myeloid or lymphoid development. The transformed cell proliferates but fails to differentiate normally, leading to accumulation of leukaemic blast cells in the bone marrow and consequently bone marrow failure. Eventually peripheral blood involvement occurs with infiltration of the liver, spleen and lymph nodes. The predisposing factors for developing acute leukaemia are listed in Table 12.15.

Classification

Classification systems are important in the management of acute leukaemia. Accurate subtyping promotes specific treatment, facilitates the comparison of results in clinical trials and improves the accuracy of determining patient prognosis in these groups of heterogenous disease.

The WHO criteria[1] classify AML into four main categories: AML with recurrent genetic abnormalities, multilineage dysplasia, treatment-related disease or not otherwise specified (Table 12.16).

The French–American–British (FAB) classification system[2] is widely used for ALL, and is divided into three main subtypes (L$_1$, L$_2$, L$_3$) according to cytology (Table 12.17).

RECENT ADVANCES

Patients' responsiveness to individual drug therapy may be predicted by genetic subtyping.[3] Karyotyping of the leukaemic blasts is important in identifying cytogenetic abnormalities of prognostic significance, and increasingly molecular techniques are being applied to identify specific genetic abnormalities and to use them for minimal residual disease monitoring.

Scope of disease

Proliferation of blast cells can lead to bone marrow failure and infiltration of the brain (leading to neurological symptoms), lymph nodes, the liver and spleen (leading to hepatosplenomegaly).

Table 12.16	World Health Organization classification of acute myeloid leukaemia*
Acute myeloid leukaemia with recurrent genetic abnormalities	
Acute myeloid leukaemia with abnormal bone marrow eosinophils and inv(16)(p13q22) or t(16;16)(p13;q22), (CBF^β/MYH11)	
Acute promyelocytic leukaemia with t(15;17)(q22;q12), (PML/RAR α) and variants	
Acute myeloid leukaemia with 11q23 (MLL) abnormalities	
Acute myeloid leukaemia with multilineage dysplasia	
Following MDS or MDS/MPD	
Without antecedent MDS or MDS/MPD, but with dysplasia in at least 50% of cells in 2 or more myeloid lineages	
Acute myeloid leukaemia and myelodysplastic syndromes, therapy related	
Alkylating agent/radiation-related type	
Topoisomerase II inhibitor-related type (some may be lymphoid)	
Others	
Acute myeloid leukaemia, not otherwise categorized	
Acute myeloid leukaemia, minimally differentiated	
Acute myeloid leukaemia without maturation	
Acute myeloid leukaemia with maturation	
Acute myelomonocytic leukaemia	
Acute monoblastic/acute monocytic leukaemia	
Acute erythroid leukaemia (erythroid/myeloid and pure erythroleukaemia)	
Acute megakaryoblastic leukaemia	
Acute basophilic leukaemia	
Acute panmyelosis with myelofibrosis	
Myeloid sarcoma	

* From Vardiman JW, Harris NL, Brunning RD. The World Health Organization (WHO) classification of the myeloid neoplasms. Blood 2002; 100: 2292–2302.

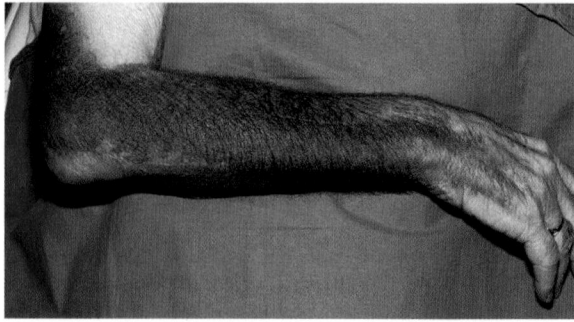

Fig. 12.4 Extensive ecchymosis in acute myeloid leukaemia.

Clinical features

Bone marrow failure is the hallmark presentation of acute leukaemia with anaemia, thrombocytopenia and neutropenia. Pallor, lethargy and dyspnoea are typical symptoms of anaemia. Spontaneous bleeding from thrombocytopenia or fibrinolysis can occur in the skin (Fig. 12.4), mucous membranes (Fig. 12.5), gastrointestinal tract and urogenital tract (haematuria). Neutropenia predisposes to bacterial and fungal infections leading to fever (pyrexia of unknown origin), septicaemic shock, pneumonia, urinary tract infection and cellulitis (Fig. 12.6). Symptoms from hyperviscosity are confusion and blurred vision.

On examination, there may be a petechial rash or bruising (Fig. 12.4). Features of leukaemic infiltration include gum infiltration (Fig. 12.7) and hypertrophy, lymphadenopathy and hepatosplenomegaly.

Initial investigations

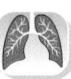

Full blood count and blood film

A normochromic normocytic anaemia is usually present with thrombocytopenia and neutropenia. Although the total white cell count is often raised, it can be normal or low. Circulating leukaemic blast cells are often detected on the blood film (Fig. 12.8).

Serum uric acid

Uric acid levels may be elevated from high cell turnover.

High cell turnover can lead to hyperuricaemia causing acute renal failure or gout, especially at the start of treatment. Very high white counts can lead to hyperviscosity, and leukaemic blast cells can activate fibrinolysis causing bleeding that is disproportionate with the platelet count.

Table 12.17	French–American–British classification of acute lymphoblastic leukaemia*	
FAB type	**Appearance**	**Cell types**
L₁	Small blast cells, almost no cytoplasm (high nuclear to cytoplasmic ratio), rounded cleaved nucleoli	T cell or B cell
L₂	Larger blast cells, approximately 20% cytoplasm, prominent nucleoli	T cell or B cell
L₃	Basophilic cytoplasm, cytoplasmic vacuolization	Usually B cell

Each type may be subdivided into early pre-B, common, pre-B-cell, mature B-cell, pre-T-cell and mature T-cell ALL.
* Adapted from Bennett JM, Catovsky D, Daniel MT, Flandrin G, Galton DA, Gralnick HR, Sultan C. Proposals for the classification of the acute leukaemias. French-American-British (FAB) co-operative group. British Journal of Haematology 1976; 33: 451–458.

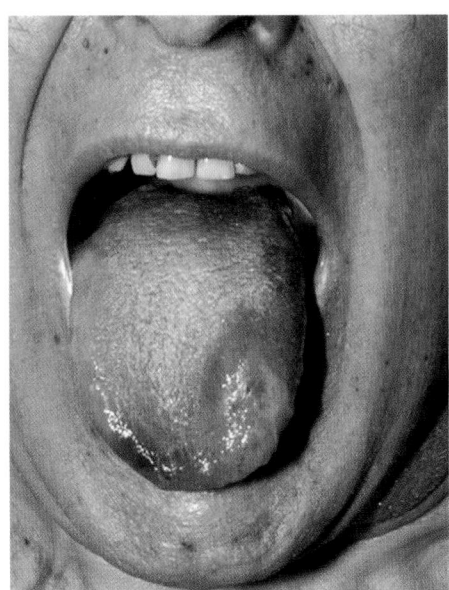

Fig. 12.5 Spontaneous tongue haematoma.

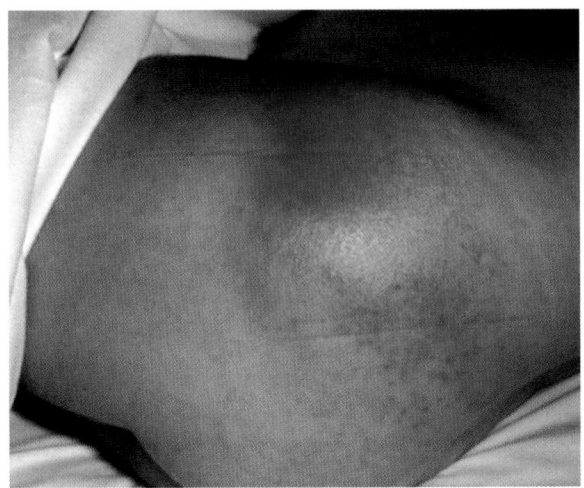

Fig. 12.6 *Staphylococcus aureus* cellulitis.

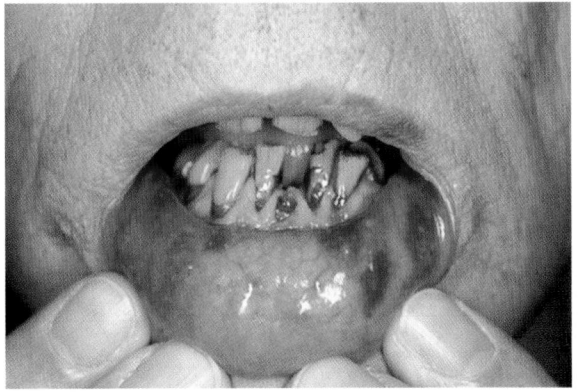

Fig. 12.7 Gum infiltration and oral ulceration in a patient with monocytic subtype acute myeloid leukaemia.

may show features of both AML and ALL (hybrid acute leukaemia).

Further investigations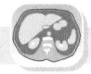

Disseminated intravascular coagulation screen
Patients with severe bleeding will require screening for disseminated intravascular coagulation (DIC, p. 820).

Lumbar puncture
Symptoms of meningism or neurological deficit warrant a lumbar puncture to screen for leukaemic blasts in the cerebrospinal fluid from meningeal leukaemia.

Specific imaging
Organ-specific symptoms (bone pain) require organ-specific imaging (plain film X-rays).

Initial management
A crucial part of treatment is supportive care in specialized units.

Central venous access
Long-term central venous access is obtained for multiple transfusions, administration of chemotherapy, antibiotics and antiemetics and occasionally intravenous feeding.

Packed cells and platelet transfusion
Blood and platelet transfusions are required to alleviate symptomatic anaemia and bleeding from thrombocytopenia. They are also essential to support patients through prolonged periods of chemotherapy-induced bone marrow failure.

Management of infection
Ideally patients are nursed in single rooms with careful attention to hygiene to reduce the risk of nosocomial infection. Air filtration, if available, may reduce the risk of fungal infection. Some leukaemia units give patients prophylactic

Serum lactate dehydrogenase
LDH may be elevated.

Serum calcium
Occasionally serum calcium levels are raised.

Bone marrow aspiration
A bone marrow aspirate is required to confirm the diagnosis. The normal marrow is replaced by blast cells. The WHO classification defines leukaemia as acute when more than 20% of the marrow is replaced by blast cells, but this is often more than 90% at initial diagnosis. Often routine staining cannot reliably differentiate AML from ALL, and the use of immunological markers (monoclonal antibodies), or cytochemical stains is required. Rarely, the blast cells

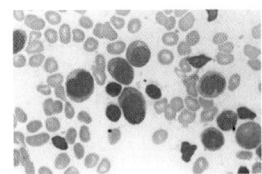

Fig. 12.8 Blast cells of acute monoblastic leukaemia.

801

ciprofloxacin to reduce the incidence of Gram-negative sepsis,[4] and antifungal prophylaxis.

In the patient with a fever or more localized symptoms of infection, broad-spectrum antibacterial therapy (aminoglycoside and an antipseudomonal penicillin or cephalosporin) is initiated after microbiological cultures. The treatment is then tailored according to the sensitivities of any identified organism. Resistant fever is treated with empiric antifungal therapy since failure of resolution of symptoms or signs of infection may indicate a fungal infection or less commonly a viral infection.

Medical management

Chemotherapy

Treatment is different for AML and ALL and is increasingly tailored to specific subtypes. It is usually given in the following stages: induction, consolidation and maintenance chemotherapy.

The aim of the induction therapy is to reduce the number of leukaemic cells to a morphologically undetectable level, allowing normal haemopoiesis to recover. Disease remission is defined as the return of normal blood counts and <5% blasts in the marrow. The specific regimen varies according to AML, ALL and their subtypes. Therapy is often trial based.

When disease remission is achieved, consolidation treatment is administered to further reduce leukaemic cells to very low levels that can be controlled or eradicated by the patient's own immune system. This is usually administered as multiple blocks (1–3 cycles) of combination chemotherapy. Prophylactic cranial irradiation and intrathecal chemotherapy are administered to most patients aged under 60 years with ALL due to the high risk of central nervous system disease.

Low-intensity maintenance chemotherapy to prevent recurrence is given to all patients with ALL not undergoing stem cell transplantation for 2 years; it is not usually given to patients with AML.

Stem cell transplantation (bone marrow or peripheral blood)

Allogeneic stem cell transplantation is used in first remission for certain subgroups of young patients deemed to have a poor prognosis with conventional chemotherapy. Examples include Philadelphia chromosome positive ALL and AML with poor prognosis cytogenetics such as monosomy 7. Allogeneic transplantation is the considered treatment of choice for all young patients with relapsed AML who achieve a second remission. The fatal complications of the transplant procedure, such as graft-versus-host disease, have made the benefit of allogeneic transplantation in other situations unclear. The role of autologous transplantation remains unproven in acute leukaemia.

All-*trans* retinoic acid

Patients with the subgroup of AML known as acute promyelocytic leukaemia benefit from all-*trans* retinoic acid (ATRA), a vitamin A analogue that induces the leukaemic cells to mature to neutrophils.

Prognosis

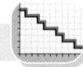

Prognosis in AML depends on age, cytogenetic risk group and achievement of prompt remission. In younger patients a good risk group is defined with a 70% long-term survival whilst a poor risk group is defined with only 10–20% long-term survival. The majority fall into an intermediate group with a survival of 40–50%. Older people fare badly because of poor tolerance of chemotherapy and increased incidence of treatment-resistant leukaemia.

Approximately 80% of children with ALL are cured with chemotherapy; in the remaining 20% salvage therapy with stem cell transplantation or participation in clinical trials may be required. Adults with ALL have a poorer survival, as a higher proportion have more aggressive disease such as Philadelphia chromosome positive ALL. Approximately 30–40% of young adults become long-term survivors. Old age carries a very poor prognosis.

REFERENCES

(1) Vardiman JW, Harris NL, Brunning RD. *The World Health Organization (WHO) classification of the myeloid neoplasms.* Blood 2002; 100: 2292–2302.

(2) Bennett JM, Catovsky D, Daniel MT, Flandrin G, Galton DA, Gralnick HR, Sultan C. *Proposals for the classification of the acute leukaemias. French-American-British (FAB) co-operative group.* British Journal of Haematology 1976; 33: 451–458.

(3) Holleman A, Cheok MH, den Boer ML, et al. *Gene-expression patterns in drug-resistant acute lymphoblastic leukemia cells and response to treatment.* New England Journal of Medicine 2004; 351: 533–542.

(4) Cortellaro M, Cofrancesco E, Pasargiklian I, et al. *Ciprofloxacin for infection prophylaxis in granulocytopenic patients with acute leukemia.* Haematologica 1990; 75: 541–545.

Chronic leukaemias

The difference between chronic and acute leukaemias is that in the former the malignant cells retain their differentiating capability, at least during the early period of the disease. Hence patients are less likely to present with bone marrow failure. There are two principal chronic leukaemias: chronic myeloid leukaemia and chronic lymphocytic leukaemia.

Chronic lymphocytic leukaemia

Epidemiology

Chronic lymphocytic leukaemia (CLL) is the most common leukaemia in the Western world accounting for one third of all leukaemias. In the West, 95% of CLL is due to B-CLL. The estimated incidence in the West is 2.3 per 100 000 per year.[1] CLL is twice as common in men and is predominantly a disease of old age. It is rare before the age of 30 years and almost never occurs in children.

Pathology

Chronic lymphocytic leukaemia is a slowly progressive disease that arises from a relentless accumulation of malignant B cells in blood, marrow, liver and spleen.

There are two forms of disease: the leukaemic equivalent of memory B cells and the leukaemic equivalent of a naive B cell. In the first type, the malignant B cell has undergone rearrangement of its immunoglobulin genes, passed through the germinal centre of the lymph node, and been selected for antigen by hypermutation of its rearranged immunoglobulin genes.

In the second type of disease, the leukaemic B cell has not been selected for antigen by hypermutation of the immunoglobulin genes (leukaemic equivalent of a naive B cell). This form of disease is much more aggressive and resistant to chemotherapy, and patients with this disease have a shorter survival.

Clinical features

The early stage of this disease is asymptomatic, and may be diagnosed on a routine full blood count (approximately 50%). Anaemia, bacterial infections (leukopenia) and prolonged bleeding (thrombocytopenia) can result from progressive marrow infiltration, and patients with advanced disease may complain of weight loss and drenching night sweats.

On examination, patients may have features of organ infiltration such as lymphadenopathy, splenomegaly or hepatomegaly with progressive disease.

Investigations

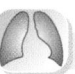

Full blood count and blood film
Leukocytosis is present: up to 99% of nucleated cells are small lymphocytes of B-cell origin. The lymphocyte count ranges between 5 and more than 300×10^9/L. Chronic lymphocytic leukaemia cells tend to fragment during preparation of the blood film, producing 'smear cells'. Anaemia (normocytic) and thrombocytopenia are late developments.

In approximately 10%, a secondary autoimmune haemolytic anaemia develops, with reticulocytosis, microspherocytes and a positive direct antiglobulin test.

Serum immunoglobulins
Serum immunoglobulins are low in the later stages of the disease.

Immunophenotyping
B-CLL cells stain positive for the antigens CD19, CD5 and CD 23 and weakly for surface immunoglobulin. This pattern of staining is useful for helping to distinguish CLL from B-non Hodgkin lymphoma.

Cytogenetic analysis
Fluorescent in situ hybridization (FISH) is able to detect cytogenetic abnormalities such as deletions of 13q and 11q and trisomy 12.

Bone marrow aspiration
The bone marrow is hypercellular, with progressive replacement of normal tissue by small lymphocytes.

Initial management

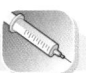

Staging
The results from clinical assessment and initial investigations form the basis for staging. The two most commonly used systems are listed in Table 12.18. The Rai[2] system is more commonly used in the USA and the Binet system[3] is more commonly used in Europe.

Patient education
At present, CLL is still incurable. However, many patients with early stage disease do not require treatment at all or for many years. Randomized trials have shown no overall survival benefit for treating early stage disease (Binet A)[4] therefore a watch and wait policy is adopted.

Medical management

Treatment is indicated for progressive disease identified by the development of significant cytopenia, bulky lymphadenopathy, hepatosplenomegaly or systemic symptoms (weight loss and night sweats).

First-line treatment
Treatment is usually initiated with single agent chlorambucil or fludarabine, a purine analogue that inhibits DNA synthesis or fludarabine and cyclophosphamide. The UK CLL4 trial has shown that this combination is the most effective. It has previously been suggested that fludarabine yields higher response rates (20% versus 4% complete remission) and a longer duration of remission (median of 25 months versus 14 months) compared to chlorambucil, but no significant differences in overall survival are evident.[5] Combination chemotherapy regimens such as cyclophosphamide, vincristine and prednisone (CVP) and cyclophosphamide, doxorubicin, vincristine and prednisone (CHOP) have not proved to be superior to single agent therapy.

Second-line treatment
At relapse, patients can be treated with the same regimen again or progress to second- and third-line therapies, for example fludarabine if they have had chlorambucil as first-line therapy. Aggressive forms of the disease in younger patients may respond to intensive chemotherapy using combinations such as fludarabine and cyclophosphamide (with or without rituximab). The results of these therapies

803

are still currently under evaluation. Stem cell transplantation may be an option, although its precise role is still to be defined.

RECENT ADVANCES

Monoclonal antibody therapy with rituximab[6] (anti-CD20) in combination with chemotherapy and alemtuzumab[7] (anti-CD52) alone or in combination is being evaluated for use in CLL.

Prognosis

The disease usually follows a predictable clinical course with a median survival of 25 years from diagnosis for the immunoglobulin hypermutated form of the disease, but only 8 years for the unmutated form. Elderly patients with good prognosis disease often die from an unrelated cause. The stage-related prognosis is provided in Table 12.18.

i **FURTHER INFORMATION**

Oscier D, Fegan C, Hillmen P, et al. Guidelines on the diagnosis and management of chronic lymphocytic leukaemia. British Journal of Haematology 2004; 125: 294–317.

REFERENCES

(1) Kalil N, Cheson BD. Chronic lymphocytic leukemia. Oncologist 1999; 4: 352–369.
(2) Rai KR, Sawitsky A, Cronkite EP, Chanana AD, Levy RN, Pasternack BS. Clinical staging of chronic lymphocytic leukemia. Blood 1975; 46: 219–234.
(3) Binet JL, Auquier A, Dighiero G, et al. A new prognostic classification of chronic lymphocytic leukemia derived from a multivariate survival analysis. Cancer 1981; 48: 198–206.
(4) Dighiero G, Maloum K, Desablens B, et al, The French Cooperative Group on Chronic Lymphocytic Leukemia. Chlorambucil in indolent chronic lymphocytic leukemia. New England Journal of Medicine 1998; 338: 1506–1514.
(5) Rai KR, Peterson BL, Appelbaum FR, et al. Fludarabine compared with chlorambucil as primary therapy for chronic lymphocytic leukemia. New England Journal of Medicine 2000; 343: 1750–1757.
(6) Byrd JC, Rai K, Peterson BL, et al. Addition of rituximab to fludarabine may prolong progression-free survival and overall survival in patients with previously untreated chronic lymphocytic leukemia: an updated retrospective comparative analysis of CALGB 9712 and CALGB 9011. Blood 2005; 105: 49–53.
(7) Osterborg A, Dyer M, Bunjes D, Pangalis G, Bastion Y, Catovsky D, Mellstedt H. Phase II multicenter study of human CD52 antibody in previously treated chronic lymphocytic leukemia. European Study Group of CAMPATH-1H Treatment in Chronic Lymphocytic Leukemia. Journal of Clinical Oncology 1997; 15: 1567–1574.
(8) Damle RN, Wasil T, Fais F, et al. Ig V gene mutation status and CD38 expression as novel prognostic indicators in chronic lymphocytic leukemia. Blood 1999; 94: 1840–1847.

Chronic myeloid leukaemia

Epidemiology

Chronic myeloid leukaemia (CML) can occur in either sex and in any age group. The most common age at presentation is between 40 and 60 years.

Pathology

In CML, the normal bone marrow is replaced by a clone of cells of pluripotential stem cell origin. In 95% of cases there is a reciprocal translocation between chromosomes 9 and 22, which in 95% of cases can be recognized in standard karyotypes as a Philadelphia chromosome (small chromosome 22, Fig. 12.9). This translocation results in a new fusion gene called *BCR–ABL*. Due to the pluripotent stem cell origin, erythroid, megakaryocytic, granulocytic and B-lymphocyte cell lines all carry the defect.

The protein product of this gene behaves as an abnormal tyrosine kinase, promoting myeloid progenitor cell expansion. Knowledge of the pathogenesis has been utilized to develop novel therapeutic agents such as tyrosine kinase inhibitors (see below).

The disease runs a chronic phase for a number of years. In patients who have not undergone successful stem cell transplantation the disease eventually enters an aggressive phase due to the emergence and dominance of a clone of myeloid cells which have lost the ability to differentiate. At this stage, the disease resembles acute myeloid leukaemia (or less commonly acute lymphoblastic leukaemia) and this 'blast crisis' is always fatal.

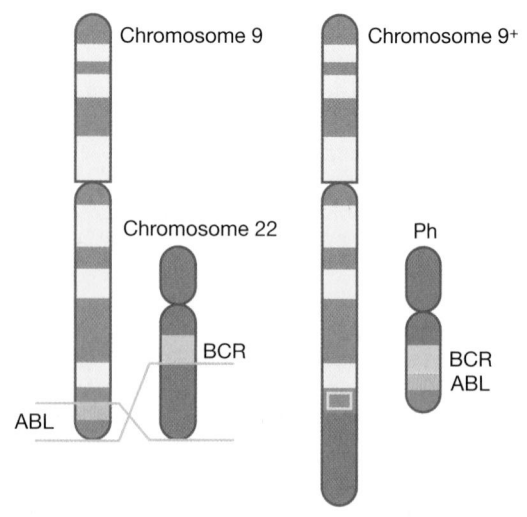

Fig. 12.9 Philadelphia chromosome (Ph) resulting from t(9;22) translocation. The Ph chromosome is the small derivative chromosome 22.

Table 12.18	Staging of chronic lymphocytic leukaemia	
Rai stage[a]		**Median survival**
Stage 0	Bone marrow and blood lymphocytosis only	>150 months
Stage 1	Lymphocytosis with enlarged nodes	101 months
Stage II	Lymphocytosis with enlarged spleen or liver or both	71 months
Stage III	Lymphocytosis with anaemia	19 months
Stage IV	Lymphocytosis with thrombocytopenia	19 months
Binet stage[b]		**Median survival**
Stage A	No anaemia, no thrombopenia, less than three involved areas (axillary, cervical, inguinal lymph nodes, spleen and liver)	Same as the age and sex matched general population
Stage B	No anaemia, no thrombopenia, three or more involved areas (axillary, cervical, inguinal lymph nodes, spleen and liver)	84 months
Stage C	Anaemia (Hb less than 10 g) and/or thrombopenia (platelets less than 100×10^9/L)	24 months

[a] From Rai KR, Sawitsky A, Cronkite EP, Chanana AD, Levy RN, Pasternack BS. Clinical staging of chronic lymphocytic leukaemia. Blood 1975; 46: 219–234.
[b] From Binet JL, Auquier A, Dighiero G, et al. A new prognostic classification of chronic lymphocytic leukaemia derived from a multivariate survival analysis. Cancer 1981; 48: 198–206.

Hypermetabolism from the high turnover of white cells can occur with hyperuricaemia as a complication. Rarely hyperviscosity can result from extreme elevations of the white cell count. Splenomegaly is almost always present.

Clinical features

In the chronic phase, the presenting symptoms are those of anaemia, weight loss and abdominal fullness or pain (splenic infarction) due to massive splenomegaly.

Symptoms of hypermetabolism include weight loss and excess sweating. Rarely, altered consciousness, blurred vision and cardio-respiratory failure can occur from hyperviscosity. Joint pains and other symptoms of gout are listed on page 506.

The clinical features during blast crises are those of an acute leukaemia (p. 799).

Investigations

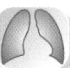

Full blood count, blood film

Leukocytosis is a uniform feature, and the white cell count can be in excess of 300×10^9/L. A normochromic anaemia is usually present whilst platelets can be increased (sometimes over 1000×10^9/L), normal or reduced.

The blood film resembles a bone marrow aspirate, with myelocytes, promyelocytes, myeloblasts and normoblasts present as well as large numbers of band cells and mature polymorphonuclear granulocytes. Basophilia is common.

Karyotyping

Approximately 95% of patients have the Philadelphia chromosome on routine G-banding, and a further 2.5% will have an occult t(9;22) translocation identified by a positive polymerase chain reaction (PCR) for the BCR–ABL transcript.

Approximately 2.5% are negative for the t(9;22) translocation (by G-banding and PCR) and are termed atypical Philadelphia negative CML.

Bone marrow aspirate

The bone marrow is hypercellular with predominant granulocytopoiesis and marked reduction of the fat spaces. In blast crises, increased numbers of blast cells become evident in blood and bone marrow. Correspondingly anaemia and thrombocytopenia are more marked.

Management

Chronic disease

Allogeneic stem cell transplantation

Allogeneic stem cell/bone marrow transplantation offers a potential cure for CML. The precise role of allogeneic transplantation following the introduction of imatinib therapy is controversial. Transplantation is generally reserved for patients who fail to respond to imatinib mesylate. The best results are achieved in young (less than 30 years) fit patients with a suitable donor. The transplant-related mortality ranges from 20% to 40%. The relapse rates are usually less than 20% with a survival that stabilizes at 3–7 years.[1]

Imatinib mesylate

Imatinib is standard therapy in all patients unsuitable for allogeneic transplantation. In present practice virtually all new patients have a trial of imatinib mesylate therapy. This drug binds to the ATP binding site of BCR–ABL and inhibits the function of the tyrosine kinase protein. Complete haematological response was achieved in 95% of patients at a median time interval of 1 month, and freedom from progression to accelerated phase or blast crisis was 99% at

1 year.[2] Common side effects of treatment in a third of patients include oedema, nausea, muscle cramps, bone and joint pains, resulting in discontinuation of treatment in 14%.

Interferon-alfa and cytarabine

The current best second-line treatment is recombinant interferon-alfa and low-dose cytarabine. This regimen led to complete haematological response in 56% at a median time interval of 2.5 months and freedom from progression to accelerated phase or blast crisis was 93% at 1 year.[2]

Accelerated and blast crisis phase disease

Combination chemotherapy

Imatinib is as an agent for use in the advanced phase; currently, the benefits are short lived. Combination chemotherapy may return the patient to chronic phase, especially from lymphoid blast crises. Allogeneic or autologous transplantation may prolong the second chronic phase but for most patients the second chronic phase is short lived. The new kinase inhibitors Dasatinib and Nilotanib show promise in advanced disease and imatinib resistance.

Prognosis

Prognosis in CML has been determined by the Sokal index which is based on age, spleen size, platelet count and percentage of blast cells.[3] However, it has been of limited use for individual patients and its significance in the era of imatinib therapy is unclear.

REFERENCES

(1) Silver RT, Woolf SH, Hehlmann R, et al. An evidence-based analysis of the effect of busulfan, hydroxyurea, interferon, and allogeneic bone marrow transplantation in treating the chronic phase of chronic myeloid leukemia: developed for the American Society of Hematology. Blood 1999; 94: 1517–1536.

(2) O'Brien SG, Guilhot F, Larson RA, et al, the IRIS Investigators. Imatinib compared with interferon and low-dose cytarabine for newly diagnosed chronic-phase chronic myeloid leukemia. New England Journal of Medicine 2003; 348: 994–1004.

(3) Bacigalupo A, Gualandi F, Van Lint MT, et al. Multivariate analysis of risk factors for survival and relapse in chronic granulocytic leukemia following allogeneic marrow transplantation: impact of disease related variables (Sokal score). Bone Marrow Transplantation 1993; 12: 443–448.

Chronic myeloid neoplasms

Chronic myeloproliferative diseases

Polycythaemia

Polycythaemia is an increase in red cell concentration above the normal limit, usually accompanied by a corresponding increase in haematocrit and haemoglobin concentration.

Epidemiology

The prevalence of polycythaemia is approximately 8.8 per 100 000, but the majority is due to secondary polycythaemia (especially smoking related). The prevalence of polycythaemia vera (primary polycythaemia) is approximately 0.3 per 100 000.[1] The incidence increases with age and the disorder is equally common in both sexes.

Pathology

Polycythaemia is not a diagnosis but a manifestation of disease (Table 12.19). It can be 'true' due to a real increase in red cell concentration, or 'apparent' due to low plasma volume (e.g. dehydration). 'True' polycythaemia is divided into primary and secondary causes.

Primary polycythaemia (polycythaemia vera) is due to a neoplasm of the myeloid series. An acquired mutation in the gene for the tyrosine kinase JAK2 has been identified recently in a high proportion of cases of myeloproliferative disease, especially polycythaemia vera.

Secondary polycythaemia is due to raised erythropoietin levels and may be appropriate (chronic low oxygenation) or inappropriate (erythropoietin production from renal tumours).

The management of secondary polycythaemia involves the identification and treatment of the underlying cause where possible. In the remainder of this section, the diag-

Table 12.19	Classification and causes of polycythaemia

True polycythaemia (increased red cell mass)

Primary polycythaemia
Polycythaemia vera

Secondary polycythaemia
Appropriate erythropoietin production (hypoxia)
    Smoking (due carbon monoxide exposure)
    Chronic respiratory disease
    Long-term exposure to high altitude
    Cyanotic heart disease
    High-affinity haemoglobinopathy

Inappropriate erythropoietin production
    Renal carcinoma or cysts
    Renal artery stenosis
    Renal amyloidosis
    Massive uterine fibroids
    Hepatocellular carcinoma
    Cerebellar haemangioblastoma

Apparent polycythaemia (reduced plasma volume, normal red cell mass)

Low plasma volume polycythaemia (dehydration, burns, enteropathy)

Gaisböck's syndrome*

* Gaisböck's syndrome tends to occur in middle-aged, overweight male heavy smokers. The pathogenesis is obscure and it is associated with increased risk of arterial occlusion causing myocardial infarction and stroke. The management involves lifestyle change (weight reduction, quitting smoking, reduced alcohol consumption) and avoidance of diuretics which may worsen the plasma contraction.

nosis and management of polycythaemia vera, a myeloproliferative disease, is described.

Scope of disease

High red cell concentration predisposes to thrombosis, and extreme elevations can lead to hyperviscosity syndrome. As polycythaemia is part of the myeloid family of neoplasms, progression to acute myeloid leukaemia and myelofibrosis can occur. There may also be increased bleeding due to the production of functionally abnormal platelets.

Clinical features

The condition may be asymptomatic for months or years. Presenting features of polycythaemia vera are fatigue, aquagenic pruritus (skin itching after a hot bath), sweating and, occasionally, weight loss. Patients may also present with complications such as stroke, deep vein thrombosis or hyperviscosity (headache, blurred vision and confusion).

On examination there is plethora and, occasionally, cyanosis. Scratch marks or spontaneous bruising may be visible on the skin. The conjunctival vessels are engorged and dilated retinal veins may be evident on fundoscopy. Splenomegaly may be palpable on examination of the abdomen.

Initial investigations

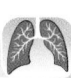

Full blood count, blood film

Polycythaemia is diagnosed when the haemoglobin concentration is increased to more than around 17.5 g/dL in men and 15.5 g/dL in women with an accompanying rise in red cell count. The corresponding increase in haematocrit is more than around 55% in men and 47% in women.

In polycythaemia vera, thrombocytosis and neutrophil leukocytosis are present in up to 50% of cases.

Serum uric acid

Serum uric acid is increased in polycythaemia vera due to increased cell turnover.

Arterial blood gas

Arterial blood gas estimation on air is useful to evaluate the oxygen concentration in the blood. It is normal in primary polycythaemia but reduced in secondary polycythaemia due to respiratory failure or cardiac disease with right to left shunt.

Further investigations

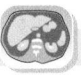

Total red cell volume

Red cells in a sample of blood from the patient are tagged with ^{51}Cr, and the labelled red cells are reinjected. The dilution of the isotope in a subsequent venous blood sample is used to calculate the red cell mass. The normal range is between 25 and 35 mL/kg in men and 22 and 32 mL/kg in women.

In the presence of ongoing blood loss (there is a predisposition to bleeding and peptic ulceration), iron-deficient

polycythaemia results and the haemoglobin and haematocrit may be normal or low. The condition should be suspected when there are obviously iron deficient red cells (low MCV) without anaemia and with a very high red cell count.

Plasma volume

^{125}I-albumin is used to estimate total plasma volume; the normal range is between 35 and 45 mL/kg. This is usually performed in conjunction with the estimation of total red cell volume to distinguish between real and apparent polycythaemia (the latter is due to low plasma volume).

Bone marrow aspiration

In polycythaemia vera there is a hypercellular bone marrow with erythroid hyperplasia. Megakaryocytes may be prominent and increased reticulin deposition is common.

Initial management

Aspirin

Treatment with aspirin reduces the risk of thrombotic complications (myocardial infarction, stroke and death from cardiovascular causes) without significantly increasing the risk of major bleeding.[2]

Medical management

Venesection

Venesection is the mainstay of treatment and is performed, for example weekly, to lower the haematocrit to less than 45%. Subsequently less frequent venesections are performed as maintenance therapy.

Chemotherapy

Myelosuppression with hydroxyurea is used to control thrombocytosis. Radioactive phosphorus and alkylating agents are rarely used now.

Prognosis

The life expectancy of patients with polycythaemia vera is reduced compared with the general population. The overall 15-year survival probability from diagnosis is 65%.[3] Progression to a myelofibrotic state is common and transformation to acute myeloid leukaemia can occur, especially after radiophosphorus treatment.

REFERENCES

(1) *Ruggeri M, Tosetto A, Frezzato M, Rodeghiero F. The rate of progression to polycythemia vera or essential thrombocythemia in patients with erythrocytosis or thrombocytosis. Annals of Internal Medicine 2003; 139: 470–475.*
(2) *Landolfi R, Marchioli R, Kutti J, Gisslinger H, Tognoni G, Patrono C, Barbui T. Efficacy and safety of low-dose aspirin in polycythemia vera. New England Journal of Medicine 2004; 350: 114–124.*
(3) *Passamonti F, Rumi E, Pungolino E, et al. Life expectancy and prognostic factors for survival in patients with polycythemia vera and essential thrombocythemia. American Journal of Medicine 2004; 117: 755–761.*

Essential thrombocythaemia

Essential thrombocythaemia is a myeloproliferative disorder and an important cause of thrombocytosis.

Epidemiology

The prevalence of essential thrombocythaemia has been estimated at 0.4 per 100 000.[1] It is generally a disorder of older adults.

Pathology

Abnormal proliferation of megakaryocytes leading to a high platelet count is the dominant feature. An acquired mutation in the gene for the tyrosine kinase JAK2 has been identified recently in a high proportion of cases of myeloproliferative disease, including essential thrombocythaemia. Paradoxically, there can be a predisposition to either thrombosis (due to excess number and increased function of platelets) or haemorrhage (functionally defective platelets).

Clinical features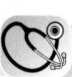

The disorder may be asymptomatic for many years, and the diagnosis is frequently suspected due to the incidental finding of thrombocytosis on a blood count performed as part of investigations for another complaint. Alternatively the presentation may be with arterial thrombosis, including ischaemic stroke or venous thromboembolism. Painful ischaemic lesions of the digits are an occasional feature. Presentation with bleeding tends to occur in those with platelet counts over 1500×10^9/L. It may be difficult to distinguish essential thrombocythaemia from reactive thrombocytosis, for example due to chronic inflammatory disease, malignancy or chronic blood loss; therefore the clinical assessment is invaluable.

Investigations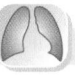

Full blood count, blood film

The platelet count is elevated, ranging from 400 to >3000 $\times 10^9$/L, although there is often diagnostic uncertainty if the count is 400–600 $\times 10^9$/L and there are no clinical features. Neutrophil leukocytosis may also be present. Anaemia, when present, is usually due to iron deficiency from chronic blood loss. The blood film may reveal 'giant' platelets and megakaryocyte fragments. Howell–Jolly bodies and other features of hyposplenism may be apparent due to splenic infarction.

Bone marrow aspiration

Bone marrow cellularity is normal or increased, megakaryocytes predominate, and some increase in marrow reticulin is common.

Management

Chemotherapy

The platelet count can be rendered normal by continuous treatment with hydroxycarbamide. To avoid prolonged exposure to the drug, which can theoretically increase the risk of transformation to leukaemia, thromboprophylaxis with low-dose aspirin without cytoreductive therapy is used in younger subjects, especially if there are no additional risk factors for thrombosis.

Prognosis

The life expectancy of patients with essential thrombocythaemia is normal.[2] Transformation to polycythaemia vera, myelofibrosis or acute myeloid leukaemia can occur.

REFERENCES

(1) *Ruggeri M, Tosetto A, Frezzato M, Rodeghiero F. The rate of progression to polycythemia vera or essential thrombocythemia in patients with erythrocytosis or thrombocytosis. Annals of Internal Medicine 2003; 139: 470–475.*
(2) *Passamonti F, Rumi E, Pungolino E, et al. Life expectancy and prognostic factors for survival in patients with polycythemia vera and essential thrombocythemia. American Journal of Medicine 2004; 117: 755–761.*

Chronic idiopathic myelofibrosis

Chronic idiopathic myelofibrosis is a myeloproliferative disease characterized by gross bone marrow fibrosis with massive extramedullary haemopoiesis in liver and spleen. This condition is also known as myelofibrosis with myeloid metaplasia and myelosclerosis.

Epidemiology

The incidence of chronic idiopathic myelofibrosis has been estimated at 0.4 per 100 000 per year.[1] The average age of diagnosis is 60 years, and it is slightly more common in men (1.4 times).[2]

Pathology

The pathogenesis is thought to be the release of platelet-derived growth factor from abnormal megakaryocyte hyperplasia, which in turn stimulates a polyclonal proliferation of fibroblasts leading to reactive fibrosis in the bone marrow.

Clinical features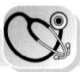

Symptoms mainly relate to anaemia and splenomegaly. Pallor, lethargy and dyspnoea are common presenting features of anaemia, with a dragging sensation in the abdomen due to massive splenomegaly. Symptoms of hypermetabolism such as weight loss and night sweats may also be present.

In some patients the onset is insidious, but usually patients have a past medical history of polycythaemia vera or essential thrombocythaemia that has transformed into myelofibrosis.

Investigations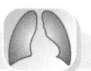

Full blood count, blood film
Anaemia is usually present, initially with elevated platelets and white cell counts that gradually decline with progressive disease. The blood film is typically leukoerythroblastic, and the characteristic teardrop-shaped poikilocytes are a consistent finding.

Bone marrow trephine biopsy
Bone marrow cannot be aspirated due to the fibrotic process. Trephine biopsy reveals variable cellularity with increased reticulin, progressing to massive deposition of collagen. Megakaryocytes are often increased. Bony trabeculae may be expanded.

Management

Blood transfusions
Supportive therapy with regular blood transfusion may be required for patients with recurrent anaemia.

Allopurinol
Allopurinol is recommended to prevent gout and urate nephropathy that results from high cell turnover.

Splenectomy
Splenectomy is indicated for patients with unacceptably high transfusion requirement, severe thrombocytopenia and symptomatic splenomegaly. The effect of splenectomy on the blood count in patients with concomitant hepatomegaly is less predictable.

> **RECENT ADVANCES**
>
> Currently, thalidomide (an angiogenesis inhibitor) is being investigated for the treatment of myelofibrosis. An early trial reported elimination of transfusions in 22%, increase in platelet counts in 22% and reduction of splenomegaly in 19% of patients. Reduction of an overall disease severity score occurred in 31%.[3] Allogeneic stem cell transplantation can lead to remission and resolution of fibrosis in some patients.

Prognosis

The median survival after diagnosis is 10 years. Features associated with poor survival are anaemia, leukocytosis, leukocytopenia, thrombocytopenia, increased blasts in the peripheral blood, male sex, age over 60, and symptomatic disease.[2]

REFERENCES

(1) *Kutti J, Ridell B. Epidemiology of the myeloproliferative disorders: essential thrombocythaemia, polycythaemia vera and idiopathic myelofibrosis. Pathologie et Biologie 2001; 49: 164–166.*
(2) *Okamura T, Kinukawa N, Niho Y, Mizoguchi H. Primary chronic myelofibrosis: clinical and prognostic evaluation in 336 Japanese patients. International Journal of Hematology 2001; 73: 194–198.*
(3) *Marchetti M, Barosi G, Balestri F, et al. Low-dose thalidomide ameliorates cytopenias and splenomegaly in myelofibrosis with myeloid metaplasia: a phase II trial. Journal of Clinical Oncology 2004; 22: 424–431.*

Plasma cell neoplasms

Plasma cells are the immunoglobulin-producing cells and are normally identifiable in the bone marrow. Diffuse neoplastic, monoclonal proliferation of plasma cells throughout the red marrow is characteristic of *plasma cell myeloma*, previously known as multiple myeloma. When the proliferation is more localized and discrete, a plasma cell tumour develops. This usually occurs in the bone and is termed a *solitary plasmacytoma of bone*. Monoclonal proliferation of IgM-producing plasma cells and lymphoplasmacytoid cells in the reticuloendothelial organs, bone marrow, liver and spleen is present in a third type of plasma cell neoplasm known as *Waldenström's macroglobulinaemia*.

Plasma cell myeloma

Plasma cell myeloma (previously known as multiple myeloma) is a neoplastic monoclonal proliferation of bone marrow plasma cells.

Epidemiology

The incidence is estimated to be 0.4 per 100 000 per year in the UK, and the median age of diagnosis is approximately 60 years.[1] Less than 2% occur before the age of 40 years.

Pathology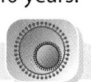

The causes of myeloma are not known; most arise as new cases and some have evolved from monoclonal gammopathy of undetermined significance.

The proliferation of malignant plasma cells leads to the erosion of the bones of the axial skeleton. In the majority (99%), the plasma cells synthesize paraprotein, a monoclonal immunoglobulin. This consists of IgG (60%), IgA 20%, light chain only 20%, and rarely IgM or IgD. In two thirds of IgG and IgA myeloma, monoclonal free light chains (κ or λ) are produced in addition to the complete immunoglobulin molecule. Due to the molecular weight, immunoglobulins cannot pass through the glomerular filter, but the free light chains are small enough to enter into the urine, where they are called Bence Jones protein. Plasma concentrations of unaffected immunoglobulins are often markedly suppressed leading to 'immune paresis'.

Scope of disease

Proliferation of plasma cells can result in lytic destruction of the skeleton by inappropriate activation of osteoclasts and predispose to pathological fractures of proximal long bones, ribs, sternum or vertebrae. Spinal compression can result from malignant infiltration of the vertebrae or paravertebral tissues. Anaemia can result from chronic disease, low erythropoietin (renal failure) or bone marrow failure in patients with end-stage myeloma. Hyperviscosity is associated with IgA paraproteins due to the physical characteristics of IgA. Renal failure is common and results from free light chain in the urine. Chronic disease also predisposes to amyloidosis.

Clinical features

Patients typically present with any combination of bone pain, anaemia or renal impairment. Bone pain is common and is often severe: patients may complain of backache and occasionally present with pathological fractures. Dyspnoea, lethargy and pallor can occur with anaemia. Polydipsia, polyuria, anorexia and vomiting can occur with renal failure.

Complications of amyloidosis can present as carpal tunnel syndrome or macroglossia. Hyperviscosity syndrome is rare and presents with confusion and blurred vision.

Initial investigations

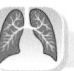

The diagnosis of myeloma is confirmed by two out of three criteria of serum or urine paraprotein, lytic lesions on X-ray and over 10% plasma cells in the bone marrow.

Full blood count

The full blood count tends to show a normochromic normocytic anaemia.

Erythrocyte sedimentation rate

The ESR is usually elevated.

Urea and electrolytes and serum calcium

Serum urea and creatinine may be elevated from renal failure, and hypercalcaemia (with a normal alkaline phosphatase) may also occur.

Protein electrophoresis

Protein electrophoresis of serum will identify an intact paraprotein and identify the isotype as usually IgG or IgA. In a proportion of cases there is no intact paraprotein, only free light chain; in approximately 1% neither intact paraprotein nor free light chain is produced (non-secretory myeloma).

Urine analysis

The urine contains Bence Jones protein in over 50% of cases.

Plain film skeletal survey

Plain X-rays are the best way of identifying lytic lesions. A 'skeletal survey' consists of images of the skull, chest, pelvis and proximal long bones.

Bone marrow aspiration

The bone marrow shows patchy and variable levels of infiltration by plasma cells, usually in the range of 10–40%.

> **RECENT ADVANCES**
>
> *New nephelometric-based assays of serum free light chain may make Bence Jones testing of urine obsolete. This test is more sensitive, and a significant proportion of non-secretory cases are recognized as low-level secretors of light chain using this new test.[2]*

Further investigations

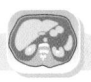

Prognostic markers

Serum prognostic markers include β_2-microglobulin, lactate dehydrogenase and C-reactive protein.

MRI scanning

MRI can be useful in identifying myeloma bone disease, marrow infiltration and suspected cord compression.

Initial management

Initial management consists of supportive measures in patients who present with complications of the disease.

Hydration

Adequate hydration is required for patients with new-onset renal impairment or hypercalcaemia.

Packed cells transfusion

Transfusion of packed cells may be required for patients with severe anaemia.

Antibiotics

Hospital admission and treatment with broad-spectrum intravenous antibiotics may be required for patients who present with severe infection.

Patient education and support

Information about the disease should be conveyed to the patient. Simple measures such as analgesia and aids such as spinal supports may be required for painful bony lesions.

Medical management

Treatment is not required in asymptomatic patients with no bony lesions, but regular surveillance is required.

Chemotherapy

Single agent melphalan with or without prednisolone is the initial chemotherapeutic agent of choice for elderly patients with symptomatic disease with acceptable neutrophil ($>1 \times 10^9$/L) and platelet counts ($>75 \times 10^9$/L).

If the neutrophil or platelet count is too low, an alternative agent is cyclophosphamide.

High-dose chemotherapy and stem cell transplantation

In younger patients (<65 years) chemotherapy with vincristine, doxorubicin (Adriamycin) and dexamethasone (VAD) followed by high dose melphalan and stem cell transplantation may be offered. This regimen achieved a response rate of 81% compared to 57% on conventional therapy, with a 5-year survival probability of 52% compared to 12% respectively.[3]

Bisphosphonates

Bisphosphonates are powerful inhibitors of osteoclasts and should be prescribed routinely for treatment of hypercalcaemia, prevention of pathological vertebral fractures (25% versus 35%) and reduction in bone-related pain (51% to 42%).[4]

Localized radiotherapy

Localized radiotherapy may be required for patients with localized disease, and also for the treatment of spinal cord compression and malignant infiltration of the vertebrae.

RECENT ADVANCES

Thalidomide and the proteasome inhibitor Batezomib have demonstrated significant activity in both resistant and previously untreated myeloma.[5] Up to a third of relapsed patients respond to treatment with thalidomide and its derivatives. Trials are currently underway to evaluate these treatments.

Surgical management

Orthopaedic surgery

Orthopaedic surgery (long bone fixation) is usually reserved for patients with pathological fractures and prophylactically for patients with impending fractures.

Prognosis

Adverse risk factors for survival include age over 80 years and elevated serum LDH and β_2-microglobulin and low albumin. The mitotic activity (percentage of cells in the S phase) of the bone marrow plasma cells has proved to be a powerful prognostic factor. S-phase values of 1% or less, 1–3% and more than 3% are associated with median survivals of 34, 22 and 12 months respectively.[6] New international staging system for myeloma:

CRITERIA	MEDIAN SURVIVAL (months)
I B2M < 3.5 mg/l and albumin > 35 g/l	62
II Neither I or III	45
III Serum B2M > 5.5 mg/l	29

ⓘ FURTHER INFORMATION

UK myeloma forum. British Committee for Standards in Haematology. Diagnosis and management of multiple myeloma. British Journal of Haematology 2001; 115: 522–540.

REFERENCES

(1) *UK myeloma forum. British Committee for Standards in Haematology. Diagnosis and management of multiple myeloma. British Journal of Haematology 2001; 115: 522–540.*
(2) *Mead GP, Carr-Smith HD, Drayson MT, Morgan GJ, Child JA, Bradwell AR. Serum free light chains for monitoring multiple myeloma. British Journal of Haematology 2004; 126: 348–354.*
(3) *Attal M, Harousseau J-L, Stoppa A-M, et al, The Intergroupe Francais du Myelome. A prospective, randomized trial of autologous bone marrow transplantation and chemotherapy in multiple myeloma. New England Journal of Medicine 1996; 335: 91–97.*
(4) *Djulbegovic B, Wheatley K, Ross J, et al. Bisphosphonates in multiple myeloma. The Cochrane Database of Systematic Reviews 2002: CD003188.*
(5) *Weber D. Thalidomide and its derivatives: new promise for multiple myeloma. Cancer Control 2003; 10: 375–383.*
(6) *Garcia-Sanz R, Gonzalez-Fraile MI, Mateo G, et al. Proliferative activity of plasma cells is the most relevant prognostic factor in elderly multiple myeloma patients. International Journal of Cancer 2004; 112: 884–889.*

Myelodysplastic syndromes

The myelodysplastic syndromes (MDS) are a group of neoplastic disorders of the bone marrow (Table 12.20) characterized by dysplastic haemopoiesis and peripheral blood cytopenia. As part of the family of myeloid neoplasms, there is a tendency for the disease to progress to acute myeloid leukaemia. Some patients may have features common to both MDS and myeloproliferative disease (Table 12.21), classified as myelodysplastic/myeloproliferative disease (MDS/MPD).

Table 12.20	World Health Organization classification of myelodysplastic syndromes*
Refractory anaemia	
Refractory anaemia with ring sideroblasts (RARS)	
Refractory cytopenia with multilineage dysplasia (RCMD)	
Refractory cytopenia with multilineage dysplasia and ringed sideroblasts (RCMD-RS)	
Refractory anaemia with excess blasts-1 (RAEB-1)	
Refractory anaemia with excess blasts-2 (RAEB-2)	
Myelodysplastic syndrome unclassified (MDS-U)	
MDS associated with isolated del(5q)	

* Adapted from Vardiman JW, Harris NL, Brunning RD. The World Health Organization (WHO) classification of the myeloid neoplasms. Blood 2002; 100: 2292–2302.

811

Table 12.21	World Health Organization classification of myelodysplastic/myeloproliferative syndromes*
Chronic myelomonocytic leukaemia (CMML)	
Atypical chronic myelomonocytic leukaemia (aCMML)	
Juvenile myelomonocytic leukaemia (JMML)	

* Adapted from Vardiman JW, Harris NL, Brunning RD. The World Health Organization (WHO) classification of the myeloid neoplasms. Blood 2002; 100: 2292–2302.

Epidemiology

The incidence of MDS is 4.9 per 100 000 per year, and is rare before 60 years. The sex distribution is approximately equal at the age of 60 and increases to become twice as common in men after the age of 70.[1]

Pathology

The causes of MDS are unknown but recognized risk factors are similar to those for acute myeloid leukaemia and include old age and exposure to chemotherapy, radiation and chemicals such as benzene.

The hallmarks of these diseases are hypercellular bone marrow with dysplastic cell morphology and paradoxical peripheral blood cytopenia. The paradox may result from apoptosis of dysplastic bone marrow progenitor cells, in turn leading to ineffective production of differentiated cells for release into the blood.

Clinical features

Symptomatic anaemia is the most common presentation, but patients may also present with bleeding from thrombocytopenia or with recurrent infections due to neutropenia. Patients with chronic myelomonocytic leukaemia (CMML) may have hepatosplenomegaly or other evidence of tissue infiltration by leukaemic cells.

Investigations

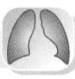

Full blood count and blood film
A macrocytic anaemia is usual, and neutropenia, thrombocytopenia and monocytosis may also be evident. The peripheral blood film shows evidence of dysplasia including misshapen red cells, agranular neutrophils and circulating blast cells.

Bone marrow aspiration
The bone marrow is usually hypercellular with dysplasia in one or more cell lines. Ring sideroblasts may be present, and the blast count may be increased to 5–20%. Bone marrow cytogenetics often demonstrates a clonal cytogenetic abnormality of prognostic importance.

Management

Blood and platelet transfusion
The mainstay of management is supportive care with blood and platelet transfusions as required. Iron chelation therapy may be required for excessive iron loading with repeated transfusions.

Erythropoietin and colony-stimulating factors
Treatment with the growth factors erythropoietin and G-CSF can improve the anaemia in a proportion of patients and the neutrophil count in the majority, which may help at the time of infections.

Chemotherapy
Selected patients with increased blast cells may achieve temporary remission with AML-type chemotherapy.

Prognosis

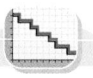

The prognosis depends on the subtype of disease and ranges from a few months (patients with excess blasts) to several years (refractory anaemia with ring sideroblasts). Patients die either from transformation to acute myeloid leukaemia or from the effects of bone marrow failure and its treatment.

REFERENCE

(1) Germing U, Strupp C, Kundgen A, Bowen D, Aul C, Haas R, Gattermann N. No increase in age-specific incidence of myelodysplastic syndromes. Haematologica 2004; 89: 905–910.

The lymphomas

The lymphomas are a group of malignant diseases arising from lymphocytes and their precursor cells. They are broadly divided into Hodgkin and non-Hodgkin lymphoma.

Hodgkin lymphoma

Epidemiology

Hodgkin lymphoma is rare. The annual incidence in the West is approximately 3 per 100 000 with a bimodal age distribution. Most cases occur in young adults (18–35) and a second peak occurs in the over 60s.

Pathology

The cause of Hodgkin lymphoma is unknown. There have been reported associations with clinical glandular fever. A third of cases seem to have an association with Epstein–Barr virus, with viral DNA present in the malignant cell.

In 97%, the malignant cell is a transformed B lymphocyte with a characteristic binucleate appearance, known as a Reed–Sternberg (RS) cell. Interestingly, the bulk of the malignant lymph nodes are composed of reactive T lymphocytes and polymorphs, suggesting an ineffective immune response to the malignant RS cells.

Recently the recognition of a subgroup characterized by a nodular lymphocyte predominant appearance and a clinical course that was characterized by multiple relapses and remissions and a tendency in 5–10% of cases to progress to large B-NHL led the WHO[1] to separate this subtype from classical Hodgkin's disease (Table 12.22).

Clinical features

The most common presentation is painless asymmetrical lymphadenopathy, usually in the cervical region, but potentially involving any lymph node area. Mediastinal lymphadenopathy is more common in young adults with the nodular sclerosing subtype, whilst extranodal involvement (skin, brain, lung disease) tends to be a late manifestation.

Patients may also experience systemic symptoms (B symptoms) such as drenching night sweats, swinging fever and weight loss (of 10% body weight) that are important in staging. Other constitutional symptoms include pruritus, alcohol-induced pain, weakness and cachexia.

On examination, localized lymphadenopathy may be evident, and the spleen is enlarged in approximately 50%.

Initial investigations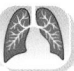

Full blood count and blood film
A normochromic normocytic anaemia is common, accompanied by a leukocytosis in a third of patients. The platelet count is normal in the early stages but declines with disease progression.

Erythrocyte sedimentation rate
The ESR is usually elevated.

Lymph node excision biopsy
The most important investigation is a lymph node biopsy that should be analyzed by a haemato-pathologist. The diagnosis is usually established by identification of the Reed–Sternberg cell and classified according to the subtype listed in Table 12.22.

Table 12.22	World Health Organization 2001 classification of Hodgkin lymphoma

Nodular lymphocyte predominant Hodgkin lymphoma

Classical Hodgkin lymphoma
   Nodular sclerosis
   Mixed cellularity
   Lymphocyte-depleted
   Lymphocyte-rich

Further investigations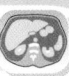

Liver profile
Serum alkaline phosphatase and gamma GT may be elevated with liver involvement. Bilirubin may be elevated with biliary obstruction by lymphadenopathy at the porta hepatis.

Calcium
Serum calcium levels may be elevated.

Serum lactate dehydrogenase
Elevated LDH carries a poorer prognosis.

Staging CT of the chest, abdomen and pelvis
A CT scan is required to establish the extent of disease and stage according to the Ann Arbor system[2] (Table 12.23).

Bone marrow trephine biopsy
Bone marrow involvement is rare in early disease; occasionally a trephine biopsy may be necessary for diagnosis.

Table 12.23	Modified Ann Arbor staging of Hodgkin lymphoma*

Stage I
Involvement of a single lymph node region or of a single extranodal organ or site (I E)

Stage II
Involvement of two or more lymph node regions on the same side of the diaphragm or localized involvement of an extranodal organ or site and one or more lymph nodes on the same side of the diaphragm (II E)

Stage III
Involvement of lymph node regions on both sides of the diaphragm, which may be accompanied by localized involvement of an extranodal organ or site (III E), spleen (III S) or both (III E,S)

Stage IV
Diffuse or disseminated involvement of one or more extralymphatic organs, or isolated extranodal organ involvement with distant lymph node involvement such as the marrow (M), liver (H), lung (L), pleura (P) or skin (D)

Symptoms
Each stage is further classified into A (asymptomatic) or B depending on the presence of

Fevers:	Unexplained temperature more than 38°C
Night sweats:	Drenching sweats that require the change of bed clothes
Weight loss:	Unexplained weight loss of 10% or more of the body weight in the 6 months prior to diagnosis

* Modified from Lister TA, Crowther D, Sutcliffe SB, et al. Report of a committee convened to discuss the evaluation and staging of patients with Hodgkin's disease: Cotswolds meeting. Journal of Clinical Oncology 1989; 7: 1630–1636.

Medical management

Treatment of Hodgkin lymphoma has been extremely successful over the last 30 years and the majority of younger patients can now be cured. Treatment planning is complex and must take into account the long-term complications of therapy in a group of young patients destined to be cured. For this reason extensive single modality radiotherapy is rarely, if ever, used now because of long-term side effects, particularly breast cancer and other cancers in the radiation field.

Early stage disease

Patients in stage I to IIA represent the most favourable subgroup, and the aim of multimodality therapy is to reduce the total radiation exposure whilst maintaining equivalent efficacy. Currently, modified involved field radiotherapy is used with 2–4 cycles of combination chemotherapy.

Locally extensive, limited stage disease

Patients with bulky mediastinal masses or extranodal extension into the mediastinal structures usually receive radiotherapy and combination chemotherapy with either MOPP (mechlorethamine, vincristine, procarbazine and prednisone) or ABVD (doxorubicin, bleomycin, vinblastine and dacarbazine) regimens. The latter combination achieves a higher survival rate at 7 years (77% versus 68%).[3]

Advanced disease

Currently the ABVD regimen is the treatment of choice for patients with advanced disease, although other multi-agent chemotherapy regimens such as Stanford V and bleomycin, etoposide, doxorubicin, cyclophosphamide, vincristine, procarbazine and prednisone (BEACOPP) or escalated BEACOPP may offer better remission rates.[4]

Recurrent disease

Patients who relapse can still be cured, especially if the relapse is late (greater than 1 year). Early relapses are treated with intensive salvage chemotherapy followed by high-dose chemotherapy and autologous stem cell rescue.

Prognosis

The overall 5-year survival is 78%. In advanced disease a poor prognosis is related to increasing Ann Arbor stage, low serum albumin, low haemoglobin, male sex, older age, high white cell count, and low lymphocyte count.[5]

REFERENCES

(1) *Jaffe ES, Harris NL, Stein H, Vardiman JW. World Health Organization Classification of tumours of haematopoietic and lymphoid tissues. Lyon: IARC Press, 2001.*
(2) *Carbone PP, Kaplan HS, Musshoff K, Smithers DW, Tubiana M. Report of the Committee on Hodgkin's Disease Staging Classification. Cancer Research 1971; 31: 1860–1861.*

REFERENCES—cont'd

(3) *Santoro A, Bonadonna G, Valagussa P, et al. Long-term results of combined chemotherapy-radiotherapy approach in Hodgkin's disease: superiority of ABVD plus radiotherapy versus MOPP plus radiotherapy. Journal of Clinical Oncology 1987; 5 :27–37.*
(4) *Horning SJ, Hoppe RT, Breslin S, Bartlett NL, Brown BW, Rosenberg SA. Stanford V and radiotherapy for locally extensive and advanced Hodgkin's disease: mature results of a prospective clinical trial. Journal of Clinical Oncology 2002; 20: 630–637.*
(5) *Hasenclever D, Diehl V, Armitage JO, et al. The International Prognostic Factors Project on Advanced Hodgkin's Disease. A prognostic score for advanced Hodgkin's disease. New England Journal of Medicine 1998; 339: 1506–1514.*

Non-Hodgkin lymphomas

The spectrum of non-Hodgkin lymphomas (NHL) ranges from indolent low-grade lymphomas that are incurable yet compatible with long-term survival, to aggressive high-grade lymphomas that can be rapidly fatal if untreated, but can also be cured.

Epidemiology

The global age-standardized incidence of NHL is 5.6 (men) and 3.8 (women) per 100 000 per year. The areas with the highest incidence are North America, Australia, Western Africa and Europe.[1]

Pathology

In most cases, the causes of NHL are unknown. Risk factors associated with NHL include older age, Epstein–Barr virus infection (Burkitt's lymphoma), HTLV-1 infection (adult T-cell leukaemia/lymphoma), *Helicobacter pylori* infection (gut lymphoma), prolonged immunosuppression (congenital immunodeficiencies, HIV, transplant-associated lymphoproliferative disease), and autoimmune disorders such as Hashimoto's thyroiditis and coeliac disease.

Classification

The majority of NHL in the West are of B-cell type, and the current pathological classification by the WHO 2001 (Table 12.24) has superseded the Keil (1992) and REAL (1994) classifications. The WHO separates lymphoid malignancy into B lymphocyte or T lymphocyte, the perceived cell of origin, recognized acquired genetic abnormalities and whether or not the lymphoma can be reproducibly identified as a distinct entity.

In clinical practice, the grade determines the behaviour of the lymphoma and it remains the most useful classification for treatment. Low-grade lymphomas are incurable with present therapy but have an indolent clinical course with non-destructive growth patterns, rarely involving the central nervous system, and are compatible with a long patient survival. High-grade lymphomas on the other hand have an aggressive clinical course with destructive growth patterns, often involving the central

Table 12.24	World Health Organization 2001 classification of lymphoid neoplasms*

B-cell neoplasms	T-cell and NK-cell neoplasms
Precursor B-cell neoplasm	**Precursor T-cell and NK-cell neoplasms**
Precursor B lymphoblastic leukaemia/lymphoma	Precursor T lymphoblastic leukaemia/lymphoma
	Blastic NK-cell lymphoma
Mature B-cell neoplasms	**Mature T-cell and NK-cell neoplasms**
Chronic lymphocytic leukaemia/small cell lymphocytic lymphoma	T-cell prolymphocytic leukaemia
B-cell prolymphocytic leukaemia	T-cell large granular lymphocytic leukaemia
Lymphoplasmacytic lymphoma	Aggressive NK-cell leukaemia
Splenic marginal zone lymphoma	Adult T-cell leukaemia/lymphoma
Hairy cell leukaemia	Extranodal NK/T-cell lymphoma nasal type
Plasma cell neoplasms	Enteropathy-type T-cell lymphoma
Extranodal marginal zone B-cell lymphoma of mucosa-associated lymphoid tissue (MALT lymphoma)	Hepatosplenic T-cell lymphoma
Follicular lymphoma	Subcutaneous panniculitis-like T-cell lymphoma
Diffuse follicle centric lymphoma	Mycosis fungoides
Mantle cell lymphoma	Sézary syndrome
Diffuse large B-cell lymphoma	Primary anaplastic large cell lymphoma
Mediastinal thymic large B-cell lymphoma	Peripheral T-cell lymphoma, unspecified
Intravascular large B-cell lymphoma	Angioimmunoblastic T-cell lymphoma
Primary effusion lymphoma	Anaplastic large cell lymphoma
Burkitt lymphoma	
B-cell proliferation of uncertain malignant potential	**T-cell proliferation of uncertain malignant potential**
Lymphomatoid granulomatosis	Nodular lymphocyte predominant Hodgkin lymphoma
Post transplant lymphoproliferative disorder	Classical Hodgkin lymphoma

*Adapted from Jaffe ES, Harris NL, Stein H, Vardiman JW. World Health Organization Classification of tumours of haematopoietic and lymphoid tissues. Lyon: IARC Press, 2001.

nervous system and extranodal tissue. They are curable in a significant proportion but can be rapidly fatal without treatment.

Scope of disease

Accumulation of lymphoid tissue can lead to mediastinal obstruction, obstructive nephropathy, spinal cord compression, meningeal lymphoma and bone marrow failure. Paraneoplastic effects include hypercalcaemia and other metabolic derangements. Low-grade non-Hodgkin lymphoma can also cause immune-mediated haemolysis or thrombocytopenia.

Clinical features

The majority of adults (70%) present with nodal disease, usually with one or more areas of painlessly enlarged lymph nodes (Fig. 12.10). The majority of children present with extranodal disease in locations that include the gut, testes, thyroid, bone (Fig. 12.11), muscle, lung, central nervous system, facial sinuses and skin (Fig. 12.12). Hepatosplenomegaly is common to both adults and children.

Systemic symptoms include drenching night sweats, loss of weight and culture-negative fever. Ascites and pleural effusions (sometimes chylous) are usually end-stage features of high-grade NHL.

Initial investigations

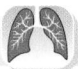

Full blood count, blood film
A normochromic normocytic anaemia is usually present, and with progressive marrow infiltration, neutropenia and thrombocytopenia develop. Lymphoma cells may be found in the peripheral blood in some patients.

Liver profile, serum calcium, serum uric acid
Elevated alkaline phosphatase and gamma GT may suggest liver involvement. Elevated calcium and uric acid levels may also occur.

Lymph node or extranodal biopsy
Confirmatory diagnosis requires a lymph node or extranodal tissue biopsy for histopathological examination, often aided by immunohistochemistry, cytogenetic and molecular techniques.

815

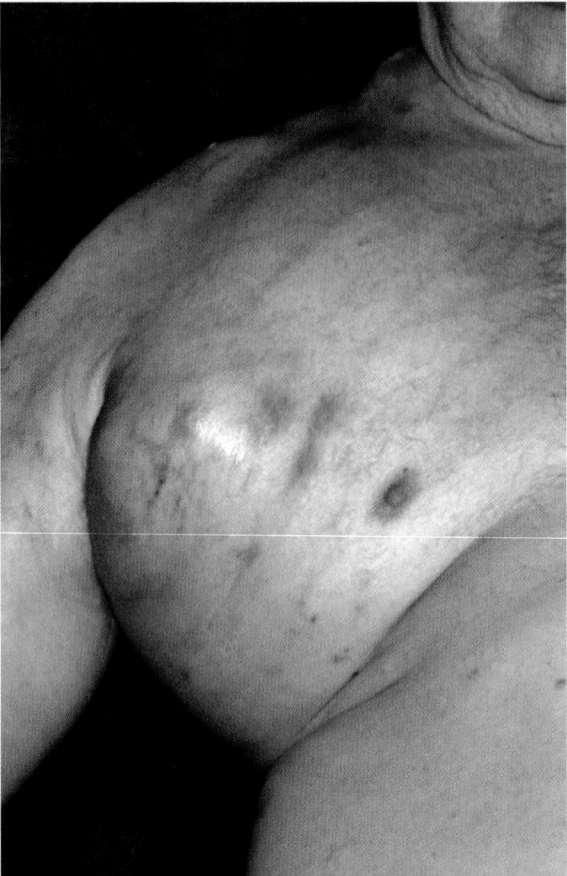

Fig. 12.10 Massive axillary lymphadenopathy resulting from high-grade diffuse large B-cell lymphoma.

Further investigations

Serum lactate dehydrogenase and β₂-microglobulin

Elevation of these biochemical indices often indicates a large tumour burden.

Chest X-ray

A plain chest film may reveal evidence of mediastinal involvement.

CT of the chest, abdomen and pelvis

Staging CT is required to assess the extent of nodal and extranodal involvement.

Bone marrow aspiration and trephine biopsy

Bone marrow aspiration and trephine biopsy is performed to assess the morphology of the lymphoma, and to perform immunophenotyping and cytogenetic analysis.

Other diagnostic imaging

Depending on the clinical features, further anatomical imaging such as CT of the head (or lumbar puncture), MRI of the spine, or a bone scan may be required.

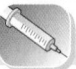

Initial management

Staging

After the diagnosis is established, the stage, grade of the disease and cell type need to be determined to plan further treatment. The Ann Arbor system as described for Hodgkin lymphoma (p. 813) is also applied to stage NHL, and the management is detailed accordingly.

Medical management

The medical management of this large group of disorders is detailed by grade and cell type.

Low-grade NHL

The low-grade lymphomas comprise up to 45% of NHL and tend to be disseminated at the time of presentation with widespread lymphadenopathy, hepatosplenomegaly and bone marrow involvement.

B-cell follicular lymphoma

This is a typical low-grade NHL, presenting in the older age group. Stage I disease may be cured by radiotherapy, but more commonly the disease presents as stage III or IV when it remains incurable with present treatments.

In general, patients are observed until symptoms warrant intervention. Historically, initial treatments have included local radiotherapy to sites of bulk disease, single agent chemotherapy such as chlorambucil, or combination chemotherapy such as CVP or CHOP. These treatments produce good initial clinical responses, including complete remissions, but relapse is inevitable. Despite the indolent nature of follicle centre cell lymphoma, it is a fatal disease with a median survival of 8–10 years.

> **RECENT ADVANCES**
>
> *Recent randomized trial data have shown that the addition of rituximab (anti-CD20) to either CVP or CHOP chemotherapy significantly improves the response rate and the time to progression compared to chemotherapy alone. An apparent survival advantage has also been demonstrated. Trials of maintenance rituximab in remission are also encouraging. Other useful treatments include the purine analogues fludarabine and 2-chlorodeoxyadenosine (2-CDA). In younger patients the role of allogeneic transplantation and autologous transplantation with immunologically purged progenitor cells is being explored. Interferon-alfa may prolong chemotherapy- or transplant-induced remissions. Finally, the understanding of the molecular basis of this lymphoma has led to the initiation of antisense therapy aimed at suppressing the production of the Bcl-2 protein.*

High-grade NHL

High-grade NHL are best considered as those with a strong tendency to involve the central nervous system, and this includes the subtypes of lymphoblastic, Burkitt's lymphoma, adult T-cell lymphoma/leukaemia and primary central

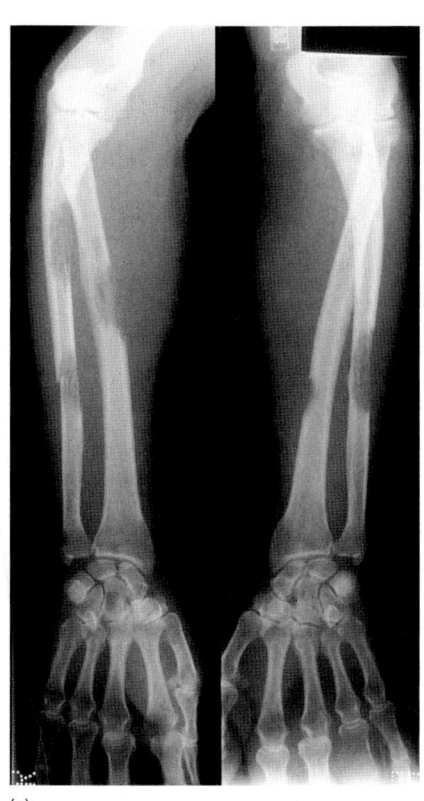

(a)

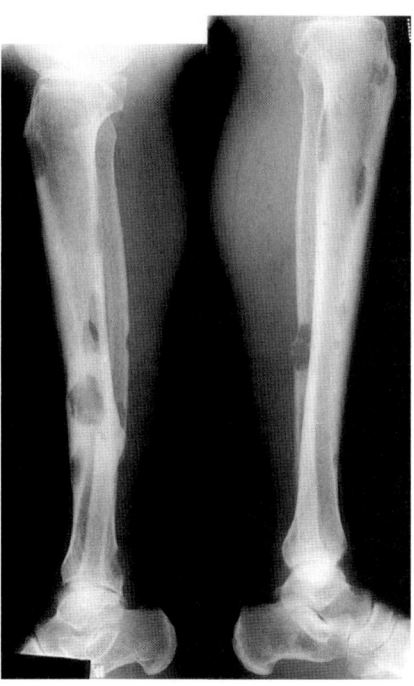

(b)

Fig. 12.11 Multifocal lytic bone lesions from extranodal lymphoma of bone. Note the peripheral distribution compared to the axial distribution of lytic lesions in myeloma.

nervous system lymphoma (PCL). The risk of central nervous system disease also increases if the testes, breast and sinuses are involved or there is extensive extranodal involvement or a high LDH.

Burkitt's lymphoma

This is endemic in equatorial Africa where 90% of cases are associated with EBV infection. Children and young adults present with destructive head and neck tumours. Non-endemic Burkitt's lymphoma is associated with EBV in 20% of cases, more commonly presents with abdominal disease, and is in some cases associated with HIV infection.

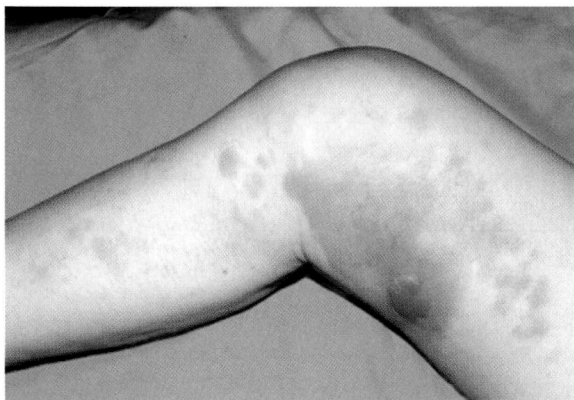

Fig. 12.12 Cutaneous extranodal diffuse large B non-Hodgkin lymphoma of the leg.

Treatment success has improved considerably with short courses of intensive chemotherapy that include high-dose methotrexate, cyclophosphamide/ifosfamide with intrathecal therapy.

Precursor T/B lymphoblastic leukaemia/lymphoma

Lymphoblastic lymphomas are more common in children and often of T-cell type. The typical presentation is that of a mediastinal mass and pleural effusion. Urgent or emergency management may be required for mediastinal obstruction and the prevention of tumour lysis syndrome (acute renal failure with hyperuricaemia, hyperphosphataemia and hyperkalaemia as a result of rapid tumour breakdown on initiation of therapy).

Intensive combination chemotherapy with schedules similar to those used for ALL, including CNS directed therapy, has improved the outlook in children. Results in adults, however, are not as good. Poor prognostic features include bone marrow or CNS involvement, raised LDH (over 300 i.u./L), age over 30 years and delayed achievement of complete remission. In this poor prognostic group, allogeneic and autologous progenitor cell transplantation may improve survival.

Diffuse large B-cell lymphoma

Diffuse large B-cell lymphoma is the most common high-grade NHL that presents with nodal or extranodal disease. A short course of combination chemotherapy (CHOP) followed by radiotherapy can cure 90% of patients with non-bulky stage IA disease.

For more advanced stage disease, combination chemo-therapy (CHOP) in conjunction with rituximab (anti-CD20 monoclonal antibody) confers a clear survival advantage over CHOP alone.

Autologous progenitor cell transplantation confers a survival benefit to relapsed patients who respond to salvage chemotherapy.

Prognosis

The prognosis of NHL is complex and relates to disease subtype. For diffuse large B-cell lymphoma, the Inter-national Prognostic Index has provided a useful clinical prognostic scoring system based on age, performance status, stage, number of extranodal sites and LDH, predict-ing 5-year survivals between 30% and 75%. However, this is likely to be superseded by gene expression profiling

which uses patterns of expressed genes to identify prog-nostic groups.

For follicular lymphoma a clinical index called the Follicular Lymphoma Prognostic Index (FLIPI) has recently been developed based on number of nodal areas, LDH, age, stage and haemoglobin level. Three prognostic groups are identified with 10-year survivals ranging from 33% to 70%. However, again gene expression profiling is likely to supersede this in the future. Interestingly, the gene expres-sion pattern of the infiltrating T cells may be as or more important prognostically than the tumour gene expression pattern in follicular lymphoma.

REFERENCE

(1) *Parkin DM, Pisani P, Ferlay J. Global cancer statistics. CA Cancer Journal for Clinicians 1999; 49: 33–64.*

SECTION 12.7   Platelet disorders

Thrombocytosis

Thrombocytosis is a frequent incidental finding as blood counts are increasingly performed for the investigation of systemic disease. Thrombocytosis does not necessarily indicate the presence of a primary disease of the blood or bone marrow. It can be reactive, in response to blood loss, iron deficiency, chronic inflammation, tissue trauma and malignancy. Thrombocytosis as a result of haematological malignancies of the myeloproliferative group (p. 812) is less common, and is more likely to cause thrombosis than is reactive thrombocytosis.

Thrombocytopenia

Thrombocytopenia is a platelet count that is below 150×10^9/L. The causes of a low platelet count can be grouped according to reduced production, increased destruction/consumption, or pooling in the spleen (Table 12.25).

History

Mucosal bleeding, petechial rash and easy bruising are manifestations of thrombocytopenia. However, primary haemostasis is only impaired when the count falls below around 80×10^9/L. Unless there is also a defect of platelet function, spontaneous purpura and mucosal bleeding are unusual until the count falls below $10–20 \times 10^9$/L.

Table 12.25	Causes of thrombocytopenia
Impaired production	
Bone marrow infiltration: malignancy or fibrosis	
Megaloblastic anaemia	
Chemotherapy	
Aplastic anaemia	
Alcohol abuse	
Congenital	
Increased losses	
Increased destruction	
Autoimmune thrombocytopenia	
Alloimmune thrombocytopenia Post-transfusion purpura Neonatal alloimmune thrombocytopenia	
Increased consumption	
Disseminated intravascular coagulation	
Thrombotic thrombocytopenic purpura	
Haemolytic uraemic syndrome	
Massive haemorrhage	
Mixed	
HIV infection	
Dilutional/pooling	
Massive blood transfusion	
Hypersplenism	

A detailed history and examination is required to determine underlying causes of a low platelet count. The drug history, including over-the-counter drugs, is important, as some cases of immune thrombocytopenia are drug-induced, for example due to quinine. Heavy alcohol intake causes moderate degrees of thrombocytopenia, and dietary deficiency of folate, which is common in alcoholics, may exacerbate the low platelet count. Hypersplenism in cirrhosis also predisposes to thrombocytopenia. Occasionally thrombocytopenia is part of a heritable condition such as Wiskott–Aldrich syndrome, a rare X-linked disorder with thrombocytopenia, recurrent infection and eczema.

Examination may suggest other causes of thrombocytopenia, for example malignancy complicated by marrow infiltration or disseminated intravascular coagulation.

Examination

On examination, there may be evidence of abnormal bleeding with petechiae (Fig. 12.13) and bruising.

Investigations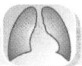

Full blood count

Thrombocytopenia alone (with normal haemoglobin and white cell counts) is usually due to increased destruction, whereas failure of platelet production due to bone marrow failure is usually associated with abnormalities in the other blood cell counts.

Bleeding time

Bleeding time is an investigation of platelet function and therefore primary haemostasis. It is a useful screening investigation in patients with symptoms of abnormal bleeding but is rarely indicated in thrombocytopenia as it is predictably prolonged if the platelet count is $<80 \times 10^9$/L. The normal bleeding time is between 3 and 8 minutes.

Coagulation screen

Clotting times are normal in autoimmune thrombocytopenia but may be useful to exclude other causes of low platelet count, in particular disseminated intravascular coagulation.

Alloimmune thrombocytopenia

Two rare but serious bleeding disorders are due to platelet alloantibody: neonatal alloimmune thrombocytopenia and post-transfusion purpura. Neonatal alloimmune thrombocytopenia is analogous to rhesus haemolytic disease as it is due to transplacental passage of an antibody following sensitization of the mother. In most cases the mother is negative for a platelet antigen (HPA1a), and the fetal platelets are positive for the antigen. Immunization with fetal platelets leads to anti-HPA1a in the maternal plasma. HPA1a is present in 98% of Caucasians. The

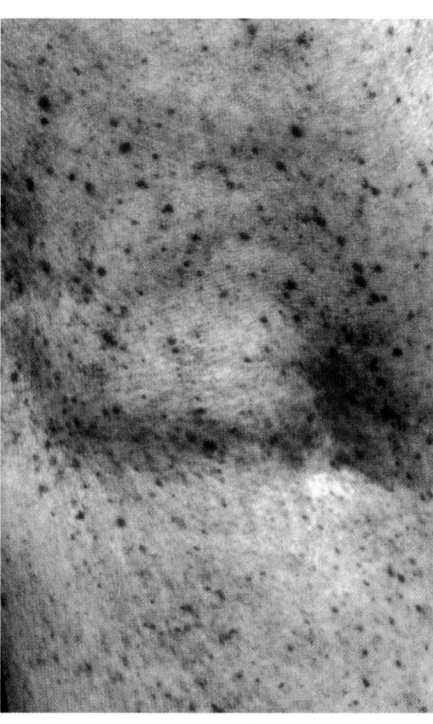

Fig. 12.13 Purpuric rash caused by thrombocytopenia.

affected fetus often has severe thrombocytopenia and is at risk of intracranial haemorrhage in utero or during delivery. This disorder may occur in the first pregnancy and subsequent fetuses tend to be increasingly severely affected. When an at-risk pregnancy has been identified, the diagnosis can be confirmed by sampling of fetal blood in utero. If severe thrombocytopenia is confirmed, it can be managed by repeated intrauterine transfusion of platelets (lacking the relevant antigen). In less severe cases, intravenous infusion of high-dose human IgG into the mother may improve the fetal platelet count.

In post-transfusion purpura, sudden, severe but transient thrombocytopenia with bleeding develops after blood transfusion due to the formation of platelet alloantibodies to an antigen in the transfused blood which is absent in the recipient, usually HPA1a. There is transient severe thrombocytopenia, often with life-threatening bleeding.

Autoimmune thrombocytopenic purpura

Epidemiology

Autoimmune thrombocytopenic purpura (ITP) is a common cause of isolated thrombocytopenia. There are two peaks in the incidence: the first in childhood, and the second between 15 and 50 years. It tends to be more common in females.

Pathology

There are three principal manifestations of this disease: an acute spontaneously remitting form (in children), a chronic idiopathic state (all ages), and drug-induced (all ages). The acute childhood variety may follow an infection such as measles, whilst the chronic type may occur in association with other autoimmune disease (such as rheumatoid arthritis) or as a complication of lymphoproliferative disease (chronic lymphocytic leukaemia or lymphoma).

In autoimmune thrombocytopenic purpura, an IgG autoantibody develops against one of the major receptor glycoproteins on the platelet plasma membrane. Bound antibody is recognized by macrophages through their Fc receptors, and platelets are destroyed in the reticuloendothelial system, especially the spleen.

Where the condition is drug-induced an immune complex mechanism is involved in most cases, similar to that in some instances of drug-induced immune haemolytic anaemia. Many drugs have been associated with autoimmune thrombocytopenic purpura, such as quinine and sulphonamides. A clinically unique form, associated with thrombosis rather than bleeding, is an occasional complication of heparin use.

In pregnant women with immune thrombocytopenic purpura there is a risk of fetal and transient neonatal thrombocytopenia due to transplacental passage of IgG platelet antibody.

Clinical features
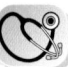

Increased bleeding is the main clinical feature, with a severity that is dictated by the platelet count. Patients with mild reductions in platelet counts ($>40 \times 10^9$/L) may have no symptoms or easy bruising only.

In severe thrombocytopenia (platelets $<10 \times 10^9$/L) there may be petechiae, especially on the skin of the lower legs, spontaneous bruising and mucosal bleeding (gums and epistaxis), serious internal bleeding and a risk of death from spontaneous intracranial haemorrhage.

Unlike immune haemolytic anaemia, splenomegaly is not a usual feature.

Investigations
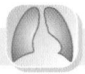

There is no reliable platelet antibody test available to confirm ITP at present and diagnosis rests largely on the exclusion of other causes of isolated thrombocytopenia.

Full blood count

The full blood count is generally normal apart from thrombocytopenia. However, anaemia may develop from external bleeding in severe cases.

Bone marrow aspiration

Where there is doubt regarding the aetiology of a low platelet count, a bone marrow examination may be helpful to exclude malignant infiltration or hypoplasia. In immune thrombocytopenia, the marrow has plentiful megakaryocytes with no abnormal cells.

Management

The management depends upon the presentation and severity of bleeding.

Conservative management

Immunomodulation is not always required. The acute form in childhood is usually self-limiting over days or weeks and there is no indication for specific therapy in many cases. Drug-induced immune thrombocytopenia usually responds to withdrawal of the causal agent. In mildly affected patients with the adult form where the platelet count remains above 20×10^9/L, conservative therapy is often the best approach, with avoidance of immunosuppressive agents unless serious bleeding occurs or if there is a need for surgery.

Immunomodulation therapy

Immune thrombocytopenia often responds to immunosuppressive therapy. Oral prednisolone (1 mg/kg/day) may lead to complete recovery over days or weeks. However, relapse frequently occurs on withdrawal of treatment.

Intravenous infusion of a concentrate of normal human IgG prepared from plasma is an alternative therapy but has to be repeated every few weeks to maintain any effect. It may act through blockade of the reticuloendothelial Fc receptors responsible for binding of antibody-coated platelets, or possibly through anti-idiotype activity (the presence of IgG molecules in the concentrate which block the binding site of the causative autoantibody). In some cases other immunomodulatory treatments are employed in the long term, for example azathioprine.

Splenectomy

Splenectomy may result in long-term remission and is a preferred option in resistant cases or those in whom side effects of long-term immunosuppressive therapy are unacceptable. It may be achieved by a laparoscopic procedure. Immunization against encapsulated bacteria (meningococcus, pneumococcus and *Haemophilus influenzae*) before the procedure is mandatory, with lifelong prophylaxis using oral penicillin or erythromycin to reduce the risk of life-threatening infection secondary to hyposplenism.

Prognosis

In general, the acute childhood form and that associated with drugs are self limiting. The adult form of immune thrombocytopenia is often a chronic relapsing condition.

Disseminated intravascular coagulation

Disseminated intravascular coagulation (DIC) is a condition in which systemic activation of coagulation is triggered by disease, resulting in fibrin deposition in the microvasculature. Small vessel occlusion and the consumption of platelets and coagulation factors result in a clinical picture of tissue and organ ischaemia with systemic bleeding.

Epidemiology

Fulminating DIC with widespread organ ischaemia and/or major bleeding is uncommon, but lesser degrees are common among hospitalized patients.

Pathology

DIC results from a systemic trigger that activates the coagulation cascade in a manner that overwhelms the physiological antithrombotic control mechanisms. Such triggers include tissue factor from the placenta or amniotic fluid that enters the maternal circulation in placental abruption, secretion of procoagulant substances by tumours (especially mucin-secreting adenocarcinomas) and unregulated tissue factor expression by monocytes during septicaemia (Table 12.26).

In DIC, the fibrinolytic system is activated and plasmin is generated. Excess amounts of plasmin result in the digestion of fibrinogen, coagulation factors (V and VIII) and fibrin. Fibrin degradation products that result from this process can be measured in plasma to assist in the diagnosis of DIC.

Clinical features

Fibrin deposition in the microvasculature results in ischaemia and organ dysfunction. There may be gangrene of digits, focal cerebral ischaemia causing confusion, motor or sensory dysfunction and coma. In up to a third of patients organ dysfunction is present, of which the most common are renal and hepatic impairment.[1] Mucosal bleeding, bruising and haemorrhage from skin puncture sites may occur.

Investigations
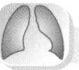

Full blood count, blood film

There is thrombocytopenia, and schistocytes may be seen on a blood film.

Disseminated intravascular coagulation screen

The DIC screen consists of estimation of the plasma fibrinogen concentration, thrombin time (TT), prothrombin time (PT), activated partial thromboplastin time (APTT) and fibrin degradation products (D-dimers).

In overt DIC typically the plasma fibrinogen concentration is reduced, the TT, PT and APTT are prolonged due to consumption of clotting factors, and the plasma concentration of fibrin degradation products is markedly increased. More subtle changes are present in many cases, for example slight prolongation of the PT with increased fibrin degradation products only.

Table 12.26	Causes of disseminated intravascular coagulation	
Precipitating cause		**Example**
Infection		Bacterial septicaemia Falciparum malaria
Neoplasm		Adenocarcinoma
Tissue trauma		Major burns Massive injury
Shock		Acute blood loss
Massive intravascular haemolysis transfusion		ABO mismatched
Pregnancy complications		Abruptio placentae Eclampsia Retained dead fetus

Management

Identify and treat precipitating cause

Coagulation activation will continue until the trigger is removed, therefore the main aspect of management centres on identification and management of the precipitating cause. Antibiotic therapy is instituted for septicaemia, and delivery of fetus and placenta is required in eclampsia. Anticoagulants appear to be ineffective in most cases and may exacerbate bleeding.

Transfusion of blood products

If bleeding is uncontrolled, transfusion of plasma, cryoprecipitate and platelets may be indicated as supportive therapy.

Prognosis

DIC carries a poor prognosis; the mortality has been reported to be as high as 42%.[2]

REFERENCES

(1) Okajima K, Sakamoto Y, Uchiba M. Heterogeneity in the incidence and clinical manifestations of disseminated intravascular coagulation: a study of 204 cases. American Journal of Hematology 2000; 65: 215–222.
(2) Chuansumrit A, Hotrakitya S, Sirinavin S, et al. Disseminated intravascular coagulation findings in 100 patients. Journal of the Medical Association of Thailand 1999; 82 Suppl 1: S63–8.

Thrombotic thrombocytopenic purpura and haemolytic-uraemic syndrome

The principal features of thrombotic thrombocytopenic purpura (TTP) and haemolytic-uraemic syndrome (HUS) are thrombocytopenia due to platelet consumption in micro-vascular occlusive platelet plugs and a microangiopathic haemolytic anaemia (haemolysis due to physical damage to red cells). Unlike disseminated intravascular coagulation (DIC), fibrin deposition is not a major feature. In HUS the vascular lesions occur mainly in the renal circulation whereas in TTP they are more diffuse, including in the cerebral circulation.

Epidemiology

HUS often occurs in epidemics in children, as it is associated with an infection. TTP is usually sporadic, but familial forms are recognized.

Pathology

In many cases HUS is associated with a prodromal acute haemorrhagic colitis due to pathogenic *E. coli*, usually strain O157. In *E. coli* related HUS, the bacteria produce a toxin which damages the endothelium of the renal micro-circulation resulting in platelet adhesion, erythrocyte fragmentation in the renal circulation and impaired renal function.

Sporadic TTP appears to be an autoimmune disease. An autoantibody develops which interferes with the activity of a protease responsible for processing von Willebrand factor secreted from endothelial cells. When this protease activity is inhibited, abnormally high molecular weight forms of von Willebrand factor persist in the circulation to activate the platelets, resulting in systemic microvascular occlusion, ischaemia, thrombocytopenia and microangiopathic haemolysis. In familial TTP there is an inherited deficiency of the protease.

Clinical features

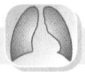

In HUS there is renal failure and anaemia with features of microangiopathic haemolysis. In most cases it is a self-limiting disorder.

In fully developed TTP there is a pentad of clinical features: thrombocytopenia, microangiopathic haemolysis, central nervous system dysfunction, renal impairment and fever. The presenting neurological feature may be only headache, but fluctuating motor dysfunction, confusion, fits and coma often ensue if treatment is not instituted promptly.

Investigations

Full blood count, blood film
In both TTP and HUS the diagnosis rests upon the finding of thrombocytopenia and haemolysis with schistocytes in the appropriate clinical context.

Coagulation screen
Although DIC is associated with similar haematological features, the coagulation times are normal in TTP and HUS.

Fibrin degradation products
In contrast to DIC, fibrin degradation products are not markedly increased.

Management

In general, platelet transfusion is avoided for both TTP and HUS as it may exacerbate microvascular occlusion.

Haemolytic-uraemic syndrome
Supportive treatment, with dialysis if necessary, is the main-stay of management in HUS.

Thrombotic thrombocytopenic purpura

Fresh frozen plasma and corticosteroids
In TTP, corticosteroids and high-volume plasma exchange with fresh frozen plasma replacement have been shown to reduce mortality from the condition. This should be insti-tuted as emergency therapy once the diagnosis is made. The mechanism of action is presumed to be the removal of abnormally high molecular weight von Willebrand factor and the pathogenic autoantibody whilst also supplying a source of protease. The response rate to this treatment is approximately 80%.[1] In chronic relapsing TTP, immuno-suppression may help, including the anti CD20 antibody rituximab.

Aspirin
Aspirin is administered in some centres, but the evidence for the efficacy of aspirin remains to be proven.

Prognosis

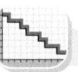

In HUS, recovery is often complete although there may be chronic renal impairment. In TTP, there may be complete remission but some cases follow a relapsing course.

REFERENCE

(1) de la Rubia J, Lopez A, Arriaga F, Cid AR, Vicente AI, Marty ML, Sanz MA. Response to plasma exchange and steroids as combined therapy for patients with thrombotic thrombocytopenic purpura. Acta Haematologica 1999; 102: 12–16.

Heparin-induced thrombocytopenia

Heparin-induced thrombocytopenia (HIT) is an unusual subtype of drug-induced immune thrombocytopenia in which there is thrombosis rather than bleeding.

Epidemiology

The risk of developing HIT is low; less than 1% of patients receiving heparin develop the clinical syndrome.

Pathology

The pathogenesis is an IgG antibody that forms a complex with heparin and platelet factor 4 (a protein from platelet granules). The immune complex activates platelets through their Fc receptors leading to aggregation, thrombocytopenia and thrombosis.

Clinical features

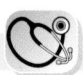

Patients typically present with new thrombosis or thrombosis extension after 5–10 days of exposure to heparin. This condition is important because fatal thrombosis can occur if heparin is not discontinued and replaced with an alternative anticoagulant.

HIT must be suspected when there is an otherwise unexpected progressive fall in platelet count beginning 5–21 days after heparin prophylaxis or treatment is commenced, especially if there is evidence of new thrombosis also. The fall in platelet count may occur before 5 days if there has been previous recent exposure to heparin. In some cases there is skin necrosis at the site of heparin injection or systemic symptoms such as rigors and fever.[1] Despite thrombocytopenia, increased bleeding rarely occurs.

> **CLINICAL ALERT**
>
> *In order to facilitate diagnosis before thrombosis occurs, the platelet count should be closely monitored for developing thrombocytopenia in any subject continuing heparin, including prophylactic doses, for longer than 5 days.*

Investigations

Full blood count
Although the platelet count falls, severe thrombocytopenia is uncommon.

Heparin-induced thrombocytopenia antibody screen
There are two commonly used assays: a platelet activation assay in which washed normal platelets are activated in the presence of a low concentration of heparin and plasma from the patient, due to the presence of HIT antibody, and a platelet factor 4-dependent enzyme immunoassay, which is more sensitive but less specific.

Management

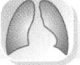

Stop heparin
All exposure to heparin, including heparin flushes into indwelling devices, must cease as soon as the diagnosis is strongly suspected.

Alternative anticoagulants
Unless alternative anticoagulant therapy is introduced there is a high risk of thrombosis, which persists for several days. The antithrombotic of choice is the thrombin inhibitor lepirudin, because it is effective and there is no cross-reaction by the HIT antibody. The heparinoid danaparoid has also been used but there is a small risk of failure due to cross-reacting antibody.

Warfarin alone is not effective in prevention of thrombosis in the first few days of treatment of HIT and is contraindicated. Platelet transfusion should be avoided.

Prognosis

Cessation of heparin alone is not associated with improved outcome as death from thrombosis still occurs in approximately 5%.

> **REFERENCE**
>
> (1) *Warkentin TE, Greinacher A. Heparin-induced thrombocytopenia: recognition, treatment, and prevention: the seventh ACCP conference on antithrombotic and thrombolytic therapy. Chest 2004; 126: 311S–337.*

Disorders of platelet function

Platelet function abnormalities cause defective platelet adhesion or aggregation. They result in prolongation of the skin bleeding time despite a normal or only moderately reduced platelet count.

Epidemiology

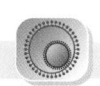

Causes of abnormal platelet function are listed in Table 12.27. Congenital disorders are rare. Qualitative platelet disorders are usually acquired and are very common (such as the mild iatrogenic bleeding tendency from aspirin use).

Pathology

Congenital disorders include Bernard–Soulier syndrome, a recessively inherited deficiency of platelet membrane glycoprotein complex Ib/IX, a receptor for von Willebrand factor. As a result there is failure of platelet adhesion. Glanzmann's disease is a recessively inherited deficiency of platelet membrane glycoproteins IIb and IIIa. The IIb/IIIa complex is the principal platelet fibrinogen receptor. An inability to bind fibrinogen precludes platelet aggregation. Inherited metabolic disorders of platelets include: deficiency of adenine nucleotides due to an abnormality of platelet storage granules (dense bodies): platelet storage pool deficiencies; and defects in the enzymes responsible for the synthesis of the pro-aggregatory prostanoid thromboxane A_2, including cyclo-oxygenase.

Table 12.27	Causes of abnormal platelet function
Congenital platelet function disorders	
Glanzmann's disease	
Bernard–Soulier syndrome	
Storage pool disease	
Enzymopathies	
Acquired platelet function disorders	
Drugs	
Non-steroidal anti-inflammatory agents	
Clopidogrel	
Metabolic disease	
Severe uraemia	
Hepatic failure	
Myeloproliferative disease	
Paraproteinaemias	

The most common acquired disorder of platelet function is drug induced, due to the inhibition of cyclo-oxygenase by aspirin and other non-steroidal anti-inflammatory drugs. In uraemia and liver failure platelet interaction with subendothelium is defective, and in myeloproliferative disease the clonal haemopoiesis results in functionally abnormal platelets. In paraproteinaemias such as plasma cell myeloma, platelets become coated with immunoglobulin that blocks surface receptors and prevents platelet aggregation.

Clinical features

The main presenting feature is abnormal bleeding (typically bruising and mucosal haemorrhage). Severity is variable, for example aspirin use results in a mild prolongation of the skin bleeding time and a tendency to increased skin bruising and bleeding from surgical wounds, whereas in Glanzmann's disease there is complete failure of platelet aggregation with a hugely prolonged bleeding time and a life-long risk of fatal haemorrhage.

Investigations

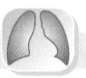

Full blood count
The platelet count is usually normal or mildly reduced, for example in liver failure and Bernard–Soulier syndrome.

Platelet function tests
Skin bleeding time is prolonged in patients with disorders of platelet function. Platelet aggregation tests are employed to determine the nature of the functional deficit. Flow cytometry employing antibodies specific for platelet membrane glycoprotein receptors is useful to confirm Bernard–Soulier syndrome and Glanzmann's disease.

Management

No intervention is usually required for the acquired conditions.

Platelet transfusion
In Glanzmann's disease and Bernard–Soulier syndrome treatment is supportive but transfusion of donor platelets may be necessary for the treatment of serious bleeding episodes. Platelet transfusion carries the risk of antibody formation to the missing platelet glycoprotein and subsequent refractoriness to platelet transfusion. Recombinant factor VIIa is a novel but expensive treatment which appears to be effective in a range of bleeding disorders.

Prognosis

Congenital disorders of platelet function are irreversible and carry the life-long risk of severe haemorrhage. Acquired disorders of platelet function are usually mild and may be reversible by identifying and correcting the precipitating cause if possible.

SECTION 12.8   Disorders of coagulation and thrombosis

Coagulation disorders

Bleeding disorders result from defects of primary haemostasis or defects of blood coagulation (Table 12.28). Defects of primary haemostasis are principally due to quantitative (thrombocytopenia) or qualitative (platelet function defects) platelet disorders or von Willebrand disease (p. 825). Defects of blood coagulation (below) are usually due to deficiencies in clotting factors or the presence of coagulation inhibitors, including the anticoagulant medication heparin.

Conditions that mimic bleeding disorders without increased bleeding tendency include senile purpura and skin purpura from corticosteroid therapy. In both cases the bruising results from dermal vascular instability due to collagen degradation. There is no systemic bleeding tendency.

In Henoch–Schönlein purpura, the rash is due to vasculitis affecting cutaneous vessels. It resembles throm-

Haemophilia

Von Willebrand disease

Vitamin K deficiency

Heritable thrombophilia

Antiphospholipid syndrome

Table 12.28	Disorders of coagulation

Congenital

Factor VIII deficiency (haemophilia A)

Factor IX deficiency (haemophilia B)

Von Willebrand factor deficiency (von Willebrand disease)

Other rare factor deficiencies (e.g. factor XI, XIII)

Acquired

Drugs
 Oral vitamin K inhibitor (warfarin)
 Parenteral anticoagulant (heparin)
 Thrombolytics

Vitamin K deficiency
 Haemorrhagic disease of the newborn
 Obstructive jaundice

Reduced coagulation factors
 Liver failure (reduced synthesis)
 Disseminated intravascular coagulation (increased consumption)
 Massive blood transfusion (dilutional)

Coagulation factor inhibitors (antibodies)
 Acquired haemophilia (factor VIII autoantibodies)
 Acquired von Willebrand disease (vWF autoantibodies)

bocytopenic purpura in distribution but the purpuric rash is slightly raised and palpable, the platelet count is normal and there is no systemic bleeding disorder. In hereditary haemorrhagic telangiectasia severe epistaxis occurs from telangiectatic vascular lesions in the nasal mucosa without any systemic bleeding tendency.

History

In bleeding disorders due to defects in primary haemostasis, the skin and mucous membranes are principally involved. The pattern of bleeding from coagulation disorders is somewhat distinct, in that mucosal bleeding is less prominent and soft tissue bleeding is more common. Severe coagulation factor deficiencies can lead to spontaneous bleeding into the joints (acute haemarthrosis).

A drug and past medical history is important, as acquired coagulation disorders are commonly due to drugs (warfarin, heparin) or underlying disease (obstructive jaundice or liver failure).

Age of onset and family history are important as a guide to the likelihood of a bleeding disorder being due to congenital deficiency of a coagulation factor. Deficiency of every clotting factor has been reported but all are very uncommon. Haemophilia A and B, due to deficiency of factor VIII and factor IX respectively, are the least rare. Factor XII deficiency is a relatively common abnormality but is not accompanied by increased bleeding.

Examination

On examination, bruising, purpura or mucosal bleeding may be evident and in severe cases joint deformities from haemarthrosis.

Investigations
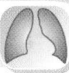

Coagulation screen

The first-line tests in the investigation of abnormal bleeding are the activated partial thromboplastin time (APTT), the prothrombin time (PT), the thrombin time (TT), fibrinogen concentration, skin bleeding time and platelet count. It must be recognized that some significant bleeding disorders may be present in the face of normal screening tests. These include mild von Willebrand disease and deficiency of factor XIII. Therefore the range of investigations employed must be guided by the persuasiveness of the clinical history of bleeding symptoms.

In disseminated intravascular coagulation there is always a precipitating illness such as septicaemia, cancer or pre-eclampsia. Diffuse coagulation activation typically results in consumption of platelets, coagulation factors and fibrinogen. In the full syndrome there is thrombocytopenia, prolonged clotting times and reduced fibrinogen concentration. Tests for fibrin degradation products, such as D-dimer, are positive.

In liver failure there is diminished synthesis of most clotting factors with prolongation of clotting times and reduced fibrinogen concentration. Thrombocytopenia may be present due to hypersplenism. The pattern of test results resembles DIC. In obstructive jaundice the coagulopathy is due to vitamin K deficiency. There may be isolated prolongation of the PT, with otherwise normal coagulation screening tests.

Coagulation factor assays

Specific coagulation factor assays may be indicated by the pattern of abnormal clotting times, for example assay of factors VIII and IX when there is a bleeding history and isolated prolongation of the APTT.

Platelet function tests and von Willebrand factor assay

If the history suggests a defect of primary haemostasis and the skin bleeding time is prolonged with normal platelet numbers, a platelet function defect or von Willebrand disease must be suspected.

Haemophilia

Deficiencies of factor VIII (haemophilia A) and factor IX (haemophilia B or Christmas disease) are the most common bleeding disorders due to inherited coagulation factor deficiency, excluding von Willebrand disease.

Epidemiology

Haemophilia A is rare, with a similar prevalence in all ethnic groups. Haemophilia B is approximately 5 times less common than haemophilia A.

Pathology

Both factor VIII and factor IX are essential for thrombin generation during the coagulation cascade. Factor VIII has a plasma half-life of 12 hours and requires von Willebrand factor (a carrier protein) to maintain the half-life duration. The plasma half-life of factor IX is approximately 24 hours.

As the production of both factor VIII and IX is controlled by genes on the X chromosome, deficiencies are inherited as sex-linked disorders. Affected males manifest the full bleeding disorder; female carriers are usually asymptomatic but may have mild bleeding symptoms. In approximately 30% of affected subjects, the gene mutation occurs de novo and there is no family history of bleeding.

A variety of defects in the factor VIII gene have been recognized in haemophilia A. These include partial or complete deletions of the factor VIII gene and single base changes. They result in the absence of the coagulation factor or in the synthesis of a truncated protein which is functionally ineffective and rapidly degraded. Comparable defects in the factor IX gene are seen in haemophilia B.

Acquired haemophilia is rare, and can occur in either sex from the development of an autoantibody that results in diminished function and rapid clearance of factor VIII.

Scope of disease

In severely affected subjects there is painful bleeding into weight-bearing joints. Recurrent bleeds cause massive synovial hypertrophy and severe arthropathy. Debilitating bleeding into muscles can also occur, such as in the iliopsoas. Complications of repeated blood product transfusions in haemophilia include the acquisition of HIV and hepatitis.

Clinical features

The severity of bleeding is related to the plasma concentration of factor VIII or IX (Table 12.29), and is constant within a kindred.

Severe disease may present in early infancy with umbilical stump bleeding, whilst less severe cases may remain undiagnosed, for example until marked bruising from minor trauma occurs at the toddler stage. Spontaneous haemorrhage into major joints, especially knees, hips, elbows and shoulders, occurring several times each month, was typical of the severe disease before effective

Table 12.29	Classification of severity of haemophilia A	
Severity	**Factor levels (normal range 50–150%)**	**Clinical features**
Mild	>3%	Bleeding after trauma only
Moderate	1–3%	Serious bleeding after trauma, including surgery, spontaneous skin bruising
Severe	<1%	Spontaneous joint and life-threatening soft tissue bleeding

treatment was available. Prolonged episodes of haematuria, massive retroperitoneal or intracranial haemorrhage can occur and may be fatal. Any surgical intervention (e.g. dental surgery) results in protracted and severe bleeding unless treatment is given.

Initial investigations

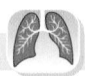

Coagulation screen
The APTT is prolonged in both factor VIII and IX deficiency; other coagulation tests are normal. In severe disease the blood does not coagulate.

Further investigations

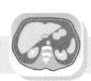

Coagulation factor assay
The diagnosis is confirmed by assay of factor VIII or IX. The concentration of von Willebrand factor is normal, as is the skin bleeding time.

Molecular genetic analysis
Molecular genetic analysis has facilitated genetic counselling and prenatal diagnosis in affected kindreds.

Initial management

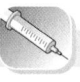

Patient education
The management of haemophilia should be undertaken in specialized centres, and is delivered by specialist clinicians and nurses with access to support from physiotherapists, orthopaedic surgeons and other specialists. Information about the disease should be provided to the parents of the affected child. The clinical course and treatment modalities should be explained. In addition, genetic counselling and screening of relatives for the haemophilia gene should be offered. Immunization against hepatitis B is recommended.

Medical management

Factor VIII/IX replacement
Normalization of the clotting factor level is possible through repeated intravenous infusion of factor VIII (haemophilia A) or IX (haemophilia B). The concentrated clotting factor is prepared from pooled donated plasma, but products manufactured by recombinant technology are now available.

Severe haemophilia can be managed effectively in infancy and childhood with regular prophylactic infusion of clotting factors every few days. Only a modest increase in the plasma factor level is required to prevent spontaneous bleeding. In older children and adults, self-administration of factor concentrate at the first sign of an acute bleed is an effective strategy to prevent the onset of crippling arthropathy.

Correction of the plasma concentration of factor VIII or IX before surgical procedures is essential. This is achieved by repeated or continuous intravenous administration of factor concentrates until wound healing has occurred.

Approximately 16% of patients with haemophilia A develop antibodies (inhibitors) to factor VIII by the age of 5 (6% of patients with haemophilia B), and the rate gradually increases with time.[1] The development of an inhibitor is a serious complication as it limits the effectiveness of treatment.

Desmopressin

In mild haemophilia A, an alternative approach to treatment is administration of des-diamino-vasopressin (DDAVP). This analogue of vasopressin increases the factor VIII level in plasma after intravenous infusion or nasal instillation, but is not effective for severe disease or haemophilia B.

Prognosis

Many older subjects with haemophilia are chronic carriers of hepatitis and there have been numerous deaths from AIDS due to the previously unrecognized contamination of plasma concentrates with viruses. Modern products appear to be much safer.

In the absence of HIV infection, the life expectancy of patients with haemophilia is 64 years, and the median age at death is 67 years. The overall life expectancy including patients with HIV infection is approximately 39 years, with the median age at death of 35 years.[2]

REFERENCES

(1) *Darby SC, Keeling DM, Spooner RJ, et al. The incidence of factor VIII and factor IX inhibitors in the hemophilia population of the UK and their effect on subsequent mortality, 1977–99. Journal of Thrombosis and Haemostasis 2004;2:1047–1054.*
(2) *Soucie JM, Nuss R, Evatt B, et al, the Hemophilia Surveillance System Project Investigators. Mortality among males with hemophilia: relations with source of medical care. Blood 2000; 96: 437–442.*

Von Willebrand disease

Von Willebrand disease is generally a mild to moderate bleeding disorder due to reduced synthesis of, or the production of functionally abnormal, von Willebrand factor (vWF).

Epidemiology

Von Willebrand disease is an autosomal dominant disorder with variable expression. The prevalence has been reported as 821 per 100 000.[1] However, discrimination between mild disease and normality is problematic, so estimates of prevalence vary. In contrast to factor VIII, vWF synthesis is under autosomal control therefore males and females are equally affected.

Pathology

Von Willebrand factor is a large multimeric protein that is synthesized and assembled by vascular endothelial cells as well as megakaryocytes. It is an essential cofactor for primary haemostasis (facilitating platelet adhesion to exposed subendothelium) and functions as a carrier protein for factor VIII. Therefore reduced plasma concentration of vWF is accompanied by reduced factor VIII concentration.

The majority of von Willebrand disease is caused by a quantitative deficiency of vWF (type I); in approximately 20%, the disorder is due to synthesis of a dysfunctional vWF (type II). In both types, the plasma concentrations of functional vWF and factor VIII are low, but rarely less than 20% of normal. Homozygous disease (type III) is rare and results in much more severe bleeding.

Clinical features

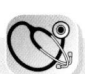

Features of von Willebrand disease include easy bruising, bleeding after minor trauma and, in women, menorrhagia. However, these symptoms are common in healthy subjects, and the range of normal von Willebrand factor concentration in plasma is wide, making diagnosis of mild disease problematic. In contrast to haemophilia, haemarthrosis is not a feature, other than in type III disease.

RECENT ADVANCES

Some patients previously diagnosed with type I von Willebrand disease do not have a specific hemorrhagic disorder. Modification of the interpretation of a modest reduction in von Willebrand factor concentration has been proposed, in that it should be considered as a modest risk factor for bleeding that exists on a continuous scale, analogous to the relationship between blood pressure and the risk of stroke.[2] Population studies which will identify genetic variants underlying type I von Willebrand disease are in progress.

Investigations

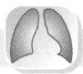

Coagulation screen
The APTT may be modestly prolonged due to low factor VIII, but may be normal in mild deficiency.

Bleeding time
Although platelets are normal, platelet adhesion requires the presence of fully functional vWF. As a result, the skin bleeding time is typically increased. In vitro surrogate assays for bleeding time which depend upon platelet adhesion are being introduced.

Factor VIII and vWF assay
The diagnosis is confirmed by use of specific assays for factor VIII and vWF, both of which are low in von Willebrand disease. Repeat testing may be necessary if initial factor levels are low normal, as a transient increase in vWF can

827

occur after physical exertion, psychological stress and in pregnancy. Moreover, subjects of blood group O normally have approximately 30% lower levels of vWF than do those of groups A, B and AB, adding to the difficulty in diagnosing mild type I disease.

Management

Avoiding precipitating factors of bleeding

In mild cases no intervention may be necessary. As in all bleeding disorders, aspirin and non-steroidal anti-inflammatory drugs should be avoided if possible as their platelet inhibitory effect exacerbates the bleeding tendency.

Tranexamic acid

The oral antifibrinolytic drug tranexamic acid is effective in some women with menorrhagia due to vWD.

Desmopressin

Most cases respond transiently to DDAVP. This is useful in the preparation of patients for surgical interventions. Side effects include water retention, including severe hyponatraemia on occasions. DDAVP is contraindicated in subjects with arteriosclerosis.

vWF rich concentrates

vWF-rich concentrates are reserved for serious bleeding and to prevent excessive blood loss during major surgery when DDAVP therapy is inadequate.

Prognosis

The prognosis of patients with von Willebrand disease is related to the severity of the disease. Life expectancy is normal in most cases.

REFERENCES

(1) Rodeghiero F, Castaman G, Dini E. Epidemiological investigation of the prevalence of von Willebrand's disease. Blood 1987; 69: 454–459.
(2) Sadler JE. Von Willebrand disease type 1: a diagnosis in search of a disease. Blood 2003; 101: 2089–2093.

Vitamin K deficiency

Vitamin K is essential for the synthesis of several coagulation factors. Deficiency can be congenital (haemorrhagic disease of the newborn) or acquired due to intestinal disorders and obstructive jaundice.

Epidemiology

The exact prevalence of vitamin K deficiency in adults is unknown, but it commonly coexists in patients with jaundice, cancer and the critically ill.[1] The incidence of unexpected bleeding due to haemorrhagic disease of the newborn is up to 1700 per 100 000 per year.[2]

Pathology

Vitamin K is an essential vitamin for the completed synthesis of coagulation factors II, VII, IX and X. It is obtained from green vegetables and bacterial synthesis in the gut. Being a fat-soluble vitamin, it requires bile to facilitate absorption. Therefore deficiency can develop from inadequate intake, abnormalities of the bowel (blind loop syndrome) and obstructive jaundice.

Vitamin K deficiency can also occur in the breast-fed neonate, as neonates lack gut bacteria (for vitamin K synthesis) and the concentration of vitamin K is low in breast milk. The resulting coagulopathy is termed haemorrhagic disease of the newborn and was common prior to routine vitamin K supplementation to neonates.

Clinical features

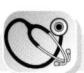

Easy bruising and soft tissue bleeding are common features. Accompanying deep jaundice suggests bile duct obstruction as the underlying cause of vitamin K deficiency.

In classical haemorrhagic disease of the newborn, a bleeding tendency develops 2–5 weeks after birth with bruising, gastrointestinal bleeding and (rarely) fatal intracranial haemorrhage. A variant of the condition occurs even earlier in the neonates of women treated with anticonvulsants during pregnancy.

Investigations

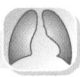

Coagulation screen

The prothrombin time is most sensitive to deficiency of factors II, VII and X and is prolonged in vitamin K deficiency. The anticoagulant effect of vitamin K deficiency is analogous to that induced by warfarin, a competitive inhibitor of vitamin K. The APTT may be normal or prolonged.

Management

Vitamin K supplementation

In obstructive jaundice 5 mg of intravenous vitamin K is usually sufficient to reverse any coagulopathy within a few hours. Haemorrhagic disease of the newborn can be prevented by use of oral or intramuscular supplementation of vitamin K.

Clotting factor concentrates and fresh frozen plasma

In life-threatening bleeding, immediate improvement in coagulation can be achieved by infusion of appropriate clotting factor concentrates or (less efficiently) fresh frozen plasma.

Prognosis

Treatment with intravenous vitamin K results in correction of the coagulation abnormalities within 6–12 hours.

REFERENCES

(1) Crowther MA, McDonald E, Johnston M, Cook D. Vitamin K deficiency and D-dimer levels in the intensive care unit: a prospective cohort study. Blood Coagulation and Fibrinolysis 2002; 13: 49–52.
(2) Committee on Fetus and Newborn. Controversies concerning vitamin K and the newborn. Pediatrics 2003; 112: 191–192.

Thrombophilia

Thrombophilia is a term used to describe a predisposition to thrombosis. The causes are congenital or acquired (Table 12.30).

Heritable thrombophilia is a term used to describe inherited conditions in which there is a life-long predisposition to thrombosis, principally affecting the venous system. Some conditions are known to increase thrombotic risk, but are only partly determined by inheritance, such as increased plasma coagulation factors VIII, IX, XI and fibrinogen.

In acquired thrombophilia, the arteries, veins and microcirculation may be affected, in contrast to predominantly venous thrombosis in heritable thrombophilia.

Table 12.30	Causes of thrombophilia
Congenital	
Common gene mutations Factor V Leiden mutation Prothrombin G20210A mutation	
Rare inherited deficiencies of physiological anticoagulants Antithrombin deficiency Protein C deficiency Protein S deficiency	
Acquired	
Myeloproliferative disease Essential thrombocythaemia Polycythaemia vera	
Other haematological malignancies Acute promyelocytic leukaemia Lymphoma Plasma cell myeloma	
Non-haematological malignancies	
Paroxysmal nocturnal haemoglobinuria	
Antiphospholipid syndrome	
Drugs Heparin-induced thrombocytopenia Chemotherapy	
Disseminated intravascular coagulation (microvascular thrombosis)	
Microangiopathic haemolytic anaemia	
Haemolytic-uraemic syndrome	
Thrombotic thrombocytopenic purpura	

Heritable thrombophilia

Epidemiology

In patients presenting with venous thromboembolism, up to 30% have a detectable inherited pro-thrombotic state. The most common is factor V Leiden mutation with a prevalence of 1% to over 5% (up to 5000 per 100 000). Countries with the highest prevalence are those of Northern Europe, Poland and Argentina.[1] In some families few clinical events occur, suggesting the need for interaction with other genes for penetrance.

Pathology

The point mutation in the gene for coagulation factor V renders the product resistant to the anticoagulant effect of protein C, a physiological coagulation inhibitor. The result is a chronic hypercoagulable state. A point mutation in the prothrombin gene (prothrombin G20210A) is associated with increased prothrombin in plasma and a similar hypercoagulable state and is present in around 1% of some populations.

Other recognized heritable thrombophilias are due to deficiency or defect of one of the physiological anticoagulant proteins (antithrombin, protein C and its cofactor protein S) and are genetically heterogeneous and less common. These conditions are all autosomally inherited and heterozygotes are clinically affected. In the case of antithrombin deficiency, the homozygous state appears to be incompatible with life, and homozygous protein C deficiency may cause life-threatening thrombosis in neonatal life.

Clinical features
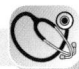

There is a predisposition to venous thromboembolism but no significantly increased risk of arterial thrombosis. The incidence of thrombosis increases with age and is rare in childhood. Not all individuals with a heritable thrombophilia will suffer thrombosis. Although venous thromboembolism can occur apparently without provocation, more usually thrombosis is precipitated by an environmental or acquired factor against a background genetic predisposition. For example, a young woman who is heterozygous for factor V Leiden has an overall increased risk of venous thromboembolism of around 4-fold but the absolute risk is low because venous thromboembolism is relatively uncommon during the first four decades. However if such a woman uses the combined oral contraceptive, which carries its own increased risk of venous thromboembolism of around 4-fold, the effect is multiplicative and her relative risk increases to around 30-fold.

The principal acquired factors that predispose to venous thromboembolism and presenting clinical features are provided on page 159.

Investigation

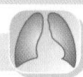

Thrombophilia screen

PCR-based tests for factor V Leiden and prothrombin G20210A are easily accessible and reliable. Deficiencies of protein C, protein S or antithrombin are identified through assay of the relevant protein and functional assays.

Management

Heparin

The acute and longer-term management of venous thromboembolism in a subject with heritable thrombophilia is identical to that for other patients with venous thromboembolism. Low molecular weight heparin is administered for at least 5 days and until adequate anticoagulation is achieved with warfarin.

Warfarin

Warfarin therapy may be initiated at the same time as heparin. Warfarin should not be introduced without initial heparin in protein C and S deficiency as these are vitamin K dependent proteins and warfarin may induce a transient procoagulant state causing thrombosis. A target INR of 2.5 (range 2.0–3.0) is maintained for 3–6 months. In recurrent venous thromboembolism, long-term warfarin therapy should be considered.

Prognosis

Patients with thrombophilia have a life-long risk of thrombosis that increases with age. The median age at which an individual either experiences an episode of thrombosis or death is 34 years for antithrombin deficiency, 37 years for protein S deficiency, 50 years for the factor V Leiden mutation and 62 years for protein C deficiency.[2]

Case finding

In families with a clear history of venous thromboembolism in two or more first-degree relatives testing can be considered for young family members to facilitate counselling and education to minimize the risk of venous thromboembolism (e.g. the choice of contraceptive). As this represents genetic testing for a late-onset disorder with incomplete penetrance it is essential that the proband and relatives are fully informed by a knowledgeable practitioner before testing is performed. Population screening is not considered to be a useful strategy.

REFERENCES

(1) Herrmann FH, Koesling M, Schroder W, et al. Prevalence of factor V Leiden mutation in various populations. Genetic Epidemiology 1997;14:403–411.

(2) Tirado I, Mateo J, Soria JM, et al. Contribution of prothrombin 20210A allele and factor V Leiden mutation to thrombosis risk in thrombophilic families with other hemostatic deficiencies. Haematologica 2001; 86: 1200–1208.

Antiphospholipid syndrome

The antiphospholipid syndrome is a clinical syndrome defined by pregnancy morbidity (mostly fetal loss) and/or thrombosis (venous, arterial or microvascular) in the presence of persistently positive tests for antiphospholipid antibodies, usually anticardiolipin antibodies and lupus anticoagulant.[1]

Epidemiology

The prevalence of the antiphospholipid syndrome is not known, in part because there is a large variability in the presence of antiphospholipid antibodies in the normal population.[2]

Antiphospholipid syndrome is a significant acquired thrombophilic state in patients presenting with venous or arterial thromboembolism. It is 4 times more commonly identified in women, and the average age at diagnosis is 42 years.[3] In approximately half of cases, antiphospholipid syndrome occurs against the background of another disease, most commonly systemic lupus erythematosus (secondary antiphospholipid syndrome). In the remainder it occurs in isolation (primary antiphospholipid syndrome).[3]

Pathology

Antiphospholipid syndrome is an autoimmune disease, with an antibody reactivity that is not directly against phospholipids but against plasma proteins which have the property of binding to negatively-charged phospholipids such as cardiolipin, and most prominently β2 glycoprotein I and prothrombin. Some such antibodies result in prolongation of the clotting time, especially the APTT, referred to as lupus anticoagulant activity. Paradoxically there is thrombosis in vivo, not bleeding. How the antibodies induce a pro-thrombotic state is complex and appears to include endothelial cell activation and enhanced thrombin formation. The pathogenesis of pregnancy failure is also incompletely understood.

Antiphospholipid syndrome is an important acquired thrombophilia, as it carries a high risk of recurrent thrombosis.

Clinical features

Women may have a predisposition to recurrent miscarriages, fetal death and early severe pre-eclampsia, as well as thrombosis. Limb deep vein thrombosis and visceral vessel thrombosis also occur. In the arterial circulation ischaemic stroke is predominant. Other manifestations of the syndrome include livedo reticularis, a characteristic skin rash, and mild thrombocytopenia.

Investigations

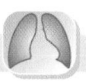

Coagulation screen

The APTT may be prolonged, but in many cases more sophisticated coagulation tests are required to detect lupus anticoagulant.

Autoantibody tests

In immunoassays, antibody activity in serum is typically detected against cardiolipin, a negatively charged phospholipid. In antiphospholipid syndrome there may be lupus anticoagulant, anticardiolipin antibody or both.

Management

Anticoagulation and antiplatelet therapy

Patients with venous thromboembolism are treated with heparin and warfarin, target INR 2.5. Patients with stroke may be treated with aspirin, although many clinicians recommend warfarin prophylaxis against further events. Although a high risk of thrombosis recurrence after first stroke has been suggested in antiphospholipid syndrome, recent evidence does not support this supposition.[4]

In women with pregnancy failure, aspirin and low-dose heparin have been used to attempt to improve pregnancy outcome.

Prognosis

The survival of patients with primary antiphospholipid syndrome is not well documented. In those with secondary antiphospholipid syndrome, the 15-year survival probability is 65%.[5]

REFERENCES

(1) *Wilson WA, Gharavi AE, Koike T, et al. International consensus statement on preliminary classification criteria for definite antiphospholipid syndrome: report of an international workshop. Arthritis and Rheumatism 1999; 42: 1309–1311.*
(2) *Petri M. Epidemiology of the antiphospholipid antibody syndrome. Journal of Autoimmunity 2000; 15: 145–151.*
(3) *Cervera R, Piette JC, Font J, et al. Antiphospholipid syndrome: clinical and immunologic manifestations and patterns of disease expression in a cohort of 1,000 patients. Arthritis and Rheumatism 2002; 46: 1019–1027.*
(4) *Crowther MA, Wisloff F. Evidence based treatment of the antiphospholipid syndrome II. Optimal anticoagulant therapy for thrombosis. Thrombosis Research 2005; 115: 3–8.*
(5) *Ruiz-Irastorza G, Egurbide MV, Ugalde J, Aguirre C. High impact of antiphospholipid syndrome on irreversible organ damage and survival of patients with systemic lupus erythematosus. Archives of Internal Medicine 2004; 164: 77–82.*

Antiphospholipid syndrome

SECTION 12.9   Transfusion medicine

Knowledge of the use of blood and blood products is important for the treatment of a wide range of disorders, and can be life saving. Whole blood is rarely required. Donated blood is fractionated into separate components for use.

CLINICAL ALERT

Transfusion of blood products carries a significant risk of morbidity and mortality. Each and every transfusion must be fully justified on clinical grounds and alternatives evaluated. Patient misidentification is a principal cause of fatalities from haemolytic transfusion reactions. The importance of careful identification and blood sample labelling cannot be overemphasized.

Red cells

Preparation

Red cells are prepared from donated whole blood and stored at 2–6°C. The shelf life is 35 days, and the red cells must be transfused within 5 hours of leaving storage conditions. A unit of packed red cells will increase the haemoglobin concentration by 1 g/dL in an average adult.

Indication

Transfusion may be life saving in resuscitation after acute haemorrhage. Transfusion of red cells is considered in symptomatic anaemia when no alternative, such as correction of haematinic deficiency, is appropriate and when the symptomatic benefit outweighs the risks. In addition, availability of red cells for transfusion is essential for the safe performance of many surgical procedures.

Administration

ABO compatibility is a prerequisite for red cell transfusion. In conditions of extreme urgency, O negative red cells may be used while awaiting crossmatched red cells. Administration is via a large-bore cannula with a blood administration set. Care must be taken to avoid volume overload in patients with a history of cardiac failure.

Complications

A list of general complications is provided in Table 12.31. Among these, allergic and febrile reactions are common, although the latter have been reduced in frequency by routine filtration of red cell products to remove leukocytes. Haemolytic reactions are relatively common, potentially lethal and avoidable (p. 834).

Other complications are rare. The risk of virus transmission has been substantially reduced by improved donor selection, screening of the donated blood and virucidal treatment of pooled plasma concentrates. Transmission of cytomegalovirus still occurs and has serious consequences in the immunocompromised recipient. Parvovirus is also transmitted by blood products and can severely exacerbate anaemia in haemolysis or bone marrow failure.

Transfusion-related acute lung injury presents as non-cardiac pulmonary oedema due to pulmonary capillary damage from components of neutrophil leukocytes, and may be lethal. Transfusion-associated graft-versus-host disease is usually fatal and most likely to occur when the recipient has a cellular immune deficiency (premature infants, bone marrow transplant recipients). Fever, skin rash, diarrhoea and liver dysfunction develop several weeks after transfusion. It can be prevented by gamma-irradiation of blood products prior to transfusion to high-risk patients.

Platelets

Preparation

Platelets are prepared from donated whole blood or by donor apheresis, and stored at 20–24°C on agitator racks. The shelf life is 5 days.

Indications

Platelets can be usefully transfused to treat bleeding in severely thrombocytopenic patients. Support of patients rendered thrombocytopenic temporarily by combination chemotherapy for haematological malignancies is the principal use of bank platelets.

In general, the threshold for prophylactic transfusion in stable patients is a platelet count below 10×10^9/L. To cover invasive procedures the platelet count should be raised to above 50×10^9/L, and to 100×10^9/L if the invasive procedure involves the central nervous system.

Administration

ABO compatibility is preferable. Administration is via a large-bore cannula with a blood administration set. Care must be taken to avoid contamination of the blood administration set with previously transfused blood, and a fresh administration set should be used for platelet transfusion.

Table 12.31	Complications of blood transfusion	
Complication	**Cause**
Immune mediated	
Acute haemolytic transfusion reaction	ABO mismatch
Delayed transfusion reaction	Atypical antibodies
Febrile non-haemolytic transfusion reaction	HLA antibodies after multiple transfusions or in multigravida
Allergic reaction	Hypersensitivity or anaphylaxis in response to a component of transfused plasma
Graft-versus-host disease	Engraftment of donor T lymphocytes in the recipient
Transfusion-related acute lung injury	Leukocyte antibodies or other activators in the donor
Post-transfusion purpura	Sensitization to transfused platelet antigens
Infection	
Viral infection	HIV, hepatitis B and C, cytomegalovirus and parvovirus in donor blood product
Other infections	Bacterial contamination of the blood product, malaria parasites in the donor red cells
Volume related	
Circulatory overload	Excessive transfused volume
Coagulopathy	Massive red cell transfusion leading to dilutional coagulopathy
Other complications	
Tissue iron overload	Repeated red cell transfusion for indications other than blood loss
Haemolytic disease of the newborn	Transfusion of D-positive red cells to a D-negative female of child-bearing age

Complications

The greatest risk is infection transmission such as viruses and contaminating bacteria.

Fresh frozen plasma and cryoprecipitate

Preparation

Fresh frozen plasma (FFP) and cryoprecipitate (derived from fresh frozen plasma) is obtained from donated whole blood and stored at –30°C. The shelf life is 1 year, and products must be transfused within 4 hours of leaving storage conditions. A pool (unit) of fresh frozen plasma contains approximately 180–300 mL, cryoprecipitate between 10 and 20 mL.

The content of fibrinogen in fresh frozen plasma is between 2 and 5 mg/L and the concentrations of factor VIII and other clotting factors are usually more than 0.7 i.u./mL. In cryoprecipitate, the concentration of fibrinogen is between 150 and 300 mg per pack and the factor VIII and von Willebrand concentration is 80–120 i.u/pack.

Indications

The main indications for FFP are replacement of coagulation factors in the management of bleeding due to fibrinogen and clotting factor depletion in disseminated intravascular coagulation and massive blood transfusion and for plasma exchange in thrombotic thrombocytopenic purpura. Cryoprecipitate is principally used as a source of fibrinogen in DIC.

Administration

ABO compatibility is required, and administration is via a large-bore cannula with a blood administration set. Care must be taken to avoid volume overload in the case of FFP.

Complications

There are risks of infection due to viral transmission.

Haemolytic transfusion reactions

In red cell transfusion it is essential to ensure compatibility between antigens on the donor erythrocytes and antibodies present in the recipient's plasma in order to avoid acute haemolysis of the donor cells, which may be fatal.

Epidemiology

Deaths from ABO incompatible blood transfusions are rare but still occur despite being avoidable.

Pathology

A common cause of incompatible blood transfusion is clerical or administrative error leading to patient misidentification. This can occur at any stage from the venepuncture for blood sampling, through the screening procedure to the administration of red cells.

Acute massive intravascular haemolysis occurs when complement-activating antibodies, usually anti-A and anti-B, interact with the relevant antigen on transfused red cells. The immune reaction leads to circulatory shock whilst the red cell stroma and free haemoglobin cause renal impairment.

Delayed transfusion reactions occur when there are low titres of antibodies to one of the non-ABO blood group antigens in the recipient. Often, the low antibody levels are undetectable in the antibody screening procedure and do not cause lysis at the time of transfusion. Immune stimulation by the incompatible red cells leads to increasing antibody titres over a few days and eventual haemolysis of the incompatible transfused red cells.

Clinical features

In major haemolytic transfusion reaction, shock develops within minutes of starting an incompatible blood transfusion. There may be apprehension, flushing, agitation and pain at the infusion site and abdominal, flank or chest pain. On examination there is hypotension and fever. If disseminated intravascular coagulation ensues, generalized oozing can occur. Haemoglobinuria is a prominent feature but anuria may develop.

In delayed reactions, red cell lysis occurs after a delay of a few days producing anaemia and jaundice.

> **⚡ CLINICAL ALERT**
>
> *If there is any clinical suspicion of haemolytic transfusion reaction, the transfusion must be discontinued immediately and no further blood product administered until the diagnosis has been excluded, or, if confirmed, the cause identified and compatible blood issued.*

Investigations

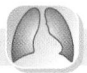

Returning of the suspected incompatible blood

The red cell pack and administration set and a sample of venous blood must be sent to the transfusion laboratory for urgent investigation to confirm the presence of acute haemolysis and determine the cause.

Full blood count and coagulation screen

Disseminated intravascular coagulation may develop leading to prolongation of clotting times and thrombocytopenia.

Urea and electrolytes

Monitoring of renal function is required.

Blood cultures

Bacterial contamination of the transfused blood product is a differential diagnosis.

Management

The management is largely supportive.

Fluid administration

Shock should be treated initially by intravenous administration of crystalloid or colloid. High fluid volume is required to maintain a good urine output (more than 30 mL/h) to minimize the risk of acute renal failure.

Furosemide

Intravenous furosemide may be required to maintain a good urine output.

Corticosteroids and anti-inflammatory agents

Chlorphenamine and intravenous hydrocortisone are administered if there is evidence of anaphylaxis. Inotrope may be required to maintain the blood pressure.

Dialysis

In established renal failure, dialysis may be required.

Antibiotics

Broad-spectrum antibiotics are reserved for patients with suspected bacterial contamination of the transfused blood.

Prognosis

Death is uncommon but can occur following incompatible blood transfusion.

Diseases of the breast

13

John Dewar, Alastair Thompson, Colin Purdie

SECTION 13.1 Introduction

Breast conditions are extremely common. Two thirds of women experience breast pain, and a third have changes in the consistency, shape or size of the breast during their life. General practitioners see the majority of women with breast problems. Only 1 in 10 are referred to hospital, of which 1 in 10 turn out to have malignancy.

Applied basic sciences of the breast

The breast is an adapted sweat gland composed microscopically of duct lobular units capable of manufacturing milk, transported via ducts to the nipple. The breast epithelium is subject to development and cyclical changes under the influence of oestrogen, progesterone and other hormones.

The breast lies on the pectoral fascia. The base extends from the second to the sixth rib and the sternal edge to the midaxillary line. When a mastectomy is performed, the extent of dissection to remove the adipose tissue extends from the clavicle to the rectus sheath (superior to inferior), and from the sternal edge to the anterior border of the latissimus dorsi (medial to lateral); in addition, the axillary tail of the breast is dissected and excised. As the base of the breast lies in close proximity to chest wall, during fine-needle aspiration there is a risk of puncturing the intercostal space and producing a pneumothorax.

The blood supply to the breast is from the axillary artery, internal thoracic artery and the second to the fourth intercostal arteries. The venous drainage accompanies the arterial supply. The breast is well-vascularized tissue and many perforating arteries are encountered during breast surgery.

The lymphatic drainage from the breast is principally to the axillary lymph nodes and thence to the supraclavicular and cervical nodes, although some drainage from the medial part of the breast goes to the internal mammary chain. The presence of lymph node metastasis is a very important clinical feature in breast cancer as it influences surgical management and the decision for postoperative adjuvant therapy and is an important predictor of survival.

The internal architecture of the breast consists of glandular tissue, stroma and adipose tissue. The glandular tissue consists of branching ducts and terminal lobules. The lobules consist of the portion of the glands that secrete milk. In breast cancer, the tumour type is classified according to the cell of origin, and may be ductal or lobular. The integrity of the basement membrane determines whether a cancer is in situ or invasive.

Symptoms of breast disease

There are a limited number of breast symptoms, which may be caused by a range of breast conditions. An important aim is to distinguish between benign and malignant disease. Apart from eliciting features that support the diagnosis of a benign condition, the history is invaluable to assess the risk of cancer.

Lump

The breast lump detected on self-examination is a very common presenting complaint. From Table 13.1, it is easy to appreciate that the majority of breast lumps are due to benign disease. However, significant proportions (26%) are due to breast cancer. The age of the patient is important, as benign disease is the most common cause before the age of 30, and breast cancer is uncommon before the age of 50 years (Fig. 13.1). Assessment of the risk for cancer is also important (see Past medical history, below).

Changes in the size of the lump with menstruation would favour the diagnosis of an aberration of normal development or involution, and multiple well-circumscribed spherical lumps are usually due to benign cysts. Precipitating causes such as localized trauma would suggest fat necrosis. Associated symptoms of tenderness, erythema and fever in a breast-feeding mother would suggest an abscess. Rarely, an inflammatory cancer may present in a similar manner.

Table 13.1	Diagnosis of patients with a breast lump*
Localized benign	38%
Carcinoma	26%
Cysts	15%
Fibroadenoma	13%
Periductal mastitis	1%
Duct ectasia	1%
Abscess	1%
Others	5%

* From Dixon JM, Mansel RE. ABC of breast diseases: congenital problems and aberrations of normal breast development and involution. BMJ 1994; 309: 797–800.

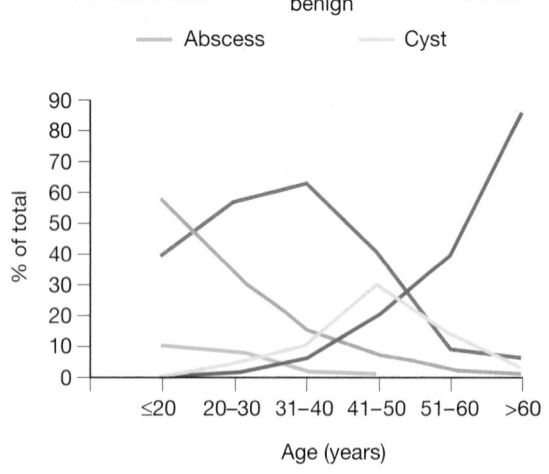

Fig. 13.1 Incidence of breast disorders with age.

Pain

Pain in the breast (mastalgia) is classified into cyclic (varies with menstruation), non-cyclic (does not vary with menstruation) or extramammary (pain that is not localized within breast tissue). Cyclic mastalgia is usually benign, and may be associated with a lump in aberrations of normal development or involution. Trauma (fat necrosis) and breast abscess are two common causes of non-cyclic mastalgia, usually associated with a breast lump.

In general, the risk of cancer in a woman presenting with breast pain as her only symptom is extremely low, and the management of breast pain is detailed on page 839.

Nipple discharge

Nipple discharge is usually milk, blood or pus. The discharge of milk is a normal process in lactating mothers; abnormal lactation is termed galactorrhoea. As the breast is also under endocrine control, galactorrhoea may be a symptom of underlying endocrine disease or (more commonly) a side effect of medication (Table 13.2).

Discharge of blood from the nipple is often worrying. A common cause is periductal mastitis, but it may uncommonly be a presenting feature of breast cancer.

Pus from the nipple is usually due to an underlying infection or a breast abscess that communicates with a duct.

Nipple retraction

Nipple retraction may be a congenital abnormality. When it develops later in life, it may be the result of tethering from an underlying breast cancer.

Skin changes

Any systemic disorder of the skin can affect the breast. One important symptom is new-onset eczema around the nipple, as Paget's disease of the breast due to malignant infiltration may present in this way.

Past medical history

The past medical history provides a lot of information on the breast cancer risk. Important risk factors are a previous history of breast cancer, post-menopausal status, a first-degree relative with breast cancer and a history of the use of hormone replacement therapy.

Table 13.2	Causes of galactorrhoea
Drug induced	
Phenothiazine	
Tricyclic antidepressants	
Opiates	
Verapamil	
Hypothalamic and pituitary stalk lesions	
Prolactinomas	
Null cell adenomas	

Examination of the breast

Inspection

Clinical examination should take place in a warm room with a chaperone. The woman should be examined sitting, naked to the waist, to look for any changes in the contour of the skin or nipples. Asking the woman to raise her arms above her head and subsequently push her hands in towards her hips helps when looking for any tethering of lesions within the breast to the underlying muscles or skin.

Palpation

It is often helpful to ask the patient where any localized problems lie and to avoid these until the end of the examination to exclude lesions elsewhere, then to focus on the specific problem.

With the patient lying comfortably on her back with arms behind her head, further inspection is undertaken to screen for any abnormalities in this different position. Palpation is performed by flattening the patient's breast tissue against the chest and, if necessary, the patient should turn to either side to ensure that the minimum amount of breast tissue is between the examiner's hand and the chest wall (Fig. 13.2).

Palpation may begin in the axillary tail of the breast and proceed to the midaxillary line, then progress medially in a superior to inferior direction. Palpation should be undertaken using the pulp of the fingers with varying degrees of pressure to detect lumps that are lying in different depths of the breast tissue.[1]

The regional lymph nodes should be examined (for the left axilla) by supporting the patient's right arm with the examiner's right arm and then gently palpating using the left hand in the axilla to seek any lumps or masses. A similar process on the other side should be followed by palpating the infraclavicular, supraclavicular and cervical regions for lymphadenopathy.

If a nipple discharge has been reported, ask the patient to squeeze the nipple to elicit any discharge, which should be tested using urinary dipsticks for blood to complete the breast examination. All examination findings should be meticulously recorded using diagrams.

The overall sensitivity of the clinical examination to detect (rule out) breast cancer is 54% and the specificity (to rule in breast cancer) is 94%.[1]

FURTHER INFORMATION

Saslow D, Hannan J, Osuch J, et al. Clinical breast examination: practical recommendations for optimizing performance and reporting. CA Cancer Journal for Clinicians 2004; 54: 327–344.

REFERENCE

(1) *Barton MB, Harris R, Fletcher SW. Does this patient have breast cancer?: The screening clinical breast examination: should it be done? How? JAMA 1999; 282: 1270–1280.*

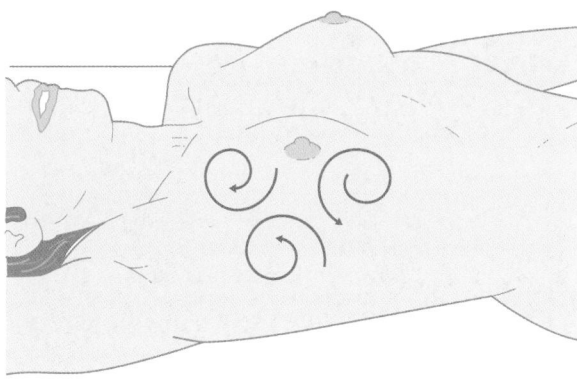

Fig. 13.2 Positioning and direction of palpation for breast examination.

SECTION 13.2 Investigations for breast disease

Fine-needle aspiration and core biopsy

Palpable lesions may undergo fine-needle aspiration cytology. A 21 or 23 gauge needle is used to aspirate cells from within the lump; the cells are spread on a slide and then stained for examination by a skilled cytologist.

When malignancy is suspected, a core biopsy using a 4 mm needle can be performed under local anaesthetic to yield tissue for histological confirmation.

The advantages of the fine-needle aspirate are that it can be spread, stained and reported on within 20 minutes in the clinic. A core biopsy, although it takes longer to process, shows architectural features lacking in a fine-needle aspirate. A core biopsy can distinguish between invasive and in situ carcinoma, which a fine-needle aspirate cannot.

Ultrasound scan

Ultrasound of the breast is particularly effective in younger women (under the age of 35 years) where the breast is often too radiologically dense for successful mammographic interpretation. Ultrasound is useful to distinguish solid from cystic lumps and can also be used to supplement mammography.

Mammography

Mammography (see Fig. 13.6, p. 842) is conducted using soft tissue X-rays through the breast, which is squashed between plates in a craniocaudal and then oblique view. It may be supplemented by additional localized or magnification views. Radiological imaging should localize any abnormalities which, if impalpable, can be followed up by ultrasound or mammographically guided fine-needle aspirate or core biopsy.

> ### RECENT ADVANCES
>
> *Increasingly, magnetic resonance imaging is used where mammography and ultrasound are inconclusive or to investigate young women at risk of breast cancer or those who have reconstructed breasts or implants.*[1]

> **REFERENCE**
>
> (1) *Bluemke DA, Gatsonis CA, Chen MH, et al. Magnetic resonance imaging of the breast prior to biopsy. JAMA 2004; 292: 2735–2742.*

SECTION 13.3 Benign breast conditions

Epidemiology

Benign breast changes are extremely common: a third of women at any one time may have features suggestive of benign breast conditions, and 90% of patients attending breast clinics in developed countries have benign conditions.

Pathology

There are a number of benign breast conditions, but the majority are due to aberrations of normal development and involution (ANDI), resulting in tiny focal areas of adenosis, apocrine metaplasia, sclerosis and microcysts (Table 13.3).

Infection of the breast normally occurs during lactation or in middle-aged smokers. Common organisms include *Staphylococcus aureus* and anaerobic bacteria.

Benign intraductal papilloma may imitate breast cancer by presenting as a bloodstained nipple discharge from a single duct. Fat necrosis secondary to trauma may imitate breast cancer as an ill-defined lump appearing radiologically similar to a carcinoma. Phyllodes tumour (a biphasic stromal and epithelial lesion) may have features ranging from benign through borderline to frankly sarcomatous (malignant).

Sclerosing adenosis and radial scars (disordered epithelial and stromal lesions) may mimic carcinoma and are often detected on breast screening.

Table 13.3	Common benign breast conditions			
	Usual age (years)	Features	Management	
Breast pain (mastalgia)	15–50	Cyclical (related to menses) or non-cyclic	Correct fitting bra Tamoxifen or danazol, bromocriptine if severe	
Fibroadenoma	<30	Smooth mobile lump	Excision if patient wants	
Cyst	35–55	One or multiple well-circumscribed lumps	Aspiration	
Infection	Breast-feeding mother, middle-aged smoker	Staphylococcal or anaerobic abscess	Aspiration or incision and drainage + antibiotics	
Gynaecomastia	Men <30	Unilateral swelling, usually physiological	Reassurance ± surgical excision if patient prefers	
	Men >50	Usually secondary to medication or liver disease		

Clinical features

The main presenting features are a breast lump, pain and discharge. The evaluation of these symptoms is detailed on page 835 and examination features are detailed on page 837. As previously mentioned, an important aim of clinical assessment is to establish the risk of underlying breast cancer, as it influences subsequent investigation and management.

Low-risk patients

Young patients with a clear precipitating cause such as trauma-induced fat necrosis or breast abscess need not undergo any further investigations, and the management is directed to the underlying cause. This group also includes young patients with a clear history of a painful breast lump that varies with menstruation without any other risk factors for breast cancer.

Intermediate and high-risk patients

Most patients fall into the category of intermediate to high risk and should undergo triple assessment to evaluate the possibility of breast cancer (clinical, radiological and pathological assessment). This group also contains those with asymptomatic lesions that are detected on routine breast screening.

Investigations

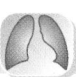

The common radiological assessment modalities are mammography and ultrasound, and pathological assessment is usually performed on breast tissue obtained using fine-needle aspiration or core biopsy. Magnetic resonance imaging (MRI) may play a role where there are diagnostic difficulties.

Mammography

Mammography is a useful investigation to screen for breast cancer, however the performance of the test is related to patient age. In young women, dense breast tissue renders the mammogram more difficult to interpret. As a result, the sensitivity to rule out cancer is lower before the age of 50.[1]

Ultrasound scan

The ultrasound scan is a useful modality to investigate patients with suspected breast cysts.

Fine-needle aspiration and core biopsy

Fine-needle aspiration (p. 838) can obtain tissue for cytology in patients with suspected malignant disease. It can be diagnostic and therapeutic for patients with simple breast cysts. The overall sensitivity and specificity to detect cancer is 93%.[2]

The sensitivity of fine-needle aspiration to detect cancer is 91%, compared to 95% for core biopsies (when 4 or more cores were obtained) for clinically suspicious lesions greater than 2 cm.[3]

Initial management

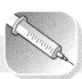

Reassurance

Reassurance is only appropriate for patients with a clear history of a benign condition and low risk of breast cancer. Often, the results of radiological and pathological examination are required before reassurance can be provided, and under these circumstances, the performance of the test needs to be considered as approximately 7% can have false negative results.

Medical management

Mastalgia

A simple initial step in the management of mastalgia is to ensure that the patient has a correctly fitted bra. Tamoxifen and danazol are two agents used to treat severe cyclical mastalgia. Tamoxifen treatment is associated with 53% of patients being free from breast pain, compared to 37% of patients receiving danazol.[4]

839

A second-line agent is bromocriptine. This also improves symptoms of breast pain but has a high non-compliance rate due to the side effects of nausea and dizziness in 45%.[5]

Evening primrose oil is a popular natural remedy, but unfortunately has not proven to be better than placebo.[6]

Surgical management

Excision biopsy

The main indications for excision biopsy are a suspicious but indeterminate lesion on triple assessment or a strong patient preference. Lesions that are positive for cancer should be managed as detailed on page 842.

Aspiration or incision and drainage of breast abscess

Initial aspiration may be attempted to drain a breast abscess under local or general anaesthetic. If the abscess is loculated, aspiration may not be effective. Formal incision and drainage will be required and the wound is packed to facilitate healing from the base to the skin surface to obliterate the abscess cavity.

Mastectomy

Mastectomy for benign disease is usually reserved for men with gynaecomastia for cosmetic reasons.

Prognosis

The prognosis for patients with confirmed benign breast disease is no different to that of the normal population.

REFERENCES

(1) *Mushlin AI, Kouides RW, Shapiro DE. Estimating the accuracy of screening mammography: a meta-analysis. American Journal of Preventive Medicine 1998; 14: 143–153.*
(2) *Vetrani A, Fulciniti F, Di Benedetto G, et al. Fine-needle aspiration biopsies of breast masses. An additional experience with 1153 cases (1985 to 1988) and a meta-analysis. Cancer 1992; 69: 736–740.*
(3) *Dennison G, Anand R, Makar SH, Pain JA. A prospective study of the use of fine-needle aspiration cytology and core biopsy in the diagnosis of breast cancer. Breast Journal 2003; 9: 491–493.*
(4) *Kontostolis E, Stefanidis K, Navrozoglou I, Lolis D. Comparison of tamoxifen with danazol for treatment of cyclical mastalgia. Gynecological Endocrinology 1997; 11: 393–397.*
(5) *Mansel RE, Dogliotti L. European multicentre trial of bromocriptine in cyclical mastalgia. Lancet 1990; 335: 190–193.*
(6) *Blommers J, de Lange-De Klerk ES, Kuik DJ, Bezemer PD, Meijer S. Evening primrose oil and fish oil for severe chronic mastalgia: a randomized, double-blind, controlled trial. American Journal of Obstetrics and Gynecology 2002; 187: 1389–1394.*

SECTION 13.4 Breast cancer

Breast cancer is the third most frequent cancer in the world. The lifetime risk of developing breast cancer is 1 in every 11 women.

Epidemiology

Breast cancer is common in all developed countries. The incidence is highest at 86 per 100 000 in the United States and 68 per 100 000 in Europe.[1] The incidence of breast cancer increases with age; it is rare in men (200 times less common).

Pathology

Predisposing factors

Breast cancer arises due to a combination of environmental and genetic factors. The environmental factors relate to the internal endocrine environment of the woman. Increased risk is associated with early age of menarche, late age first pregnancy, late menopause and prolonged use (more than 5 years) of hormone replacement therapy. Rarely, previous radiation exposure may be a feature, and other environ-mental factors such as alcohol, smoking and pesticides have all been implicated. In 5–10% of women who develop breast cancer, a strong genetic component can be found with the *BRCA1* gene (breast and ovarian cancer families) or *BRCA2* gene (breast and other cancers in families); the ataxia telangiectasia and *p53* genes are implicated in a small number of families. In most women the precise cause of breast cancer is uncertain.

Pathologic classification

Breast cancer arises in the terminal duct/lobular units: 80% are described as being ductal carcinoma of no special type (Fig. 13.3), 10% show lobular features, and a further 10% show special differentiation to tubular, medullary or other special types. In general, lobular carcinoma is difficult to detect radiologically and special types of invasive breast cancer have a better prognosis than ductal carcinoma of no special type. Ductal carcinoma in situ (DCIS, Fig. 13.4) is often detected adjacent to invasive ductal carcinoma although some patients (particularly those who are detected on screening) present with ductal carcinoma in situ alone and require surgical excision of these areas.

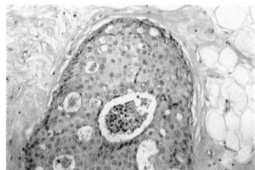

Fig. 13.3 Ductal carcinoma (no special type).

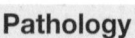

Fig. 13.4 Ductal carcinoma in situ.

The cancer itself can be graded (1–3) according to the cytological features, organization of the tumour cells and size. Staging is performed according to the TNM classification. In addition, the tumour size, lymph node status and grade can be combined to obtain prognostic information as in the Nottingham prognostic index in Table 13.4. Tumour oestrogen, progesterone receptor and HER2 status are extremely useful in guiding subsequent endocrine and biological therapy.

Table 13.4	The Nottingham prognostic index		

The Nottingham prognostic index (NPI) is calculated from: 0.2 × pathology tumour size (in cm) + pathology tumour grade (1, 2 or 3) + axillary node status (score 1 for no nodes involved, 2 for 1–3 nodes involved, 3 for 4 or more nodes involved)

Prognostic group	Index value	10-year survival (%)
Excellent	≤2.4	91
Good	≤3.4	82
Moderate I	≤4.4	73
Moderate II	≤5.4	55
Poor	>5.4	26

TNM staging of breast cancer (clinical stage)

T—Primary tumour

TX   Primary tumour cannot be assessed

T0   No evidence of primary tumour

Tis   Carcinoma in situ

    Intraductal carcinoma

    Lobular carcinoma in situ

    Paget's disease of the nipple with no tumour

T1   Tumour 2 cm or less in greatest dimension

    T1a   0.5 cm or less in greatest dimension

    T1b   More than 0.5 cm but not more than 1 cm in greatest dimension

    T1c   More than 1 cm but not more than 2 cm in greatest dimension

T2   Tumour more than 2 cm but not more than 5 cm in greatest dimension

T3   Tumour more than 5 cm in greatest dimension

T4   Tumour of any size with direct extension to chest wall or skin

    T4a   Extension to chest wall

    T4b   Oedema (including peau d'orange),

        or ulceration of the skin of the breast

        or satellite skin nodules confined to the same breast

    T4c   Both 4a and 4b

    T4d   Inflammatory carcinoma

N—Lymph nodes

NX   Regional lymph nodes cannot be assessed (e.g. previously removed)

N0   No regional lymph node metastasis

N1   Metastasis to movable ipsilateral axillary node(s)

N2   Metastasis to ipsilateral axillary node(s) fixed to one another or to other structures

N3   Metastasis to ipsilateral internal mammary lymph node(s)

M—Metastasis

MX   Distant metastases cannot be assessed

M0   No distant metastasis

M1   Distant metastasis

Scope of disease

Most patients present with disease that is apparently localized to the breast and regional lymph nodes. Despite staging investigations, only 7% will have distant metastases detected at first presentation. However, many more patients have systemic involvement, and occult metastases only become apparent in time. Therefore it is difficult to make an accurate prediction for survival. Apart from regional treatments, adjuvant systemic treatment is administered to target any undetected disease that may be present.

Local disease

This usually presents as a lump. Local infiltration into the chest wall can occur, resulting in a fixed mass.

Metastatic disease

The main sites for metastatic disease are bone, lung, brain and liver. Distant spread can give rise to pathological fractures, pleural effusions, localizing neurological abnormalities, jaundice, hepatomegaly or ascites.

Paraneoplastic disease

Apart from hypercalcaemia, paraneoplastic effects are uncommon.

Clinical features

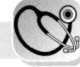

Most patients with breast cancer present with a recently noticed lump on the breast. A detailed history is required to evaluate the risk for breast cancer (p. 835). The two most important risk factors are age and a positive family history. A small proportion of patients present with the complications of metastatic disease such as a pathological fracture or liver metastases.

On examination, features of a breast lump associated with increased risk of cancer are tethering (Fig. 13.5), a large size (more than 2 cm) and a fixed, hard or irregular appearance.[2] Features of more advanced disease include axillary

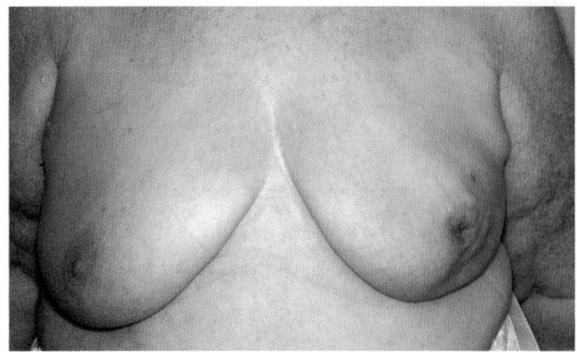

Fig. 13.5 Left-sided breast cancer with tethering, nipple retraction and visible axillary lymphadenopathy.

or supraclavicular lymphadenopathy, the presence of a fungating mass, cachexia, jaundice, hepatomegaly or a pleural effusion.

Initial investigations

Clinical examination, radiological imaging and pathological analysis form the standard triple assessment for breast cancer.

Mammography
Mammography is undertaken of both breasts (Fig. 13.6). The performance of this investigation has been detailed on page 838. Features suggestive of cancer are a mass with ill-defined or spiculated borders, microcalcifications or distortion of the adjacent breast tissue.

Fine-needle aspiration cytology or core needle biopsy
Multiple repeated aspirations are undertaken and the cells are smeared on a slide for cytological analysis. When malignancy is suspected a core biopsy is undertaken (p. 838).

Further investigations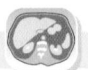

Following diagnosis of breast cancer by triple assessment, the patient undergoes further staging investigations to determine the clinical TNM stage for subsequent management.

Full blood count
FBC may reveal anaemia from chronic disease, or less commonly as a result of bone marrow infiltration.

Liver profile
Raised liver enzymes may indicate liver metastasis, and raised alkaline phosphatase bony metastases.

Serum calcium
Serum calcium levels may be raised from bony metastases.

Chest X-ray
A CXR is required to screen for pulmonary metastatic disease.

Ultrasound of the liver
A liver ultrasound scan is required for patients with hepatomegaly or irregularity on clinical examination or patients with abnormal liver function tests.

Bone scan
A technetium-99m (^{99m}Tc) labelled phosphate bone scan (Fig. 13.7) should be performed for patients with localized bony tenderness, raised serum alkaline phosphatase or raised serum calcium.

Initial management

Patient education and counselling
Having acquired a histopathological diagnosis confirming breast cancer, it is necessary to communicate with the patient to discuss the management options and determine the optimum treatment strategy.

The multidisciplinary management of patients in the diagnosis and decision-making process (at the clinical pathology conference) at each stage of treatment has contributed to a marked improvement in the prognosis of patients with breast cancer in the last decade.

Surgical management

Surgery for breast cancer aims to establish local and regional control and to provide information (e.g. nodal

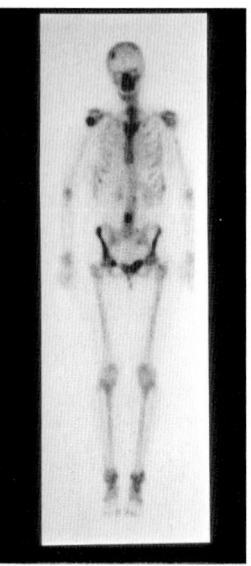

Fig. 13.7 A bone scan revealing 'hotspots' in the cranium, right shoulder and vertebrae, suggestive of metastatic disease.

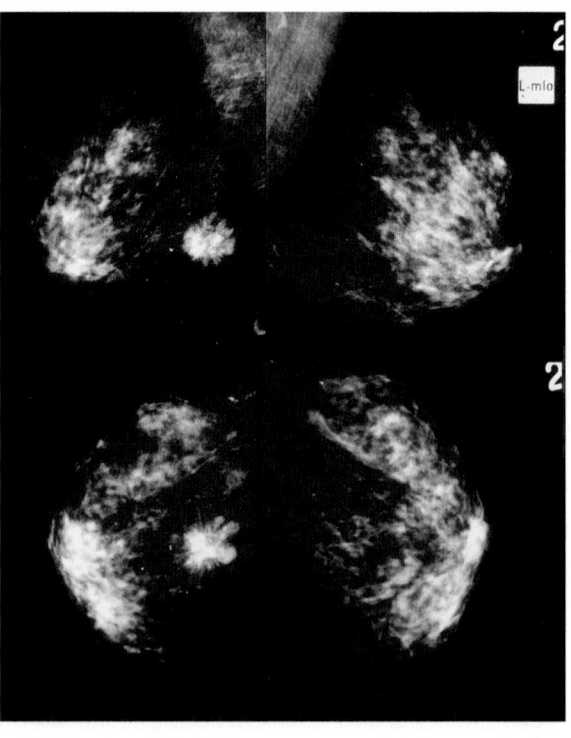
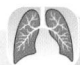

Fig. 13.6 A mammogram showing a densely calcified spiculated lesion in the right breast.

status) to guide further therapy. There are three important aspects to breast surgery: management of the tumour, management of the axillary nodes, and breast reconstruction (where required).

Management of the tumour

The extent of the surgery will depend on the apparent size of the lesion, as an adequate resection margin is important. Wide local excision is a suitable option for a small lump in a large breast, whereas mastectomy is more appropriate for more extensive disease.

Needle localization biopsy

Impalpable (usually screen-detected) cancers require guide-wire placement to direct surgical excision.

Wide local excision and quadrantectomy

Local excision is a reasonable option for patients with a small lump (less than 4 cm) and an adequate amount of surrounding breast tissue. A circumferential incision is made over the lump and the mass excised with a surrounding cuff of normal breast tissue (Fig. 13.8).

Mastectomy

A transverse elliptical incision is made, and excision of all breast tissue is undertaken from the clavicle (superior) to the anterior border of the latissimus dorsi (lateral) to the rectus sheath (inferior) and midline (medial). In addition, the axillary tail of the breast is dissected and excised. Suction drains are left at the end of the procedure, and the skin flaps are closed.

Complications of breast surgery include haematoma, infection and seroma formation. The cosmetic appearance can vary widely according to the extent of surgery.

Management of the axillary lymph nodes

Ideally tissue diagnosis is made on core biopsy before any surgery so a single operation can be performed to deal with the tumour in the breast and at the same time regional lymph node assessment, either through a sampling technique (sentinel node biopsy, axillary sample) or axillary clearance.

Sentinel node biopsy or axillary node sampling

Sentinel node biopsy entails injection of radiolabelled dye plus visible blue dye around the tumour which, at the time of surgery, can then be traced to the first or sentinel node to which the tumour drains (Fig. 13.9). Following pathological examination, if the sentinel node is free of tumour it is likely that the rest of the axilla is free and therefore can be left alone. Similarly, a four-node axillary sample performed without the aid of dyes can indicate the axillary status.

Axillary clearance

If tumour is found on sentinel or sampling techniques, either radiotherapy to the axilla or an axillary clearance may be performed. An axillary clearance aims to excise all lymph nodes and adjacent tissue inferior to the axillary vein and deep to the pectoralis muscles. Axillary surgery provides evidence for prognosis and to guide adjuvant therapy but importantly can establish local control in the axilla if the cancer has metastasized to the axillary tissues.

The complications of axillary lymph node surgery include damage to the intercostal brachial nerve, seroma formation, infection and, in the medium to long term, upper limb lymphoedema.

Breast reconstruction

Approximately 50% of women do not require a mastectomy, and undergo breast conservation surgery with excellent cosmetic results (Fig. 13.8). Women who undergo mastectomy or quadrantectomy may seek to improve the appearance of the chest wall, and it is an individual choice whether to use an external prosthesis to fit inside a bra or to undergo breast reconstruction.

Breast reconstructive surgery

Breast reconstruction can be performed either at the time of mastectomy or at a later date and can be performed using a breast implant with or without autologous flap reconstruction.

Breast reconstruction using a tissue expander following mastectomy allows stretching of the skin and pectoral

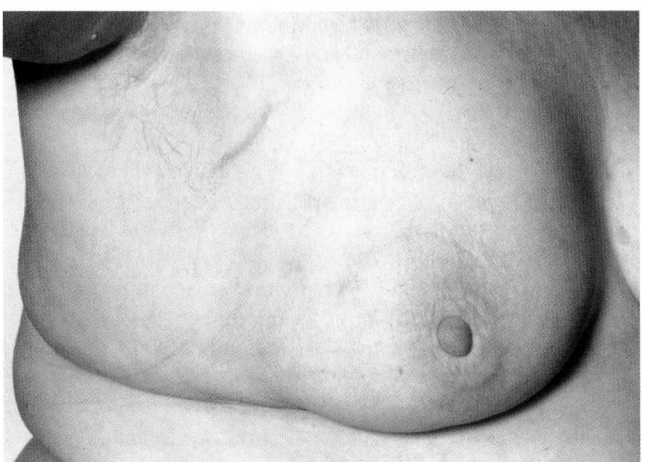

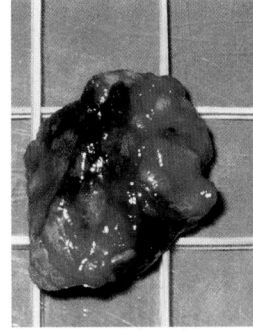

Fig. 13.8 Breast conservation surgery.

Fig. 13.9 The blue dye uptake can be seen in this sentinel node.

843

muscles over a balloon which can then be partly deflated or replaced with a shaped silicon prosthesis.

Autologous flap reconstruction is performed with either a unilateral latissimus dorsi flap (which may be supplemented by a silicon or saline implant) or by using the tissue that lies transversely over rectus abdominis muscle (TRAM flap) either as a free flap or as a pedicled flap hinging on the superior epigastric pedicle. Both techniques can give excellent cosmetic results in terms of appearance and the feel of the tissue (Fig. 13.10).

Non-surgical management

Neoadjuvant therapy

Large tumours (more than 3 cm) and locally advanced tumours (T4) may be treated with chemotherapy or endocrine therapy prior to surgery to reduce the size and tumour burden. In 8–12%, this results in complete disappearance of the tumour (on pathological review) and improves the prognosis. In other patients it may allow breast conservation surgery instead of mastectomy.

Adjuvant radiotherapy

Radiotherapy is used to reduce local recurrence after surgery. The indications are patients who have had breast conservation surgery, patients at increased risk of local relapse after mastectomy (involved margins, extensive lymphovascular invasion, extensive axillary lymph node involvement, tumour size >4 cm), and locally to the axilla where a sample of lymph nodes contained tumour.

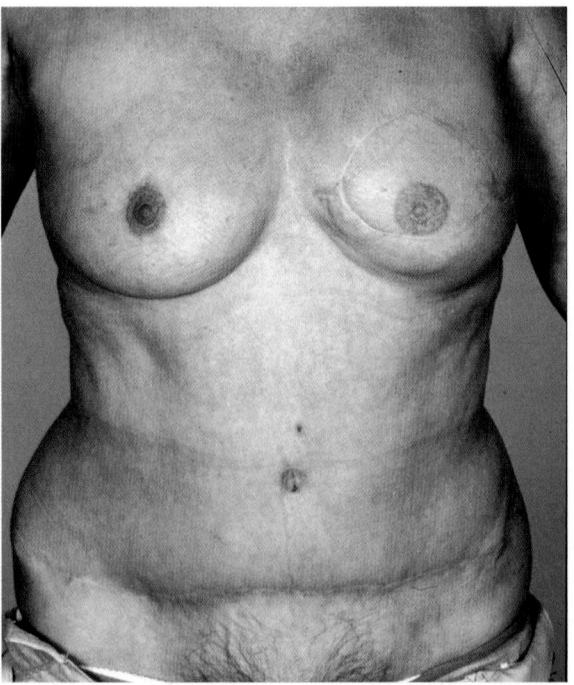

Fig. 13.10 Breast reconstruction after mastectomy.

Radiotherapy is administered to the breast or chest wall, usually by two fields that enter either side of the breast (medial and lateral), thus including the chest wall but minimizing the dose to the underlying lung and heart. The latter is important since in the long term radiation to the heart can be associated with subsequent ischaemic heart disease.

Radiotherapy following surgery for breast cancer (mastectomy or lumpectomy) reduces the risk of local recurrence in the breast or chest wall by about two thirds.[3] Thus, if the risk of recurrence is 60%, radiotherapy will reduce it to 20%, which is clearly useful. If, however, the risk is only 3%, then the risk of recurrence is reduced to 1%, which is less useful.

The main side effects of radiotherapy are erythema of the skin, which in a small number of cases may amount to moist desquamation (most frequently seen in the inframammary fold) and fatigue. Both are often most marked after completion of the radiotherapy; discomfort on swallowing (supraclavicular radiotherapy) or a dry cough may also occur. In contrast to chemotherapy, nausea and vomiting do not usually occur and there is no alopecia. If the lymph node areas (supraclavicular fossa and axilla) are irradiated, there is an increased risk (<5%) of lymphoedema of the ipsilateral arm and usually some reduction of mobility of the glenohumeral joint. For patients who have had an axillary clearance, radiotherapy to the axilla increases the risk of lymphoedema to about 30%, without any improvement in local control; radiotherapy should therefore be avoided in these patients.

Systemic adjuvant therapy

Systemic therapy following surgery aims to reduce the risk of distant relapse and improve survival. Both hormone therapy and chemotherapy reduce the risk of disease relapse by 20–25%, but the absolute benefit is greatest in those patients at the greatest risk of relapse. Thus the absolute benefit in terms of reduction of risk of death will be about 10–12% in high-risk patients, but may only be 1–2% in patients with good-prognosis tumours.

Hormone therapy

Hormone therapy (tamoxifen, ovarian ablation—surgical or medical, aromatase inhibitors) is only of benefit for patients with tumours that express oestrogen receptor or progesterone receptor.[4,5]

Cytotoxic chemotherapy

Cytotoxic chemotherapy is of potential benefit to all groups of patients but is relatively more effective in younger patients (under 50 vs over 50 years). There are few data for patients aged over 70.

Originally, the main chemotherapy regimen used was a combination of the drugs cyclophosphamide, methotrexate and 5-fluoruracil (CMF), but subsequent studies have shown that regimens containing an anthracycline (doxorubicin or epirubicin) are more effective.[6] Trials are ongoing to discover whether adding a taxane (docetaxel or paclitaxel) confers any further benefit.

Combination therapy

Combinations of hormone therapy and chemotherapy for patients with oestrogen receptor positive tumours are more effective than one agent alone, but by less than the simple addition of their individual benefits.

The main side effects of systemic adjuvant therapy are summarized in Table 13.5.

Management of localized recurrence

Local recurrence of breast cancer is distressing to the patient and can be difficult to control. In a small number of patients who have local recurrence as the only site of disease, the local recurrence acts as the nidus for metastatic spread and so is associated with an increased mortality.

Table 13.5	Main side effects of systemic treatments

Ovarian ablation

Infertility if performed surgically (usually laparoscopically), but reversible if performed medically (by monthly injection of an LHRH agonist)

Menopausal symptoms (hot flushes, atrophic vaginitis), which are usually more marked compared with a physiological menopause

Tamoxifen and aromatase inhibitors*

Hot flushes

Weight gain

Increased risk of deep venous thrombosis and hence pulmonary embolus

Long-term use is associated with an increased risk of endometrial cancer

In post-menopausal women, it provides a measure of protection against osteoporosis

Cytotoxic chemotherapy

Nausea and vomiting, although current antiemetic regimens are reasonably effective

Neutropenia, risk of neutropenic sepsis (particularly at 10–14 days post therapy)

Alopecia, particularly with anthracyclines

Induction of an early menopause (in premenopausal women, especially if over 40)

Lassitude, especially in the latter cycles and after completion of chemotherapy

*From this list, only hot flushes are associated with the use of aromatase inhibitors.

The treatment options for localized recurrence include surgical resection, radical radiotherapy and systemic therapy. The choice will depend on operability, prior treatment and the patient's overall medical state.

Management of systemic metastasis

The most common sites for local spread of breast cancer are the skin and subcutaneous tissues; the most common sites for distant metastasis are bone (Fig. 13.7), pleura, liver, lung and brain, although any organ can be affected. Once breast cancer has spread to distant sites the patient is incurable but not untreatable. The aim of therapy is to maintain a good quality of life for as long as possible. This can usually be best achieved by controlling the metastatic disease with effective systemic therapy.

Endocrine therapy

Endocrine therapy includes ovarian ablation (for pre-menopausal women), anti-oestrogen (tamoxifen), aromatase inhibitors (anastrozole, letrozole and exemestane for post-menopausal women) and progestogens (megestrol acetate, medroxyprogesterone acetate).

For patients whose tumour is oestrogen receptive and/or progesterone receptor positive, endocrine therapy can give effective control in about 60% with modest side effects. In view of the relative lack of toxicity, endocrine therapy is usually first-line treatment, although chemotherapy would normally be given for patients with liver metastases or lymphangitis carcinomatosis of the lungs since the response to endocrine therapy at these sites is poor. The choice of endocrine therapy is influenced by menopausal status and prior use of adjuvant endocrine therapy. If the patient responds to one agent, then on relapse a further response may be obtained with a different class of agent.

Cytotoxic chemotherapy

Breast cancer responds well to chemotherapy, and response is not influenced by menopausal status or the presence of hormone receptors in the cancer. Chemotherapy is generally used for patients with hormone receptor negative disease or hormone receptor positive disease that is refractory to hormones. A wide variety of chemotherapy agents can be used, although the mainstay remains anthracycline-based combinations. The choice depends mainly on prior adjuvant chemotherapy, toxicity profile and the patient's overall condition. Drug combinations or single agents can be used sequentially, with each agent being used on failure of the previous regimen.

Treatment of bone metastasis

Bone is a frequent site of metastases from breast cancer. Pain from these lesions can be helped not only by analgesics but also by local radiotherapy. Regular administration of bisphosphonates, either intravenously or orally, can reduce the morbidity of bony metastatic disease by reducing the amount of pain and decreasing the risk of fracture. Pathological fractures, especially in long bones (humerus, femur) may require orthopaedic intervention and those at risk may need this prophylactically.

Other specific treatments

Pleural effusion should be drained and pleurodesis obtained. Ascites may also require drainage. High-dose steroids and radiotherapy may help in patients with brain metastases. Occasionally, a single brain metastasis may be resected.

RECENT ADVANCES

In patients with tumours that express the erbB-2 oncogene (about 20% of breast cancers), the use of an antibody (trastuzumab) is another therapeutic option. In future, targeting the epidermal growth factor receptor may also be beneficial.

Prognosis

In most developed countries the average 5- and 10-year survival probability is approximately 80% and 60% respectively. The median survival of patients with metastatic breast cancer is 2 years.

A more accurate prediction for survival for patients with operable disease can be obtained with the Nottingham prognostic index, a formula that summates the histological grade, axillary nodal status and the tumour size (Table 13.4).

REFERENCES

(1) *Parkin DM, Pisani P, Ferlay J. Global cancer statistics. CA Cancer Journal for Clinicians 1999; 49: 33–64.*
(2) *Barton MB, Harris R, Fletcher SW. Does this patient have breast cancer?: the screening clinical breast examination: Should it be done? How? JAMA 1999; 282: 1270–1280.*
(3) *Favourable and unfavourable effects on long-term survival of radiotherapy for early breast cancer: an overview of the randomised trials. Early Breast Cancer Trialists' Collaborative Group. Lancet 2000; 355: 1757–1770.*
(4) *Ovarian ablation in early breast cancer: overview of the randomised trials. Early Breast Cancer Trialists' Collaborative Group. Lancet 1996; 348: 1189–1196.*
(5) *Tamoxifen for early breast cancer: an overview of the randomised trials. Early Breast Cancer Trialists' Collaborative Group. Lancet 1998; 351: 1451–1467.*
(6) *Polychemotherapy for early breast cancer: an overview of the randomised trials. Early Breast Cancer Trialists' Collaborative Group. Lancet 1998; 352: 930–942.*
(7) *Piccart-Gebhart MJ, Procter M, Leyland-Jones B, et al, the Herceptin Adjuvant (HERA) Trial Study Team. Trastuzumab after adjuvant chemotherapy in HER2-positive breast cancer. New England Journal of Medicine 2005; 353: 1659–1672.*

SECTION 13.5 Breast cancer screening

Large studies in Sweden, UK and North America have demonstrated that mammographic screening detects small cancers and improves survival in women aged 40–74. As a consequence, national screening programmes have been implemented in some developed countries.[1]

Based on cost effectiveness calculations, in the UK women aged 50–70 are invited to participate in the breast cancer screening programme with the aim of detecting 6 cancers for every 1000 women screened.

Currently breast cancer screening consists of mammography, performed on a 3-yearly basis. Women with abnormalities on the mammogram undergo triple assessment (clinical, radiological and pathological) to further evaluate the abnormality and if necessary receive the appropriate treatment.

REFERENCE

(1) *Humphrey LL, Helfand M, Chan BKS, Woolf SH. Breast Cancer Screening: A Summary of the Evidence for the U.S. Preventive Services Task Force. Annals of Internal Medicine 2002; 137: 347–360.*

Diseases of the skin

14

Hiva Fassihi, Ian White

Introduction

Applied basic sciences of the skin

Anatomy

The skin consists of three distinctive layers: the epidermis, dermis and subcutaneous fat. All normal skin has this same basic structure (Fig. 14.1). However, there is considerable morphological variation in different regions of the body, reflecting different functional demands. Normal skin can vary in thickness, colour and presence of hairs, glands and nails.

The epidermis

The epidermis is a stratified squamous keratinizing epithelium. It is composed of different morphological layers (Table 14.1, Fig. 14.2). The principal cells in the epidermis are the keratinocytes. They arise in the stratum basale (germinal/basal layer) adjacent to the dermis, as a result of mitosis of the resident stem cells. They undergo maturation and gradually migrate through the spinous and granular layers until they reach the most superficial layer, the stratum corneum (horny layer). This outermost mature keratinized layer is shed continuously and is replaced by progressive movement of keratinocytes up from the germinal layer. In humans the process of maturation of a basal cell through to desquamation takes from 25 to 50 days in normal skin.

Keratins are intermediate filament proteins produced by keratinocytes. They form the major component of the keratinocytes' cytoskeleton. There are two main groups, type I (acidic) and type II (neutral and basic). Keratin intermediate filament formation involves the dimerization of a keratin pair, with one of the pair having type I keratin and the other type II. In normal basal epidermis the predominant keratins are K5 and K14, compared to the suprabasal spinous layer where K1 and K10 are preferentially expressed.

Adjacent keratinocytes are linked by a series of junctional complexes, principally desmosomes, adherens junctions, gap junctions and tight junctions. Desmosomes consist of transmembrane glycoproteins, the cadherins (desmocollin and desmoglein) as well as other components such as desmoplakins and plakoglobulins that link the desmosomal plaque to the keratin filament cytoskeleton.

In addition to the keratinocytes, three other cell types are found in the epidermis. These are the melanocytes, Merkel cells and Langerhans' cells.

Melanocytes are dendritic cells that are usually located along the basal layer of the epidermis. They are of neuroectodermal origin (neural crest) and are responsible for skin pigmentation through production of melanin. Numbers

Table 14.1	Layers of the skin
1. The stratum corneum (horny layer)	
2. The stratum lucidum, only present in extremely thick skin	
3. The stratum granulosum (granular layer)	
4. The stratum spinosum (prickle cell layer)	
5. The stratum basale (germinal/basal layer)	

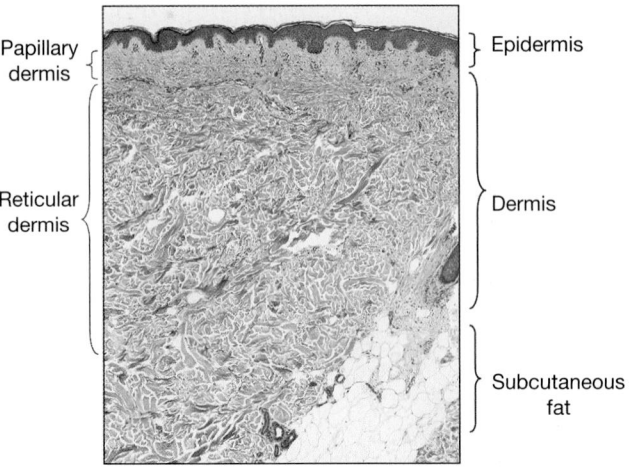

Papillary dermis

Epidermis

Reticular dermis

Dermis

Subcutaneous fat

Fig. 14.1 Histology of normal skin.
Courtesy of Dr Alistair Robson, Consultant Dermatopathologist, St John's Institute of Dermatology, St Thomas' Hospital, London, UK.

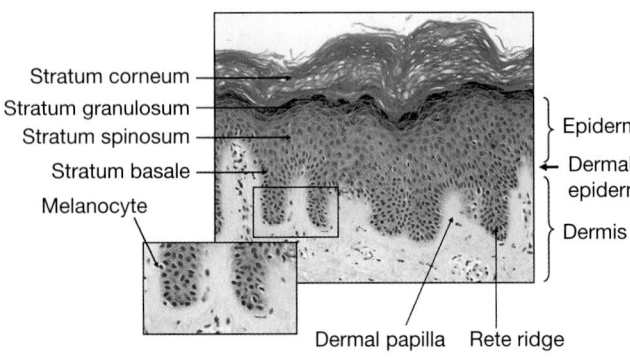

Stratum corneum
Stratum granulosum
Stratum spinosum
Stratum basale
Melanocyte

Epidermis

Dermal-epidermal

Dermis

Dermal papilla   Rete ridge

Fig. 14.2 Histology of normal epidermis showing the cell layers.
Courtesy of Dr Alistair Robson, Consultant Dermatopathologist, St John's Institute of Dermatology, St Thomas' Hospital, London, UK.

of melanocytes vary between different parts of the body, ranging from one in four to one in ten basal keratinocytes, being highest on the skin of the face and the external genitalia. The number of melanocytes is relatively constant between individuals of different race; the differences in skin colour are due to the amount of melanin produced and not the number of melanocytes present.

Melanin is synthesized from the amino acid tyrosine within melanocytes. It accumulates within secretory vesicles known as melanosomes and is then transferred through the long dendritic processes to the surrounding keratinocytes in the basal layer. The size and rate of production of melanosomes vary between individuals of one race and between racial groups. Sunlight promotes melanin synthesis, as does the pituitary hormone melanocyte-stimulating hormone (MSH), although the physiological importance of this is not well understood.

Merkel cells are associated with free nerve endings in thick skin (such as on the fingers) and are presumed to serve as sensory receptors.

Langerhans' cells have long dendritic processes and are of particular importance in antigen processing. When stimulated they migrate via dermal lymphatics to regional lymph nodes for presentation of the antigen to T lymphocytes. They are typically found in the upper layers of the epidermis.

The dermal–epidermal junction

The dermal–epidermal junction separates the epidermis from the dermis. It is characterized by downward folds of epidermis called rete ridges which interdigitate with upward projections of the dermis called dermal papillae (Fig. 14.2). At the interface between the epidermis and dermis is the basement membrane zone. Hemidesmosomes are the major adhesion units at the dermal–epidermal junction. Ultrastructurally, they are composed of electron-dense inner and outer plaques that bind to intracellular keratin intermediate filaments and also connect to the epidermal basement membrane via anchoring filaments, which in turn bind to the lamina densa and anchoring fibrils in the superficial papillary dermis (Fig. 14.3). Keratin intermediate filaments are made up of K5 and K14 and are within the keratinocyte cytoplasm. They are capable of binding both plectin and the 230 kDa bullous pemphigoid antigen within the hemidesmosomal inner plaque. They interact with the two major transmembrane molecules, integrin $\alpha6\beta4$ and type XVII collagen (also known as the 180 kDa bullous pemphigoid antigen). Integrin $\alpha6\beta4$ is the receptor for the extracellular ligand laminin 5 which in turn binds to type VII collagen, the major component of anchoring fibrils. Antibodies to any of these structural proteins or mutations of the genes encoding these proteins result in the different types of blistering skin disorders (p. 882).

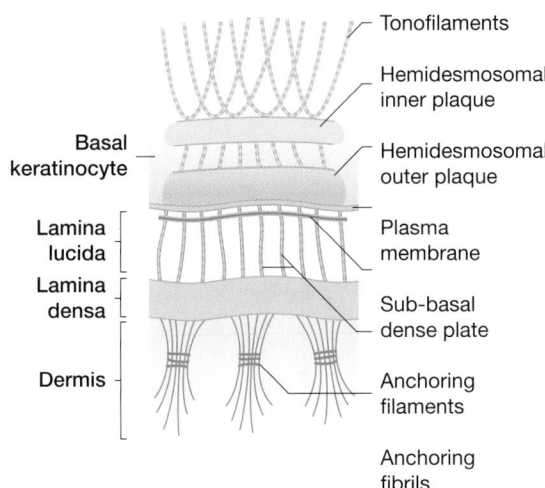

Basal keratinocyte — Tonofilaments — Hemidesmosomal inner plaque — Hemidesmosomal outer plaque — Plasma membrane — Sub-basal dense plate — Anchoring filaments — Anchoring fibrils

Lamina lucida — Lamina densa — Dermis

Fig. 14.3 The cutaneous basement membrane zone. Courtesy of Prof John McGrath and the Genetic Skin Disease Group, St John's Institute of Dermatology, St Thomas' Hospital, London, UK.

The dermis

The dermis is a thick layer of dense fibroelastic tissue which is highly vascular and contains many sensory receptors. It provides nutrition to the avascular epidermis. The dermis is divided into two zones. Superficially, the dermal papillae and the tissue immediately below them comprise the papillary dermis. The main bulk of the dermis below is the reticular layer (Fig. 14.1).

There are two main proteins in the dermis. The first is collagen, which is the major component of the dermal fibrous connective tissue and provides strength. A number of subtypes of collagen are recognized and the dermis consists predominantly of type I mixed with smaller amounts of type III and type V collagen, all of which can be demonstrated by Masson's trichrome stain. In the papillary dermis there is fine interlacing of collagen fibres. However, in the reticular layer the collagen fibres are coarse and arranged in thick irregular bundles. The other protein is elastin (demonstrated by elastic van Gieson stain), which constitutes only a minor component of the dermal fibrous connective tissue and gives the skin its elasticity. It forms a fine interlacing network of fibres in the papillary dermis, whereas in the reticular layer the elastin forms long thick fibres which follow the path of the coarse collagen bundles. The main type of cell in the dermis is the fibroblast, and this is responsible for the synthesis of collagen, elastin and the ground substance. The latter is composed of hyaluronic acid, chondroitin-4-sulphate and dermatan sulphate in addition to fibronectin.

Meissner's corpuscle is an encapsulated nerve ending responsible for touch reception. It is found in the dermal papillae and consists of nerve fibres and stacked Schwann cells surrounded by a perineural fibrous capsule.

The Pacinian corpuscle is responsible for deep pressure and vibration sensation. It is usually located in the deep dermis and subcutaneous fat. Greatest numbers are present on the palms, soles and around the external genitalia. It is composed of concentric Schwann cell lamellae surrounding a nerve terminal.

Epidermal appendages

Sweat glands, sebaceous glands, hair follicles and nails are epithelial structures termed epidermal appendages since they originate during embryological development from downgrowth of epidermal epithelium into the dermis and subcutaneous fat.

The sweat glands

Eccrine sweat glands are distributed in the skin of most parts of the body but are especially numerous on the palms, soles, axillae and forehead. They are simple coiled tubular glands which secrete a watery fluid onto the skin surface. The ducts consist of an outer layer of contractile myoepithelial cells and an inner layer of secretory cells. The coiled, secretory portions of these glands are important for thermoregulation. When the body needs to lose heat, skin blood flow and sweat production increases. Sweat evaporation causes cooling of the skin surface and loss of heat from the underlying vascular bed. These glands are innervated by cholinergic fibres of the sympathetic nervous system.

Apocrine sweat glands are mainly confined to the axillae, groins and anogenital regions and produce a viscid, milky secretion. They are composed of an outer layer of myoepithelial cells and an inner layer of cuboidal to columnar cells which display so-called 'decapitation secretion'. They are innervated by adrenergic fibres of the sympathetic nervous system.

Hair

Hairs are highly modified keratinized structures produced by hair follicles, which are cylindrical downgrowths of the surface epithelium surrounded by a connective tissue sheath. Hair growth takes place at the terminal bulbous expansion of the follicle called the hair bulb. This consists of actively dividing epithelial cells, the hair root, enclosing a network of capillaries, the dermal papillae. The hair follicle consists of five concentric layers of epithelial cells. The epithelial cells surrounding the dermal papilla proliferate to form the four inner layers of the follicle whilst the outermost layer merely represents a downward continuation of the stratum basale of the surface epithelium. The innermost three layers form the hair shaft (medulla, cortex forming the bulk of the hair, and the cuticle). The fourth layer of the follicle constitutes the internal root sheath. This layer disintegrates at the level of the sebaceous gland ducts. The outermost layer is the external root sheath. This layer is separated from the connective tissue sheath by a specialized basement membrane known as the glassy membrane (Fig. 14.4).

A bundle of smooth muscle cells, the arrector pili muscle, is inserted obliquely into the perifollicular connective tissue sheath. This muscle is innervated by the sympathetic nervous system. Contraction of this muscle causes the hair to become erect.

849

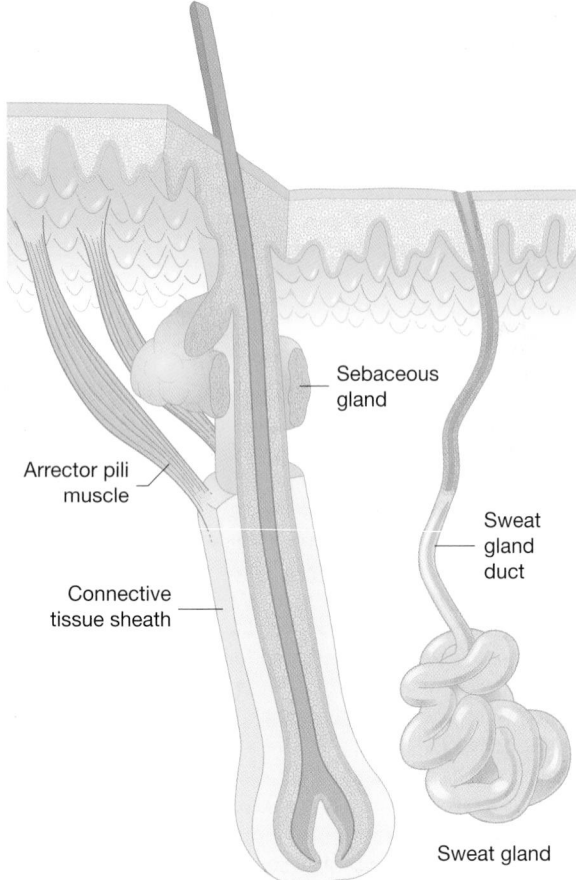

Fig. 14.4 A hair and its follicle.

Three terms are used to describe hair. Lanugo hairs are long, unmedullated hair grown in utero and shed during the end of pregnancy and the first few months after birth. In infancy, childhood and females, body hair is fine and soft and known as vellus. These hairs are short, non-pigmented hairs produced by follicles that penetrate only into the papillary dermis. They are medullated and the hair shafts are no longer than the inner root sheath of the follicle that produces them. In contrast, terminal hairs are coarse and found on the scalp. They are produced by follicles that penetrate to the reticular dermis. They are medullated and wider than the inner root sheath of the follicle that produces them. Male sex hormone production at puberty is responsible for the development of further terminal pubic and axillary hair in both sexes.

Hair shaft diameter, colour and density vary according to race, age, sex and region of the body. Hairs grow discontinuously with periods of growth followed by periods of rest. Hair follicles cycle through three stages: anagen refers to the active growth phase, during catagen the growth stops and the cycling portion of the follicle undergoes apoptosis, and in telogen the hair is shed. The duration of

these growth and rest periods varies in different parts of the body.

The sebaceous glands
Sebaceous glands are especially numerous on the face (particularly the nose), scalp, midline of back and perineum. They are usually associated with a hair follicle, although occasionally they drain directly onto the skin surface. These glands secrete an oily substance called sebum which acts as a waterproofing and moisturizing agent for the hair and skin surface.

Nails
The nail consists of a dense keratinized plate, the nail plate, which rests on a stratified squamous epithelium called the nail bed. The proximal end of the nail, the nail root, and the underlying nail bed, extend deeply into the dermis to lie close to the distal interphalangeal joint. Nail growth occurs by proliferation and differentiation of the epithelium under the nail root, the nail matrix, and the nail plate then slides distally over the rest of the nail bed. Normal nail grows at about 0.5–1.2 mm a week for the fingernails and 0.2–0.5 mm for the toenails. The lunula underlies the proximal nail fold. It represents the most distal region of the nail matrix and is normally white. The skin over the root of the nail is known as the nail fold and its free edge is known as the eponychium. The hyponychium is the most distal region of the nail bed and marks the transition to normal skin. Nails serve for protection of the distal phalanx and they enhance the tactile capacity of the hands (Fig. 14.5).

The subcutaneous layer or hypodermis
The subcutaneous layer contains variable amounts of adipose tissue and attaches the dermis to the underlying tissue.

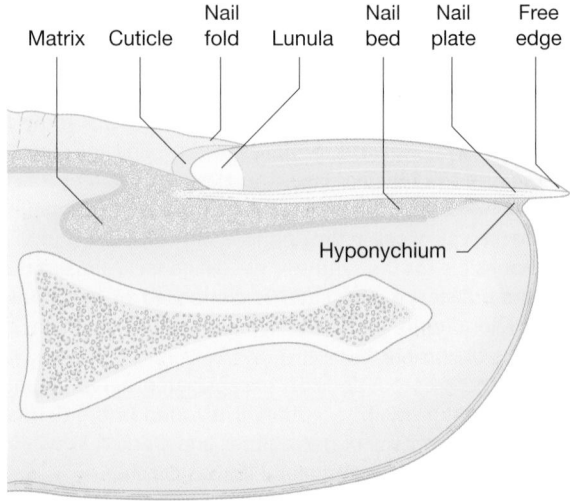

Fig. 14.5 Cross-section drawing of normal nail.

Physiology

The skin circulation

The blood supply of the skin is important for nutrition and thermoregulation. The main arteries supplying the skin are located in the hypodermis and give rise to branches passing upwards to two plexuses of anastomosing vessels. The deeper plexus lies at the junction of the hypodermis and the dermis and is known as the cutaneous plexus. The more superficial plexus lies just beneath the dermal papillae and is known as the subpapillary plexus. The venous drainage is arranged into plexuses broadly corresponding to the arterial supply. There are numerous arterio-venous shunts, which play an important role in thermoregulation. Glomus bodies are structures that control the flow in arterio-venous shunts. They are found in the deep dermis of peripheral sites, in particular the fingertips and the external ear.

Skin pigmentation

The colour of the skin depends on the following three main factors. The skin has an inherent yellowish colour due, in part, to the presence of carotene-derived pigments in the subcutaneous fat. The degree of haemoglobin oxygenation and the presence of other pigments such as bile pigments in the blood are also reflected in the skin colour. In addition, the amount of the pigment, melanin, present in the epidermis determines the skin colour.

Function of the skin

The skin is the largest organ of the body, constituting almost one sixth of the total body weight. It has four major functions:

Protection

The skin provides protection against mechanical, chemical and thermal insults. Its main defence against ultraviolet radiation is the production of melanin. The epidermis forms a relatively impermeable surface, preventing the inward and outward passage of water and electrolytes. In this way, it prevents dehydration. An intact stratum corneum acts as a physical barrier and prevents invasion by normal skin flora and pathogenic microorganisms. The skin is also an important component of the immune system, containing an organized arrangement of immunocompetent cells, in particular epidermal Langerhans' cells, which mediate specific and non-specific immune responses.

Sensation

The skin is the largest sensory organ of the body and contains a variety of receptors for touch, pressure, pain and temperature.

Thermoregulation

The skin is a major organ of thermoregulation. The body is insulated against heat loss by the presence of hairs and subcutaneous adipose tissue. In contrast, heat loss is facilitated by evaporation of sweat from the skin surface and increased blood flow through the rich vascular plexuses of the dermis.

Metabolic functions

The skin has a number of metabolic functions. Subcutaneous adipose tissue constitutes a major store of energy. Following exposure to ultraviolet B radiation, vitamin D_3 is synthesized in the epidermis from provitamin D_3.

Symptoms of skin disease

A full medical history, together with a thorough clinical examination and appropriate laboratory investigations, are important for an accurate diagnosis in dermatology.

A thorough history should include the details of the presenting complaint, including the time and site of onset of skin lesions. It is also important to note the character and duration of individual lesions, as well as their course, rate of change and pattern of spread. Provoking or alleviating factors such as sunlight, temperature, drugs, and occupation may give clues to the underlying aetiology. It is essential to enquire about associated features such as itch or pain, in addition to constitutional symptoms. Any previous treatments for the skin disorder, either topical or systemic, should also be noted.

A detailed past medical history should include previous general medical or surgical problems, past dermatological conditions and recent infections (viral or bacterial). A complete drug history, both past and present, is important as a number of medications can trigger certain skin disorders. In addition, all allergies, particularly drug allergies, should be documented carefully.

Enquiries should be made about a family history of atopy (asthma, eczema or hay fever) and of dermatological conditions. The social history is very important. Occasionally skin diseases are associated with places of residence, exposure to environmental agents, travel, occupation and other leisure activities (sports, hobbies). Finally, a sexual history may need to be obtained, as well as risk factors for human immunodeficiency virus (HIV).

Examination of the skin

As well as examining the area of skin involved, a dermatological examination should include visual assessment of the whole skin with adequate illumination. During the examination, the morphology, shape, arrangement and distribution of the skin lesions should be recorded. In addition, it is always important to palpate skin lesions in order to assess their consistency, temperature, mobility, tenderness and depth of involvement.

Morphology

Table 14.2 lists the various morphologies of common primary skin lesions, which in turn can have additional, superimposed features (Table 14.3).

Applied basic sciences of the skin

Symptoms of skin disease

Examination of the skin

851

Table 14.2	Morphology of skin lesions
Macule	A flat, non-palpable lesion less than 5 mm in diameter, distinguished from the adjacent normal skin by a change in colour
Patch	A flat, non-palpable lesion greater than 5 mm in diameter
Papule	A solid raised lesion less than 5 mm in diameter
Nodule	A larger, raised lesion greater than 5 mm in diameter
Plaque	A flat-topped lesion with a diameter considerably greater than its height
Wheal	A transient swelling of the skin of any size, often associated with surrounding, localized erythema (the flare)
Vesicle	A blister less than 5 mm in diameter
Bulla	A blister greater than 5 mm in diameter
Pustule	A visible accumulation of pus
Erosion	An area of skin from which the epidermis alone has been lost
Ulcer	An area of skin from which the epidermis and part of the dermis has been lost
Fissure	A cleft-shaped ulcer
Telangiectasia	Visibly dilated, small dermal blood vessels
Comedone	Accumulation of keratin and sebum lodged in a dilated pilosebaceous orifice

Table 14.3	Associated features of skin lesions
Scale	A flake of keratinized epidermal cells lying on the skin surface
Exudate	Material escaped from blood vessels with a high content of protein, cells and cellular debris
Crust	Dried serous and sanguinous exudates
Hyperkeratosis	An area of thickened stratum corneum
Atrophy	Thinning of the skin due to the partial loss of one or more of the tissue layers (epidermis, dermis or subcutis)
Sclerosis	Hardening of the skin due to dermal pathological change characterized by induration
Excoriation	Scratch or abrasion of the skin
Lichenification	Thickened skin with increased markings usually due to prolonged scratching
Warty	Horny excrescence

Table 14.4	Colour of skin lesions
Erythema	Redness due to microvascular dilatation (blanched by pressure)
Erythroderma	Refers to a particular dermatosis that has resulted in confluent erythema affecting >90% of the body surface area
Purpura	Darker redness due to extravasation of blood into the skin (does not blanch on pressure)

Table 14.5	Shape of skin lesions
Linear	Resembling a line
Discoid	Coin shaped
Annular	Ring shaped
Targetoid	A lesion consisting of concentric rings
Arcuate	Arc shaped
Serpiginous	Wavy or snake-like in shape
Whorled	Lesions which follow the developmental lines of Blaschko* and are curved or spiral
Digitate	Finger-like in shape
Zosteriform	Resembling herpes zoster
Umbilicated	Papule with a central depression

*Lines of Blaschko represent a pattern followed by many skin disorders. The cause of the pattern is unknown; the lines do not follow nerves, vessels or lymphatics. In contrast to dermatomes, Blaschko's lines form a V shape over the spine and an S shape on the lateral and anterior aspects of the trunk. These lines, which are invisible under normal conditions, may indicate the normal embryonic movements of the skin that occur during embryogenesis.

Table 14.6	Arrangement and distribution of skin lesions
Grouped	Discrete lesions occurring in a localized area
Scattered	Multiple lesions distributed over a wide area
Confluent	Coalescence of individual lesions
Centrifugal	Mostly affecting extremities
Centripetal	Mostly affecting the trunk
Palmoplantar	Affecting palms and soles
Flexural	Involving flexural skin
Extensor	Involving extensor skin
Dermatomal	Affecting skin of one or more dermatomes
Light-exposed	Involving skin routinely exposed to sunlight

Skin lesions can be a variety of different colours (Table 14.4). Commonly they are flesh-coloured, have increased or decreased pigmentation compared to the normal surrounding skin (hyper- or hypo-pigmentation), or are characterized by redness.

Shape

The shape of lesions can give important clues to the clinical diagnosis in certain conditions (Table 14.5).

Arrangement and distribution

The majority of skin diseases have a characteristic distribution or a predilection for particular sites, and therefore the recognition of a particular configuration is also important for diagnosis (Table 14.6).

General physical examination

Patients should also have a general physical examination, as indicated by the clinical presentation and differential diagnosis, with particular attention to the hair and nails, mucous membranes, lymph nodes and any sensory changes.

Examination of the skin

Investigations for skin disease

Wood's lamp examination

Wood's lamp emits ultraviolet long-wave light in the 320–365 nm range of the spectrum and is valuable in the diagnosis of certain skin and hair diseases. Normal hair and skin fluoresce bluish-white. When shone on hair infected with certain dermatophyte species (*Microsporum audouinii* and *M. canis*) an apple-green fluorescence is observed. Erythrasma, caused by the bacterium *Corynebacterium minutissimum*, produces a characteristic coral red colour. Pityriasis versicolor may be detected by pale yellow fluorescence.

Excess porphyrins in the urine (porphyrinuria) will make it fluoresce pink under Wood's light, and this is most striking in porphyria cutanea tarda and in congenital erythropoietic porphyria or Günther's disease. However, this has no value as a diagnostic tool since the concentration of porphyrins has to be very high before there is any visible fluorescence. Wood's light is a very insensitive method of detecting porphyrinuria; for a clinical diagnosis one requires accurate quantitation of urinary porphyrins by an experienced laboratory.

Wood's light can also be used to determine the depth of melanin in the skin.

Dermoscopy

The dermoscope is a hand-held lens with built-in lighting and a magnification of 10×–30×. It allows observation of a lesion covered with a drop of oil and so permits inspection of the deeper layers of the skin. This is called epiluminescence microscopy and, although operator dependent, may allow the distinction of benign and malignant growth patterns in pigmented lesions.

Diascopy

Diascopy consists of firmly pressing a microscopic slide over a skin lesion. This helps to differentiate the red colour of a lesion caused by capillary dilatation (erythema) from that caused by extravasation of blood (purpura) which does not blanch with pressure. In addition, the red-brown papules of lupus vulgaris have a diagnostic yellow-brown 'apple-jelly' colour on diascopy.

Biopsy of the skin

Biopsy of the skin is a simple and helpful diagnostic tool. A number of techniques can be used to study the excised specimen including histopathology, immunopathology and electron microscopy. A variety of methods are used to obtain a diagnostic biopsy of the skin. Commonly, a punch biopsy, a tubular knife which varies in size from 3 to 8 mm in diameter, is used. Larger lesions can be removed in the shape of an ellipse with the long axis parallel to crease lines. This reduces the tension along the suture line, resulting in a cosmetically more acceptable scar. In certain circumstances skin lesions can be simply shaved or curetted and the base cauterized. Biopsies should either be fixed in formalin for histopathology with appropriate special stains or transported in Michel's medium and frozen for immunofluorescence. Skin biopsies can also be sent for bacteriological and mycological cultures.

Immunofluorescence techniques

Immunofluorescence techniques are the mainstay of diagnosis and classification of bullous diseases, and are valuable in suspected cases of lupus erythematosus. Direct immunofluorescence of skin or mucosal surface demonstrates the sites where immunoglobulins, components of complement (C3) and fibrinogen are deposited. This technique uses antibodies raised against these human components conjugated with a fluorescent dye. Indirect immunofluorescence of the serum detects circulating autoantibodies in two steps. Antibodies in the patient's serum bind to antigens in a section of normal skin, and then antibodies raised against human immunoglobulin, conjugated with a fluorescent dye, are used to stain these bound antibodies. Split skin techniques, which artificially cleave the lamina lucida of the basement membrane zone, improve the sensitivity of indirect immunofluorescence and aid diagnosis of subepidermal bullous diseases.

Patch tests

Patch testing is essential if an allergic contact dermatitis (p. 867) is suspected. In very small children it may be difficult to perform. Most dermatology departments use the standard European series of contact allergens. More specialized patch-test series (including a separate series for medicaments, hairdressers, etc.) are used for refining the diagnosis as required. The allergen, suitably diluted, is introduced into an aluminium chamber that is then applied to the back of the patient and left in place for 2 days (Fig. 14.6). When removed, positive reactions will show

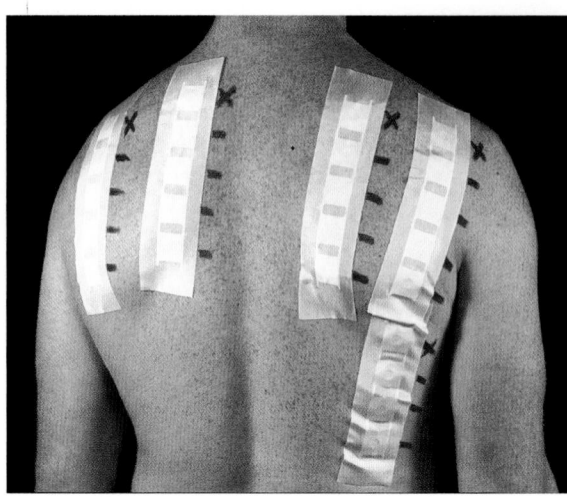

Fig. 14.6 Patch testing.

grades of erythema, induration or vesiculation depending on degree of reactivity. Patients should be re-examined after 4 days because some will show a slower response. In addition, irritant contact reaction (a non-immunological reaction giving an early false positive result) should have lessened by this time.

Photopatch testing

This is used to identify a potential photoallergen. The application of the test substance is followed by irradiation with ultraviolet light (UVA) at 5 J/cm^2.

Tests of immediate hypersensitivity

Serum IgE

Serum IgE measurements greater than 100 i.u. are sugges-tive of atopy, a genetic tendency to develop allergic diseases, which includes atopic dermatitis, allergic rhinitis (hay fever) and asthma. However a normal IgE does not rule out atopy.

Skin prick tests

A small amount of antigen in solution is introduced into the skin with a lancet, and if it is recognized by the IgE on mast cells in the skin a wheal will develop. Appropriate positive and negative controls are required for interpretation of results (a positive response should be at least the same size as the positive control).

The IgE radioallergosorbent test (RAST)

RASTs measure antigen-specific IgE in the blood and are commercially available. The results should be interpreted with caution as a positive RAST does not indicate causality, and a negative result does not rule out allergy.

Bacteriology, viral and mycology

Bacteriology

Gram stains and cultures of exudates and tissue samples are done if bacterial infections are suspected.

Viral swabs

Microscopic examination of cells obtained from the base of vesicles by gentle curettage with a scalpel (Tzanck smear) and staining with Giemsa's stain may reveal giant epithelial and multinucleated giant cells seen in herpes infections. In addition, culture, immunofluorescent tests or polymerase chain reaction (PCR) for herpes are now available.

Mycology

Skin scrapings, nail clippings and hairs from involved areas are placed on a slide with 20% potassium hydroxide and warmed gently. Fungal mycelia may be seen under the microscope. These initial tests are usually formalized by fungal cultures.

General laboratory investigations

Blood and urine tests

Routine blood tests including full blood count, renal and liver function tests, fasting glucose, erythrocyte sedi-mentation rate (ESR), as well as thyroid function tests, autoimmune screen and urinalysis are performed when appropriate.

SECTION 14.3 Papulosquamous and eczematous dermatoses

Psoriasis

Psoriasis is a common inflammatory dermatosis, most frequently characterized by red scaly plaques on extensor aspects of limbs and scalp.

Epidemiology

Psoriasis has a worldwide prevalence of up to 3000 per 100 000. It is estimated to affect 2% of the UK population.[1] It is uncommon in Native Americans and the Inuit population (500 per 100 000).

Pathology

There is a genetic predisposition to psoriasis. Approximately 30% of those with chronic plaque psoriasis have a family member with the disease and twin studies indicate a 70% concordance in monozygotic twins and 30% in dizygotic twins. Current research groups are attempting to identify the gene(s) linked to psoriasis. Independent genome-wide scans have identified at least nine disease susceptibility loci (PSORS1–9, psoriasis susceptibility 1–9) (Table 14.7). Of these, the PSORS1 region on chromosome 6p21 may account for up to 50% of psoriasis familial clustering. Within this region reside at least three potential candidate genes for psoriasis susceptibility: human leukocyte antigen C (*HLA-C*), α-helical coiled coil rod (*HCR*) and corneodesmosin (*CDSN*) genes.[2] The relatively low concordance rate in monozygotic twins together with the heterogeneity of chromosomal loci indicate that psoriasis is probably a polygenic disease expressed only in the presence of certain stimuli (such as streptococcal infection).

Type 1 (early-onset) psoriasis presenting before the age of 40 (peak age 20), has an aggressive course and is more likely to be familial. This subtype is associated with PSORS1. Type 2 (late-onset) psoriasis occurs after the age of 40 (peak 55–60), has a more indolent course and is less likely to be familial. In this subtype, the association with PSORS1 is not significantly different from that observed in the normal population,[3] suggesting that PSORS1 is not a major inheritance risk factor in the pathogenesis of late-onset psoriasis. Other variants include guttate psoriasis and palmoplantar pustular psoriasis. Guttate psoriasis is strongly associated with PSORS1 but palmoplantar pustular psoriasis shows no association with this locus. This suggests that chronic plaque psoriasis and guttate psoriasis have a similar genetic basis, whereas palmoplantar pustular psoriasis may be a distinct disorder.[4]

The three key pathological features of a psoriasis plaque are epidermal keratinocyte hyperproliferation with loss of differentiation, vascular endothelial cell proliferation and enhanced vascular permeability, and inflammation of the epidermis and dermis (T cells and neutrophils). The inflammatory infiltrate is the primary event with epidermal keratinocyte changes being secondary.

Epidermal keratinocytes

In the epidermis of normal skin, keratinocyte migration from basal layer to stratum corneum takes about 28 days; in psoriasis there is significant hyperproliferation and this process only takes 4 days. Epidermal stem cells in psoriasis are more susceptible to the growth-promoting effects of T lymphocyte-derived cytokines such as interferon-γ (IFN-γ).

Histological appearances include parakeratosis (nucleated keratinocytes persisting in the stratum corneum) coupled with the formation of Munro's microabscesses (sterile collections of neutrophils). Although the epidermis is greatly thickened (acanthotic) there is significant extension of dermal papillae into the epidermis, to the extent that the epidermis directly above such dermal papillae is thin and fragile.

Endothelial cells

Early in the development of a psoriatic plaque there is vascular endothelial cell proliferation and enhanced vascular permeability. This process occurs in the capillary loop in the dermal papilla and is coupled with the expression of the angiogenesis-associated antigen αvβ3. It appears to be partly dependent on keratinocyte-derived angiogenic factors such as vascular endothelial growth factors (VEGF). Circulating VEGF in severe psoriasis is associated with disease activity and the presence of arthritis.

Other early changes that occur on endothelial cells are induction and upregulation of adhesion molecules, including E-selectin, vascular cell adhesion molecule-1 (VCAM-1) and intercellular adhesion molecule-1 (ICAM-1). Expression of these molecules facilitates binding and subsequent trafficking of leukocytes from peripheral blood into the skin.

Table 14.7	Main psoriasis susceptibility loci
Locus name	**Chromosome location**
PSORS1	6p21
PSORS2	17q25
PSORS3	4q34

Inflammatory infiltrate

Psoriasis is a T cell-mediated disease and an evolving plaque is characterized by an influx of T lymphocytes. It is thought that antigen presentation to lymphocytes, for example from streptococci in the tonsils, results in preferential migration to the skin. These lymphocytes express the cutaneous lymphocyte-associated antigen (CLA). CLA is the natural ligand for E-selectin on endothelial cells and expression of CLA on T lymphocytes allows adherence to cutaneous cells and consequent migration into the skin.[5] The cytokine profile of psoriatic plaques is predominantly of the Th1 subset (IFN-γ, IL-2 and IL-12) in contrast to the Th2 profile of atopic dermatitis (IL-4, IL-5, IL-6 and IL-10). This cytokine polarization of these two diseases is demonstrated clinically, in that severe psoriasis and severe atopic eczema rarely occur in the same individual.

RECENT ADVANCES

There have been case reports of patients with psoriasis who have gone into prolonged remission after receiving bone marrow from a non-psoriatic sibling, and also development of psoriasis following transplantation from a psoriatic donor.

Scope of disease

Psoriasis can affect any area of the skin. Severe disease can be life threatening with fluid losses, temperature dysregulation and sepsis. Up to 25% of patients with chronic plaque psoriasis have associated arthritis (p. 490): in 15%, skin and joint disease begin simultaneously; in 60% the skin disease precedes the arthritis; in the remaining 25% the arthritis precedes the skin disease. Certain subtypes of psoriasis may also be related to an underlying precipitating condition, such as streptococcal infection in guttate psoriasis. A degree of psychological and social disability accompanies psoriasis and may be disproportionate to the severity of disease.[6]

Clinical features

Psoriasis is most commonly characterized by well-defined, salmon pink plaques with silvery white scales on the extensor aspects of limbs, scalp, navel and natal cleft. Psoriasis does not scar the skin but may be itchy. The severity and duration of the disease are variable and a wide variety of clinical patterns are recognized. Different forms of the disease may occur in the same patient at different times.

Sunshine can exacerbate psoriasis in a few patients, but in the majority natural sunshine is beneficial. Psoriasis exhibits the Köbner phenomenon—psoriasis appears at sites of trauma. Other precipitating or exacerbating factors are listed in Table 14.8.

Chronic plaque psoriasis

Chronic plaque psoriasis is also known as psoriasis vulgaris. It is the most common form, accounting for 80% of disease, and is equally common in both sexes. It is characterized by

Table 14.8	Precipitating and exacerbating factors for psoriasis
Drugs	
Beta-blockers	
ACE inhibitors	
Lithium	
Antimalarials	
NSAIDs	
Alcohol	
Infection	
β-haemolytic streptococci	
HIV (pre-existing psoriasis may become more refractory to therapy)	
Injury to the skin	
Mechanical injury	
Sunburn	

well-demarcated, thickened, red plaques, covered by silvery scales (Fig. 14.7). 'Auspitz sign' is a characteristic diagnostic feature where light scraping of the scale with a wooden spatula produces multiple bleeding points. Although the plaques may be distributed anywhere, the most common sites are the extensor aspects of limbs (particularly knees and elbows), the lumbosacral region and scalp. The disease may be localized or widespread, covering most of the body (Fig. 14.8). When psoriasis involves

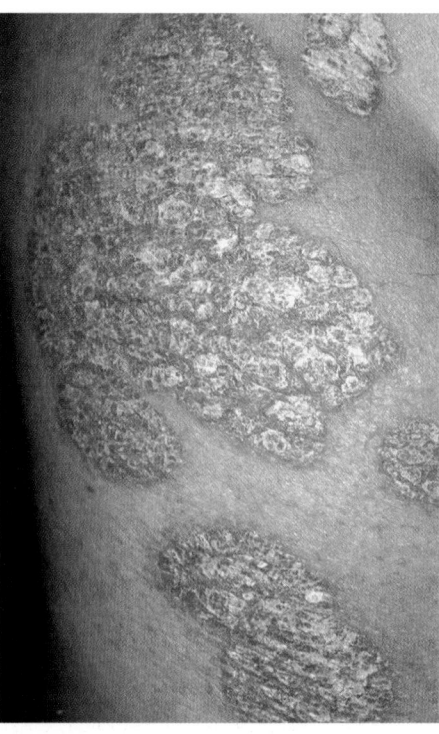

Fig. 14.7 Close-up of psoriatic plaque.

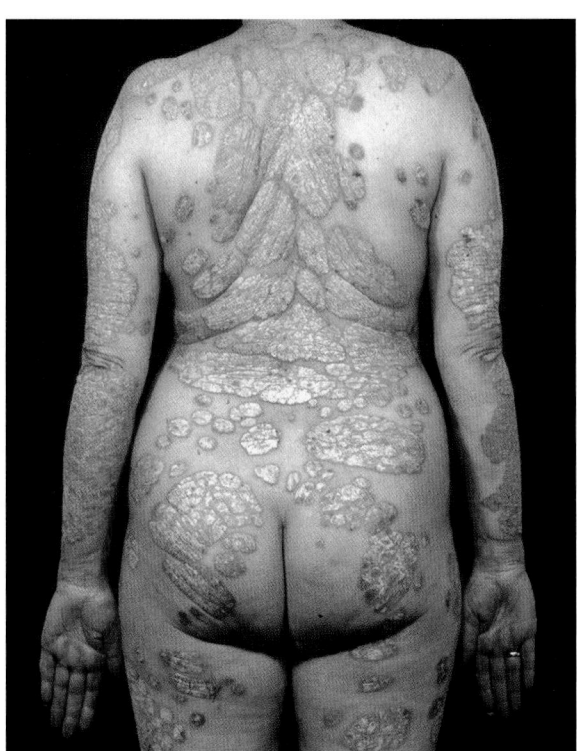

Fig. 14.8 Chronic plaque psoriasis.

flexures or the genitalia, it is frequently atypical in that there is no scaling as a result of the moist environment.

Guttate psoriasis

Guttate psoriasis is the acute onset of small droplets of psoriasis, generally on the trunk (Fig. 14.9). It classically occurs 2–3 weeks after a streptococcal throat infection in children and young adults. On examination, there are numerous red, oval or round, scaly plaques up to 1 cm in diameter. These rapidly appear on the trunk and proximal limbs, and may coalesce. Guttate psoriasis is usually self-limiting and responds readily to treatment. A short course of an antistreptococcal antibiotic in those with a proven streptococcal throat infection may also be beneficial.

Pustular psoriasis

Pustular psoriasis is rare and may be localized or generalized. Chronic, localized pustular psoriasis (also called palmoplantar pustulosis) occurs predominantly in adults and is 9 times more common in women. There is an association with tobacco use: over 90% of patients are smokers. It manifests as recurrent crops of sterile yellow pustules, 0.1–0.5 cm in diameter, on palms and soles. The pustules involute to leave red-brown stained macules which may scale before disappearing.

Generalized pustular psoriasis is a serious, unstable form of psoriasis associated with a significant mortality. Erythematous plaques studded with sterile pustules rapidly appear at any site and may become confluent. Fever and malaise are common. This pustular form may occur in patients with chronic plaque psoriasis after withdrawal of oral or potent topical steroids.

Erythrodermic psoriasis

Active psoriasis can progress to sub-erythroderma (70% body surface area involved) or erythroderma (over 90% of body surface area affected), which can be life threatening as skin fluid loss, temperature dysregulation and potential sepsis can occur. Patients need urgent admission to hospital and may require systemic therapy.

Scalp psoriasis

Scalp psoriasis describes areas of well-demarcated erythema and lumpy scaling interspersed with normal skin (Fig. 14.10). An unusual form of thick psoriasis on the scalp is pityriasis amiantacea in which the scales are adherent to the hair shaft (the same clinical appearance may also be seen in seborrhoeic dermatitis).

Nails

Nail abnormalities are present in up to 50% of patients with psoriasis, especially in those with associated psoriatic arthritis. The most common findings are pitting, onycholysis (separation of the nail plate from the nail bed), 'salmon patches' or oil spots (subungual yellow-brown areas of discolouration), and subungual hyperkeratosis (Fig. 14.11a). Severe nail dystrophy can occur and may need to be differentiated from onychomycosis (Fig. 14.11b).

Initial investigations

The diagnosis of psoriasis is made clinically and laboratory investigations are rarely helpful.

Further investigations

Skin biopsy

A skin biopsy may be required when the diagnosis is unclear or if the patient fails to respond to treatment.

Anti-streptolysin O (ASO) titres

ASO titres may be performed to screen for streptococcal infection in patients with guttate psoriasis.

HIV test

Psoriasis in the context of a modified immune response is commonly atypical, severe and refractory to treatment. An HIV test should be performed in such clinical cases.

Syphilis serology

In the case of guttate psoriasis, the differential diagnosis includes secondary syphilis. This can be ruled out by appropriate serological tests.

Nail clippings

Nail clippings for microscopy and fungal culture are performed to rule out onychomycosis (dermatophyte nail infection) in patients with severe nail dystrophy.

Psoriasis

Pityriasis rosea

Lichen planus

Endogenous dermatitis

Exogenous (contact) dermatitis

Intertrigo

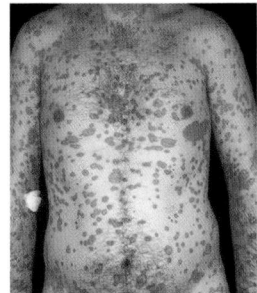

Fig. 14.9 Guttate psoriasis.

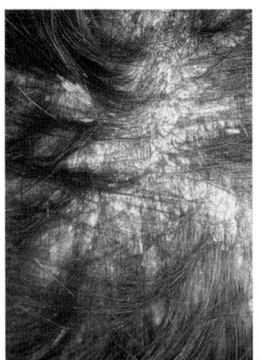

Fig. 14.10 Scalp psoriasis.

857

Initial management

Patient education

There is no cure for psoriasis. Treatment is suppressive and aimed at inducing remission or at least reducing the extent and severity, so that the disease has as minimal an impact as possible on the patient's daily routine. Response to treatment will be influenced by compliance, and so regimens should be adapted to suit each patient's circumstances. The need for treatment will often be dictated by the patient's own perception of his or her disability, and management should take these views into account. Tolerance and understanding are required in helping patients overcome the social stigma that may be associated with their disease.

Emollients

Patients with psoriasis should be encouraged to use emollients regularly to moisturize the skin and prevent fissuring.

Antihistamines

Occasionally psoriasis may be itchy, and in these cases a sedating antihistamine can be useful at night when pruritus is usually most troublesome.

Medical management

Chronic plaque psoriasis is classified as mild if less than 10% of the body surface area (BSA) is affected. Mild disease is usually treated with first-line topical treatment. Depending on the ease with which these treatments can be applied, patients may be managed in the primary care setting or in hospital. More severe disease (>15% of BSA affected) requires second-line treatments that are predominantly hospital based and supervised by a dermatologist (Table 14.9).

First-line therapy
Keratolytics

Keratolytics, such as salicylic acid, may be used in combination with one of the other first-line treatments to descale plaques.

Coal tar

The mechanism of action of coal tar is poorly understood; however, it is a keratolytic and probably possesses anti-inflammatory and antiproliferative effects. Inpatient treatment is usually started with 1% coal tar and can be gradually increased to 30%, depending on efficacy and local irritation. Crude extracts of coal tar can be made up in emulsifying ointment to be used by patients at home. There are also shampoos which contain coal tar for scalp psoriasis. The most common side effects are irritation of uninvolved skin, folliculitis, odour and staining of clothing, so compliance is often a problem. Coal tar treatments act synergistically with ultraviolet B radiation in the traditional Goeckerman regimen. There is at present no epidemiological evidence that topical tar products cause cutaneous or internal cancers when used to treat psoriasis.

Table 14.9	Medical management of psoriasis
First-line therapy	
Emollients	
Keratolytic agents	
Coal tar	
Dithranol	
Topical steroids	
Vitamin D$_3$ analogues (calcipotriol)	
Topical retinoids	
Second-line therapy	
Phototherapy Broadband UVB (wavelength 290–320 nm) Narrowband UVB (wavelength 311–313 nm)	
Photochemotherapy PUVA	
Systemic therapy Methotrexate Ciclosporin Acitretin Systemic steroids Hydroxyurea Azathioprine Mycophenolate mofetil 'Biologics'	

Dithranol

This is one of the oldest treatments available for psoriasis, and when used together with ultraviolet B radiation (Ingram regimen) it is an important management option for inpatients or those treated at day treatment centres. Dithranol has a direct antiproliferative effect on epidermal keratinocytes. It is probably the most effective and safest topical treatment available but, as with coal tar, its use is limited by cosmetic acceptability. Treatment, usually in hospital, is started at 0.1% in non-smudging zinc oxide (Lassar's) paste and gradually increased. Paste is applied to each plaque and left in place under stockinette gauze for up to 24 hours. There are also short-contact preparations of dithranol, such as Dithrocream, which can be used at home under the supervision of the general practitioner. The main side effects are irritation, burning and purple-brown discolouration of uninvolved skin, clothes and baths.

Topical corticosteroids

Topical corticosteroids have a high patient compliance because of their efficacy and cosmetic acceptability. However, patients should be warned of their potential side effects. They can be used all over but are particularly reserved for sites such as hands, feet, flexures, genitalia and scalp. Recalcitrant psoriasis, particularly on the hands and feet, usually requires treatment with potent corticosteroids, sometimes under occlusion. In areas where the skin is much thinner, such as flexural sites, the face and genitalia, only mild potency steroids should be used. Topical corticos-

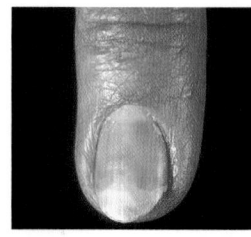

(a)

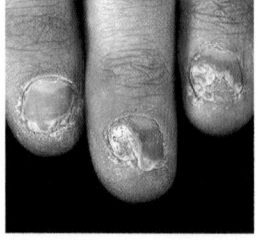

(b)

Fig. 14.11a, b (a) Psoriatic pitting, onycholysis and 'salmon patch'. (b) Psoriatic nail dystrophy.

teroids should not be used regularly for more than 4 weeks without review. Rapid relapse may occur after stopping therapy. Corticosteroids can be used as monotherapy or in conjunction with other topical agents including tar, dithranol and vitamin D_3 analogues.

Vitamin D_3 analogues

Vitamin D_3 analogues (calcipotriol and tacalcitol) directly normalize the abnormal epidermal keratinocyte proliferation and differentiation in psoriasis, and may be anti-inflammatory. They have the advantage of being cosmetically acceptable, effective and relatively safe. They are usually used once daily, in the evening, in combination with a moderate–potent corticosteroid in the mornings, for a few weeks. Their use in extensive psoriasis is limited by irritation and the potential for hypercalcaemia.

Topical retinoids

Tazarotene, a third-generation acetylenated retinoid, has been shown to have some effect in psoriasis, possibly by normalization of epidermal keratinocyte proliferation and differentiation.

Second-line therapy
Phototherapy

UVB (wavelength 290–320 nm) plays an important role in the management of psoriasis. It is effective in the treatment of guttate and thin plaque psoriasis but has little efficacy in thick chronic plaque psoriasis. The main side effects are burning and potential carcinogenicity. UVB-induced erythema is predominantly caused at wavelengths of 290–300 nm, however recent studies have shown that the therapeutic wavelengths in psoriasis are in the order of 311–315 nm. This led to the development of the TL-01 lamp which emits a wavelength of 311–313 nm, so-called 'narrowband UVB', allowing a higher dose of UVB to be delivered with less burning. TL-01 has been shown to be more effective than traditional broadband UVB. Clearance rates of 80–85% have been achieved in some studies of TL-01 therapy, and these are compatible to rates achieved with PUVA.[7] Current human use suggests that TL-01 has a similar long-term risk to the older broadband tubes[8] and a reduced risk of carcinogenicity when compared to PUVA.[9]

Photochemotherapy

Photochemotherapy is extremely effective with clearance rates of up to 90%.[10] It combines a photosensitizing agent (psoralen) with long-wave UVA (wavelength 320–400 nm) and is known as PUVA. Patients take psoralen tablets 2–3 hours before UVA. If nausea occurs, bath PUVA can be considered. Patients are advised to wear UVA protective glasses for 12 hours after taking psoralen.[11] Long-term PUVA causes photoageing and non-melanoma skin cancers, especially squamous cell carcinoma, and may possibly be related to the development of melanoma.[9] In view of these long-term effects, PUVA is now only used twice a week when attempting to clear psoriasis, and maintenance treatments are now avoided.

Methotrexate

Methotrexate is effective treatment for all forms of psoriasis. It is given as a once-weekly dose, but its use is limited by potential side effects of bone marrow toxicity and hepatic fibrosis. Patients are advised to abstain from alcohol while on the drug. Hepatic fibrosis can occur despite normal liver function tests. Recently, it has been shown that serum levels of the amino-propeptide of procollagen III, a marker of fibrosis, correlate with the results of liver biopsy in patients taking methotrexate.[12] This marker is now used instead of regular liver biopsies in patients on methotrexate to monitor hepatic fibrosis; only if the procollagen levels are repeatedly high is a liver biopsy recommended.

Ciclosporin

Ciclosporin has a known suppressive effect on T-lymphocyte function. It is a highly effective and rapidly acting systemic treatment for psoriasis. Before initiation of treatment patients should be normotensive with normal renal and hepatic function. The most common side effects are dysaesthesia, hypertrichosis, malaise and gingival hypertrophy. The main risks of prolonged treatment are hypertension and renal dysfunction, which is dose related. Ciclosporin should not be used in combination with phototherapy because of an increased risk of skin cancer.

Systemic retinoids

Acitretin is a polyaromatic retinoid. It is an antiproliferative agent that acts on keratinocytes. Although not as effective as methotrexate or ciclosporin, it is relatively safe in the long term as it is not immunosuppressive. Before treatment, liver function and fasting lipids should be measured as acitretin is occasionally hepatotoxic and may increase serum levels of cholesterol and triglycerides. It is teratogen with a long half-life and therefore should be avoided in women of child-bearing age.[13] Women should be advised not to become pregnant during and for at least 2 years after treatment with acitretin. Generalized pustular psoriasis and palmoplantar pustular psoriasis are particularly responsive to acitretin.

Other immunomodulation agents

Other systemic agents include hydroxyurea, azathioprine and mycophenolate mofetil.

Table 14.10 lists the indications for the use of systemic therapy in psoriasis.

Table 14.10	Indications for systemic treatment
Failure of topical treatment	
Repeated hospital admissions for topical treatments	
Generalized pustular or erythrodermic psoriasis	
Severe psoriatic arthropathy	
Severe psychological distress as a result of the disease	

RECENT ADVANCES

'Biologics' are a new class of selective immunomodulatory drugs for the treatment of psoriasis.[14] Patients with severe disease who have drug-related toxicity or who have become intolerant or unresponsive to standard systemic therapy should be considered eligible for treatment with biologics, as well as those who have psoriatic arthritis or unstable life-threatening disease. Currently, these therapies for psoriasis comprise two main groups: agents targeting the cytokine tumour necrosis factor-alpha (TNF-α), such as etanercept and infliximab, and agents targeting T cells or antigen-presenting cells, such as efalizumab.

Infliximab and etanercept are both already used in rheumatoid arthritis. These biologics block the effects of the pro-inflammatory cytokine TNF-α.[15] Infliximab is a humanized monoclonal antibody,[16] whereas etanercept represents the soluble TNF-α receptor.[17] Etanercept is given twice a week as a subcutaneous injection and infliximab as an intravenous infusion, just 3 times overall with intervals of several weeks. Efalizumab is a humanized form of a murine antibody directed against CD11a (a subunit of leukocyte function-associated antigen-1).[18] By binding to this, efalizumab inhibits T-cell activation, cutaneous T-cell trafficking and T-cell adhesion to keratinocytes. It is given as a weekly subcutaneous injection. Disadvantages of these immunomodulatory compounds include cost, increased risk of infections and malignancy. Figure 14.12 summarizes the immunology of psoriasis together with its management using immunomodulators.

Prognosis

Approximately 50% may remit spontaneously for varying periods of time; remission is rarely permanent.

 FURTHER INFORMATION

British Association of Dermatologists—clinical guidelines for psoriasis. www.bad.org.uk/doctors/guidelines/psoriasis.asp

Smith CH, Anstey AV, Barker JN, et al. British Association of Dermatologists guidelines for use of biological intervention in psoriasis 2005. British Journal of Dermatology 2005; 153: 486–497.

REFERENCES

(1) Rea JN, Newhouse ML, Hail T. Skin disease in Lambeth. A community study of prevalence and use of medical care. British Journal of Preventive and Social Medicine 1976; 30: 107.
(2) Capon F, Munro M, Barker J, Trembath R. Searching for the major histocompatibility complex psoriasis susceptibility gene. Journal of Investigative Dermatology 2002; 118: 745–751.
(3) Allen MH, Ameen H, Veal C, et al. The major psoriasis susceptibility locus PSORS1 is not a risk factor for late-onset psoriasis. Journal of Investigative Dermatology 2005; 124: 103–106.
(4) Asumalahti K, Ameen M, Suomela S, et al. Genetic analysis of PSORS1 distinguishes guttate psoriasis and palmoplantar pustulosis. Journal of Investigative Dermatology 2003; 120: 627–632.
(5) Griffiths CEM, Voorhees JJ. Psoriasis, T cells and autoimmunity. Journal of the Royal Society of Medicine 1996; 89: 315–319.
(6) Sampogna F, Sera F, Abeni D. Measures of clinical severity, quality of life and psychological distress in patients with psoriasis: A cluster analysis. Journal of Investigative Dermatology 2004; 122: 602–607.
(7) Picot E, Meunier I, Picot-Debeze MC, et al. Treatment of psoriasis with a 311-UVB lamp. British Journal of Dermatology 1992; 127: 509–512.
(8) Young AR. Carcinogenicity of UVB phototherapy assessed. Lancet 1995; 345: 1431–1432.
(9) Stern RS, Laird N. The carcinogenic risk of treatments for severe psoriasis. Cancer 1994; 73: 2759–2764.

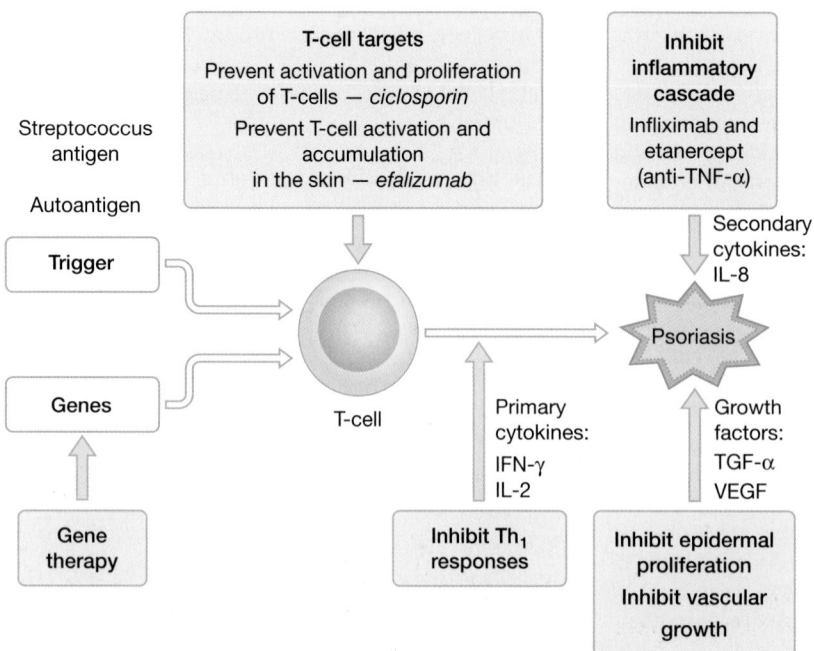

Fig. 14.12 Immunology and immunotherapy for psoriasis. TNF-α, tumour necrosis factor alpha; IL, interleukin; IFN-γ, interferon-gamma; TGF-α, transforming growth factor alpha; VEGF, vascular endothelial growth factor.

REFERENCES—cont'd

(10) British Photodermatology Group. *Guidelines for PUVA. British Journal of Dermatology* 1994; 130: 246–255.

(11) Moseley H, Jones SK. *Clear UV blocking lenses for use by PUVA patients. British Journal of Dermatology* 1990; 123: 775.

(12) Boffa MJ, Smith A, Chalmers RGJ, et al. *The place of type III procollagen aminopeptide (PIIINP) measurement in the assessment of liver damage in methotrexate-treated psoriatic patients. British Journal of Dermatology* 1995; 133 (Suppl 45): 16–17.

(13) Geiger JM, Baudin M, Saurat JH. *Teratogenic risk with etretinate and acitretin treatment. Dermatology* 1994; 189: 109–116.

(14) Asadullah K, Volk HD, Sterry W. *Novel immunotherapies for psoriasis. Trends in Immunology* 2002; 23: 47–53.

(15) Victor FC, Gottlieb AB. *TNF-alpha and apoptosis: implications for the pathogenesis and treatment of psoriasis. Journal of Drugs in Dermatology* 2002; 1: 264–275.

(16) Chaudhari U, Romano P, Mulcahy LD, et al. *Efficacy and safety of infliximab monotherapy for plaque-type psoriasis: a randomised trial. Lancet* 2001; 357: 1842–1847.

(17) Leonardi CL, Powers JL, Matheson RT, et al. *Etanercept as monotherapy in patients with psoriasis. New England Journal of Medicine* 2003; 349: 2014–2022.

(18) Lebwohl M, Tyring SK, Hamilton TK, et al. *A novel target T-cell modulator, efalizumab, for plaque psoriasis. New England Journal of Medicine* 2003; 349: 2004–2013.

Pityriasis rosea

Pityriasis rosea is a relatively common acute inflammatory skin disease. Most cases occur in the 10–35-year age group, and males and females are equally affected. The aetiology is unknown but there is considerable evidence for an infectious cause. Clinically, the first manifestation is usually a 'herald patch' on the thigh, upper arm or trunk (Fig. 14.13). This is an oval, slightly raised plaque 2–5 cm in diameter and red in colour. After an interval of 5–15 days, disseminated, smaller oval dull pink papules and plaques covered by fine, dry silvery-grey scales develop, usually confined to the trunk and proximal aspects of arms and legs. The lesions desquamate to leave the characteristic fine 'collarette' (collar-like) of scales around each lesion. The lesions are orientated parallel to the direction of the ribs giving a characteristic 'Christmas-tree' appearance on the trunk (Fig. 14.14). Diagnosis is made clinically; however, differential diagnoses include tinea corporis, drug eruption, guttate psoriasis and secondary syphilis. The eruption is often asymptomatic although sometimes it is mildly pruritic. Oral antihistamines are helpful for relief of the pruritus. The eruption fades within 6–12 weeks without treatment and recurrences are rare.

Lichen planus

Epidemiology

Lichen planus is a relatively common inflammatory mucocutaneous disorder with the greatest incidence in the 30–60-year age group.

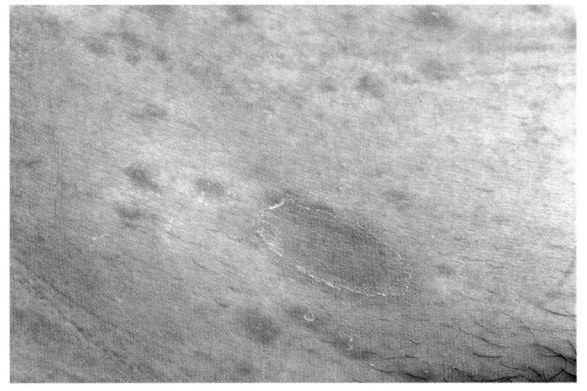

Fig. 14.13 Herald patch in pityriasis rosea.

Pathology

Most cases of lichen planus are idiopathic, however certain drugs can induce a lichen planus-like (lichenoid) eruption, and links to hepatitis C infection have also been reported.

Clinical features

Lichen planus characteristically presents as violaceous, flat-topped, shiny polygonal papules, with fine white lines on the surface (Wickham's striae). Lichen planus exhibits the Köbner phenomenon and pruritus is often severe. The lesions show a predilection for the wrists (Fig. 14.15), forearms, ankles and lower back. Hyperkeratosis is seen over lesions on palms, soles and lower legs. Lesions on the scalp result

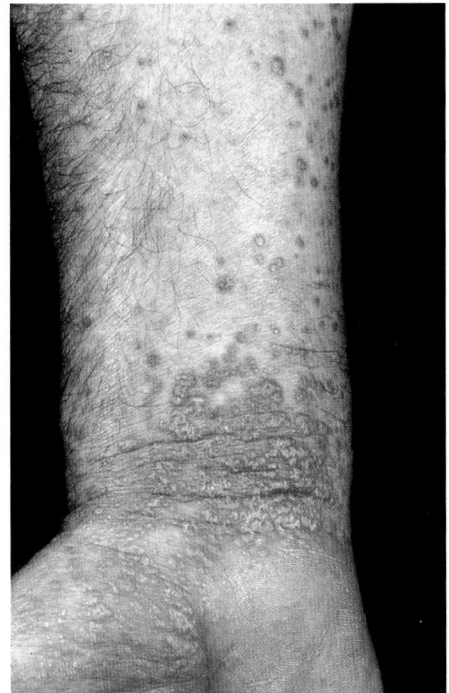

Fig. 14.15 Lichen planus.

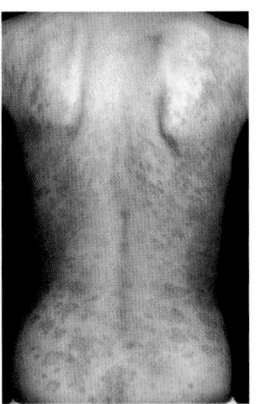

Fig. 14.14 'Christmas tree' appearance of pityriasis rosea.

in scarring alopecia, and nail involvement causes longitudinal striations, atrophy and scarring (Fig. 14.16). In 40–60% of individuals there is mucous membrane involvement. Patients present with a white lace-like appearance on the buccal mucosa (Fig. 14.17) or tongue, although erosions, ulcers and plaques are also sometimes seen. Oral lichen planus may predispose to the development of squamous cell carcinoma within lesions.

Investigations
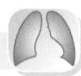

Skin biopsy
The diagnosis of lichen planus is usually made clinically and can be confirmed by histological findings of hyperkeratosis, acanthosis and a band lymphocytic (CD4-positive T cells) infiltrate in the superficial dermis.

Management

Antihistamines
Sedative antihistamines are helpful at night to control pruritus.

Immunomodulation
Potent or very potent topical corticosteroids are helpful in localized disease. In resistant or more generalized cases, systemic treatment with steroids or ciclosporin may be required.

Prognosis

Approximately 50% of lesions resolve spontaneously within 9 months and 85% by 18 months, leaving temporary post-inflammatory hyperpigmentation, more marked in dark skins. Recurrence may occur in about 20% of cases.

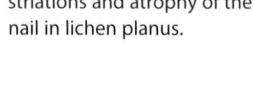

Fig. 14.16 Longitudinal striations and atrophy of the nail in lichen planus.

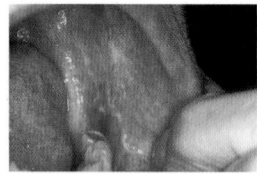

Fig. 14.17 Oral lichen planus.

Dermatitis

Dermatitis (or eczema) describes a pattern of skin inflammation characterized histologically by a lymphohistiocytic infiltrate in the upper dermis, with oedema between keratinocytes in the epidermis (spongiosis) and varying degrees of epidermal thickening (acanthosis). In general, dermatitis can be subdivided into two main groups (Table 14.11): endogenous (constitutional) and exogenous (contact). However, in practice it usually has a multifactorial aetiology.

Endogenous dermatitis

Atopic dermatitis

Epidemiology
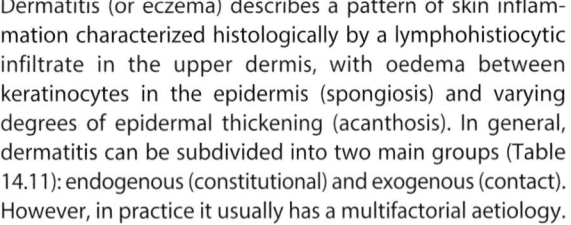

The point prevalence of dermatitis in the UK is estimated at about 20%, of which atopic dermatitis constitutes the

Table 14.11	Classification of dermatitis
Endogenous (constitutional) dermatitis	
Atopic dermatitis	
Seborrhoeic dermatitis	
Discoid (or nummular) dermatitis	
Vesicular hand and foot (dyshidrotic) dermatitis (pompholyx)	
Stasis (gravitational or varicose) dermatitis	
Lichen simplex	
Asteatotic dermatitis	
Exogenous (contact) dermatitis	
Irritant contact dermatitis	
Allergic contact dermatitis	
Photocontact dermatitis	

majority, affecting 20% of school children and 3% of adults in the UK.[1] The incidence has been increasing over the last 30 years although the reasons for this are unclear.

Pathology

The pathogenesis of atopic dermatitis is not fully understood. It has a multifactorial aetiology, with interactions between genetic and environmental factors. The tendency to develop an atopic disorder is inherited; approximately 70% of patients have a family history of atopy. A child with one parent who has eczema will have a 30% risk of developing it; this rises to 50% if both parents are affected. Allergens in house dust mites (*Dermatophagoides pteronyssinus*), pets and certain foods may play a role. Physical factors such as microbial infection and irritation from soap and textiles are also important. Stress may exacerbate atopic dermatitis.

Scope of disease

Patients with atopic dermatitis are more prone to certain cutaneous infections. Secondary infection with *Staphylococcus aureus* is common and may present with crusting, weeping or pustules. A potentially dangerous viral skin infection in atopic dermatitis is herpes simplex. This may give rise to a disseminated skin infection (eczema herpeticum). Patients can become acutely unwell and develop widespread monomorphous papules that become vesicular (Fig. 14.18).

As the clinical features of atopic dermatitis settle, the pathological features subside to normal. However in pigmented skin, pigment may be left deposited in the dermis within macrophages. This is referred to as post-inflammatory hyperpigmentation (see p. 915).

Clinical features

Clinically, atopic dermatitis has two phases: acute and chronic. The acute phase is characterized by erythema and

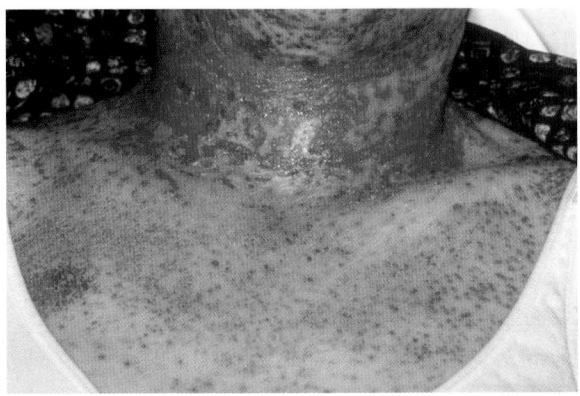

Fig. 14.18 Eczema herpeticum.

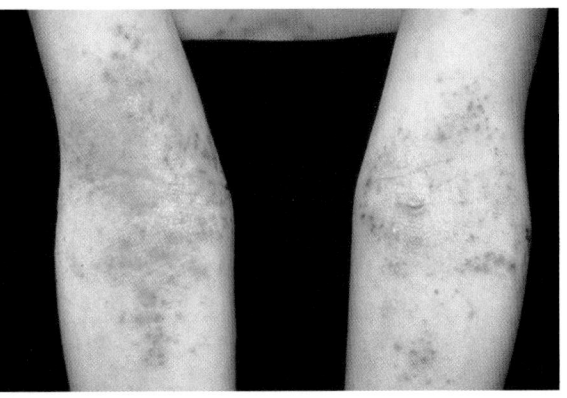

Fig. 14.19 Atopic dermatitis (flexural).

vesiculation, and the chronic phase by dryness, lichenification and fissuring. The main symptom is pruritus.

In the first two years of life, eczematous lesions are often present on exposed areas such as cheeks or outer aspects of the forearms or legs. The lesions are red and poorly defined with surface changes such as scaling, erosions, papules or vesicles. In the older child, eczema usually affects flexural sites such as the antecubital and popliteal fossae, the front of the ankles and the neck and face (Fig. 14.19). Children are often miserable as a result of intractable itching. In those whose disease continues into adult life, the flexures, limbs and face are often involved. Chronic eczematous changes are common on the face, although any site of the body may be involved.

Initial investigations

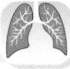

Most patients with atopic dermatitis do not require any investigations.

Further investigations

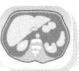

Allergy testing (type I hypersensitivity)

Allergy testing is usually not required to establish the diagnosis of atopic dermatitis and is unreliable in children under 5 years of age. There is no evidence to show any benefit from routine examination of total serum IgE or identification of specific IgE antibodies to common allergens such as house dust mite, pollen or food using skin-prick testing or a radioallergosorbent test (RAST). However, a positive skin-prick test and IgE RAST are useful supportive features in clinically difficult cases.

Patch tests (type IV hypersensitivity)

Patch testing should also be considered in cases of atopic dermatitis unresponsive to treatment as sensitization to topical medicaments may have developed.

Bacterial swabs

Bacterial swabs should be sent for microscopy, sensitivity and culture if secondary bacterial infection is suspected.

Viral swabs

Viral swabs should be taken for virology screening and a smear for electron microscopy if the patient is thought to have eczema herpeticum.

Skin scrapings

Scabies must be excluded in a widespread pruritic eruption of recent onset.

Initial management

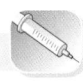

Patient education

Atopic dermatitis can have a profound effect on the quality of life of both sufferers and their families. One of the most important aspects of management is the need for adequate time for explanation, education and discussion.

Atopic dermatitis may cause considerable psychological suffering for the patient. Support services such as the National Eczema Society are invaluable. Patients may also be helped by various cognitive behavioural techniques.

Identify and address any precipitating factors

Patients should be advised to avoid any exacerbating factors, emotional stress and temperature change. Irritants should also be avoided. To date, trials of allergen avoidance have often given inconclusive or negative results.

The role of diet in atopic dermatitis has been investigated repeatedly with no clear conclusion. In general, dietary restriction is of little or no benefit in adults, and in children it is worth trying only in selected infants under expert supervision.

Emollients

In atopic dermatitis, the natural barrier function of the skin is impaired, resulting in loss of fluid and drying of the skin. Dry skin is irritable and exacerbates the symptoms of dermatitis. Emollients have a pivotal role in the treatment of dermatitis. Most normal soaps and shampoos are based on detergents and remove natural lipids from the skin. These will potentially dry the skin further and therefore should be avoided. Daily bathing with bath oils or emollients will rehydrate the skin and leave a lipid layer on the surface which will trap the water and prevent its evaporation. Patients should be advised to apply further emollients or moisturizers after bathing and regularly throughout the day.

Potassium permanganate soaks

Atopic dermatitis may also present with exudative lesions, especially when superinfected. In these cases, daily potassium permanganate soaks (1 in 8000 dilution, described as 'pink gin') help dry the skin.

Antihistamines

Sedating antihistamines may be used at night to reduce pruritus and help patients sleep.

Medical management

Topical corticosteroids

Topical steroids are the mainstay in the treatment of atopic dermatitis. To minimize potential side effects the least potent preparation required to keep the dermatitis under control should be used (Table 14.12). Treatment should not be applied more than twice a day and the 'fingertip unit' (one fingertip equals 0.5 g) is a convenient way to advise the patient how much should be applied (Table 14.13).

Only mild potency topical steroids (1% hydrocortisone) should be used routinely in children as the side effects are minimal. In adults, mild potency topical steroids should be used on the face and in the flexures, as steroid absorption is increased at these sites. Flexural sites are prone to candidal intertrigo and a combination of topical steroids and antifungal agents is useful. On the thick skin of the palms

Table 14.13	Recommended amount of topical corticosteroid by body region
Site	**Fingertip unit**
Face	1
Trunk (front and back)	14
One arm	3
One hand	1
One leg	6
One foot	1

and soles, percutaneous absorption is reduced and so potent preparations can be used until the dermatitis is well controlled. Response rates on lichenified skin may be accelerated with keratolytic agents in combination with topical steroids or with topical steroids under occlusion. Steroid therapy should not be stopped suddenly as rebound flare may occur. Once the dermatitis is controlled, the potency of the steroids should be reduced.

Systemic side effects are rare with the use of topical steroids. Topical therapy under occlusive dressings, however, will result in increased systemic absorption. Children and the elderly are particularly susceptible. Adrenal suppression and subsequent growth retardation can occur in children.

Topical macrolides

Tacrolimus and pimecrolimus are immunosuppressive macrolides which act on T lymphocytes to inhibit interleukin-2 transcription, resulting in decreased responsiveness to foreign antigens.[2] Pimecrolimus is licensed for topical use in mild to moderate atopic eczema and tacrolimus is an effective treatment for moderate or severe disease.[3] The use of these agents avoids some of the side effects of topical steroids and they are particularly useful for atopic dermatitis affecting the areas where skin is thin, such as the face. Treatment should be supervised by a specialist and long-term studies are still awaited.

Systemic therapy

Ciclosporin, azathioprine and mycophenolate mofetil have been reported to be effective in atopic dermatitis and can be used in severe refractory cases. Systemic corticosteroids have an important role in the management of patients with severe atopic dermatitis during an acute flare. They should not be used for maintenance treatment until all other avenues have been explored.

Phototherapy and photochemotherapy

PUVA and UVB have been found to be helpful in selected patients. There are concerns about the long-term adverse effects such as cutaneous malignancies. Narrowband ultraviolet B has recently been introduced and appears safer than PUVA but is equally as effective.

Table 14.12	Local side effects of topical corticosteroids

Epidermal
  Thinning
  Hypopigmentation

Dermal
  Reduced collagen synthesis
  Thinning
  Striae distensae
  Haemorrhage/purpura after minor skin trauma
  Telangiectasia and thread veins

Infection
  Worsening fungal and viral infections
  Folliculitis

Eyes
  Glaucoma and cataracts with prolonged use of potent topical steroids around the eyes

Other
  Rosacea with use of moderate and potent steroids on the face
  Contact dermatitis because of contact allergy to topical steroids

Antibiotics and antiviral agents

Atopic dermatitis, particularly when excoriated, is very susceptible to secondary infection. Bacterial infection of the skin, if mild to moderate can be treated with a topical antibiotic such as fusidic acid, usually in combination with a topical steroid. If the infection is severe a concomitant systemic antibiotic should be used. Flucloxacillin (or erythromycin in penicillin-allergic patients) is usually the most appropriate antibiotic for treating *Staphylococcus aureus*, which is the most common pathogen. Phenoxy-methylpenicillin should be given if β-haemolytic strepto-cocci are isolated. Eczema herpeticum responds to oral aciclovir, and this should be given early in the course of disease.

Prognosis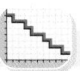

Most patients with atopic dermatitis should expect to keep their eczema under control if managed correctly. Approximately 75% of children with atopic dermatitis are clear of their condition by their early teens but relapses may occur.

i FURTHER INFORMATION

Hanifin JM, Cooper KD, Ho VC, et al. Guidelines of care for atopic dermatitis, developed in accordance with the American Academy of Dermatology/American Academy of Dermatology Association 'Administrative Regulations for Evidence-based Clinical Practice Guidelines'. Journal of the American Academy of Dermatology 2004; 50: 391–404.

REFERENCES

(1) *Charman C. Clinical evidence. Atopic eczema. BMJ 1999; 318: 1600–1604.*
(2) *Reitamo S, Remitz A, Kyllonen H, Saarikko J. Topical noncorticosteroid immunomodulation in the treatment of atopic dermatitis. American Journal of Clinical Dermatology 2002; 3: 381–388.*
(3) *Alomar A, Berth-Jones J, Bos JD, et al. The role of topical calcineurin inhibitors in atopic dermatitis. British Journal of Dermatology 2004; 151 (Suppl 70): 3–27.*

Seborrhoeic dermatitis

Epidemiology

Seborrhoeic dermatitis is a common relapsing dermatitis.

Pathology

Seborrhoeic dermatitis affects regions where sebaceous glands are most active such as the scalp, face and upper trunk. Although the exact pathogenesis is unknown, there is strong evidence to link it with the presence of the *Malassezia* yeasts and the condition responds to antifungal therapies. There is seasonal variation with aggravation in winter. Widespread seborrhoeic dermatitis is very common in HIV infection and may be due to altered cellular immunity.

Clinical features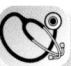

Patients usually complain of the cosmetic effects of scaling and redness rather than itching. Lesions are covered with fine scale and are often well demarcated. The scalp may be diffusely involved or lesions may be localized to the scalp margins. On the face, the paranasal areas, eyebrows and external ears are commonly affected (Fig. 14.20). Elsewhere, the presternal area, interscapular area, axillae and groins may be involved.

Seborrhoeic dermatitis of infancy can appear during the first 18 months of life. There is a non-pruritic, well-demarcated eczema of the scalp and intertriginous areas. Greasy thick yellowish scales cover the scalp ('cradle cap'). This can spread to the face and trunk. Lesions of the axillae and inguinal folds are acutely inflamed and sharply demarcated. Superimposed infection with *Candida* species may occur. Symptoms are usually mild and this condition has an excellent prognosis. Its precise relationship with adult seborrhoeic dermatitis is unclear.

Investigations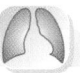

The diagnosis is clinical and investigations are not usually required.

Management

Antifungal shampoo
Scalp involvement is usually treated with a shampoo containing antifungal agents.

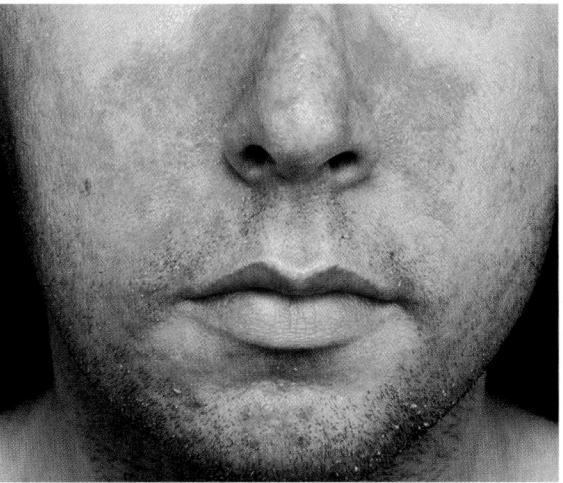
Fig. 14.20 Seborrhoeic dermatitis.

Topical antifungals and immunomodulation

Facial and other glabrous skin lesions are treated with topical antifungals or a combination of a mild topical steroid and an antifungal cream. Short courses of oral antifungal therapy have been shown to be useful in severe cases.

Prognosis

In general there is a good response to treatment.

Discoid or nummular dermatitis

Discoid dermatitis is a chronic condition that is more common in men and occurs predominantly in persons over 50 years of age. The pathogenesis is unknown. It is characterized by sharply demarcated, erythematous coin-shaped lesions which are extremely pruritic (Fig. 14.21). The centre of the lesions can contain vesicles, crusts and scales. Secondary infection with *Staphylococcus aureus* is common. The lesions require treatment with potent topical steroids.

Vesicular hand and foot (dyshidrotic) dermatitis (pompholyx)

Endogenous vesicular hand and foot dermatitis is common and affects both sexes, usually before the age of 40. The pathogenesis is unknown. It is an intensely pruritic condition that presents with crops of clear vesicles or blisters on the palms (Fig. 14.22), soles and sides of fingers and toes. The lesions slowly resolve over a few weeks but recurrence is common, especially in the summer. Secondary infection may occur with pustule formation. The treatment of the

acute condition requires potent topical steroids and in severe attacks a short course of systemic steroids may be necessary. In addition, potassium permanganate soaks are used to dry the lesions initially. Emollients should be used during the healing phase.

Stasis (gravitational or varicose) dermatitis

Stasis dermatitis is a common condition of the lower legs, more common in middle-aged and elderly women. It is caused by venous hypertension and so is seen in association with varicose veins and following deep venous thrombosis. Increased venous pressure results in an increase in the escape of fibrinogen from capillaries, leading to deposition of a fibrin sheath around them. This impedes diffusion of oxygen and other nutrients into the tissues, leading to the inflammatory response characteristic of this condition. Stasis dermatitis commonly affects the inner lower leg, characterized by erythema and scaling. It can result in oedema, haemosiderin deposition, small white areas of atrophy (atrophie blanche) and ulceration (Fig. 14.23). In some patients, lipodermatosclerosis may be evident, with woody hardness of the legs. This condition is managed with leg elevation, pressure bandages or support stockings and moderately potent topical steroids.

Lichen simplex

Lichen simplex is not associated with underlying skin disease. The skin becomes thickened or lichenified by repeated rubbing, as a habit secondary to stress. Areas typically affected include the nape and sides of the neck, lower legs and ankles and anogenital regions. Reduction of underlying emotional stress and potent topical steroids under occlusion are useful in treatment.

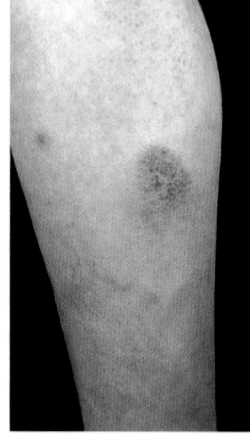

Fig. 14.21 Discoid dermatitis.

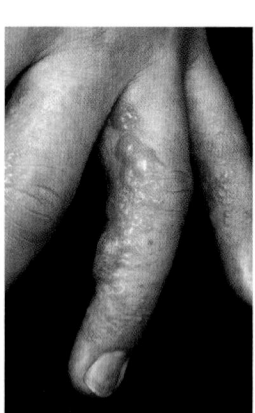

Fig. 14.22 Endogenous vesicular hand dermatitis.

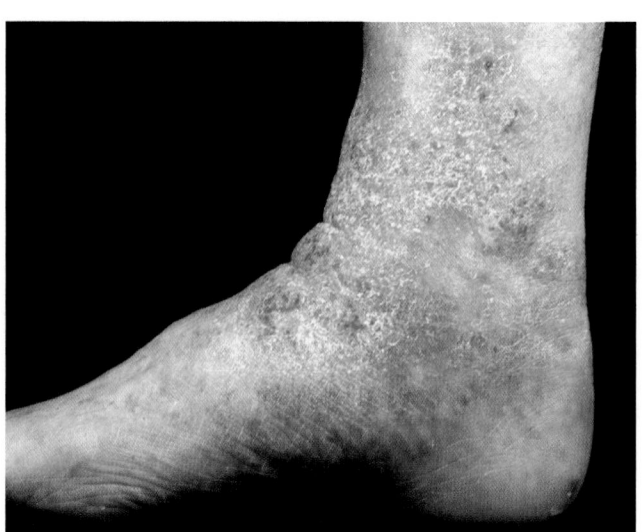

Fig. 14.23 Stasis dermatitis.

Asteatotic dermatitis

Asteatotic dermatitis results when there is excessive loss of skin lipids. It usually occurs on the shins of elderly patients. The skin is generally dry and in some areas cracks appear which become red (eczema craquelé). It is precipitated by excessive washing and is usually worse in the winter (low humidity and drying effect of central heating). The use of soap substitutes and emollients treats and prevents this condition.

Prurigo nodularis

Prurigo nodularis is a chronic condition characterized by a papulonodular dermatitis which is very pruritic. Its aetiology is unknown. This condition is difficult to treat. Topical corticosteroids are the treatment of choice. Oral treatments with ciclosporin and thalidomide have been shown to improve both the appearance of the skin and the pruritus.

Exogenous (contact) dermatitis

Exogenous dermatitis, also known as contact dermatitis, is caused by exposure to external substances. It may be irritant or allergic. Although patients may suffer with these subtypes separately, in practice it is not uncommon for endogenous, irritant and allergic aetiologies to coexist, particularly in hand dermatitis (Fig. 14.24).

The prevalence of contact dermatitis has been estimated at 5% in the general population and 10% in patients with high-risk occupations. Occupational contact dermatitis is the most common of all occupational diseases.

Irritant contact dermatitis

Irritant dermatitis is the most common form of contact dermatitis, accounting for up to 75% of exogenous dermatitis. It is a non-immunological process and results from direct chemical or physical damage to the skin by offending agents such as detergents or organic solvents. All individuals are susceptible to the development of an irritant contact dermatitis if exposure to irritant agent(s) is sufficient. The most common site affected is the hands (Fig. 14.25).

There are two principal types of irritant contact dermatitis: acute and chronic. The acute form is caused by exposure to an agent causing early impairment in the stratum corneum function followed by an inflammatory reaction. The chronic form is caused by repeated exposure to the same or different factors resulting in cumulative damage until an inflammatory reaction ensues which persists for a long period, even after further exposure is stopped. Those with a history of atopic dermatitis, especially atopic hand dermatitis, are particularly at risk of developing a chronic irritant contact dermatitis.

The main aim of management is to identify and avoid or control exposure to the irritant(s). Topical steroids can help in the acute stage and healing should occur within 2 weeks. Cases of chronic irritant dermatitis may last many months and tend to have a poor prognosis. These patients benefit from regular use of emollients.

Allergic contact dermatitis

Allergic contact dermatitis is caused by exposure to an allergen that has previously sensitized the patient.

Epidemiology

Allergic contact dermatitis is common and may develop in response to a vast range of substances. Approximately

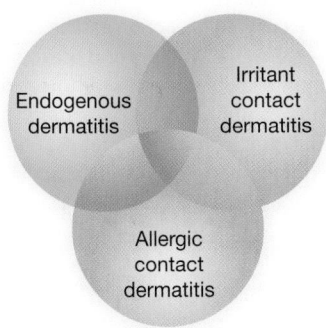

Fig. 14.24 Possible multifactorial aetiology of dermatitis.

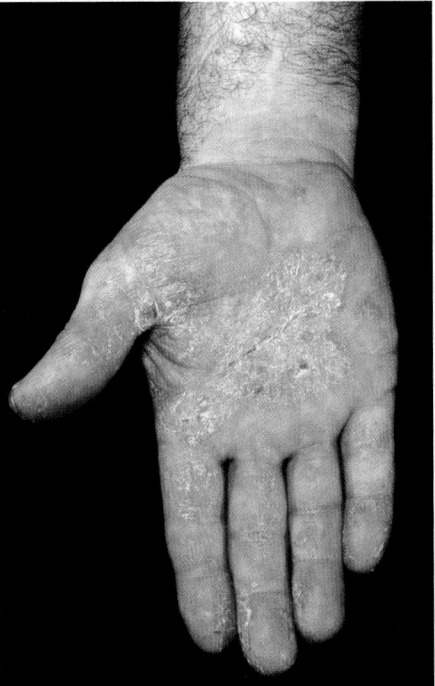

Fig. 14.25 Irritant contact hand dermatitis.

867

10% of women are allergic to nickel, which used to be found in some jewellery (Fig. 14.26).

Pathology

Allergic contact dermatitis is caused by a type IV hypersensitivity reaction. There are two phases: induction and elicitation. The induction phase occurs when an antigen placed on the skin penetrates the epidermis and is recognized as foreign by Langerhans' cells. They transport the antigen to the T-cell areas of the draining lymph node, where they present it to T cells and generate T-cell clones. No clinical abnormality is observed during the induction phase. The elicitation phase refers to the process whereby the same antigen placed on the skin is recognized by Langerhans' cells, leading to an influx of sensitized T cells into the skin. The resulting delayed-type hypersensitivity reaction, which is mediated by a variety of cytokines produced by the T cells, typically takes 48–72 hours to develop and leads to the histological and clinical features of dermatitis.

The probability of developing hypersensitivity depends on the sensitizing capacity of the chemical and exposure to it (exposure is assessed in terms of dose per unit area applied to the skin).

Clinical features

On exposure to the allergen, a delayed-type hypersensitivity reaction (type IV) occurs, giving rise to an eczematous rash at the site of contact several hours later (Fig. 14.26).

Investigations

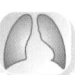

Patch tests (type IV hypersensitivity)
Patch testing (see investigations, p. 853) is the only method for objective evaluation of an exogenous dermatitis. It is essential if an allergic contact dermatitis is suspected, particularly in cases where the hands or the face are affected. It should also be considered in cases of atopic dermatitis, stasis dermatitis or otitis externa unresponsive to treatment as sensitization to topical medicaments may have developed.

Management

Patients need to avoid the offending allergen and when necessary use topical steroids.

Prognosis

Although hypersensitivity may be lost over a long time, once acquired it should be considered to last indefinitely.

i FURTHER INFORMATION

Bourke J, Coulson I, English J, British Association of Dermatologists. Guidelines for care of contact dermatitis. British Journal of Dermatology 2001; 145: 877–885.

REFERENCE

(1) *White IR. ABC of work related disorders. Occupational dermatitis. BMJ 1996; 313: 487–489.*

Photocontact dermatitis

The term photocontact dermatitis is used to describe a local eczematous reaction in the skin caused by exposure of a topically applied chemical to sunlight. It is divided into photo-irritant (phototoxic) and photoallergic contact dermatitis. Reactions are restricted to sun-exposed areas such as the face (typically sparing areas under the nose and chin), neck and forearms. Photo-irritant (phototoxic) reactions clinically resemble exaggerated sunburn and can be caused by essential oils such as citron, lavender and lime. Phytophototoxic contact dermatitis is a type of photo-irritant reaction and is caused by contact with furocoumarins (psoralens) in plants, followed by light exposure. Photoallergic contact dermatitis is clinically similar to a simple allergic contact dermatitis. If it becomes chronic, lichenification occurs. This reaction can be seen in response to certain ingredients in UV filters and used to be seen with halogenated antimicrobial agents. Photopatch tests are used to identify potential photoallergens in suspected cases of photoallergic contact dermatitis. Patients need to avoid the offending allergen as well as sunlight and when necessary use topical steroids.

Intertrigo

Intertrigo is a non-specific inflammation of opposed skin, occurring in the submammary region, axillae, groins and

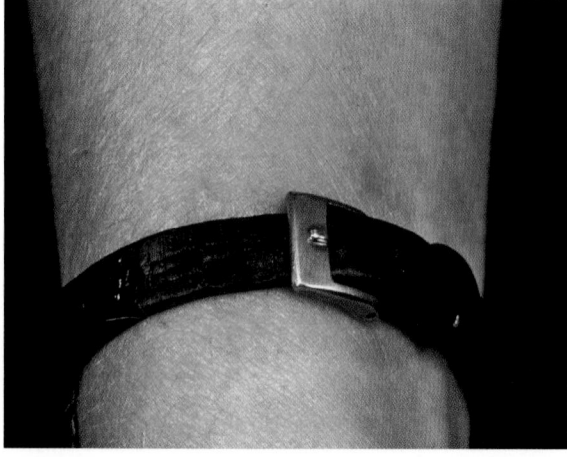

Fig. 14.26 Allergic contact dermatitis from nickel.

gluteal folds. With increased moisture and maceration, the stratum corneum becomes eroded. This problem is more common in obese individuals. It presents with erythema and symptoms of pruritus and tenderness. Intertriginous infections caused by bacteria and yeasts must be ruled out (p. 890). Dermatoses such as psoriasis vulgaris, seborrhoeic

dermatitis and atopic dermatitis also occur in body folds and these need to be considered in the differential diagnosis. A moderate topical steroid containing antimicrobials (such as clobetasone with oxytetracycline and nystatin) is often helpful.

SECTION 14.4 Urticaria and other inflammatory dermatoses

Urticaria

Urticaria encompasses two main entities, wheals and angio-oedema. Wheals are transient, superficial, pruritic swellings of the skin due to plasma leakage from small blood vessels, whilst angio-oedema is deeper swellings of the skin and the gastrointestinal tract. Urticaria has a spectrum of clinical presentations and causes (Table 14.14).

Epidemiology

Urticaria is a common disorder that affects 20% of all people at some stage during their lifetime.

Pathology

Urticaria and angio-oedema result from the degranulation of mast cells and basophils. This results in the release of histamine and other vasoactive compounds such as bradykinin and prostaglandins. Urticaria is characterized by oedema, vascular dilatation with endothelial swelling and

a perivascular infiltrate consisting of lymphocytes and variable number of eosinophils.

Urticaria can be triggered by a number of physical factors (such pressure on the skin), biological or chemical contact on the skin, as well as foods and drugs. However, in the majority of cases an external cause cannot be identified,[1] and this is referred to as ordinary urticaria (Table 14.14). This 'ordinary' pattern of urticaria may have diverse aetiologies including autoimmunity, allergy and infection, although the majority will remain idiopathic after investigation (Table 14.15).

Overall, the aetiology of urticaria can be subdivided into idiopathic, immunological and non-immunological (Table 14.15).

Immunological urticaria

In approximately 33% of patients with chronic ordinary urticaria, histamine-releasing autoantibodies are found which degranulate mast cells by binding either to IgE receptors or to IgE bound to them. These cases are now referred to as autoimmune urticaria; some are associated with autoimmune thyroid disease.

Cross-linking of specific IgE on mast cells by allergens (immediate type I hypersensitivity reactions) can cause allergic contact urticaria, anaphylaxis and some cases of acute ordinary urticaria.

Table 14.14	Clinical classification of urticaria and angio-oedema*

Ordinary urticaria (76%)
  Acute (up to 6 weeks of continuous activity)
  Chronic (6 weeks or more of continuous activity)

Physical urticarias (defined by the triggering stimulus) (14%)
  Dermographism
  Cholinergic urticaria
  Delayed pressure urticaria
  Cold urticaria
  Aquagenic urticaria
  Solar urticaria
  Localized heat urticaria
  Acquired vibratory angio-oedema

Contact urticaria (induced by biological or chemical skin contact) (1%)

Urticarial vasculitis (defined by vasculitis on skin biopsy) (0.5%)

Angio-oedema (without wheals) (9%)

* Grattan C, Powell S, Humphreys F. Management and diagnostic guidelines for urticaria and angio-oedema. British Journal of Dermatology 2001; 144: 708–714.

Table 14.15	Aetiology of urticaria and angio-oedema*

Idiopathic

Immunological
  Autoimmune (autoantibodies against IgE receptors or IgE bound to them)
  IgE dependent (type I hypersensitivity reactions)
  Immune complex (urticarial vasculitis)
  Complement dependent (C1 esterase inhibitor deficiency)

Non-immunological
  Direct mast cell releasing agents (e.g. opiates)
  Aspirin, non-steroidal anti-inflammatories and dietary pseudo-allergens
  Angiotensin-converting enzyme inhibitors

* Grattan C, Powell S, Humphreys F. Management and diagnostic guidelines for urticaria and angio-oedema. British Journal of Dermatology 2001; 144: 708–714.

In urticarial vasculitis, circulating immune complexes are deposited in the dermal vessels of the skin resulting in a type III hypersensitivity reaction.

The angio-oedema of C1 esterase deficiency results from uncontrolled complement activation (consumption causes low levels of C2 and C4) and generation of vasoactive mediators. Trauma to the skin can trigger an attack because C1 esterase inhibitor activity is involved in the fibrinolytic cascade as well as in complement pathways.

Non-immunological urticaria

Certain agents can result in degranulation of mast cells without involvement of the IgE receptor. These include certain drugs such as codeine and radiocontrast media.

Aspirin, non-steroidal anti-inflammatories and dietary pseudo-allergens may possibly precipitate urticaria through leukotriene formation although the exact mechanism is unknown. Angiotensin-converting enzyme (ACE) inhibitors inhibit kinin breakdown and may result in urticaria and angio-oedema.

In a small proportion of cases, underlying infection such as bowel helminths may be found, although there is little evidence to support this association.

Scope of disease

Urticaria is normally uncomplicated with no systemic manifestations. Although wheals and angio-oedema are often a feature of anaphylactic reactions, which may result in glottal and laryngeal swelling and potential fatal airway obstruction, urticaria only very occasionally progresses to anaphylaxis.

Clinical features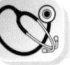

Wheals are transient, oedematous, pink or red papules or plaques, of sudden onset, often pruritic. Clearing of the central area may leave an annular pattern (Fig. 14.27) that often resolves leaving normal appearing skin. Angio-oedema consists of dermal and subcutaneous swelling, often in a perioral and periorbital distribution (Fig. 14.28).

Urticaria is classified according to clinical presentation, duration of activity and time taken for individual wheals to resolve (Table 14.14).

Ordinary urticaria

Ordinary urticaria is the most common form of urticaria (76%).[1] Individual wheals may occur anywhere on the body and last from 2 to 24 hours. In the acute form the signs and symptoms last a few days and often no cause can be found. Occasionally it may be associated with a recent infection, medication (antibiotics such as penicillins, aspirin, codeine) or certain foods (including nuts, fish, eggs, milk and vegetables). In chronic cases, wheals occur daily for longer than 6 weeks and a cause is almost never found (chronic idiopathic urticaria). Angio-oedema is common and frequently a component of ordinary urticaria.

Physical urticaria

Physical factors that precipitate urticaria usually result in wheals that appear in minutes and last for less than an hour (except in delayed pressure urticaria where they take longer to develop and fade). Dermographism is the most common physical urticaria and consists of the development of pruritic, linear wheals at sites where the skin is firmly stroked. In delayed pressure urticaria, painful wheals appear after a delay of hours at sites of sustained pressure on the skin (such as from tight clothing or from gripping tools) and can occur in association with chronic ordinary urticaria. Cholinergic urticaria occurs under conditions which cause sweating such as exertion, heat, emotional stress and eating spicy foods. Small wheals occur within minutes, usually on the trunk. Antihistamines are helpful and are best taken prophylactically before the triggering event. Cold urticaria is precipitated by cold wind and water, leading to pruritic wheals at exposed sites that can also be reproduced by the application of an ice cube to the forearm. Aquagenic urticaria is an extremely rare type of urticaria. Wheals occur on the skin at sites of contact with water at any temperature. Solar urticaria is rare and presents with wheals immediately after exposure to sunlight.

Contact urticaria

Contact urticaria can be allergic (IgE-mediated immediate) or non-immunological. Allergic contact urticaria is clinically the more common type. It is precipitated by allergens in contact with the skin and may present with symptoms ranging from burning and stinging at the site of contact to localized wheals (typically lasting up to 2 hours). Common causes include natural rubber latex proteins and fruits.

Urticarial vasculitis

The lesions of urticarial vasculitis persist for days but may look indistinguishable from ordinary urticaria. They resolve to leave post-inflammatory hyperpigmentation. Wheals show histological features of venulitis and can be accompanied with arthralgia and abdominal pain. The majority of cases are idiopathic, although in some patients urticarial vasculitis may be the presenting feature of underlying

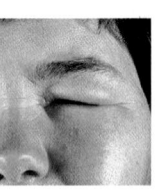

Fig. 14.28 Angio-oedema.

Fig. 14.27 Urticaria.

connective tissue disease such as systemic lupus erythematosus (SLE) and Sjögren's syndrome. Patients need a full vasculitis screen, and possible infective precipitants of the process such as a recent streptococcal infection or hepatitis infection should be sought.

Hereditary angio-oedema

Hereditary angio-oedema is a rare autosomal dominant disorder. It occurs as a result of C1 esterase inhibitor deficiency. Patients suffer with recurrent acute episodes of intestinal colic, or facial, orbital and laryngeal oedema. A characteristic feature is the absence of pruritus and urticarial lesions. Of affected patients, 15% have normal levels of C1 inhibitor but functional assays show it to be inactive in these cases. A severe attack of angio-oedema may result in fatal obstruction of the airway.

Initial investigations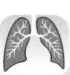

Urticaria is usually diagnosed and classified clinically. In general, there is little value in laboratory investigations, and patients with mild to moderate urticaria do not require investigation.

Further investigations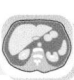

Allergy tests

IgE-mediated reactions to environmental allergens such as nuts in acute ordinary urticaria and latex in contact urticaria can be confirmed by skin-prick testing and radioallergosorbent (RAST) tests.

Full blood count (FBC)

FBC and white cell differential may be abnormal in cases of urticaria associated with infection (eosinophilia in bowel helminth infections).

Markers of inflammation

The ESR is raised in cases of urticarial vasculitis.

Vasculitic screen

A full vasculitic screen including complement assays should be conducted in suspected cases of urticarial vasculitis.

Thyroid function tests

Thyroid function tests (and autoantibodies) are performed in patients with autoimmune urticaria to screen for thyroid dysfunction.

Autologous serum skin test

An autologous serum skin test involves intradermal injection of autologous serum and is a relatively sensitive and specific screening test in centres with experience for histamine-releasing autoantibodies.

Challenge tests

There are proposed international standards and challenge tests for the diagnosis of physical urticaria.

Skin biopsy

A skin biopsy is essential for the diagnosis of urticarial vasculitis.

Complement levels and C1 esterase inhibitor assay

C1 esterase inhibitor (level and function) deficiency should be screened for in patients with recurrent angio-oedema. Usually C1, C2 and C4 levels are low.

Initial management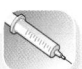

Identify and address any precipitating cause

Precipitating factors such as drugs (codeine, aspirin, NSAIDs, ACE inhibitors), dietary pseudo-allergens and physical factors should be avoided or minimized.

Patient education

It is important to explain to the patient that in the majority of cases the underlying cause cannot be found.

> ### ⚡ CLINICAL ALERT
>
> *In patients who develop laryngeal oedema or anaphylaxis, intravenous hydrocortisone is given with intramuscular adrenaline (1:1000). Although the effects of intravenous hydrocortisone are not immediate, it is given to limit the swelling once the crisis is over. Patients with a history of severe oral angio-oedema should carry an adrenaline self-injection device with them at all times.*

Medical management

Antihistamines

Non-sedating H_1 receptor antagonists, for example fexofenadine and loratadine, are the mainstay of treatment for urticaria. Combination with an H_2 antagonist (such as cimetidine) and sedating antihistamines at night may be useful in resistant cases. Of the treated patients, over 50% show a good response.[1] Conditions in which prolonged wheals are present (delayed pressure urticaria and urticarial vasculitis) do not respond well to antihistamine therapy.

Corticosteroids

Oral corticosteroids may shorten the duration of acute urticaria. Short tapering courses of oral steroids may be necessary for urticarial vasculitis and severe delayed pressure urticaria.

Immunomodulation

Plasmapheresis and intravenous immunoglobulin may be effective in severe autoimmune chronic urticaria. Ciclosporin has recently been shown to be effective in patients with severe autoimmune disease resistant to antihistamines.

Management of C1 esterase inhibitor deficiency

Attenuated androgens (stanozolol, danazol) and tranexamic acid may be used for long-term treatment of C1 esterase inhibitor deficiency. Maintenance treatment is only required in cases with recurrent angio-oedema or abdominal pain. Stanozolol and danazol have virilizing side effects when used long term, and patients require regular monitoring for hepatic inflammation and tumours. Tranexamic acid can also be given as prophylaxis for a few days before planned surgery; however, it is contraindicated in patients with a history of thrombosis, and regular liver function tests are recommended. C1 esterase concentrate or fresh frozen plasma can be given as emergency treatment for angio-oedema or as prophylaxis before emergency surgery. In severe cases adrenaline and hydrocortisone are required.

Prognosis

Approximately 50% of patients with chronic urticaria with wheals alone are clear in 6 months. However, over 50% of patients with wheals and angio-oedema still have severe disease after 5 years.[2]

> **_i_ FURTHER INFORMATION**
>
> Grattan CEH. The urticaria spectrum: recognition of clinical patterns can help management. Clinical and Experimental Dermatology 2004; 29: 217–221.

REFERENCES

(1) *Nettis E, Pannofino A, D'Aprile C, Ferrannini A, Tursi A. Clinical and aetiological aspects in urticaria and angio-oedema. British Journal of Dermatology 2003; 148: 501–506.*
(2) *Grattan C, Powell S, Humphreys. Management and diagnostic guidelines for urticaria and angio-oedema. British Journal of Dermatology 2001; 144: 708–714.*

Erythema nodosum

Erythema nodosum is the most common form of panniculitis (inflammation of the subcutaneous fat).

Epidemiology

Erythema nodosum commonly presents in the third decade and has a higher incidence in females.

Pathology

Erythema nodosum probably results from the formation of immune complexes and their deposition in and around venules of connective tissue septa in the subcutaneous fat. Circulating immune complexes and complement activation have been recorded in some patients. This immunological reaction is elicited by various infections, systemic disorders and drugs (Table 14.16).

Histologically, erythema nodosum is a septal panniculitis. The septa of subcutaneous fat are thickened and infiltrated by inflammatory cells that extend to the peri-septal areas of fat lobules. In early lesions oedema, fibrin exudation and neutrophils are responsible for the septal thickening, whereas fibrosis, peri-septal granulation tissue, lymphocytes and multinucleated giant cells are the main findings in the late-stage lesions of erythema nodosum.

Clinical features

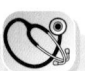

The main clinical features are tender, poorly defined, erythematous warm nodules usually located bilaterally on the shins (Fig. 14.29). At first the nodules are bright red in colour, but within a few days they become purplish and finally exhibit a greenish yellow appearance resembling a bruise. The patient may also be systemically unwell with fever, malaise and arthralgia.

Investigations

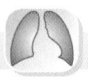

Full blood count/markers of inflammation
Investigations reveal an elevated ESR, CRP and a leukocytosis.

Table 14.16	Causes of erythema nodosum

Infection

Bacterial infections
  Streptococcal infection
  Tuberculosis
  Leprosy
  Salmonella gastroenteritis
  Yersinia enterocolitis
  Campylobacter colitis
  Chlamydia pneumoniae

Fungal infections
  Histoplasmosis
  Coccidioidomycosis
  Dermatophytes

Viruses
  Infectious mononucleosis
  Hepatitis B

Drugs

Sulphonamides

Oral contraceptive pill

Penicillin

Bromides

Other

Sarcoidosis

Inflammatory bowel disease

Malignancy

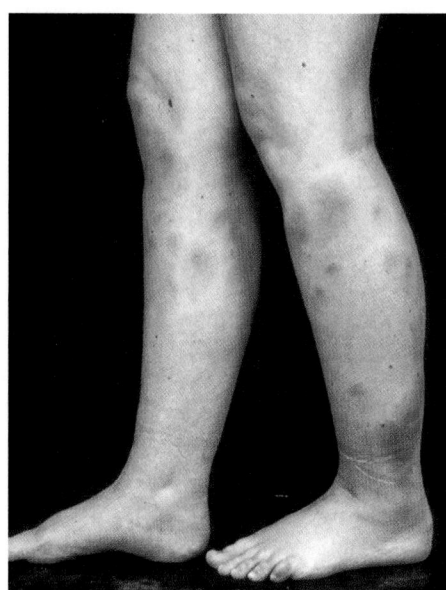

Fig. 14.29 Erythema nodosum.

Antistreptolysin O titres

ASO titres are raised in streptococcal infection.

Throat swab

Throat swabs should be taken for group A β-haemolytic streptococcus.

Stool sample

A stool sample should be sent when there are gastroenterological symptoms.

Chest X-ray

A chest X-ray is important to look for bilateral hilar lymphadenopathy in sarcoidosis.

Skin biopsy

The diagnosis is made clinically but may be supported by characteristic histopathological appearances. A deep wedge biopsy of the tissue is required.

Management

Identify and address any underlying condition

Treatment should be directed to the underlying associated condition, if known.

Symptomatic treatment

Symptoms can be reduced with compressive bandages to the legs and bed rest. Non-steroidal anti-inflammatories can be helpful.

Immunomodulation

Systemic steroids are rarely indicated but can be given in severe cases (once underlying infection is ruled out), with rapid resolution of lesions.

Prognosis

Individual lesions last a few days and heal without atrophy or scarring but new lesions erupt in their place. Spontaneous resolution occurs in about 6 weeks, however the actual course depends on aetiology.

i FURTHER INFORMATION

Requena L, Requena C. Erythema nodosum. Dermatology Online Journal 2002; 8: 4.

Erythema multiforme and Stevens–Johnson syndrome

Erythema multiforme is an acute self-limiting disorder caused by inflammation of the skin and mucous membranes, and presents with characteristic target lesions. Stevens–Johnson syndrome is a severe variant of erythema multiforme associated with fever and extensive mucous membrane lesions.

Epidemiology

Erythema multiforme is uncommon and tends to occur in the young: 50% of patients are under 20 years of age. It is more frequent in males than females.

Pathology

Erythema multiforme is a cell-mediated hypersensitivity reaction to many different immunological triggers, in particular drugs and infectious agents. In over 50% no cause is found (Table 14.17). Histologically, there is epidermal necrosis and subepidermal bulla formation with a lymphohistiocytic infiltrate and oedema of the upper dermis.

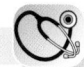

Clinical features

Patients present with a polymorphic eruption of erythematous macules, papules, blisters, erosions and target lesions (Fig. 14.30). This is often most severe on the palms, soles and face but can become widespread. Mucous membrane involvement, in particular the eyes, mouth and occasionally the larynx and trachea, is often seen in cases of erythema multiforme triggered by a drug reaction. The patient may also be systemically unwell with fever and malaise.

In Stevens–Johnson syndrome, the oral mucosa, lips and conjunctivae are most commonly affected, although the genital mucosa and the respiratory tract may also be involved. Ophthalmological complications involve conjunctival/corneal erosions, synechiae formation and keratitis, and therefore an ophthalmologist should be involved early on in the management of these patients.

873

Table 14.17	Causes of erythema multiforme

Idiopathic

Infections
  Herpes simplex
  Mycoplasma
  HIV
  Hepatitis B
  Tuberculosis
  Orf

Drugs
  Barbiturates
  Penicillin
  Sulphonamides

Collagen vascular disorder
  Systemic lupus erythematosus
  Dermatomyositis
  Polyarteritis nodosa
  Wegener's granulomatosis

Other
  Underlying malignancy
  Sarcoidosis

Management

Identify and address any precipitating cause

Mild disease is self-limiting and the first line of management is withdrawal of the offending drug and prompt treatment of any associated disease.

Immunomodulation

Systemic corticosteroids may have a role in severe cases, though their effectiveness has not been established by controlled studies.

Aciclovir

Recurrent erythema multiforme is usually associated with outbreaks of herpes simplex infection and in these cases chronic suppressive aciclovir therapy is helpful.

Prognosis

The prognosis depends on the severity of disease, the underlying trigger and the appropriateness and promptness of management.

Toxic epidermal necrolysis

Toxic epidermal necrolysis is a rare disorder characterized by extensive epidermal death.

Epidemiology

Toxic epidermal necrolysis has an incidence of 0.2 per 100 000 per year.

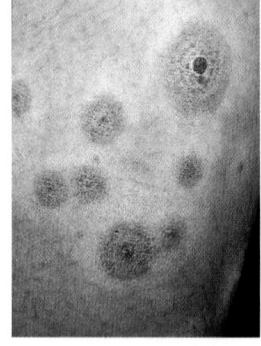

Fig. 14.30 Erythema multiforme.

Pathology

Toxic epidermal necrolysis is almost invariably due to drugs, with sulphonamides, anticonvulsants, thiazide diuretics, antimalarials and non-steroidal anti-inflammatories being the most common precipitating agents. The median time of the illness following first exposure to a candidate drug is 10–14 days, but may be as long as 6 weeks. The eruption is immediate on second exposure to a previous trigger. Histopathology shows subepidermal blisters and keratinocyte necrosis progressing to full thickness epidermal necrosis. Damage to the skin is thought to be mediated by cytotoxic T cells and mononuclear cells which induce apoptosis in keratinocytes expressing drug-derived antigens at their surface.

Scope of disease

The main mechanism of death is overwhelming infection, often after several weeks of recurrent episodes of infection. The causative organism is usually *Staphylococcus aureus* early on, and Gram-negative infections later in the course of the disease.

Clinical features

There is initially a prodromal phase of fever, cough and malaise. About 3 days later, there is widespread erythema which is rapidly followed by blister formation with confluence and eventual sloughing of large sheets of epidermis involving more than 30% of body surface area (Fig. 14.31). The cutaneous lesions resemble superficial burns and show a positive Nikolsky sign (epidermal separation induced by gentle lateral pressure on the surface of the skin). Oral, conjunctival and anogenital mucous membranes are prominently involved. Ophthalmological complications involve conjunctival/corneal erosions, synechiae formation, keratitis and sicca syndrome. In some cases there may be extensive involvement of the gastrointestinal tract, and respiratory involvement occurs in up to 30% of cases. Other target organs include bone marrow, liver, pancreas and kidney.

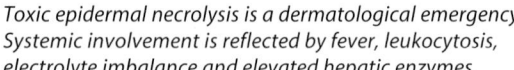

CLINICAL ALERT

Toxic epidermal necrolysis is a dermatological emergency. Systemic involvement is reflected by fever, leukocytosis, electrolyte imbalance and elevated hepatic enzymes.

Initial investigations

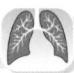

The diagnosis is clinical and investigations are not usually required.

Further investigations

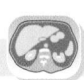

Skin biopsy

A skin biopsy may be helpful if the diagnosis is in doubt.

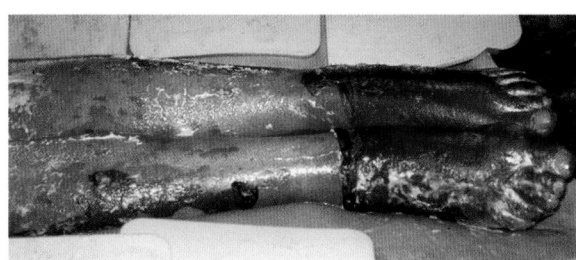

Fig. 14.31 Toxic epidermal necrolysis.

Blood tests
Full blood count, renal and liver function tests, amylase and inflammatory markers are all useful in assessing systemic involvement.

Bacterial swabs
Bacterial skin swabs should be sent for microscopy, sensitivity and culture.

Blood and line cultures
Blood cultures must be sent if there is any evidence of infection. Any lines or catheters must also be cultured.

Initial management

Identify and address any precipitating cause
The suspected drugs must be promptly withdrawn. All drugs started within 7–21 days of the first manifestation of the skin eruption should be stopped.

Supportive treatment
Early referral to a high-dependency or intensive-care unit for supportive management is appropriate. As the main mechanism of death is overwhelming infection, meticulous attention to minimizing infection is essential. Renal failure, pulmonary failure, fluid and electrolyte imbalance and nutritional deficiencies are other contributing factors. Early nutritional support (nasogastric or parental feeding) with high-protein supplements should be initiated. Patients require adequate pain relief and may even need general anaesthesia for pain control and often for dressing change.

Skin and oral care
Careful skin management with particular emphasis on aseptic techniques is essential. Emollients must be applied to all non-eroded areas 2–3 times daily and patients should be nursed on greased padded sheets. Topical antiseptic creams should be applied to all eroded sites and the skin covered with non-adhesive dressings. The dressings should be changed every 24 hours initially and then every 2–3 days as the skin starts to re-epithelialize. Antiseptic and analgesic mouth rinses 4–5 times a day are necessary.

Medical management

Immunomodulation
The opinions on immunomodulation treatment are controversial. Systemic corticosteroids and immunosuppressive drugs (ciclosporin) have been used to suppress progression of disease, together with symptomatic and supportive therapy, but some consider immunomodulation drugs harmful as they greatly enhance the risk of infection. More recently intravenous immunoglobulin treatment has been used with inconclusive results.[1]

Multidisciplinary approach
A multidisciplinary team approach is favoured. Patients require full assessment of skin, mouth, eyes, genital area and urethra, and all possible target organs. Ophthalmologists should be involved early on.

Prognosis

Increasing age, significant comorbidity, neutropenia and greater extent of skin involvement correlate with a worse prognosis. Toxic epidermal necrolysis has an overall mortality of 25% and there is frequent disability from ophthalmological and mucous membrane sequelae in survivors.

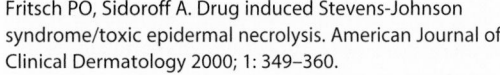

i FURTHER INFORMATION

Fritsch PO, Sidoroff A. Drug induced Stevens-Johnson syndrome/toxic epidermal necrolysis. American Journal of Clinical Dermatology 2000; 1: 349–360.

Chave TA, Mortimer NJ, Sladden MJ, et al. Toxic epidermal necrolysis: current evidence, practical management and future directions. British Journal of Dermatology 2005; 153: 241–253.

REFERENCE

(1) *Bachot N, Revuz J, Roujeau JC. Intravenous immunoglobulin treatment for Stevens-Johnson syndrome and toxic epidermal necrolysis. Archives of Dermatology 2003; 139: 33–36.*

Pyoderma gangrenosum

Pyoderma gangrenosum is an uncommon condition characterized by non-infectious inflammatory necrosis of the skin.

Epidemiology

The incidence of pyoderma gangrenosum is uncertain. It most commonly affects the 30–50-year age group.

Pathology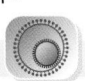

The aetiology is unknown but in the majority of cases pyoderma gangrenosum is associated with an underlying disease, most commonly inflammatory bowel disease, rheumatoid and seronegative arthritis, monoclonal gammopathy, haematological malignancy or following surgery.

Clinical features

Patients present with rapidly spreading, painful and tender ulcers which classically have an undermined violaceous border (Fig. 14.32). The lower limb is most frequently affected although lesions can occur at any site. Patients are often unwell with general malaise and fever.

Investigations
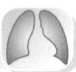

Skin biopsy
Diagnosis is based on typical clinical presentation, history of an underlying disease and histopathological findings (a neutrophilic infiltrate in the dermis and vasculitic change thought to be secondary to the ulceration).

Management

Identify and address underlying cause
The underlying systemic disorder should be recognized and managed.

Immunomodulation
Systemic steroids are needed for rapidly advancing or widespread disease. In refractory cases immunosuppression, most commonly with ciclosporin or azathioprine, may be warranted. Sulfa drugs such as dapsone, or clofazimine, minocycline and thalidomide, have been used in combination with corticosteroids as a corticosteroid-sparing alternative. Alternative treatments include local application of granulocyte–macrophage colony-stimulating factor and intravenous immunoglobulin.

Antibiotics
Systemic antibiotics may be needed for secondary bacterial infections.

Surgical debridement
Surgery rarely has a role as debridement or skin grafting carries a risk of tissue pathergy, a key feature of the disease in which any traumatized skin develops additional necrosis and ulceration.

RECENT ADVANCES
Recently there have been reports of larger wounds being managed surgically in conjunction with immunosuppression with promising results.[1]

Prognosis

Despite recent advances in therapy, the prognosis of pyoderma gangrenosum remains unpredictable.

i FURTHER INFORMATION

Crowson AN, Mihm MC Jr, Magro C. Pyoderma gangrenosum: a review. Journal of Cutaneous Pathology 2003; 30: 97–107.

Powell FC, O'Kane M. Management of pyoderma gangrenosum. Dermatologic Clinics 2002; 20: 347–355.

REFERENCE

(1) *Kaddoura IL, Amm C. A rationale for adjuvant surgical intervention in pyoderma gangrenosum. Annals of Plastic Surgery 2001; 46: 23–28.*

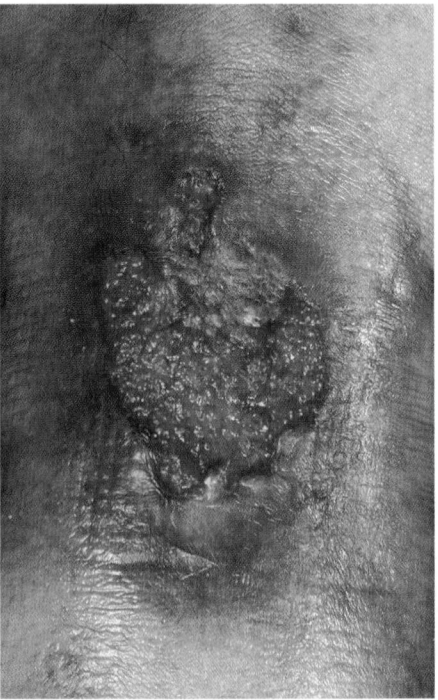

Fig. 14.32 Pyoderma gangrenosum.

Granuloma annulare

Granuloma annulare is a common chronic inflammatory dermatosis.

Epidemiology

Granuloma annulare most commonly affects children and young adults and is more common in females.

Pathology

The aetiology is unknown. Granuloma annulare is characterized by the degeneration of dermal collagen and an associated lymphohistiocytic infiltrate.

Clinical features

Clinically, granuloma annulare can be localized or diffuse and presents as flesh-coloured, erythematous or violaceous papules arranged in an annular pattern (Fig. 14.33). The lesions are most commonly found on the dorsum of hands and feet and are usually asymptomatic. They enlarge centrifugally and may last months to years before resolving without scarring. There may be an association between diffuse granuloma annulare and diabetes mellitus, although this has not been clearly established. Several studies support the view that generalized granuloma annulare, especially in the elderly, is associated with impaired glucose tolerance.

Investigations

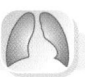

Skin biopsy

Physical signs are often characteristic, however if the diagnosis is in doubt, it can be confirmed on skin histology.

Management

Expectant management

Granuloma annulare is a self-limiting disorder and no treatment is required in the majority of patients.

Immunomodulation

Topical or intralesional steroids can be effective when lesions result in cosmetic disfigurement.

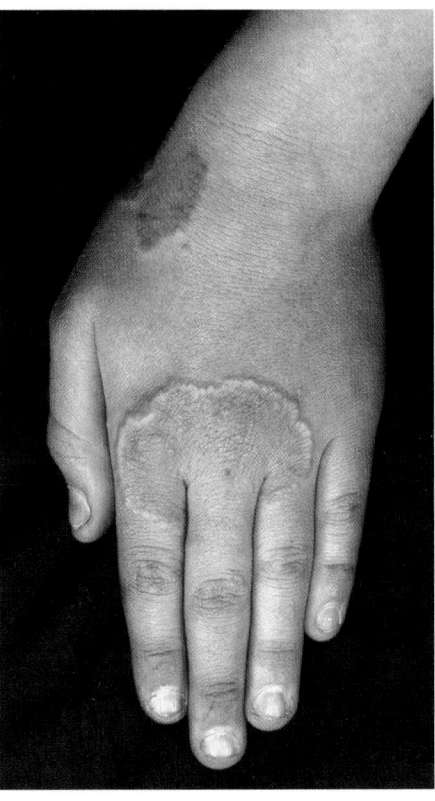

Fig. 14.33 Granuloma annulare.

PUVA photochemotherapy

In generalized granuloma annulare, PUVA photochemotherapy may be effective.

Prognosis

In general, granuloma annulare is a self-limiting disorder but recurrences can occur in up to 40%.

Disorders of sebaceous and apocrine glands

Acne vulgaris

Acne is a chronic inflammatory condition of pilosebaceous units and manifests itself as comedones, papules, pustules and eventually scarring.

Epidemiology

Acne vulgaris is a common disease affecting around 40% of 16–18-year-olds.[1] Minor degrees are an almost universal finding throughout puberty in both sexes. All races may be affected, although there is a lower incidence in Asians and blacks.

Pathology

The aetiology of acne involves abnormal keratinization, hormonal activity, bacterial growth and immune hypersensitivity. The disease is limited to the pilosebaceous units of the head and upper trunk. The primary lesion arises from a change in the keratinization of the hair follicle and results in a micro-comedone due to impaction and distension of the follicle with improperly desquamated keratinocytes and sebum.

At puberty, androgens stimulate sebaceous glands to produce larger amounts of sebum, and pre-existing comedones become filled with lipids and enlarge. *Propionibacterium acnes*, a usually harmless commensal bacterium in the pilosebaceous units, contains bacterial lipases that convert lipid into fatty acids. Together with sebum, it causes an inflammatory response in the pilosebaceous unit resulting in the hyperkeratinization and plugging of the follicle.

The enlarging follicular lumen that contains keratin and lipid debris is known as a whitehead (closed comedone). A follicle with a port of entry at the skin with oxidized sebum forming a black tip is known as a blackhead (open comedone). The distended follicle may rupture releasing its contents into the dermis. This provokes a foreign body response resulting in papules, pustules or nodules. Scarring can follow this intense inflammation.

Clinical features

The lesions of acne vulgaris almost always occur on the face. The upper back and chest are involved in approximately 70%. The main skin lesions are comedones, both open and closed. Papules, pustules and nodules may also be present (Fig. 14.34). Nodulocystic acne is a variant consisting of large tender nodules and cysts, which eventually form deep scars (Fig. 14.35). It is important to

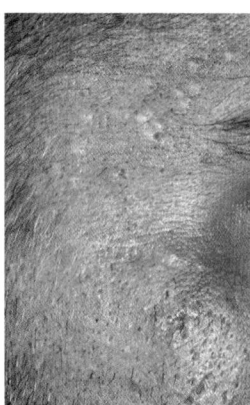

Fig. 14.34 Acne vulgaris.

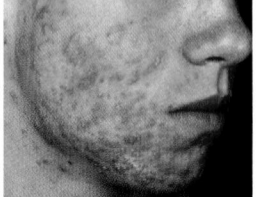

Fig. 14.35 Nodulocystic acne.

recognize and treat this form of acne early in life before extensive scarring has occurred. The severity of disease can be assessed using the revised Leeds grading system.[2] This is a pictorial grading approach which looks at the extent of inflammation, range and size of inflamed lesions, and associated erythema.

A number of factors, including endocrine disorders and drugs, can exacerbate acne vulgaris (Table 14.18).

Initial investigations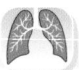

Acne is a clinical diagnosis.

Further investigations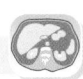

Investigations may be required to rule out underlying causes such as hyperandrogenism and polycystic ovary syndrome.

Testosterone, follicle-stimulating hormone (FSH), luteinizing hormone (LH) and dehydroepiandrosterone sulphate (DHEA-S) levels

In the overwhelming majority of acne patients, hormone levels are normal and, unless clinically indicated, do not need to be checked. Raised free testosterone and DHEA-S levels indicate hyperandrogenism. In polycystic ovary syndrome, the ratio of LH to FSH is increased and the levels of testosterone, oestradiol and androstenedione are raised.

Medical management

Treatment should be commenced early to prevent scarring. The choice of treatment depends on whether the acne is

Table 14.18	Exacerbating factors for acne
Oils or cosmetics (pomade acne)	
Occlusion and pressure on the skin (acne mechanica)	

Endocrine disease
    Polycystic ovarian disease
    Cushing's disease
    Congenital adrenal hyperplasia	

Drugs
    Lithium
    Isoniazid
    Phenytoin
    Topical and systemic glucocorticoids
    Oral contraceptives
    Androgens	

predominantly comedonal or inflammatory, and its severity (Fig. 14.36).

Patient education

The psychological impact of acne should be assessed in each patient and therapy modified accordingly. Patients should be warned that an improvement might not be seen for at least a couple of months.

Topical preparations

Benzoyl peroxide is effective in mild to moderate acne and can be used for both comedones and inflamed lesions. Adverse effects include local skin irritation, particularly when treatment is initiated. Azelaic acid has both antimicrobial and anticomedonal properties. It is less likely to cause local irritation and may be an alternative to benzoyl peroxide.

Topical antibacterials

For mild–moderate inflammatory acne, topical antibacterials such as erythromycin and clindamycin can be used together with benzoyl peroxide. This treatment should be continued for at least 6 months before its benefits can be fully assessed. Antibacterial resistance of *P. acnes* has increased over the last 20 years. Failure to respond to topical treatment after 8 weeks should prompt a change of treatment.

Topical retinoids

Tretinoin and isotretinoin are effective in comedonal and inflammatory acne. Patients should be warned that some redness and peeling might occur but will settle with time.

Improvement occurs over a period of months but may take longer for non-inflamed comedones.

Oral antibiotics

Systemic antibacterial treatment should be considered for all cases of moderate–severe inflammatory acne, and in cases of mild–moderate inflammatory acne where topical treatments used over a period of 3–6 months have been ineffective. Anticomedonal treatment such as benzoyl peroxide or topical retinoids can be used in conjunction with oral antibiotics. Oxytetracycline or tetracycline 500 mg twice a day is usually used. If there is no response after the first 3 months another oral antibiotic should be given. Maximum benefit usually occurs after 4–6 months. Doxycycline and minocycline both at 100 mg daily are alternative antibiotics. Erythromycin can also be used; however, there are now widespread resistant propionibacterium strains and so the response is often poor.

Hormone treatment

Co-cyprindiol (cyproterone acetate with ethinylestradiol) contains an antiandrogen that decreases sebum secretion. It is useful in women who need treatment for acne and also wish to receive oral contraception.[3]

Oral retinoids

Isotretinoin is a synthetic retinoid that inhibits sebaceous gland function and keratinization, and also has some anti-inflammatory activity. It is extremely effective treatment for severe acne (including nodulocystic acne) and disease which has not responded to an adequate course

Acne vulgaris

Rosacea

Hidradenitis suppurativa

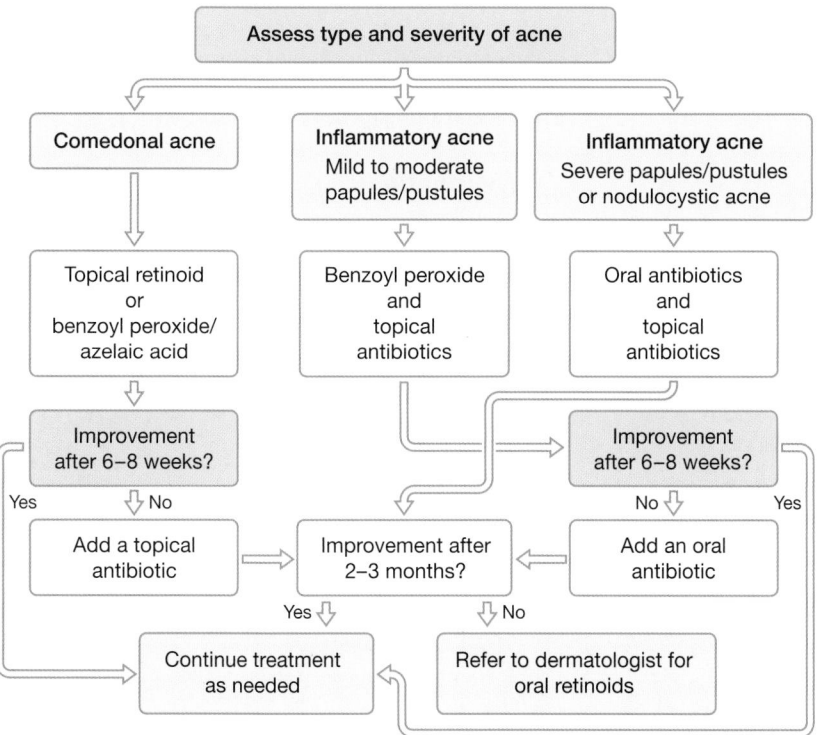

Fig. 14.36 Management of acne vulgaris.

of a systemic antibacterial. Isotretinoin, 0.5–1 mg/kg, is given for about 16 weeks. Although it has revolutionized the management of acne, it is a toxic drug that is prescribed only by, or under the supervision of, a consultant dermatologist. The drug is teratogenic and must not be given to women of child-bearing age unless they practise effective contraception. Pre-treatment tests should include a lipid profile, liver function tests, full blood count and, in the case of women, a negative pregnancy test. These tests should be repeated at 1 month and then every 3 months until the treatment is completed. Concerns have been raised that oral isotretinoin may occasionally cause depression, psychotic symptoms and rarely suicide attempts. However, retrospective studies have failed to demonstrate a relationship. Nevertheless, particular care needs to be taken in patients with a history of depression (Table 14.19).

After successful control of disease, maintenance treatment with topical agents is essential with reintroduction of oral antibiotics if acne recurs.

Prognosis

Most cases of acne clear spontaneously by the early twenties but around 5% of cases may persist into the third decade. With the appropriate treatment 90% of patients show a 50% improvement in 3 months and an 80% improvement within 6 months, but continuous treatment may be necessary for many years.

i FURTHER INFORMATION

Webster GF. Acne vulgaris. BMJ 2002; 325: 475–479.

British Association of Dermatologists. Isotretinoin. Advice on safe introduction and continued use of isotretinoin in acne. http://www.bad.org.uk/healthcare/guidelines/acne.asp

REFERENCES

(1) Cordain L, Lindeberg S, Hurtado M, Hill K, Eaton SB, Brand-Miller J. Acne vulgaris. A disease of Western civilization. Archives of Dermatology 2002; 138: 1584–1590.
(2) O'Brien SC, Lewis JB, Cunliffe WJ. The revised acne grading system. Journal of Dermatological Treatment 1998; 9: 215–220.
(3) Shaw JC. Acne: effect of hormones on pathogenesis and management. American Journal of Clinical Dermatology 2002; 3: 571–578.

Table 14.19	Adverse effects of isotretinoin
Dry skin and mucous membranes	
Myalgia	
Epistaxis	
Thinning of hair	
Hepatitis	
Night blindness	
Possible association with depression	

Rosacea

Rosacea is a chronic inflammatory facial eruption characterized by papules and pustules on a background of erythema and telangiectasia.

Epidemiology

Rosacea is common. An epidemiological study from Sweden reported a prevalence of 10 000 per 100 000.[1] The peak age at presentation is the third or fourth decade and the condition has been more frequently observed in patients with fair skin. It has an equal sex incidence but men often have more severe disease.

Pathology

The pathogenesis of rosacea is unknown. Histologically there is a non-specific perifollicular and perivascular inflammatory infiltrate with dilated capillaries in the superficial dermis.

Clinical features

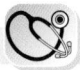

Rosacea is a persistent disease with episodic inflammatory flares. Patients usually have a long history of episodic facial flushing, which may be exacerbated by heat, emotional upset, hot drinks, spicy foods and alcohol. During these episodes, there is intense erythema symmetrically over the cheeks, nose, forehead and chin. There are three stages in the evolution of this disease (Table 14.20).

Chronic rosacea can be associated with marked sebaceous hyperplasia, most commonly on the nose giving a bulbous craggy appearance. This is known as rhinophyma (Fig. 14.38). There may also be lymphoedema resulting in swelling of the central part of the face. Approximately 50% of patients have minor degrees of ocular involvement, most commonly conjunctivitis, blepharitis and keratitis leading to corneal scarring (p. 651).

Investigations

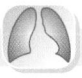

Rosacea can be diagnosed clinically; investigations are not usually required.

Skin biopsy

If the diagnosis is in doubt a skin biopsy may be required for histopathology.

Table 14.20	Stages in the evolution of rosacea
Stage	**Clinical features**
I	Persistent erythema with telangiectasia
II	Persistent erythema, telangiectasia, papules and tiny pustules (Fig. 14.37)
III	Persistent deep erythema, dense telangiectasia, papules, pustules and nodules

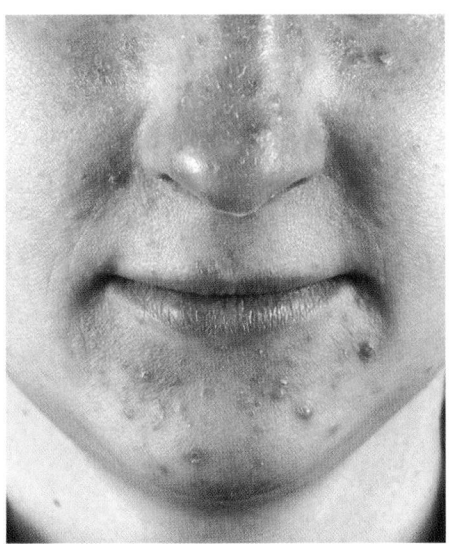

 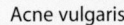
Acne vulgaris

Rosacea

Hidradenitis suppurativa

Fig. 14.37 Stage II rosacea.

Surgery

Rhinophyma is treated by surgery or laser surgery, shaving the hypertrophic tissue from the nose. Unfortunately regrowth of this tissue frequently occurs.

Prognosis

Despite optimal treatment, recurrences are common.

FURTHER INFORMATION

Rebora A. The management of rosacea. American Journal of Clinical Dermatology 2002; 3: 489–496.

REFERENCE

(1) *Berg M, Liden S. An epidemiological study of rosacea. Acta Dermato-venereologica 1989; 69: 419–423.*

Management

Identify and address precipitating factors

Patients are advised to avoid factors that provoke facial flushing. Reduction of alcoholic and hot beverages is helpful in some cases.

Concealing agents

Camouflages can be used for the erythema, and laser treatment is helpful in the treatment of telangiectasia.

Antibiotic therapy

Papules and pustules of rosacea respond well to topical metronidazole or to oral oxytetracycline or tetracycline 500 mg twice daily. Courses usually last 6–12 weeks and are repeated intermittently. Alternatively doxycycline or minocycline 100 mg daily can be given.

Oral retinoids

Isotretinoin is occasionally given in refractory or severe cases. Despite topical and systemic treatment the redness and telangiectasia may not improve.

Hidradenitis suppurativa

Hidradenitis suppurativa is a chronic inflammatory and suppurative disease of apocrine gland-bearing skin in the axillae, inguinal areas, perianally and on the perineum. It usually occurs alone but may be associated with severe nodulocystic acne, pilonidal sinuses and Crohn's disease. The exact pathogenesis is unknown. Initial papules, pustules and cysts go on to form sinus tracts with considerable scarring. Management is difficult and most patients require a combination of systemic antibiotics, intralesional gluco-corticoids and oral isotretinoin. Surgery may be required for severe disease and this can range from incision and drainage to excision of the involved area and split skin grafting.

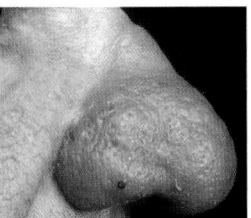

Fig. 14.38 Rhinophyma.

Vesicular and bullous diseases

Blistering may be a feature of a wide range of skin disorders (Table 14.21). A blister less than 5 mm in diameter is called a vesicle and one greater than 5 mm is referred to as a bulla.

Autoimmune bullous diseases

The autoimmune bullous diseases are a rare group of disorders characterized by blistering of the skin and mucous membranes. They are classified according to the level of split within the skin. Subcorneal (beneath the stratum corneum) and intraepidermal blisters (within the stratum spinosum) rupture easily, whereas subepidermal ones (at the dermal–epidermal junction) are less fragile. Direct and indirect immunofluorescence techniques demonstrate the autoantibodies involved (see p. 853) and are the mainstay of diagnosis and classification (Table 14.22).

Table 14.21	Causes of vesicular and bullous eruptions
Trauma	
Friction	
Burns	
Drugs	
Barbiturates	
D-penicillamine	
Infections	
Impetigo	
Herpes simplex virus	
Varicella zoster virus	
Autoimmune	
Pemphigus	
Pemphigoid	
Pemphigoid gestationis	
Epidermolysis bullosa acquisita	
Dermatitis herpetiformis	
Linear IgA disease	
Congenital	
Epidermolysis bullosa	
Other	
Insect bites	
Eczema	
Erythema multiforme	
Toxic epidermal necrolysis	
Porphyria cutanea tarda	
Paraneoplastic pemphigus	

Pemphigus

Pemphigus is a group of uncommon but potentially life-threatening autoimmune bullous disorders caused by circulating IgG against epidermal antigens. There are several forms of pemphigus, varying in their epidemiology, clinical presentation and target antigen. Pemphigus vulgaris and pemphigus foliaceus are the two main subtypes.

Epidemiology

Pemphigus is a disease of all ages. The most common age of onset is in the fifth and sixth decades. It has an equal incidence in males and females but shows marked racial and geographical variation.

Pathology

In patients with pemphigus, there is a loss of normal cell to cell adhesion in the epidermis as a result of circulating IgG autoantibodies. These antibodies bind to cell surface desmosomal glycoproteins and induce acantholysis (disruption of epidermal intercellular connections resulting in separation of keratinocytes).

In pemphigus vulgaris this antigen is desmoglein 3 (Dsg3), whereas in pemphigus foliaceus the target antigen is desmoglein 1 (Dsg1). However, at least 50% of pemphigus vulgaris patients have additional autoantibodies to Dsg1. Dsg3 is more prevalent in the deeper layers of the epidermis, in contrast to Dsg 1 which is localized more superficially. The differences in the position of these antigens explain the different sites of acantholysis histologically, and the clinical appearance in the two conditions.

A pemphigus vulgaris or pemphigus foliaceus like syndrome can be induced by D-penicillamine and less frequently by captopril and other drugs. In most, but not all, instances the eruption resolves after stopping the offending drug.

Scope of disease

Painful mouth lesions may prevent adequate food intake, resulting in weakness and weight loss. There are often secondary bacterial infections and when large areas of skin are denuded, fluid loss and catabolic changes produce severe metabolic disturbances. In mothers with pemphigus, transient neonatal disease may occur in the offspring due to placental transfer of IgG autoantibodies.

Table 14.22   Classification of autoimmune bullous diseases according to the level of split within the skin

Level of cleavage	Disease	Direct IF	Indirect IF
Subcorneal	Pemphigus foliaceus	Intercellular IgG/C3	Intercellular IgG
Intraepidermal	Pemphigus vulgaris	Intercellular IgG/C3	Intercellular IgG
	Pemphigus vegetans	Intercellular IgG/C3	Intercellular IgG
Subepidermal	Bullous pemphigoid	Linear BMZ IgG/C3	Anti-BMZ IgG Binding to roof of SS
	Cicatricial pemphigoid	Linear BMZ IgG/C3	Anti-BMZ IgG Binding to roof of SS
	Pemphigoid gestationis	Linear BMZ C3	Complement and anti-BMZ IgG Binding to roof of SS
	Epidermolysis bullosa acquisita	Linear BMZ IgG	Anti-BMZ IgG Binding to base of SS
	Dermatitis herpetiformis	Granular deposits of IgA in dermal papillae	No circulating antibodies to BMZ or dermal papillae IgA endomysial antibodies
	Linear IgA disease	Linear BMZ IgA	Anti-BMZ IgA Binding to roof on SS

IF, immunofluorescence; BMZ, basement membrane zone; SS, split skin.

Clinical features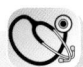

Pemphigus affects the skin and the mucous membranes. It is characterized by widespread flaccid blisters which rapidly rupture forming erosions and crusts. Shearing stresses on normal skin may cause superficial separation of the skin and new lesions to form (Nikolsky's sign). The oral cavity is the most common mucous membrane involved and in a third of cases the mouth is affected before the skin.

Pemphigus vulgaris is the most common type, with widespread blisters and erosions. Lesions usually start in the oral mucosa and many months elapse before skin lesions occur (Fig. 14.39). Pemphigus vegetans is a more localized form of this with vegetating purulent plaques at flexural sites. In pemphigus foliaceus, widespread more superficial blisters rupture, leaving predominantly erosions and crusts. This is because the target antigen, Dsg1, is located more superficially in the epidermis. There is no mucosal involvement. A distinctive form of pemphigus foliaceus (Brazilian pemphigus) is endemic in Brazil, where it affects all age groups and is thought to be related to an arthropod-borne infectious agent.

Investigations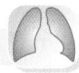

Skin biopsy

Skin biopsies should be sent for histology and (fresh) for immunofluorescence staining. Histology shows intraepidermal blisters high in the epidermis in pemphigus foliaceus and in a suprabasal location in pemphigus vulgaris. Acantholysis (disruption of epidermal intercellular connections) of the epidermis is seen in both forms.

Direct immunofluorescence of uninvolved skin shows characteristic intercellular epidermal deposits of IgG and C3 beneath the stratum corneum in pemphigus foliaceus and within the stratum spinosum in pemphigus vulgaris and pemphigus vegetans. Around 90% of patients also have circulating IgG autoantibody demonstrated on indirect immunofluorescence. The titre of circulating antibodies often correlates with disease activity.

Initial management

Antibiotics

General measures include antibiotics for bacterial skin infections.

Fluid and electrolytes

Replacement of fluid and correction of any electrolyte imbalances are important.

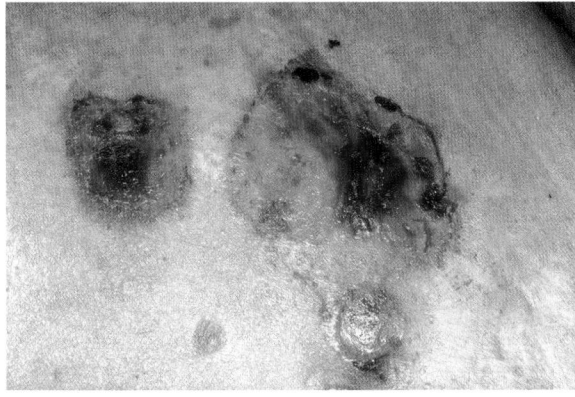
Fig. 14.39 Pemphigus vulgaris.

Medical management

Systemic corticosteroids

Systemic corticosteroids are the mainstay of treatment in pemphigus, initially given at high doses (1 mg/kg body weight of prednisolone) until new blister formation ceases. This is followed by gradual tapering to a minimum effective maintenance dose. Treatment successes are often associated with profound corticosteroid-related complications (p. 425).

Other immunomodulatory agents

Many patients require a second immunosuppressive drug either for its corticosteroid-sparing effect or to achieve complete remission. Azathioprine can be given in doses up to 2.5 mg/kg daily until complete clearing. The risk of myelosuppression should be assessed by measurement of thiopurine methyltransferase (TPMT) activity prior to its use. Azathioprine may be continued for months after cessation of corticosteroids. Treatment should only be stopped if there is clinical freedom from disease and a negative pemphigus antibody titre for at least 3 months. Methotrexate and cyclophosphamide can also be given as adjuvant or alternatives to corticosteroids. Mycophenolate mofetil and high-dose intravenous immunoglobulin have been reported to be beneficial and clinical studies are ongoing.

Monitoring for haematological and biochemical indicators of immunosuppressive-induced adverse effects is necessary.

Plasmapheresis

Plasmapheresis (removal of pathogenic antibodies and inflammatory mediators) is used in severe or resistant cases unresponsive to conventional therapy and with high titres of pemphigus autoantibodies.

Management of mucosal lesions

Patients should be advised to use a mouthwash regularly. They may require steroid ointments for mucosal lesions and amphotericin B or nystatin for oral candidiasis.

Prognosis

The mortality rate with pemphigus is high unless it is diagnosed early and treated aggressively with immunosuppressive agents. The use of systemic corticosteroids has dramatically reduced mortality rates, from approximately 90% to less than 5%.

i **FURTHER INFORMATION**

Harman KE, Albert S, Black MM. Guidelines for the management of pemphigus vulgaris. British Journal of Dermatology 2003; 149: 926–937.

Bullous pemphigoid

Bullous pemphigoid is a chronic acquired autoimmune disorder in which subepidermal blisters develop as a result of circulating IgG antibodies directed against the basement membrane zone.

Epidemiology

Although bullous pemphigoid is the most common autoimmune blistering disease of the skin, it is rare with an estimated incidence of 0.6 per 100 000 per year in Europe. It predominantly affects the elderly and occurs equally in both sexes. There is no racial or geographical predilection.

Pathology

Pemphigoid is an autoimmune disease in which circulating IgG autoantibodies recognize two types of antigen, both components of the hemidesmosome adhesion complex. The first is a 230 kDa glycoprotein that is part of hemidesmosomes (BP230). The other is a 180 kDa transmembranous polypeptide (BP180). This results in junctional cleavage through the lamina lucida of the basement membrane zone.

An association with malignancies has previously been suggested, but large series have concluded that there is no significant increased risk of malignancy when compared to age- and sex-matched controls.[1]

Clinical features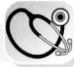

In bullous pemphigoid the eruption may be localized or generalized. Characteristically blisters develop on the flexural aspects of the extremities and the abdomen (Fig. 14.40), and may have been preceded by an urticarial or eczematous rash. They may become large and stay intact for several days (Fig. 14.40). Nikolsky's sign (p. 874) is negative. The degree of itch is variable and may precede the

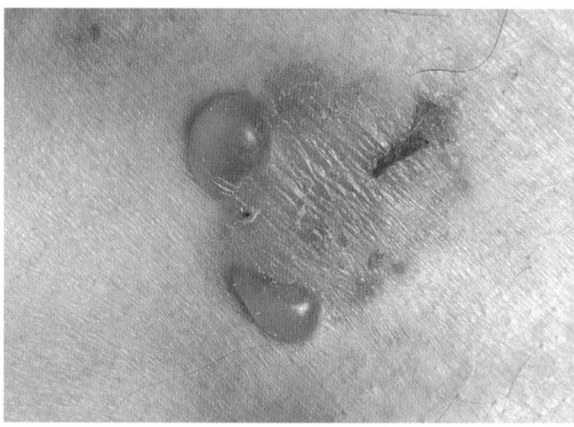

Fig. 14.40 Bullous pemphigoid.

appearance of blisters by weeks, months or occasionally years. The mucous membranes are involved in approximately 50%.

Investigations

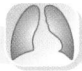

Skin biopsy

Biopsy of a fresh lesion shows a subepidermal blister with a mixed dermal inflammatory infiltrate containing eosinophils.

Direct immunofluorescence of uninvolved skin shows characteristic linear deposits of IgG and C3 at the basement membrane zone. Indirect immunofluorescence demonstrates circulating autoantibodies, which bind to the roof of salt-split skin. The titre of circulating antibody does not correlate with disease activity.

Management

There are two approaches to the management of bullous pemphigoid: either to start with a minimum dose of systemic treatment to control the disease, or to start with high-dose therapy and reduce the dose once control has been achieved. With either regimen, after initial control has been achieved, patients should be reviewed regularly until they are in complete remission.

Systemic corticosteroids

Systemic corticosteroids are the most established first-line treatment in bullous pemphigoid (Table 14.23). The initial doses are continued until new blister formation ceases and then gradually decreased according to the clinical response.

Topical corticosteroids may be effective in patients with localized disease and are also useful in generalized disease.

Other immunomodulatory agents

Many patients require a second immunosuppressive drug either for its corticosteroid-sparing effect or to achieve complete remission. Azathioprine is the best-established drug and can be given in doses up to 2.5 mg/kg daily. The risk of myelosuppression should be assessed by measurement of thiopurine methyltransferase (TPMT) activity prior to its use. There are numerous other immunosuppressive treatments that may be useful in resistant cases. These include dapsone and sulphonamides, cyclophosphamide, methotrexate, ciclosporin and mycophenolate mofetil. Tetracycline and nicotinamide have been reported to be effective in some cases of mild–moderate disease. As yet, there are no controlled clinical trials in the literature to assess the effectiveness of these other treatments.

Prognosis

Bullous pemphigoid is a chronic but self-limiting condition. Associated mortality rates can be as high as 41%.[2]

i FURTHER INFORMATION

Wojnarowska F, Kirtschig G, Highet AS, Venning VA, Khumalo NP. Guidelines for the management of bullous pemphigoid. British Journal of Dermatology 2002; 147: 214–221.

REFERENCES

(1) *Venning VA, Wojnarowska F. The association of bullous pemphigoid and malignant disease: a case control study. British Journal of Dermatology 1990; 123: 439–445.*
(2) *Korman NJ. Bullous pemphigoid. The latest in diagnosis, prognosis and therapy. Archives of Dermatology 1998; 134: 1137–1141.*

Dermatitis herpetiformis

Dermatitis herpetiformis is an acquired predominantly IgA-mediated subepidermal bullous disorder.

Epidemiology

Dermatitis herpetiformis is rare. It affects both sexes equally and has a predilection for Europeans and those of European descent.

Pathology

The exact pathogenesis is unknown; however, the majority of patients also have an asymptomatic gluten-sensitive enteropathy. There is a high incidence of HLA B8 and DR3, and association with other autoimmune disorders such as thyroid disease and pernicious anaemia. Dermatitis herpetiformis is also associated with an increased incidence of gastrointestinal lymphoma.

Clinical features

Dermatitis herpetiformis most commonly presents in young adults as an intensely pruritic eruption composed of grouped papules and vesicles distributed symmetrically on the extensor aspects of the elbows, knees and buttocks (Fig. 14.41). Mucosal involvement is minor.

Table 14.23	Initial prednisolone dose in bullous pemphigoid*		
Severity	**Mild**	**Moderate**	**Severe**
Initial dose of prednisolone	20 mg	40 mg	50–70 mg
Initial daily dose by weight	0.3 mg/kg	0.6 mg/kg	0.75 mg/kg

* Wojnarowska F, Kirtschig G, Highet AS, Venning VA, Khumalo NP. Guidelines for the management of bullous pemphigoid. British Journal of Dermatology 2002; 147: 214–221.

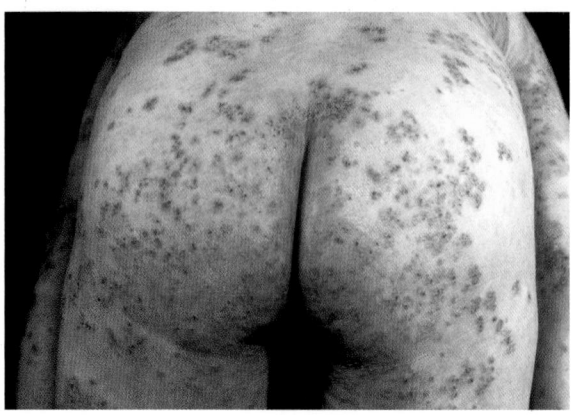

Fig. 14.41 Dermatitis herpetiformis.

Investigations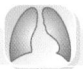

Skin biopsy

Skin biopsy shows subepidermal vesicles and microabscesses at the tips of dermal papillae. Direct immunofluorescence of normal skin shows granular deposits of IgA in the upper papillary dermis. There are no circulating antibodies to the basement membrane zone or dermal papillae.

Endomysial antibodies

Approximately 80% of patients have endomysial antibodies, a specific marker for underlying gluten-sensitive enteropathy.

Small intestinal biopsy

On small intestinal biopsy, these patients demonstrate partial or subtotal villous atrophy histologically.

Management

Gluten-free diet

A gluten-free diet may completely suppress the disease or allow reduction of the dose of systemic treatment, but the response is very slow.

Dapsone

There is often a rapid response to dapsone, which is the systemic drug of choice. Most lesions resolve within 48–72 hours. G6PD levels should be checked before starting dapsone as it may precipitate haemolytic anaemia in patients who are G6PD deficient. The full blood count is monitored carefully for the first few months.

Prognosis

The condition may persist for years with a third of the patients eventually undergoing spontaneous remission.

 FURTHER INFORMATION

Fry L. Dermatitis herpetiformis: problems, progress and prospects. European Journal of Dermatology 2002; 12: 523–531.

Congenital blistering diseases—epidermolysis bullosa

Epidermolysis bullosa (EB) is a group of inherited heterogeneous disorders characterized by the development of blisters after minor mechanical trauma to the skin (mechanobullous disease). There are three major subtypes—simplex, junctional and dystrophic—determined according to the level in the skin within which blisters develop (Fig. 14.42). Recent studies have identified specific protein and genetic abnormalities for most epidermolysis bullosa subtypes (Fig. 14.43).

A multidisciplinary team approach is required in the management of epidermolysis bullosa and should be tailored to the severity and extent of disease. This consists of supportive care for skin and other organ systems and entails a combination of wound management including surgical input as needed, nutritional support and preventative screening for squamous cell carcinoma in recessive dystrophic epidermolysis bullosa. New advances in the understanding of molecular pathophysiology have provided much of the basis for prenatal and pre-implantation genetic diagnosis, and current efforts to develop effective gene and protein therapy.

i **FURTHER INFORMATION**

Fine JD, Eady RAJ, Bauer EA, et al. Revised classification system for inherited epidermolysis bullosa: Report of the Second International Consensus Meeting on Diagnosis and Classification of Epidermolysis Bullosa. Journal of the American Academy of Dermatology 2000; 42: 1051–1066.

Uitto J, Richard G. Progress in epidermolysis bullosa: genetic classification and clinical implication. American Journal of Medical Genetics Part C, Seminars in Medical Genetics 2004: 131C; 61–74.

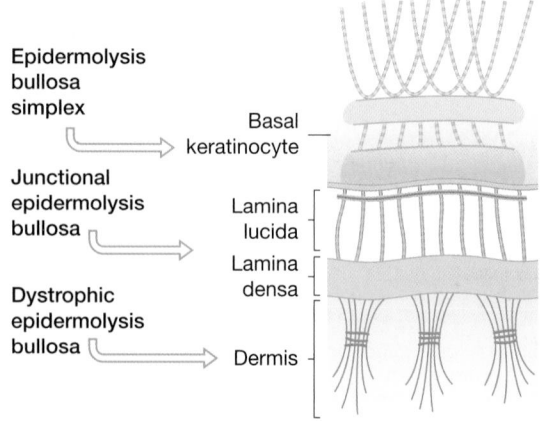

Fig. 14.42 Level of cleavage at the basement membrane zone in the three major subtypes of epidermolysis bullosa (see Fig. 14.3).

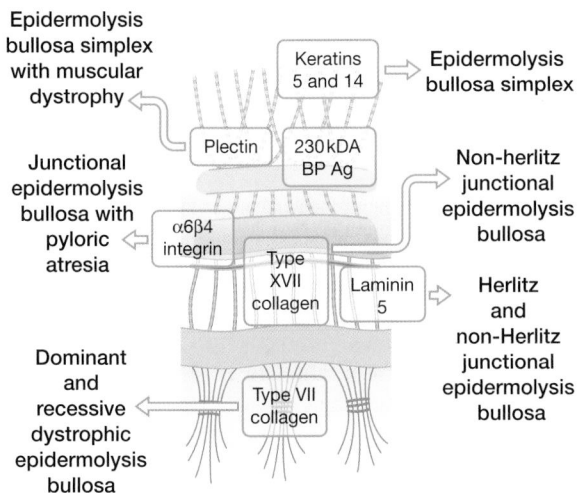

Fig. 14.43 Proteins involved in the different subtypes of epidermolysis bullosa.
Courtesy of Prof John McGrath and the Genetic Skin Disease Group, St John's Institute of Dermatology, St Thomas' Hospital, London, UK.

Epidermolysis bullosa simplex

Epidermolysis bullosa simplex is the most common subtype and is inherited as an autosomal dominant condition in the majority of cases. In this subtype, the plane of cleavage is through the basal keratinocytes (Fig. 14.42). This results from mutations in the genes encoding keratins 5 and keratin 14 which form the intracytoplasmic network of filaments of the basal keratinocytes (Fig. 14.43). There are several variants, the most common of which is Weber–Cockayne disease with localized involvement of the palms and soles. The more generalized variants include Köbner and Dowling–Meara. There is no significant extra-cutaneous involvement and blisters generally heal with no scarring.

Junctional epidermolysis bullosa

Junctional epidermolysis bullosa is inherited as an auto-somal recessive condition. In this subtype the plane of cleavage is at the level of the lamina lucida (Fig. 14.42) and results from mutations in the genes encoding components of the hemidesmosome-anchoring filament complex, laminin-5 and type XVII collagen (Fig. 14.43). There are two main variants. The more severe Herlitz form of junctional epidermolysis bullosa is characterized by widespread blistering of the skin and mucous membranes and is usually fatal within the neonatal period. In contrast, non-Herlitz junctional epidermolysis bullosa is less severe and generally carries a better prognosis. Blisters heal with atrophic scars and there are nail and teeth abnormalities.

Dystrophic epidermolysis bullosa

In the dystrophic form of the disease, separation occurs beneath the lamina densa (Fig. 14.42) because of mutations in the gene encoding type VII collagen, the major component of anchoring fibrils at the cutaneous basement membrane zone (Fig. 14.43). There are two main variants, autosomal dominant and autosomal recessive dystrophic epidermolysis bullosa. Those with the autosomal dominant form have milder disease. In both types there is widespread blistering and scarring with nail and teeth abnormalities. In the recessive form patients end up with mitten deformities because of fusion and scarring of skin on their hands and feet. There is extensive mucous membrane involvement which may lead to oesophageal strictures. Other complications include anaemia, growth retardation and squamous cell carcinomas in areas of repeated blistering and scarring.

Scleroderma, morphoea and lichen sclerosus

Scleroderma

The term scleroderma describes 'thickening of the skin' characterized by excess deposition of collagen in the dermis and fibrosis. It can be a feature of a number of disorders and occurs in both localized and systemic forms. The localized form of scleroderma is referred to as morphoea, described below. The systemic form is called systemic sclerosis (p. 495), in which the cutaneous involvement can be limited or diffuse (Table 14.24). Morphoea and systemic sclerosis are two separate entities, not a spectrum of disease.

Morphoea

Morphoea (localized scleroderma) is a disorder of unknown aetiology in which there is localized dermal fibrosis.

Epidemiology

The disease is three times more common in women and is more likely to present later in life.

Pathology

The aetiology is unknown but it is thought that complex interactions between genetic and environmental factors (local triggers) are responsible.

Clinical features

There are four main clinical variants: plaque morphoea, linear morphoea, Parry–Romberg syndrome and generalized morphoea.

Plaque morphoea

Plaque morphoea is the most common presentation with asymmetrical, well-circumscribed, indurated plaques between 2 and 15 cm in diameter, often with an active, violaceous border and an ivory coloured centre (Fig. 14.44).

Linear morphoea

Linear morphoea has a more indolent course, usually affecting the limbs in childhood. It can involve the underlying fascia, muscles and tendons, impairing joint mobility. There is no gender preference.

Parry–Romberg syndrome

Patients with Parry–Romberg syndrome present with hemifacial atrophy, often in childhood or as young adults. This is probably a severe variant of linear morphoea.

Generalized morphoea

Generalized morphoea is a further subtype of localized scleroderma. In this entity, although the skin involvement is widespread, there is a lack of any systemic manifestations. However, the disease may result in severe scars and functional disability.

Table 14.24	Skin changes in systemic sclerosis
Facial telangiectasia	
Restricted mouth opening	
Perioral puckering	
Smooth shiny pigmented indurated skin	
Raynaud's phenomenon	
Sclerodactyly	
Pulp atrophy	
Dilated nail fold capillaries	
Ragged cuticles	
Calcinosis cutis	
Livedo reticularis	
Leg ulcers	

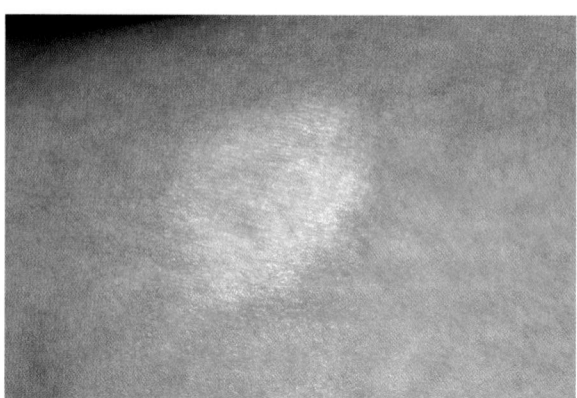

Fig. 14.44 Plaque morphoea.

Investigations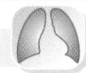

Skin biopsy

The clinical diagnosis can be confirmed by a skin biopsy. Histologically, there is localized dermal fibrosis with associated atrophy of epidermal appendages.

Serology

There are high titres of anti-nuclear antibodies (ANA) in 40–80% of young patients with linear or generalized morphoea.

Management

Topical immunomodulatory agents

Various treatment modalities have been reported for morphoea, particularly for the more severe variants of linear and generalized morphoea. These include high-potency topical glucocorticoids or intralesional injections of triamcinolone. Systemic glucocorticoids and antimalarials are usually ineffective. High doses of oral methotrexate may provide some benefit in adult patients with generalized morphoea.

Disease-modifying antirheumatic agents

D-penicillamine may halt the formation of new lesions and induce the softening of older lesions.

Phototherapy

Both UVA1 phototherapy (340–450 nm) and photochemotherapy (PUVA) have been reported to be helpful.

Prognosis

The course of morphoea is variable. In the majority of patients it progresses for several years and then regresses. Patients do not have any associated systemic disease.

Lichen sclerosus

Lichen sclerosus is a common acquired inflammatory disorder of the skin and mucous membranes.

Epidemiology

Lichen sclerosus has a prevalence of about 125 in 100 000 and it is more common in females. It can occur at any age, but in the female population there is a bimodal peak in prepubertal children and after the menopause, and in the male population the disorder is most common at 30–50 years of age.

Pathology

The aetiology is unknown, although disease association with the class II HLA antigen DQ7 and high rates of autoimmune disorders suggests that autoantibodies to specific mucocutaneous antigens are involved. Recently there has been evidence for a specific humoral immune response to extracellular matrix protein 1 (ECM1) in this condition.[1] Infective agents such as the human papillomavirus have also been implicated in the aetiology of lichen sclerosus, but the exact pathogenesis is not known. In addition, at sites of trauma, the Köbner phenomenon can trigger this condition.

Scope of disease

Some long-standing cases of lichen sclerosus are complicated by malignant disease, most commonly squamous cell carcinoma, and therefore these patients require long-term monitoring.

Clinical features

Lichen sclerosus presents as ivory-white macules that coalesce into plaques. It has a predilection for anogenital skin but can also affect extragenital sites. Symptoms can include itching and soreness. Chronic skin and mucous membrane inflammation can lead to scarring. In men, the term balanitis xerotica obliterans is used to describe late and severe lichen planus of the penis. Extragenital disease commonly occurs on the head and neck, axillae and thighs and is generally asymptomatic.

Initial investigations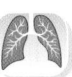

In many cases, the diagnosis can be made on clinical grounds.

Further investigations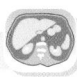

Skin biopsy

The diagnosis is made on clinical grounds; however, a skin biopsy may be helpful if the diagnosis is in doubt or there are concerns about malignant change. Histologically, there is basal cell degeneration, upper dermal oedema, homogenization of collagen and a chronic inflammatory infiltrate.

Medical management

Immunomodulation

The most effective treatment for lichen sclerosus is the very potent topical corticosteroid, clobetasol propionate. Extragenital lesions are less responsive than genital disease to this treatment. Topical testosterone and progesterone have also been used in genital disease but are not as effective as corticosteroids.

Surgical management

Scarring of the female genitalia can result in labial adhesions and introital stenosis, which can be managed surgically. In men, circumcision is helpful in lichen sclerosus of the foreskin, and meatal dilatation or meatotomy may be needed for meatal stenosis.

Prognosis

The condition tends to be remitting and relapsing, with spontaneous regression reported in a few. Scarring and progression to squamous cell carcinomas can occur in chronic disease, resulting in significant morbidity.

ɩ̇ FURTHER INFORMATION

Neill SM, Tatnall FM, Cox NH. Guidelines for the management of lichen sclerosus. British Journal of Dermatology 2002; 147: 640–649.

REFERENCE

(1) Oyama N, Chan I, Neill SM, et al. Autoantibodies to extracellular matrix protein 1 in lichen sclerosus. Lancet 2003; 362: 118–123.

SECTION 14.8 Skin infections and infestations

Bacterial infections

Cutaneous bacterial infections can be classified according to the histological layer of the skin affected and the organism involved.

Superficial cutaneous infections

Superficial infections of the stratum corneum and hair follicles occur as a result of overgrowth of normal flora at sites of occlusion and high surface humidity.

Erythrasma

Erythrasma is a chronic superficial infection with *Corynebacterium minutissimum*, a Gram-positive rod (diphtheroid) and part of the normal skin flora. It presents as asymptomatic, well-marginated, brownish-red and slightly scaly macules affecting intertriginous areas of toes, groins and axillae. Adults are more often affected than children and it is more common in warm and humid climates and in diabetics. The diagnosis is made by coral red fluorescence under Wood's lamp and skin swabs show a heavy growth of *Corynebacterium*. Differentiation from dermatophyte infection can be difficult; however, there is an absence of fungi on direct microscopy. Topical antibiotics such as erythromycin or fusidic acid are usually effective unless the infection is extensive. Relapses are common.

Pyoderma

Normal skin is heavily colonized by bacterial flora. *Staphylococcus epidermidis* predominates on the skin surface and anaerobic diphtheroids in the hair follicle. A small percent-

age of people are colonized with *Staphylococcus aureus* and group A β-haemolytic streptococcus (*Streptococcus pyogenes*) which are not part of the normal flora of skin. These carriers are at increased risk for pyoderma (impetigo, ecthyma, furuncles, carbuncles, abscesses and folliculitis) and soft tissue infections (erysipelas, cellulitis and necrotizing fasciitis).

Impetigo and ecthyma

Staphylococcus aureus and *Streptococcus pyogenes* can cause infections of the epidermis (impetigo) that can extend into the dermis (ecthyma). Impetigo is an acute infection of the skin most often caused by *S. aureus*. It presents with transient small vesicles that rupture, resulting in erosions, usually affecting the face. Golden-yellow crusts form from the exuding serum (Fig. 14.45). The lesions spread locally and may coalesce. Children are more commonly affected than adults. Impetigo can arise in minor superficial breaks in the skin, especially in individuals with pre-existing dermatoses such as atopic dermatitis. Streptococcal impetigo may trigger acute glomerulonephritis (p. 713). Impetigo is contagious and frequent hand washing reduces the risk

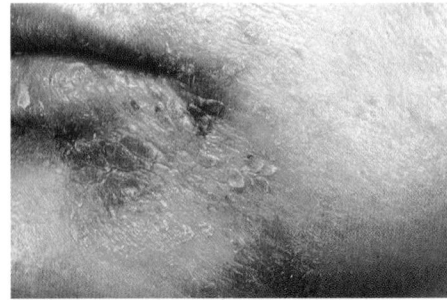

Fig. 14.45 Impetigo.

of person to person transmission. Treatment with topical fusidic acid or mupirocin is effective for localized disease. Oral flucloxacillin (and phenoxymethylpenicillin if streptococcal infection is suspected) or erythromycin can be given in extensive disease. Untreated lesions of impetigo can progress to ecthyma, a deeper more prolonged infection, usually on the limbs and characterized by chronic ulceration with thick adherent crusts (Fig. 14.46). Ecthyma develops as a result of poor hygiene, skin trauma and crowded living conditions and most commonly occurs in homeless people and intravenous drug users. Systemic antibiotics are required. In contrast to impetigo, ecthyma heals with scarring.

Infectious folliculitis

Folliculitis is commonly caused by an infection in the upper portion of the hair follicle. It is more common in young adults although any age group can be affected. It is characterized by papules or pustules centred on the hair follicle, occasionally surrounded by an erythematous halo (Figure 14.47). The most common infecting organisms are *Staphylococcus aureus*, *Pseudomonas aeruginosa* and *Malassezia* yeasts. Investigations should include a skin swab for microscopy and culture and scrapings for fungal culture. Treatment with topical antimicrobial therapy as well as avoidance of predisposing factors such as occlusion of hair-bearing areas, high temperatures or humidity, is effective.

Furuncle and carbuncle

Staphylococcus aureus folliculitis can progress to a deeper infection within a single hair follicle with the formation of a furuncle. This typically affects healthy young adults and presents as a red, hot, tender nodule, on any hair-bearing region. The nodule becomes fluctuant with abscess formation, pointing to a central pustule and eventually discharging. Furuncles are often multiple. Carbuncles are more extensive lesions with infection of multiple contiguous follicles and surrounding soft tissue. Patients may be systemically unwell with a low-grade fever and malaise. Swabs for direct microscopy (Gram stain) and bacterial culture should be taken. Sensitivities to antibiotics can guide management. Early furuncles can be treated with topical antibiotics but more established lesions and carbuncles require incision and drainage and systemic antibiotics (flucloxacillin). Recurrent furunculosis is more common in individuals with chronic *S. aureus* carrier state, diabetes mellitus and poor hygiene. Their management should involve identification and eradication of *S. aureus* from carriage sites (nostrils, axilla, perineum) and treatment with antiseptics and antibiotics. Lesions heal leaving a scar.

Soft tissue infections

Soft tissue infections (cellulitides) are acute, diffuse, spreading infections of the dermis and subcutaneous tissue, usually caused by *Streptococcus pyogenes*. They can be divided into non-necrotizing and necrotizing soft tissue infections. The non-necrotizing types are treated with systemic antibiotics and drainage of abscess. The necrotizing types are often life threatening and require urgent extensive surgical debridement and broad-spectrum intravenous antibiotics.

Erysipelas and cellulitis

Erysipelas and cellulitis are non-necrotizing soft tissue infections.

Epidemiology

Erysipelas and cellulitis are common conditions.

Pathology

Both conditions are usually caused by group A β-haemolytic streptococcus (*Streptococcus pyogenes*) and more rarely by *Staphylococcus aureus*. The causative organism may gain entry through a split in any mucocutaneous site. Pre-existing underlying dermatoses, chronic lymphoedema and any cause of immunosuppression are important predisposing factors and can lead to recurrent attacks.

Clinical features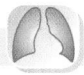

Erysipelas is superficial and characterized by a hot, bright-red, oedematous and indurated, sharply demarcated, tender plaque with an advancing raised border. Cellulitis has many features of erysipelas but extends into the subcutaneous tissues. Clinically it can be differentiated from erysipelas as the lesions are not raised or well demarcated. Red streaks of lymphangitis and tender lymphadenopathy are common. Blisters, occasionally haemorrhagic, can appear in acute cases. Patients may be systemically unwell, with fever and malaise, before the cutaneous changes present.

Investigations

Skin swabs
Skin swabs of the affected skin for direct microscopy and culture should be performed but are often negative.

Blood cultures
Blood cultures should be taken, especially if the patient is pyrexial, although the yield is very low.

ASO titres
Measurement of antistreptolysin O titre (ASOT) and anti-DNAase B may identify a streptococcal cause.

Management

Leg elevation and support stockings
Bed rest with leg elevation is important. With recurrent disease the affected area may become lymphoedematous and support stockings are beneficial.

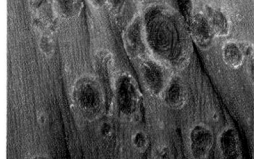
Fig. 14.46 Ecthyma.

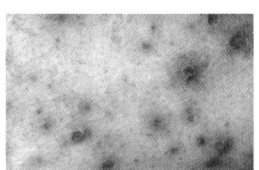
Fig. 14.47 Folliculitis.

891

Antibiotics

Treatment is with systemic antibiotics, phenoxymethyl-penicillin and flucloxacillin (or erythromycin alone if the patient is allergic to penicillin). If the infection is severe, intravenous benzylpenicillin and flucloxacillin may be required. Recurrent cellulitis may require long-term antibiotics and skin care to avoid portals of entry.

Prognosis

Most infections will respond to antibiotics in the early stages of the disease.

 FURTHER INFORMATION

Bonnetblanc JM, Bedane C. Erysipelas: recognition and management. American Journal of Dermatology 2003; 4: 157–163.

Erysipeloid

Erysipeloid is a non-necrotizing soft tissue infection caused by *Erysipelothrix rhusiopathiae*. This organism affects a wide range of animals, in particular birds and fish. In humans, infections are most common in butchers, fishmongers and cooks, usually localized to the finger or hand, spreading to wrist and forearm. The lesions are purplish-red and oedematous, and enlarge with central fading. The infection is usually mild with no systemic symptoms. It responds well to penicillin.

Necrotizing fasciitis

Necrotizing fasciitis is characterized by necrosis of the dermis, subcutaneous fat, fascia or muscle. A mixture of pathogens including streptococci and anaerobes are responsible. It starts with erythema and painful induration, followed by rapid development of black eschar which transforms into a liquefied black and malodorous necrotic mass. In necrotizing fasciitis the erythema is often dusky when compared to cellulitis, and deep haemorrhagic bullae can develop with necrosis of the skin and soft tissues. Necrotizing fasciitis is a dermatological emergency and requires early and complete surgical debridement of the necrotic tissue in combination with high-dose intravenous antibiotics.

Gram-negative infections

Pseudomonas aeruginosa

Pseudomonas aeruginosa is an aerobic Gram-negative bacillus which exists in moist environments associated with hospitals. Patients can become colonized, and local invasion of mucocutaneous sites is possible with haematogenous spread in compromised individuals. Rarely necrotic skin lesions develop when septic vasculitis, vascular occlusion and infarction of tissue follow *Ps. aeruginosa* septicaemia. Systemic antibiotics (ceftazidime, piperacillin, ciprofloxacin) or surgical debridement may be required in severe infection.

Cat-scratch disease

Cat-scratch disease is a benign, self-limited infection caused by the Gram-negative bacillus *Bartonella henselae*. A few days after a cat bite or scratch, a red papule appears at the site of inoculation. Tender regional lymphadenopathy as well as a mild fever follows a few weeks later and lasts several weeks. The glands may discharge before settling spontaneously. Occasionally, surgical drainage of the suppurative node is indicated. Systemic antibiotics have not proved to be effective.

Mycobacterial infections

Leprosy

Epidemiology

The geographical distribution of leprosy has varied greatly with time and it is now endemic in only 15 countries (where prevalence rates are above 0.1 per 100 000). The majority of cases are present in six countries: India, Brazil, Myanmar, Indonesia, Madagascar and Nepal. The young are most susceptible to acquiring the infection and spread occurs mainly through the oronasal route.

Pathology

Leprosy is a slowly progressive, chronic infectious disease caused by the bacillus *Mycobacterium leprae*, primarily affecting the peripheral nerves and secondarily involving the skin and other organs. Nerve involvement typically occurs after an incubation period of 3–5 years.

Clinical features

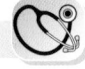

Leprosy has a number of distinct clinical presentations and the features are dependent on the underlying state of immunity (Table 14.25). Tuberculoid leprosy is seen in those with high immunity. Lesions are few and consist of a well-defined plaque with an erythematous raised border and a hypopigmented, dry, anaesthetic centre, commonly on the face (Fig. 14.48). Thickened peripheral nerves may be palpated. Lepromatous leprosy is the more contagious form and occurs in individuals with poor cell-mediated immunity. Multiple infiltrated dermal papules, nodules and plaques favour the peripheries. In addition, some peripheral nerves may be thickened. There is also a borderline form between the lepromatous and tuberculoid subtypes (Fig. 14.49).

Table 14.25	Tuberculoid versus lepromatous leprosy	
	Tuberculoid	**Lepromatous**
Immunity	High degree of cellular immunity	Poor cellular immunity
Involves	Skin and nerves	Many tissues
Lesions	Few lesions Commonly on face Sharply demarcated Hypopigmented macules	Numerous lesions Widespread Macules, papules, nodules and plaques
Histology	Absence of acid-fast bacilli Epithelioid cell granulomas forming around dermal nerves	Presence of acid-fast bacilli Extensive cellular infiltrate Macrophages filled with *M. leprae*
Nerves	Thickened near lesions Hypoaesthesia of lesion Hypohidrosis of lesion	Most peripheral nerves thickened Glove and stocking anaesthesia Trophic ulcers of periphery

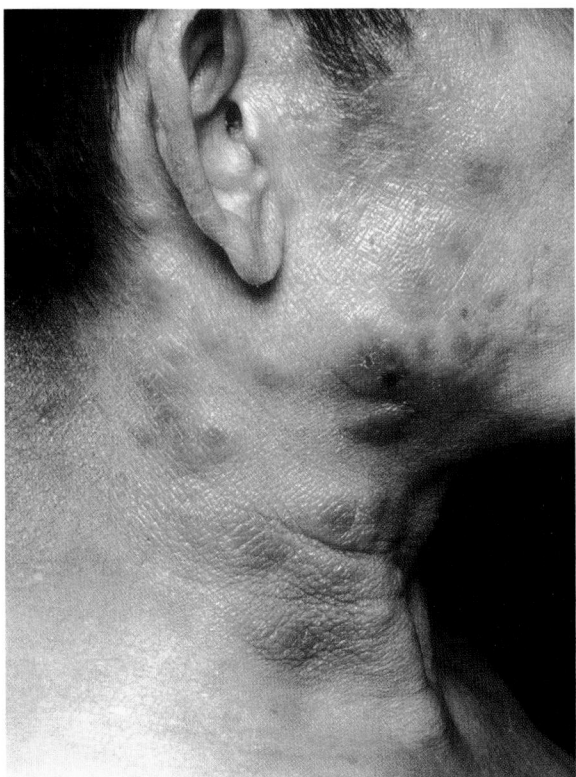

Fig. 14.48 Tuberculoid leprosy.

Investigations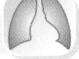

The lepromin skin test

The lepromin skin test is not a diagnostic test for leprosy but a measure of host resistance to it. Heat-killed organism is injected intradermally and granulomatous reactions develop in those capable of developing cell-mediated immunity to the bacillus.

Skin biopsy

M. leprae DNA detection by PCR has been reported by many researchers to be both sensitive and specific. This technique may become very important as an aid in the diagnosis of tuberculoid disease.

Management

Isolation

A brief period of isolation is needed for patients with infectious lepromatous leprosy.

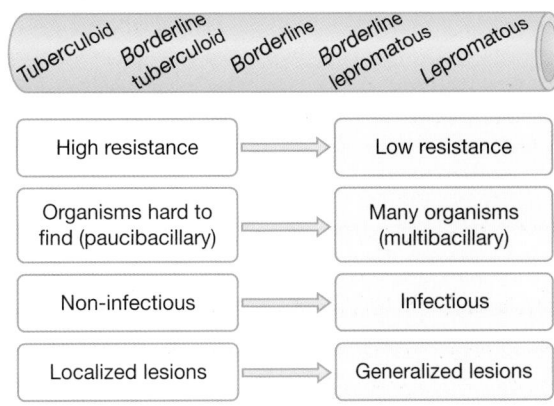

Fig. 14.49 Spectrum of leprosy: tuberculoid to lepromatous.

There is no single diagnostic laboratory test for leprosy, and the diagnosis remains clinical. The World Health Organization has designated diagnostic criteria as one or more hypopigmented or reddish skin patches with definite loss of sensation, thickened peripheral nerves and acid-fast bacilli seen on skin smears/biopsies.

Antibiotics

Current treatment involves rifampicin, clofazimine and dapsone for 12 months. Oral corticosteroids are sometimes needed to prevent nerve damage when initiating therapy. Multidrug therapy aims to effectively eliminate *M. leprae* in the shortest possible time to prevent resistance from occurring.

Prognosis

Leprosy is a mutilating and stigmatizing disease in many parts of the world and early diagnosis and therapy is the most important strategy for its control. Intervention at an early stage will avoid the onset of more serious nerve damage and disability.

---

i **FURTHER INFORMATION**

Ustianowski AP, Lockwood DNJ. Leprosy: current diagnostic and treatment approaches. Current Opinion in Infectious Diseases 2003; 16: 421–427.

Viral infections

Viral warts

Cutaneous warts are common, benign and usually self-limiting skin lesions that commonly occur on the hands and feet due to infection of the epidermis with human papillomavirus (HPV).

Epidemiology

Infection with HPV is very common. Most people will experience HPV infection at some point in their life. The prevalence of viral warts in children and adolescents in the UK has been reported as up to 4.9%.[1] Visible warts are twice as common in white Europeans compared to other ethnic groups but there is no evidence of a sex difference.

Pathology

There are a number of different HPV types (Table 14.26), subdivided on the basis of their genotype, which preferentially infect either the cornified stratified squamous epithelium of the skin or the uncornified mucous membranes. Viral warts are spread by direct contact, especially to abraded or damaged skin.

Clinical features

The clinical manifestations of mucocutaneous HPV infection are influenced not only by the viral type but also by environmental and host factors. Table 14.29 summarizes the different clinical types of warts and the associated HPV type.

Common, flat and plantar warts are the three most common clinical manifestations of cutaneous HPV infections. Approximately 70% of all cutaneous warts are of the common type (Fig. 14.50), occurring in up to 20% of all school-aged children. These are usually found on the hands but may develop on any area. Lesions are hard, rough, skin-coloured lumps that range from a few millimetres to large confluent masses. Plantar warts are common in older children and young adults, accounting for 30% of cutaneous warts. These are often found on the soles of the feet (called verrucas) and sometimes cause pain (Fig. 14.51). Flat warts occur in children and adults and account for about 5% of cutaneous warts. They are smaller and flatter than the other types and may spread widely, usually on the face and dorsal surfaces of the hands.

HPV infection can also result in genital warts (condylomata acuminata), the most prevalent sexually transmitted disease. Some HPV types (16,18) are high risk for the development of invasive squamous cell carcinoma of anogenital epithelium. Viral warts are especially common in immunocompromised and transplant patients. Approximately 50% of renal transplant patients develop warts

Table 14.26	Morphology of warts and associated HPV types	
Clinical manifestation	**Appearance**	**HPV subtype**
Common warts	Rough, hard and keratotic papules	1, 2, 4, 57
Plane (flat) warts	Flat-topped papules (2–4 mm in diameter) Skin-coloured or light brown	3, 10
Intermediate	Features of both common and plane warts	2, 3, 10, 28
Plantar warts	Firm, keratotic papules with a collar of thickened keratin Studded with brown/black dots (thrombosed capillaries)	1, 2, 4, 57
Mosaic warts	Coalescence of palmar/plantar warts into plaques	2
Myrmecia	Deep burrowing wart	1
Anogenital/venereal warts (condylomata acuminata)	Papules in the perineum and on the genitalia	6, 11
Oral warts	White/pink papules on the oral mucosa	6, 11, 32

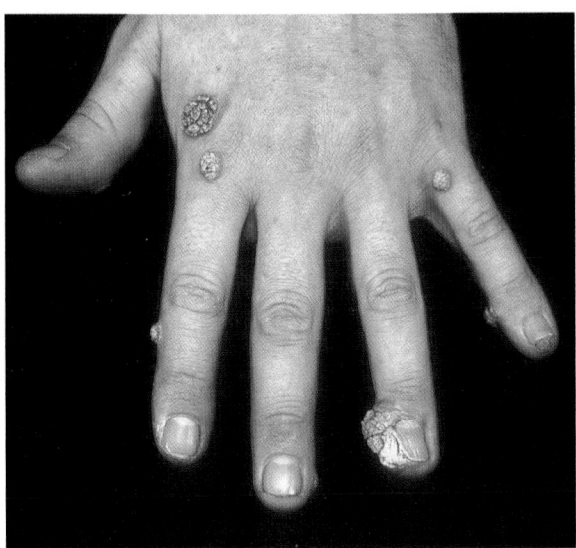
Fig. 14.50 Common warts.

within 5 years of transplantation. In these patients dysplastic change of warty lesions may progress to malignant squamous lesions.

Investigations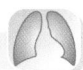

Diagnosis of viral warts is usually clinical.

Skin biopsy

Rarely a confirmatory biopsy is required. Histology shows an acanthotic epidermis with hyperkeratosis and papillomatosis. There are large keratinocytes with eccentric condensed nuclei surrounded by a perinuclear halo (referred to as koilocytes, characteristic of viral warts). Typing of HPV is only available in a few centres and can be useful in cases of genital warts in children suspected to have been sexually abused.

Management

There are a number of treatment options, and different methods can be combined for increased efficacy. The main aim of treatment is removal of the wart with no scarring or recurrence. It is important to note that not all warts need to be treated, as the majority will spontaneously clear. The indications for treatment include pain, interference with function, cosmetic embarrassment and risk of malignancy.

Viral warts in immunosuppressed patients are more recalcitrant to treatment as an immune response is usually essential for effective treatment and clearance.

Local treatments used for viral warts can be destructive, virucidal, antimitotic or immunomodulating. However, no one treatment is strikingly effective and little is known about the absolute and relative efficacy of the different treatment modalities.[2]

Destructive
Salicylic acid
Salicylic acid (daily application of 15–20% salicylic acid) is a keratolytic agent that gradually destroys the virus-infected epidermis and induces an immune response. Cure rates of 75% in cases compared with 48% in controls have been reported.[2]

Cryotherapy
Cryotherapy with liquid nitrogen (using a cotton wool-tipped applicator or cryospray) is commonly used. It is thought that this treatment either causes necrotic destruction of HPV-infected keratinocytes or possibly induces local inflammation and an effective cell-mediated response. Destruction of warts by freezing every 3 weeks can give a clearance rate of 69% at 12 weeks.[3] Pain and blistering are commonly reported side effects. No significant differences have been found between treatments at intervals of 2, 3 or 4 weeks, however a higher rate of adverse effects is reported with a short interval between treatments.

Other destructive therapy
Other local destructive options include curettage and cautery, chemical cautery with daily use of silver nitrate stick, carbon dioxide laser, pulse dye laser and photodynamic therapy.

Virucidal
Formaldehyde and glutaraldehyde
Formaldehyde and glutaraldehyde are both virucidal and available as a gel or solution. However, they are not commonly used in the treatment of viral warts.

Antimitotic
Podophyllin
Podophyllin/podophyllotoxin acts as an antimitotic agent by binding to the spindle during mitosis. It is extensively used for anogenital warts but it is much less effective for the treatment of cutaneous warts as penetration of the thick stratum corneum is poor.

Bleomycin
Intralesional bleomycin is cytotoxic and is used in cases that have failed to respond to other modalities of treatment. Pain is the main limiting factor and local anaesthetic is routinely used before injection of bleomycin.

Retinoids
Retinoids (tretinoin cream) disrupt epidermal growth and differentiation and can help reduce the bulk of warty lesions.

Immunomodulation
Imiquimod cream is an immune modulator and is licensed for the treatment of external anogenital warts. It can be applied to lesions that are not thickly keratinized, up to 3 times a week.

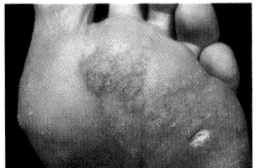
Fig. 14.51 Plantar warts.

895

The induction of delayed hypersensitivity with the potent contact sensitizer dinitrochlorobenzene has also been used as a treatment for viral warts.

Prognosis

Extragenital viral warts in patients who are immuno-competent are harmless and usually resolve spontaneously owing to natural immunity. Several studies have suggested clearance rates of 23% at 2 months, 30% at 3 months and 65–78% at 2 years. Viral warts in immunocompromised patients are less likely to resolve spontaneously.

i **FURTHER INFORMATION**

Sterling JC, Handfield-Jones S, Hudson PM, et al. Guidelines for the management of cutaneous warts. British Journal of Dermatology 2001; 144: 4–11.

REFERENCES

(1) *Williams HC, Pottier A, Strachan D, et al. The descriptive epidemiology of warts in British schoolchildren. British Journal of Dermatology 1993; 128: 504–511.*
(2) *Gibbs S, Harvey I, Sterling J, et al. Local treatments for cutaneous warts: systematic review. BMJ 2002; 325: 461–463.*
(3) *Bunney MH, Nolan MW, Williams DA. An assessment of methods of treating viral warts by comparative treatment trials based on standard design. British Journal of Dermatology 1976; 94: 667–669.*

Varicella

Primary infection with the herpes varicella virus gives rise to a widespread vesicular eruption (chicken pox). Chicken pox is very common and occurs in epidemics in young people. Spread is by droplet infection rather than from skin contact and there is an incubation period of 2–3 weeks. There is initially mild fever and malaise followed by the development of a pruritic papular rash that rapidly becomes vesicular. The lesions appear in crops and tend to be centripetal. They usually heal with scarring. No active treatment is usually needed, only rest and symptomatic therapy. Immunosuppressed patients can be treated with aciclovir for pneumonitis or encephalitis. Varicella zoster immunoglobulin may be administered to pregnant women or immunocompromised patients exposed to the virus. Live attenuated virus is preventative in the healthy individuals who may become infected, and it modifies the infection in those at risk.

Herpes zoster

Herpes zoster (shingles) is an acute dermatomal infection associated with the reactivation of varicella zoster virus.

Epidemiology

Over 90% of adults have serological evidence of varicella zoster virus and are at risk for herpes zoster; the lifetime risk is estimated at 20%. The incidence of herpes zoster increases with age.

Pathology

Shingles results from the reactivation of the latent herpes varicella virus from the sensory ganglia. Herpes zoster is contagious, giving rise to chicken pox in those who have not previously had chicken pox. Declining virus-specific cell-mediated immune responses, which occur naturally as a result of ageing but can also be induced by immunosuppression from malignancy (leukaemia/lymphoma), medications and HIV infection, increase the incidence and severity of disease.

Patients over the age of 50 and those who are immunocompromised are at increased risk of severe complications. The pain and dysaesthesia may persist after cutaneous healing; this is referred to as post-herpetic neuralgia. Involvement of the ophthalmic region (the nasociliary ganglion of the ophthalmic branch of the trigeminal nerve) results in unilateral pain and lesions on the forehead, periocular area and the nose. This is often associated with ocular complications (keratitis, episcleritis and iritis) which may be sight threatening. Facial palsy can result from the involvement of the geniculate ganglion (Ramsay Hunt syndrome). Rarely there is retention of urine or faeces following involvement of sacral nerves. In immunosuppressed patients the infection is often more severe and may become disseminated resulting in encephalitis or pneumonitis.

Clinical features
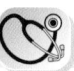

Shingles presents as a vesicular eruption along a dermatome (usually thoracic/lumbar or facial, Fig. 14.52). The eruption is often preceded by pain or paraesthesia within the affected dermatome. These symptoms, prior to the development of the eruption, can result in

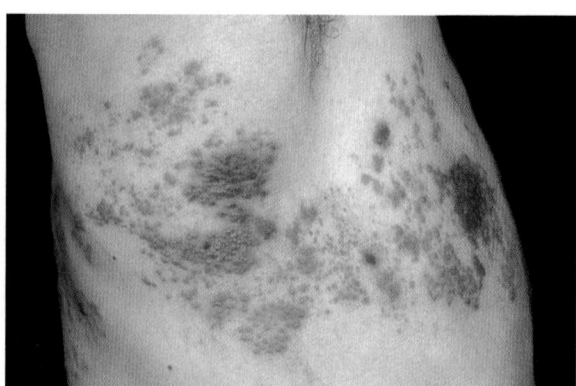

Fig. 14.52 Herpes zoster.

diagnostic difficulties, especially on the thorax as they can mimic cardiac and pleural pain. Occasionally patients also report headache, photophobia and malaise. After 3–4 days, grouped red papules appear in one or more adjacent dermatomes, becoming vesicular and pustular, then ulcerating and eventually crusting over. The lesions are unilateral dermatomal in distribution and do not cross the midline. Fever and pain are common and there is usually enlargement of the draining lymph nodes. Lesions usually clear in a few weeks but tend to heal with scarring, particularly if secondarily infected.

Investigations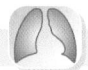

The diagnosis is primarily clinical and investigations are not usually necessary.

Blister swabs

If the clinical presentation is atypical, electron microscopy and direct immunofluorescence assays, or viral culture can be used to confirm the diagnosis. PCR techniques are also useful.

Management

Antiviral agents

There is no role for topical antiviral drugs in the management of herpes zoster. Three oral antivirals that are available for the treatment of herpes zoster are aciclovir, its derivative valaciclovir, and famciclovir. Initiation of early treatment (48–72 hours after onset of rash) with oral aciclovir (800 mg 5 times a day for 7–10 days) significantly reduces symptoms as well as the duration and intensity of the outbreak. However it does not influence post-herpetic neuralgia. The newer agents, valaciclovir (1000 mg 3 times daily) and famciclovir (500 mg 3 times daily), have better oral bioavailability and require less frequent administration than aciclovir but there is no difference with regards to their efficacy and safety.

Analgesia

Adequate analgesia should be prescribed as the neuralgic pain is usually very severe and should not be underestimated.

Management of ocular complications

Ocular complications should be evaluated by an ophthalmologist and treated with oral antivirals. Ramsay Hunt syndrome can be managed with systemic steroids as well as aciclovir in order to reduce inflammation.

Management of post-herpetic neuralgia

Post-herpetic neuralgia is difficult to manage. Opioids, tricyclic antidepressants (amitriptyline) and gabapentin can reduce the severity and duration either as single agents or in combination. Topical capsaicin 0.025% can also be helpful but the intense burning sensation during initial treatment may limit its use.

Prognosis

Most lesions resolve spontaneously over 3–5 weeks; however, antiviral agents shorten the course of disease. Only a small proportion of patients develop complications.

ℹ FURTHER INFORMATION

Gnann JW, Whitley RJ. Herpes zoster. New England Journal of Medicine 2002; 347: 340–346.

Herpes simplex

Epidemiology

Primary infection with type 1 herpes simplex virus (HSV) occurs in about 50% of individuals by the time they reach adult life.

Pathology

Herpes simplex hominis is a double-stranded DNA virus which can be divided into types 1 and 2. Primary infections with type 1 HSV usually cause a gingivostomatitis, and although both types 1 and 2 can affect the genital mucosa, up to 90% of genital infections are caused by type 2. Both types can produce primary and recurrent mucocutaneous infections, and transmission is usually by direct contact.

The primary attack tends to be more severe than the recurrences, which occur without re-exposure to the virus. Recurrent attacks are due to reactivation of the virus which is dormant in the dorsal root ganglion. For example, reactivation of the latent virus type 1 in the trigeminal ganglia produces grouped vesicles on the face, usually on the lips (referred to as 'cold sores', Fig. 14.53). This is often preceded by symptoms of itch or tingling. Recurrences occur at an unpredictable rate and are commonly precipitated by fever, stress, concurrent illness, skin or

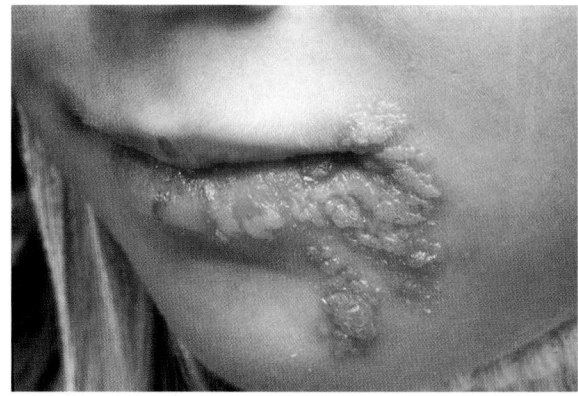

Fig. 14.53 Herpes simplex infection type 1.

mucosal irritation, sunlight or altered hormonal milieu (menstruation).

Scope of disease

When the skin is damaged as in atopic dermatitis, herpes can spread and become life threatening (eczema herpeticum). Immunosuppression due to HIV infection, malignancy (leukaemia/lymphoma) and drugs can result in disseminated infection. Spread of infection to the eye can cause potentially blinding keratoconjunctivitis. Neonates can be infected during delivery or in the perinatal period, usually from the mother but also from individuals around the infant after birthing. Herpes simplex infection is one of the most common triggers of erythema multiforme. Other complications include pneumonitis and encephalitis.

Clinical features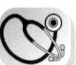

Herpes simplex infection, whether primary or recurrent, typically presents as grouped macules which progress to vesicles surrounded by erythema or vesiculopustules (Fig. 14.53). These then crust before healing in about a week. There is occasional post-inflammatory hyperpigmentation.

Primary infection with type 1 HSV usually causes gingivostomatitis. There is often a febrile illness and painful vesicles and ulcers on the hard and soft palate. Genital lesions, most commonly caused by type 2 HSV, start as vesicles which are usually bilateral and coalesce to produce eroded areas which are very painful. There may be oedema and secondary urinary retention. The majority of genital infections are sexually acquired. Herpes infection can also develop following direct contact. On the finger this results in deep painful, grouped vesicles known as herpetic whitlow.

Investigations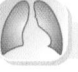

Blister swabs

A Tzanck smear from the base of a blister will show multinucleated giant cells. Swabs can also be taken from the de-roofed blister for culture, and smears for electron microscopy and immunofluorescent tests (monoclonal antibodies specific for HSV type 1 and 2 antigens detect and differentiate between HSV antigens on smears taken from the lesions). PCR may also be helpful.

Management

Minimize contact

Transmission of HSV infection is by direct contact and this should be avoided during an outbreak of infection.

Aciclovir

Aciclovir is the drug of choice in herpes infection. It is active against the virus but does not eradicate it. It is effective only if started at the onset of an episode. For minor recurrences, topical aciclovir (5% cream) is used. Systemic aciclovir can

be used in the primary attack, which is usually most severe, and in eczema herpeticum and neonatal infections. Regular low-dose aciclovir prophylaxis should be considered if there are frequent (>5 episodes/year) and severe recurrences, particularly in the immunocompromised. Famciclovir and valaciclovir are alternative antivirals to aciclovir.

Prognosis

The majority of the lesions resolve spontaneously in immunocompetent individuals. Treatment with antivirals shortens the course of the disease.

i FURTHER INFORMATION

Nikkels AF, Pierard GE. Treatment of mucocutaneous presentations of herpes simplex virus infections. American Journal of Clinical Dermatology 2002; 3: 475–487.

Molluscum contagiosum

Molluscum contagiosum is a benign epidermal viral infection caused by a poxvirus (molluscum contagiosum virus—MCV). Infection is spread by direct skin to skin contact with an incubation period of several months. It is characterized by multiple rounded, dome-shaped, waxy papules that are 2–5 mm in diameter and contain a central umbilication (Fig. 14.54). They can occur at any site but are commonly found on the head, neck and flexures in preadolescent children. In adults, lesions are more often found on the lower abdomen and genitals, and are usually sexually transmitted. Lesions are more widespread, larger and hyperkeratotic in immunosuppressed patients, in particular in HIV-infected individuals. Treatment in childhood is often not necessary as in the majority the lesions spontaneously resolve in 6 months. Troublesome lesions are commonly treated with cryotherapy, curettage or electrodesiccation. In HIV-infected patients the lesions usually resolve with antiretroviral therapy.

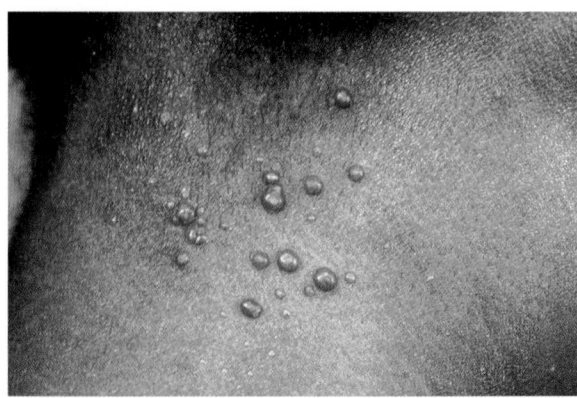

Fig. 14.54 Molluscum contagiosum.

FURTHER INFORMATION

Smith KJ, Skelton H. Molluscum contagiosum: recent advances in pathogenic mechanism, and new therapies. American Journal of Clinical Dermatology 2002; 3: 535–545.

Orf

Orf is a poxvirus infection common in sheep, goats and deer. Infection in humans is most commonly seen in farmers and is typically caused through contact with lambs. Human to human infection does not occur. Orf commonly presents as a solitary purplish papule on the hand which gradually enlarges over the next few days to become umbilicated, haemorrhagic and vesicopustular with central crusting. Investigations are often not necessary, as the diagnosis is made on the history and clinical findings, although electron microscopy of the vesicular fluid can confirm the diagnosis. The lesions heal spontaneously in 3–5 weeks and treatment of any secondary infection is all that is required.

Fungal infections

Superficial fungal infections are the most common of all mucocutaneous infections. They are usually caused by either dermatophytes or *Candida* species.

Dermatophyte infections

Dermatophytes (or ringworm) are fungi that are capable of infecting keratinized epithelium including hair, nails and the stratum corneum of the skin. They can affect the scalp (tinea capitis), body (tinea corporis), groin (tinea cruris), hands (tinea manuum), feet (tinea pedis) or nails (tinea unguium).

Epidemiology

Dermatophyte infections are very common. Tinea capitis is seen predominantly in pre-adolescent children (in particular Afro-Caribbean children) and this infection can become epidemic in schools and institutions. Dermatophyte infection at other body sites occurs more commonly in adults. The endemic species of fungi varies from country to country.

Pathology

Dermatophytes consist of branching hyphae that mat together to form mycelia. They synthesize keratinases that digest keratin and sustain existence of the fungi in keratinized structures. There are three genera: *Microsporum*, *Trichophyton* and *Epidermophyton*. They may be acquired from three sources, most commonly from another person (anthropophilic), from animals (zoophilic), and occasionally from soil (geophilic). Fungi transmitted from animals usually produce more inflammation than those that are exclusively human pathogens. A number of factors facilitate dermatophyte infections including atopy, immunosuppression, high humidity and sweating.

Clinical features

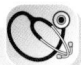

Tinea corporis

Tinea corporis is infection of non-hair bearing skin and is commonly caused by *Trichophyton rubrum* and *Microsporum canis*. Clinically, any part of the body can be affected. Tinea corporis presents as a spreading itchy rash. The lesions are circular red patches with a scaly edge that gradually spread outwards with central clearing (Fig. 14.55). Often there is post-inflammatory hyperpigmentation.

Tinea cruris

Tinea cruris presents as an itchy rash in the groins that gradually advances down the inner thigh. Clinically it is similar to tinea corporis.

Tinea pedis

Tinea pedis, also known as 'athlete's foot', is extremely common and is caused by *Trichophyton interdigitale, T. rubrum* and *Epidermophyton floccosum*. It can be transmitted by walking barefoot on contaminated floors. It presents with itching and scaling of the feet and web spaces (Fig. 14.56). In the acute form there are vesicles and bullae, usually on the sole of the foot. When the infection is chronic, clinically there is crescentic scaling of the soles and webs of toes, and there may be associated fungal infection of the toenails. Dry fissuring of the infected area may provide a site for bacterial entry and subsequent cellulitis.

Tinea capitis

Tinea capitis is the result of *Microsporum canis, M. audouinii* and some species of *Trichophyton* invading the hair shaft

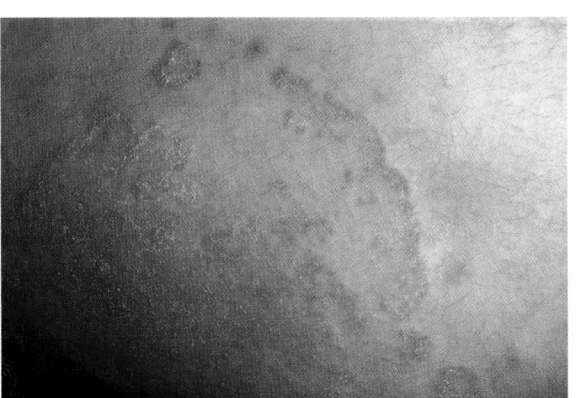

Fig. 14.55 Tinea corporis.

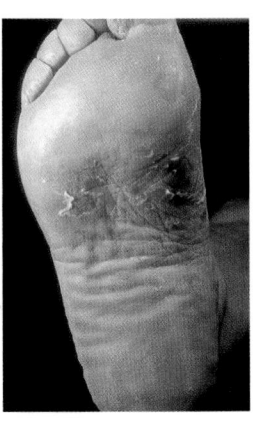

Fig. 14.56 Tinea pedis.

and surrounding skin. *Trichophyton tonsurans* now accounts for more than 90% of cases in the UK and North America.[1] Infection frequently spreads among family members and classmates. Clinically there is patchy loss of scalp hair, usually with underlying red and inflamed skin (Fig. 14.57). Animal dermatophytes such as *T. verrucosum* cause the most inflammation, producing a painful, swollen, boggy, purulent plaque known as a kerion. In these cases malaise, lymphadenopathy and scarring alopecia are common.

Tinea manuum

Tinea manuum presents as a dry and scaly rash, usually on one hand only. It is most commonly caused by *T. rubrum*. There is hyperkeratosis and scaling confined to the palmar creases and inflammation is minimal. There is often associated fungal infection of the fingernails.

Investigations

Skin scrapings

The clinical diagnosis should be confirmed by mycological examination. Direct microscopy and culture of skin scrapings, nail clippings and brushed hair samples (including the hair root) are performed.

Wood's light examination

Microsporum species exhibit a brilliant green fluorescence under Wood's light.

Management

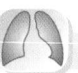

Topical antifungals

Most dermatophyte infections can be treated adequately with topical antifungal preparations, which should be applied twice daily to affected areas for about 4 weeks. The imidazole antifungals such as clotrimazole, miconazole and ketoconazole are all effective, as is terbinafine cream, an allylamine. Tinea manuum and pedis tend to recur unless concurrent fungal infections of the fingernails and toenails are also eradicated.

Compound benzoic acid

Compound benzoic acid ointment (Whitfield's ointment) has been used for ringworm infections but is cosmetically less acceptable.

Systemic antifungals

Systemic therapy is required for tinea capitis, tinea of the nails, and when topical treatment has failed in other types of infection.

Tinea capitis should be treated with oral griseofulvin (10–25 mg/kg daily in divided doses for an 8–10-week course) or terbinafine (<20 kg 62.5 mg, 20–40 kg 125 mg, >40 kg 250 mg daily for a 4-week course). Adjuvant therapy with antifungal shampoo (selenium sulphide, ketoconazole) increases the rate of eradication of scalp infection, which may reduce the transmissibility of the organism. It is also important to examine all home and school contacts of affected children for asymptomatic carriers and mild cases of disease. Antifungal shampoos may also be helpful in eradicating the asymptomatic carrier state.

Prognosis

Most infections respond to antifungal therapy although recurrent disease can be troublesome.

ℹ FURTHER INFORMATION

Higgins EM, Fuller LC, Smith CH. Guidelines for the management of tinea capitis. British Journal of Dermatology 2000; 143: 53–58.

Fuller LC, Child FJ, Midgley G, Higgins EM. Diagnosis and management of scalp ringworm. BMJ 2003; 326: 539–541.

REFERENCE

(1) *Hay RJ, Clayton YM, de Silva N, Midgley G, Rosser E. Tinea capitis in south east London—a new pattern of infection with public health implications. British Journal of Dermatology 1996; 135: 955–958.*

Candidiasis

Epidemiology

Candidiasis is a common fungal infection.

Pathology

Candidiasis is an infection caused by *Candida* (most frequently *C. albicans*), a yeast that is normally an asymptomatic non-pathogenic colonizer of mucosal surfaces. The sites that are most commonly affected are the mouth, genitalia, nail folds and flexural/intertriginous skin.

Clinical features

Oral candidiasis

Patients with oral candidiasis present with a sore mouth. On examination there are cream or whitish plaques on the tongue or palate which become confluent, raw and eroded. This can be associated with dentures, poor oral hygiene, and incorrect use of inhaled glucocorticoids and is commonly seen in immunosuppressed patients.

Candida vulvovaginitis

Candida vulvovaginitis causes vaginal irritation, soreness and a thick creamy discharge. Lesions are present around the vulva and may spread perianally and onto the inner

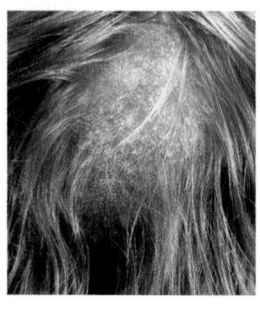

Fig. 14.57 Tinea capitis.

thigh. On examination there are plaques that coalesce with redness and swelling. Satellite curd-like lesions peripheral to the main site of the eruption are often seen. Candida vulvovaginitis is associated with pregnancy, oral contraceptives, antibiotics and diabetes mellitus.

Cutaneous candidiasis

Cutaneous candidiasis occurs on moist occluded surfaces. Flexural areas such as the groins (Fig. 14.58), axillae and under the breast are commonly affected and this is referred to as candida intertrigo. Small cream-coloured plaques are present on an erythematous base. They coalesce, erode, and are often surrounded by maceration. Affected areas become very sore and itchy.

Other sites

Nail fold infection (paronychia) with *Candida* results in painful swelling of the nail folds and fingers. Infections of the oesophagus and/or the tracheobronchial tree occur in the setting of malignancy or significant immunosuppression, in particular HIV infection and AIDS. This can lead to disseminated disease, which may be fatal.

Investigations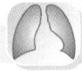

Skin scrapings

The clinical diagnosis of candidiasis should be confirmed by mycological examination. Direct microscopy demonstrates pseudohyphae and yeast forms.

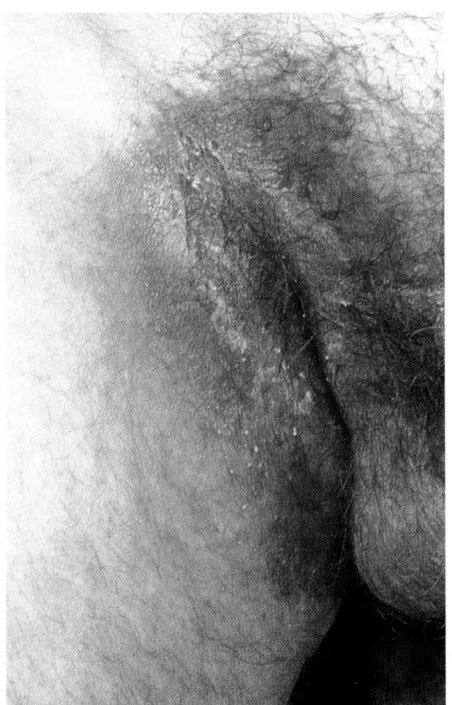

Fig. 14.58 Candida intertrigo.

Management

Topical antifungal agents

Positive culture alone in an asymptomatic individual does not warrant treatment as *Candida* is a normal inhabitant of mucosal surfaces. Cutaneous candidiasis can be treated with topical imidazole antifungal drugs such as clotrimazole, ketoconazole and miconazole (cream, powder or spray). Topical terbinafine is an alternative. Nystatin is also effective for candidiasis but is ineffective against dermatophyte infections. By keeping intertriginous areas dry, recurrence of infection can be prevented. Candida vulvovaginitis should be treated with both cream around the vulva and intravaginal antifungal pessaries or cream.

Oral antifungal suspensions

Oral candidiasis is treated with lozenges, pastilles or oral suspensions of antifungals. Amphotericin and nystatin are not absorbed from the gastrointestinal tract and can be applied locally to the mouth.

Systemic antifungal agents

Fluconazole and itraconazole are absorbed when taken by mouth and are available for oropharyngeal or vaginal candidiasis and serious disseminated disease. Immuno compromised patients with recurrent infections are often given antifungal drugs prophylactically. In all cases treatment of an underlying cause should also be considered.

Prognosis

Unless severely immunocompromised, most patients respond to antifungal therapy.

Pityriasis versicolor

Pityriasis versicolor is a chronic asymptomatic superficial cutaneous infection with the yeast *Malassezia furfur*. This is a colonizer of normal skin and thrives on warm, moist, oily skin. Pityriasis versicolor is characterized by well-demarcated scaling patches with variable pigmentation, occurring most commonly on the trunk (Fig. 14.59).

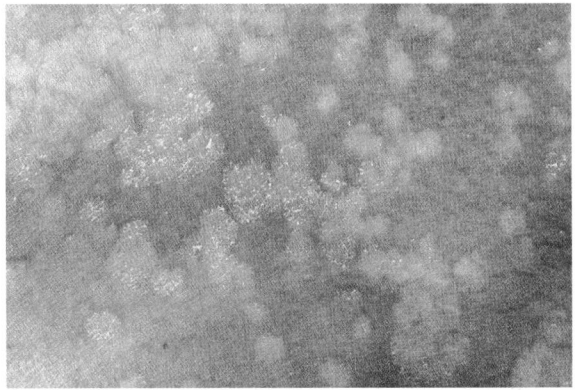

Fig. 14.59 Pityriasis versicolor.

The lesions fail to tan on sun exposure. Direct microscopy of the scales demonstrates filamentous hyphae and round yeast, termed 'spaghetti and meatballs'. Topical antifungals (such as ketoconazole) and oral antifungals (itraconazole 200 mg daily for 1 week) are both effective therapies.

Infestations

Scabies

Scabies is a common, highly pruritic infestation of the skin caused by the skin mite *Sarcoptes scabiei* var. *hominis*.

Epidemiology

The incidence of scabies has been rising: the estimated incidence is 100 per 100 000 per year.[1] Outbreaks in facilities for care of the elderly and nursing homes are common.

Pathology

The female mite burrows into the stratum corneum within 30 minutes of mating, tunnels at 2–3 mm a day, lays 1–3 eggs per day and lives for a total of 4–6 weeks. Each egg hatches within 3–4 days, releasing a larva that escapes to the skin surface where it remains until maturity.

Scabies gives rise to an intensely pruritic eruption which is caused by an immune reaction to the burrowed mites and their products (saliva and faeces). It is contagious and passes from one person to another by direct contact. Its spread is facilitated by the latent period of 2–6 weeks during which the scabies mite is carried asymptomatically.

Clinical features

The diagnosis of scabies is usually considered immediately in a patient with intractable generalized pruritus and papules, vesicles and excoriations distributed characteristically on the flexor aspects of the wrists, in the finger webs (Fig. 14.60) and on the buttocks and genitalia. The burrows are white/grey linear or serpiginous papules in the form of a ridge, up to 5 mm in length, with dark vesicles containing the female mites at one end. They are commonly found on the hands and genitalia. Itching is often worse at night in bed when the patient is warm and mite activity is increased. Untreated scabies may be associated with secondary bacterial infection.

Crusted scabies (formerly called Norwegian scabies) is an uncommon subtype characterized by crusts on the hands, feet, scalp and ears, loaded with scabies mites. It is highly contagious. This subtype may not be particularly itchy and is more common in immunocompromised or institutionalized patients.

Investigations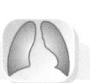

Scabies is usually diagnosed from the history and clinical findings.

Skin scrapings

If there is any doubt, microscopic examination for the mite in skin scrapings or from burrows is necessary.

Management

> **CLINICAL ALERT**
>
> *Treatment should be administered if scabies is suspected clinically, even if the diagnosis cannot be confirmed by microscopy.*

Topical acaricide agents

Permethrin 5% cream and Malathion 0.5% liquid are most commonly used. They should be applied to the whole body twice, 1 week apart.

Systemic therapy

Oral ivermectin is the most recently developed treatment for scabies. A single oral dose of ivermectin 200 µg/kg of body weight is well tolerated and very effective. It is has been used in combination with topical agents for the treatment of crusted scabies, scabies in immunocompromised hosts and infestations in crowded communities.

Contact tracing and treatment

Recurrence is inevitable unless all contacts and members of the affected household are treated simultaneously. Re-infestation can provoke symptoms within 24–48 hours.

Symptomatic treatment

Because the itching and dermatitis of scabies may persist for several weeks after successful elimination of the mites, patients may also need symptomatic treatment in the form of emollients, sedating antihistamines at night-time, crotamiton lotion or mild-potency topical corticosteroids.

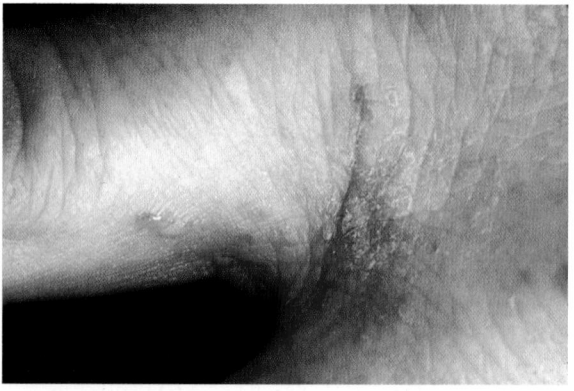
Fig. 14.60 Scabies.

Prognosis

Correct treatment of patients and their contacts with topical acaricides is usually very effective.

 FURTHER INFORMATION

Scott GR. European guidelines for the management of scabies. International Journal of STD & AIDS 2001; 12 (Suppl 3): 58–61.

REFERENCE

(1) *Downs AM, Harvey I, Kennedy CTC. The epidemiology of head lice and scabies in the UK. Epidemiology and Infection 1999; 122: 471–477.*

Head lice

Head lice or pediculosis capitis is an infestation of the scalp by the head louse *Phthirus humanus capitis*. It occurs most commonly in schoolchildren. Pruritus may lead to excoriations and secondary infection. The lice themselves are usually scanty but their nits, which are white oval eggs, can be found adhering to hair shafts. Carbaryl, Malathion and the pyrethroids (permethrin and phenothrin) are effective but lice in some districts have developed resistance. To overcome the development of resistance, a mosaic strategy is required whereby, if a course of treatment fails, a different insecticide should be used for the next course. Lotion, liquid or cream rinse formulations should be applied twice for 12 hours or overnight, 7 days apart. This prevents the emergence of lice from any eggs that survive the first application. Thorough regular combing has been shown to be equally effective.[1]

REFERENCE

(1) *Hill N, Moor G, Cameron MM, Butlin A, Preston S, Williamson MS, Bass C. Single blind, randomised, comparative study of the Bug Buster kit and over the counter pediculicide treatments against head lice in the United Kingdom. BMJ 2005; 331: 384–387.*

Skin tumours

Benign tumours arising from the epidermis

Seborrhoeic keratosis

Seborrhoeic keratosis is one of the most common benign epithelial tumours and results from a proliferation of keratinocytes. These lesions are common in individuals over 40 years of age, and the numbers of lesions tend to increase with age. Classically there are multiple brown, warty papules or plaques with a stuck-on appearance (Fig. 14.61). They mostly arise on the trunk and face. The sudden appearance of multiple seborrhoeic keratoses may be associated with underlying malignancy (sign of Leser–Trélat). Cryotherapy with liquid nitrogen or curettage is first line of treatment, although recurrences are frequent. If the diagnosis is in doubt and a melanoma cannot be excluded, a biopsy should be performed for histopathological confirmation.

Keratoacanthoma

Keratoacanthoma arises from rapid proliferation of keratinocytes, giving rise to a squamo-proliferative nodule. It is an uncommon lesion that tends to occur on sun-exposed skin, particularly the head and upper limbs of middle-aged men. Clinically, a solitary, firm, skin-coloured nodule with a central keratin plug enlarges over a period of days to weeks (Fig. 14.62). Distinction between a keratoacanthoma and an invasive squamous cell carcinoma may be difficult. A surgical excision biopsy should always be performed and the lesion sent for histopathological examination.

Epidermal naevus

An epidermal naevus is a developmental disorder characterized by hyperplasia of epidermal structures. It is usually present at birth or occurs early in infancy. There are several variants. Verrucous epidermal naevus is usually localized

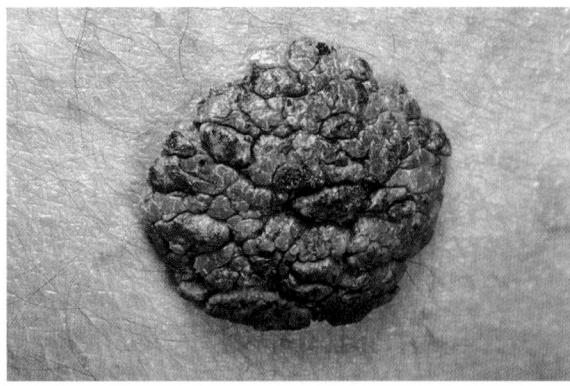

Fig. 14.61 Verruciform seborrhoeic keratosis.

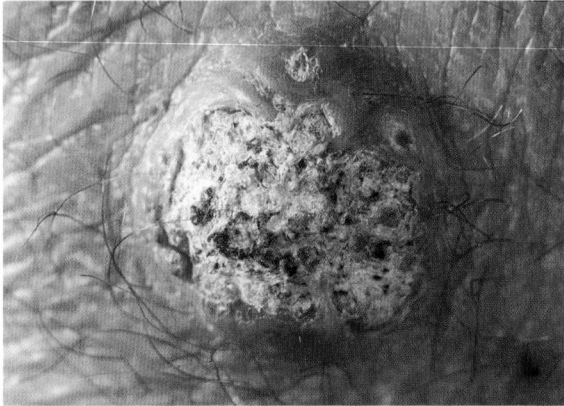

Fig. 14.62 Keratoacanthoma.

and may be excised for cosmetic reasons. Extensive lesions are called systematized epidermal naevi; when localized on half the body, they are referred to as naevus unius lateris. The lesions may also exhibit erythema, scaling and crusting (referred to as inflammatory linear verrucous epidermal naevus). All lesions gradually enlarge and in adolescence become stable. In general, they are difficult to treat.

Benign tumours arising from the dermis and subcutis

Lipoma

A lipoma is a benign subcutaneous fatty tumour. It is a common finding in either sex. Histologically it consists of an encapsulated, usually lobulated, discrete collection of uniform mature adipocytes. Familial multiple lipomata is an autosomal dominant trait that appears in early adulthood and consists of a number of slowly growing non-tender lesions. Adipositas dolorosa or Dercum's disease occurs

most commonly in middle-aged women and results in multiple tender lipomas that arise in adulthood. On examination, a lipoma is soft, rounded and movable against the overlying skin. The trunk and proximal extremities are common sites. Lipomas can be excised if they enlarge rapidly or are of functional significance for the patient.

Dermatofibroma

A dermatofibroma, also known as a benign fibrous histiocytoma, is an extremely common benign tumour and may represent an abnormal reaction to insect bites or other trauma. Histologically, there is a dermal nodule comprised of whirling fascicles of spindle cells with eosinophilic cytoplasm and vesicular nuclei, mixed with histiocytes. There is overlying epidermal hyperplasia. Clinically, dermatofibroma presents most commonly on the limbs of middle-aged individuals as a red-brown nodule (Fig. 14.63). On palpation it feels like 'a dried pea beneath the skin' and pinching the lesion between two fingers usually results in an apparent downward movement, known as the dimple sign. Surgical removal is not indicated unless the lesions are cosmetically unacceptable or they undergo repeated trauma. In general, lesions appear over several months, persist for many years and tend to regress spontaneously.

Skin tags

Skin tags are very common, soft, skin-coloured or brown pedunculated papillomas that are variable in size. They occur more often in the middle-aged and in the elderly, and are more common in obese females. Histologically, they are composed of normal or hyperplastic epidermis overlying a fibrovascular connective tissue core. Characteristically they are present in intertriginous areas and on the neck. The lesions are asymptomatic but occasionally may become tender following trauma or torsion. They can be simply shaved off or electrodesiccated if they are problematic.

Malignant neoplasms and their precursors

Actinic keratosis

Actinic keratoses (solar keratoses) are lesions that result from cumulative damage to keratinocytes by ultraviolet radiation. They are common lesions, particularly in individuals with skin phototypes I and II (see Table 14.34, p. 919) who are over the age of 40 and give a history of chronic sun exposure. On examination, they appear as multiple red, scaly plaques on sun-exposed skin. All patients should be strongly advised to minimize their sun exposure. Cryotherapy is effective in most cases; otherwise topical 5-fluorouracil

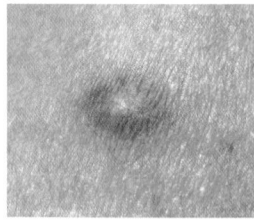

Fig. 14.63 Dermatofibroma.

cream or retinoids can be used. The presence of actinic keratoses is an indicator of increased risk of non-melanoma skin cancers. They occasionally disappear spontaneously but in general remain for many years.

Bowen's disease

Bowen's disease (squamous cell carcinoma in situ) presents as a fixed red plaque and represents an intraepidermal squamous cell carcinoma.

Epidemiology

Bowen's disease may occur at any age but is rare before the age of 30; most patients are aged over 60 at presentation. In the UK, it occurs predominantly in women (85% of cases).[1]

Pathology

A number of different factors have been implicated in the aetiology of Bowen's disease. The age group and body sites affected are suggestive of a relationship with chronic exposure to ultraviolet radiation.

Histologically, keratinocytes show loss of polarity, atypia and increased mitotic rate with involvement of the entire thickness of the epidermis from basal layer to stratum corneum. The basement membrane remains intact.

Clinical features

Bowen's disease presents as solitary or multiple, gradually enlarging, well-demarcated erythematous macules, papules or plaques. The lesions usually have an irregular border with surface crusting or scaling (Fig. 14.64). Approximately 75% of lesions are on the lower legs. They are most often asymptomatic, but may bleed. In the uncircumcised male, the lesions can present as smooth, red, velvety plaques on the glans penis (erythroplasia of Queyrat).

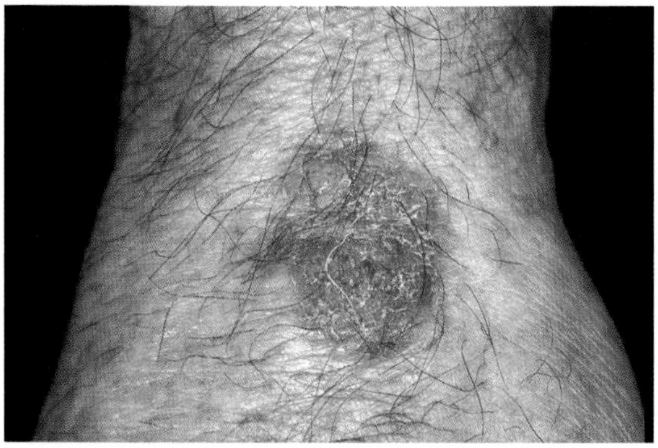

Fig. 14.64 Bowen's disease.

Investigations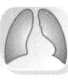

The diagnosis is suggested on the basis of clinical features.

Skin biopsy
Histology is required to confirm the diagnosis.

Management

Ablation of the lesion
Treatment options for Bowen's disease include cryotherapy, curettage and cautery, excision, laser (CO_2, argon and Nd:YAG) and topical 5-fluorouracil (applied once or twice daily as 5% cream for up to 2 months). All have recurrence rates of up to 10% and no treatment modality appears to be superior.[2]

Prognosis
If Bowen's disease is untreated, most studies suggest a 3% risk of progression to invasive squamous cell carcinoma.[3] Up to 50% of patients have other previous or subsequent skin malignancies, most commonly basal cell carcinoma. Genital Bowen's disease carries a higher risk of invasive cancer.

ℹ️ FURTHER INFORMATION

Cox NH, Eedy DJ, Morton CA. Guidelines for management of Bowen's disease. British Journal of Dermatology 1999; 141: 633–641.

REFERENCES

(1) *Eedy DJ, Gavin AT. Thirteen-year retrospective study of Bowen's disease. British Journal of Dermatology 1987; 117: 715–720.*
(2) *Cox NH, Eedy DJ, Morton CA. Guidelines for management of Bowen's disease. British Journal of Dermatology 1999; 141: 633–641.*
(3) *Kao GF. Carcinoma arising in Bowen's disease. Archives of Dermatology 1986; 122: 1124–1126.*

Squamous cell carcinoma

Squamous cell carcinoma is a malignant invasive proliferation of epidermal keratinocytes.

Epidemiology

Squamous cell carcinoma is the second most common type of skin cancer. It is more common in men and in the elderly population.[1]

Pathology

There is a relationship with chronic ultraviolet exposure. Squamous cell carcinoma is especially common in individuals with skin phototypes I and II (see Table 14.34, p. 919). Other aetiological factors include topical and systemic carcinogens such as arsenic, photochemotherapy (PUVA) and chronic immunosuppression (following allogeneic organ transplantation or in those with lymphoma or leukaemia). The lesions may also arise at sites of long-standing radiation dermatitis, scarring (discoid lupus erythematosus), ulceration and pre-existing lesions such as Bowen's disease. Some squamous cell carcinomas are associated with human papillomavirus infection. Smoking is associated with lesions on the lip.

Scope of disease

Squamous cell carcinoma is locally invasive and has the potential to metastasize to lymph nodes and other organs of the body.

Clinical features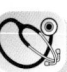

Squamous cell carcinoma usually presents as an expanding plaque or nodule with an ill-defined, indurated base and surface crusting (Fig. 14.65). The lesion may ulcerate. It is most often seen on sun-exposed sites (face, neck, forearms and dorsum of hands) in association with solar elastosis and multiple actinic keratoses. Local lymph nodes may be enlarged with metastatic involvement.

Investigations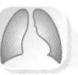

Skin biopsy
A skin biopsy is required to establish a histopathological diagnosis and to gain information on the degree of differentiation, grade, depth and level of dermal invasion, the presence of perineural, vascular or lymphatic invasion, and clearance margins of the excised tissue.

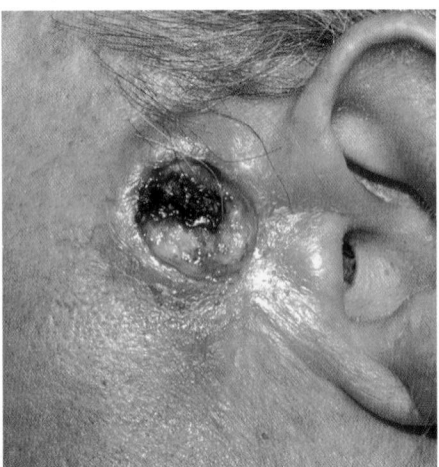

Fig. 14.65 Squamous cell carcinoma.

Lymph node biopsies
Squamous cell carcinomas usually spread to local lymph nodes; therefore clinically enlarged nodes should be excised and submitted for histopathological analysis.

Initial management

Patient education
Sun avoidance, the use of sunscreen and protective clothing are the main steps in the prevention of actinic keratoses and further squamous cell carcinomas, particularly in patients receiving immunosuppression.

Multidisciplinary team approach
There is overlap between dermatologists, clinical oncologists and plastic surgeons in the management of patients with squamous cell carcinoma, and therefore a multidisciplinary approach is favoured.

Surgical management

Curettage and cautery
Curettage and cautery may be feasible treatment options for small, well-defined, low-risk tumours.[2]

Excision biopsy and regional node dissection
Surgical excision or Mohs' micrographic surgery is the treatment of choice for the majority of lesions. For low-risk tumours (less than 2 cm in diameter), excision with a 4 mm margin is expected to achieve complete cure in 95%.

Mohs' micrographic surgery is indicated for larger, higher-risk tumours. With this technique, each section is examined with frozen section analysis to determine the completeness of resection. It is particularly useful in difficult sites where wide surgical margins may be technically difficult to achieve without functional impairment.

Tumour-positive lymph nodes are usually managed by regional node dissection.

Medical management

Radiotherapy
Other treatment options include radiotherapy for non-resectable tumours or lymph node disease.

Prognosis

Squamous cell carcinoma has an overall remission rate after therapy of 90%. The factors that influence metastatic potential include anatomical site, tumour size, degree of differentiation and immunosuppression.[3] Tumours arising in areas of radiation injury, chronic inflammation or chronic ulcers have the highest metastatic potential when compared to those from sun-exposed sites. Tumours more than 2 cm in diameter are 3 times as likely to metastasize compared to smaller tumours. Tumours more than 4 mm in depth or extending down to the subcutaneous tissue are more likely to recur and metastasize compared to thinner tumours. Poorer prognosis is associated with less well differentiated tumours, and tumours arising in patients who are immunosuppressed.

 FURTHER INFORMATION

Motley R, Kersey P, Lawrence C. Multiprofessional guidelines for the management of the patient with primary cutaneous squamous cell carcinoma. British Journal of Dermatology 2002; 146: 18–25.

REFERENCES

(1) *Marks R. Squamous cell carcinoma. Lancet 1996; 347: 735–738.*
(2) *Motley R, Kersey P, Lawrence C. Multiprofessional guidelines for the management of the patient with primary cutaneous squamous cell carcinoma. British Journal of Dermatology 2002; 146: 18–25.*
(3) *Friedman NR. Prognostic factors for local recurrences, metastases and survival rates in SCC of the skin, ear and lip. Journal of the American Academy of Dermatology 1993; 28: 281–282.*

Basal cell carcinoma

Basal cell carcinoma (rodent ulcer) is a slow-growing, locally invasive tumour with virtually no capacity to metastasize.

Epidemiology

Basal cell carcinoma is the most common type of skin cancer, approximately 4 times more common than squamous cell carcinoma.

Pathology

The most significant aetiological factor is chronic excess ultraviolet radiation exposure. As a result, exposed areas such as the head and neck are most commonly involved. Other risk factors include increasing age, male sex, and skin phototypes I and II (see Table 14.34, p. 919). Histologically there is a proliferation of atypical basal keratinocytes.

Clinical features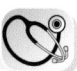

The clinical appearances and morphology are diverse and include nodular, morphoeic, superficial multifocal, keratotic and pigmented varieties.

The nodular basal cell carcinoma tends to arise on the forehead, nose or adjacent to the inner canthus of the eye as a skin-coloured or pigmented, translucent nodule with surface telangiectasia (Fig. 14.66). Gradual enlargement leads to central ulceration (ulcerated basal cell carcinoma) with a peripheral, 'rolled' pearly edge. There may also be cystic change (cystic or nodulocystic basal cell carcinoma).

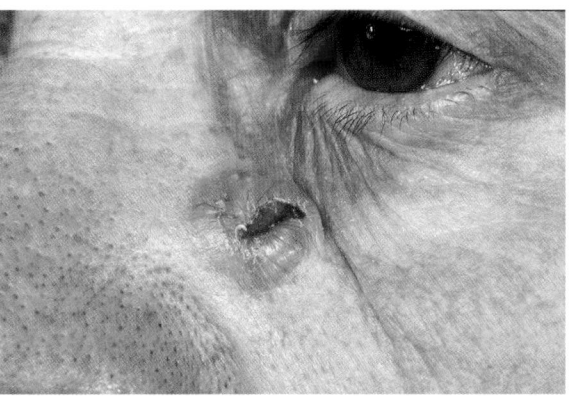
Fig. 14.66 Basal cell carcinoma.

The morphoeic (sclerosing) basal cell carcinoma presents as a firm, indurated, skin-coloured, scar-like plaque with ill-defined edges, commonly on the nasolabial fold or forehead. Superficial multifocal basal cell carcinomas tend to arise on extrafacial sites as red, scaly plaques and have no relation to sun exposure. Pigmented basal cell carcinomas may be brown, blue or black with a smooth glistening surface. Keratotic basal cell carcinomas have evidence of keratinization on histology.

Initial investigations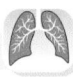

Skin biopsy
A skin biopsy confirms the diagnosis and determines the histological subtype. Alternatively, cytology can be performed on skin scrapings.

Initial management

Multidisciplinary team approach
Depending on the size and site of the basal cell carcinoma, dermatologists, clinical oncologists and plastic surgeons may all be involved in the management. Therefore, a multidisciplinary approach is favoured.

Surgical management

Curettage and cautery
Curettage and cautery is a suitable option for patients with low-risk lesions (small, well-defined, primary lesion) and can achieve 5-year cure rates of up to 97%. Patients with recurrent morphoeic tumours in high-risk sites such as the nose, nasolabial folds and around the eyes should undergo formal surgical excision.

Cryotherapy
Cryotherapy can be used on low-risk lesions with non-aggressive histology that are not recurrent lesions.

Surgical excision

The main aim of surgery is complete excision with a clear surgical margin. For small (<2 cm) well-defined basal cell carcinomas, a 3 mm surgical margin achieves cure in 85% and a 5 mm margin will increase the cure rate to 95%. Morphoeic, large or recurrent basal cell carcinomas require a larger margin or Mohs' micrographic technique (Table 14.27). Excision of a lesion may require primary closure, skin flaps or grafts. Mohs' micrographic surgery offers a 5-year cure rate of 99% together with maximal preservation of normal tissues for primary basal cell carcinoma. It is a specialized, expensive and time-consuming procedure.

Medical management

Radiotherapy

Radiotherapy is useful for treatment of basal cell carcinoma in locations where disfigurement results from surgical excision (although atrophy telangiectasia may develop in the long term and affect the cosmetic results). The 5-year cure is approximately 90%. Patients with recurrent lesions after radiotherapy should undergo surgical excision.

Topical 5-fluorouracil

Topical 5-fluorouracil is usually the treatment of choice for multiple superficial basal cell carcinomas on the trunk and lower limbs.

Palliative management options

Aggressive treatment can be inappropriate in elderly debilitated patients, especially for asymptomatic low-risk lesions. Palliative treatment such as debulking the tumour or radiotherapy may be more appropriate.

> **RECENT ADVANCES**
>
> *Intralesional interferon and photodynamic therapy are still under investigation with some early promising results.*

Prognosis

Table 14.28 lists the factors affecting prognosis. Metastasis is extremely rare and the morbidity is related to local tissue invasion and destruction. Patients with a single tumour are at a significant increased risk of developing subsequent basal cell carcinomas.

i FURTHER INFORMATION

Wong CSM, Strange RC, Lear JT. Basal cell carcinoma. BMJ 2003; 327: 794–798.

Telfer NR, Colver GB, Bowers PW. Guidelines for management of basal cell carcinoma. British Journal of Dermatology 1999; 141: 415–423.

Table 14.27	Indications for Mohs' micrographic surgery
Site (eyes, ears, lips, nose, nasolabial folds)	
Histological subtypes (morphoeic)	
Recurrent basal cell carcinoma	
Size (>2 cm, especially in high-risk sites)	

Table 14.28	Factors affecting the prognosis of basal cell carcinoma
Tumour size	
Tumour site	
Tumour type and definition of tumour margins	
Growth pattern	
Histological subtype	
Failure of previous treatment	
Immunocompromised patients	

Disorders of melanocytes

Lentigo

A lentigo is a common lesion that presents as a small, pigmented macule due to an increase in the number of melanocytes within the basal layer of the epidermis. These are unaffected by sunlight. Solar lentigines develop on sun-exposed sites following either acute severe sunburn in young adults or chronic ultraviolet exposure in the elderly. Multiple lentigines may rarely be a manifestation of Peutz–Jeghers syndrome, particularly when distributed on the lips, buccal mucosa and acral sites.

Acquired melanocytic naevi

Acquired melanocytic naevi are common benign proliferations of melanocytes. They can be classified according to the site of the cluster of melanocytes. Junctional naevi describe the position of the cells at the dermal–epidermal junction above the basement membrane. Intradermal naevi describe cells that are exclusively in the dermis. Compound naevi have histological features of both junctional and intradermal naevi.

Junctional naevi present as small, dark brown, evenly pigmented, symmetrical macules (Fig. 14.67). The majority of naevi in children are junctional and occur on any body site. Compound naevi (where melanocytes are present in both the epidermis and dermis) occur at any site and vary from light brown papules to dark brown papillomatous plaques (Fig. 14.68). Intradermal naevi are usually detected in the third decade, frequently on the face, and may be devoid of pigment (Fig. 14.69). They may be dome-shaped

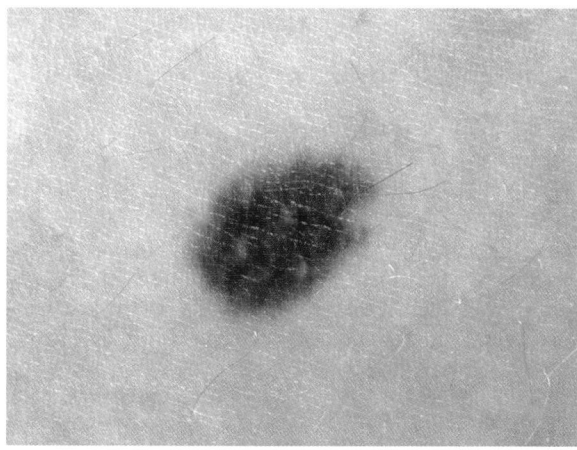

Fig. 14.67 Junctional naevus.

or pedunculated skin tags. These lesions appear in early childhood and reach a maximum in young adulthood. There is then a gradual involution, and most lesions disappear by the age of 60. A skin biopsy is only required when clinical differentiation from malignant melanoma is difficult.

Blue naevus

A blue naevus is an acquired, benign, firm, dark blue to black, sharply defined papule representing a deep dermal aggregate of melanocytes. The dermal melanocytes are thought to represent melanocytes which have failed to migrate from the neural crest to the epidermis during fetal life. Blue naevus is most common on the dorsum of hands or feet of older children and young adults. Malignant change is very rare.

Spitz naevus

A Spitz naevus is a benign melanocytic tumour that is distinct from acquired melanocytic naevi on both clinical and pathological grounds. The majority occur in children as a discrete, red-brown or pink papule on the face. The clinical presentation is distinctive and there is often a history of recent rapid growth. Differentiation from malignant melanoma may be difficult and in these cases complete excision is recommended.

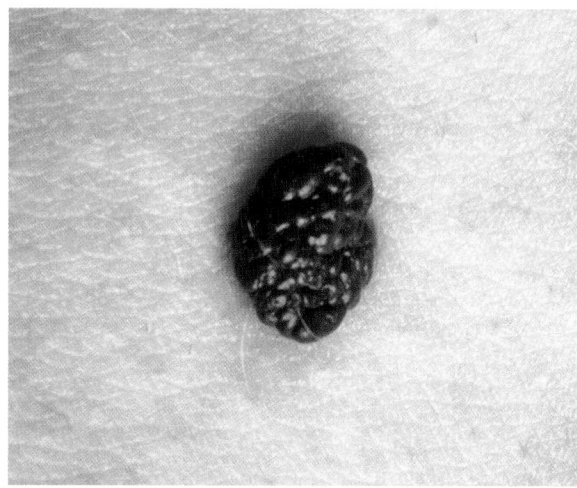

Fig. 14.68 Compound naevus.

Mongolian spot

A Mongolian spot is a congenital grey-blue macular lesion that can occur anywhere on the skin but is characteristically located on the lumbosacral area. Histologically there are ectopic melanocytes in the dermis, possibly interrupted in their migration from the neural crest to the epidermis. Mongolian spots disappear in early childhood. No melanomas have been reported in these lesions.

Naevus spilus

A naevus spilus is a common lesion consisting of a light brown macule, varying in size from a few centimetres to a very large area, with many darker small macules (2–3 mm) or papules scattered throughout. Histologically, the background macule shows an increased number of melanocytes and the scattered lesions are either junctional or compound naevi. Malignant melanoma very rarely arises in these lesions.

Dysplastic melanocytic naevus

Dysplastic melanocytic naevi are melanocytic lesions with atypical clinical and histological features. They are regarded

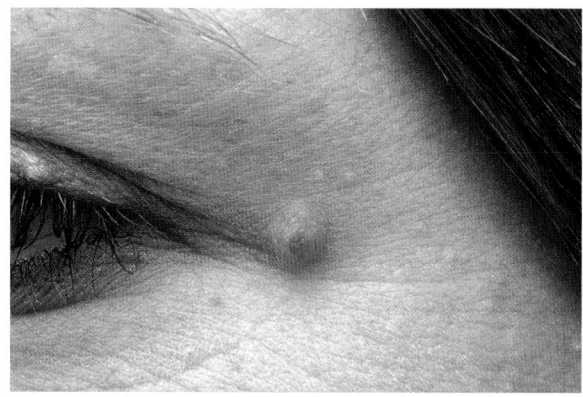

Fig. 14.69 Intradermal naevus.

Benign tumours arising from the epidermis

Benign tumours arising from the dermis and subcutis

Malignant neoplasms and their precursors

Disorders of melanocytes

Cutaneous lymphomas and sarcomas

as potential precursors of superficial spreading melanoma and also as markers of persons at risk for developing primary malignant melanoma. These pigmented lesions are clinically distinct from acquired melanocytic naevi, being larger and more variegated in colour, with an asymmetrical outline and irregular border. Lesions may occur sporadically or may arise against a background of dysplastic naevus syndrome, an autosomal dominant condition with multiple atypical naevi. Surgical excision of lesions with minimal margins is recommended, especially in lesions that are changing or those that cannot be closely followed by the patient (on the scalp or back).

> ### ⚡ CLINICAL ALERT
>
> **Six signs of malignant melanoma**
> A   Asymmetry in shape
> B   Border is irregular
> C   Colour variegation—shades of brown, black, grey, red and white
> D   Diameter is usually large, >6 mm
> E   Elevation is almost always present
>   Enlargement—a history of growth in size of the lesion

Malignant melanoma

Melanoma arises from malignant proliferation of melanocytes.

Epidemiology

The incidence of and mortality from melanoma are increasing. The incidence in the UK is approximately 10 per 100 000 per year.[1] The highest incidence occurs in white-skinned individuals in Australia and New Zealand. Melanoma is more common in women than in men.

Pathology

Ultraviolet exposure is a major aetiological factor, particularly short, intense exposure resulting in sunburn during childhood. Phenotypic factors associated with melanoma include fair skin, red or blonde hair, blue eyes, inability to tan, freckles, lentigines, large numbers of benign melanocytic naevi and the presence of dysplastic naevi (Table 14.29).

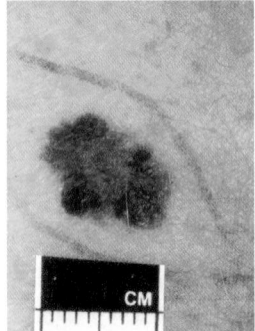

Fig. 14.70 Superficial spreading malignant melanoma.

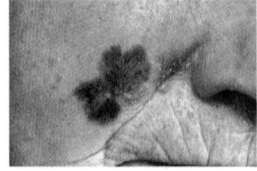

Fig. 14.71 Lentigo maligna.

Table 14.29	Important risk factors for malignant melanoma
Presence of precursor lesions (dysplastic melanocytic naevi)	
Family history of melanoma in parents or siblings	
Skin phototypes I and II with an inability to tan	
Excess sun exposure, especially during childhood	

Clinical features

Malignant melanoma has two patterns of growth, radial and vertical. Radial growth is horizontal within the epidermis and superficial dermal layers, as in the lentigo maligna, acral/mucosal lentiginous and superficial spreading types. During this stage of growth the tumour does not have the capacity to metastasize. Vertical growth occurs with time, and the melanoma grows downwards into the deeper dermal layers as an expansile mass, lacking cellular maturation. This correlates with the emergence of a clone of cells with metastatic potential. The nature and extent of this vertical growth phase determine the biological behaviour of malignant melanoma. The different types of malignant melanoma are categorized on morphology and histological findings.

Superficial spreading

Superficial spreading is the most common variant of melanoma (70%), presenting as a macule or papule, usually greater than 0.5 cm in diameter. There is variable pigmentation (from pale brown to blue-black), an irregular edge, and surface oozing or crusting (Fig. 14.70). In males it most frequently presents on the back, while in females the leg is the most common site. In the radial growth phase it is characterized by atypical melanocytes, singly and in clusters, widely scattered throughout the layers of the epidermis. Left untreated it may progress to the vertical growth phase over months to years.

Nodular melanoma

Nodular melanoma is the second most common variant (14%) and, by definition, presents in the vertical growth phase. It classically presents as a rapidly enlarging, frequently ulcerated, blue-black nodule.

Lentigo maligna

Lentigo maligna presents as an irregularly pigmented macule, slowly enlarging over many years, commonly on the cheek or temple of an elderly person (Fig. 14.71). It is characterized by basally located atypical melanocytes. Development of a more rapidly growing, deeply pigmented papule or nodule indicates dermal invasion by malignant melanocytes (lentigo maligna melanoma).

Acral lentiginous melanoma

Acral lentiginous melanoma is an uncommon subtype, although it is the predominant variant in the Afro-Caribbean population. The sole of the foot is most often affected and lesions may also arise on the digits. Subungual or periungual melanoma, a variant of acral lentiginous melanoma, occurs either as a linear pigmented streak in the nail or an isolated nail dystrophy, accompanied by the pigmentation of the proximal nail fold (Hutchinson's sign).

Amelanotic melanoma

Amelanotic melanoma is a non-pigmented variant of melanoma.

Malignant melanoma on mucous membranes

Malignant melanoma on mucous membranes is very rare and may affect the vulva, urethra and anus. It has a poor prognosis, due in part to its often advanced stage at presentation.

Investigations

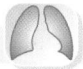

Skin biopsy

An excision skin biopsy must be performed to confirm the diagnosis. This will give important histological data (Table 14.30) and provide valuable staging information (Table 14.31).

Management

The management of malignant melanoma varies according to the stage at presentation, and ranges from surgical excision to radiotherapy and chemotherapy. A summary of the management is presented in Figure 14.72.

Prognosis

Melanoma has a mortality rate of 25% and therefore early diagnosis and treatment is essential. Prognostic factors include thickness, level of invasion, sex and site of tumour.

Table 14.30	Histological data from melanoma

Clarke's level

I	melanoma cells confined to epidermis
II	melanoma cells invade papillary dermis
III	melanoma cells completely occupy papillary dermis
IV	melanoma cells invade mid-reticular dermis
V	melanoma cells invade subcutaneous fat

Tumour thickness in mm from granular layer of the epidermis to maximum depth (Breslow thickness)

Presence of radial or vertical growth

Tumour infiltrating lymphocytes

Mitoses per mm^2

Presence or absence of tumour regression (mitosis, inflammatory infiltrate, pigmentary incontinence, fibrosis and dermal scarring, and vascular proliferation)

Microsatellites

Evidence of perineural infiltrate

Evidence of vascular and lymphatic invasion

Whether excision is complete

Pathological staging (Table 14.31)

Table 14.31	TNM staging system for melanoma		
Stage (T)	**Primary tumour**	**Lymph node (N)**	**Distant metastases (M)**
0	In situ tumours	No nodes	None
IA	<1 mm, no ulceration	No nodes	None
IB	<1 mm with ulceration	No nodes	None
	1.01–2 mm, no ulceration	No nodes	None
IIA	1.01–2 mm with ulceration	No nodes	None
	2.01–4 mm, no ulceration	No nodes	None
IIB	2.01–4 mm with ulceration	No nodes	None
	>4 mm, no ulceration	No nodes	None
IIC	>4 mm with ulceration	No nodes	None
IIIA	Any Breslow thickness, no ulceration	Micrometastases in nodes	None
IIIB	Any Breslow thickness with ulceration	Micrometastases in nodes	None
	Any Breslow thickness, no ulceration	Up to 3 palpable nodes	None
	Any Breslow thickness ± ulceration	No nodes but in-transit metastases or satellites	None
IIIC	Any Breslow thickness with ulceration	Up to 3 palpable nodes	None
	Any Breslow thickness ± ulceration	4 or more palpable nodes or matted nodes or in-transit metastases with nodes	None
IV			M1: skin, subcutaneous or distant lymph nodes
			M2: lung
			M3: all other sites or any site with raised lactate dehydrogenase

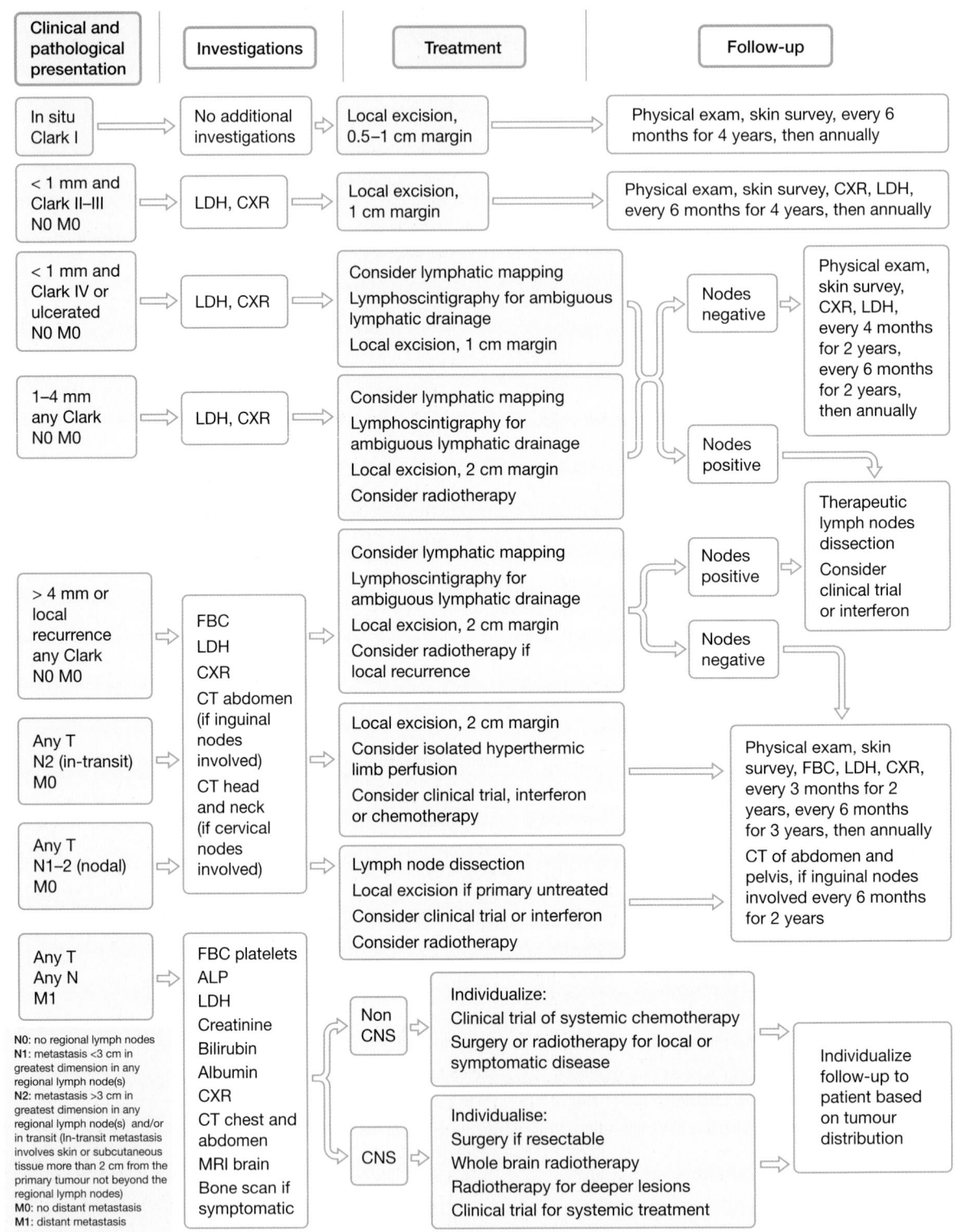

Fig. 14.72 Management of malignant melanoma. LDH, lactate dehydrogenase; CXR, chest X-ray; FBC, full blood count; ALP, alkaline phosphatase.

Benign tumours arising
from the epidermis

Benign tumours arising
from the dermis
and subcutis

Malignant neoplasms
and their precursors

Disorders of melanocytes

**Cutaneous lymphomas
and sarcomas**

FURTHER INFORMATION

Roberts DLL, Anstey AV, Barlow RJ. UK guidelines for the management of cutaneous melanoma. British Journal of Dermatology 2002; 146: 7–17.

Thomas JM, Newton-Bishop J, A'Hern R, et al. Excision margins in high-risk malignant melanoma. New England Journal of Medicine 2004; 350: 757–766.

Tsao H, Atkins MB, Sober AJ. Management of cutaneous melanoma. New England Journal of Medicine 2004; 351: 998–1012.

REFERENCE

(1) *Melia J. Changing incidence and mortality from cutaneous malignant melanoma. BMJ 1997; 315: 1106–1107.*

Cutaneous lymphomas and sarcomas

Cutaneous lymphomas

Primary cutaneous T-cell lymphoma

Epidemiology

Primary cutaneous T-cell lymphoma is a rare, low-grade, cutaneous T-cell lymphoma that is most frequently seen in males in the sixth to seventh decades.

Pathology

The most common form of primary cutaneous T-cell lymphoma is mycosis fungoides. There are also other rarer types, each with a different prognosis. Proposed aetiological factors include HTLV1 infection. This form of lymphoma generally runs a slow course remaining confined to the skin; however, rarely it can spread further to involve lymph node and internal organs.

Clinical features
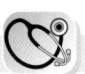

Mycoses fungoides tends to give rise to a chronic erythematous scaly dermatosis. The lesions may be distributed anywhere but mostly occur on the trunk and buttocks. Cutaneous lesions may progress from patch to plaque to tumour stage disease. It can be difficult to differentiate the early patch stage from eczema or psoriasis.

Investigations
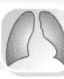

Skin biopsy
Diagnosis is made by a skin biopsy sent for histology and T-cell receptor gene rearrangement studies.

Staging investigations
Blood tests, a staging CT scan, bone marrow and lymph node biopsy may be required to confirm the disease subtype and decide on the most appropriate course of treatment.

Management

Localized disease
Treatment options include PUVA, topical steroids and chemotherapy, and localized superficial radiotherapy.

Widespread disease
More widespread disease requires systemic therapy such as interferon-alfa, oral or intravenous chemotherapy, total body electron-beam radiotherapy and extracorporeal photophoresis (treating blood with ultraviolet light).

Prognosis

All treatments improve the skin but none has been shown to alter the natural history of the disease.

FURTHER INFORMATION

Whittaker SJ, Marsden JR, Spittle M, et al. Joint British Association of Dermatologists and UK Cutaneous Lymphoma Group guidelines for the management of primary cutaneous T-cell lymphomas. British Journal of Dermatology 2003; 149: 1095–1107.

Willemze R, Jaffe ES, Burg G, et al. WHO-EORTC classification for cutaneous lymphomas. Blood 2005; 105: 3768–3785.

Cutaneous B-cell lymphomas

Cutaneous B-cell lymphomas are rare malignant proliferations of B lymphocytes within the skin that present as nodules or groups of nodules with a predilection for the trunk. Diagnosis is made by a skin biopsy sent for histology and immunoglobulin gene rearrangement studies. Routine blood tests, a staging CT scan, bone marrow and lymph node biopsies are usually required to decide on the course of treatment. The majority respond well to local superficial radiotherapy to the nodules. If disease is more widespread, oral chemotherapy may be required. The disease usually has a slow course, remaining confined to the skin. In some patients the lesions resolve spontaneously. Most have an excellent prognosis.

Diseases of the skin

i FURTHER INFORMATION

Fung MA, Murphy MJ, Hoss DM, Grant-Kels JM. Practical evaluation and management of cutaneous lymphomas. Journal of the American Academy of Dermatology 2002; 46: 325–359.

Willemze R, Jaffe ES, Burg G, et al. WHO-EORTC classification for cutaneous lymphomas. Blood 2005; 105: 3768–3785.

Kaposi's sarcoma

Kaposi's sarcoma is a multisystem vascular neoplasia characterized by mucocutaneous violaceous lesions as well as multiorgan involvement.

Epidemiology

Kaposi's sarcoma is a rare tumour but has an increasing incidence due to the association with HIV infection. In HIV-positive patients, the development of Kaposi's sarcoma is an AIDS-defining illness.

Pathology

Kaposi's sarcoma cells are derived from the endothelium of the blood and lymphatic microvasculature. This is now generally regarded as widespread cellular proliferation in response to angiogenic substances rather than a true malignancy. The aetiology is not known but epidemiological data support a viral infection, possibly human herpesvirus 8 (HHV-8).

Clinical features

Classic Kaposi's sarcoma was initially reported in Jews and is classically found on the legs of elderly men of Eastern European heritage. It is slowly progressive and usually responds well to radiotherapy of involved skin (Fig. 14.73). AIDS-associated Kaposi's sarcoma is found in approximately one third of AIDS patients and is more common in homo-

sexual men. There is early involvement of the face and widespread distribution on the trunk. The disease progresses rapidly with extensive systemic involvement (lymph nodes, lungs, urogenital tract, gastrointestinal tract). Approximately one third develop a second malignancy such as lymphoma or leukaemia. Patients with the African variety of Kaposi's sarcoma present with violaceous skin plaques. This variant occurs in children and younger men. Transplantation-associated Kaposi's sarcoma is rare and occurs particularly in patients on high-dose immunosuppressive therapy.

Investigations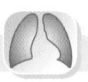

Skin biopsy

The diagnosis of Kaposi's sarcoma should be confirmed histologically in all patients. All variants have similar histology. The early or 'patch' stage is characterized by thin-walled dilated vascular spaces in the epidermis with inflammatory cells and extravasated red cells. Later or 'nodular' lesions comprise spindle-shaped stromal cells with irregular slit-like spaces filled with red blood cells and lined by recognizable endothelium, intertwined with normal vascular channels.

Management

Identify and address any underlying cause

Patients may develop Kaposi's sarcoma as the first presenting symptom of AIDS. Alternatively, it may be related to immunosuppression, and lesions may regress with a change or attenuation in the intensity of immunosuppression.

Interferon-alfa and cytotoxic chemotherapy

Interferon-alfa and cytotoxic chemotherapy (liposomal anthracycline) may be administered to patients with AIDS-associated Kaposi's sarcoma.

Prognosis

The prognosis depends on the subtype. Patients with classic disease tend to die of unrelated causes. Patients with AIDS-related Kaposi's sarcoma usually die from secondary infection seen in AIDS rather than as a direct consequence of Kaposi's sarcoma. The African variety is an aggressive tumour that is ultimately fatal, whereas immunosuppression-related lesions often regress when immunosuppression is stopped.

i FURTHER INFORMATION

Buonaguro FM, Tomesello ML, Buonaguro L, Satriano RA, Ruocco E, Castello G, Ruocco V. Kaposi's sarcoma: aetiopathogenesis, histology and clinical features. Journal of the European Academy of Dermatology and Venereology 2003; 17: 138–154.

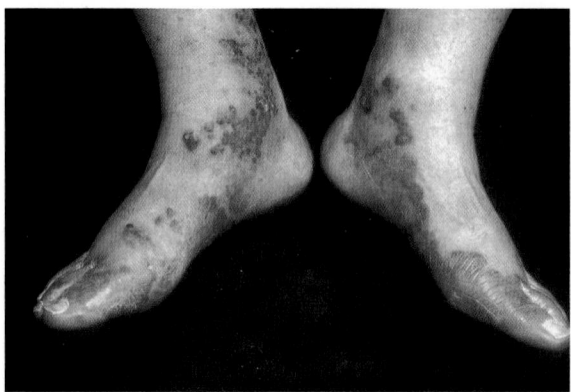

Fig. 14.73 Classic Kaposi's sarcoma.

914

Disorders of pigmentation

Hyperpigmentation

A number of disorders result in hyperpigmentation of the skin (Table 14.32) with two main patterns that differ based on the location of melanin deposition. Brown pigmentation or hypermelanosis results from increased melanin in the basal keratinocytes of the epidermis (as seen after sun exposure). However, melanin may also be deposited in macrophages in the deep dermis, resulting in a blue discolouration of the skin. Non-melanin pigmentation results from deposition of pigment other than melanin in the dermis.

Hypermelanosis

Melasma

Melasma is characterized by symmetrical irregular brown hyperpigmentation of the skin over light-exposed areas (Fig. 14.74). It results from an increase in epidermal and dermal pigmentation and is most commonly seen in women during pregnancy or as a result of the oral contraceptive pill. The pigmentation occurs on the cheeks, forehead and chin, and becomes more marked following sun exposure. Therapy for melasma begins with the identification and elimination of causative factors such as the oral contraceptive pill or other hormone-containing drugs. Broad-spectrum sunscreen and sun protection are essential. Application of a depigmenting cream (hydroquinone 5% with retinoic acid 0.1% and hydrocortisone 1%) may be beneficial.

Café-au-lait macules

Café-au-lait macules are well-circumscribed tan-coloured macules, unrelated to ultraviolet exposure, which can vary in size and number (see Fig. 14.81, p. 931). They may be present at birth or acquired in early childhood. The pigmentation is due to an increased number of melanocytes in the epidermis as well as increased melanin, and is enhanced by Wood's light. The presence of 6 or more café-au-lait macules greater than 1.5 cm in diameter is usually a sign of neurofibromatosis.

Albright's syndrome

Albright's syndrome is a genetic condition with unilateral hyperpigmented macules, fibrous dysplasia of bone and endocrine dysfunction. The brown macules in this condi-

tion can be differentiated from café-au-lait macules because in Albright's syndrome the lesions have irregular contours and the hairs within tend to be darker.

Incontinentia pigmenti

Incontinentia pigmenti is an autosomal dominant X-linked disorder that is lethal in males. Mutations in the *NEMO* gene, on the X chromosome, have been described. A variety of skin lesions are associated with developmental defects of the eye, teeth, skeleton and central nervous system. Three clinical stages of cutaneous changes are seen in females. Soon after birth, linear groups of tense blisters are seen on the limbs or trunk. These may be accompanied by red nodules or plaques. Within days to weeks, these lesions dry up leaving warty or verrucous streaks. After a few weeks, these are replaced by irregular brown or blue-grey pigmentation, classically in a 'Chinese figure' distribution. This pigmentation slowly fades and is usually undetectable by the third decade.

Post-inflammatory hyperpigmentation

Post-inflammatory hyperpigmentation is very common and can occur after any inflammatory condition of the skin, either endogenous such as atopic dermatitis, lichen planus, discoid lupus erythematosus and acne vulgaris, or exogenous such as trauma or thermal injury. The brown discolouration results from accumulation of melanin and iron pigments in the dermis, with or without increased melanin in the epidermis. The hyperpigmentation persists after the primary lesions have resolved and is much more likely to occur in dark-skinned individuals. Treatment is difficult.

Other hypermelanotic lesions

Other hypermelanotic lesions include freckles (ephelides), lentigines, lentigo maligna, Mongolian spot, and naevus of Ota and of Ito.

Non-melanin pigmentation

Haemosiderosis

Haemosiderosis is the deposition of the iron-containing pigment haemosiderin within the skin and often results

Table 14.32 Disorders of hyperpigmentation

Hereditary or developmental disorders

Incontinentia pigmenti

Albright's syndrome

Epidermal naevi

Dermal melanocytosis
   Naevus of Ota and naevus of Ito
   Mongolian spot

Metabolic disorders

Haemochromatosis

Niemann–Pick disease

Gaucher's disease

Macular and lichenoid amyloidosis

Ochronosis

Porphyria cutanea tarda

Wilson's disease

Endocrine disorders

Melasma

Addison's disease

Melanocyte-stimulating hormone (MSH)-producing neoplasm

Cushing's syndrome

Exogenous ACTH therapy

Inflammatory disorders

Post-inflammatory hyperpigmentation

Lichen planus

Lupus erythematosus

Fixed drug eruption

Chemically induced disorders

Antimalarial agents—brown or blue-black pigmentation

Tetracyclines—blue-black pigmentation, particularly at sites of previous inflammation

Amiodarone—blue-grey pigmentation of sun-exposed area

Chlorpromazine—blue-grey pigmentation of sun-exposed area

Oral contraceptive pill—may induce melasma

Arsenic intoxication—macular hyperpigmentation with areas of hypopigmentation

Heavy metals
   Silver (argyria)
   Gold (chrysiasis)
   Lead—blue/black line at gingival margin, grey discolouration of the skin

Nutritional disorders

Pellegra

Vitamin B_{12} deficiency

Kwashiorkor

Neoplastic disorders

Metastatic melanoma

Mastocytosis (urticaria pigmentosa)

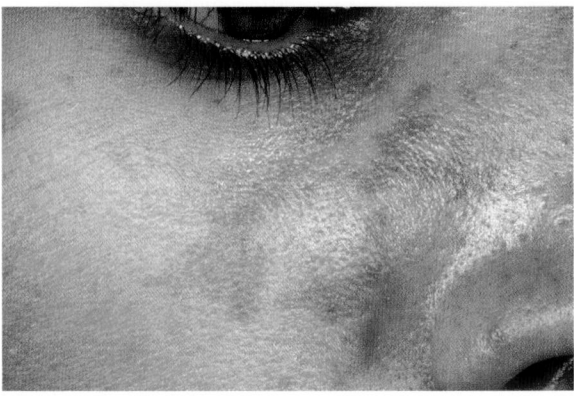

Fig. 14.74 Melasma.

from loss and destruction of red blood cells in the dermis. Haemosiderin deposition also stimulates melanogenesis and therefore there is often some associated hyper-melanosis. Haemosiderosis is most commonly seen on the lower legs in individuals with venous hypertension. Clinically, specks of orange-red pigment gradually become brown and more uniform with increasing hypermelanosis.

Carotenaemia

Carotenaemia is excess blood carotene levels and results in yellow discolouration of the skin (carotenoderma). This is most obvious on the palms and soles. It is seen in patients taking β-carotene (the natural provitamin of vitamin A) or in those eating excessive amounts of carotene-containing foods such as carrots or oranges. Other than reducing the amount of carotene intake, no treatment is required.

Ochronosis

Ochronosis is the deposition of a brownish-black pigment, derived from polymerized homogentisic acid, in the skin and sclera. It occurs in the inherited metabolic disorder alkaptonuria but is more commonly seen in an acquired form from long-term application of skin-lightening creams containing hydroquinone, an inhibitor of tyrosinase. Ochronosis presents as a dusky, cutaneous pigmentation (described as 'confetti pigmentation') that is most marked over cheeks and forehead but may also be seen in the axillae, genitalia and buccal mucosa.

Argyria

Argyria is the deposition of silver within the skin, either from occupational exposure or from medication. It presents as slate blue-grey pigmentation following many years of accumulation in the skin, and is most obvious in sun-exposed areas. Silver granules are seen in the dermis on skin biopsy.

Drug-induced pigmentation

Drug-induced skin pigmentation can be caused by a number of mechanisms, including increased melanin synthesis, post-inflammatory hyperpigmentation, and deposition of a drug-related material.

FURTHER INFORMATION

Dereure O. Drug-induced skin pigmentation. Epidemiology, diagnosis and treatment. American Journal of Clinical Dermatology 2001; 2: 253–262.

Hypopigmentation

There are a number of disorders that can present with hypopigmentation of the skin (Table 14.33). This results from a reduction of melanin and melanocytes in the epidermis and is referred to as hypomelanosis.

Vitiligo

Vitiligo is an acquired idiopathic pigmentary disorder characterized by areas of depigmented skin, resulting from loss of epidermal melanocytes.

Epidemiology

Vitiligo is relatively common with a prevalence of up to 2000 per 100 000 worldwide. The onset of disease may be at any age but the incidence peaks in the second and third decades of life. There is no gender predominance or racial predilection.

Table 14.33	Disorders with depigmentation or hypopigmentation
Vitiligo	
Oculocutaneous albinism	
Idiopathic guttate hypomelanosis	
Post-inflammatory hypopigmentation	
Pityriasis alba	
Piebaldism	
Pityriasis versicolor	
Scleroderma	
Tuberous sclerosis	
Naevus depigmentosus	

Pathology

Genetic studies suggest that vitiligo is a multifactorial, polygenic disorder. The cause of loss of epidermal melanocytes is unknown but it is thought to involve an autoimmune process. Patients with more extensive disease tend to have a higher incidence of other autoimmune diseases such as thyroid disease, diabetes mellitus and pernicious anaemia.

Clinical features

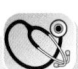

The depigmented lesions of vitiligo are discrete, well-circumscribed, white patches, often symmetrically distributed (Fig. 14.75). The lack of melanin pigment makes lesional skin more sensitive to sunburn. The disease can be focal (with only a few patches), segmental (patches on one side of the body), acral or acrofacial, or generalized (widespread patches). The generalized distribution is the most common pattern with symmetrical areas of depigmentation. Progression of disease can result in widespread depigmentation that is cosmetically debilitating and psychologically devastating, especially in darker-skinned individuals.

Investigations

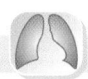

Skin biopsy
The diagnosis is made clinically but can be confirmed by a skin biopsy.

Thyroid-stimulating hormone (TSH)
In view of the association with other autoimmune conditions, in particular thyroid disease, routine thyroid function screening tests may be valuable.

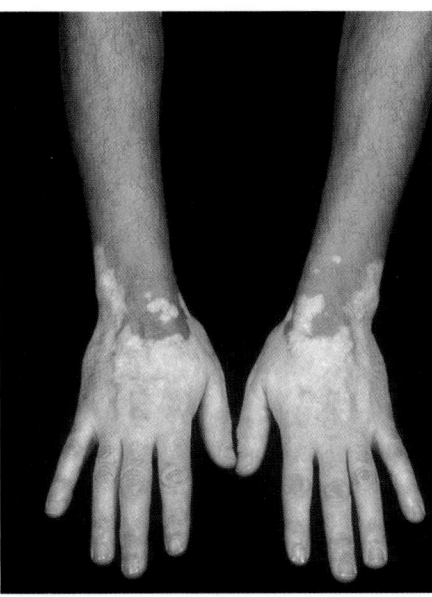

Fig. 14.75 Vitiligo.

Management

Camouflage products

For more localized disease, particularly on the face, camouflage products can be very helpful.

Topical steroids and tacrolimus

Topical steroids and tacrolimus can be effective as repigmenting agents by inhibiting T-cell activation and thereby blocking the production and release of pro-inflammatory cytokines.

Phototherapy

Narrowband UVB is now the treatment of choice for patients with moderate to severe vitiligo, particularly in skin phototypes II and III (see Table 14.34, p. 919). It causes repigmentation by local immunosuppression, production of melanocyte-stimulating hormone, and an increase in melanocyte proliferation and melanogenesis.

Depigmentation agents

In widespread vitiligo, residual pigment can be removed by depigmentation agents.

Prognosis

The course of disease is unpredictable. Lesions may remain stable or slowly progress over years. Occasionally spontaneous remission can occur, but it is unusual.

ℹ FURTHER INFORMATION

Grimes PE. New insights and new therapies in vitiligo. JAMA 2005; 293: 731–735.

Oculocutaneous albinism

Oculocutaneous albinism is a clinically heterogeneous autosomal recessive disorder. It is characterized by hypomelanosis in most tissues including the skin, hair and eyes, accompanied by reduced visual acuity with nystagmus and photophobia. Oculocutaneous albinism is a disorder of melanin synthesis. There are six different subtypes caused by different underlying genetic defects.

There is no specific treatment; however, sunscreens and sun avoidance are crucial in patients with minimal or no pigmentation as they are at high risk of photocarcinogenesis. Those in tropical regions are particularly at risk of developing squamous cell carcinomas, associated with significant morbidity and mortality.

ℹ FURTHER INFORMATION

Tomita Y, Suzuki T. Genetics of pigmentary disorders. American Journal of Medical Genetics Part C, Seminars in Medical Genetics 2004; 131C: 75–81.

Post-inflammatory hypopigmentation

Just as hyperpigmentation can occur after any inflammatory condition of the skin, hypopigmentation may also occur. This may be a feature in children with a form of low-grade eczema, where it presents as poorly circumscribed scaly macules on the face and is referred to as pityriasis alba.

Sunlight and the skin

Ultraviolet radiation (UVR) comprises only about 5% of terrestrial sunlight, with visible light and infrared radiation making up the remaining 95%. However, it is UVR which is chiefly responsible for the harmful effects of sunlight exposure. On a sunny day, UVA (315–400 nm) accounts for at least 95% of terrestrial UVR, and UVB (280–315 nm) no more than 5%. UVR has acute and chronic effects on the skin.

Acute effects

Erythema (sunburn)

Sunburn or erythema can vary in intensity from mild redness to oedema, blistering and peeling. Susceptibility to sunburn and tanning depends on the skin phototype of the individual (Table 14.34). UVB is much more effective at inducing erythema than UVA. UVB accounts for only about 5% of solar radiation but it contributes to about 80% of the erythema caused by sunlight. Experiments suggest that the synthesis and release of prostaglandin E_2 (PGE_2), following cyclooxygenase-2 (*cox-2*) gene activation, and nitric oxide within the dermis are responsible for UV-induced erythema.

Melanogenesis (tanning)

Skin colour is genetically controlled but can be enhanced by UVR exposure. Table 14.34 lists the different skin phototypes and the ability to tan. Tanning and epidermal hyperplasia following UVR exposure protects against erythema and burning, but maintaining this requires repeated exposures, which can result in the chronic effects of photodamage.

Immunosuppression

Both UVA and UVB exposure suppress cutaneous cell-mediated immunity in humans. This effect is significantly higher in skin types I/II than in types III/IV. UVR-induced immunosuppression is thought to play an important role in the emergence of skin cancer, which explains the increased risk of skin cancer in individuals with skin types I/II who have a history of repetitive and intense UVR exposure.

Vitamin D synthesis

The only benefit of UVR exposure is the production of vitamin D_3, essential for optimal bone mineralization. Receptors for vitamin D are expressed on keratinocytes and immune cells.

Chronic effects

Photoageing

Photoageing results in dry, deeply wrinkled, inelastic, leathery skin with telangiectasia, mottled pigmentation, freckling and lentigines. Repeated long-term UVR exposure, especially UVB, results in changes within the dermal connective tissue. There is elastosis and degradation and disorganization of collagen fibrils. It is thought that UVR-induced metalloproteinases (endopeptidases that degrade structural proteins) degrade the dermal matrix, which then undergoes imperfect repair.

Photocarcinogenesis

Skin cancer is the long-term result of a complex interaction between UVR exposure and genetics. Genetic factors include skin phototype, DNA repair capacity and immuno-competence. DNA damage occurs following UVR, and this is repaired by nucleotide excision repair. Repeated UV exposure together with suboptimal repair results in the clonal expansion of cells with mutated oncogenes leading to melanoma and non-melanoma skin cancer. Studies have shown that squamous cell carcinomas develop as the consequence of accumulated sun exposure, whereas melanoma and basal cell carcinomas are more dependent on specific patterns of childhood and intermittent high-dose sun exposure. Other important risk factors for the development of skin cancer include UVR-induced immunosuppression as well as immunosuppressant drugs as seen in organ transplant patients.

Photodermatoses

Photodermatoses (diseases caused by sunlight) can be divided into two main categories, those in which the sunlight has a primary role in the condition (primary photosensitivity) and those in which the sunlight acts as an exacerbating factor (secondary photosensitivity).

Table 14.34	Skin phototypes
Skin phototype	**Response to UVR exposure**
I	White skin, always burns, never tans (Celtic)
II	White skin, burns initially, tans with difficulty
III	White skin, rarely burns, tans easily
IV	White skin, never burns always tans (Mediterranean)
V	Brown skin (Asian)
VI	Black skin

919

Primary photosensitivity

Polymorphic light eruption

Epidemiology

Polymorphic light eruption is a common photodermatosis affecting 15% of the UK population, and is most often seen in young women.

Pathology

Polymorphic light eruption is most severe in the spring and early summer, and improves with continuing exposure as the summer progresses. Studies suggest that this eruption is most commonly induced by UVA (315–400 nm), although UVB (280–315 nm) and, more rarely, visible light (400–800 nm) wavelengths may also be involved. The pathogenesis of polymorphic light eruption is not fully understood. It is thought to be the result of a delayed-type hypersensitivity reaction to an ultraviolet-induced endogenous cutaneous antigen in individuals with a reduced capacity for normal ultraviolet radiation-induced cutaneous immunosuppression. It improves over the summer with gradual immunosuppression and development of tolerance.

Clinical features

The eruption tends to be polymorphic; however, it most commonly presents as erythematous papular, sometimes papulovesicular, itchy lesions within hours of significant sunlight exposure, and usually resolves over a number of days without scarring. The eruption is symmetrically distributed and affects some, or less frequently all, exposed areas. Occasionally covered sites may also be affected. Chronically exposed sites such as the face and back of hands are often spared.

Investigations

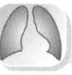

The diagnosis is made on a characteristic history and clinical findings, and investigations are not routinely required.

Management

Patient education
In the majority of cases, simple measures such as sensible sun avoidance and regular application of highly protective combined UVA/UVB sunscreens adequately control the condition.

Phototherapy
More severely affected patients may need annual, month-long, twice-weekly courses of low-dose narrowband UVB phototherapy or photochemotherapy (PUVA) at the beginning of spring.

Prognosis

Polymorphic light eruption may be life-long, but occasionally improves or completely ceases with time.

Chronic actinic dermatitis

Chronic actinic dermatitis is an uncommon eczematous photodermatosis, particularly affecting the sun-exposed skin of middle-aged and elderly men. The rash is pruritic, patchy or confluent, and eczematous. Lichenification is commonly seen. Photosensitivity can be mild, and in fact about half of all patients are unaware of this aspect. Photo-testing usually reveals UVA, UVB and sometimes visible wavelength sensitivity. Coexistent allergic contact sensitivity to widespread, often airborne, chemicals such as plant allergens, fragrances or rubber chemicals is also common. Treatment involves avoidance of light and contact allergens, protective clothing, broad-spectrum sunscreens and topical steroids. In those who fail to respond to simple measures, photochemotherapy (PUVA), azathioprine or ciclosporin should be considered. Chronic actinic dermatitis persists for many years, but thereafter not infrequently gradually resolves.

Actinic prurigo

Epidemiology

Actinic prurigo is a rare photodermatosis that presents before puberty and most commonly occurs in females. It is predominantly seen in American Indians but has also been described in Caucasians.

Pathology

In 40% of patients there is a personal or family history of atopy. Recently, an association with HLA-DR4 has been found in over 80% of cases, in particular with the rare DR4 subtype DRB1*0407 in approximately 60% of cases.

Clinical features

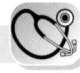

Clinically, there are intensely itchy papules, plaques, nodules and excoriations on sun-exposed areas, although covered sites may also be affected. Patients often describe seasonal variations with exacerbations at the beginning of spring and improvement in the autumn.

Investigations

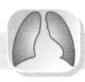

Phototesting
The diagnosis is made clinically, but if there is any doubt phototesting may be helpful. Although phototest results

are variable, abnormal responses tend to occur more frequently in the UVB range.

Management

Patient education
Simple measures such as sun avoidance, protective clothing, broad-spectrum sunscreens and topical steroids tend to be ineffective.

Photochemotherapy
Induction of tolerance with photochemotherapy (PUVA) can be beneficial, and in uncontrolled cases immunomodulatory therapy with thalidomide (with close monitoring) has been reported to be helpful.

Prognosis

Actinic prurigo may run a chronic course, however most cases resolve spontaneously in adolescence.

Secondary photosensitivity

Photosensitivity from topical agents

Photosensitivity from topical agents can be divided into photoallergic or phototoxic contact reactions. Phototoxicity is a direct cutaneous response induced by ultraviolet radiation in the presence of an adequate amount of a specific radiation-absorbing compound, referred to as the photosensitizer. Examples include phytophotodermatitis from plants, fruit and vegetables, the photosensitizer often being a furocoumarin (psoralen), which is also used in PUVA. Coal tar derivatives also act as photosensitizers and are used routinely in the Goeckerman regimen for the treatment of psoriasis. Although now prohibited, the presence of oil of bergamot in perfumes was also implicated. Aromatherapy oils such as citron, lavender, lime and sandalwood may also produce a phototoxic reaction.

Photoallergic contact dermatitis is a cell-mediated hypersensitivity reaction during which an ultraviolet-induced photoactivated product acts as an antigen. In the 1970s, halogenated salicylanilides and chlorinated phenols were used in antibacterial soaps and caused severe photoallergy reactions. These compounds are now all banned. Photoallergy to non-steroidal anti-inflammatory drugs as well as sunscreen ultraviolet filters (such as benzophenone-3 and PABA) has also been reported. Photopatch testing is required if this is suspected.

Oral drug photosensitivity

A number of systemic agents can cause drug photosensitivity. Phototoxic reactions are often seen with thiazide diuretics, quinine, amiodarone, non-steroidal anti-inflammatory agents, chlorpromazine, calcium channel antagonists, retinoids and psoralens.

Light-exacerbated dermatoses

Ultraviolet radiation exposure can exacerbate a number of skin conditions. Photosensitivity can occur in seborrhoeic and atopic eczema. Sunburn in psoriasis may lead to Köbnerization and deterioration of the condition. Sunlight can exacerbate systemic lupus erythematosus, and in porphyria, porphyrins deposited in the skin are activated by ultraviolet radiation.

SECTION 14.12   Diseases of collagen and elastic tissue

Disorders of connective tissue are a diverse group of conditions involving cutaneous, musculoskeletal, cardiovascular, ocular, gastrointestinal and pulmonary systems.

Ehlers–Danlos syndrome

Ehlers–Danlos syndrome is a common inherited connective tissue disorder. The prevalence has been estimated at 20 per 100 000. There are a number of subtypes, and different classifications have been used (Table 14.35). The syndrome may be inherited as an autosomal dominant, recessive or X-linked recessive trait. There is a wide spectrum of clinical manifestations and for many the symptoms are so minimal that the condition remains undiagnosed. The cardinal manifestations include skin hyperextensibility, atrophic scars, easy bruising, joint laxity and variable involvement of internal organs. In general, the skin is soft and velvety with a doughy texture, and although hyperextensible, it retains its normal elastic recoil. Redundant skin (acquired cutis laxa) may be evident over the elbows and knees. Trauma and laceration of the skin lead to tissue-paper scars and poor wound healing (Fig. 14.76). Fibrous lumps (molluscoid pseudotumours) may occur over the elbows and knees.

Table 14.35 Classification of the Ehlers-Danlos syndrome*

New classification	EDS type	Clinical features	Inheritance	Molecular defect
Classical	I	Widespread scarring, bruising Skin hyperextensibility Joint laxity	Autosomal dominant	COL5A1 and COL5A2 mutations
Classical	II	Less severe than type I	Autosomal dominant	COL5A1 and COL5A2 mutations
Hypermobility	III	Marked joint laxity Minimal skin involvement	Autosomal dominant	?
Vascular	IV	Thin, translucent skin, bruising Vascular rupture Colonic perforation Premature death	Autosomal dominant and recessive	COL3A1 mutations
Kyphoscoliosis	VI	Severe cardinal manifestations Ocular involvement Scoliosis	Autosomal recessive	Lysyl hydroxylase mutations
Arthrochalasis	VII (A, B)	Short stature Extreme joint laxity Congenital hip dislocation	Autosomal dominant	COL1A1 and COL1A2 mutations
Dermatosparaxis	VII (C)	Skin fragility and cutis laxa	Autosomal recessive	Procollagen peptidase deficiency
Others	V	Similar to EDS I/ II	X-linked	?
Others	VIII	Similar to EDS II Gum resorption Pigmented pretibial plaques	Autosomal dominant	Occasionally collagen III deficient
Others	X	Cardinal manifestations Normal skin texture	Autosomal recessive	Fibronectin deficiency

* Beighton P, De Paepe A, Steinmann B, et al. Ehlers-Danlos syndromes: Revised nosology, Villefranche, 1997. American Journal of Medical Genetics 1998; 77: 31–37.

Subcutaneous firm, small, cyst-like nodules (spheroids), which can become calcified, develop in a third of patients over the shins or forearms. In five of the six main subtypes, gene defects have been elucidated facilitating a molecular diagnosis. As there is no cure, management is largely restricted to the complications that develop. The prognosis is dependent on the subtype of disease; for example patients with classical Ehlers–Danlos syndrome have a normal lifespan but those with the vascular subtype tend to die prematurely from vascular rupture.

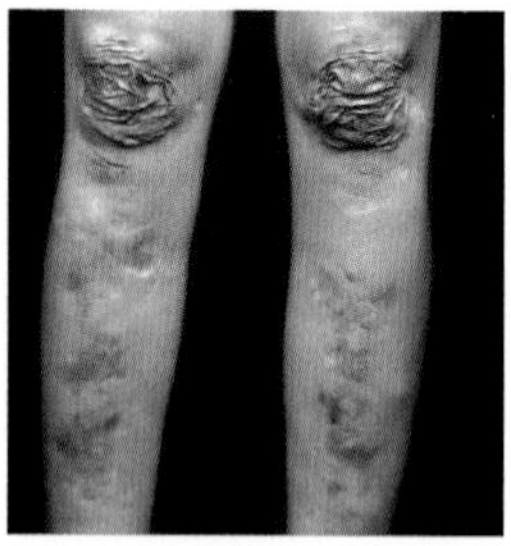

Fig. 14.76 Tissue paper scars in Ehlers–Danlos syndrome.

922

i FURTHER INFORMATION

Burrows N. The molecular genetics of the Ehlers-Danlos syndrome. Clinical and Experimental Dermatology 1999; 24: 99–106.

Congenital cutis laxa

Congenital cutis laxa refers to a rare heterogeneous group of connective tissue disorders. Generalized elastolysis (destruction and loss of elastic fibres) results in inelastic, redundant, loose-hanging skin, giving the appearance of premature ageing, together with variable systemic involvement. These changes may be present at birth or may develop during infancy. An autosomal dominant and two autosomal recessive forms of cutis laxa have been described. A previously defined X-linked form, caused by mutations in the ATP7A gene, is now classified within the group of copper deficiency syndromes. The autosomal dominant form is a relatively mild condition without systemic involvement. Some dominant forms are caused by mutations in the elastin gene. Type I autosomal recessive cutis laxa is characterized by more severe skin involvement, pulmonary and cardiovascular disease, umbilical and inguinal hernias, and gastrointestinal diverticula. This type has the poorest prognosis. The type II recessive form is called cutis laxa with joint laxity and developmental delay. The genetic defect in the recessive forms has not yet been identified.

Pseudoxanthoma elasticum

Pseudoxanthoma elasticum is a heritable connective tissue disorder characterized by degeneration and progressive calcification of elastic structures in the skin, the eyes and the cardiovascular system.

Epidemiology

Pseudoxanthoma elasticum has an estimated prevalence of 1 per 100 000 live births.

Pathology

Recently, mutations in the *ABCC6* gene, located on chromosome 16p13.1, have been implicated in the aetiology of pseudoxanthoma elasticum. *ABCC6* encodes the sixth member of the ATP-binding cassette (ABC) transporter protein, MRP6. As yet, the substrates transported by the MRP6 protein and its physiological role in the aetiology of pseudoxanthoma elasticum are unknown.

Apart from skin lesions, degeneration and calcification of the elastic fibres of Bruch's membrane in the retina result in angioid streaks, choroidal neovascularization, and consequently loss of visual acuity. Elastin-rich arterial blood vessels become progressively calcified, resulting in abnormal brittleness and vascular occlusion. Patients most commonly suffer from intermittent claudication, myocardial infarctions at a relatively early age, mitral valve prolapse and gastrointestinal bleeding.

Clinical features

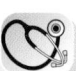

There is considerable variability in the clinical manifestations of pseudoxanthoma elasticum. Within families, significant differences exist in onset, progression and severity of disease. Pseudoxanthoma elasticum is usually not present at birth, and the early cutaneous findings often do not become noticeable until the second decade of life.

The primary skin lesions are small yellow papules and nodules, usually at the antecubital fossae, axillae and sides of the neck. These lesions coalesce to form a distinctive peau d'orange surface pattern. Changes in the connective tissue lead to redundant, inelastic hanging folds of skin (Fig. 14.77). The mucous membranes may also be affected.

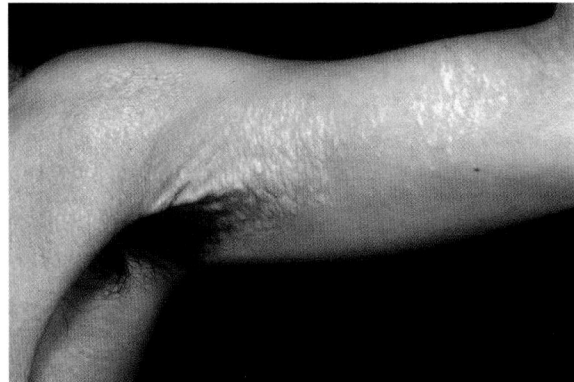

Fig. 14.77 Pseudoxanthoma elasticum.

Skin involvement is usually associated with pathological changes in the eyes and the cardiovascular system.

Investigations

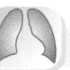

The diagnosis of pseudoxanthoma elasticum is clinical.

Genetic analysis

Identification of mutations in the *ABCC6* gene provides a means for prenatal and presymptomatic testing in families at risk for recurrence.

Management

Symptomatic treatment

There is no cure for pseudoxanthoma elasticum. Management is usually directed to any complications that arise.

Prognosis

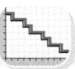

Cardiovascular complications occur in about a quarter of all patients with pseudoxanthoma elasticum and are the major cause of morbidity.

ι FURTHER INFORMATION

Ohtani T, Furukawa F. Pseudoxanthoma elasticum. Journal of Dermatology 2002; 29: 615–620.

Marfan's syndrome

Marfan's syndrome is an autosomal dominant disorder of connective tissue with an estimated prevalence of 20 per 100 000. Mutations in the gene for fibrillin-1 (*FBN1*), located on chromosome 15q21.1, have been shown to cause Marfan's syndrome as well as a series of other related disorders collectively termed type-1 fibrillinopathies. Fibrillin-1 is one of the major structural components of the elastin-associated 10–12 nm microfibrils, and is important for elastogenesis and homeostasis of elastic fibres. Marfan's syndrome has highly variable clinical manifestations, primarily cardiac, ocular, and a range of skeletal anomalies (Table 14.36). The diagnosis is dependent on a set of clinical criteria, termed 'Ghent nosology'.[1] Aortic dissection is the major cause of mortality, and without treatment most patients die in their twenties. Early diagnosis and treatment of existing thoracic aortic disease is therefore crucial. Over the past 30 years, the evolution of aggressive medical and surgical management of the cardiovascular problems has resulted in considerable improvement in life expectancy.

FURTHER INFORMATION

Pyeritz R. The Marfan syndrome. Annual Review of Medicine 2000; 51: 481–510.

REFERENCE

(1) *De Paepe A, Devereux RB, Dietz HC, Hennekam RC, Pyeritz RE. Revised diagnostic criteria for Marfan syndrome. American Journal of Medical Genetics 1996; 62: 417–426.*

Table 14.36	Clinical manifestations of Marfan's syndrome
Skeletal system	
Tall stature	
Pectus carinatum or pectus excavatum	
Arm span to height ratio >1.05	
Reduced upper (pubis to vertex) to lower (soles to pubis) segment ratio	
Scoliosis of >20° or spondylolisthesis	
Joint hypermobility	
Positive Steinberg's sign (thumbs adducted over the palm cross the ulnar border of the hand)	
Acetabular protrusions	
Facial appearance (elongation and asymmetry)	
High-arched palate	
The eye	
Ectopia lentis (lens dislocation)	
Abnormally flat cornea	
Increased axial length of globe	
Cardiovascular system	
Aortic dilatation	
Aortic dissection	
Mitral valve prolapse	
Respiratory system	
Spontaneous pneumothorax	
Apical blebs	
Skin and integument	
Lumbosacral dural ectasia	
Striae atrophicae	
Inguinal and femoral herniae	

SECTION 14.13   Disorders of hair and nails

Hair loss

Hair loss is a common problem that may affect both males and females in all age groups. It can have a significant social and psychological impact. Loss of hair is called alopecia; it can be subdivided into scarring and non-scarring types. Scarring alopecia is permanent loss of hair due to destruction of the hair follicles by an inflammatory and scarring cutaneous disorder (Table 14.37). The skin is usually scarred and atrophic and there is no potential for re-growth. Any underlying disorder should be identified and treated. In contrast, non-scarring alopecia is loss of hair with preserved hair follicles and there is therefore potential for re-growth (Table 14.38).

FURTHER INFORMATION

Chartier MB, Hoss DM, Grant-Kels JM. Approach to the adult female patient with diffuse nonscarring alopecia. Journal of the American Academy of Dermatology 2002; 47: 809–818.

Telogen effluvium

Telogen effluvium is sudden extensive hair loss occurring 1–2 months after a precipitating event such as pyrexia, surgery, haemorrhage, crash dieting or nutritional deficiencies. It can also occur in the post partum period and

Table 14.37	Causes of scarring alopecia

Physical injury
  *Burns
  *Radiotherapy

Infection
  *Fungal kerion
  Staphylococcal infection
  Tuberculosis

Hereditary
  Ichthyosis

Other
  *Discoid lupus erythematosus
  Lichen planopilaris
  Morphoea
  Sarcoidosis

*Most common causes

Table 14.38	Causes of non-scarring alopecia

Endocrine
  Hypopituitarism
  Hypo- and hyperthyroidism
  Hypoparathyroidism
  Pregnancy

Infection
  Tinea capitis

Drugs
  Carbimazole
  Thiouracil
  Heparin
  Warfarin
  Lithium
  Oral contraceptive pill
  Cytotoxics (especially cyclophosphamide)

Malnutrition
  Iron and zinc deficiency
  Malabsorption
  Vegetarians
  Marasmus

Other
  Telogen effluvium
  Androgenic alopecia
  Alopecia areata
  Trichotillomania
  Traction alopecia

following a change in hormonal therapy. Although it can occur at any age, it is more common in young adults, and females are twice as likely to be affected. It is characterized by the loss of 'handfuls' of hair, and clinically there is a diffuse alopecia affecting the entire scalp. Other hair-bearing areas may also be involved. There is an increase in the number of telogen hairs (follicle undergoing apoptosis—programmed cell death) and a reduction in anagen hairs (follicles in active growth phase). These patients should be reassured as recovery usually occurs within 6 months, although the duration may be variable.

Androgenic alopecia

Androgenic alopecia (male pattern baldness) is caused by the miniaturization of the hair follicle through successive cycles, affecting the fronto-vertex and crown of the scalp.

Epidemiology

Androgenic alopecia is one of the most common forms of hair loss in both men and women. There appears to be a genetic predisposition, and it affects all races worldwide. In men, it can occur from the late teens to the early 50s (affecting 50% of men by the age of 50). In women, it is more commonly seen after the menopause.

Pathology

The hair follicles undergo miniaturization, with a gradual conversion of terminal to vellus hairs through successive cycles.

Clinical features

The scalp hair loss begins with recession at the temples and the frontal hairline in men (Hamilton pattern) followed by thinning over the crown and vertex. This progresses over several years and in severe cases hair only remains at the occiput and sides of the scalp. Vellus hair may remain on the vertex.

In women (Ludwig pattern), the frontal hairline is frequently kept but a diffuse thinning occurs over the top of the scalp. If, in conjunction with this pattern of hair loss, there is also hirsutism, acne vulgaris, obesity and irregular menstruation, the possibility of polycystic ovarian syndrome should be investigated.

Investigations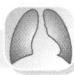

No routine investigations are required.

Hormone profile

In women, a hormone profile and ovarian ultrasound scan may confirm a diagnosis of polycystic ovarian syndrome.

Management

Although this is a medically benign condition, it is a significant psychosocial issue for many patients.

Topical minoxidil

Treatments for women include topical minoxidil solution and systemic antiandrogens if topical measures fail. In men, minoxidil or finasteride therapy is offered.

Hair transplantation

Hair transplantation can be considered in severe cases unresponsive to other forms of treatment.

Hair loss

Excessive hair growth

925

Prognosis

Hair loss in androgenic alopecia is progressive and permanent.

FURTHER INFORMATION

Bolduc C, Shapiro J. Management of androgenetic alopecia. American Journal of Clinical Dermatology 2000; 1: 151–158.

Alopecia areata

Alopecia areata is a chronic non-scarring inflammatory condition that can affect any hair-bearing area.

Epidemiology

Alopecia areata is common. It affects all races with an equal incidence in males and females. It can occur at any age, with a peak age at presentation of 10–30 years.

Pathology

Approximately 20% of people with alopecia areata have a family history of disease, indicating a genetic predisposition. Alopecia areata has been linked with human leukocyte antigen (HLA) class II alleles, as well as cytokine and immunoglobulin genes, suggesting that the genetic predisposition is multifactorial. An association with autoimmune diseases (such as vitiligo, autoimmune thyroid disease, pernicious anaemia) and organ-specific auto-antibodies suggests an autoimmune pathogenesis.

Clinical features

Clinically there is a sudden onset of solitary or multiple circular or oval bald areas, usually affecting the scalp, although any hair-bearing area may be affected. Residual hair follicles are visible, confirming a lack of scarring. Diagnostic 'exclamation mark hairs' may be visible at the margins of an expanding lesion. The affected scalp may be slightly erythematous but otherwise appears normal. The affected areas may spread and involve the whole scalp (alopecia totalis) and eventually the facial and body hair (alopecia universalis). Characteristic nail changes may also accompany hair loss, including fine regular pitting or a roughened, sandpaper appearance (trachyonychia).

Investigations

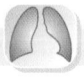

Scalp biopsy

The diagnosis of alopecia areata is usually made clinically, although the appearance on a scalp biopsy can be supportive.

Management

A number of treatments can induce hair growth in alopecia areata but none has been shown to alter the course of the disease.

Patient education

Localized disease has a good prognosis and therefore in many cases it can be managed by reassurance alone. Long-standing extensive hair loss has a poor prognosis with a high treatment failure rate. Some patients in this group prefer not to be treated, and for many female patients with extensive alopecia areata a wig or hairpiece is the most effective solution. As with all forms of hair loss, all treatment strategies should address the significant psychological and social impact of this condition. Contact with other sufferers and patient support groups may be of help.

Immunomodulation

Topical, intralesional and systemic corticosteroids can produce temporary re-growth. The dual properties of ciclosporin as an immunomodulation drug and a hyper-trichotic agent make it a potential treatment for alopecia areata, and this has been supported by animal studies.

Other therapy

Irritants (dithranol), allergens (diphenylcyclopropenone or squaric acid dibutylester) and PUVA have also been used. Topical minoxidil may be clinically efficacious.

Prognosis

Approximately 50% of patients recover within a year, although almost all will experience more than one episode of disease. Spontaneous recovery occurs more frequently in localized disease, and re-growth hairs are commonly white in colour. Remission is seen in 80% of patients with limited patchy hair loss of less than 1 year's duration. Poor prognostic factors include extensive involvement, onset in childhood, rapid rate of hair loss, other autoimmune diseases and nail involvement.

FURTHER INFORMATION

MacDonald Hull SP, Wood ML, Hutchinson PE, et al. Guidelines for the management of alopecia areata. British Journal of Dermatology 2003; 149: 692–699.

Trichotillomania

Trichotillomania is self-induced hair loss in which the patient chronically pulls hair from the scalp and/or other sites. It occurs more frequently in females than in males and may occur at any age. It is most commonly seen in children as a habit tic but occasionally occurs in adult life in association with depression or psychosis. Anxiety and emotional stress are precipitating factors. On examination there are localized patches of thinned hair with poorly defined margins, more commonly found on one side of the scalp corresponding with the handedness of the patient. The scalp skin is normal with no evidence of inflammation. The hairs in the affected area are broken off at varying lengths above the surface. The scalp is the most common area affected but hair loss may also occur in the eyebrows, eyelashes or body hair. Patients may show other evidence of self-mutilation (dermatitis artefacta). In children the condition is often benign and self-limiting and all that is required is reassurance. In adults the condition tends to persist and management is difficult. The tricyclic antidepressant, clomipramine, is the most useful drug although the treatment response may not be maintained over the long-term. Habit reversal psychotherapy is also recommended. Treatment of the underlying psychosis or depression in adults has also been shown to be beneficial.

Excessive hair growth

The growth of an excessive amount of hair on any area of the body is referred to as 'hypertrichosis'. The term 'hirsutism' should only be applied to women with excess growth of terminal hairs in a 'male pattern' due to androgen overproduction or increased end-organ sensitivity to androgens.

Hypertrichosis

Androgen-independent hypertrichosis is defined as increased body hair beyond the normal variation for a patient's reference growth, i.e. hair growth that is abnormal for the age, sex, or race of an individual, or for a particular part of the body. Abnormal hair growth can result in considerable emotional stress and social ostracism. There are a number of mechanisms for hypertrichosis, although the triggers that initiate these mechanisms are largely unknown. These include conversion of vellus to terminal hairs, increased percentage of follicles in anagen stage of the hair growth cycle, and increase in hair follicle density. Hypertrichosis is usually a cosmetic problem, but may also be the presenting symptom of an associated condition that requires further investigation and treatment. It can be classified into congenital and acquired conditions with generalized versus localized hair growth. When hypertrichosis is a cosmetic or psychosocial problem, there are various temporary and permanent methods of effective hair removal (Table 14.39). Epilatory methods last longer than depilation. Some forms cause sufficient damage to the follicle to provide long-term or permanent hair removal and include electrolysis (destruction of dermal papilla through production of hydroxide ions in the follicle by a direct electric current) and thermolysis (destruction by the heat produced by an alternating electric current). At the moment, laser-assisted hair removal is the most efficient method available. A new formulation that may be beneficial in hypertrichosis is eflornithine hydrochloride 13.9% cream. This probably works by inhibiting cell synthetic or mitotic functions. In general, treatment of hypertrichosis

is more satisfactory for those with localized rather than generalized involvement.

 FURTHER INFORMATION

Wendelin DS, Pope DN, Mallory SB. Hypertrichosis. Journal of the American Academy of Dermatology 2003; 48: 161–179.

Hirsutism

The term 'hirsutism' defines the presence of terminal hairs in a male pattern, in a woman. It is related to an increase in androgen levels or to an increased end-organ response to androgens. There are a number of causes (Table 14.40). The management of hirsutism depends on the cause. Increased production of ovarian androgens is controlled by contraceptives containing an oestrogen and a progestogen, resulting in ovarian suppression. In cases of increased production of adrenal androgens, there are a number of treatment options including adrenal suppression with glucocorticoids, and antiandrogen therapy with cyproterone acetate, spironolactone, flutamide and finasteride. In addition, in cases of ovarian or adrenal tumours, surgical intervention is often required.

Table 14.39	Management options for hypertrichosis

Bleach
Commercial bleach or 6% hydrogen peroxide.

Hair removal
Depilation—removal of the hair at some point along its shaft
  Mechanical shaving
  Cutting the hair
  Chemically dissolving it (commercial sulphide or alkali
    metal preparation)

Epilation—a process that removes the entire hair shaft
  Tweezing
  Waxing
  Electrolysis
  Thermolysis
  Laser-assisted hair removal

Table 14.40	Causes of hirsutism

Increased production of ovarian androgens
  Polycystic ovary syndrome
  Ovarian tumours

Ovarian failure
  Post-oophorectomy
  Post-menopausal

Increased production of adrenal androgens
  Adrenal tumours or hyperplasia
  Hyperpituitarism

Inborn error of steroid metabolism
  Androgenital syndrome

Androgenic drugs
  Testosterone
  Danazol
  Progestogens
  Systemic steroids

SECTION 14.14 Systemic disease and the skin

Connective tissue disorders

Cutaneous lupus erythematosus

Lupus erythematosus is an autoimmune disease with variable clinical presentations ranging from cutaneous changes only to progressive multisystem disease, systemic lupus erythematosus (SLE). The majority of patients with SLE (p. 492) have cutaneous manifestations.

Epidemiology

The prevalence of cutaneous lupus varies from 14.6 to 68 per 100 000 people. It can occur at any age, although it is more common in young women.

Pathology

Cutaneous lupus erythematosus (CLE) can be divided into acute, subacute and chronic forms, based on clinical morphology, average duration of skin lesions and histopathological findings (Table 14.41).

The histological features of acute cutaneous lupus erythematosus (ACLE) are often subtle with mild basal cell degeneration and patchy chronic inflammatory cell infiltrate. In subacute cutaneous lupus erythematosus (SCLE) the epidermis is atrophic with evidence of hyperkeratosis. There is often marked basal cell degeneration with lymphocytic exocytosis (lymphocytes migrating up from the dermis into the epidermis). The dermal infiltrate is usually superficial and band-like in distribution. Histology from patients with discoid cutaneous lupus erythematosus (DLE) shows hyperkeratosis with follicular plugging and epidermal atrophy. There is basal cell degeneration and a lymphohistiocytic infiltrate is distributed around blood vessels and the adnexa.

Table 14.41	Subclasses of cutaneous lupus erythematosus
Acute cutaneous lupus erythematosus (ACLE)	
Subacute cutaneous lupus erythematosus (SCLE)	

Chronic cutaneous lupus erythematosus (CCLE)
    Discoid lupus (DLE)
    Lupus panniculitis
    Chilblain lupus	

Drug-induced lupus (DIL)	

Clinical features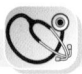

Acute cutaneous lupus erythematosus

Acute cutaneous lupus erythematosus (ACLE) commonly presents as a localized malar 'butterfly rash', although patients may also have generalized photosensitive lupus dermatitis or a maculopapular rash. Often there is diffuse hair thinning, mucosal ulceration and nail fold erythema. Less commonly patients have a bullous or toxic epidermal necrolysis type eruption. All patients with acute cutaneous lupus erythematosus develop SLE.

Subacute cutaneous lupus erythematosus

Subacute cutaneous lupus erythematosus (SCLE) is a photosensitive subset of cutaneous lupus. It presents as a widespread non-scarring papulosquamous or annular, polycyclic eruption (Fig. 14.78) particularly on sun-exposed areas, most commonly the upper chest and back. The lesions are long lasting. Extracutaneous involvement is normally very mild.

Chronic cutaneous lupus erythematosus

Chronic cutaneous lupus erythematosus (CCLE) is 2–3 times more common than SLE but has a less severe course. Systemic symptoms are more likely if there is generalized skin involvement.

Discoid lupus erythematosus

Discoid lupus erythematosus (DLE) is the most common form of CCLE and presents as sharply demarcated, erythematous scaly plaques which are often exacerbated by sunlight and heal with atrophic scarring (Fig. 14.79). The

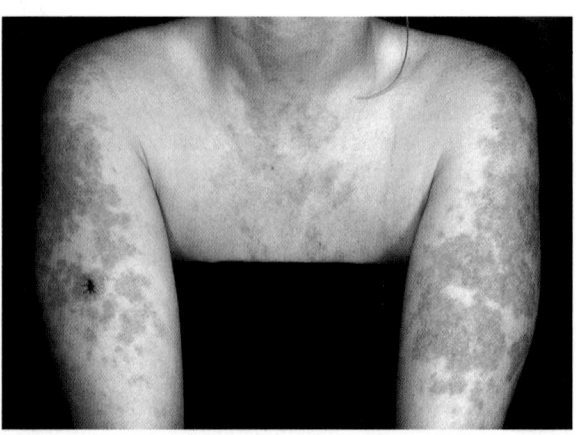

Fig. 14.78 Subacute cutaneous lupus erythematosus.

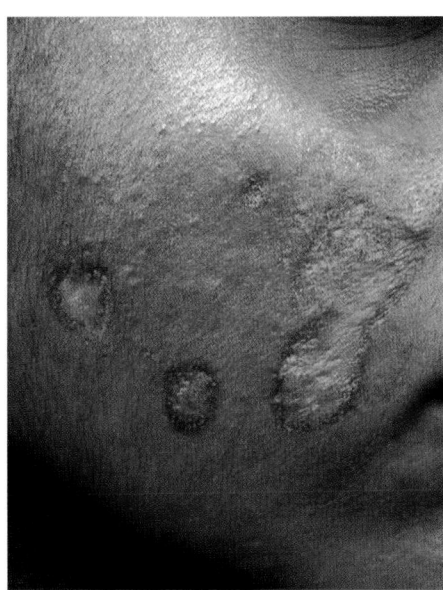

Fig. 14.79 Discoid lupus erythematosus.

lesions are commonly present on the head, neck, and hands but occasionally may be more generalized. Plaques on the scalp result in scarring alopecia (p. 925). Approximately 20% of patients with generalized discoid lupus erythematosus and 5% of those with localized disease develop SLE. There are associations with complement deficiencies (C1q, C3 and C5), and 15% have a history of Raynaud's. The diagnosis is made clinically and supported by histopathology and direct immunofluorescence.

Lupus panniculitis

Lupus panniculitis occurs in 1–2% of patients with lupus erythematosus. Tan or violaceous plaques are most often found symmetrically on the head and neck area, upper arms, trunk and buttocks. Lesions may ulcerate and heal with atrophy. There is a weak association with SLE and 50% of patients have no other signs of lupus erythematosus.

Chilblain lupus

Chilblain lupus is a rare form of CCLE. The lesions are found on the extremities (fingers, toes, heels, knees, nose and ears) and are aggravated by cold exposure. Serology shows increased immunoglobulin levels and positive rheumatoid factor. Cold agglutinins, cryoglobulins and anticoagulants are negative.

Drug-induced lupus

Drug-induced lupus (DIL) should be considered in all patients who have been commenced on a new drug and develop signs of lupus erythematosus with positive antinuclear antibodies (ANA). Males and females are equally affected but the condition is 6 times more common in Caucasians than in Afro-Caribbeans. In this subgroup, skin disease is less frequent (only 20% of cases) but pulmonary involvement is more common. Drug-induced lupus has been reported with chlorpromazine and hydralazine, and with these drugs there is a 90% association with anti-histone antibodies. Other drugs involved are isoniazid and procainamide. Although rare, drug-induced cases of subacute cutaneous lupus erythematosus have been reported with griseofulvin, diuretics and carbamazepine.

Investigations

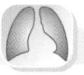

Skin biopsy

Skin biopsy facilitates the diagnosis and is able to characterize the subset of disease.

Serology

With acute cutaneous lupus erythematosus 95% of patients have positive ANA. Anti-double stranded DNA and anti-Sm antibodies are specific for SLE (p. 493). In subacute cutaneous lupus erythematosus, ANA is present in approximately 80% of patients. There is an association with the presence of anti-Ro (80%) and anti-La (50%) antibodies. Serology is often negative in discoid lupus erythematosus, which also excludes systemic disease.

Immunofluorescence of skin

The lupus band test (LBT) detects deposits of immunoglobulins (IgM>IgG>IgA) and/or complement in a band-like pattern along the dermal–epidermal junction in lupus erythematosus. In systemic lupus, a positive LBT can be found in lesional skin (90%) as well as clinically normal skin (70–80% of sun-exposed skin and 50% of sun-protected skin). The latter has a worse prognosis. In discoid lupus erythematosus, deposits of IgM are found in 90% of lesional skin biopsies. The LBT is negative in normal, non-lesional skin of patients with discoid and subacute cutaneous lupus erythematosus.

Management

Patient education

Effective sun protection is the first rule of management of CLE as most patients are very photosensitive. High-factor sunscreens with UVA and UVB protection must be used.

Topical corticosteroids and antimalarial agents

Topical corticosteroids are the mainstay of treatment, and antimalarial agents are first-line systemic agents in discoid and subacute cutaneous lupus erythematosus. Hydroxychloroquine and mepacrine give protection from sunlight and are also anti-inflammatory.

Retinoids

Retinoids may be used to treat chronic forms of cutaneous lupus erythematosus, in particular hyperkeratotic cases.

Systemic immunomodulatory agents

Immunomodulatory agents, such as azathioprine, methotrexate and ciclosporin, are required to manage underlying systemic disease activity in acute cutaneous lupus erythematosus, together with corticosteroids. High-dose oral prednisolone or pulsed intravenous methylprednisolone is used in exacerbations of disease.

Prognosis

Cutaneous lupus is a chronic and recurrent disease. There is very little evidence-based data on its treatment; however, topical corticosteroids and oral antimalarials are the standard therapies and are effective in a majority of patients.

i **FURTHER INFORMATION**

Patel P, Werth V. Cutaneous lupus erythematosus: a review. Dermatologic Clinics 2002; 20: 373–385, v.

Callen JP. Update on the management of cutaneous lupus erythematosus. British Journal of Dermatology 2004; 151: 731–736.

Cutaneous sarcoidosis

Epidemiology

Cutaneous involvement occurs in about 25% of patients with systemic sarcoidosis and is most likely to be seen at the onset of the disease process. Skin lesions can also occur in the absence of systemic disease.

Pathology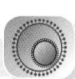

There is a wide range of cutaneous presentations in sarcoidosis and these can be classified as specific or non-specific. Specific lesions contain non-caseating granulomas, and non-specific lesions are reactive processes.

Clinical features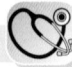

Common specific sarcoidosis skin lesions include papules, nodules, plaques, infiltrative scars and lupus pernio. Papules, nodules and plaques tend to be red-brown to purple in colour. Papular lesions are commonly found on the face, nape of the neck, upper back and extremities. Nodules can be found at any site although they have a predilection for periocular skin. Plaques occur on the face, scalp, back, shoulders, arms and buttocks. Annular plaques can occur on the scalp and result in scarring alopecia.

Inactive scars can also become infiltrated with sarcoidosis and develop a red or purple hue with induration. Lupus pernio is the most characteristic skin lesion of sarcoidosis and consists of red-brown to purple, indurated, swollen, shiny skin changes on the nose, cheeks, lips and ears (Fig. 14.80). This is commonly associated with chronic disease of the upper respiratory tract, pulmonary fibrosis, chronic uveitis and bone cysts. Some of the more uncommon specific sarcoidosis skin lesions include ulcers, hypopigmented patches and ichthyosis. The most common non-specific lesion associated with acute, benign and self-limiting sarcoidosis is erythema nodosum. When this coexists with bilateral hilar adenopathy, migratory polyarthritis, fever and iritis, it is called Löfgren's syndrome. This carries a good prognosis.

Investigations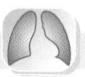

Skin biopsy
The diagnosis of cutaneous sarcoidosis rests on the presence of non-caseating granulomas on skin biopsy and the exclusion of other granulomatous skin diseases.

Management

Immunomodulation
Cutaneous sarcoidosis generally responds to therapy given for systemic involvement. For purely cutaneous disease there are many therapeutic options, including simple observation or intralesional steroids. Patients with severe lesions or widespread involvement may require oral corticosteroids or antimalarial drugs such as hydroxychloroquine, although the lesions tend to recur once systemic therapy is discontinued.

Other therapeutic options reported in the literature include low-dose methotrexate, retinoids and thalidomide. Up to 60% of patients with systemic sarcoidosis experience spontaneous resolution and an additional 15% undergo resolution with corticosteroid use.

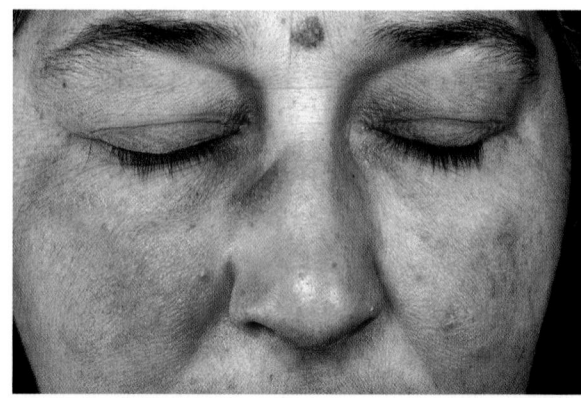

Fig. 14.80 Lupus pernio in sarcoidosis.

Prognosis

The overall prognosis of cutaneous prognosis depends primarily on the degree of systemic involvement.

 FURTHER INFORMATION

English JC, Purvisha JP, Kenneth EG. Sarcoidosis. Journal of the American Academy of Dermatology 2001; 44: 725–743.

Giuffrida TJ, Kerdel FA. Sarcoidosis. Dermatologic Clinics 2002; 20: 435–447.

Neurocutaneous syndromes

Neurocutaneous disorders are characterized by the involvement of organs of ectodermal origin (nervous system, eyes and skin). They are rare and include neurofibromatosis, tuberous sclerosis, Sturge–Weber syndrome and von Hippel–Lindau disease. In other conditions, skin lesions may be seen in conjunction with neurological disease. For example, in epidermal naevus syndrome, pigmented linear naevi may be associated with epilepsy or mental retardation.

Neurofibromatosis

There are two distinct types of neurofibromatosis, type 1 (von Recklinghausen's neurofibromatosis) and type 2.

Epidemiology

Neurofibromatosis type 1 has an incidence of 33 per 100 000 per year, whereas neurofibromatosis type 2 has an incidence of about 2.86 per 100 000 per year.

Pathology

Both types of neurofibromatosis are inherited in an autosomal dominant manner with almost 100% penetrance but variable expression. Up to 50% of cases are due to sporadic gene mutations.

Neurofibromatosis type 1 is caused by mutations in the gene *NF1*, located on chromosome 17q11.2, which encodes the protein neurofibromin, known to have a role in tumour suppression. Inactivation of the gene results in the loss of function of neurofibromin and subsequent development of the tumours seen in neurofibromatosis type 1.

Neurofibromatosis type 2 results from mutations in the gene *NF2*, located on chromosome 22q12.1, which encodes the cytoskeletal protein merlin or schwannomin, also known to have a role in tumour suppression.

Scope of disease

Phaeochromocytoma is a rare association seen in about 3% of patients with neurofibromatosis type 1. Patients presenting with abdominal pain, haematemesis or melaena should be investigated for intestinal tumours. About 6% develop hypertension secondary to renovascular disease or coarctation of the aorta. Learning disabilities are present in 50% of patients.

Clinical features

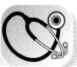

The most common clinical features in neurofibromatosis type 1 are café-au-lait spots, hyperpigmented macules seen in 90% of patients (Fig. 14.81), and axillary or groin freckling (70%). Neurofibromas (flesh-coloured smooth polypoid swellings) are a typical characteristic and there are three subtypes. The majority of patients have discrete benign neurofibromas in the dermis (Fig. 14.82). Others develop nodular neurofibromas in peripheral nerves which can grow large but do not infiltrate the surrounding tissues. Thirty per cent of patients have plexiform neurofibromas which affect long portions of nerves, infiltrate the surrounding tissues, cause widespread disfigurement and are the major cause of morbidity and mortality in neurofibromatosis type 1. In about 2–16% of patients, these neurofibromas transform to malignant peripheral nerve sheath tumours. Other clinical manifestations include optic nerve gliomas, Lisch nodules (benign multiple melanotic hamartomas of the iris), and bony lesions (dysplasia of the sphenoid wing, thinning of the long bones). The diagnostic criteria for neurofibromatosis type 1 are listed in Table 14.42.

In neurofibromatosis type 2, the main clinical feature is bilateral vestibular schwannomas; cutaneous involvement is minimal.

Investigations

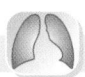

Genetic testing
Although genetic testing is now available, the diagnosis is based on clinical findings.

Investigations of complications
Investigations are not routinely required, but may be needed when looking into potential complications.

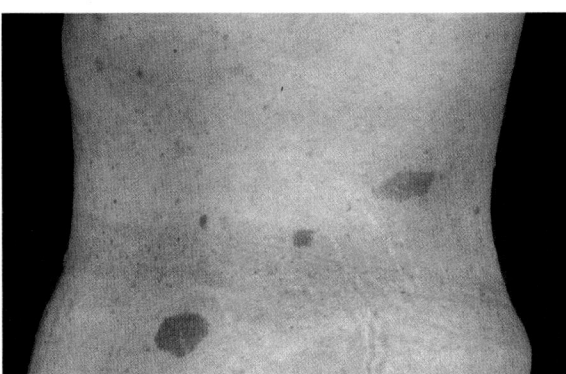

Fig. 14.81 Café-au-lait spots.

931

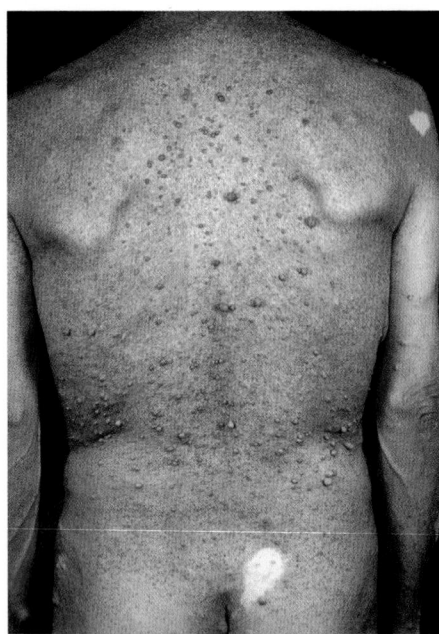

Fig. 14.82 Neurofibromatosis type 1.

Table 14.42	Diagnostic criteria for neurofibromatosis type 1

Two or more of the following:
   Six or more café-au-lait spots
      >1.5 cm in post-pubertal individuals
      >0.5 cm in pre-pubertal individuals
   Two or more neurofibromas of any type, or one or more
      plexiform neurofibromas
   Axillary or groin freckling
   Two or more Lisch nodules
   First-degree relative with neurofibromatosis type 1

Management

Supportive

There is no cure for the disease, and management is directed to the complications that may develop.

Prognosis

Patients with neurofibromatosis type 1 may have a reduced life expectancy resulting from malignant neoplasm or vascular disease.

i **FURTHER INFORMATION**

Reynolds RM, Browning GG, Nawroz I, Campbell IW. Von Recklinghausen's neurofibromatosis: neurofibromatosis type 1. Lancet 2003; 361: 1552–1554.

Tuberous sclerosis

Tuberous sclerosis (tuberous sclerosis complex—TSC) is an autosomal dominant neurocutaneous disorder with variable clinical manifestations.

Epidemiology

Tuberous sclerosis has an incidence of 17 per 100 000 per year with over half the cases being sporadic. Tuberous sclerosis is characterized by the widespread development of benign tumours termed hamartomas (Table 14.43).

Pathology

Tuberous sclerosis is caused by mutations in either the *TSC1* or *TSC2* tumour suppression gene (located on chromosome 9q34 and 16p13). The *TSC1* and *TSC2* proteins are referred to as hamartin and tuberin, respectively, and form the TSC1–TSC2 complex.[1] The mechanism of hamartomatous growth is not completely understood.

Clinical features

The principal early manifestations are the triad of seizures, mental retardation and congenital hypomelanotic macules. These macules are leaf-like in shape (ashleaf macules) and are commonly present on the trunk. Wood's light examination demonstrates decreased melanin pigmentation. Facial angiofibromas (adenoma sebaceum) occur in 70% of

Table 14.43	Clinical manifestations of tuberous sclerosis complex

Skin
   Hypomelanotic (ashleaf) macules
   Shagreen patch
   Subungual fibromas
   Facial angiofibromas (adenoma sebaceum)

Brain
   Cortical tubers (gliomas)
   Subependymal nodules
   Subependymal giant cell astrocytomas

Eye
   Retinal hamartomas

Heart
   Cardiac rhabdomyomas

Kidney
   Benign and malignant angiomyolipomas
   Renal cell carcinoma

Lung
   Lymphangioleiomyomatosis

Behaviour
   Mental retardation
   Seizures
   Autism
   Manic depression

affected individuals. They are characterized by erythematous papules or nodules in the centre of the face, appearing in the third or fourth year. Periungual fibromas arise late in childhood and have the same pathology as the facial papules. Shagreen patches are skin-coloured plaques, most frequently seen on the back and buttocks (Table 14.43).

Investigations
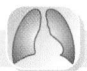

Genetic testing
Although genetic testing is now available, the diagnosis is usually made on clinical findings. Other family members may be screened, and genetic counselling is imperative.

Investigation of complications
Various types of imaging (CT and MRI of the head, renal ultrasound) as well as electroencephalography are required to evaluate the patient further.

Management

Management is directed to any complications that develop.

CO$_2$ laser
Facial angiofibromas may be treated with the CO$_2$ laser to improve cosmesis.

Prognosis

Over 50% of patients with severe disease die before reaching the second decade.

Table 14.44	Dermatological disorders and infections in HIV

General
Psoriasis
Eczema
Seborrhoeic dermatitis
Folliculitis

Fungal
Malassezia ovale
Candidiasis

Bacterial
Staphylococcus aureus
Tuberculosis
Syphilis

Viral
Human papillomavirus
Molluscum contagiosum
Herpes zoster

Malignancy
Kaposi's sarcoma
Lymphomas
Intraoral squamous cell carcinoma

FURTHER INFORMATION

Barron RP, Kainulainen VT, Forrest CR, et al. Tuberous sclerosis: clinicopathological features and review of the literature. Journal of Craniomaxillofacial Surgery 2002; 30: 361–366.

REFERENCE

(1) Pan D, Dong J, Zhang Y, Gao X. Tuberous sclerosis complex: from Drosophila to human disease. Trends in Cell Biology 2004; 14:[2] 78-85.

Table 14.45	Genetically determined syndromes with cutaneous manifestations
Syndrome	**Cutaneous manifestations**
Ataxia telangiectasia	Mucocutaneous telangiectasia associated with an increased risk of lymphoma, leukaemia and breast carcinoma
Cowden's disease	Tricholemmomas (facial nodules), papules of mucous membranes and punctate keratoses of palms and soles associated with breast and thyroid carcinoma
Familial adenomatous polyposis (incl. Gardner's syndrome)	Epidermal cysts, lipomata and fibromata associated with gastrointestinal polyposis
Gorlin syndrome	Jaw cysts, bifid ribs and palmar pits associated with aggressive basal cell carcinomas
Howel–Evans syndrome	Palmoplantar kertoderma associated with oesophageal carcinoma
Neurofibromatosis type 1	Café-au-lait macules, axillary freckling and neurofibromas associated with malignant peripheral nerve sheath tumours
Peutz–Jeghers syndrome	Mucocutaneous pigmentation associated with gastrointestinal polyposis
Sturge–Weber syndrome	Port-wine stain associated with ipsilateral vascular malformations in the eye and leptomeninges
Torre–Muir syndrome	Sebaceous tumours associated with gastrointestinal malignancy
Tuberous sclerosis	Angiofibromas, periungual fibromas, shagreen patches and ash-leaf macules associated with rhabdomyomas, malignant angiomyolipomas and gliomas
von Hippel–Lindau syndrome	Haemangiomas associated with vascular tumours of the central nervous system, phaeochromocytoma, renal and pancreatic carcinoma
Wiskott–Aldrich syndrome	Eczema and immunodeficiency associated with increased risk of lymphoma and leukaemia

Malignancy and skin disease

There are numerous cutaneous markers of malignant disease. Skin changes can either be manifestations of genetically determined syndromes (Table 14.45) or present as paraneoplastic features associated with certain types of malignancy (Table 14.46).

Table 14.46	Dermatological features and common associated malignancies
Dermatological feature	**Most commonly associated neoplasm**
Acanthosis nigricans	Gastrointestinal adenocarcinoma
Acanthosis palmaris	Bronchial carcinoma
Generalized pruritus	Lymphoma
Dermatomyositis	Breast and ovarian malignancy
Erythema gyratum repens	Bronchial carcinoma
Acquired hypertrichosis lanuginosa	Gastrointestinal and bronchial carcinoma
Migratory thrombophlebitis	Pancreatic or gastric carcinoma
Pyoderma gangrenosum	Myeloproliferative disorders
Paraneoplastic pemphigus	Lymphoma
Erythroderma	Lymphoma and leukaemia
Necrolytic migratory erythema	Glucagonoma

Acknowledgements

We would like to thank St John's Institute of Dermatology and Stuart Robertson for supplying all the clinical photographs.

Infectious diseases

15

Kathleen Bamford

Introduction

Applied basic sciences of infectious disease

Innate immunity and normal flora

The innate immune response provides the first lines of defence against infection. It consists of a combination of physical barriers such as the skin and mucociliary escalator, antibacterial proteins, phagocytic cells, a range of sensing and response molecules such as Toll-like receptors and interleukin (IL)-1, as well as the host's normal flora.

Physical barriers and mechanisms

The skin is an excellent physical barrier to invasion which, when compromised, increases the risk of a number of infections (Fig. 15.1).

Physical 'flushing' in the urinary tract dislodges bacteria. In the respiratory tract, humidification and warming of inhaled air in the nasal turbinates and sinuses causes particles to settle and become trapped in the sticky mucus coating. These are then transported by the upward-beating cilia to the oropharynx and swallowed so that the respiratory tract is effectively sterile below the carina.

Antimicrobial substances

Sebum, fatty acids and a variety of antibacterial peptides all help to inhibit bacterial growth.

Mucous membranes are a potential route of access for microorganisms. A variety of mechanisms protect against this. Polysaccharides in mucus are identical to, or mimic, many epithelial surface structures. This provides a 'decoy' that binds and traps pathogens.

The body secretes a variety of antibacterial compounds, e.g. lysozyme in tears, that can degrade Gram-positive bacterial peptidoglycan; lactoferrin in breast milk and different iron-binding compounds at other mucosal surfaces can inhibit bacterial growth by sequestering iron.

The complement system

The complement system is made up of about 30 proteins that are activated by a classical or alternative pathway, the latter being particularly important for innate defence. The net result is the ability to opsonize, i.e. to render bacteria more susceptible to being engulfed and killed by phagocytic cells, and to activate host response cells to lyse cells or bacteria. Deficiencies in the function of the complement system are associated with infection with *Neisseria meningitidis* and *N. gonorrhoeae*.

Phagocytosis

Phagocytic cells, principally macrophages and neutrophils, are attracted to sites of infection and engulf (phagocytose) organisms which are then killed by a variety of mechanisms. Impairment of phagocytosis or intracellular killing is characteristically associated with recurrent staphylococcal, fungal and other infections.

The normal flora

The normal flora provides protection against infection at sites such as the oropharynx, gut, vagina and skin. Here, the

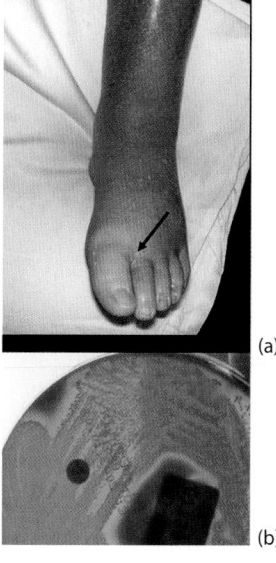

Fig. 15.1 (a) Cellulitis is usually caused by *S. pyogenes*. Here, cracks between the toes caused by athlete's foot (arrow) are the likely portal of entry. (b) Growth on blood agar showing complete haemolysis.

normal flora forms a 'pavement' which occupies attachment sites, competes for nutrients, and secretes bacteriocins or other molecules that inhibit potential invaders. Composition of the flora is very varied, and there are frequently small numbers of a wide range of potential pathogens. The most important components of the normal flora at different sites are shown in Table 15.1.

Disturbance of the normal flora in illness increases the risk of a variety of infections. It should also be recognized that the normal flora itself can cause disease if other measures such as the adaptive immune response and antiphagocytic activity are breached or compromised.

Pathogenicity and transmission of microorganisms

Definitions

Colonization is the presence of microorganisms without causing harm (e.g. the normal flora). Potential pathogens may be part of the normal flora, and are termed pathogens when they cause disease or infection.

Pathogens that have capacity to cause disease may also be virulent, that is they have the capacity to cause serious disease, and to cause disease in otherwise healthy individuals. The ability to cause disease depends on pathogenicity (Fig. 15.2) or virulence determinants (Table 15.2).

Sources and spread of infection

Infections may be endogenous and arise from the normal (or transient) flora, or exogenous (arising from external sources).

Endogenous infections are frequently associated with other illnesses or particular susceptibilities. Surgical wound infections may be endogenous, arising from staphylococci in the individual's nose, or from *E. coli* and *Bacteroides* species in the patient's bowel. Neutropenic patients are susceptible to Gram-negative bacteraemia because their immune systems are unable to control the normal gut flora. Exogenous infection may take a variety of routes (Table 15.3).

Organisms may arise from a variety of sources, for instance from other people (*Salmonella typhi*, *Treponema pallidum*, epidemic MRSA), from the environment (*Naegleria*

Table 15.1	Components of the normal flora
Site	**Predominant normal flora**
Nasopharynx	*Staphylococci* *Streptococci* *Haemophilus* *Neisseria* Mixed anaerobes *Actinomyces* *Candida*
Skin	*Staphylococci* *Corynebacteria* *Propionibacterium* Yeasts *Streptococci* *Acinetobacter* spp.
Small bowel	*Enterobacteria* *Enterococci* *Candida* Mixed anaerobes
Colon/rectum	*Bacteroides* spp. *Bifidobacterium* *Clostridia* *Peptostreptococci* *Enterobacteria*
Vagina	*Lactobacilli* *Corynebacteria* *Streptococci* *Candida* *Actinomyces* *Mycoplasma/ureaplasmas*

Table 15.2	Determinants of pathogenicity or virulence
Ability to colonize	Microorganisms employ a variety of adhesins that interact with structures on the host epithelium or other cells. Examples: influenza virus adheres to respiratory epithelium via haemagglutinin and neuraminidase, while *E. coli* adheres to urinary epithelium via P-fimbriae
Ability to gain nutrients and divide	Many bacteria use iron-scavenging mechanisms, or cause cellular damage that makes nutrients more available, e.g. bacterial siderophores chelate iron from surrounding tissue while cytolysins disrupt cells releasing their contents
Ability to invade tissues or cells	All viruses, and many bacteria such as salmonella, listeria and *Mycobacterium tuberculosis*, gain access to the intracellular compartment
Ability to evade host defences	*Haemophilus influenzae*, *Helicobacter pylori* and *Neisseria meningitidis* destroy IgA via IgA proteases. *Streptococcus pneumoniae* and *Cryptococcus neoformans* produce capsules that interfere with different host functions Bacteria can evade intracellular killing by preventing lysosomal fusion (*M. tuberculosis*, *L. monocytogenes*), producing catalase (e.g. *S. aureus*), or preventing oxygen-dependent killing (e.g. *Salmonella typhi*)
Production of damage via toxins	Protein exotoxins produced by bacteria affect intestinal fluid balance and nerve conduction. Many cause shock and sepsis syndrome
Endotoxin-mediated damage	Shock and sepsis syndrome are mediated by endotoxin, a major component of the Gram-negative bacterial cell wall. Gram-positive peptidoglycan may have similar effects

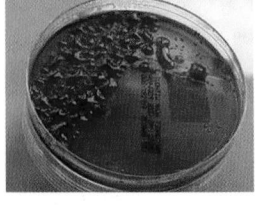

Fig. 15.2 The mucoid colonies on blood agar indicate that this organism produces a lot of capsular polysaccharide, which will help it evade host defences and is often associated with antibiotic resistance.

Table 15.3	Routes of exogenous infection

Mucous membranes

Respiratory tract
Influenza, measles, *Neisseria meningitidis*

Gastrointestinal tract
Campylobacter jejuni, poliovirus, *salmonella*, hepatitis A

Genital tract (sexual intercourse)
Neisseria gonorrhoeae, herpes simplex type II, *Treponema pallidum*, HIV, hepatitis B

Wounds

Clostridium tetani and *C. perfringens*, *Pasteurella multocida*, *S. aureus*, *S. pyogenes*

By inoculation

Arthropod bites
Plasmodium falciparum, yellow fever

Intravenous drug/blood products
Hepatitis B, HIV

Animal bites
Rabies, *Pasteurella multocida*, cat-scratch disease

Contaminated surgical or other instruments
HIV, hepatitis B, Creutzfeldt–Jakob disease

and *Acanthamoeba, Legionella pneumophila, Clostridium tetani*) or from animals (zoonoses such as salmonella food poisoning, *Campylobacter*, brucellosis and leptospirosis). Organisms such as *T. pallidum*, HIV, *Neisseria gonorrhoeae* are obligate pathogens (they always cause disease).

More frequently, the likelihood of disease depends on a range of circumstances; for example, *S. aureus* may be part of normal skin flora but can also cause a wound infection. These infections are 'conditional' on the circumstances around the event. Opportunistic pathogens are those which would not usually cause infection in healthy individuals but are pathogens in the immunocompromised; for example, *Aspergillus fumigatus* causes infection in neutropenic patients, *Pseudomonas aeruginosa* causes lung infection in cystic fibrosis, and cytomegalovirus infections occur in patients with HIV and those with renal or bone marrow transplants. Indwelling vascular cannulae and endotracheal tubes are a common entry point for infections such as *Staphylococcus epidermidis* and *Pseudomonas aeruginosa* in hospitalized or dialysis patients.

Survival and transmission

Survival and transmission of microorganisms in the environment, or ability to adapt to a particular niche, are crucial determinants in an organism's spread. Sexually transmitted organisms rarely survive in the environment and require close personal contact for transmission. In contrast, clostridia and *Bacillus anthracis* can survive for years in an inhospitable environment because of their ability to form environmentally resistant spores. The spores are thick-walled structures that can start germinating when inoculated into suitable areas such as wounds.

Helminth eggs also have a tough shell that allows them to survive until they are ingested, e.g. ascaris and taenia. In many diseases the organisms are adapted to a life cycle involving arthropods or other animals, e.g. trypanosomiasis, hydatid disease, malaria.

Food and water may act as a source for many pathogens, some of which have their effects at sites other than the gastrointestinal tract (e.g. toxoplasmosis and cysticercosis).

Investigations for infectious disease

The laboratory investigation of infection

Infections may be multisystem or localized. There may be potential for dissemination, even with localized infections. Investigations may involve testing of samples specific to a particular body system, or samples applicable to generalized infection. Indirect methods of diagnosis may rely on the detection of a host response to a suspected pathogen. Interpretation is wholly dependent on taking an appropriate sample, handling it (transport, investigation) in an appropriate and timely way, and having the relevant clinical information. Clinicians should liaise with the laboratory to make best use of the systems available.

While viral diagnosis has become largely nucleic acid based, diagnosis of bacterial and fungal infections is still largely culture based. Many human pathogens are fastidious and require special transport media for swabs.

Blood cultures

One of the most important specimens for the diagnosis of infection is the blood culture (Fig. 15.3). This must be taken aseptically. Most laboratories use semi-automated, continuous monitoring systems with two bottles. About 5–10 mL of blood are added to culture media that are designed for the isolation of bacteria (including fastidious organisms such as brucella and neisseria), with one bottle for aerobic and the other for anaerobic bacteria. In addition to this, there are single bottle systems for paediatrics to make best use of smaller samples, as well as semi-automated systems for detection of mycobacteria in the blood.

Nucleic acid and antigen detection in blood

Blood samples can be used for direct antigen (e.g. HbsAg) or nucleic acid amplification tests (NAAT e.g. HIV,

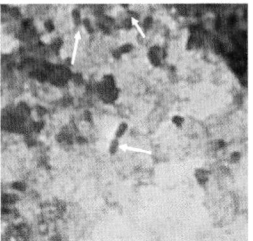

Fig. 15.3 Gram-negative bacilli (arrows) in a blood culture.

937

N. meningitidis). Serological evaluation based on detection of host antibodies is also available, but there may be a diagnostic delay due to the time taken for the host to mount an antibody response.

Investigation of specific organs or sites of infection

Localized infections are investigated using specimens from that site. Appropriate specimens will depend on the suspected site of infection, e.g. expectorated sputum or bronchoalveolar lavage for lower respiratory infection, midstream urine for acute urinary tract infection, and first-pass urine for urethritis. Sexually transmitted diseases can be evaluated with throat, rectal, cervical and urethral swabs, with separate specimens to diagnose chlamydia and *N. gonorrhoeae* infections. Depending on the pathogens being sought, specimens can be investigated using a wide range of techniques, e.g. direct microscopy, Gram stain, specialized stains (auramine, Ziehl–Neelsen, iodine, India ink), direct or indirect immunofluorescence, dark ground microscopy, culture, direct antigen detection, NAAT or probing.

A sample of pus is always better than a swab. Solid and liquid (broth) media culture is used for swabs from infected sites. Most specimens are incubated at 37°C in air plus CO_2, and anaerobically.

The role of the normal flora

The specific technique used by the laboratory depends on whether the site of the specimen has a normal flora. Selective media may be needed to differentiate or reduce overgrowth of normal flora so that the relevant pathogens can be detected.

Identification of pathogens

Pathogens can be identified based on a variety of bio-chemical (Fig. 15.4), antigenic and nucleic acid features. In many cases, particularly with bacteria, identification will depend on a series of tests, e.g. *Helicobacter pylori* can be identified by atmospheric requirement, Gram stain and oxidase and urease activity. Conversely, nucleic acid amplification and sequencing is used to detect and identify organisms that are slow, difficult or not possible to grow, e.g. hepatitis C genotypes and *Tropheryma whipplei*.

Antimicrobial susceptibility testing

Accurate assessment of susceptibility to antimicrobial agents is increasingly important for many viruses and fungi,

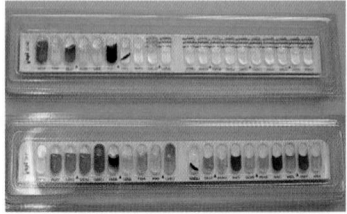

Fig. 15.4 Different batteries of biochemical tests can be used to identify different groups of organisms.

as well as bacteria. A susceptible organism is one where a normal dose of an antibiotic is likely to result in cure; a resistant organism is one where antibiotic therapy is likely to fail. Testing methods include disc diffusion agar or broth dilution, inhibition of cytopathic effects in tissue culture, probe and NAAT.

Serological diagnosis

A variety of serological techniques such as agglutination, complement fixation, virus neutralization and enzyme immunoassay (EIA) can be used to diagnose infection by detecting the host's immune response to pathogens. Different patterns of antibody response reflect different stages of infection. For instance, acute infection may be detected by elevated IgM in a single acute sample or by a 4-fold rise in IgG in paired acute and convalescent samples taken a few weeks apart.

Choice of method

The choice of diagnostic method depends on a combination of the ease and speed with which different pathogens can be detected. For example, treponemes may be seen in an exudate from a chancre in primary syphilis, but the pathogen is almost impossible to detect in latent or tertiary syphilis and the diagnosis rests on the detection of antibody. Hepatitis B cannot be cultured, but viral antigen, DNA and antibody may be detected. By contrast, *S. aureus* will grow easily within 24 hours in the laboratory from a swab taken from pus at a wound. Sensitivity data will then be available the next day.

> **RECENT ADVANCES**
>
> *Rapid diagnosis is increasingly being sought, with the aim of achieving same-day diagnostic and therapeutic interventions. Widening arrays of rapid molecular diagnostic tests are particularly useful in viral diagnosis, which relied until recently on lengthy tissue culture or serology. Rapid testing is likely to be extended to common and important bacteria in the next 10 years, with a broad range of techniques likely to enter commercial development.*

Other clinical investigations

Accurate diagnosis and evaluation of the therapeutic response depends on the full history and examination, as well as ancillary investigations. It is crucial to consider the evidence for infection as a whole rather than to rely on any single modality. The history of the development of illness and potential exposure to pathogens is of utmost importance: specific enquiries about travel, occupation, agriculture, hobbies, and others who are or have been ill should be made. The differential diagnosis and laboratory investigation of fever in a 30-year-old who visited rural Sierra Leone 4 days ago are quite different from those for a 95-year-old who has been in residential care in the UK for 4 years.

Fever pattern and height, localizing or generalized pain, respiratory rate and changes in urine, stool or exudates are all important. The appearance of the skin, response to blanching, presence of rashes, temperature of extremities, character of pulse and heart rate are all useful clues that may support the diagnosis of sepsis. Leukocyte count and differential may be helpful: some infections are associated with neutrophilia or lymphocytosis, while patients with typhoid may have lymphopenia or eosinophilia. The C-reactive protein (CRP) is usually very high (>300) in pneumococcal sepsis and will be raised in most bacterial infections. Lactate levels may be raised in severe sepsis. Imaging may be very useful in the diagnosis of localized infection. This may include chest X-ray, abdominal ultrasound, computed tomography (CT) scanning (Fig. 15.5) or magnetic resonance imaging (MRI) of brain, spinal cord, bone or joints, echocardiography to visualize heart valves, and diagnostic taps to obtain specimens from deep-seated collections.

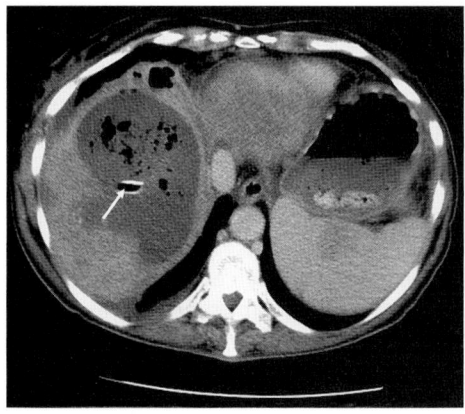

Fig. 15.5 CT scan of the liver. A large multiloculated liver abscess containing gas developed following embolizations of liver metastases. The arrow denotes a drain in situ.
Courtesy of Dr Nicola Strickland, Department of Imaging, Hammersmith Hospital, UK.

Manifestations of infectious disease

Pyrexia of uncertain origin

Pyrexia of unknown origin (PUO) is an unexplained intermittent or persistent fever greater than 38.2°C that lasts for more than 2 weeks. This term is increasingly used to refer to fever of shorter duration. In general, the longer a PUO lasts, the less likely it is to have an infectious origin.

Epidemiology

PUO is a relatively common clinical presentation.

Pathology

The main causes are infections, malignancy and connective tissue disease (Table 15.4). In a proportion of patients the diagnosis remains uncertain despite investigations. It is important to consider drug hypersensitivity, especially to β-lactams such as the penicillins and cephalosporins, as it may be the antibiotic therapy that is causing the fever rather than the presumed infection.

Clinical features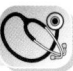

The detailed history of the presenting illness should include occupational details and potential exposure to animals or animal products. A social and sexual history of the patient is important: cross-country runners have contracted hepatitis B from scratches caused by thorny vegetation, windsurfers are at risk of leptospirosis and waterborne enteroviruses, and veterinarians and farmers may acquire zoonotic infections such as brucellosis and Q fever. Recent travel may indicate possible exposure to a variety of tropical infections and parasites. A detailed sexual history may indicate potential exposure to HIV or related risks.

Table 15.4	Causes of pyrexia of uncertain origin
Infection (55%)	
Localized abscesses or dental sepsis	
Tuberculosis (pulmonary or other sites)	
Endocarditis	
Brucellosis	
Enteric fevers	
Zoonoses	
Malaria	
Hepatitis	
Infectious mononucleosis	
Malignancy (20%)	
Lymphoma	
Renal carcinoma	
Lung carcinomas	
Connective tissue disorders (15%)	
Rheumatoid disease	
Systemic lupus erythematosus	
Polyarteritis nodosum	
Polymyalgia rheumatica	
Rare causes (10%)	
Drug hypersensitivity (penicillins and cephalosporins)	

939

Many drugs and health products can potentially cause fever, and the patient should be asked about prescribed, alternative and over-the-counter medications. It is quite easy for doctors, nurses and patients to overlook vital information or to miss the significance of some facts at the first interview (such as a liking for unpasteurized fresh cheeses from a local market). Further opportunities for reviewing the possibility of exposure to infectious agents are often necessary.

A complete and thorough examination is crucial. Identification of localized discomfort or swelling, bone or joint pain, unusual, new or subtle rashes, lymphadenopathy, abdominal masses, cardiac murmurs, mild neurological signs and mild meningism may provide important clues. A complete physical examination should be repeated regularly and by more than one individual to detect changes or intermittent or developing features, for example a new soft systolic murmur or increasing abdominal tenderness, fleeting rashes or joint swelling. Splenomegaly and hepatomegaly are important signs that may emerge as the illness progresses (endocarditis, enteric fever).

Initial investigations

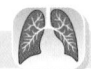

The most important aspect in investigating PUO is to regularly review and repeat the history and key investigations.

Full blood count
FBC and blood film (Fig. 15.6) are obtained together with red cell indices and differential white count. The differential white cell count may point to a specific aetiology such as an eosinophilia with parasitic infection.

Markers of inflammation
C-reactive protein and erythrocyte sedimentation rate (ESR) are performed to monitor the course of the disease.

Antibody screen
Serum samples that are taken during the acute phase of disease should be saved for future antibody detection.

Blood cultures
At least three blood cultures should be taken at different times.

Urinalysis and cultures
Urine dipstick testing and culture of the urine should be performed.

Stool cultures
Stools are examined for ova and cysts.

Sputum cultures
Early morning sputum cultures should be performed routinely.

Chest X-ray
A chest film is performed to screen for pulmonary disease.

Further investigations

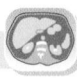

These are guided by the findings of history and physical examination and will be prompted by specific features; for example, exposure to agricultural animals or animal products will lead to investigations for brucella, Q fever, psittacosis and chlamydia, leptospirosis and salmonella. Haematuria and an appropriate travel history will lead to investigation for schistosomiasis.

Specific serological investigations
Additional screening tests may be useful in narrowing down the differential diagnosis or excluding potential pathogens. For example, tests for *Coxiella burnetii* or Bartonella may be helpful in excluding these pathogens as a cause of endocarditis.

Further imaging
Additional tests may include investigations such as abdominal ultrasound, echocardiography, sinus and dental X-ray, CT or MRI scanning of head and neck, thorax, abdomen, pelvis or spine.

Medical management

Trial of antibiotic therapy
A diagnosis should usually be made before any antimicrobial therapy is commenced. However, a trial of therapy may occasionally be considered where a diagnosis is suspected but confirmation is not readily available, e.g. tuberculosis or brucellosis.

Prognosis

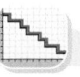

Prognosis is strongly determined by the underlying cause of the pyrexia.

Septicaemia

Bacteraemia refers to 'bacteria in the blood stream' which may, or may not, have any clinical consequences. Transient bacteraemia occurs with tooth brushing, as well as without any obvious cause, and can lead to infection of a prosthetic device or valve. Bacteraemia may also result from shedding of bacteria from a focus of infection, or arise from a generalized invasive infection.

When bacteraemia is associated with systemic signs of severe infection and ongoing multiplication of the pathogen, it is known as septicaemia. It is generally not useful to distinguish between bacteraemia and septicaemia, but to refer to the clinical syndrome of sepsis (Table 15.5) and severe sepsis (with or without septic shock).

Epidemiology

The point prevalence of sepsis is approximately 21 000 per year in England and Wales. Patients with severe sepsis

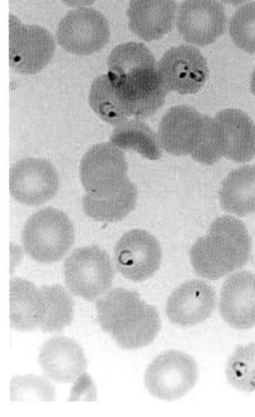

Fig. 15.6 *Plasmodium falciparum* in a blood film showing ring forms.

Table 15.5	Definition and grading of severity of sepsis

Sepsis is defined as clinical evidence of infection and a systemic response with 2 or more of the following:

1. Temperature >38°C or <36°C

2. Heart rate >90 beats/min

3. Respiratory rate >20 breaths/min or arterial CO_2 <4.3 kPa

4. White cell count >12 or <4 × 10^3 cells/mm^3

Sepsis is defined as severe when this is associated with one of the following:

1. Hypotension

2. Lactic acidosis

3. Oliguria

4. Confusion

5. Hepatic dysfunction

Septic shock is when the inadequate tissue perfusion persists despite fluid resuscitation in a patient with sepsis

make up about a quarter of admissions to intensive care units.

Pathology

Sepsis is most likely to develop in those who are immunocompromised, and in patients who are very young or very old.

Bacteraemia may arise from many sources including infections of skin and soft tissue, oropharynx and respiratory tract, biliary and gastrointestinal tracts, urinary or genital tract, as well as via intravascular devices (Table 15.6). Although the term 'Gram-negative shock' is widely used, sepsis syndrome can actually be due to both Gram-positive or Gram-negative organisms.

Table 15.6	Causes of sepsis

Organism	Common associations or sites of infection
E. coli and S. aureus	The most frequent causes of sepsis in patients admitted via A&E
Anaerobes and mixed enterobacteria	Disease involving obstruction of a viscus or the biliary tract
E. coli and Gram-negative infection	Urinary tract
S. pyogenes or S. aureus	Skin and soft tissue infections
Gonococcus	Ascending pelvic infection, may be accompanied by arthritis in women
N. meningitidis or S. pneumoniae	Invasion via the oropharynx, may be accompanied by meningitis (both organisms) or respiratory tract infection (S. pneumoniae)
Fungi, anaerobes	Immunosuppression

Septicaemia following surgery may be caused by a wide range of organisms, including contamination by skin flora. This problem is particularly important in orthopaedic, cardiovascular and surgical surgery involving prosthetic devices.

Sepsis is caused by a combination of active infection and the host response to components of the pathogen. A systemic inflammatory response syndrome (SIRS) may develop in response to a variety of stimuli, of which infection is one (Table 15.7). These substances cause activation of complement, neutrophils, monocytic cells, macrophages and endothelial cells and trigger the clotting cascade. This, in turn, results in further cellular activation and initiation of a cytokine cascade involving IL-6, tumour necrosis factor (TNF)-α and IL-1, increases in tissue factors, reactive oxygen and mediators involving the nitric oxide pathways, activation of coagulation and fibrinolysis, and increases in bradykinin.

The net result of these interrelated pathways is capillary leaking, neutrophil accumulation, fever, metabolic and hormonal changes, vasodilatation and disseminated intravascular coagulation. If untreated, these progress to shock, vascular insufficiency, organ dysfunction and eventually multi-organ failure and death.

Clinical features

Patients with sepsis may present with clinical features relating to the site of infection. Patients with severe sepsis are usually ill with fever and shock, sometimes aggravated by depressed consciousness. Atypical presentation can occur at extremes of age and in the immunocompromised. Fever may be absent in children and the elderly, and shock may not have developed. As such, these patients may simply appear confused, drowsy or non-specifically unwell. It is impossible to determine from clinical assessment alone whether the sepsis is due to Gram-positive or Gram-negative bacteria.

Some organisms may have characteristic associated clinical signs, e.g. the purpuric rash associated with *N. meningitidis*, or others that suggest a particular aetiology, e.g. gastrointestinal upset and rash associated with toxic shock syndrome.

Investigations

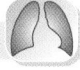

Full blood count

FBC with a differential white cell count should be performed.

Table 15.7	Precipitants of the host inflammatory response

Microbial products
  Endotoxin (lipopolysaccharide and protein A)
  Peptidoglycan
  Lipoteichoic acid
  Variety of toxins (streptolysin)
  Superantigens (toxic shock syndrome toxin-1)
  Enzymes (phospholipase C)

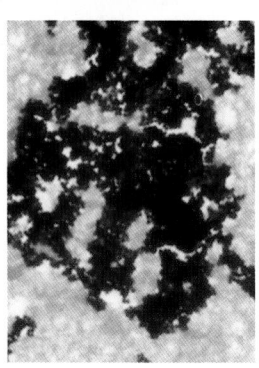

Fig. 15.7 Light microscopy of Gram-positive cocci in clusters in a positive blood culture.

C-reactive protein

CRP is measured to determine the trend.

Arterial blood gases

Arterial blood gases are performed and serum lactate estimated to estimate the severity of sepsis.

Clotting screen

A clotting screen should be performed with measurement of fibrin and fibrin degradation products to screen for disseminated intravascular coagulation (p. 820).

Blood cultures

Blood culture is the mainstay of diagnosis (Fig. 15.7). Whenever possible this should be carried out before antimicrobials are given.

Other specific cultures

Other investigations are directed to finding the source of the sepsis, e.g. urine culture, cerebrospinal fluid (CSF), abdominal ultrasound, sputum culture and skin swabs.

Chest and abdominal X-ray

A chest and abdominal film should be performed to screen for changes associated with infection (Fig. 15.8).

Management

Supportive therapy

Supportive therapy is the most important initial step and should include careful management of fluid balance, blood pressure and oxygenation (in an intensive care setting for those with severe sepsis). Some patients may present early on with relatively uncomplicated illness that responds well to therapy. In other patients, the condition progresses rapidly to septic shock, and aggressive management in the intensive care unit is needed.

Antibiotics

Empirical parenteral therapy with a broad-spectrum antibiotic should be started promptly. The choice of drug should be based on an assessment of the probable source of infection and the most likely pathogens.

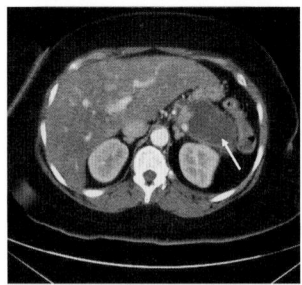

Fig. 15.8 CT scan of the abdomen. A large infected pseudocyst replaces most of the tail of the pancreas. Courtesy of Dr Nicola Strickland, Department of Imaging, Hammersmith Hospital, UK.

Drotrecogin alfa

Recombinant human activated protein C may be used in the treatment of patients with severe sepsis. The drug appears to promote fibrinolysis and attenuate the inflammatory response in severe sepsis. Drotrecogin achieved an absolute reduction of 6.5% in the 28-day mortality rate for patients with severe sepsis and multi-organ failure.[1]

Prognosis

The mortality rate for severe sepsis ranges from 30% to 50%, despite intensive medical management. Survivors of sepsis may experience long-term health problems as severe sepsis can cause permanent organ damage.

RECENT ADVANCES

The role of corticosteroids in sepsis remains controversial, although benefit has been demonstrated in meningitis in developing countries. The clinical effect of anticytokine therapies has been disappointing. Further work in vaccines and immune modulation is likely to be developed in the near future.

REFERENCE

(1) *Green C, Dinnes J, Takeda A, et al. Clinical effectiveness and cost-effectiveness of drotrecogin alfa (activated) (Xigris) for the treatment of severe sepsis in adults: a systematic review and economic evaluation. Health Technology Assessment 2005; 11: 1–126, iii–iv.*

Bacterial infection

SECTION 15.4 Gram-positive bacteria

Staphylococci

Staphylococci are Gram-positive, non-sporing, non-motile, cluster-forming cocci. Up to 40% of healthy people carry *S. aureus* asymptomatically in the nose, skin, axilla or perineum. Other important species in this family are *S. epidermidis, S. saprophyticus* and *S. haemolyticus*.

Pathology

The main determinant of virulence of *S. aureus* is the production of coagulase, an enzyme that converts fibrinogen to fibrin, and helps wall off infection from the host defences. This also provides the principal method of identifying it. Other determinants of virulence include DNAse, lipase, adhesion molecules including fibrinectin-binding proteins and a number of highly active exotoxins with superantigenic properties—enterotoxins, toxic shock syndrome toxins and epidermolytic toxin.

Coagulase-negative staphylococci, principally *S. epidermidis*, produce extracellular slime. Many can adhere to prosthetic material and are associated with device-related infection.

S. saprophyticus, distinguished by novobiocin sensitivity, is associated with urinary tract infection. *S. haemolyticus* is associated with high levels of antibiotic resistance.

> *RECENT ADVANCES*
>
> *Currently, potential outbreaks are investigated using phage, pulsed field electrophoresis and multi locus sequence typing.*

Scope of disease

S. aureus is the most common cause of skin, soft tissue and wound infections including folliculitis, boils, furuncles, impetigo and cellulitis (p. 801), osteomyelitis and septic arthritis (p. 510). Infections associated with surgical sites and intravenous lines are hospital acquired. Cross-infection may be important, particularly with 'outbreak' meticillin-resistant *S. aureus* (MRSA) strains. Invasive infection can occur resulting in deep-seated abscesses in any organ and septicaemia. Endocarditis can result from the bacteraemia or may be acquired from cannula site infection (p. 33). *S. aureus* pneumonia also progresses rapidly with cavity formation and carries a high mortality rate. *S aureus* pneumonia can be a hospital-acquired infection or develop as a complication of viral pneumonia. Enterotoxin-mediated diseases include food poisoning, scalded skin syndrome and toxic shock syndrome.

The coagulase-negative staphylococci also cause endocarditis (*S. epidermidis*), urinary tract infections (*S. saprophyticus*), and infections in premature neonates and patients with indwelling devices such as urinary catheters.

Clinical features

Toxic shock syndrome

Toxic shock syndrome is described in menstruating women. It occurs through vaginal carriage of specific toxin (TSST-1) producing strains of *S. aureus* and is exacerbated by the use of hyperabsorbent tampons that act as a rich source of culture medium for the growth and multiplication of bacteria. Clinical features are a diffuse rash followed by desquamation of the skin, including that of the palms and soles. Septicaemia can ensue giving rise to fever, hypotension and multiple organ failure due to disease involvement.

Scalded skin syndrome

Staphylococcal scalded skin syndrome is characterized by red blistering skin resembling a burn or scald (Fig. 15.9). It is caused by the release of epidermolytic toxins A and B from toxigenic strains and often starts from a localized staphylococcal infection in infants and young children.

Medical management

The choice of antibiotic agent for staphylococcal disease depends on the type, extent and severity of the illness. In addition, regional variation in antibiotic resistance also influences the choice for initial therapy.

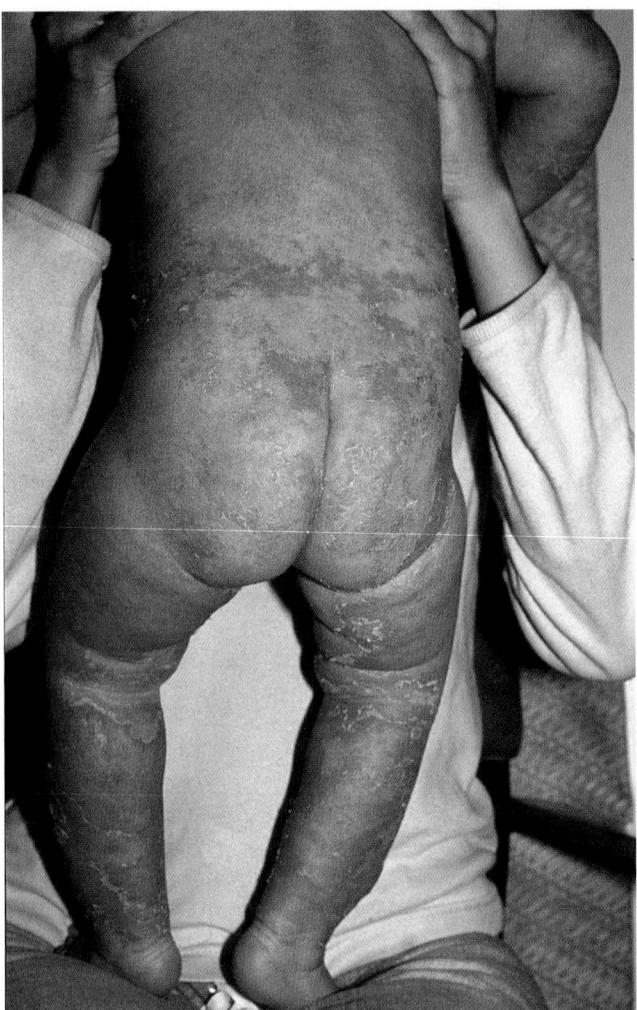

Fig. 15.9 A baby with staphylococcal scalded skin syndrome.

Penicillin-resistant organisms

Most staphylococci produce β-lactamase and are penicillin resistant. Therefore the treatment of choice for *S. aureus* is flucloxacillin or oxacillin. In penicillin allergy erythromycin or clindamycin may be used. Glycopeptides and gentamicin are also effective.

Meticillin-resistant organisms

Meticillin resistance is conferred by the *mec A* gene which codes for a low-affinity penicillin-binding protein. If the organism is meticillin resistant a glycopeptide such as vancomycin may be required.

Streptococci

Streptococci and the related enterococci are catalase-negative, chain-forming Gram-positive cocci that can be found in the normal flora of the oropharynx and gastro-intestinal tract. They are classified in Table 15.8.

Table 15.8	Classification of streptococci
Streptococci can be classified based on haemolysis (beta-complete, alpha-incomplete), Lancefield grouping and by biochemical reactions	
Beta-haemolytic streptococcus	
Lancefield group A streptococcus (*Streptococcus pyogenes*)	
Lancefield group B streptococcus (*Streptococcus agalactiae*)	
Lancefield group C streptococcus	
Lancefield group G streptococcus	
Alpha-haemolytic streptococcus	
Streptococcus pneumoniae (pneumococcus)	
Viridans streptococci (bacterial endocarditis)	
Non-haemolytic streptococcus	
Lancefield group D (*Enterococcus faecalis*)	
Certain members of Lancefield groups B, C, D, H, and O	

Pathology

The streptococci are fastidious, facultative anaerobes that require rich blood-containing media. Many are present in the normal flora.

Streptococcus pyogenes (Lancefield group A, beta-haemolytic) is present in the pharynx in 5–30% of the population. The viridans group (which comprises many species) is found in the mouth, and the enterococci are found in the gut. *S. pneumoniae* is present in small numbers in the oropharynx. *S. pyogenes* and other beta-haemolytic streptococci produce hyaluronidases, collagenases and other enzymes that break down connective tissue. The surface polysaccharide interferes with phagocytosis, particularly with *S. pneumoniae*. Different surface M proteins are associated with different diseases or tissue affiliations. Haemolytic streptococci produce a variety of super-antigenic toxins associated with streptococcal toxic shock, and also an erythrogenic toxin that causes scarlet fever. *S. mutans* produces a glycan that aids adherence to teeth and contributes to cavity development. *S. pneumoniae* produces a number of different polysaccharide capsules which confer virulence, and also produces pneumolysin and other toxins. Diseases associated with streptococci are listed in Table 15.9.

Clinical features

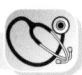

The clinical presentation of haemolytic streptococcal infections varies with the site of infection. *S. pyogenes* infections are typically rapidly spreading and associated with significant toxicity.

Rheumatic fever has been rare over the past 25 years but its incidence has increased recently. It is an inflammatory process that affects the joints (arthritis), heart (carditis), central nervous system (chorea) and skin (erythema marginatum and nodules).

Pneumococcal pneumonia (Fig. 15.10) presents with fever, confusion, respiratory signs including cough with a characteristic 'rusty' bloodstained sputum, and very high CRP.

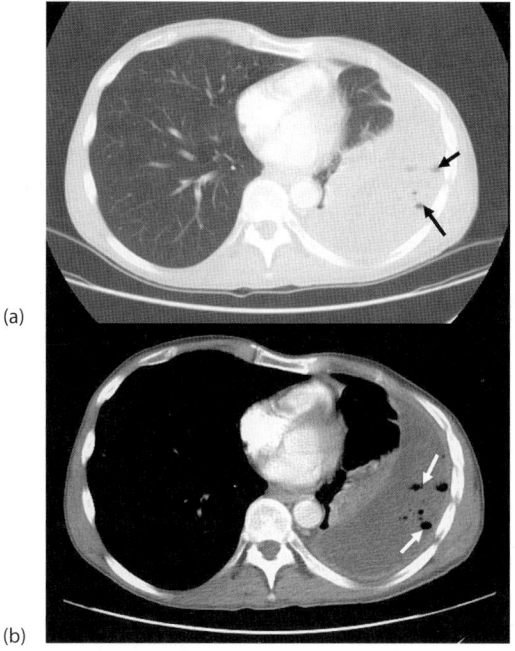

(a)

(b)

Fig. 15.10 CT scan of left pneumonia. (a) Lung and (b) soft tissue fields showing a large empyema which followed pneumococcal pneumonia. The gas in the empyema is indicated by arrows. (a) and (b) courtesy of Dr Nicola Strickland, Department of Imaging, Hammersmith Hospital, UK.

Management

Isolation

S. pyogenes can spread rapidly in surgical and obstetric wards; infected or colonized patients should be isolated in a side-room until 48 hours after initiation of effective antibiotic therapy.

Benzylpenicillin

Prompt treatment prevents secondary immune disease, e.g. rheumatic fever. Benzylpenicillin is the treatment of choice.

Staphylococci

Streptococci

Bacillus anthracis

Bacillus cereus

Corynebacteria

Listeria monocytogenes

Table 15.9	Diseases associated with streptococci	
Organism	**Pathogenesis of disease**	**Disease states**
S. pyogenes	Infection	Bacterial pharyngitis, cellulitis, erysipelas, wound infections, necrotizing fasciitis
	Toxin mediated	Scarlet fever, streptococcal shock
	Immune-mediated post-infectious syndromes	Rheumatic fever, glomerulonephritis, erythema nodosum
S. agalactiae	Infection	Neonatal sepsis, meningitis
Viridans streptococci and enterococci	Infection	Endocarditis
Enterococci	Infection	Urinary tract infection
S. pneumoniae	Infection	Pneumonia, respiratory tract infections, otitis media, bacteraemia, meningitis, endocarditis
The milleri group (often group C)	Infection	Deep abscesses in liver, lung and brain

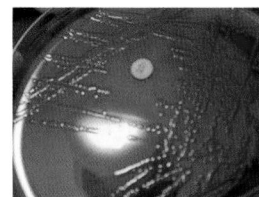

(c)

Fig. 15.10 *Cont'd* (c) *Streptococcus pneumoniae* growing on blood agar.

945

Macrolides

Macrolides (erythromycin) are an alternative for patients with allergy.

Cephalosporins and glycopeptides

As penicillin resistance in *S. pneumoniae* is increasing, cefotaxime or a glycopeptide (vancomycin) may be needed in serious infections.

Combination therapy

Bacteraemia and endocarditis due to enterococci and group B streptococci are treated with penicillin and gentamicin.

Vaccination

Vaccination against *S. pneumoniae* using a 23-valent polysaccharide vaccine is indicated in susceptible individuals (splenectomized patients, those with chronic organ failure or sickle cell disease and the elderly). Vaccination reduces the incidence of severe diseases such as meningitis and septicaemia. Future vaccines are now being developed using protein–polysaccharide conjugates, which are made up of 7–11 selected polysaccharides bound to a protein carrier.

RECENT ADVANCES

Antimicrobial resistance in enterococci is an emerging problem. Many teaching hospitals and tertiary referral centres have problems with vancomycin-resistant enterococci (VRE).

Bacillus species

The genus *Bacillus* consists of a group of large, blunt-ended, spore-forming Gram-positive bacilli that grow readily on most non-selective media. The two main pathogens in this genus are *B. anthracis* and *B. cereus*. Clinical specimens may occasionally be contaminated by other non-pathogenic *Bacillus* species from the environment unrelated to the disease.

Bacillus anthracis

This is a soil organism that causes anthrax. It has recently emerged as an agent of bioterrorism.

Pathology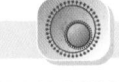

Anthrax is not usually transmitted from person to person as the organism has relatively low infectivity. Its pathogenicity is conferred by a capsule comprising a polypeptide of D-glutamic acid which inhibits phagocytosis, and a plasmid-encoded toxin made up of protective antigen, oedema factor and lethal factor. These three components cause shock by increasing vascular permeability.

Clinical features

Cutaneous anthrax

Cutaneous anthrax is the most common form and may be seen in farmers and hide sorters. This is the least severe form of infection (mortality rate <20%) and occurs when the spores have gained entry to the skin via a pre-existing lesion. A pustule may be seen at the site of inoculation and develops into a black eschar with severe local swelling.

Inhalation anthrax

Inhalation anthrax follows inhalation of spores. This is the form seen today in bioterrorism and in the past as wool-sorter's disease. The fatality rate is high (>80%) once symptoms develop. Inhalation anthrax develops 2–4 days after spores are inhaled, with a rapid onset of fever and catastrophic inflammatory reaction, associated with respiratory failure and a widened mediastinum.

Intestinal anthrax

Intestinal anthrax is a rare form that follows ingestion of contaminated food. Fatality rates may be up to 75%. It is characterized by severe abdominal pain, vomiting and watery or bloody diarrhoea developing into bacteraemia in 2–3 days. Gram-positive bacilli may be seen in blood.

Investigations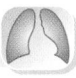

Blood cultures

Investigation involves Gram stain of blood and blood cultures.

Management

Containment

Special containment and public health measures are required where anthrax is suspected. Local and national public health experts must be involved early, particularly in a possible deliberate release scenario (see www.cdc.gov and www.hpa.org.uk).

Antibiotics

The antibiotic of choice is ciprofloxacin. This should be given for 60 days for inhalation anthrax, or where deliberate release may be a possibility.

Bacillus cereus

Bacillus cereus is similar to *B. anthracis* in culture but lacks the D-glutamic acid capsule. Food poisoning arises from exotoxins that are produced when spores germinate in improperly stored food (rice and grain dishes). Patients may present with vomiting about 6 hours after ingestion of preformed acid- and heat-stable toxin. Alternatively, a predominantly diarrhoeal form develops after 8–24 hours caused by a heat-labile enterotoxin that develops in the intestine. *B. cereus* may also cause post-traumatic ophthalmitis, requiring aggressive local and intraocular therapy to save the eye.

Corynebacterium and Listeria

Corynebacteria

Corynebacteria are non-sporing, non-motile and non-capsulate Gram-positive pleomorphic bacilli arranged in irregular patterns. There are many species, most of which are skin commensals that can, on rare occasions, cause prosthetic infections.

Pathology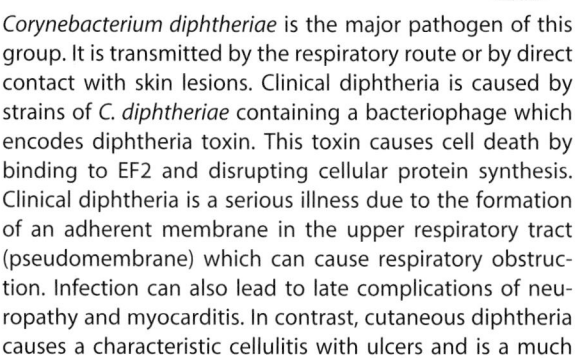

Corynebacterium diphtheriae is the major pathogen of this group. It is transmitted by the respiratory route or by direct contact with skin lesions. Clinical diphtheria is caused by strains of *C. diphtheriae* containing a bacteriophage which encodes diphtheria toxin. This toxin causes cell death by binding to EF2 and disrupting cellular protein synthesis. Clinical diphtheria is a serious illness due to the formation of an adherent membrane in the upper respiratory tract (pseudomembrane) which can cause respiratory obstruction. Infection can also lead to late complications of neuropathy and myocarditis. In contrast, cutaneous diphtheria causes a characteristic cellulitis with ulcers and is a much less severe illness. Non-toxigenic strains may cause mild sore throat.

C. ulcerans and C. pseudotuberculosis rarely cause pharyngitis and granulomatous lymphadenitis respectively. *C. jeikeium* is associated with bacteraemia in the immuno-compromised and is highly resistant to most antibiotics except vancomycin.

Clinical features

Clinical diphtheria usually presents as a nasopharyngeal infection with sore throat and fever. Acute inflammation and necrosis occurs, with necrotic exudates and a pseudo-membrane that forms over the tonsils and posterior wall of the pharynx. Severe toxaemia can develop, with complications such as myocarditis, neuropathies and paralysis occurring later on. A cutaneous form with typical 'punched-out' lesions can also develop.

Investigations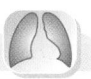

Nasopharyngeal swabs
The nasopharynx and membrane should be swabbed, and the laboratory notified so that special culture media can be used.

Specific laboratory procedures are required for the isolation and identification of *C. diphtheriae*. The organism hydrolyses tellurite to produce black colonies on Hoyle's or Tindale's medium. Speciation is by biochemical tests and toxin detection by Elek's test and PCR.

Management

Isolation
Patients suspected of having diphtheria should be isolated and given antitoxin.

Supportive care
Intensive care support may be needed to maintain a patent airway or if the illness is complicated by paralysis or heart failure.

Erythromycin
Erythromycin is used to reduce toxin production, to eliminate local infection, and to minimize the potential for transmission. Treatment should be continued until two successive cultures are negative.

Contact tracing and vaccination
Household and other contacts should receive vaccination if they have not already done so. They should also be given antibiotic prophylaxis with oral erythromycin for 7 days.

Clinical diphtheria in the population is prevented by vaccination with a toxoid as part of the childhood immunization schedule. As the duration of immunity is unclear, adults will require a booster if they run the risk of being, or have been, exposed to diphtheria.

Other corynebacterial infections
Other corynebacterial infections are managed according to the clinical picture as well as other investigations to determine the significance of particular isolates and anti-microbial sensitivity testing. Vancomycin is likely to be needed for infections caused by *C. jeikeium*.

Listeria monocytogenes

Listeria monocytogenes is a Gram-positive, non-sporing, motile, facultative anaerobic psychrotroph (grows at 40°C) that is found in soil and in the gut of animals.

Pathology

Listeria contaminates the human food chain from the gut of agricultural and other animals. The organism is able to grow at 4°C, and foods that are consumed without further cooking are a recognized risk, e.g. soft cheeses, coleslaw and ready meals.

Infection is usually mild and self-limiting. Listeria is a recognized cause of meningitis and meningoencephalitis with septicaemia in the immunocompromised, the elderly, neonates and pregnant women. Bacteraemia in pregnancy causes intrauterine death, premature labour with early or late onset neonatal septicaemia, and meningitis.

The organism is isolated from blood, CSF or products of conception.

Clinical features

Clinical presentation may be as a "flu" like illness or as acute pyogenic meningitis, bacteraemia or encephalitis (with a high mortality) in patients with reduced cell-mediated immunity.

Investigations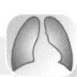

Cultures

Cultures of sites that are appropriate to the clinical features should be obtained.

Management

Ampicillin and gentamicin

The combination of ampicillin and gentamicin is the treatment of choice.

Other antibiotics

Vancomycin or co-trimoxazole may also be effective. *Listeria monocytogenes* is resistant to the cephalosporins.

Prevention

Prevention is by good food hygiene and handling. High-risk foods (rinded soft cheese) should be avoided by pregnant women and the immunocompromised.

SECTION 15.5   Anaerobes

Anaerobic bacteria

A range of bacteria thrive in an environment in which there is no or little oxygen. These bacteria can cause infections and toxin-mediated disease in humans.

Pathology

The anaerobes can be divided into two main groups based on their spore-forming ability.

The non-sporing anaerobes inhabit the oral cavity, female genital tract and gastrointestinal tract, with the greatest concentration in the large bowel. Infection arises when the organisms are able to multiply outside the confines of the bowel, or invade locally within damaged tissue. This group includes the *Bacteroides* species, of which the fragilis group is most commonly associated with disease.

Spore-forming anaerobes are members of the genus *Clostridium*. Members of this group cause disease by direct invasion and by production of a variety of destructive and neurological toxins which are described in Table 15.10.

Non-sporing anaerobes can cause intra-abdominal and dental abscesses, and abscesses in a number of sites such as lung, brain and liver. *Actinomyces* is an uncommon cause of chronic discharging sinus and abscess formation in the mouth, lung or abdomen.

Clostridium species produce a wide range of diseases, ranging from diarrhoea and food poisoning to fatal neurological or muscular illness.

Clinical features

Abscesses that involve anaerobes may present with a wide variety of signs and symptoms, but they are commonly

Table 15.10	Pathogenesis of clostridial diseases				
Organism	*C. botulinum*	*C. tetani*	*C. perfringens*	*C. difficile*	*C. perfringens*
Source	Environment	Environment	Environment and endogenous	Environment and endogenous	Environment
Pathogenesis	Ingested preformed toxins A–G. Inhibits neurotransmitter release	Tetanospasmin disseminates from site of production in localized wound. Prevents release of the inhibitory neurotransmitter GABA	α-toxin (and others) produced by infecting organisms in devitalized tissue. Further tissue destruction leads to progression	Overgrowth and displacement of normal flora. Enterotoxin A and/or B produced in gut.	Enterotoxin produced when organism sporulates in gut

associated with fever, which may be swinging, and a raised CRP level. There may be localizing signs with swelling and tenderness, or a collection may only be detectable using more sophisticated imaging such as CT, MRI or technetium-labelled white cell scanning.

Clostridium perfringens causes wound infections, gas gangrene and gastroenteritis. Gas gangrene presents with severe pain, swelling, discolouration and crepitus associated with a wound. This is accompanied by generalized toxicity and raised creatine kinase from muscle necrosis. Exploration of the wound reveals devitalized tissue.

C. botulinum causes adult and infant botulism, and certain forms of food poisoning. Botulism presents with an advancing, descending flaccid paralysis, often beginning with the cranial nerves and manifesting as blurring of vision with difficulty in swallowing. Respiratory difficulty develops with progression and usually requires ventilatory support. Sensation remains intact. This is a form of food poisoning that may be associated with household or larger outbreaks.

C. tetani causes tetanus, which presents with spastic paralysis and muscle spasms. These symptoms may start around the site of an infected wound and then become more generalized with motor excitability triggered by minimal stimuli. There may be signs and symptoms due to spasms of the perioral muscles (risus sardonicus) or legs and spinal muscles (opisthotonos). In developed countries, tetanus is most frequent in middle-aged and elderly women who sustain penetrating gardening injuries that are not optimally managed.

C. difficile causes pseudomembranous colitis and antibiotic-associated diarrhoea. Pseudomembranous colitis usually occurs in patients who have had broad-spectrum antibiotics, especially in association with bowel surgery. Symptoms include diarrhoea, which is offensive, copious and often bloody with mucus streaks. Disease may progress from pseudomembrane formation to extensive colonic ulceration, toxic megacolon and perforation.

C. perfringens food poisoning typically presents with abdominal pain and diarrhoea 8–12 hours after ingestion of contaminated food. It is usually self-limiting.

Investigations
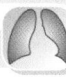

Cultures
Cultures appropriate to the site of infection should be performed.

Management

Metronidazole or tinidazole
Metronidazole or tinidazole is the treatment of choice for most non-sporing anaerobic infections.

Other antibiotics
Antibiotics such as clindamicin, co-amoxiclav and carbapenems also have good anti-anaerobic activity and can be considered for use as second-line options (e.g. if there is failure to respond, or intolerance to the initial agent).

Specific infections
Antitoxin for tetanus or botulism

Antitoxin should be given to patients with tetanus or botulism. Intensive care with ventilatory support may be required for neuromuscular paralysis.

Penicillin for actinomyces or tetanus

Penicillin is used in treatment of *Actinomyces*, tetanus (to prevent further toxin development) and also gas gangrene (together with metronidazole and surgical therapy).

Oral metronidazole or vancomycin

Pseudomembranous colitis is treated with oral metronidazole or oral vancomycin. Vancomycin is increasingly reserved for second-line therapy to reduce the acquisition of vancomycin-resistant enterococci.

Management of abscess
Incision and drainage

Abscesses should be drained and anti-anaerobic antimicrobials administered.

The treatment of gas gangrene is surgical. All devitalized tissue must be removed, e.g. by amputation.

Anaerobic bacteria

Gram-negative bacteria

Neisseria

Neisseria are oxidase-positive, Gram-negative diplococci. The pathogenic neisseria are fastidious intracellular organisms; there are other non-pathogenic commensal neisseria that are less fastidious.

Neisseria gonorrhoeae

Pathology

Neisseria gonorrhoeae infection is spread by sexual contact and most commonly occurs in patients aged between 15 and 35 years. The organism adheres to the genitourinary epithelium via pili. It then gains access to the intracellular compartment and causes local inflammation and pus formation. Bacteraemia with dissemination to joints is a recognized problem. Extension to the uterus and fallopian tubes may occur in women, while local infection in men may resolve with urethral stricture developing as a late complication. *N. gonorrhoeae* (gonococcus) causes purulent urethritis, septic arthritis and pelvic inflammatory disease. Pharyngeal and rectal infections also occur.

Clinical features

Urethral infection with *N. gonorrhoeae* causes an acute inflammation with pus formation resulting in acute urethritis and urethral discharge with pain on micturition. In women, cervicitis may be asymptomatic but this can develop into salpingitis and may disseminate to cause bacteraemia. Septic arthritis, which is a well recognized complication, may be chronic and flitting with a pustular rash.

Investigations

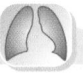

As the pathogens are fastidious organisms, specialist and enriched media are used for isolation and identification.

Urethral swabs

Diagnosis is made from swabs of pus from the urethra, cervix, rectum and throat. These should be plated directly in the clinic or into transport medium for rapid delivery to the laboratory. Speciation is based on biochemical tests and serological methods.

Management

Ciprofloxacin

In *N. gonorrhoeae* infection, antibiotics, usually ciprofloxacin, are given after specimens are taken. Penicillin is seldom used due to resistance; ceftriaxone or spectinomycin are alternative choices. Sensitivity testing is important.

Contact tracing

Sexual contacts in *N. gonorrhoeae* infection should be reviewed and treated. Prior infection does not confer immunity and there is no vaccine. Prevention is by avoidance of sexual contact and barrier contraception.

Neisseria meningitidis

Pathology

Neisseria meningitidis infection occurs predominantly in winter and early spring. Although asymptomatic carriage of *N. meningitidis* is common, disease develops in relatively few people. Pathogenicity is related to the polysaccharide capsule that is used in grouping the species. Meningococci cross the mucosal epithelium by endocytosis; the capsule allows survival in the blood stream. The group B capsular polysaccharide mimics antigens found in human brain. Lipo-oligosaccharide induces complement activation and a cytokine cascade leading to shock and disseminated intravascular coagulation. *N. meningitidis* (meningococcus) causes life-threatening meningitis and septicaemia which is fatal without rapid, appropriate treatment. Complications include loss of digits, deafness and cranial nerve palsies.

Clinical features

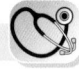

Meningococcal meningitis presents with fever, neck stiffness and a lowering of consciousness. A non-blanching petechial rash is a sign of septicaemia, which has a worse prognosis and may be present without other signs of meningitis. Septicaemia develops rapidly into a full-blown sepsis syndrome with shock and disseminated intravascular coagulation. Disease may progress very rapidly from a completely non-specific febrile illness to full-blown sepsis syndrome.

Investigations

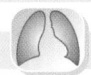

Blood, petechial and CSF cultures

Diagnosis is clinical but must be confirmed by culture and PCR of blood, petechial fluid and CSF (if there is no sign of raised intracranial pressure that precludes lumbar puncture from being performed).

Management

Immediate benzylpenicillin

Patients suspected of having meningococcal meningitis should immediately be given a dose of intravenous benzylpenicillin prior to transfer to hospital. Fluid resuscitation and intensive care support may be required for those with sepsis syndrome.

Cefotaxime or ceftriaxone

Acute *N. meningitidis* infection is life threatening and rapidly progressive. High-dose cefotaxime or ceftriaxone should be given as initial blind therapy, without waiting for results of investigations. Benzylpenicillin is an alternative. Chloramphenicol may be used in patients who have a history of anaphylaxis to penicillin or cephalosporins.

Contact tracing

Antibiotic prophylaxis should be given to household contacts of patients with *N. meningitidis* infection. In parts of Africa and Asia, the attack rate is very high, particularly with group A strains.

RECENT ADVANCES

There is increasing evidence that short-course, high-dose steroids may improve prognosis in meningococcal sepsis. Disease due to serogroup C strains has been significantly reduced by the introduction of a new conjugate vaccine. Serogroup B now causes most cases of the disease in developed countries. As yet there is no effective vaccine for this group.

Escherichia coli and related bacteria

E. coli is the most common pathogenic member of the Enterobacteriaceae, a large family of ubiquitous organisms containing over 20 genera and 100 species of facultatively anaerobic (able to grow in either the presence or absence of oxygen), Gram-negative bacilli. These organisms inhabit the human and animal intestine, and can be characterized by a series of biochemical tests.

Pathology

Infection arises endogenously (from the patient's own flora) when the flora is disturbed or following surgical, traumatic or medical intervention. Infection can also occur by transmission from other people and the environment. *E. coli* has a range of virulence determinants that enable it to cause a wide variety of different diseases. Enterobacteriaceae are classified by their antigenic structure. This is based on O (somatic), K (capsular) and H (flagellar) antigens. In many cases a particular O serotype has been associated with a particular characteristic virulence determinant and disease type. *E. coli* O157 has been associated with non-fermentation of sorbitol, haemorrhagic colitis and haemolytic-uraemic syndrome, while capsular types KI and K10 are associated with neonatal meningitis.

Clinical features

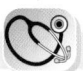

Urinary tract infection

E. coli is the most common cause of urinary tract infection. Most cases are caused by a limited number of *E. coli* serotypes that are adapted to this role. Strains that cause pyelonephritis are more likely to have haemolysin, and increased amounts of K antigen and P-pili that mediate adherence to uro-epithelium. Another member of the Enterobacteriaceae, *Proteus* spp., can also cause urinary tract infection. The ability to split urea raises the urinary pH, promoting calcium precipitation and stone formation, which, in turn, increases the susceptibility to further infection and makes treatment more difficult.

Meningitis

E. coli is the second most common cause of neonatal meningitis, and it carries a high mortality rate, particularly with KI capsular strains.

Intra-abdominal abscess

E. coli and a variety of other Enterobacteriaceae contribute to polymicrobial intra-abdominal, biliary tract, liver and other organ abscesses, particularly following bowel surgery.

Diarrhoea and food poisoning

Different strains of *E. coli* cause diarrhoea by a variety of mechanisms. In general, *E. coli* diarrhoeal diseases are self-limiting, although enterohaemorrhagic *E. coli* (EHEC) can cause serious, life-threatening disease.

Enterotoxigenic *E. coli* (ETEC) produce heat-labile or -stable toxin (LT and/or ST) that interacts with adenyl or guanyl cyclase in the enterocyte in a similar way to that of cholera toxin. This leads to increased fluid secretion into the lumen and causes traveller's diarrhoea, which is usually self-limiting.

Enteropathogenic *E. coli* (EPEC) adhere to the microvilli of the mucosa and cause flattening and loss of villous structure. Particular O serotypes have been associated with outbreaks in nurseries, schools and the under 5s.

Recent strains of enterohaemorrhagic *E. coli* (EHEC) can produce verotoxin (toxic to Vero cells) and are associated with bloody diarrhoea, sometimes complicated by haemolytic-uraemic syndrome. Acquisition is usually from food or water contaminated by animal faeces, or from direct contact with animals in which the pathogen is a commensal. The toxin is very similar to that produced by *Shigella dysenteriae* (Shiga toxin).

Enteroaggregative *E. coli* (EAggEC) can cause chronic diarrhoea. These strains of *E. coli* can attach to, and aggregate, enteric cells, without invading the mucosa. These strains possess fimbriae, which may be involved in the aggregation, and the pathogens may also express toxins.

Bacteraemia

E. coli is one of the most common causes of bacteraemia, which often follows a urinary tract infection or intra-abdominal and surgical infection. It may be associated with shock and sepsis syndrome.

Other infections

A variety of other related bacteria such as *Klebsiella, Enterobacter, Serratia* and *Citrobacter* are associated with similar infections to those caused by *E. coli,* but are more often acquired in the hospital environment and are more likely to be antibiotic resistant. They also cause ventilator-associated pneumonia, urinary tract infection, wound infection and bacteraemia.

Management

Supportive care

Fluid replacement and supportive care are important, particularly in cases of severe diarrhoea or septic shock.

> ⚡ **CLINICAL ALERT**
>
> *Antibiotics do not alter the course of E. coli-induced diarrhoea and may prolong carriage of the organism. As such, antibiotics are only prescribed if the patient develops bacteraemia.*

Antibiotics

Where treatment is required (non-gastroenteric and systemic infection), aminoglycosides, ureidopenicillin, cephalosporins or fluoroquinolones should be considered. Sensitivity testing is important, particularly with hospital-acquired infections where resistance may have developed as a result of widespread antibiotic exposure.

Four species of *Shigella* cause dysenteric illnesses with invasion of the colonic mucosa, ulceration and diarrhoea with blood and mucus. Disease with *S. sonnei* is usually self-limiting. *S. dysenteriae* may cause severe haemorrhagic colitis due to production of Shiga toxin. Antibiotics are seldom indicated, but ciprofloxacin may be used in patients with severe systemic upset.

Drainage of abscesses

Surgical drainage is indicated for intra-abdominal and other collections of pus or infected fluids.

Salmonella

The salmonellae are bile-tolerant, Gram-negative facultative anaerobes that are members of the Enterobacteriaceae. They are now classified as a single species, *Salmonella enterica*. There are a number of subtypes: *enterica, salamae, arizonae, diarizonae, houtenae* and *bongori*. These are further divided into different serotypes, according to the antigenic composition of their O and H antigens. Serotypes of *S. enterica* subsp. *enterica* are responsible for most human and mammalian infections. Salmonellae are generally referred to by naming the subtype, e.g. *Salmonella enterica* subsp. *enterica* subtype enteritidis is usually known as *S. enteritidis*.

Pathology

Salmonellae are commensals and pathogens in the bowel of many animals, and frequently colonize agricultural animals, poultry and wild birds. Humans are exposed and infected by consuming contaminated and undercooked foodstuffs. Poultry products, including eggs, are particularly implicated as sources.

Salmonellae use a variety of mechanisms to enter M cells in the gut and survive inside phagocytes. In enteric fever, the bacteria invade the intestinal wall after ingestion and spread to the local draining lymph nodes. Here, they multiply and cause a primary bacteraemia, followed by generalized infection of the reticuloendothelial system. The organisms are then excreted from the gallbladder, from where they re-enter the bloodstream and gut to multiply in Peyer's patches.

Infection by enteric salmonellae leads to gastroenteritis. In some cases, invasive disease causes bacteraemia with complications such as osteomyelitis or septic arthritis. These are important complications in patients with sickle cell disease or with HIV.

The enteric fevers (typhoid and paratyphoid) are life-threatening, invasive bacteraemic infections caused by *Salmonella typhi* and *S. paratyphi* type A, B and C respectively. Mortality is approximately 20% in untreated typhoid.

Reactive arthritis or a chronic carrier state can complicate salmonella infection. Renal and gallbladder involvement also occurs, and this increases the risk of chronic carriage.

Clinical features

Gastroenteritis

Gastroenteritis usually presents 6–18 hours after ingestion with nausea, vomiting, diarrhoea and fever. Severe disease and life-threatening septicaemia are more common in the very young, the elderly or debilitated.

Enteric fever

The enteric fevers usually present about 2 weeks after exposure with mild respiratory symptoms, anorexia and vague abdominal symptoms (usually constipation) followed by a stepwise increase in fever. During the bacteraemic period patients present with fever, alteration of bowel habit (diarrhoea or constipation) and the classical but rare rash (rose spots on the abdomen). Fever escalates and intestinal signs may worsen with reinfection of the bowel. Involvement of the Peyer's patches results in ulceration that may progress to perforation or cause severe intestinal haemorrhage. Hepatosplenomegaly may also develop and there may be lymphopenia. Relapse may follow apparent recovery. As with other salmonella infections, enteric fever may be complicated by osteomyelitis and (rarely) meningitis.

Investigations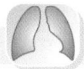

Stool cultures

The organisms can be isolated from stool samples using specialized selective and enrichment media (Fig. 15.11).

Blood cultures

Blood culture in the first 7–10 days of a typhoid or paratyphoid like illness, or during relapse, is the mainstay of diagnosis of enteric fever.

Bone marrow cultures

Culture of bone marrow can improve the detection rate.

Investigations for late infection

Organisms may also be isolated from faeces or urine later in the infection. Serological tests are available but are unreliable and of limited use.

Management

Antibiotics

While the salmonellae responsible for gastroenteritis may be sensitive in vitro to many antibiotics, treatment may prolong excretion of pathogens and increase the risk of chronic carriage. If septicaemia is present, the most effective treatment is with a fluoroquinolone such as ciprofloxacin, which also penetrates into bony tissue.

Ciprofloxacin is also the treatment of choice for typhoid and paratyphoid. Sensitivity testing should be carried out, and resistance is an emerging problem. Cefotaxime and co-trimoxazole are alternatives. Chronic carriage is more likely with typhoid and paratyphoid than in other forms of salmonellosis.

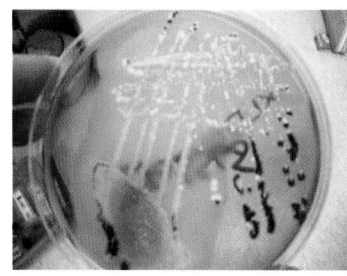

Fig. 15.11 *Salmonella* spp., including typhoid and paratyphoid, produce non-lactose-fermenting (yellow) colonies on XLD agar.

Contact tracing and reporting

Management includes investigation of household contacts and food history to monitor food poisoning. Food poisoning should be notified to the proper officer or communicable disease control specialist.

Vaccination

Vaccines for typhoid and paratyphoid have partial efficacy and are available for travellers and those in endemic areas.

Pseudomonas

Pseudomonas spp. are obligately aerobic (must have oxygen to survive), oxidase-positive, non-fermentative, Gram-negative bacilli that are ubiquitous in the environment.

Pathology

The most frequent human pathogen, *Pseudomonas aeruginosa,* causes opportunistic infections. It is found in damp areas including sink traps, taps, flower vases, mop heads and many detergent or disinfectant solutions that have been diluted and used over 24 hours.

P. aeruginosa produces cytotoxins and proteases, haemolysin and elastase (exotoxin A and S) which cause tissue damage and help it to spread. A mucoid form with a copious polysaccharide alginate occurs in infected cystic fibrosis patients. This protects the organisms from the host response, interferes with opsonization and phagocytosis, and reduces antibiotic penetration.

Infections are usually opportunistic. Typical infections include ventilator-associated pneumonia (due to contamination of ventilator equipment), respiratory tract infection in patients with cystic fibrosis and bronchiectasis, and bacteraemia in neutropenic patients which rapidly progresses to fatal septicaemia.

Superficial infections include corneal infection, often of preceding corneal ulcers. This can progress rapidly to destruction and involvement of the anterior chamber of the eye. Otitis externa, particularly in diabetics, may lead to mastoiditis. Infection of burns may lead to secondary septicaemia or failure of skin grafts. *P. aeruginosa* may also cause an irritating and painful skin infection (folliculitis) associated with hot tubs or Jacuzzis, painful nail infections in those who have persistently wet hands, and can be a rare cause of urinary tract infection (Fig. 15.12).

Burkholderia cepacia, Stenotrophomonas maltophilia and *Acinetobacter* spp. are frequently multiresistant and may cause hospital-acquired infections in similar situations to *P. aeruginosa.*

Clinical features

Ventilator-associated pneumonia presents with deterioration in pulmonary function, raised inflammatory markers, increasing and more purulent tracheal secretions, and new chest X-ray abnormalities.

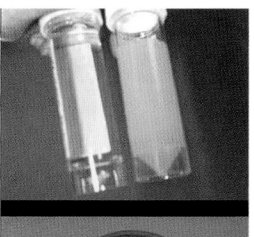
(a)

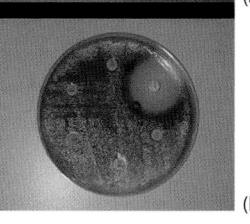
(b)

Fig. 15.12a, b Urinary tract infection by *Pseudomonas.* (a) Cloudy urine is a good indicator of the presence of infection, which in this example was caused by a multiresistant *Pseudomonas aeruginosa* (b).

In neutropenic sepsis, an embolic vasculitis (ecthyma gangrenosum) can cause necrotic patches to appear on the skin.

Investigations

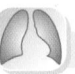

Cultures

Pseudomonas aeruginosa grows easily in the laboratory. Importantly, many disinfectants including cetrimide are used to select its growth. It produces blue-green and fluorescent pigments and can grow at 42°C. Outbreaks can be detected by a variety of typing methods.

Management

Antipseudomonal antibiotics

Treatment is with antipseudomonal antibiotics, which are often used in combination. These include aminoglycosides, carbapenems, ureidopenicillins, expanded-spectrum (antipseudomonal) cephalosporins or fluoroquinolones. Antibiotic resistance is frequently a problem, and good hospital infection control measures are needed to prevent infection.

Vibrios and *Campylobacter*

These are all curved, motile, oxidase-positive, Gram-negative bacilli. *Campylobacter* and *Helicobacter*, which is also in the same family, are microaerophilic, i.e. they flourish at low oxygen tensions.

Vibrios

Pathology

Cholera is a human infection transmitted by contaminated water and food. It is a disease of developing countries with poor sanitation and unsafe water supplies. Epidemics are associated with environmental change (flooding, refugee movements, mass migration) and associated reduced hygiene. Pandemics occur regularly and sweep across South East Asia, India, Africa and South and Central America.

Cholera is caused by infection with toxigenic strains of *Vibrio cholerae* with O1 and O139 somatic antigens. The vibrio survives gastric acid to attach to the G_{M1} ganglioside on intestinal epithelial cells via the five B subunits of its toxin. The A subunit is inserted into the cytoplasm where it irreversibly activates adenyl cyclase to increase cAMP. This inhibits Na^+ and Cl^- uptake, increases Cl^- and HCO_3^- secretion, and results in the inhibition of water uptake. Massive water excretion results in watery diarrhoea and acute water and electrolyte depletion.

There are more than eight vibrio species. Some, such as *V. vulnificus*, cause rapidly spreading cellulitis in wounds exposed to contaminated warm waters (Gulf of Mexico estuaries). *V. parahaemolyticus* causes gastroenteritis and food poisoning often associated with shellfish.

Clinical features

In endemic areas, the diagnosis of cholera is made clinically. Infection ranges from mild asymptomatic illness to the cholera syndrome. Excretion of up to 20 litres per day of painless, fluid diarrhoea may be accompanied by vomiting. Death occurs due to severe dehydration and electrolyte imbalance, particularly with depletion of potassium.

V. parahaemolyticus gastroenteritis presents with vomiting, diarrhoea and abdominal pain.

Investigations

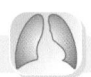

Stool cultures

Immobilization of cholera bacteria in a diarrhoeal stool with specific antiserum yields a rapid diagnosis. The organism can be enriched in samples using alkaline peptone water and cultured on special media—thiosulphate citrate bile-salt sucrose. It is identified using biochemical and serological tests to confirm the diagnosis.

Management

Rehydration

Oral rehydration solution (salt and glucose mix) is the mainstay of treatment and is usually effective. Intravenous fluid replacement may be necessary in very severe disease.

Tetracycline or ciprofloxacin

Tetracycline or ciprofloxacin will shorten the duration and severity of symptoms. Safe water and education is the key to prevention. In future, some of the vaccines under trial may be useful in prevention. *V. parahaemolyticus* infection is usually self-limiting and antibiotics are not usually required.

Campylobacter

Pathology

Campylobacter spp. (principally *C. jejuni*) is the most common cause of bacterial diarrhoea. It is a zoonotic infection (acquired from animal sources) and is usually transmitted in contaminated meat, poultry, water or unpasteurized milk. The organisms cause an intracellular infection of the small intestinal epithelium.

Cross-reactivity of some strains with nerve tissue is thought to be involved in the pathogenesis of Guillain–Barré syndrome.

Clinical features

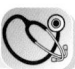

Disease usually presents following a prodrome with fever, aches and pains followed by 7–10 days of cramping abdominal pain and often bloodstained diarrhoea. A self-limiting bacteraemia is common.

Investigations

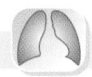

Stool cultures

Diagnosis is made by isolating the seagull-shaped, Gram-negative, oxidase and catalase positive organisms on *Campylobacter*-specific medium incubated at 42°C in a microaerophilic atmosphere.

Blood cultures

In severe disease, blood cultures are performed to screen for bacteraemia.

Management

Erythromycin or fluoroquinolones

Diarrhoea is often self-limiting. However, erythromycin or fluoroquinolones (e.g. ciprofloxacin) can shorten the duration of symptoms. Aminoglycosides are used when bacteraemia is evident (blood culture positive).

Prevention

Prevention of campylobacteriosis depends on good animal husbandry and abattoir practices, and good food hygiene in shops, dairies and the home.

Legionella spp.

Legionella are fastidious, small, Gram-negative bacilli. Over 39 species of *Legionella* are found in the aqueous environment where they multiply at temperatures between 20 and 40°C.

Pathology

Legionella are found in association with other organisms including amoebae and Cyanobacteria (algae), and this serves to increase multiplication and protect *Legionella* from more extreme environmental conditions such as chemical or heat stress. The main habitat of *Legionella* spp. is wet areas such as rivers, lakes, domestic water supplies, fountains, swimming pools and Jacuzzis. *Legionella* are transmitted to humans sporadically and in outbreaks associated with air cooling and water handling plants such as those seen in institutional air-conditioning and hot water systems. Travellers may be exposed to the organism through hotel air-conditioning or water supply (e.g. by taking a shower).

Although previously healthy individuals may develop *Legionella* infection, smokers, the elderly, those with underlying lung or heart disease, and the immunocompromised are particularly susceptible.

Legionella pneumophila causes legionnaires' disease (a multisystem infection with pneumonia) and Pontiac fever (a mild self-limiting disease associated with outbreaks of legionellosis whose pathogenesis is unclear).

Clinical features

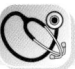

L. pneumophila is the principal cause of legionnaires' disease. The symptoms are non-specific and after a 2–10-day incubation period patients may present with fever, influenza-like symptoms or confusion from hyponatraemia due to inappropriate antidiuretic hormone (ADH) production. Gastrointestinal features and transient hepatic disturbance are also common. Milder illness may also occur, particularly in younger adults. Features suggestive of pneumonia are an unproductive cough and progressive shortness of breath. Mortality in previously healthy subjects may be as high as 10%.

Pontiac fever is a milder, self-limiting, non-pneumonic fever associated with exposure to *Legionella*.

Investigations

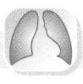

Urine testing

Diagnosis is made by detecting antigen in urine.

Serology

A rising serum antibody titre is confirmatory but of less immediate use.

Chest X-ray

Pneumonia may initially be atypical, affecting middle and upper lobes.

Bronchoscopy and lavage

Diagnosis can also be achieved by direct immunofluorescence on bronchoalveolar lavage fluid. Culture of lavage fluid or respiratory secretions on specialized media is also available.

Management

Erythromycin

The infection is principally intracellular and does not respond to β-lactam antibiotics. Legionnaires' disease is effectively treated with macrolides (erythromycin) plus rifampicin or ciprofloxacin.

Prevention

Prevention is by effective maintenance of water and air-conditioning systems. The gradual phasing out of water cooling towers as well as the development of biocide and maintenance programmes have reduced the number of outbreaks.

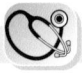

SECTION 15.7 Mycobacteria

Mycobacteria are important, worldwide bacteria that are known as acid-fast bacilli because of their lipid-rich cell wall that resists decolourization with acid.

Pathology

There are more than 50 species, and most are environmental organisms that rarely cause human infection. The main human pathogens are *Mycobacterium tuberculosis*, causing tuberculosis, and *M. leprae*, which causes leprosy.

Mycobacterium tuberculosis

M. tuberculosis is ingested by macrophages but escapes from the phagolysosome to multiply in the cytoplasm. The intense immune response causes local tissue destruction (cavitation in the lung) and cytokine-mediated systemic effects (fever and weight loss). Many antigens have been identified as possible virulence determinants, including lipoarabinomannan (stimulates cytokines) and superoxide dismutase (promotes intramacrophage survival).

Tuberculosis is spread from person to person by the aerosol route. The lung is the first site of infection and most infections resolve with local scarring, which forms the primary complex. Infection may disseminate from the primary focus throughout the body (miliary spread); this may resolve spontaneously or develop into localized infection, e.g. meningitis. Resistance to tuberculosis depends on T-cell function, and disease may reactivate if immunity falls (estimated 10% lifetime risk of reactivation). Immunocompromised individuals such as patients with AIDS are more likely to develop symptomatic disease.

Mycobacterium leprae

Mycobacterium leprae cannot be cultivated in artificial medium. The organism attacks peripheral nerves causing anaesthesia. Digital destruction and deformity follow, leaving the patient severely disabled. The scope of disease ranges from tuberculoid to lepromatous depending on the immune response.

Mycobacterium avium-intracellulare

Mycobacterium avium-intracellulare complex (MAIC) includes *Mycobacterium avium*, *M. intracellulare* and *M. scrofulaceum*. Some are natural pathogens of birds; others are environmental saprophytes.

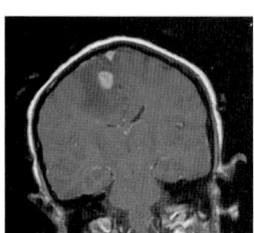

Fig. 15.13 MRI showing a tuberculoma in the brain with surrounding oedema. Courtesy of Dr Nicola Strickland, Department of Imaging, Hammersmith Hospital, UK.

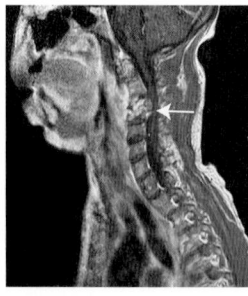

Fig. 15.14 Sagittal MRI of the head and neck showing destruction of C3 and cord compression (arrow) due to tuberculous osteomyelitis. Courtesy of Dr Nicola Strickland, Department of Imaging, Hammersmith Hospital, UK.

Clinical features

Mycobacterium tuberculosis

M. tuberculosis may affect every organ of the body and can mimic both inflammatory and malignant diseases. Pulmonary tuberculosis may present with a chronic cough, haemoptysis, fever and weight loss, or as recurrent bacterial pneumonia (p. 122). Untreated, the infection follows a chronic, deteriorating course. Tuberculous meningitis presents with fever and slowly deteriorating level of consciousness, and tuberculosis can also manifest as a tuberculoma in the brain (Fig. 15.13). Kidney infection may lead to signs of local infection, fever and weight loss, complicated by ureteric fibrosis and hydronephrosis. The lumbosacral spine is a common site of bone infection and progression may cause vertebral collapse and nerve compression (Fig. 15.14). Additionally, pus may spread under the psoas sheath to appear as a groin swelling (psoas abscess). Infection of large joints may lead to a destructive arthritis. In abdominal infection, mesenteric lymphadenopathy and chronic peritonitis may present as fever, weight loss, ascites and intestinal malabsorption. Disseminated infection (miliary disease) can occur without evidence of active lung infection.

Mycobacterium leprae

In leprosy the clinical picture varies depending on the immune response. The tuberculoid form has a strong Th_1 immune response and is associated with nerve thickening, loss of sensation and trophic injury but few bacteria. In contrast, the lepromatous form is associated with a Th_2 type of response. Patients with this form of disease have poor cell-mediated immunity, generalized disease (leonine facies, depigmentation and anaesthesia) and no granulomas.

Atypical mycobacteria

A number of 'atypical' mycobacteria such as *M. avium-intracellulare* complex (MAIC) are associated with systemic and pulmonary tuberculosis-like infections in the immunocompromised. They may also cause prosthetic infections, particularly in association with vascular grafts. MAIC are a common cause of mycobacterial lymphadenitis in children. They cause osteomyelitis in immunocompromised patients and chronic pulmonary infection in the elderly. In advanced HIV disease, they cause disseminated infection and bacteraemia.

Mycobacterium kansasii, *M. malmoense* and *M. xenopi* also cause pulmonary infection resembling tuberculosis in those with underlying chronic lung disease and in the severely immunosuppressed.

Mycobacterium marinum and *M. ulcerans* cause chronic granulomatous ulcers. The bacteria can be found in rivers, poorly maintained swimming pools and agricultural fish tanks (Africa and Australia).

Investigations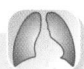

Site-specific cultures are performed.

Mycobacterium tuberculosis
Specimens are stained by the Ziehl–Neelsen method, then cultured on lipid-rich (egg-containing) medium with malachite green (Löwenstein–Jensen) to suppress other organisms. It may take up to 8 weeks for the organism to grow in such cultures.

Mycobacterium leprae
Diagnosis is by Ziehl–Neelsen stain and histological examination of split-skin smears and nerve and skin biopsies.

Management

Tuberculosis
The standard regimen for pulmonary infection is rifampicin and isoniazid for 6 months with ethambutol and pyrazinamide for the first 2 months. Regimens for other sites are similar, taking into account drug penetration (p. 125).

Vaccination with attenuated bacille Calmette–Guérin (BCG) strain may protect against miliary spread but trials in some countries have shown no benefit. Patients at high risk of developing tuberculosis may be given prophylaxis with isoniazid and rifampicin.

Leprosy
Treatment with rifampicin, dapsone and clofazimine is effective in rapidly rendering the patient non-infectious. However, the drugs must be continued for many months to ensure cure, and they do not alter nerve damage and deformity, which must be managed by remedial surgery.

Mycobacterium avium-intracellulare
MAIC are naturally resistant to many antituberculosis agents. Multidrug regimens should be used including rifabutin, clarithromycin and ethambutol. Lymphadenitis may require surgery.

> **RECENT ADVANCES**
>
> Growth of M. tuberculosis and atypical mycobacteria can be detected more quickly in broth culture by radiometric or fluorescence methods. Susceptibility is tested on slopes of Löwenstein–Jensen medium or in automated systems.
>
> Polymerase chain reaction can be used in rapid diagnosis, and also in detection of rifampicin resistance when used together with sequence determination of the rpoB gene. Restriction fragment length polymorphism (RFLP) enables the typing of M. tuberculosis and is a useful tool for the epidemiological evaluation of clusters of infection.

Leptospira

Borrelia

SECTION 15.8   Spirochaetes

Three genera of spiral bacteria—*Leptospira*, *Borrelia* and *Treponema*—are associated with important human infections. *Treponema pallidum* causes syphilis.

Leptospira

Leptospira interrogans is the species associated with human infection (leptospirosis). It has more than 200 serovariants, which are generally given a species name (e.g. *L. icterohaemorrhagiae*). *Leptospira* are tightly coiled, motile bacteria with characteristic flexion at each end, and are fastidious and difficult to culture aerobically.

Pathology

Different serovars of *L. interrogans* have different preferred mammalian hosts. For instance, the natural host of *L. icterohaemorrhagiae* is the rat. The bacteria colonize the rat's renal tubules and are excreted in the urine. Humans become infected by direct or indirect contact with animal urine, for example via contaminated water or soil. This may occur occupationally, e.g. in agricultural and abattoir workers, or sewage workers. Knowledge of the sources of infection and use of personal protective equipment should prevent this source of infection. Others at risk are those who engage in outdoor recreational or sporting activities that expose them to contaminated water.

Leptospirosis is a generalized infection involving the central nervous system (meningitis), liver (hepatitis and jaundice) and kidneys. Different serovars may be associated with disease of differing severity, e.g. *L. icterohaemorrhagiae* infection is usually more severe than *L. copenhageni* infection.

Clinical features

Leptospirosis has a bacteraemic phase with fever, headache, myalgia, conjunctivitis and abdominal pain,

957

following which fever, uveitis and aseptic meningitis predominate. At this stage, leptospires disappear from the blood stream. In severe disease, jaundice, haemorrhage, renal failure and myocarditis may develop with a significant mortality.

Investigations
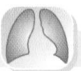

Blood cultures
Leptospires can be cultured from the blood using specialist techniques during the first week of illness. An antibody response is mounted following the disappearance of the organisms from the blood stream. Diagnosis is then made by detecting rising IgG antibody titres or specific IgM.

Management

Penicillin
Penicillin or doxycycline should be commenced as soon as possible. Doxycycline is used prophylactically when exposure is known or thought to have occurred.

Borrelia

Borrelia are a Gram-negative spiral bacterium coiled with a longer wavelength than *Leptospira*. *Borrelia* are fastidious, but some can be cultured using specialist techniques.

Pathology

Some *Borrelia* constitute part of the normal flora of the mouth and intestine, while others contribute to local infection in the oral cavity. Louse and tick bites are responsible for the human transmission of other important pathogenic *Borrelia*.

Borrelia recurrentis
Louse-borne relapsing fever is caused by *B. recurrentis*. Endemic tick-borne relapsing fever is caused by a number of species, including *B. duttoni*, and is transmitted by soft *Ornithodoros* ticks. In relapsing fever, *Borrelia* invade the blood stream, producing fever. The host produces antibodies to clear the organism from the blood, but antigenic variations of the bacteria lead to relapse. If left untreated, the relapsing fever resolves when the organism exhausts its repertoire of antigenic variation. Infections occur worldwide but tend to be sporadic. Humans are the only host of epidemic or louse-borne relapsing fever (*B. recurrentis*), which may arise during war or refugee mass migration. Endemic tick-borne relapsing fever is a zoonosis transmitted from rodents. It occurs worldwide with a distribution that reflects the habitat of the vector.

Borrelia burgdorferi
Borrelia burgdorferi causes Lyme disease. The infection is transmitted by hard *Ixodes* ticks to humans who are accidental hosts. It is endemic in the eastern USA and Europe. The New Forest area is particularly affected in the UK. Initial, localized skin infection is followed by migration through the skin and dissemination throughout the body. This causes chronic inflammation involving the heart, joints, central nervous system and skin. The early symptoms of Lyme disease are due to the acute infective process; later manifestations are thought to be related to the host immune response.

Borrelia vincentii
B. vincentii causes necrotizing gingivitis and oral co-infection with fusobacteria (Vincent's angina, p. 959).

Clinical features

Relapsing fever
Patients with relapsing fever experience headaches, myalgia, tachycardia and rigors; examination may reveal hepatosplenomegaly and a petechial rash. Episodes last for 3–6 days; relapses are approximately a week apart. Louse-borne relapsing fever has a high mortality (up to 40%); tick-borne disease mortality rarely exceeds 5%. Dysrhythmias (secondary to myocarditis), cerebral haemorrhage or hepatic failure are the usual causes of death.

Lyme disease
In Lyme disease, an expanding rash that starts as a red macule or papule may develop (erythema chronicum migrans). This is followed by chronic manifestations including headache, conjunctivitis, fever and regional lymphadenopathy. New skin lesions, myocarditis, arthritis, aseptic meningitis with cranial nerve palsies and radiculitis may occur.

Vincent's angina
Vincent's angina presents as a painful ulcerative lesion in the mouth.

Investigations
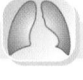

Blood cultures
The diagnosis of relapsing fever is made by visualizing *Borrelia* in the peripheral blood.

Serology
Lyme disease is most appropriately diagnosed by detecting specific antibody using EIA.

Throat swabs
Gram stain of oral swabs is diagnostic in Vincent's angina.

Management

Relapsing fever

Doxycycline is used to treat relapsing fever.

Lyme disease

Doxycycline or amoxicillin is used for treatment of early Lyme disease. Cefotaxime or ceftriaxone is more appropriate for late or recurrent disease.

Arthritis and myocarditis may have permanent sequelae, and treatment should be directed at alleviating symptoms that arise.

Vincent's angina

Vincent's angina can be treated with phenoxymethyl-penicillin.

Leptospira

Borrelia

Viral infection

Adenoviruses

Adenoviruses are a large group of icosahedral, double-stranded DNA viruses. There are approximately 50 different human adenoviruses, divided into groups A–F on the basis of DNA homology with type-specific and common antigens.

Pathology

Infections occur worldwide and throughout the year. Some are transmitted by the respiratory route and others by the faecal–oral route. Eye infections are transmitted by hand and by contact with infected lacrimal secretions. The nature of the illness depends on the group of adenovirus (Table 15.11).

Clinical features

The presentation varies according to the system involved. Infections generally occur in childhood or relatively early in life, and are mild and self-limiting illnesses such as pharyngitis, pharyngoconjunctival fever, other upper respiratory infections, and enteritis. However, adenoviruses occasionally cause a severe pneumonia or unpleasant and painful keratoconjunctivitis, particularly in immunocompromised patients who may also develop pneumonia, acute haemorrhagic cystitis and hepatitis (especially those with transplants).

Investigations

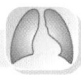

Stool, throat and conjunctival swab cultures
Diagnosis is by virus isolation in tissue culture, visualization on electron microscopy of stool samples, or by culture from respiratory secretions, throat or conjunctival swabs.

Serology
Immunological assays and NAAT are increasingly used to detect adenovirus in these samples as well. Antibodies can also be detected in acute and convalescent serum.

Management

Treatment is symptomatic.

Vaccination
Vaccines against a limited number of types are available and used in military settings.

Prevention
Outbreaks can be prevented by good hygiene, particularly in ophthalmology clinics, nurseries and swimming pools (chlorination of water supplies).

Table 15.11	Disease associations of different adenovirus groups	
Group	**Disease**
A	Asymptomatic enteric infection
B	Respiratory disease
C	Respiratory disease
D	Keratoconjunctivitis
E	Conjunctivitis and respiratory disease
F	Infant diarrhoea

SECTION 15.10 Herpesviruses

Herpesviruses are large, complex, enveloped, icosahedral double-stranded DNA viruses. They cause life-long infection with latency and relapses or reactivation later in life, especially if immunosuppression develops. Classification is based on DNA homology, viral characteristics and tissue of latency (Table 15.12). All are antigenically diverse except for herpes simplex 1 and 2.

Herpes simplex virus

Herpes simplex virus (HSV) is transmitted by direct contact. Primary HSV 1 infection is often asymptomatic but may present as acute keratoconjunctivitis, herpetic whitlow (usually on a finger), or as fever, vesicular gingivostomatitis and lymphadenopathy; in adults, pharyngitis or tonsillitis may occur. Virus may remain latent in the sensory ganglia, reactivating to cause cold sores in response to triggers such as infection, sunlight or psychological stress. Severe infection may occur in immunosuppressive conditions. Rarely, the infection causes fatal encephalitis (Fig. 15.15) particularly involving the temporal lobes. Perinatal exposure can result in neonatal encephalitis. HSV 2 infections cause painful genital ulceration that can be transmitted to sexual partners. HSV 2 is an important cofactor in HIV transmission. HSV can be visualized in vesicle fluid using electron microscopy or immunofluorescence. Polymerase chain reaction is used to detect virus in cerebrospinal fluid. Management consists of topical, oral and intravenous aciclovir. Valaciclovir is an alternative with better oral absorption.

Varicella-zoster virus

Pathology

The primary infection with varicella-zoster virus (VZV) results in chicken pox, is the recurrent form (shinges). VZV causes vesicular infections. Vesicle rupture releases large numbers of VZV, which is then transmitted by airborne/respiratory routes. Attack rates in non-immune individuals are more than 90%.

Clinical features

VZV generally causes a mild but potentially uncomfortable primary infection in childhood following a 14–21-day incubation period. Individuals are infectious for 2 days before the rash appears, and until the vesicles have crusted. Life-long immunity generally follows natural infection. The vesicles are mostly concentrated centrally, and appear in crops lasting up to 10 days.

Rarely, haemorrhagic skin lesions and varicella pneumonia, which is more common in adults, the pregnant, and the immunocompromised, can be life threatening. Mild post-infectious encephalitis develops in rare instances. Neonatal infection is serious and associated with maternal infection within 10 days of birth.

VZV may become latent in the posterior root ganglion. Shingles develops when VZV reactivates and travels down the axon to produce lesions. An acutely painful vesicular rash develops in the affected dermatome. Ocular damage

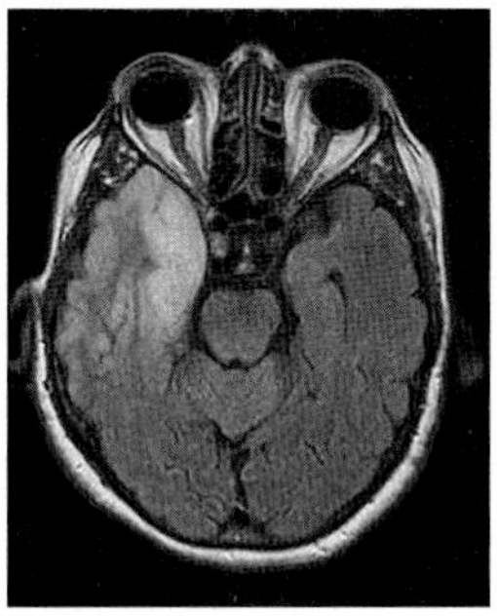

Fig. 15.15 MRI of the head. Herpes simplex encephalitis affecting the right temporal lobe.
Courtesy of Dr Nicola Strickland, Department of Imaging, Hammersmith Hospital, UK.

Table 15.12	Classification of herpesviruses	
Group	**Characteristics**	**Viruses**
α-Herpesviruses	Fast growing, latent in neurones	Herpes simplex 1 and 2 Varicella-zoster virus
β-Herpesviruses	Slow growing, latent in secretory glands (salivary, kidney)	Cytomegalovirus HHV 6 and 7
γ-Herpesviruses	Latent in lymphoid tissue	Epstein–Barr virus HHV 8 (Kaposi's sarcoma)

may follow the involvement of the ophthalmic division of the trigeminal nerve. Up to 10% of episodes are followed by post-herpetic neuralgia, which can last for years and is associated with a risk of suicide.

Investigations

Vesicle fluid analysis

Diagnosis is made clinically and can be confirmed by electron microscopy immunofluorescence or PCR of CSF in the case of encephalitis.

Management

Aciclovir

Management of severe (pneumonic) primary infection, infection in neonates or the immunocompromised is with aciclovir. Topical and systemic aciclovir reduces pain and post-herpetic neuralgia.

Zoster immune globulin

Primary infection can be prevented in exposed immuno-compromised seronegative individuals by zoster immune globulin.

Vaccination

A live attenuated virus vaccine is available but is not currently part of the routine immunization schedule in many countries. Management of VZV exposure in the health-care setting and among health-care workers is important.

Cytomegalovirus

Cytomegalovirus (CMV) is transmitted vertically, by blood products, by organ donation or by close contact and may shed in the urine and saliva. Infection is usually asymptomatic and rapidly spreads among people living in crowded housing conditions. Approximately 50% of adults in the UK have been infected. Rarely, a mononucleosis syndrome similar to glandular fever develops. Neonates congenitally infected either have severe generalized effects or are apparently not affected. In some patients, hearing defects or delay in developmental milestones may manifest late. Acquisition or reactivation may result in severe pneumonitis, retinitis or gut infection in the immunocompromised HIV-positive or transplant patient. Diagnosis is confirmed by PCR. Viral load measurement is useful to monitor therapy. Management is with ganciclovir in serious disease in the immunocompromised. Retinitis may cause blindness. Gut perforation may also occur. Foscarnet is an alternative if resistance is demonstrated. Organ donor and blood product screening reduces transmission.

Epstein–Barr virus

Epstein–Barr virus (EBV) infects the young in developing countries and adults in developed countries. Following respiratory secretion and transmission, the virus infects and disseminates in B cells. Immortalization of B cells may lead to neoplasia: Burkitt's lymphoma (sub-Saharan Africa), nasopharyngeal carcinoma (China), and lymphoma (immunocompromised). Clinical infection is usually asymptomatic. Glandular fever presents with sore throat, which may be membranous, lymphadenopathy, fever, malaise, fatigue, and occasionally hepatitis lasting about 2 weeks. It may be followed by persistent symptoms. Rare complications include respiratory obstruction due to lymphadenopathy (this generally responds to steroids), meningitis or encephalitis, and Guillain–Barré syndrome. Provisional diagnosis is by rapid slide agglutination (Paul–Bunnell test) and confirmed by detecting IgM to the EBV viral capsid antigen.

Human herpesviruses 6 and 7

Human herpesviruses (HHV) 6 and 7 are associated with febrile illness in children, including roseola infantum. They may reactivate in immunocompromised patients.

Human Kaposi sarcoma virus

Human Kaposi sarcoma virus (HHV 8) is transmitted vertically or by mucosal contact. Immunocompromised patients, especially those with HIV, develop Kaposi's sarcoma with reddish purple or brownish lesions on the skin, mucosal membranes and gastrointestinal tract. Virus is detected by PCR in suspicious tissues. Management of underlying HIV or immune status, chemotherapy and local radiotherapy are used in treatment.

SECTION 15.11 Orthomyxoviruses

The orthomyxoviruses are single-stranded RNA viruses. They are packaged with a viral RNA-dependent RNA polymerase, surrounded by a protein shell.

Influenza

Pathology

Influenza viruses are divided into A, B and C, depending on the nucleoprotein. The RNA genome is divided into eight segments that re-assort to produce different viral surface antigens. These antigens project as two types of spike from the envelope: the haemagglutinin (H—15 types) that binds to sialic acid and promotes binding of envelope to cell membrane; and the mushroom-shaped neuraminidase (N—9 types) that assists with mucin penetration and cleaves sialic acid to release virus from infected cells.

Influenza viruses are typed based on the haemagglutinin (H) and neuraminidase (N) antigens. The viruses are also described by their type or host of origin (human, swine, avian), country of isolation, strain number and year of isolation (H type and N type), for example A/swine/Iowa/3/70(H_1N_1). Antigenic shift (major change) is principally confined to influenza A. Both influenza A and B may also display antigenic drift (minor change). Immunity is strain specific, based on H and N type.

Investigations

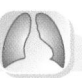

Diagnosis is clinical, particularly in outbreak periods. Confirmation is by virus isolation and typing. Virus can be directly detected in respiratory secretions using immunofluorescence or NAAT. Serology (haemagglutination inhibition) provides a retrospective diagnosis.

Scope of disease

The influenza viruses cause influenza, a generalized viral illness with respiratory symptoms. Influenza A is usually more severe.

Local influenza epidemics occur every winter. The size depends on the degree of antigenic drift or shift. Pandemics occur at intervals of 10–40 years following antigenic shift and may follow species jumping, e.g. 'Spanish flu' killed 20 million in the 1919 epidemic. In 1997 an avian H_5N_1 strain outbreak which spread from chickens was halted by mass slaughter of chickens.

Clinical features

Influenza A infection is transmitted by the respiratory route. Symptoms develop after a 2-day (range 1–4) incubation period. Patients are infectious from 1 day before onset and for the initial 3 days of symptoms. Headache, myalgia, anorexia and fever develop. Respiratory symptoms with dry cough are common. Fever rise is rapid and high (38–41°C). Up to 20% of cases may be subclinical.

Complications are more common in the very young, the elderly, and patients with cardiopulmonary disease. These groups may develop primary viral and secondary bacterial (classically *S. aureus*) pneumonia which often manifests after initial regression of influenza symptoms, thus resulting in a biphasic illness.

Influenza B behaves in a similar way but is generally slightly milder with more gastrointestinal involvement ('gastric flu').

Influenza C is generally a mild, afebrile, coryzal childhood infection.

Management

Management is generally symptomatic.

Amantadine

Influenza A can be prevented or modified in susceptible or immunocompromised patients with amantadine.

Neuraminidase inhibitors

Neuraminidase inhibitors such as zanamivir and oseltamivir also reduce the duration of symptoms, if given early enough.

Oseltamivir

Oseltamivir can be used for post-exposure prophylaxis in the elderly and susceptible (e.g. those with underlying cardiac or respiratory disease or diabetes) who have had close contact with an influenza patient within the previous 48 hours.

Antibiotics

Secondary bacterial infections require urgent appropriate antibiotics. Staphylococcal pneumonia in association with influenza may be fatal.

Vaccination

Influenza can be prevented or modified by inactivated viral vaccines. These are prepared annually to correspond to the currently circulating viruses H and N types. Annual vaccination is recommended for at-risk individuals, such as those with cardiopulmonary disease and asthma, and health-care workers. The World Health Organization is responsible for coordinating worldwide surveillance to detect new strains and direct production of relevant vaccine stocks each year.

SECTION 15.12 Paramyxoviruses

Paramyxoviruses are single-stranded enveloped RNA viruses that cause infections involving the respiratory tract. The most important viruses are parainfluenza, measles, mumps and pneumovirus (respiratory syncytial virus).

Parainfluenza

Parainfluenza viruses usually cause minor upper respiratory tract infections but can also cause more severe manifestations, such as croup and bronchiolitis, in younger children. Seasonality varies with type.

Measles

Measles is highly infectious (95–100% attack rate) and is transmitted by the aerosol route with a 9–12-day incubation period.

Pathology

Measles virus attaches to respiratory epithelium via transmembrane glycoproteins and a haemagglutinin. Invasion of local lymphoid tissue is followed by primary viraemia and general involvement of the reticuloendothelial system. A secondary viraemia then occurs, with dissemination and symptomatic manifestations. There is only one serotype. Natural infection is followed by life-long immunity.

Clinical features

A 2–4-day coryzal (flu-like) illness with small white papules (Koplik's spots) on the buccal mucosa is followed by the development of a morbilliform rash. This usually starts at the ears, spreads over the body, and then becomes browner and often desquamates. Clinical features may be atypical in those who have previously been vaccinated.

Complications include a giant cell pneumonia, secondary bacterial pneumonia and otitis media. Mortality is highest in developing countries in adults and those under 2 years. Fatalities are rare in developed countries, except in those who are immunocompromised.

Approximately 1 in 1000 patients develop immunologically mediated acute encephalitis with a high mortality. This usually develops 7–10 days after the onset of measles and is more frequent in older children and adults.

Subacute sclerosing panencephalitis (SSPE) is a rare, late-onset, progressive, fatal encephalitis that may manifest about 7 years after the initial illness. It occurs when measles virus persists in the brain and is most common in those who contracted the initial infection at a young age.

Investigations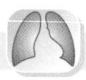

Serology

Initial diagnosis is clinical and can be confirmed by demonstrating a rise in haemagglutination inhibition titres or specific IgM. Antibody is present in CSF in SSPE.

Management

Supportive management

Therapy is essentially supportive, with antibiotics for bacterial superinfection if needed.

Vaccination

Effective vaccines are now in use, although it is unclear how long protection will last.

Mumps

Pathology

Mumps infection usually occurs in childhood but has a relatively low attack rate so there is a significant risk that adults are susceptible. Infection is more severe in adulthood and carries an increased risk of complications. Lifelong immunity follows natural infection.

Clinical features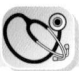

Respiratory transmission is followed by a 14–18-day incubation period. Infection is commonly subclinical, especially in children. Those who do develop symptoms may present with fever, malaise, myalgia and parotid gland inflammation. Approximately 10% of those with parotitis develop mumps meningitis, from which recovery is almost invariable. Rare complications include death and deafness from meningitis. Infection of testes, ovaries, central nervous system and pancreas is more common in adolescents and adults. Testicular involvement may result in infertility.

Investigations

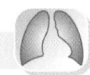

Serology

Rising antibody titres or specific IgM will confirm clinical diagnosis.

Saliva samples

Viral isolation or PCR may detect virus in saliva.

Management

Management is supportive.

Vaccination

Mumps is prevented by childhood vaccination.

Pneumovirus

Respiratory syncytial virus (RSV) principally causes bronchiolitis in infants. Minor respiratory infections may occur in adults, and adults may have symptoms from reinfections by RSV. It is increasingly recognized as a cause of epidemics and severe disease (typically pneumonia) in the elderly. Severe disease also occurs in neutropenic, transplant and immunocompromised patients. Much of the damage associated with pneumovirus is mediated by the host response. Diagnosis is by direct detection in respiratory secretions using immunofluorescence. Ribavirin can be given by nebulizer for those who are at risk of severe disease, usually premature or immunocompromised infants. There are currently no effective vaccines.

Nipah and Hendra viruses

These newly recognized viruses, currently classified as paramyxoviruses, have been associated with outbreaks in animals and transmission to humans with high fatality rates, often from encephalitis.

Togaviruses

Rubella

Rubella virus is a single-stranded RNA Togavirus with a single antigenic type. It is icosahedral in shape, and has a pleomorphic envelope derived from the host cell membrane.

Pathology

Rubella (German measles) is a worldwide infection and is endemic in countries that do not have comprehensive vaccination policies. Childhood infection is common in such settings, with major outbreaks approximately every 6 years. Screening for antibody is carried out as part of antenatal follow-up in those countries with vaccination programmes.

Rubella infection is transmitted by the respiratory route and is most common in winter. Affected patients shed virus and are therefore infectious from 7 days before and up to 14 days after rash develops. Recurrence is very rare; there is a high level of post-infection natural immunity.

Rubella itself is a mild illness with few complications. However, rubella is a cause of congenital malformations when associated with infection in pregnancy (congenital rubella syndrome). The risk of congenital rubella syndrome depends on the stage of pregnancy at the time of infection. Over 70% of babies infected in the first trimester will be affected whereas infection-related abnormalities are rare if infection takes place after the 16th week of pregnancy (Table 15.13).

Clinical features

In postnatal primary rubella, symptoms develop following an incubation period of between 12 and 21 days. Patients have a macular rash that usually starts on the face and then spreads to the rest of the body. There may be mild fever,

Table 15.13	Congenital abnormalities associated with rubella infection in the first trimester of pregnancy
System	**Common abnormalities in congenital rubella syndrome**
Eyes	Bilateral or unilateral cataracts, microphthalmia, glaucoma, retinopathies
Ears	Sensorineural deafness at birth or developing later in life
Heart	Patent ductus arteriosus, pulmonary artery and outlet abnormalities including valve and artery stenosis, ventricular septal defects

malaise, and suboccipital or generalized lymphadenopathy. Symptoms can be more severe in adults. Women, in particular, may experience arthralgia; this may be transitory but can also persist for some time. Children who develop rubella are often asymptomatic. Rare complications include encephalitis and thrombocytopenia. Full recovery is usual.

Congenital infection occurs when the fetus is infected during a primary maternal infection. Infections in the first trimester of pregnancy may be associated with fetal death or a wide spectrum of severe abnormalities. A frequent triad occurring in congenital rubella syndrome consists of abnormalities of the eyes, ears and heart (Table 15.13). As well as physical defects, there is frequently intrauterine growth retardation resulting in low birth weight. Babies may be born with thrombocytopenic purpura and hepatosplenomegaly.

Central nervous system effects include microcephaly and psychomotor retardation. In rare instances, progressive central nervous system infection results in a syndrome similar to subacute sclerosing panencephalitis. Diabetes mellitus, growth and thyroid hormone deficiencies may develop later in life.

Investigations

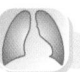

Serology
Diagnosis of primary postnatal rubella is usually based on clinical suspicion and it may be difficult to be certain about the diagnosis. If a non-immune pregnant woman is involved, or is a household contact, there is a vital need to reach an accurate diagnosis, and this can be made by detecting rubella-specific IgM and IgG.

IgM becomes detectable around the time the rash develops. It then increases and lasts for up to 3 months. In congenital infection the baby will have rubella-specific IgM antibodies that persist for more than 6 months. Virus may also be isolated from the baby.

Management

Patient education
Counselling regarding possible termination and accurate diagnosis are required if primary infection occurs in the first 16 weeks of pregnancy.

Supportive care
Supportive care is all that is required for postnatal primary infection.

Vaccination
Rubella is readily prevented by immunization. Sexually active women should be screened for immunity and offered rubella vaccination before they consider pregnancy. Alternatively, vaccination can be given postnatally if they are found to be non-immune during their first pregnancy. Elimination of congenital rubella in a community requires 90% vaccine uptake.

In the UK the vaccination involves the use of a combined live attenuated vaccine to measles, mumps and rubella (MMR). This is given as a single dose at 13–15 months, followed by a booster dose at school entry. Although postulated links between vaccination and autism have now been discredited, the reduction in uptake of vaccine has led to a resurgence of mumps and measles.

SECTION 15.14   **Picornaviridae**

Enteroviruses and rhinoviruses

Picornaviridae are small, icosahedral, single-stranded RNA viruses. They include the enteroviruses, rhinoviruses and hepatovirus (hepatitis A, p. 324). These viruses generally code four antigenic proteins, VP1–4. They generate type-specific antibodies, as well as some that cross-react with other enteroviruses.

Pathology

Enteroviruses
Enteroviruses are acid stable, found in the intestine and excreted in the faeces. New viruses are given numbers, e.g. enterovirus 68-71, but viruses identified earlier are divided into the polioviruses, Coxsackie viruses and enteric cytopathic human orphan (ECHO) viruses. Enterovirus 72, which was hepatitis A virus, is now classified as a hepatovirus.

Different enteroviruses display different tissue trophism, but usually enter via the gastrointestinal tract where they may just cause a local immunizing infection that is seldom symptomatic. Others replicate and cause viraemia, and then invade or localize in different target organs such as the brain or meninges, myocardium or muscle. Important examples include the polioviruses which localize in the dorsal root ganglia, destroy the nerves and cause motor paralysis.

Enteroviruses are spread by the faecal–oral route, usually via contaminated food and water. Swimming pool outbreaks have occurred as these viruses are generally relatively robust and can persist in the environment. Infection in developing countries is widespread and occurs earlier in childhood than in developed countries.

Polioviruses

Polioviruses cause polio, which ranges in severity from asymptomatic infection to a mild uncomplicated illness to aseptic meningitis (non-paralytic polio) and to paralytic polio, the most severe form. Paralytic polio is the least common manifestation (1:1000 infections) and occurs as a result of dorsal root involvement, with subsequent lower motor neurone loss and flaccid paralysis. This may be complicated by progressive post-poliomyelitis muscle atrophy.

Clinical features

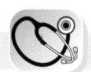

Rhinoviruses

Rhinoviruses typically cause self-limiting, common cold-like syndromes that have significant socioeconomic impact due to loss of working days.

Polio

Older children and adults are at greater risk of developing paralytic polio. Symptoms generally develop about 14 days after exposure, and paralysis develops early. Some improvement may be seen over 6 months. Involvement of the bulbar nerves leads to paralysis of muscles involved in swallowing and breathing. Muscle involvement in paralytic polio is maximal within a few days after commencement of paralysis; recovery may occur within 6 months. The outcome is generally worse if infection is associated with severe muscle activity (exercise), if it occurs late in pregnancy, or if polio is contracted within a month of receiving adjuvant-containing vaccinations.

Paralytic polio is a rare complication of vaccination or contact with someone who has been vaccinated. Rarely other meningitis-causing enteroviruses cause a paralytic infection.

Echovirus infection

Echovirus infection is common, but most patients have no symptoms or only develop mild episodes of fever, fleeting rashes and diarrhoea. The virus can occasionally cause aseptic meningitis with sudden onset of severe headache and vomiting with signs of meningism (neck stiffness, positive Kernig's sign, and photophobia). These features resolve spontaneously and with no sequelae. Rarely paralytic

infections occur. Occasionally more severe infections occur in neonates.

Coxsackie virus infection

Coxsackie viruses are divided into two groups, A and B. Group A viruses cause herpangina (vesicles in the mouth, fever and rash) and hand, foot and mouth disease (vesicular lesions on hands, feet, mouth and tongue). These illnesses usually last about a week.

Group B viruses also cause epidemic myalgia which affects the intercostal muscles and may be complicated by pleurisy and pericarditis. Coxsackie B viruses also cause myocarditis which presents as heart disease 7–10 days after an influenza-like illness.

Investigations

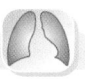

Tissue cultures

Accurate diagnosis of rhinovirus requires viral isolation or molecular identification but is rarely carried out, given the mild, self-limiting nature of the illness. Enterovirus infection diagnosis is usually by viral isolation in tissue culture from throat, faeces or CSF. RT-PCR assays are increasingly being developed. Serodiagnosis is confounded by the large number of enteroviral types.

Management

Supportive care

Supportive care may be necessary for symptomatic enteroviral infections. This may include respiratory support with assisted ventilation in paralytic disease.

Prevention of transmission

Prevention of transmission of all enteroviral infections depends on precautions against faecal–oral spread.

Vaccination

Polio is prevented by vaccination. Use of the oral live attenuated polio Sabin vaccine has been very successful worldwide. WHO enhanced surveillance is currently in operation in attempts to eliminate polio.

Rhabdoviruses

Rabies

Rhabdoviruses (rabies) are helical bullet-shaped structures surrounded by a membrane containing glycoprotein spikes. These viruses contain negative-sense single-stranded RNA and infect mammals in many regions of the world.

There have been approximately 20 cases of rabies in the UK in the past 50 years. Almost all were acquired following bites abroad. Worldwide there are over 40 000 cases annually, principally in Asia, with the majority resulting from dog bites. Rabies persists in sylvatic (in the forests) mode in North America and Europe, within small wild carnivores, foxes, raccoons and skunks, from which spread to humans is unusual. On the other hand, rabies in developing countries spreads in urban mode, via scavenger and feral dogs and cats, where there is a much higher risk of humans being bitten. Bats are emerging as a reservoir in the Americas and Europe.

Pathology

The virus is present in saliva of infected mammals. Humans become infected through the bite of such animals. Dogs are the most frequent cause, but a wide range of animals including bats have been involved. Following the bite, rabies virus enters the motor end-plates of motor neurones and travels up the axons to the brain. The incubation period depends on the length of the axon (the distance it has to travel). Sites with short neural connections to the central nervous system have the shortest incubation period (7 days), whereas a bite on the foot may have an incubation period of 100 days.

Clinical features

Clinical rabies results from an acute rhabdovirus infection. Patients may present with fever, nausea and vomiting. The central nervous system manifestations may be 'furious' (hyperexcitability, hyper-reactivity and encephalitis) or 'dumb' (ascending paralysis). Both forms are progressive and almost inevitably fatal.

Investigation

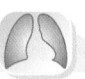

Saliva samples or corneal scrapings

Clinical features can be confirmed by specific immuno-fluorescence in salivary or corneal scrapings, by virus isolation from the same sources, or by detection of specific rabies antibody. Rabies is a hazard group 4 virus and should be treated and investigated in a designated high-containment unit.

Management

Supportive care

There is no effective therapy and supportive care is required.

Wound debridement and post-exposure vaccination

Post-exposure management includes wound debridement, injection of local antiserum, systemic hyperimmunoglobulin and a post-exposure vaccination course using the human diploid cell vaccine. Animal vaccination and management reduces the risk of human infection.

Vaccination

Rabies is effectively prevented by vaccination with a human diploid cell vaccine.

> **RECENT ADVANCES**
>
> *There is one reported case of a patient surviving rabies infection after being treated with antivirals and therapeutic induction of coma.*[1]

REFERENCE

(1) *Willoughby RE Jr, Tieves KS, Hoffman GM, et al. Survival after treatment of rabies with induction of coma. New England Journal of Medicine 2005; 352: 2508–2514.*

SECTION 15.16 Retroviruses

Human immunodeficiency virus infection and AIDS

Human immunodeficiency virus (HIV) is the first identified human retrovirus associated with acquired immune deficiency syndrome AIDS. HIV-1 is most common; HIV-2 is found mainly in West Africa.

Pathology

HIV is a spherical, enveloped RNA retrovirus that binds to the lymphocyte CD4 receptor. It uses reverse transcriptase to produce a DNA copy from viral RNA. This DNA copy is then incorporated into the host nucleus, which goes on to generate further viral RNA production and viral replication. Replication of virus results in progressive CD4+ cell depletion. HIV encephalitis and gastrointestinal infection also occur. Clinical signs may not develop until there is significant immunosuppression, with the manifestations of secondary infection or AIDS-defining illnesses.

HIV infection is transmitted by parenteral, sexual and vertical routes. It is most common in patients with a high risk of sexually transmitted disease, especially if genital ulceration is present. In developed countries, groups at greatest risk are homosexuals and intravenous drug abusers, although heterosexual transmission is increasing. HIV transmission in developing countries commonly occurs via heterosexual contact, unscreened blood transfusion and contaminated multiple-use medical equipment.

A related virus, HTLV-1, causes acute T-cell leukaemia and tropical spastic paraparesis.

Clinical features

Primary infection

Primary infection, or a seroconversion illness, may develop a few weeks after exposure. This is characteristically a mononucleosis-like syndrome with rash, fever and lymphadenopathy. HIV infection should be considered in any sexually active individual presenting in this way.

Latent phase

An asymptomatic latent period develops which may last 10–15 years until immunosuppression occurs. Persistent generalized lymphadenopathy is present in 25–30% of otherwise asymptomatic, infected individuals.

AIDS

AIDS presents in many ways due to the host's inability to respond to infections and to control tumours. AIDS-defining illnesses are listed in Table 15.14.

Investigations

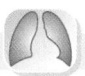

Serology

Informed consent should be obtained, and counselling offered before testing.

Detection of HIV-specific antibody confirms the diagnosis. A repeat test is needed to validate the results. Negative results may sometimes need to be repeated, depending on the interval between test and exposure, as seroconversion takes up to 3 months. RT-PCR detects viral RNA quantitatively and is used to monitor treatment.

Table 15.14	AIDS-defining illnesses
Bacterial infections	Disseminated or extrapulmonary *M. tuberculosis* *M. avium-intracellulare* Recurrent *Salmonella* septicaemia Recurrent bacterial infection in a child under 12 years
Viral infections	Cytomegalovirus retinitis Persistent herpes simplex or varicella-zoster virus JC virus infection Human papovavirus infection
Protozoal infections	Cerebral toxoplasmosis Cryptosporidiosis Isosporiasis
Fungal infections	Oesophageal candidiasis Cryptococcosis Coccidioidomycosis Histoplasmosis *Pneumocystis carinii*
Malignancy	Kaposi's sarcoma Non-Hodgkin's lymphoma
Wasting disease	
HIV dementia	
Failure to thrive or pulmonary lymphoid hyperplasia in children less than 12 years old	

Management

Antiretroviral treatment

Highly active antiretroviral treatment (HAART) is very effective in controlling progression to AIDS. Initially, two reverse transcriptase inhibitors (RTIs) and a protease inhibitor should be used before immunosuppression develops (Table 15.15).

Plasma viral load is the best way to monitor therapy. The aim is to keep the viral load below detectable levels as this helps to preserve immune function, reduces clinical manifestations and infectivity, and prolongs life. Failure of therapy is principally due to drug resistance and intolerance. Specialist advice and review must be sought.

Prevention

Transmission of HIV is prevented by avoidance of exposure to body fluids (sexual intercourse) and blood products. Blood donors and blood products must be screened, and potentially HIV-infected donations discarded. Health education programmes are directed towards the promotion of barrier contraception (condoms), and needle exchange programmes are used to help reduce the risk of transmission between drug abusers. Health-care transmission is documented but rare and is reduced by stringent needle-stick policies and immediate post-exposure prophylaxis.

Table 15.15	Drugs used to treat HIV infection
Type of drug	**Example**
Nucleoside reverse transcriptase inhibitors	Zidovudine, lamivudine, abacavir, stavudine
Non-nucleoside reverse transcriptase inhibitors	Nevirapine, delavirdine, efavirenz
Protease inhibitors	Indinavir, ritonavir, nelfinavir, amprenavir

RECENT ADVANCES

Vaccine development is ongoing but problematic due to extensive antigenic variability but remains a goal. Protease inhibitors reduce vertical transmission from mother to fetus.

Fungal infection

Candida

Candida spp. are yeast-like fungi that are widely distributed in the environment. They also form part of the human normal flora, with small numbers living in the bowel, oropharynx, vagina and skin.

Pathology

Disease develops when the balance between the yeasts and the normal flora is disrupted, with subsequent overgrowth of *Candida* spp. The use of broad-spectrum antimicrobials is the most frequent cause of this disturbance, with the resultant complication of post-antibiotic oral or vaginal 'thrush'. *Candida albicans* is the most common pathogen involved, but others such as *C. glabrata, C. tropicalis, C. parapsilosis*, and *C. cruzei* are increasing in frequency due to resistance to some antifungal agents. Little is known about the pathogenesis of these infections.

Candida and related species often cause oral and vaginal thrush following antibiotic therapy, but are also associated with infections in diabetics and in immunocompromised patients who may also have oesophageal and intestinal candidiasis. Infection of the urinary tract may occur, particularly if the patient is catheterized. Systemic infection develops following systemic broad-spectrum antibiotic therapy in intensive care patients and in the immunocompromised. Prosthetic endocarditis may occur from colonization of intravenous catheters and prosthetic valve infection, often necessitating further valve surgery. Pulmonary and systemic infection may also occur following broad-spectrum antimicrobial use in intensive care and high-dependency units.

Clinical features

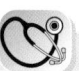

Candida infection frequently presents with white, curdy plaques on mucous membranes that lead to symptoms of redness, burning, pain and itching. The mucosa may bleed when plaques are scraped. Vaginitis and oral infection are the most common. More extensive and recurrent infections develop in immunocompromised patients, leading to pharyngitis and oesophagitis. Such patients may be troubled by dysphagia and retrosternal pain, thus causing weight loss. Cutaneous infection can manifest in moist skin folds and may involve nail beds.

Invasion of the blood stream may occur in severely immunocompromised patients, especially in the presence of prosthetic intravascular devices. These patients may have a septicaemia-like illness with fever and shock.

Investigations

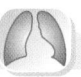

Tissue cultures

Candida spp. grow readily on most laboratory media and can be selected on specialized agar (Sabouraud's). As they form part of the normal flora, the significance of any isolates must be interpreted in the context of the clinical picture. Demonstration of germ tube formation is useful to identify *C. albicans* as this can be a guide to appropriate empirical therapy before sensitivity test results are available.

Management

Topical clotrimazole or miconazole

Less severe or localized infection in the female genital tract can be adequately treated with topical clotrimazole or miconazole.

Imidazoles

C. albicans is susceptible to imidazoles such as fluconazole. This is effective in systemic and mucosal infection.

Fluconazole-resistant isolates

Amphotericin B or one of the newer imidazoles (e.g. voriconazole) or caspofungin may be required for fluconazole-resistant isolates of other species such as *C. glabrata*.

Aspergillus

Aspergillus species are saprophytic organisms that are widely found in the environment. There are four species that commonly infect humans: *A. fumigatus, A. niger, A. flavus* and *A. terreus*.

Pathology

Aspergillus species cause disease as a byproduct of an immune response or by direct invasion.

The most common is an allergic response due to repeated inhalation of *Aspergillus* spores which stimulates a type III hypersensitivity reaction or incites a type I reaction from colonization of the airways. Allergic aspergillosis can cause progressive immunological damage to the lungs.

In contrast, invasive infection is characterized by invasion of blood vessels with embolic dissemination; there is seldom an inflammatory reaction. Invasive infections usually occur in the immunocompromised host. An aspergilloma or 'fungal ball' can develop in healed cavities following tuberculosis or bronchiectasis. Invasion of blood vessels may cause pulmonary haemorrhage. *Aspergillus* species can also cause systemic invasive infections in neutropenic patients from injections or skin punctures with a contaminated foreign body.

A. niger may be associated with otitis externa or superficial infection in burns.

Clinical features

Allergic aspergillosis causes fever, dyspnoea and progressive lung fibrosis—farmer's lung. Type I reactions (bronchopulmonary allergic aspergillosis) present with bronchospasm.

Patients with invasive disease present with haemoptysis. Invasion of blood vessels may be followed by dissemination of infected emboli to other sites, including the skin, central nervous system and eye, with a resulting poor prognosis. Systemic infection in neutropenic patients may manifest as fever that has failed to respond to other antimicrobials. Otitis externa presents with painful inflammation in the outer ear canal.

Investigations

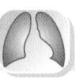

Chest X-ray and CT scan
Occasionally a cavitating lesion may be seen on a chest X-ray. Systemic infections usually begin in the lungs or paranasal sinuses, with peripheral 'wedge' sections on CT scan.

Serology
Allergic manifestations are diagnosed by detecting raised antibodies (precipitins) to cell wall components.

Bronchoscopy and lavage
Diagnosis of invasive infection is based on clinical suspicion, imaging of the respiratory tract and isolation of *Aspergillus* from bronchoalveolar lavage, sinus washout or tissue biopsies. Detection of galactomannan and PCR are emerging as useful diagnostic procedures.

Management

Allergic disease
Where possible, exposure should be avoided. Bronchodilators and corticosteroids should be used where necessary.

Otitis externa
Otitis externa is treated with topical amphotericin.

Systemic disease
Treatment of colonized patients and those with invasive disease is with systemic antifungal agents. Amphotericin B is the usual first-line agent. *A. terreus* may be resistant, and

newer agents such as caspofungin and voriconazole should be considered.

Aspergilloma
Surgical removal of an aspergilloma should be considered if possible; this involves pulmonary resection. Arterial embolization with adjuvant antifungal therapy is a good alternative.

Cryptococcus neoformans

Cryptococcus neoformans is a yeast that causes opportunistic, systemic infections in the immunocompromised. It is a saprophytic organism that is found in the environment and as a commensal in many animals. It is particularly concentrated in bird faeces (pigeon lofts). Infection with *Cryptococcus* is an AIDS-defining illness.

Pathology

The organism infects humans via the respiratory tract. In most instances, this leads to a mild self-limiting illness. Pathogenic cryptococci produce a large polysaccharide capsule which is antiphagocytic but the presence of intact host T-cell-mediated immunity is usually sufficient to overcome the pathogen.

Clinical features of disease vary widely. *Cryptococcus* causes chronic indolent meningitis which may be accompanied by pneumonia and systemic infection. Cutaneous manifestations include cellulitis, pustules and abscesses. Fungaemia and shock also occur, particularly in a late presentation, but are less common.

Clinical features

Meningitis
The most frequent presentation is of meningitis with headache, fever and confusion. The neurological symptoms may develop gradually over several days or weeks, and can appear to present suddenly with acute deterioration in consciousness.

Skin infection
Dermatological manifestations include papules, pustules and cellulitic areas from which yeasts can be isolated.

Systemic infection
The features of fulminant infection are similar to those of acute bacteraemia, with fever, shock and signs of poor tissue perfusion. *Cryptococcus* should be considered in any

immunocompromised patient with neurological deficits or confusion.

Investigations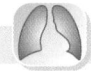

Meningitis

Lumbar puncture
Diagnosis is confirmed by direct visualization of the organisms in CSF by Gram stain, or in an Indian ink preparation that demonstrates the capsule (Fig. 15.16).

Serology
Measurement of the cryptococcal antigen level (capsular polysaccharide) in CSF and serum is also useful. The organism grows well in 2–4 days in most blood culture systems or on specialized fungal isolation media (Sabouraud's agar).

Other infections

Tissue cultures
Skin scraping or blood cultures should be performed according to the clinical presentation.

Management

Amphotericin

Amphotericin B is the treatment of choice, with the liposomal preparations being increasingly used at the maximum tolerated doses. 5-Flucytosine may provide additional synergy and good central nervous system penetration and is usually used in HIV-positive patients.

Fluconazole

Cryptococci are usually sensitive to imidazoles such as fluconazole. These agents are used as follow-up therapy and may need to be prescribed life-long in AIDS and other immunocompromised patients whose immune function cannot be reconstituted.

Immune reconstitution

An important part of the management is immune reconstitution, which involves stopping or reducing steroids or other immunosuppression. This method of achieving microbial eradication carries risks of graft rejection or flare-ups of the underlying autoimmune disease.

Management of chronic infection

Chronic infection with multiple relapses may occur in patients with lymphoma and those receiving steroids or cytotoxic therapy. Relapses are very common in AIDS patients, and life-long antifungal therapy is necessary.

> **RECENT ADVANCES**
>
> *The role of newer agents such as voriconazole and caspofungin is as yet unproven but likely to be significant.*

Candida

Aspergillus

Cryptococcus neoformans

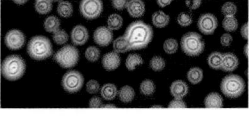

Fig. 15.16 Microscopy of cerebrospinal fluid. Budding yeast form of *Cryptococcus neoformans* in the cerebrospinal fluid of an immunocompromised patient.
Courtesy of Dr Michael Petrou, Hammersmith Hospital, UK.

Parasitic infection

SECTION 15.17 Protozoa

Amoebae

Cysts from a variety of non-pathogenic single-celled amoebae may be found in stool samples. The most important pathogenic species is *Entamoeba histolytica*.

Entamoeba histolytica

Pathology

Amoebiasis, or amoebic dysentery, is caused by *Entamoeba histolytica* infection of the large intestine. This infection is found worldwide but is most common in developing countries. Cysts are transmitted by the faecal–oral route, usually through contaminated food and water. After ingestion, the amoebae adhere to the intestinal mucosa and produce proteases and a cytotoxin that damages the epithelium. *Entamoeba histolytica* may also disseminate to cause abscesses in any organ, particularly the liver.

Clinical features

Infection of the bowel presents with abdominal pain and results in mucosal ulceration with profuse, bloody diarrhoea. The onset is often insidious with little systemic upset unless systemic infection occurs. Fever and localizing signs may indicate the presence of an abscess in the liver, abdomen, lung or brain. Features of an abscess may develop in the absence of preceding dysentery.

Investigations

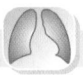

Stool cultures
Diagnosis is usually by identification of cysts in stool. Cysts of non-pathogenic amoeba are distinguished from *E. histolytica* by morphology (size, chromatin bars, nucleus) and behavioural characteristics (ingestion of red cells).

Serology
Serology can be useful in diagnosis of abscesses or chronic infection.

Sigmoidoscopy and biopsy
Ulceration of the colon can be seen on sigmoidoscopy. Active trophozoites may be detected in biopsies or occasionally on immediate examination of liquid stool where they may be seen ingesting red cells.

Imaging
Abscesses may be detected using CT, MRI or ultrasound scanning.

Management

Metronidazole
Metronidazole is the drug of choice for the treatment of amoebic dysentery and abscesses.

Diloxanide furoate or paromomycin
Diloxanide furoate or paromomycin is used to treat cysts in asymptomatic carriers, especially food handlers.

Prevention
Infections can be prevented by using a clean water supply and ensuring that food is properly cooked.

Other amoebae

In rare instances, a variety of free-living amoebae, most frequently *Naegleria fowleri*, cause meningoencephalitis in immunocompromised patients. The infection results from swimming in contaminated freshwater lakes and is frequently fatal but may respond to amphotericin

B. Acanthamoebae may cause corneal ulceration and keratitis associated with contaminated contact lens fluid.

Flagellates

Giardia lamblia

Giardia infection is a common problem throughout the world, and is acquired from water or food contaminated by cysts of this flagellate.

Pathology

Kite-shaped trophozoites develop following cyst ingestion and become attached to the duodenal and jejunal mucosa through two nucleated sucking pads. The pathogens then multiply by binary fission, thus resulting in the presence of very large numbers of the organism.

Clinical features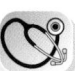

Giardia infestation causes diarrhoea. Infection is associated with anorexia, cramping abdominal pain, flatulence and bulky, offensive fatty stools. Presentation is usually acute, but chronic disease is associated with significant weight loss and malabsorption of fat-soluble vitamins.

Investigations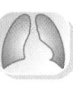

Stool cultures
The trophozoites become encysted as they pass down the intestine. The characteristic cysts may be detected by evaluating concentrated stool samples stained with iodine. Shedding is often intermittent so at least three samples should be examined if the history and symptoms are suggestive of giardiasis. Increased shedding may be seen during treatment.

Jejunal aspirates
Trophozoites may be demonstrated in jejunal aspirate if it is examined immediately.

Management

Metronidazole or tinidazole
Treatment is with metronidazole or tinidazole. Secondary malabsorption may take some time to resolve.

Prevention
Chlorination and filtration of water, and good food hygiene prevent giardiasis.

Cryptosporidium parvum

Cryptosporidium parvum is a common animal parasite that causes diarrhoea in humans who may be infected from contact with animals or contaminated water. Diarrhoea may be profuse and can be life-threatening in the immuno-compromised. Infection is prevented by water filtration or boiling. Antibiotics such as paromomycin or azithromycin may be beneficial in HIV-positive patients. Cysts found in faeces are partially acid-fast and can be detected by modified Ziehl–Neelsen stain.

Trichomonas vaginalis

Trichomonas vaginalis is a flagellate protozoan without a cyst form. It is transmitted by sexual intercourse and principally causes vaginitis with discharge that responds to metronidazole or tinidazole. Occasionally it may cause urethritis in male partners. *T. vaginalis* can be seen in fresh 'wet preparations' of vaginal fluid or can be cultured in specialized media.

Plasmodium

Malaria

Over 1.5 billion people live in areas where infection with the protozoan malaria parasite is endemic. In the UK there are over 2000 annual reports and about 10 deaths per year due to imported malaria. Four species of *Plasmodium* cause human malaria: *P. falciparum*, *P. vivax*, *P. ovale* and *P. malariae*.

Pathology

Malaria is transmitted by the bite of the female *Anopheles* mosquito that injects sporozoa into the bloodstream. The sporozoa lodge in the liver where they multiply in hepatocytes. They then invade red blood cells and multiply further. The red blood cells eventually rupture, releasing the pathogens to infect more cells and disseminate further within the blood stream.

Malaria principally causes a chronic progressive febrile illness with anaemia. This, in the case of *P. falciparum*, is associated with microcirculatory failure and multiple organ involvement. Patients in endemic areas may have a degree of immunity that reduces the severity of infection. Deaths are most common in infants and travellers from non-endemic areas.

Clinical features
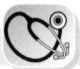

Disease usually presents as fever but may also be accompanied by abdominal and respiratory signs, or confusion. Infection with *P. falciparum* is the most severe and can progress rapidly. *P. falciparum* is particularly capable of deforming the red blood cells, causing them to block the microcirculation, and can manifest as 'black water fever'. Cerebral malaria is caused by microcirculatory failure in the kidney and brain.

Individuals who visit endemic areas on holiday or after long absences have no immunity and may progress more rapidly with shock, circulatory failure, anaemia, haemolysis and respiratory distress. *P. vivax* and *P. ovale* can develop dormant stages in the liver and cause late relapse.

Malaria must be excluded in any febrile patient returning from, or who has travelled in, an endemic area, irrespective of prophylaxis or reports of mosquito bites.

Investigations
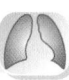

Blood films
Diagnosis is made by examining at least three blood films, both thick and thin, taken at different times. Antigen detection dipsticks should be used for rapid diagnosis, especially in situations where high levels of blood film expertise are not available.

Management

Quinine plus sulfadoxine–pyrimethamine
P. falciparum infection is usually treated with intravenous or oral quinine (depending on the level of parasitaemia) plus a sulfadoxine–pyrimethamine combination. Specialist advice should be sought in centres that do not regularly see malaria. Chloroquine is effective against *P. vivax*, *P. ovale* and *P. malariae* infection. Primaquine should be used to eradicate the liver stages (hypnozoite) of *P. vivax* and *P. ovale*.

Prevention
Prevention is of utmost importance. This includes avoidance of mosquito bites by using bed nets, use of appropriate clothing to shield the skin from mosquito bites between dusk and dawn, and application of effective mosquito repellents.

Antimalarial prophylaxis should be taken according to current expert up-to-date advice (WHO, communicable disease consultants, centres for tropical diseases) but is never completely effective even when taken assiduously.

Leishmania

Leishmaniasis

Leishmania are intracellular parasites that are transmitted by sandfly bites. A variety of clinical syndromes in different parts of the world are associated with *Leishmania* infection, depending on the species involved. Leishmaniasis is increasing in Mediterranean areas and is now more commonly associated with recreational travel.

Pathology

Sandflies bite the human host and inject infective promastigotes that are then ingested by cells of the reticulo-endothelial system. These promastigotes develop into amastigotes within the phagocytic cells and cause a variety of different diseases (Table 15.16), depending on whether there is dissemination to the viscera (spleen, liver, lymphoid tissue) or to the mucosa.

Clinical features

Visceral leishmaniasis
Visceral leishmaniasis is a systemic, life-threatening infection. There is fever and cachexia associated with cytokines from the infected macrophages, and the bone marrow may be replaced by infected cells. Anaemia and blood dyscrasias develop, accompanied by heightened susceptibility to secondary infection, which may be the presenting feature.

Mucocutaneous leishmaniasis
Mucocutaneous leishmaniasis presents with destructive sores around mucocutaneous junctions which become secondarily infected. Severe destruction of the areas around the nose and mouth (espundia) may occur.

Table 15.16	Diseases caused by *Leishmania*
***Leishmania* spp.**	**Disease**
Leishmania donovani, *L. infantum* or *L. chagasi*	Visceral leishmaniasis (kala azar)
L. braziliensis	Mucocutaneous leishmaniasis
L. major, *L. tropica* and *L. aethiopica*, *L. braziliensis*, *L. mexicana*	Cutaneous sores

Cutaneous leishmaniasis

The more widespread cutaneous form is characterized by boil-like chronic granulomatous sores that may have secondary bacterial infection.

Investigation
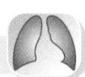

Tissue cultures

Diagnosis can be made microscopically by visualizing parasites in skin biopsies, bone marrow, blood or splenic aspirates. Samples should also be cultured in specialist media to confirm the clinical diagnosis.

Management

Liposomal amphotericin

Visceral and cutaneous leishmaniasis should be treated with liposomal amphotericin B.

Prevention

Prevention is by avoiding bites in endemic areas.

Trypanosomes

There are two geographically separated forms of trypanosomiasis, caused by different species of trypanosome and transmitted by different vectors. They have complex life cycles involving development in the insect vectors.

African trypanosomiasis

Pathology

African trypanosomiasis is caused by two main species: *Trypanosoma brucei gambiense,* an entirely human parasite, and *Trypanosoma brucei rhodesiense* which also has a reservoir in cattle and antelopes. African trypanosomiasis (sleeping sickness) is transmitted by the tsetse fly. There may be a transient chancre at the site of the insect bite, followed by parasitaemia. Parasites in the blood are partially inhibited by immune responses but the parasite overcomes this by altering its surface antigens. The parasites then continue to multiply rapidly, and central nervous system involvement (which is usually fatal) occurs.

Clinical features
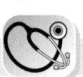

The initial symptoms are often non-specific such as a fever. Generalized lymphadenopathy may be present or there may be posterior triangle lymphadenitis—Winterbottom's sign. If left untreated, the disease worsens to involve the central nervous system with chronic progressive encephalitis. This is characterized by reduced levels of consciousness which deteriorates into coma and death. Secondary bacterial infection, especially pneumonia, is common.

Investigation
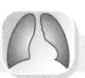

Tissue cultures

The flagellated parasites in sleeping sickness can be found in blood, CSF or lymph node aspirates. Lumbar puncture is contraindicated until circulating parasitaemia is controlled because of the danger of inoculation of the CSF. Parasites can be seen in 'wet preparations' of blood or using Giemsa stain. Serological tests are available.

Management

Suramin or pentamidine

African trypanosomiasis is treated with suramin or pentamidine in early disease.

Melarsoprol

Central nervous system disease is difficult to treat, and toxic agents such as melarsoprol are used in such circumstances.

South American trypanosomiasis

Pathology
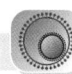

South American trypanosomiasis (Chagas' disease) is caused by *Trypanosoma cruzi*. It is transmitted by reduviid ('kissing') bugs. The trypanosomes are deposited onto human skin in the faeces of the bugs, and scratching of the skin leads to inoculation of the parasite. Trypanosomes are often scanty in peripheral blood, but they invade reticulo-endothelial cells and muscle to form non-flagellated amastigotes which multiply further. Cellular rupture releases fresh trypanosomes to be transmitted further. Patients who survive the initial infection may develop serious cardiac and muscular complications many years later.

Clinical features

Cutaneous oedema with intermittent fever develops initially. Childhood infection may be associated with significant mortality. Infection usually progresses to a latent stage followed by manifestations of chronic disease including achalasia, megacolon, cardiac dysrhythmias, cardiomyopathy and neuropathy.

Investigations
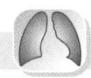

Muscle biopsy

Laboratory diagnosis is difficult in the South American variant owing to the low or absent levels of parasitaemia.

T. cruzi can be cultured in the laboratory or in reduviid bugs, where developmental stages can be detected after several weeks, but this is difficult. The amastigotes may be detected in muscle biopsies.

Serology
Serological diagnosis may be useful.

Management

Nifurtimox
Treatment of South American trypanosomiasis is not very effective. Nifurtimox is used in acute infection with some success.

Supportive management
Palliative and symptomatic treatments are required for patients with cardiac complications.

SECTION 15.18 Nematodes

Intestinal nematodes

Roundworm, whipworm and threadworm

Intestinal infection by the nematodes *Ascaris lumbricoides* (roundworm), *Trichuris trichiura* (whipworm) and *Enterobius vermicularis* (threadworm) is acquired by ingestion of the eggs. The nematodes are distributed worldwide but *Ascaris* and *Trichuris* are less common in developed countries due to improvements in hygiene.

Pathology

Ascaris has a migratory phase in which larvae from the hatched eggs migrate from the duodenum to the blood stream and gain access to the lung via the pulmonary circulation. They then travel via the trachea to the intestinal tract to live for years in the gut. The female worm can lay up to 2000 eggs per day.

Adult *Trichuris* develops in the intestine without a migratory cycle. Transmission occurs where sanitation is poor or when human faeces are used to fertilize food crops. The tough eggs, which have a characteristic appearance, are found in the faeces (three separate samples should be examined) and can survive for many years in soil.

In *Enterobius* infection, the worm, which lives in the large intestine, is principally spread within families. This occurs when fingers become contaminated by the large number of eggs laid by the adult female worm which emerges from the rectum at night. The eggs can be found by taking morning 'Sellotape' swabs from the perianal area.

Manifestations of disease depend largely on the level of infestation, but some patients may have gastrointestinal symptoms or nutrient depletion. Parasite load is an important factor as heavy worm infestation leads to increased competition for nutrients.

Clinical features

Mild infestation with these parasites is largely asymptomatic. An *Ascaris* worm may occasionally be coughed up or passed in the stool. Heavily infected children (especially with *Trichuris*) may have poor growth or impaired performance due to a dysentery syndrome with micronutrient deficiency. Heavy infection with *Ascaris* may cause bowel obstruction.

Enterobius principally causes perianal itching, leading to autoinfection from scratching.

Investigation
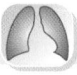

Stool cultures
Worms may occasionally be seen on examination of the stool.

Management

Albendazole or mebendazole
Intestinal nematodes are treated with albendazole or mebendazole.

Prevention
Improved sanitation is required to control the spread of infection. In endemic areas, treatment must be balanced with parasite load and likelihood of re-infection.

Families should be treated with piperazine for *Enterobius* infection.

Tissue nematodes

Filaria

The filarial worms have complex life cycles and are transmitted by biting arthropod vectors in which they have developmental stages. The disease manifestation, geographical distribution and optimal diagnostic strategy vary, depending on the species involved (Table 15.17).

Pathology

Lymphatic filariasis results from bites which usually affect the lower limbs. Adult worms develop in and block the lymphatics, thus causing lymphoedema. Over 100 million people worldwide are infected with *W. bancrofti,* which is the most important species. Larvae (microfilaria) are released and remain in the pulmonary circulation by day but circulate peripherally by night, which is a time when patients are liable to be bitten by mosquitos.

Skin filaria are transmitted by blackfly bites. Adult worms develop in subcutaneous nodules which are often found over joints and bony parts of the body. Affected areas become thickened and irritated. Adult worms may be found in excised nodules, while microfilaria may become apparent from skin slivers suspended in saline.

Filarial infections can cause serious, irreversible complications such as lymphoedema and blindness, and are an important cause of morbidity in Africa.

Clinical features

Lymphatic filarial infestation is associated with episodic acute fever and lymphoedema which may be complicated by secondary bacterial infection. In severe cases, the limb or affected part may be grossly enlarged (elephantiasis).

Skin filariasis is characterized by itching and irritation with subsequent thickening developing over joints. The most important feature is scarring and blindness that develops when the conjunctiva and eye are involved.

Loa loa presents with fleeting subcutaneous (Calabar) swellings that become apparent as the adult worm migrates in the body. Patients may give a typical history of 'a worm moving across the eye'. The infection may also be associated with fever.

Investigation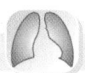

Blood and skin shavings

Either blood or skin shavings can be used for examination (Table 15.17).

Management

Diethylcarbamazine

Treatment of lymphatic filariasis is with diethylcarbamazine, but severe lymphoedema is usually irreversible. Allergic reactions may occur as worms die.

Ivermectin

Ivermectin is the treatment of choice for skin filariasis, river blindness and *Loa loa* infections.

Prevention

Vector control and bite avoidance are essential in prevention. Periodic ivermectin is useful in endemic areas.

Roundworm, whipworm and threadworm

Filaria

Table 15.17	Human filarial infections			
Species	**Tissue involved**	**Vector**	**Location**	**Diagnosis (microfilaria seen in)**
Wuchereria bancrofti, Brugia malayi	Lymphatics	*Aedes aegypti* mosquito	Throughout tropics	Night blood
Onchocerca volvulus	Skin	*Simulium damnosum*	West Africa, South and Central America	Skin shavings
Loa loa	Skin	*Chrysops* flies	West Africa	Day blood

979

Trematodes

Schistosomiasis

Schistosomiasis, or bilharzia, is caused by infection with different species of schistosome that are prevalent in different parts of the world: *Schistosoma mansoni* (Africa and South America), *S. japonicum* (Far East) and *S. haematobium* (Africa).

Pathology

Infection occurs after swimming or wading in infected water containing cercariae. These penetrate the skin and may cause swimmer's itch—a transient dermatitis. Cercariae enter the blood stream and migrate to the liver where they develop into mature worms. The male worm holds the female in the gynaecophoral canal formed from the adaptation to their integument into two long flaps. The mature worms migrate to the venous plexuses around the large intestine and rectum (*S. mansoni, S. intercalatum, S. japonicum, S. mekongi*) or bladder (*S. haematobium*). Eggs containing a miracidium are passed through the mucosa, often causing bleeding into the faeces or urine. The eggs hatch, and the released miracidia invade species of freshwater snail. After further development cercariae emerge and are able to infect humans again.

The adult worm coats itself with host antigens and causes little immune response or reaction. Egg release may be accompanied by bloody diarrhoea (schistosomal dysentery) or haematuria. Prolonged infection is associated with a fibrotic and granulomatous reaction in the liver, bladder or gut wall with a predisposition to malignant change.

Clinical features

Classically, patients may present with fever, skin rash, arthralgia, bloody diarrhoea and haematuria. On examination hepatomegaly may be evident.

Investigations

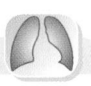

Stool and urine cultures

Ova can be demonstrated in rectal mucus or stool and terminal urine specimens. Viable ova hatch in water to produce cercariae that are visible with a hand lens.

Serology

ELISA can detect anti-schistosomal serum antibody, which falls 6 months after effective cure.

Rectal biopsies

If the diagnosis remains in doubt, rectal biopsies can be performed.

Management

Praziquantel

Praziquantel is the treatment of choice and active against all species.

Prevention

Infection is prevented by avoiding contaminated water and using protective clothing and shoes when working in wet fields. Control of the snail population can reduce exposure by interrupting the life cycle but is expensive.

Taenia

Two *Taenia* spp. commonly infect humans: *Taenia solium* is the pork tapeworm, and *Taenia saginata* the beef tapeworm.

Pathology

Tapeworms have complex life cycles involving a definitive host (where adult worms reside) and an intermediate host that contains cysts in muscle and other tissues. Humans acquire the infection by eating undercooked meat of intermediate hosts. The encysted larvae in the meat proceed to hatch in the intestine and grow into adult worms. These then shed segments containing many eggs which can be detected in the patient's stool. *T. solium* is of most concern because the eggs may hatch in the gut and the larvae disseminate around the body. This can result in multiple cysts in muscle, skin, lung, liver and brain (cysticercosis).

Infection is usually asymptomatic, except in cases of heavy infestation.

Clinical features

Infection is usually asymptomatic, but occasionally segments of worm are passed and detected. A heavy infestation may cause nutrient competition and vague abdominal symptoms.

Cysticercosis develops when *T. solium* eggs hatch in the human gut and migrate to form cysts in different tissues. This may result in inflammatory reactions and localized symptoms, depending on the site of the lesions. In endemic areas, cysticercosis is the most common cause of epilepsy, and patients may initially present with seizures.

Investigations

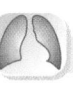

Serology
A diagnosis of cysticercosis can be made by detecting serum antibodies.

Imaging
Cysts in tissues may be imaged on X-ray, CT or MRI scanning. It is not possible to distinguish between the eggs of the different species.

Management

Praziquantel
Praziquantel is used to treat *Taenia* infection of the gut. Specialist advice should be sought before treating cysticercosis as severe inflammatory reactions may be triggered when encysted worm larvae die. This is a particular concern in patients with central nervous system disease.

Prevention
Infection is prevented by adequate cooking and food hygiene.

Other tapeworms

Diphyllobothrium latum is a large tapeworm that encysts in freshwater fish after a developmental stage in water fleas. Infestation occurs in areas where fish is eaten raw (Scandinavia and Japan) and is usually asymptomatic. However, vitamin B_{12} deficiency anaemia may occasionally occur if the patient is highly infested. *Hymenolepis nana* is a very small tapeworm that has a simple life cycle in humans and is usually asymptomatic. Diagnosis is made in both the above cases by detecting characteristic eggs in faeces. Praziquantel is used for treatment.

Echinococcus

Hydatid disease

Human hydatid disease is caused by two species of dog tapeworm: *Echinococcus granulosus* and *E. multilocularis*.

Pathology

The life cycle of *Echinococcus* is complex. Dogs and other canine species are the definitive hosts in which the organism's eggs hatch and develop into adult worms in the gut. The dog's faeces contain eggs that may be ingested by the normal intermediate hosts such as sheep and cattle. Hydatid cysts are formed in the tissues of the intermediate host, and a dog becomes infected if it preys on these animals.

Humans who live in sheep farming areas run the risk of ingesting the pathogen's eggs and may become accidental, intermediate (dead-end) hosts. Following ingestion, the eggs hatch in the large intestine. The larvae then penetrate the mucosa and travel to other organs via the blood stream, frequently ending up in the lung, liver and brain. These larvae develop into a cystic cavity—the hydatid cyst. The cysts are complex, expanding structures that develop an internal germinal layer. New 'brood capsules' develop from this and may form daughter cysts. New protoscolices, which form the heads of adult worms in the definitive host, develop inside the daughter cysts. In most cases the cysts continue to grow, although occasionally some will die and calcify. The cysts are closely attached to and enmeshed in surrounding tissues.

In some instances, disease is caused by the cysts acting as space-occupying lesions and disrupting the function of the affected organ. For instance, epilepsy may occur as a result of central nervous system involvement. Alternatively, there may be an inflammatory reaction, which usually occurs when the cyst dies.

Clinical features

Some patients may be completely asymptomatic and the disease is found incidentally when the patient is investigated for an unrelated medical problem. Cysts can produce symptoms in many cases, such as when there are space-occupying lesions in the liver, lungs, central nervous system or elsewhere in the body.

Rupture and sudden release of hydatid cyst contents can cause anaphylaxis or result in multiple seeding of the peritoneal or other cavities with subsequent cyst development.

Investigations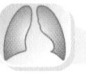

Imaging
Hydatid disease is usually diagnosed by detecting and imaging multiloculated cysts, followed by serological confirmation.

Serology
There are effective ELISA assays that can detect antibody and antigen. The Casoni skin test was used in the past to detect hypersensitivity but it lacks reliability and is no longer recommended.

 CLINICAL ALERT

Aspiration of cyst fluid for examination is contraindicated because of an associated risk of cyst rupture that triggers anaphylaxis. When accidentally aspirated on occasions where the diagnosis has not been suspected, the cyst fluid is full of scolices that can be easily identified (hydatid sand).

Management

Excision of cyst
Surgical removal is the best therapy. However this is technically demanding and the risk of anaphylaxis associated with rupture is real. This can be reduced by prior treatment with albendazole.

Albendazole
Albendazole is the drug of choice. Steroids may be needed to reduce the inflammation associated with dying cysts.

Index

Note: Page numbers in *italics* refer to tables and figures.

983

995

V

Z